Edited by
Ingrid Kohlstadt

Advancing Medicine with **Food** and **Nutrients**

Second Edition ·

Edited by
Ingrid Kohlstadt

Advancing Medicine
with **Food** and **Nutrients**

Second Edition

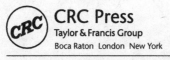

CRC Press
Taylor & Francis Group
Boca Raton London New York

CRC Press is an imprint of the
Taylor & Francis Group, an **informa** business

CRC Press
Taylor & Francis Group
6000 Broken Sound Parkway NW, Suite 300
Boca Raton, FL 33487-2742

First issued in paperback 2021

© 2012 by Taylor & Francis Group, LLC
CRC Press is an imprint of Taylor & Francis Group, an Informa business

No claim to original U.S. Government works

Version Date: 20140327

ISBN 13: 978-1-03-209914-9 (pbk)
ISBN 13: 978-1-4398-8772-1 (hbk)

Library of Congress Cataloging-in-Publication Data

Food and nutrients in disease management.
    Advancing medicine with food and nutrients / [edited by] Ingrid Kohlstadt. -- Second edition.
        pages cm
    Includes bibliographical references and index.
    ISBN 978-1-4398-8772-1 (hardback)
    1. Diet therapy. I. Kohlstadt, Ingrid, editor of compilation. II. Title.

RM216.F677 2013
615.8'54--dc23   2012043359

**Visit the Taylor & Francis Web site at
http://www.taylorandfrancis.com**

**and the CRC Press Web site at
http://www.crcpress.com**

To medical students and physicians,
who desire to make a difference
in the lives of their patients
and the practice of medicine.

Contents

SECTION I   Disorders of the Ears, Eyes, Nose, and Throat

SECTION II   Cardiovascular, Hematologic, and Pulmonary Conditions

SECTION III   Gastrointestinal Disorders

SECTION IV   Endocrine and Dermatologic Disorders

SECTION V Kidney Disorders

SECTION VI Neurologic and Psychiatric Disorders

SECTION VII Soft Tissue and Musculoskeletal Disorders

SECTION VIII Neoplasms

SECTION IX Reproductive Health and Toxicology

Preface

After decades of journeying on different paths, food and medicine are located far apart. Food has become bereft of the nutrients vital to its healing properties, and modern medicine has sought to heal with technical advances that at the outset may seem more powerful than food. The current gap between food and medicine is illustrated in our terminology, which considers food as "alternative" to modern medicine. This gap is not appropriate or healthful; in fact food and nutrients are the original medicine, the shoulders on which modern medicine stands.

Advancing Medicine with Food and Nutrients, Second Edition reunites food and medicine. Here leading physicians on the frontlines of disease management apply the latest scientific advances to the clinical practice of medicine. Each chapter offers adjuncts to standard care, fewer side effects, improved risk-reduction, or added quality of life.

PRAISE FOR THE FIRST EDITION

The first edition, entitled *Food and Nutrients in Disease Management* and published in 2009, is praised for its practical, ready-to-use, clinical applications presented by highly credentialed leaders with university affiliations such as Boston, Columbia, Johns Hopkins, Scripps, University of California, University of Washington, and Vanderbilt. Previews and reviews include *JAMA* (Vol. 302, No. 23), *Hopkins Medicine Magazine* (Spring/Summer 2009), *Pediatric Endocrinology Reviews* (Vol. 7, No. 4), and the *Chicago Tribune*.

NEW IN THIS EDITION

In this edition, patient-specific answers are buttressed with new evidence. The emerging themes have led to several new chapters.

The body increases its demand for certain nutrients when faced with toxic exposures such as molds, microbial infections, xenoestrogens, heavy metals, and inert nanoparticles. Restoring optimal nutrient levels has in some situations been shown to facilitate common detoxification pathways.

A breadth of food safety issues have emerged for patients with preexisting medical conditions: adequate labeling of food allergens such as gluten, potential adverse effects of artificial sweeteners, possible consequences of applying ionizing radiation to food, perspective on food-borne mycotoxins, critical food restrictions following bariatric surgery and certain medical conditions, precautions for preparing food in the home, and how to navigate claims of medical foods and dietary supplements.

Physical forces alter nutritional needs. Favorable effects include ultraviolet light initiating vitamin D synthesis, bright light synchronizing melatonin following jet lag or shift work, and improving biochemical markers through normalizing blood viscosity and blood pressure. Adverse physical forces include non-ionizing radiation's effects on brain glucose metabolism and excess body fat's effects on inflammation and hydration.

EXPERTS PROVIDE CONTEXT

Nutrition is a broad field. This book's 70 authors have collective experience in laboratory science, epidemiology, food anthropology, food and nutraceutical industries, medical subspecialties, international health, academic medicine, and biochemical research.

Given the diversity, it would appear likely that one chapter would conclude "black" and the other, "white." That never happened! Instead, this highly regarded team has spoken with remarkable convergence. Each chapter supports the others with varying shades of pearl, dove, and silver.

Collectively, the authors provide a discerning lens by which to interpret the evidence. Their perspectives can be particularly valuable. First of all, evidence is critically important. Today's clinicians have observed tragic consequences in their patients, stemming from false or exaggerated nutrition claims. Equally unfavorable results arise when correctable, unhealthful food choices and nutrient deficiencies contribute to disease.

These authors explain how the breadth of research informs their clinical decisions. "Omics" research such as nutrigenomics, epigenomics, and metabolomics provides new paradigms for the healing potential of food and nutrients. Since food and the human genome have evolved together, data from anthropologic research and population studies is often too meaningful to be overlooked.

Equally valuable for clinicians are the book's considerations on administering a food or nutrient intervention. Since food represents much more than mere sustenance, asking someone to change their foodways requires a commitment greater than that of taking a pill a day. Therefore, many authors elaborate on how they transition patients to more healthful choices.

ABOUT HELPING TODAY'S PATIENTS

This book is written by doctors for doctors. For medical legal purposes it is important to note that this book does not represent guidelines, recommendations, or the current standard of medical care. On behalf of the authors and editorial staff, I thank you for caring and going the extra step in finding healing answers for your patients.

Acknowledgments

Thanks to the team! This book is a gift from its 70 contributors, who have given the project long hours after clinical practice and other professional duties. They have freely shared their clinical "pears," fruits from years of patient care and research. Their work enables physicians everywhere to maximize the healing potential of food and nutrients.

I thank the families of the authors—including my own dear Ellis, Raeha, and Emmanuel—for giving time and support to this project. As the book's editor I am deeply appreciative.

About the Editor

Ingrid Kohlstadt, MD, MPH, has been elected a Fellow of the American College of Nutrition and a Fellow of the American College of Preventive Medicine. On the faculty of Johns Hopkins Bloomberg School of Public Health, Dr. Kohlstadt is researching an approach to leverage nutrition more fully in disease prevention. She directs NutriBee™ National Nutrition Competition, Inc. and founded INGRIDients™, Inc., a medical nutrition resource for colleagues, clients, and consumers.

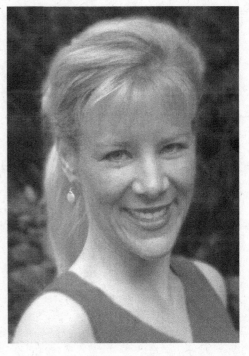

Dr. Kohlstadt is a graduate of Johns Hopkins School of Medicine, class of 1993. She earned her bachelor's degree in biochemistry at the University of Maryland and as a Rotary Club International Scholar at Universität Tübingen, Germany, in 1989.

Board certified in General Preventive Medicine and with a graduate degree in epidemiology, Dr. Kohlstadt became convinced that nutrition is powerful and underutilized in preventing disease. She therefore focused her career on nutrition through fellowships at Johns Hopkins and at the Centers for Disease Control and Prevention and as a bariatric physician with the Indian Health Service, Florida Orthopedic Institute, and Johns Hopkins Weight Management Center.

Dr. Kohlstadt maintains that clinical advances emerge at the interface between research and regulation, where she has worked as an inaugural U.S. Food and Drug Administration Commissioner's Fellow, a local health officer, a congressional intern, and a consulting physician with the U.S. Department of Agriculture.

Having practiced medicine on every continent including as station doctor in Antarctica, she is convinced that nutrition is much broader than health. "It is an expression of our interconnectedness with the earth and future generations, with each other, and those who have gone before us." Dr. Kohlstadt resides with her husband, Ellis Richman, and their children in Annapolis, Maryland.

Contributors

Daniel G. Amen, MD
Amen Clinics, Inc.
Newport Beach, California

Roger Billica, MD, FAAFP
Tri Life Health Institute
Fort Collins, Colorado

Keith I. Block, MD
Block Center for Integrative Cancer
Skokie, Illinois

Kenneth Bock, MD
Rhinebeck Health Center
Rhinebeck, New York

D. Barry Boyd, MD, MS
Yale School of Medicine
New Haven, Connecticut

David M. Brady, ND, DC, CCN, DACBN
Vice Provost, Health Sciences
Director, Human Nutrition Institute
Associate Professor of Clinical Sciences
University of Bridgeport
Bridgeport, Connecticut
Private Practice: Whole Body Medicine
Trumbull, Connecticut

Young I. Cho, PhD
Drexel University
Philadelphia, Pennsylvania

John C. Cline, MD, BSc
Cline Medical Centre
Nanaimo, British Columbia

Michael Compain, MD
Rhinebeck Health Center
Rhinebeck, New York

Nina Crowley, MS, RD
Bariatric Surgery Program
Medical University of South Carolina
Charleston, South Carolina

Ruth DeBusk, PhD, RD
Tallahassee Memorial HealthCare
Tallahassee, Florida

Mark DeLegge, MD
Division of Gastroenterology & Hepatology
Charleston, South Carolina

Beth Ellen DiLuglio, MS, RD, CCN
Nutrition Mission, LLC
Naples, Florida

Damien Downing, MBBS, MSB
New Medicine Group
London, United Kingdom

Colleen Fogarty Draper, MS, RD, LDN
Division of Gastroenterology and Hepatology
Johns Hopkins University School of Medicine
Baltimore, Maryland

Geovanni Espinosa, ND
Department of Urology
New York Langone Medical Center
New York, New York

Nicole Farmer, MD
Hyattsville, Maryland

Rodney Ford, MD, MBBS
Christchurch School of Medicine
University of Otago
Christchurch, New Zealand

Lynda Frassetto, MD
Department of Medicine/Nephrology
University of California San Francisco
San Francisco, California

Sheila George, MD
Center for Metabolic Wellness
New York, New York

Charlotte Gyllenhaal, PhD
Block Center for Integrative Cancer
Skokie, Illinois

Georges M. Halpern, MD, PhD
Distinguished Professor of Pharmaceutical
  Sciences
Hong Kong Polytechnic University
Hong Kong, China

Geoffrey R. Harris, MD
Newbury Park, California

**Leah Hechtman, MSciMed (RHHG), BHSc
(Nat), ND**
The Natural Health and Fertility Centre
Sydney, Australia

Alan R. Hirsch, MD
Smell & Taste Treatment and Research
  Foundation
Chicago, Illinois

Michael F. Holick, MD, PhD
Boston University School of Medicine
Boston, Massachusetts

Ralph E. Holsworth, Jr., DO
Tahoma Clinic
Renton, Washington

**Mark C. Houston, MD, MS, ABAARM,
FACP, FAHA, FASH, FACN**
Associate Clinical Professor of Medicine
Vanderbilt University School of Medicine
Director, Hypertension Institute and Vascular
  Biology
Saint Thomas Hospital
Nashville, Tennessee

Mark Hyman, MD
Medical Director
The UltraWellness Center
Lenox, Massachusetts

Russell Jaffe, MD, PhD, CCN
Health Studies Collegium
Ashburn, Virginia

Aaron E. Katz, MD
Chairman of Urology
Winthrop University Hospital Clinical Campus
Stony Brook University School of Medicine
Garden City, New York

David Kennedy, DDS
Past President, International Academy of Oral
  Medicine and Toxicology
San Diego, California

Dietrich Klinghardt, MD, PhD
Medical Director, Klinghardt Academy
Lead Clinician, Sophia Health Institute
Woodinville, Washington

**Ingrid Kohlstadt, MD, MPH, FACPM,
FACN**
Faculty, Johns Hopkins Bloomberg School of
  Public Health
Baltimore, Maryland
Executive Director, NutriBee National
  Nutrition Competition, Inc.
Annapolis, Maryland

Cynthia Kupper, RD
Gluten Intolerance Group of North America
Auburn, Washington

Joseph Lamb, MD
Metagenics, Inc.
Gig Harbor, Washington
KinDex Therapeutics, LLC
Seattle, Washington

Linda A. Lee, MD, AGAF
Johns Hopkins Integrative Medicine and
  Digestive Center
Johns Hopkins University School of Medicine
Baltimore, Maryland

Jay Lombard, DO
Associate Professor of Neurology
Touro College of Osteopathic Medicine
Chief Medical Officer, Genomind LLC
Chalfont, Pennsylvania

Jayashree Mani, MS, CCN
ELISA/ACT Biotechnologies, LLC
PERQUE Integrative Health, LLC
Ashburn, Virginia

Dennis Meiss, PhD
President & CEO
ProThera Inc.
Reno, Nevada

Gerard E. Mullin, MD, MHS, CNS, CNSP, FACN, FACP, AGAF, ABHM
Director of Integrative GI Nutrition Services
    Division of Gastroenterology and
    Hepatology
Director of Celiac Program
Johns Hopkins Hospital
Baltimore, Maryland

Patricia Mulready, MD
P.A. Mulready Associates, LLC
Time To Live Better.com LLC
Middletown, Connecticut

Melissa A. Munsell, MD
Division of Gastroenterology
Southern California Permanente Medical
    Group
Anaheim, California

David Musnick, MD
Peak Medical Clinic
Bellevue, Washington

Trent W. Nichols, Jr., MD, FACN, CNS, Diplomat ABIM, Gastroenterology
Hanover, Pennsylvania

Thomas O'Bryan, DC
Adjunct Faculty
Institute for Functional Medicine
Encinitas, California

Stephen Olmstead, MD
Chief Science Officer
ProThera, Inc.
Reno, Nevada

Kelly L. Olson, PhD
SleepImage
Broomfield, Colorado

Yoshiaki Omura, MD, ScD, FACA, FICAE, FRSM
Adjunct Professor of Department of Family &
    Community Medicine, New York Medical
    College
Westchester, New York
Director of Medical Research
Heart Disease Research Foundation
Brooklyn, New York

Ronald R. Parks, MD
MacroHealth Medicine
Asheville, North Carolina

David Perlmutter, MD, FACN
Perlmutter Health Center
Naples, Florida

Debbie Petitpain, MS, RD
Bariatric Surgery Program
Medical University of South Carolina
Charleston, South Carolina

Octavia Pickett-Blakely, MD, MHS
Division of Gastroenterology and Hepatology
Perelman School of Medicine
University of Pennsylvania
Philadelphia, Pennsylvania

Joseph E. Pizzorno, ND
SaluGenecists, Inc.
Seattle, Washington

Valencia Booth Porter, MD, MPH
The Chopra Center for Wellbeing
Carlsbad, California

Shideh Pouria, MBBS, BSc, MRCP (UK), PhD
Visiting Research Fellow
King's College
London, United Kingdom

Steven G. Pratt, MD, FACS, ADHM
Scripps Memorial Hospital
La Jolla, California

Scott Quarrier, MPH
Stony Brook University School of Medicine
Stony Brook, New York

Stuart Richer, OD, PhD, FAAO
Eye Clinic, Operative and Invasive Procedures
Captain James A. Lovell Federal Health Care
    Facility
North Chicago, Illinois

Jose M. Saavedra, MD
Associate Professor of Pediatrics
Johns Hopkins University School of Medicine
Baltimore, Maryland

Jyotsna Sahni, MD
Medical Director
Sleep Centers of Oro Valley
Oro Valley, Arizona

Maya Shetreat-Klein, MD
Integrative Pediatric Neurology
New York Medical College
New York, New York

Stephen T. Sinatra, MD
Assistant Clinical Professor of Medicine
University of Connecticut School of Medicine
Farmington, Connecticut

Neal Speight, MD
Center for Wellness
Matthews, North Carolina

Frederick T. Sutter, MD, MBA
Center for Wellness Medicine
Lifestyle Medicine Consultants, Inc.
Annapolis, Maryland

Jacob Teitelbaum, MD
National Fibromyalgia and Fatigue Centers

Valori Treloar, MD, FAAD
Integrative Dermatology
Newton, Massachusetts

Alan R. Vinitsky, MD
Enlightened Medicine
Gaithersburg, Maryland

Alan Weiss, MD
Annapolis Integrative Medicine
Annapolis, Maryland

Bradley W. Whitman, MD, MS
Genesis Neuroscience
Bonita Springs, Florida

Eileen Marie Wright, MD, ABIHM
Asheville, North Carolina

Section I

Disorders of the Ears, Eyes, Nose, and Throat

1 Age-Related Macular Degeneration

Geoffrey R. Harris, M.D., Steven G. Pratt, M.D.,
and Stuart Richer, Ph.D.

INTRODUCTION

Age-related macular degeneration (AMD) is an eye disease characterized by a gradual loss of central vision in people over the age of 55. While medical treatments for prevention of catastrophic loss of vision are making great strides, treatment of mild and moderate macular disease have demonstrated limited success. Nutritional interventions can make a marked difference in the prevention of disease progression and vision enhancement. Understanding the nutritional and lifestyle measures that have shown benefit against this disabling disease is important for managing an expanding older population who are at risk for developing AMD.

BACKGROUND

AMD is the leading cause of blindness in the United States in people over the age of 55. In 1992, the Beaver Dam Eye Study, a large, longitudinal study of over 5000 individuals in Wisconsin, found that the prevalence of AMD increases with age from 14.4% in patients 55 to 64 years old, to 19.4% in patients 65 to 74 years old, and 36.8% in patients over 75 years of age. Persons aged ≥ 85 years old, the fastest growing segment of the U.S. population, have a tenfold higher prevalence of late AMD than those aged 70 to 74 years [1]. With the population of individuals over the age of 55 reaching more than 66 million in the United States, the estimated number of cases of AMD there has grown to over 1.6 million. As the number of Americans over the age of 55 continues to grow, the number of cases of AMD will also continue to rise. It is estimated that there will be almost 3 million cases of AMD by 2020 [2].

AMD primarily affects both the foveal area of the retina that is used for sharp, central vision and the rod dense parafoveal region responsible for low contrast vision. There are two forms of AMD: exudative ("wet") and atrophic ("dry"). The exudative form is less common but more acutely threatening to vision and is considered an advanced form of AMD. Wet AMD accounts for only 10 to 15% of AMD cases but causes 90% of severe vision loss associated with AMD [3]. Atrophic AMD is the more common and milder form, accounting for 85 to 90% of cases. It develops gradually over time and typically causes seemingly mild vision loss in terms of traditional Snellen chart, high-contrast visual acuity. Nonetheless, patients with dry AMD have difficulty in low light and/or low contrast situations, such as twilight or night driving and reading [4].

To understand the pathophysiology of AMD, it is helpful to first review the pertinent anatomy. The macula is a small part of the retina, approximately 3 mm in diameter, which contains the fovea at its center. The center of the fovea is the thinnest part on the retina and is typically free of any blood vessels or capillaries. The macula, particularly the fovea, is responsible for detailed central vision and has a preponderance of cone-type photoreceptive cells. There are two functional layers to the macula: the photosensitive layer of rods and cones that gather light and convert it to nerve impulses and the underlying retinal pigment epithelium (RPE) with its basal lamina (Bruch's membrane) that maintains the division between the retina and the choroidal vasculature [5].

Understanding the pathophysiology helps to explain the current medical and nutritional therapies for AMD. AMD is a multi-factorial retinal and systemic disorder with multiple predisposing genetic and modifiable epigenetic factors [6,7]. Diagnosing early AMD requires the use of instruments sufficiently sensitive to distinguish the healthy aged retina from the pathologic retina. Clinically, the symptoms of early AMD are subtle with the patient complaining of 1) an area of diminished vision within the visual field (scotoma), 2) difficulty adapting to darkness (dark adaptation impairment), and 3) impaired glare recovery from photo-stress.

New, specialized commercial macular micro-perimetry instrumentation MAIA™ –Macular Integrity Assessment technology (www.elerex.com), the Nidek MP-1S Scotopic Microperimeter www.nidek.com), or combination spectral domain optical coherence tomography (SD OCT) retinal imaging microperimeter (www.opkos.com) allow early scotomas to be detected in a routine office encounter. More serious acute distortions involving deformation of the photoreceptor layer are typically self-diagnosed by the patient as distortions, or within the office with a simple Amsler Grid chart (circa 1895), Preferential Hyperacuity Perimetry, or by directly viewing the posterior photoreceptor/RPE layers of the retina for visible alterations with SD OCT imaging technology.

During the AMD disease course, the RPE/Bruch's function also deteriorates, hampering nutrient and oxygen transport to the photoreceptors. As a side effect, the photoreceptors exhibit impaired dark adaptation because they require these nutrients for replenishment of photopigments and clearance of opsin, a group of light sensitive proteins found in the photoreceptors, to regain dark vision sensitivity after light exposure. Dark adaptometry can be assessed with four clinical devices for assessment of photo-stress glare recovery: two office based, the Kowa AS 14-B (Kowa Optimed, JP) and AdaptTx (Apeliotus Vision Science, Atlanta, GA), and two portable devices (Eger Macular Stressometer, Gulden Ophthalmics, Elkins Park, PA) and MDD-2 (Health Research Sciences, Lighthouse Point, FL).

Examination of the eye typically, after age 50 years but beginning as early as the 30s in early atrophic AMD, also reveals the objective signs of retinal degeneration known as lipofuscin. This is an aging toxic RPE waste product that can be imaged with several new commercially available conventional fundus cameras (i.e., www.canonusa.com and www.topconusa.com) as well as SD OCT (i.e., Spectralis Blue Peak, www.heidelbergengineering.com).

As the AMD retina ages, expert examination of the retina reveals the accumulation of cellular debris between the retinal pigment epithelium and the basement membrane in the form of pale spots called "drusen." Atrophic ("dry") AMD causes atrophy of photoreceptors and changes to the retinal pigment epithelium, Bruch's membrane, and choroidal blood flow with calcification of the choriocapillaris. Over time, these changes worsen and overtly damage the macula and fovea through retinal pigment epithelium detachment that destroys the overlying photoreceptors. The more severe exudative ("wet") AMD is characterized by neovascularization of the fovea, which leads to capillary leakage and exudative damage to the macula. Neovascularization occurs after the integrity of Bruch's membrane is compromised [8]. It is not uncommon for a patient to have both atrophic and exudative changes in a single retina. Clinically, patients with atrophic AMD typically develop exudative AMD at a later time. The onset and progression of AMD typically follows a pattern of successive and progressive stages [9].

As mentioned, the symptoms of early AMD are subtle with the patient complaining of blurring scotoma disturbances, prolonged glare-readaptation (photo-stress recovery), a drop in contrast sensitivity (i.e., decreased vision of medium and large size objects), and the requirement of more light when reading. Central Snellen visual acuity changes occur later in the disease process compared to the early stealth-like changes that affect "cultural vision" such as driving and reading ability. Eventually, when central foveal acuity is affected, severe loss of legal-visual acuity and visual field distortions can occur.

As AMD progresses and vision worsens, patients indicate worsening disability and reduced quality of life. Central vision is critical for reading, performing basic manual tasks, driving, and even walking in an unfamiliar environment. Heightened fall risk is suggested by a study associating AMD with an increased risk for hip fracture [10]. Individuals with AMD and visual impairment rate themselves lower on quality of life surveys and questionnaires that assess activities of daily living when compared to matched, unaffected controls [11].

AMD is also a risk factor for poorer survival and cardiovascular morbidity. Data from the Copenhagen eye study identified an increased risk (RR = 1.59 with 95% confidence interval (CI) of 1.23–2.07) for all-cause mortality in women with early- and late-stage macular degeneration [12]. In this study, men did not have a significantly increased risk, but the Age-Related Eye Disease Study (AREDS) research group found an increased risk for mortality in their group of men and women with advanced AMD with a relative risk of 1.44 with a 95% CI of 1.08 to 1.86 [13]. AMD is also associated with a higher risk for developing a myocardial infarction, even when controlling for other factors like smoking and age [14]. Furthermore, a 2006 report from the Atherosclerosis Risk in Communities study found that middle-aged individuals with AMD have an increased risk for stroke, independent of other stroke risk factors [15]. While AMD may not be the direct cause of mortality or cardiovascular disease, it is a marker for other processes and diseases that affect mortality.

DIAGNOSIS OF MACULAR DEGENERATION

Signs of early AMD run the gamut from difficulty reading small type without bright lighting, color vision disturbances, and glare readaptation delays to severe central scotomas and actual loss of high contrast visual acuity on a Snellen eye chart from circa 1862 (Table 1.1). Screening for AMD can be performed using an Amsler grid from circa 1895, which looks like graph paper made from dark lines on a white background. Patients monocularly focus their vision on a small central spot about 14 inches from their face. If any of the straight lines appear wavy, broken, or distorted, a patient should be referred for a timely dilated retinal examination. Hopefully, an eye professional will perform a more detailed assessment of vision and a macular examination by fundal stereo-biomicroscopy or high-resolution SD OCT. While standard examination of the fundus can identify retinal drusen, edema, and neovascularization in exudative AMD, retinal angiography (using fluorescein dyes) and choroidal angiography (using indocyanine dyes) definitively depict the anatomic vascular outline. These dyes show the architecture (and any leakage) within the retinal vascular tree and underlying choroidal circulation, respectively. The latter high-flow choroidal vasculature system, specifically directly below the fovea, is typically the origin of pathology. Serial SD OCT imaging is increasingly being used to identify the histology of the macula, while identifying high-risk patients. The quantification of choroidal blood flow will become a routine clinical tool, allowing the clinician to evaluate the effect of nutritional intervention [5].

TABLE 1.1

Signs and Symptoms Associated with AMD

Need for Increased Illumination

Glare Sensitivity

Decreased Night Vision

Poor Color Discrimination

Difficulty Reading or Performing Activity That Requires Fine Vision

Distortion of Straight Lines

Blurred Vision

Difficulty Distinguishing Faces

Loss of Central Vision

MEDICAL TREATMENTS FOR MACULAR DEGENERATION

While there are emerging pharmaceutical treatments for atrophic AMD, the typical management is nutritionally related and will be discussed in detail here. The existing current medical treatments for AMD address only end-stage, exudative AMD and focus on inhibiting the neovascularization that leads to capillary leakage of blood and fluid in the macula. Managing neovascular AMD is sometimes a difficult, long-term process, with multiple intra-vitreal anti-VEGF (Vascular Epithelilal Growth Factor) injections, that aims to slow vision loss by preventing vessel formation. Treatments must be instituted early to prevent exudative damage, extensive neovascularization, and secondary scarring [16].

Thermal photocoagulation with a laser was the first effective therapy to show promise in neovascular AMD. Unfortunately, thermal laser was only found to be helpful when used on vessels outside of the foveal avascular zone so as to prevent any collateral damage to the crucial foveal photoreceptive cells by the laser. Older techniques have focused on foveal neovascularization using a non-thermal laser and a photosensitizing drug (verteporfin) that is more selective to blood vessels and causes less collateral photoreceptor damage [5]. Radiotherapy using fractionated radiation has also been shown to provide benefit in preserving near vision and contrast sensitivity. Other treatments being tested involve anti-angiogenic compounds (anecortave acetate and triamcinolone acetonide) injected intravitreally or administered periocularly. Recent research has focused on slowing vision loss by neutralizing epithelial growth factor using a monoclonal antibody (ranibizumab) or modified oligonucleotide (pegaptanib sodium) injected directly into the vitreous [17]. Another promising molecule is pigment epithelium derived growth factor, which prevents angiogenesis and may improve the health of the retinal pigment epithelium and restore the blood-retinal barrier [18]. Currently, no treatments are available for severe, AMD-associated central vision scarring.

RISK FACTORS FOR AGE-RELATED MACULAR DEGENERATION

MEDICAL RISK FACTORS FOR AMD

To effectively manage and prevent both the development and progression of AMD in patients, a physician must have an understanding of the associated risk factors for AMD (Table 1.2). The unmodifiable risk factors for AMD include: age, gender, race, eye color, previous AMD in one eye, and genetic predisposition or family history. However, an exciting new area of functional nutritional medicine includes modification of the expression of the genome through epigenetics and adaptive hormetic response, in which a low exposure to a noxious compound stimulates a beneficial molecular response [19]. For example, in the case of the polyphenol resveratrol, hormesis is recognized by the human body as a low-dose toxin that activates remarkable antioxidant defenses in the human body, while beneficially activating a myriad number of molecular pathways [20,21,22].

The risk for developing AMD increases with age, and individuals over 75 years old have the highest risk [2]. Women are at a higher risk for developing AMD, though many authors suggest that this may be because women have a longer life expectancy and survive to develop AMD [23]. Blue or green iris color and Caucasian race are also risk factors for developing AMD. Caucasians are at a much higher risk of losing vision to AMD than African Americans. This risk may be related to a decrease in melanin pigments or other protective mechanisms in the iris and retina that prevent high-energy light from damaging the macula [24]. Another unmodifiable risk factor for developing AMD in an eye is having AMD in the other eye, indicating that the disease is not a random occurrence, but may be related to an individual's genetic and environmental predispositions [25].

GENETIC RISK FACTORS FOR AMD

Genetic studies have shown that there is a hereditary susceptibility to developing AMD. Monozygotic twin studies have identified an increased risk for developing AMD in individuals whose identical

---

TABLE 1.2
Risk Factors for AMD

Unmodifiable Risk Factors

Advancing Age
Female Gender
Caucasian Race
Blue or Light-Colored Iris
AMD in One Eye
Family History of AMD
Previous Cataract Surgery

Modifiable and Cardiovascular Risk Factors

Smoking
Obesity
High Blood Pressure
Elevated Serum Cholesterol
Physical Inactivity
Coronary Artery Disease
Atherosclerosis
Diabetes
History of Stroke
Elevated hsCRP
High Serum Homocysteine
Increased Serum Levels of IL-6

Ocular Risk Factors

Excessive Sun Light and Blue Light Exposure
Low Macular Pigment Optical Density (MPOD)

Nutritional Risk Factors

Low Dietary Intake of Lutein and Zeaxanthin
Eating < Two Servings of Fish on a Weekly Basis
Low Long-Chain Omega-3 PUFA Intake
High Dietary Omega-6 to Omega-3 PUFA Ratio
High Fat Diet
Low Serum Vitamin D

---

twin has AMD, even when environmental factors are not shared [26]. While the development of AMD is likely multifactorial, there is particular interest in the ABCR gene which is associated with autosomal recessive Stargardt macular dystrophy. It is hypothesized that heterozygotes for ABCR mutations are at a higher risk for developing AMD [27].

More genes have been identified that are associated with an increased risk for developing advanced AMD and vision loss. Single nucleotide polymorphisms (SNPs) and specific haplotypes for multiple genes have been found to be associated with AMD. The important genes involved fall into four categories: complement factors, cholesterol metabolizing enzymes, energy metabolism genes, and extracellular matrix metabolic pathway proteins.

The first group of associated genetic risk factors is related to the complement cascade. Changes that lead to increased activation and increased inflammation are the most important. An SNP rs1061170 (T/C) in the gene for complement factor H, an inhibitor of C3 activation, was one of the first gene mutations found to be associated with AMD. Furthermore, polymorphisms in the C3 gene, which activates the complement cascade, are also associated with an increased risk for developing advanced AMD. The complement factor I, which serves as an inhibitor of activated complement factors (including C3), is another gene associated with AMD, and a genetic change in the regulation region of this gene can increase AMD risk. Other complement factor polymorphisms have also been identified that are associated with AMD [28].

The next group of genetic factors is associated with the metabolism of cholesterol. Drusen contains cholesterol, and HDL is the main transporter of the carotenoids lutein and zeaxanthin. While it is difficult to identify an association with specific serum cholesterol profiles and how they affect AMD risk, associations with AMD and the genes that control cholesterol metabolism have been identified. SNPs in the genes for the hepatic lipase gene, the lipoprotein lipase gene, cholesterol ester transferase gene, and the ABC-binding cassette A1 gene are associated with an increased risk for AMD [29].

Next, genetic alterations in the genes that repair cells from oxidative stress have also been implicated in AMD. The age-related maculopathy susceptibility 2 gene on chromosome 10q26 has an SNP site that can cause a deletion polymorphism in a gene that causes a protein not to be produced due to genetic instability. The gene protein product localizes to the mitochondria of photoreceptors where it seems to have a role in energy metabolism and oxidative stress. Also, mitochondrial DNA variations are associated with AMD. The mitochondrion genome encodes for 37 proteins that are used in energy metabolism and respiration. SNPs in the mitochondrial genome can lead to increased oxidative stress and AMD [30].

The extra cellular matrix peptidases break down the extra cellular matrix and are controlled by inhibitors. The TIMP3 gene codes for an inhibitor of metalloproteinase 3. Mutations in this gene are associated with an increased risk for developing wet AMD. It is thought that without proper inhibition that the macula can be damaged by metalloproteinase 3 and lead to exudative "wet" AMD. It is also speculated that metalloproteinase 3 can induce vascular growth, but more work is needed to completely understand its role in the eye [29].

A comprehensive genetic test has been developed by ArcticDx (www.macularisk.com). This test incorporates multiple genetic SNPs into a single test that establishes a risk profile for developing severe AMD. The test is designed for individuals with diagnosed early or intermediate AMD and is a prognostic DNA test that identifies risk of developing severe AMD. This test helps identify which individuals with early AMD need more frequent testing and nutritional interventions to thwart disease progression. The test is also being used in research studies to assess treatment outcomes [31].

Genetic risk factors for AMD are clinically relevant because they can be altered through medical and nutritional interventions. The objectives of the recent Rotterdam genetic-nutrition interaction study show the power of nutrigenomics. The purpose of this study was investigation of whether AREDS dietary nutrients can reduce the genetic risk of early AMD conferred by the genetic variants CFH Y420H and LOC387716 A69S in a nested case-control study. High dietary intake of nutrients with antioxidant properties reduced the risk of early AMD in those at high genetic risk. The authors concluded that clinicians should provide dietary advice to young susceptible individuals to postpone or prevent the vision-disturbing consequences of AMD [32].

MODIFIABLE RISK FACTORS

The most well-established modifiable risk factors for the development of AMD are smoking and obesity. Smoking is the most well-established modifiable risk factor for developing AMD, with many studies reporting a two- to threefold higher risk for current smokers compared with non-smokers [23,33]. Past smoking is also a risk, one which drops each year after quitting, although it never returns to that of age-matched individuals who never smoked [34].

Obesity has emerged as the second main modifiable risk factor behind smoking. Obesity, BMI greater than 30, higher waist circumference, and elevated waist to hip ratio have all been associated with a greater than twofold risk for the development and progression of AMD [35].

Another main set of medical risk factors associated with AMD are cardiovascular-related risks. Physical inactivity is one cardiovascular risk that is also a risk for AMD. Physically active individuals have a lower risk for developing exudative AMD (OR = 0.3, CI = 0.1 to 0.7) [36]. In addition, hypertension, elevated total cholesterol, coronary artery disease, atherosclerosis, diabetes, history of stroke, elevated C-reactive protein (specifically high-sensitivity C-reactive protein, hsCRP), high serum homocysteine, and increased levels of the systemic inflammatory marker, IL-6, are each risk factors for the development of AMD [37]. The association of AMD with elevated serum homocysteine, hsCRP, and IL-6 suggests that AMD is both an inflammatory and oxidative process [38].

OCULAR RISK FACTORS FOR AMD

Light exposure has a significant effect on ocular tissue. The sun creates full spectrum light: from ultraviolet through the visual spectrum to the infrared wavelengths. The higher energy light in the ultraviolet and blue spectrum can injure eye tissue through oxidative damage from the generation of free radicals. Ultraviolet light is absorbed by the human lens, so the only high-energy light that reaches the retina and macula is blue light [39]. There are many studies showing that exposure to blue light is toxic to retinal cells and retinal pigment epithelial cells in cell culture, rats, and monkeys [40].

Epidemiological studies of light exposure and AMD in human populations have produced conflicting results. The Pathologies Oculaires Liees a l'Age (POLA) study from France found no relationship between self-reported history of light exposure and the development of AMD [41]. However, in the Beaver Dam Eye Study, older participants who indicated that they had been exposed to the sun for more than five hours a day during their teenage years and young adulthood had a higher risk of developing AMD (RR = 2.20, CI = 1.02-4.73). In this study, participants who indicated that they had the same, high level of summer sun exposure but used hats and sunglasses at least half the time during their teenage and young adult years had a decreased risk of developing the early signs of AMD [23]. Similarly, in the Chesapeake Bay Waterman study, men exposed to increased levels of blue light were more likely to develop advanced AMD [42]. Overall, it does seem that there is an association between sunlight and blue light exposure and AMD.

Research has revealed that macular melanin and retinal pigments that absorb high-energy blue light also have a protective effect and reduce the risk of developing AMD. The macula, or macula lutea (lutea means yellow in Latin), has a yellow coloration that is attributable to the macular pigments that consist of the carotenoid xanthophyll isomers: lutein, its metabolite mesozeaxanthin, and zeaxanthin [43,44]. Xanthophylls are a type of carotenoid. There are over 600 known carotenoids, and between 40 and 50 carotenoids are available in a typical Western diet, although only 14 of these carotenoids have been detected in human blood. The two large groups of carotenoids are xanthophylls, which contain oxygen molecules in their molecular structure, and carotenes, which typically consist of only carbon and hydrogen. The most common xanthophylls in foods are lutein and zeaxanthin, while the most common carotenes are alpha-carotene, beta-carotene, and lycopene [45].

Lutein and zeaxanthin are yellow pigments that are selectively concentrated 1000 times greater in the fovea compared to other tissues [46]. Zeaxanthin being the predominant carotenoid [47]. It is generally accepted that these pigments protect the delicate macular photoreceptors and improve vision. The functions of these pigments include reduction of light scatter and color abnormalities, direct absorption of high-energy blue light that can damage the macula, and protection against free radicals created from photochemical reactions in the photoreceptor cells through lutein and zeaxanthin's antioxidant abilities. It is likely that these carotenoids perform each of these functions to protect the retina and preserve central vision [48].

All major risk factors for developing AMD are associated with the macular pigment [49]. A 2008 Japanese study identified that macular carotenoid levels decrease with age in both normal subjects and individuals with AMD. They also found that macular pigment carotenoid levels are significantly lower in patients with early AMD when compared with individuals without the signs of AMD [50]. This study confirms previous work that found that macular pigment optical density (MPOD) is inversely related to the risk of developing AMD [51].

SUNGLASSES FOR AMD

The perfect sunglasses not only block 100% of the UVA and UVB wavelengths, but also limit high-energy blue light. Sunglasses that block blue light tend to have an amber tint and can cause some minor color distortion. The amount of color distortion in amber lenses varies among different brands. The Neox lens that can be found in Callaway Golf Eyewear is a lens that blocks 100% of blue light up to 430 nm but allows the remainder of the visual spectrum to pass through causing less color distortion. Most reputable optical shops have a machine that can test the ability of a pair of sunglasses to block the appropriate wavelengths.

NUTRITIONAL RISK FACTORS FOR AMD

Intrinsic production of carotenoids does not occur in mammals, and thus macular pigment must be traced to dietary intake. Studies have shown that high dietary intake of lutein and zeaxanthin and of fruits and vegetables high in the xanthophyll carotenoids are associated with a lower risk for developing AMD [52]. Numerous studies have also shown that dietary intake of lutein and zeaxanthin has a direct association with serum levels of lutein and zeaxanthin, and that MPOD is directly related to both dietary intake of the xanthophyll carotenoids and serum levels of lutein and zeaxanthin [53,54].

Other dietary and nutritional risk factors for the development of AMD include low fish consumption, high fat diet, and low vitamin D levels. Increased intake of fish, at least two or more servings per week, reduces the risk for developing AMD [33]. Furthermore, dietary omega-3 fatty acids, which are found in high levels in fish, are also associated with a lower risk for developing AMD [55]. This reduced risk seems to be related to increased dietary intake of omega-3 polyunsaturated fatty acids (PUFAs) [56].

Recent prospective data from a large cohort of women health professionals without a diagnosis of AMD at baseline indicate that regular consumption of docosahexaenoic acid, eicosapentaenoic acid, and fish was associated with a significantly decreased risk of incident AMD and may be of benefit in primary prevention of AMD [57].

Docosahexaenoic acid (DHA), is the predominant PUFA in brain and retinal tissue, and retinal concentrations of DHA are dependent on dietary concentrations [58]. Animal studies have shown that dietary deprivation of DHA leads to lower retinal DHA levels, abnormal electroretinograms, and visual impairment [59]. Higher fish intake is associated with a lower risk for developing AMD in part because of the high concentrations of preformed DHA in fish. In order to achieve optimal retinal levels of DHA, the following dietary considerations are suggested:

1. A diet high in omega-6 PUFAs can inhibit omega-3 utilization [60]. Due to the pervasive use of vegetable oils that are high in omega-6 PUFAs, like corn and soybean oil, the relative ratio of omega-6 to omega-3 in a typical Western diet has risen to approximately 10 to 1 [61]. In non-Westernized diets and historic diets, the ratios have been estimated to be 2 to 1 and 1 to 1, respectively [62]. Studies have confirmed that high dietary intake of omega-6 PUFAs in the form of vegetable fat increases the risk of developing AMD. Vu et al. reported that individuals who ate more than 7.17 mg a day of the essential omega-6 fat linoleic acid (LA) had an increased risk of developing AMD [56]. The study found that lutein and zeaxanthin were protective for the development of AMD when LA levels were low.
2. Omega-6 fats from vegetable oils often undergo partial hydrogenation, which produces trans fats. Trans fats interfere with synthesis of DHA in several ways. One mechanism that has been well studied is the ability of trans fats to inhibit the rate-limiting enzyme

delta-6-dehydrogenase. Zinc deficiency also impedes this enzyme, presenting another mechanism by which zinc may prevent AMD.

3. Fats and oils that are processed through hydrogenation, partial hydrogenation, and several other methods lose a substantial amount of fat-soluble vitamins such as vitamin D, vitamin E, beta-carotene, lutein, and zeaxanthin. Enriched fats are those that have had the many different tocopherols and tocotrienols removed and replaced with alpha tocopherol. Oxidation in the retinal tissues is a process that requires diverse antioxidants to protect sensitive tissues like the retina. Separating fats from their antioxidant companions impairs the body's ability to safely achieve optimal protection for retinal health. How fats are processed can explain why a diet high in fat increases AMD. Consuming nuts, an unprocessed high fat food lowers risk for developing AMD [56].

The combination of high omega-6 content in the Western diet, introduction of trans fats, and processing fats to remove the natural antioxidants appears to have created a shortage of DHA usable for the retina, which can be mitigated with supplemental DHA.

Finally, vitamin D deficiency is related to the development of AMD. Serum levels of vitamin D have been shown to be inversely associated with early AMD. Furthermore, in a group of people who did not consume milk, which is fortified with vitamin D, patients who consistently took a vitamin D supplement were at lower risk (OR = 0.67, 95% CI = 0.5–0.9) of developing early AMD than individuals who did not take a vitamin D supplement [63]. Furthermore, a more recent study of vitamin D status and early AMD in 1313 postmenopausal women with complete ocular and risk factor data suggested among women younger than 75 years, intake of vitamin D from foods and supplements was related to decreased odds of early AMD in multivariate models. No relationship, however, was observed with self-reported time in direct sunlight [64].

TESTING FOR AMD IN HIGH-RISK PATIENTS

Screening for AMD is important after the age of 55. Table 1.3 summarizes screening and testing modalities for AMD. Patients can use an Amsler grid on a weekly basis to self-test for any central vision changes. An Amsler grid can easily be printed from the Internet and demonstrated in the office in only a few minutes. Unfortunately, the Amsler grid has a sensitivity of less than 50% and can miss a number of patients with AMD [65]. Additionally, most patients with early AMD have 20/20 vision by the Snellen eye chart. The best way to diagnose early AMD is through a thorough, dilated, retinal exam by an eye professional preferably using microperimetry dark adaptation and a photostress, glare recovery measurement in combination with retinal lipofuscin auto-fluorescence and SD OCT imaging. The macular pigment is typically depressed in the more involved retina and related to most risk factors.

After the age of 55, patients should have a dilated eye examination by an eye professional at least every three years and Snellen visual acuity (eye chart) testing on at least a yearly basis. The American Academy of Ophthalmology recommends that patients have a dilated eye examination every one to two years starting at the age of 65. Ideally, individuals over 55 years old should have a dilated eye examination every year by an eye professional, and this should be strongly recommended for at-risk patients.

Yearly routine physical examinations of patients over 55 years old should include questions about visual changes, problems with adapting after bright light exposure, difficulty reading, perception issues while driving, or vision loss. In addition to a thorough family history that includes eye diseases, the history should also include a social history that addresses sun exposure, utilization of sunglasses and hats, supplement usage, and dietary habits with an emphasis on fruit, vegetable, and fish consumption. Further testing should be recommended for high-risk patients. In addition to routine screening for cardiovascular disease with lipid panels, hsCRP levels, homocysteine levels, and renal and liver function panels, patients with multiple risk

TABLE 1.3

AMD Screening and Testing

Home

Amsler Grid—limited value, except in advanced disease

PHP Home Device— more effective at detecting advanced disease

Primary Care Office

Amsler Grid—limited value, except in advanced disease

Snellen Vision Testing—limited value, except in advanced disease

Thorough Ocular Review of Systems

Dietary and Sun Exposure History

BMI, Percentage of Adiposity—desirable for dosing carotenoids and fat-soluble vitamins

Low Contrast Reading Acuity—inexpensive/desirable

MDD-2 Photostress Glare Recovery Screener—inexpensive/desirable

Visual Function Questionnaire

Laboratory Tests

Renal, Liver Function

Lipid Panel—HDL especially important (macular pigment)

hsCRP

Homocysteine Level

Serum 25-Hydroxy Vitamin D

Serum Quantification of Carotenoids

Eye Professional Office

Low Contrast and Glare Recovery Vision Testing Screening

Dilated Eye Exam and Stereo Slit Lamp Biomicroscopy of the Macula

MPOD Testing (objective or subjective)—desirable

Stereo Optical Contrast Sensitivity Testing and Simulation—validated instrument

AdaptRx Glare Recovery—validated instrument

SD Optical Coherence Tomography—desirable

Autofluorescence Retinal Imaging—desirable

Fluorescein and ICG Angiography— if necessary

factors for AMD may benefit from photorecovery testing, serum carotenoid levels, and ocular testing for MPOD.

A photorecovery testing device, called the MDD-2 Macular Adaptometer, has been developed by Health Research Sciences. The MDD-2 is an office-based, FDA-approved, screening device designed for the primary care office. It is portable, non-invasive, and does not require pupillary dilation. Testing takes less than five minutes for both eyes and can be performed by a medical assistant. The results of the MDD-2 have been shown to be reproducible and photostress recovery time was shown to be statistically significant for identifying and monitoring AMD [66].

A more recent addition to photorecovery testing is the AdaptDx (MacuLogix, Hershey, PA). This is a desktop device that attempts to streamline dark adaptometry. The device performs a functional test of dark adaptation, which is the transition from being light adapted to being dark adapted [67]. Specifically, the AdaptDx measures the rate of recovery of scotopic sensitivity, or dark vision, after photobleaching. Patients are exposed to a standard camera flash and then asked to indicate when they can detect a progressively dimmer spot of light presented as a randomly timed flash at the edge of the anatomic fovea. Testing is completely non-invasive, and can be performed by an unskilled operator in < 10 minutes with a minimum of patient burden. The AdaptDx has received 510(k) clearance, based on its initial clinical trials on a small number of patients. An additional clinical trial of up to 200 people, for final validation, is currently underway at three independent sites including the Massachusetts Eye and Ear Infirmary in Boston; the Wilmer Eye Institute at Johns Hopkins University in Baltimore; and at the Penn State Hershey Eye Center in Hershey. Results are expected to be available in the third quarter of 2012. If the results follow those obtained to date, with 90% sensitivity and 100% specificity, the company hopes to begin marketing its AdaptDx as a diagnostic device by the end of 2012.

Serum quantification of carotenoids is available for clinical usage. LabCorp offers a beta-carotene level that only identifies beta-carotene, while Quest Diagnostics offers a fractionated carotene test that measures serum levels of alpha-carotene, beta-carotene, lutein, and zeaxanthin. The Quest Diagnostics test is performed by Associated Regional and University Pathologists, Inc. (ARUP) and requires an overnight fast (12 hours) and abstaining from alcohol for at least 24 hours prior to the test. The charge for the test is around $150, with the price varying based on the pricing by the local laboratory. [68] Check with your laboratory about the availability of carotenoid testing before ordering the test to ensure the proper evaluation is performed.

MPOD testing is becoming a more widely available tool for evaluating AMD risk [69]. Typically performed by an eye professional, MPOD testing is accomplished by a machine that measures the optical density of pigment in the macula, either subjectively or objectively [49]. Check with your local eye professionals as to whether they are performing MPOD determinations prior to referring a patient at high risk for developing AMD. MPOD testing and serum carotenoid levels can help guide a therapeutic plan for lowering risks and preventing AMD. Counseling and education about dietary habits, nutrient supplementation, and high-energy light avoidance and protection, are part of preventing and slowing the progression of AMD.

WHO SHOULD BE TESTED?

1. Any patient with signs or symptoms (see Table 1.1)
2. Any patient with a strong AMD risk factor, such as age over 50, smoker, obese, poor diet
3. Any patient with a family history of AMD
4. Any patient with diabetes
5. Any patient with photophobia
6. Any patient with a non-refractive reading or driving issue
7. Anyone in the transportation industry, which is 3% of the population
8. Athletes such as skiers (glare) and baseball players (fine acuity)

DIETARY AND NUTRITIONAL MANAGEMENT OF AMD

Nutritional management and prevention of AMD can be divided into two approaches: first, increasing dietary antioxidants, and second, augmenting the macular pigment by increasing the intake of xanthophyll carotenoids. Research has shown that the prevalence of AMD is higher in individuals with low antioxidant intake and low lutein intake [70]. Clearly, there is overlap between antioxidant and xanthophyll carotenoid intake because carotenoids are able to act as antioxidants, and antioxidants can increase intestinal absorption of lutein and zeaxanthin by protecting these pigmentary carotenoids [71]. However, this division is helpful when considering the scientific literature and counseling patients to make dietary changes.

ANTIOXIDANT INTAKE

Oxidative stress has been linked to AMD, and the earliest nutritional studies of AMD focused on the effects of antioxidant intake. The most commonly recognized antioxidants include vitamin C, vitamin E, and beta-carotene. Vitamin C, l-ascorbic acid, is a water-soluble, essential nutrient that can scavenge free radicals and can be regenerated (reduced) by glutathione. Vitamin E, which usually appears in supplements as alpha-tocopherol, is only one molecule in the tocopherol antioxidant family. In fact, the tocopherols, and the closely related tocotrienols, all have vitamin E activity. Tocopherols and tocotrienols are fat-soluble nutrients, as are carotenoids. The main compounds with vitamin E activity are alpha-, beta-, gamma-, and delta-tocopherol, and alpha-, beta-, gamma-, and delta-tocotrienols. Nuts, seeds, olive oil, whole-grains, and green leafy vegetables are all excellent sources of tocopherols and tocotrienols. Oxidized vitamin E, which is formed after vitamin E absorbs a free radical, is reduced back to its active form by vitamin C [72].

Beta-carotene is the most extensively studied of the carotenoids and serves as an example of both the benefit and potential risk of antioxidants. Early nutritional research found a positive correlation between consumption of foods high in beta-carotene and a lower cancer risk. This correlation led to many studies using beta-carotene supplementation as a potential means for preventing cancer. However, results of beta-carotene supplementation have been mixed, and in two large studies, beta-carotene supplementation was actually shown to increase lung cancer risk and increase mortality in smokers [73].

While most of the early studies of beta-carotene supplementation looked for a single nutritional compound for effective cancer prevention, subsequent research has discovered that the antioxidant benefit of beta-carotene involves a complicated relationship between vitamin C, vitamin E, glutathione, and other antioxidants. Beta-carotene requires other antioxidants to regenerate and prevent the development of its pro-oxidant form. To clarify this process, free radicals that are generated by oxidative stress can be absorbed by antioxidants to prevent these reactive free radicals from damaging DNA or cellular proteins and enzymes. When antioxidants absorb a free radical, they become oxidized (a pro-oxidative state) and must be reduced (regenerated). It is hypothesized that exclusive beta-carotene supplementation in individuals with low intake of other antioxidants actually causes a pro-oxidative state with oxidized beta-carotene causing further cellular damage [74].

Since antioxidants work in concert, the first antioxidant studies in AMD used a mix of compounds. One of the most publicized research studies of antioxidant supplementation in AMD is from the AREDS (Age-Related Eye Disease Study) group that is sponsored by the National Eye Institute. In their study, eleven retinal centers enrolled individuals from 55 to 80 years old and divided them into four groups based on their degree of AMD. Category 1 had no AMD and categories 2 through 4 had increasing degrees of AMD. Using a randomized, double-blinded, placebo-controlled design, participants in each category of AMD were assigned to one of four study groups: antioxidants, 80 mg of zinc (with copper to prevent anemia), antioxidants plus zinc (and copper), or placebo. In this study, the antioxidant mix included 500 mg of vitamin C, 400 IU of vitamin E, and 15 mg of beta-carotene. Average follow-up for the study was 6.3 years, with only 2.4% lost to follow-up. The outcomes that the study measured were AMD progression and change in visual acuity.

The AREDS study found no benefit of supplementation in patients with no AMD (category 1), but it did identify benefits to categories 2, 3, and 4. When categories 2, 3, and 4 were combined for analysis, there was a statistically significant decrease in risk of progression to advanced AMD for the zinc groups (when adjusted for age, sex, race, AMD category, and baseline smoking status) with an OR of 0.71 (CI = 0.51–0.98) and the antioxidant plus zinc groups with an OR of 0.72 (CI = 0.52–0.98). The risk of progression to advanced AMD was even lower when just the moderate and severe AMD groups (subjects in category 3 and 4) were analyzed. When the study looked at visual acuity loss in category 3 and 4 subjects, the only statistically significant risk decrease was achieved by subjects in the groups who took antioxidants plus zinc (OR = 0.73, CI = 0.54–0.99). It is important to note that trends toward lower risk for progression to advanced AMD and loss of visual acuity were found in categories 2, 3, and 4, for antioxidants, zinc, and antioxidants plus zinc though these did not reach statistical significance. Unfortunately, the study may not have been adequately powered to identify a benefit in the group with no AMD (category 1) [75]. Alternatively, the lack of benefit in category 1 patients may be because participants without AMD were zinc and antioxidant replete prior to supplement use or the testing used was insufficient to distinguish significant change in the macula.

Since recent research has identified the added benefit of the pigmentary carotenoids and the advantage of diets with high intake of antioxidant rich foods, studies using isolated antioxidants have been replaced by those evaluating more comprehensive supplements and dietary approaches. The AREDS has started the AREDS 2 trials that will evaluate the effects of supplemental lutein and zeaxanthin and/or omega-3 long-chain PUFAs, in combination with the original antioxidant formulation, on the development of AMD.

BETA-CAROTENE

Beta-carotene is a fat-soluble phytonutrient that is an immediate precursor of retinoic acid also known as vitamin A. While food sources are beneficial, supplements are not recommended at this time. As mentioned earlier in the antioxidant section, beta-carotene supplementation has been associated with an increased risk for developing lung cancer in smokers. Smokers, individuals with a history of smoking, and people with a higher risk for developing lung cancer, should not take beta-carotene supplements or multivitamins that contain beta-carotene. Furthermore, asbestos workers as well as individuals who abuse alcohol should avoid beta-carotene supplements. The AREDS 2 trial will also evaluate the effect of removing beta-carotene from the antioxidant formulation.

ZINC

Zinc is an antioxidant that has shown benefit in preventing the progression of AMD and has been included in antioxidant supplements for AMD. Zinc has antioxidant properties that protect proteins and tissues against free radical damage [76]. However, taking too much daily zinc can be a problem. High zinc intake can suppress copper absorption and lead to copper deficiency with subsequent immunosuppression and anemia [77]. The National Academy of Sciences–National Research Council's (NAS–NRC) recommended dietary allowance (RDA) for zinc is 8 mg/day of elemental zinc for women and 11 mg/day for men. The NAS–NRC has indicated that zinc supplementation should be limited to 40 mg a day [78].

Zinc is found in the protein component of plant and animal matter and in a variety of foods. The food sources of zinc include shellfish (especially oysters), red meat, poultry, fortified cereals, whole grains, legumes, greens, and nuts. Oysters have the highest amount of zinc per serving, but in a typical American diet most of the zinc comes from red meat and poultry. Zinc absorption is higher from animal protein than plant protein because plants contain organic acids like phytic acid and oxalic acid that bind elements like zinc and calcium and prevent their absorption. Consequently, vegetarians have a higher risk for zinc deficiency than omnivores [79]. Alcohol also decreases the absorption of zinc and increases urinary zinc excretion, and zinc deficiency is common in alcoholics [80]. Diarrhea also results in loss of zinc and zinc deficiency. Chronic diarrhea and malabsorption from celiac sprue, Crohn's disease, short bowel syndrome, pyrroluria, and bariatric surgery are risk factors for zinc deficiency [81]. Furthermore, one of the physiologic responses to emotional and physical stress is higher urinary excretion of zinc, which results in increased need of this trace mineral.

Zinc is available as a supplement, and daily multivitamins typically contain 15 mg of elemental zinc. Nutritional supplement shakes such as Ensure and Boost also contain zinc. When counseling patients about zinc intake and supplementation, it is important to understand the symptoms of zinc toxicity. High doses of zinc are associated with stomach upset, vomiting, headaches, diarrhea, fatigue, exhaustion, and a metallic taste, while copper deficiency typically presents with anemia symptoms [82]. Studies have also identified that supplementation with high levels of zinc can cause prostate enlargement [83] and increase the risk for developing Alzheimer's [84]. Continued high-dose therapy with zinc may also accelerate the development of atherosclerosis and heart disease by increasing total cholesterol and LDL, elevating serum triglycerides, and lowering HDL [85]. Zinc may also interfere with angiotensin-converting enzyme inhibitors, antibiotics, hormone replacement therapy, and non-steroidal anti-inflammatories. Zinc status can be difficult to assess in patients, and physicians must rely on a thorough dietary history and questions about supplementation to ensure patients are getting an adequate amount of zinc and avoiding excessive zinc consumption. Depleted zinc may also be suspected with certain rashes, frequent colds or viral infections, and lack of ability to taste zinc. If zinc cough drops or zinc challenge liquid taste neutral or even taste good, it is an indication that zinc stores are low. As zinc becomes replete the same cough drops and liquid taste bitter.

The effect of zinc in AREDS 1 was equivalent to the combination of the three other components. Patients should be encouraged to take a daily supplement with antioxidants including zinc, but dosages above 40 mg a day are unnecessary and potentially harmful due to the side effects and lipid effects mentioned earlier. The AREDS 2 trial will also test a lower level of zinc supplementation (25 mg) against the original high dose zinc (80 mg) that was used in the original AREDS trial.

ALPHA-LIPOIC ACID

Alpha-lipoic acid is a thiol antioxidant with an active cyclic disulfide bond that has been shown to be beneficial to retinal tissue by preventing oxidative stress and regenerating other antioxidants like glutathione, vitamin C, and vitamin E [86]. Alpha-lipoic acid is soluble in water and lipids due to its small size and chemical structure. In cell culture, retinal pigment epithelial cells are protected from oxidative damage by alpha-lipoic acid and its ability to scavenge reactive molecules [87]. Good sources of alpha-lipoic acid include broccoli and spinach. Both broccoli and spinach are also high in other antioxidants that work synergistically with alpha-lipoic acid. For example, sulforaphane, an isothiocyanate found in cruciferous vegetables like broccoli, has been shown to defend retinal tissue by working with other antioxidants to protect the macular cells from light-induced damage [88]. Furthermore, flavonoids, like luteolin, which is found in leafy vegetables like spinach, have been shown to protect retinal pigment epithelial cells from oxidative damage and decrease corneal neovascularization [89].

Alpha-lipoic acid is available as a supplement; however, recommended dosages have not been clearly established. As a nutritional supplement, the typical dosage of alpha-lipoic acid is 100–200 mg/day, although higher doses have been shown effective in treating liver disease and diabetic neuropathy. The no observed adverse effect level (NOAEL) for alpha-lipoic acid is considered to be 60 mg per kg of body weight per day [90].

LUTEIN AND ZEAXANTHIN INTAKE

Early studies revealed that increasing the dietary intake of lutein and zeaxanthin augmented the macular pigment optical density (MPOD) in study participants [91]. Furthermore, lutein supplementation of only 10 mg a day was shown to increase MPOD in individuals by 4–5% during a four-week study published in 2000 [92]. Since these studies were published, the interest in the effect of lutein and zeaxanthin on AMD has generated a large amount of exciting research.

The possibility for AMD vision improvement by macular pigment enhancement with carotenoids or nutritional cofactors has been confirmed in the Phototrop study [93]; the Lutein Xanthophyll Eye Accumulation (LUXEA) study [94]; the Lutein Nutrition effects measured by Autofluorescence study (LUNA) [95]; the Taurine, Omega-3 Fatty Acids, Zinc, Antioxidant, Lutein study [96]; the Carotenoids and Antioxidants in Age-Related Maculopathy Italian Study [97]; the Carotenoids in Age-Related Maculopathy Study [98]; and a recent macular pigment consensus paper [49].

In 2004, the LAST study (Lutein Antioxidant Supplementation Trial) published results showing improvement in visual function and MPOD in veterans with AMD taking either 10 mg of lutein alone or in combination with an antioxidant supplement [99]. In 2007, the LAST II trial showed that individuals with the lowest MPOD were the most likely to benefit from supplementation with lutein alone or lutein plus antioxidants [100]. The LAST II study results suggest that individuals with low MPOD can benefit from supplementation and actually improve their MPOD. Furthermore, the LUXEA (Lutein Xanthophyll Eye Accumulation) study published in

2007 found that supplementation with lutein (10 mg) causes pigment accumulation in the fovea, and zeaxanthin supplementation (10 mg) causes pigment accumulation over a wider area of the retina. Both xanthophyll carotenoids improved MPOD, but a mixture of lutein and zeaxanthin (10 mg/10 mg) resulted in the greatest statistically significant increase in MPOD [94]. The TOZAL study tested a multivitamin supplement that included vitamin C, vitamin E, lutein (8 mg), zeaxanthin (400 mcg), beta-carotene, zinc (70 mg), copper, and long-chain omega-3 PUFAs (120 mg DHA and 180 mg EPA, eicosapentaenoic acid, another long chain omega-3 PUFA) in patients with atrophic AMD. They found stabilization and improvement in visual acuity in 76.7% of the subjects who took the supplement over a six-month period [96].

One potentially contradictory study published in 2007 found that 6 mg of lutein supplementation in a group of 15 patients did not significantly improve contrast sensitivity in a group of AMD patients during a nine-month trial [101]. However, the small size of the study and low relative dose of lutein create more questions about the necessary study size, lutein dosage, and time to show benefit in supplement trials and AMD. The AREDS 2 trial will help clarify the appropriate supplement therapy because it is a very large, long-term (six-year) study.

More recently, the ZVF (Zeaxanthin and Vision Function) study, the only FDA approved randomized controlled trial outside the NIH/NEI/AREDS 1 and 2, was completed. They found that in older men with AMD, zeaxanthin-induced foveal macular pigment elevation mirrored that of lutein and provided complementary distinct visual benefits by improving foveal cone-based visual parameters, whereas lutein enhanced those parameters associated with gross detailed rod-based vision, with considerable overlap between the two carotenoids [102].

For now, it is reasonable to recommend an antioxidant supplement. Since many people at risk for AMD take multivitamins, the antioxidant supplement could be a multivitamin that contains lutein, zeaxanthin, alpha-lipoic acid, zinc with copper, and a full spectrum of vitamin E. This supplement should be combined with a fish oil supplement or other source of preformed DHA and EPA. We recommend patients take a total of 1 to 2 grams of a fish oil supplement daily.

CYSTEINE, GLUTATHIONE, AND TAURINE

Cysteine is an amino acid that serves double duty as a building block of proteins and precursor for glutathione and taurine, which serve as antioxidants in the retina due to their thiol group. While cysteine can be synthesized from the essential amino acid methionine, cysteine has been referred to as a "semi-essential" amino acid because humans synthesize cysteine only to a limited extent. Consequently, adequate cysteine intake is dependent on both methionine and cysteine intake [103].

In a typical Western diet, average cysteine intake is approximately 2 to 4 grams per day [104]. Despite this normal intake, studies of supplementation with cysteine have shown an added benefit to antioxidant status and health, indicating that average dietary intake may not be optimal [105]. Cysteine is easily oxidized and not shelf stable, and the disulfide form, cystine, is not well absorbed. Clinical studies of cysteine supplementation typically use N-acetylcysteine, a synthetic form of cysteine that is more stable and well absorbed, or cysteine-rich whey protein.

From an AMD standpoint, the cysteine derived antioxidants, glutathione and taurine, are found in high concentrations in the macula. In animal models of AMD, taurine deficiency leads to retinal photoreceptor degeneration and impaired visual acuity [106]. There have not been any studies that have looked at taurine for the prevention or treatment of AMD, but by ensuring that patients have an adequate intake of cysteine, taurine and glutathione will be available to the retina.

Taurine is widely distributed in animal tissues and dietary sources include eggs, seafood, and meat. Plants do not synthesize taurine and human synthesis can be limited [107]. Strict vegetarians and vegans have been shown to have significantly lower levels of taurine when compared with control groups on a typical Western diet [107]. Taurine supplementation (500 mg a day) should be considered as part of a nutritional program for vegetarians and individuals with low animal protein intake.

B VITAMINS

Elevated homocysteine levels are a risk factor for AMD. Supplementation with vitamin B6, folic acid, and vitamin B12 can lower homocysteine levels and reduce the incidence of AMD. In a long-term, double-blind study of 5205 women who had risk factors for cardiovascular disease, the incidence of developing AMD was 34% lower in the group that received 2.5 mg of folic acid, 50 mg of pyridoxine, and 1 mg of vitamin B12 on a daily basis when compared with the placebo group [108]. Managing elevated homocysteine levels with B vitamins is an essential part of AMD prevention.

THE SYNERGY OF WHOLE FOODS

To appropriately achieve a healthy dietary mix of antioxidants, carotenoids, and omega-3 PUFAs, AMD patients should receive nutritional counseling about incorporating beneficial foods and limiting harmful foods in their diet.

Whole foods are very important to the management and prevention of AMD. As scientific research expands the number of crucial nutrients that are included in the latest antioxidant AMD supplements, whole foods seem increasingly significant. Whole foods contain a mix of vitamins, minerals, and phytonutrients that act as antioxidants and anti-inflammatories. Phytonutrients are plant nutrients that work with the traditionally recognized vitamins and minerals and have therapeutic benefit. The common families of phytonutrients include: carotenoids such as lutein, zeaxanthin, lycopene, beta-carotene, and alpha-carotene; and polyphenols, which include the isoflavones, flavonoids, and tannins. The flavonoid group includes anthocyanins and catechins. Whole fruits and vegetables contain an extensive mix of these phytonutrients.

Early studies that established the benefit of antioxidants and carotenoids on AMD examined food questionnaires in epidemiological studies. The focus on individual nutrients was borne out of these studies when researchers tried to identify single vitamins, minerals, or phytonutrients from the whole foods that might be providing the benefit for AMD. Trying to discover one beneficial compound in the complicated mix of nutrients in whole foods may not be reasonable. Identifying the fruits and vegetables that prevent and slow the progression of AMD is the important issue, not the possible individual nutrients.

Intake of foods high in lutein and zeaxanthin is important to preventing AMD and slowing its progression. Studies have revealed an inverse relationship between both the volume and the frequency of carotenoid-rich food consumption and the risk of developing macular pigment abnormalities [109]. A partial list of foods that are high in lutein and zeaxanthin can be found in Table 1.4. Spinach is an excellent food for AMD because it is high in lutein and zeaxanthin, contains a mix of tocopherols, and has alpha-lipoic acid and other carotenoids and phytonutrients. Broccoli contains the xanthophyll carotenoids, alpha-lipoic acid, and sulforaphane, a phytonutrient that protects retinal cells from high-energy light induced free radicals [88]. Egg yolks are another good source of lutein, with a higher bioavailability than lutein supplements, lutein ester supplements, or spinach [110].

Furthermore, many flavonoids found in whole foods have shown benefit in preventing retinal pigment epithelial cells from oxidative stress. Fisetin found in strawberries, luteolin in oranges and spinach, quercetin from apples and red onions, and epigallocatechin gallate (EGCG) from green tea all have a protective effect against free radicals in retinal cells [89]. By including the whole food source for these phytonutrients in a typical diet, a patient will increase their dietary levels of many other vitamins and minerals that may help prevent AMD, including vitamin C, tocopherols, carotenoids, and zinc. Whole fruits and vegetables offer a nutrient synergy due to their complex mix of many vitamins, minerals, and phytonutrients that is difficult to recreate.

By increasing fruit and vegetable intake, and limiting high-fat, high-calorie, and low-nutrient foods, patients will begin to lower their risk for AMD and other medical conditions. Eating more fish, supplementing DHA, and limiting the intake of vegetable oils will positively shift the dietary ratio of omega-6 to omega-3 and improve eye health and lower cardiovascular risk.

TABLE 1.4

Lutein and Zeaxanthin Content in Select Foods

Fruit, Vegetable, or Food Source	Lutein and Zeaxanthin Amount (micrograms/100 grams edible portion)
Kale, raw	39,550
Kale, boiled and drained	15,798
Spinach, raw	11,938
Spinach, boiled and drained	7,043
Lettuce, romaine, raw	2,635
Broccoli, boiled and drained	2,226
Corn, sweet, yellow, boiled and drained	1,800
Peas, green, canned	1,350
Carrots, baby, raw	358
Oranges, raw	187
Egg, raw	55

Adapted from USDA-NCC Carotenoid Database for U.S. Foods, 1998

THE PROCESSING OF WHOLE FOODS

When recommending whole foods to patients, it is critical to consider how the foods are treated prior to arriving at the grocery or market. Nutrient content of whole foods can be diminished by the mass production of food, irradiation, and storage. The content of the nutrients discussed in this chapter are diminished by radiation of such products as meat, produce, eggs, cooking oils, flour, and spices; it is the nutrients that we want to optimize when recommending whole foods [111]. We recommend patients consider buying in-season fruits and vegetables from local growers and buying organic whenever possible.

WHOLE FOODS IN THE PREVENTION OF NEOVASCULARIZATION AND ANGIOGENESIS

There is emerging information about the beneficial effects of the phytonutrients from whole foods on the prevention of angiogenesis. Angiogenesis from the choroidal vasculature leads to neovascularization of the macula and the extremely debilitating, exudative AMD. Recent research has found that certain phytonutrients suppress endothelial cell growth and prevent angiogenesis. EGCG from green tea has been shown to block vascular endothelial growth factor (VEGF) in vitro and prevent neovascularization in an embryonic membrane and mouse corneal tissue [112]. Pomegranate extract, polyphenols from oranges, and flavonoids from berries, have all been shown to inhibit angiogenesis and inhibit VEGF [113]. Another phytonutrient—procyanidin—found in cocoa, can inhibit vascular endothelium proliferation after oxidative stimulation [114]. Furthermore, resveratrol, another phytonutrient from red wine, can prevent angiogenesis when administered orally. A 2009 case report of an 80-year-old with AMD-associated night-driving difficulties observed visual function improvements and a decrease in retinal pigment epithelial debris after five months on a daily, over-the-counter polyphenolic supplement containing resveratrol [20].

While research still needs to address the long-term effect of these phytonutrients on AMD, encouraging patients to eat berries, oranges, pomegranates, and dark chocolate is not likely to cause harm. Furthermore, eating whole fruits and vegetables and drinking green tea and red wine (in moderation) may not only benefit AMD, but prevent cancer, since the growth of solid tumors is dependent on angiogenesis. Currently, resveratrol and other phytonutrients are available as supplements and may prove beneficial as part of a comprehensive AMD management plan. We are encouraged by the potential of phytonutrients to prevent and limit angiogenesis in exudative AMD.

CARBOHYDRATES AND AMD

While whole grains that are high in nutrients and fiber are an important tool in the nutritional management of AMD, refined carbohydrates should be avoided. A 2007 study found that individuals who consumed a diet rich in refined carbohydrates with a high glycemic index had a higher risk of AMD progression when compared with individuals who consumed a diet with a low-glycemic index [115]. Physicians should encourage AMD patients to limit refined carbohydrates.

NUTRITIONAL ISSUES IN AMD MANAGEMENT

ABSORPTION AND AVAILABILITY OF DIETARY CAROTENOIDS

The two main issues with regard to carotenoid bioavailability are release of carotenoids from the food source and digestive absorption. Since carotenoids are typically intracellular in fruits and vegetables, the cell wall must be compromised for the carotenoids to be available for micellization, the process of creating a micelle, which facilitates the absorption of fat and fat-soluble nutrients. Gentle cooking, processing by chopping or shredding, and thorough mastication are the best ways to increase the availability of carotenoids from plant sources, while gastric digestion is less efficient [116]. Furthermore, there does seem to be a difference in how effectively the xanthophylls and carotenes are released. Xanthophylls seem to be more readily freed from the food matrix and more effectively micellized than carotenes, but carotenes are more efficiently absorbed by enterocytes [117]. Finally, large amounts of dietary carotene carotenoids can interfere with the absorption of xanthophyll carotenoids. Studies in which subjects were given large amounts of beta-carotene as a supplement showed declines in serum lutein levels [118].

Efficient micellization and absorption of carotenoids is also dependent on dietary fat intake because they are fat-soluble nutrients. While bile salts are important for forming micelles, fat from a meal helps the carotenoids to become soluble and allows for micelle formation and absorption [117]. Consequently, carotenoid-rich fruits and vegetables should be eaten with a small amount of dietary fat to aid intestinal absorption. An excellent way to enhance carotenoid absorption from a salad or salsa is to add avocado or avocado oil. Another important issue with regard to food preparation is cooking; while gentle cooking fractures cell walls and makes carotenoids more bioavailable, over-cooking at high heats can destroy carotenoids [119].

COOKING OIL SELECTION

In order to achieve optimal DHA from the diet, patients should evaluate their selection of cooking oils. They should avoid vegetable oils, like corn, safflower, sunflower, cottonseed, and soybean oil, which have very high relative ratios of omega-6 to omega-3 PUFAs [120]. Additionally, these oils are often hydrogenated, which generates trans fats. Margarine should also be avoided, as should cooking with high heat and deep-frying, which damage oils. Instead patients should choose olive oil and canola oil, which contain a higher proportion of omega-3 fats. Nut oils such as hazelnut, almond, avocado, macadamia, coconut, pistachio and red palm oils contain omega-9 and some short-chain saturated fats, which behave more favorably in the body than saturated animal fats. Regardless of which cooking oils are selected, the less processed the better. Extra virgin olive oil contains more antioxidants, which are the ingredients that confer the slightly green color to this oil. Some healthful oils, including walnut, flax, and pumpkinseed oil, are highly unsaturated and therefore very sensitive to heat when unprocessed. They should not be used for cooking, but can be stored in the refrigerator and added to cereal, salad, vegetables, and sauces.

Vitamin D in Older Adults

Older adults have a much higher risk for developing vitamin D deficiency. Elderly individuals typically have insufficient dietary vitamin D intake, inadequate sun exposure, and impaired renal conversion of provitamin D to calcitriol (vitamin D3) [121]. Additionally, sun exposure is not a reasonable way for older individuals to achieve appropriate vitamin D levels due to seasonal variation in the ultraviolet light levels that produce provitamin D and the risk for further macular damage from high-energy light exposure, however, 73% of the population in the United States is insufficient including nearly 50% of Floridians and Californians (www.vitaminDcouncil.org). Furthermore, ultraviolet damage to the skin from sunlight exposure is associated with an increased risk for skin cancer. Sun protection measures should be encouraged, and patients should be counseled to effectively achieve appropriate levels of vitamin D through diet and nutritional supplements.

Older individuals require more vitamin D than younger patients because of the aforementioned issues associated with achieving suitable vitamin D levels. The USDA recommends that men and women over 50 years old get 10 micrograms (400 IU) of vitamin D each day, and that people over 70 get 15 micrograms (600 IU) daily. These recommendations are not recommended dietary allowances (RDAs), but suggestions of adequate intakes (AIs). While the USDA advocates at least 600 IU per day, many nutritional experts recommend at least 2000 IU to 4000 IU per day to achieve a 25 (OH) vitamin D level of 40 to 60 ng/ml. Calcitriol, vitamin D3, is the more efficacious and preferred form of vitamin D, for adults [122].

Nutritional Health in the Elderly

Another important aspect to consider when deciding on nutritional interventions for an AMD patient is his/her general nutritional state. AMD is a disease of older individuals, and often, in an attempt to focus on AMD specific nutrients, basic nutritional education is overlooked. It is important to remember that with advancing age, nutritional status tends to decline. Changes in lifestyle, budget, and difficulty with meal preparation, combined with less efficient gastrointestinal functioning and lower caloric intake can lead to a poor nutritional state. Vitamins, amino acids, and minerals all play an important role in basic cellular functioning, management of free radicals, and tissue repair. A thorough management plan for AMD should include a discussion of diet, meal frequency, and possible difficulties with preparation or shopping.

Special Considerations for Carotenoid Intake and Absorption

Acid Blockers

The common over-the-counter drugs known as proton pump inhibitors deplete important nutrients because they alter the pH of the stomach. According to package warnings, they should not be used for more than 14 days during any four-month period. Chronic use of these medications in patients with AMD, combined with the relative achlorhydria of aging further aggravates the depletion of valuable ocular nutrients such as the carotenoids, B complex vitamins, and vitamins A, D, and E.

Warfarin

Warfarin (Coumadin) is a common oral anticoagulant that inhibits vitamin K reductase. Warfarin affects the synthesis of the vitamin K–dependent clotting factors by preventing the recycling of vitamin K. Many physicians and dieticians counsel patients on warfarin to completely avoid leafy vegetables, salads, or green vegetables due to their high vitamin K content, which can thus impair anticoagulation with warfarin. While this advice may reduce some forms of dietary vitamin K, it also prevents the dietary intake of carotenoids. Counseling and education should accompany any new prescription for warfarin. By explaining that changing dietary factors can affect warfarin's anticoagulant strength, a patient can be encouraged to maintain a diet that includes consistent amounts of carotenoid-rich vegetables. Warfarin dosage titration can be performed with the patient eating a steady and dependable amount of vegetables [123].

Obesity

Obesity is a risk factor for the development of AMD, in part because adipose tissue sequesters fat-soluble vitamins and antioxidants such as vitamin D and carotenoids (Table 1.5). Studies have shown lower plasma values of carotenoids in obese individuals [124]. Basically, obesity is associated with a relative carotenoid deficiency that may put patients at further risk for AMD [53]. It has also been established that MPOD levels are lower for obese individuals. Consequently, obese patients will require a diet with higher levels of carotenoids and more fruits and vegetables.

Gastric Bypass

It is well known that nutritional deficiencies are common in bariatric surgery patients. These nutritional deficiencies are related to both poor dietary intake and malabsorption [125]. Fat-soluble nutrient deficiency is more likely for procedures that include biliopancreatic diversion due to impaired micelle formation and lipase activity. A 1982 study found that carotenoid levels dropped rapidly and remained low in patients after jejunoileal bypass surgery [126]. To date, carotenoid level changes have not been studied for the now, more common Roux-en-Y gastric bypass. However, it is felt that overall malabsorption is less common for Roux-en-Y gastric bypass than previous procedures that diverted crucial absorptive gastrointestinal mucosa and the biliary and pancreatic digestive apparatus [127].

It is essential to understand the bypass procedure that a patient has undergone. Communication with the patient's surgeon may also be central to providing appropriate care. Furthermore, it is important to counsel gastric bypass patients to include vegetables in their diet. In addition to dietary counseling, it would be prudent to monitor carotenoid levels in bariatric surgery patients after gastric bypass to ensure they are attaining healthy levels.

Malabsorption Syndromes

Malabsorption due to decreased gastrointestinal absorptive surface area can be caused by previous bowel resection, intestinal bypass, celiac sprue, Crohn's disease, AIDS enteropathy, chemotherapy, abdominal radiation therapy, amyloidosis, and intestinal lymphoma. Malabsorption can also be caused by poor micelle formation and fat solubilization that occurs with parenchymal liver disease, cirrhosis, or biliary obstruction. Furthermore, pancreatic insufficiency from chronic pancreatitis, pancreatic resection, and cystic fibrosis can lead to malabsorption of fat-soluble nutrients due to impaired lipase activity [128]. Deficiency of fat-soluble vitamins and nutrients must be considered in patients with malabsorption syndromes, and serum carotenoid testing is warranted to monitor nutritional status.

TABLE 1.5

Fat-Soluble Vitamins and Antioxidants Can Produce Relative Deficiency in Obese Individuals Due to Fat Sequestration

Vitamin A
Vitamin D
Vitamin E (Tocopherols and Tocotrienols)
Vitamin K
Carotenoids (Alpha-Carotene, Beta-Carotene, Lycopene, Lutein, and Zeaxanthin)
Omega-3 PUFAs (DHA and EPA)

Orlistat

Orlistat, currently marketed under the brand names Xenical and Alli, is a reversible inhibitor of the lipase enzyme in the gut. By preventing lipase activity, dietary triglycerides cannot be hydrolyzed to absorbable monoglycerides and fatty acids. Undigested triglycerides pass unabsorbed into the stool. At the prescription dose of 120 mg, three times a day with meals, orlistat blocks the absorption of approximately 30% of dietary fat [129]. Fat-soluble vitamins and nutrients will also have a decreased absorption as they will pass with the undigested dietary fat. The noncaloric fat replacement olestra (brand name Olean) reduces fat-soluble vitamins by 10% when consumed in the intended amounts [130]. Since an over-the-counter formulation of orlistat is now widely available, it is important to ask patients if they are using orlistat (Alli) and might be at risk for fat-soluble nutrient deficiency. Roche, the pharmaceutical company that produces orlistat, recommends that patients using orlistat take a daily multivitamin supplement with the important fat-soluble vitamins at least two hours before taking orlistat. Furthermore, patients with malabsorption syndromes should not take orlistat because the drug will further aggravate gastrointestinal symptoms and nutrient deficiencies.

SPECIAL CONSIDERATIONS FOR OMEGA-3 FATTY ACIDS

Vegetarians

Vegans and ovo-lacto vegetarians who do not eat fish are at risk for being deficient in DHA [131]. The major dietary omega-3 PUFA in strict vegetarians is the essential fatty acid alpha linolenic acid (ALA) available from plant sources like flax and walnuts. ALA, a short-chain PUFA, must be lengthened. Studies have shown that healthy men can only convert 8% of dietary ALA to EPA and 0–4% to DHA. Due to the effects of estrogen, young women can convert about 21% of dietary ALA to EPA and 9% to DHA under optimal circumstances [132]. Because vegetarians have a relatively high intake of LA, their high ratio of omega-6 to omega-3 PUFAs can reduce elongation of ALA to DHA by 40 to 50% [131]. In summary, relying on the body to convert plant-derived ALA to DHA is not sufficient for optimum health [133].

Vegetarians should be encouraged to eat fish, take fish oil supplements, or take marine algae oil supplements to achieve appropriate levels of DHA. For strict vegetarians, the best way to get DHA is to go to the source, or at least close to it. The source of most DHA and EPA on the planet is from marine algae. Ocean microalgae make DHA and EPA naturally. Since the aquatic food chain starts with these ocean algae, fish get their DHA and EPA from eating the algae or other organisms that have eaten the algae.

Eggs yolks are another potential source of DHA. Interestingly, eggs that are high in DHA and EPA come from chickens that have been fed marine algae, fish meal, or fish oil. Please note that some eggs come from chickens fed flax meal. These eggs will have omega-3 as ALA, but much less DHA and EPA. Educate patients to read the egg cartons and choose the eggs with the highest amount of DHA and EPA.

EMERGING MOLECULAR APPROACHES

The stem cell therapies currently being researched for AMD work synergistically with the nutritional therapies described in this chapter. A limiting step for stem cell therapies in general are for the biologic treatment to migrate to the specific organ in need and take hold. For example, in the case of the red wine polyphenol resveratrol, the molecule is recognized by the human body as a low-dose toxin that activates remarkable antioxidant defenses in the human body, while beneficially activating a myriad number of molecular pathways [20,21,22]. Figure 1.1 demonstrates improvement in macular pigmentation, visual function, and retinal architecture in an octogenarian following clinical intervention with a resveratrol-based nutritional supplement [102].

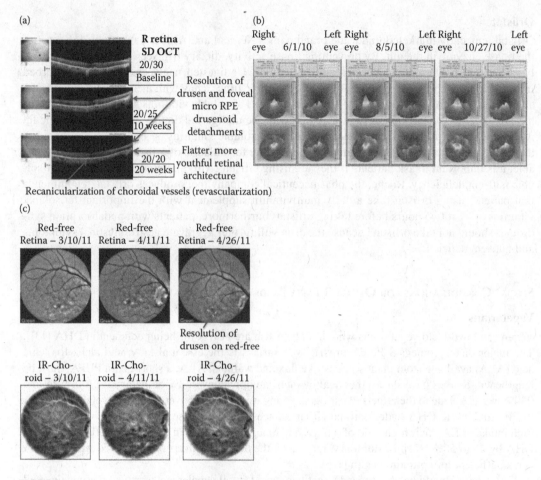

FIGURE 1.1 A resveratrol- and stem cell-based treatment reverses AMD in a case presentation.

SUMMARY

The nutritional approach to lowering the risk factors for the development of AMD and slowing the progression of the disease include:

- AMD is increasingly recognized as a disease of middle-aged and older adults who may have difficulty achieving basic nutrition. Be sure to question patients about dietary habits and access to healthy foods.
- Minimize cardiovascular risk factors, including smoking, hypertension, hyperlipidemia, hyperhomocysteinemia, and vitamin D deficiency.
- Support and promote daily exercise.
- Encourage patients to protect their eyes from high-energy light through the use of hats and sunglasses. Appropriate sunglasses should block UV wavelengths and limit high-energy blue light.
- Counsel patients to eat more fish (at least two servings a week) and take 1 to 2 grams of a fish oil supplement or marine algae supplement with DHA and EPA daily.
- Instruct high-risk patients to take an antioxidant supplement that includes vitamin C, mixed tocopherols (vitamin E), alpha-lipoic acid, zinc, copper, lutein, and zeaxanthin. Omega-3 PUFAs are also an important supplement for high-risk patients.

- Educate patients to eat whole foods that are high in lutein and zeaxanthin like spinach, kale, greens, and broccoli.
- Teach patients that whole fruits and vegetables have a mix of vitamins, minerals, and plant antioxidants that will promote eye health. Encourage berries, citrus fruits, apples, nuts, legumes, and green tea. A resveratrol or polyphenolic supplement of plant antioxidants should also be considered.
- Recommend patients optimize their 25 (OH) vitamin D liver reserve status to achieve a winter value of 40–60 ng/ml. This will likely require 2000 IU to 4000 IU of vitamin D as calcitriol (vitamin D3) daily, since they are to be avoiding sunlight for AMD prevention. Another acceptable approach is to dose supplemental vitamin D to normalize blood levels.
- Educate patients to limit processed carbohydrates, consume whole grains, and avoid iron-fortified grains if possible.
- Discourage high-fat diets and suggest patients limit their intake of fried foods and vegetable oils. Recommend patients choose lean red meats, poultry, and fish when eating meat. Encourage patients to cook with monounsaturated oils like olive oil.

REFERENCES

1. Jonasson, F., Arnarsson, A., Eiriksdottir, G., Harris, T. B., et al. 2011. Prevalence of age-related macular degeneration in old persons: Age, Gene/Environment Susceptibility Reykjavik Study. *Ophthalmology,* 118, 825–30.
2. Klein, R., Klein, B. E., and Linton, K. L. 1992. Prevalence of age-related maculopathy. The Beaver Dam Eye Study. *Ophthalmology,* 99, 933–43.
3. Friedman, D. S., O'Colmain, B. J., Munoz, B., Tomany, S. C., et al. 2004. Prevalence of age-related macular degeneration in the United States. *Arch Ophthalmol,* 122, 564–72.
4. Richer, S., Invited presentation, 10th annual Society for Free Radical Research meeting, Chennai, India, January 9, 2011.
5. Chopdar, A., Chakravarthy, U., and Verma, D. 2003. Age related macular degeneration. *BMJ,* 326, 485–88.
6. Chakravarthy, U., Wong, T. Y., Fletcher, A., Piault, E., et al. 2010. Clinical risk factors for age-related macular degeneration: Systematic review and meta-analysis. *BMC Ophthalmol,* 10, 31.
7. Chen, Y., Bedell, M., and Zhang, K. 2010b. Age-related macular degeneration: Genetic and environmental factors of disease. *Mol Interv,* 10, 271–81.
8. Zarbin, M. A. 1998. Age-related macular degeneration: Review of pathogenesis. *Eur J Ophthalmol,* 8, 199–206.
9. Sarks, J. P., Sarks, S. H., and Killingsworth, M. C. 1988. Evolution of geographic atrophy of the retinal pigment epithelium. *Eye (Lond),* 2 (Pt 5), 552–77.
10. Anastasopoulos, E., Yu, F., and Coleman, A. L. 2006. Age-related macular degeneration is associated with an increased risk of hip fractures in the Medicare database. *Am J Ophthalmol,* 142, 1081–83.
11. Knudtson, M. D., Klein, B. E., Klein, R., Cruickshanks, K. J., and Lee, K. E. 2005. Age-related eye disease, quality of life, and functional activity. *Arch Ophthalmol,* 123, 807–14.
12. Buch, H., Vinding, T., La Cour, M., Jensen, G. B., et al. 2005. Age-related maculopathy: A risk indicator for poorer survival in women: The Copenhagen City Eye Study. *Ophthalmology,* 112, 305–12.
13. Clemons, T. E., Kurinij, N., and Sperduto, R. D. 2004. Associations of mortality with ocular disorders and an intervention of high-dose antioxidants and zinc in the Age-Related Eye Disease Study: AREDS Report No. 13. *Arch Ophthalmol,* 122, 716–26.
14. Duan, Y., Mo, J., Klein, R., Scott, I. U., et al. 2007. Age-related macular degeneration is associated with incident myocardial infarction among elderly Americans. *Ophthalmology,* 114, 732–37.
15. Wong, T. Y., Klein, R., Sun, C., Mitchell, P., et al. 2006. Age-related macular degeneration and risk for stroke. *Ann Intern Med,* 145, 98–106.
16. Chakravarthy, U., Soubrane, G., Bandello, F., Chong, V., et al. 2006. Evolving European guidance on the medical management of neovascular age related macular degeneration. *Br J Ophthalmol,* 90, 1188–96.
17. Epstein, P. 2007. Trials that matter: Two faces of progress in the treatment of age-related macular degeneration. *Ann Intern Med,* 146, 532–34.
18. Lim, J. I. 2006. Macular degeneration: The latest in current medical management. *Retina,* 26, S17–20.

19. Birringer, M. 2011. Hormetics: Dietary triggers of an adaptive stress response. *Pharm Res,* 28, 2680–94.
20. Signorelli, P., and Ghidoni, R. 2005. Resveratrol as an anticancer nutrient: Molecular basis, open questions and promises. *J Nutr Biochem,* 16, 449–66.
21. Richer, S., Stiles, W., and Thomas, C. 2009. Molecular medicine in ophthalmic care. *Optometry,* 80, 695–701.
22. Vang, O., Ahmad, N., Baile, C. A., Baur, J. A., et al. 2011. What is new for an old molecule? Systematic review and recommendations on the use of resveratrol. *PLoS One,* 6, e19881.
23. Tomany, S. C., Wang, J. J., Van Leeuwen, R., Klein, R., et al. 2004. Risk factors for incident age-related macular degeneration: Pooled findings from 3 continents. *Ophthalmology,* 111, 1280–87.
24. Bressler, S. B., Munoz, B., Solomon, S. D., and West, S. K. 2008. Racial differences in the prevalence of age-related macular degeneration: The Salisbury Eye Evaluation (SEE) project. *Arch Ophthalmol,* 126, 241–45.
25. Mukesh, B. N., Dimitrov, P. N., Leikin, S., Wang, J. J., et al. 2004. Five-year incidence of age-related maculopathy: The Visual Impairment Project. *Ophthalmology,* 111, 1176–82.
26. Klein, M. L., Mauldin, W. M., and Stoumbos, V. D. 1994. Heredity and age-related macular degeneration. Observations in monozygotic twins. *Arch Ophthalmol,* 112, 932–37.
27. Baird, P. N., Robman, L. D., Richardson, A. J., Dimitrov, P. N., et al. 2008. Gene-environment interaction in progression of AMD—The CFH gene, smoking and exposure to chronic infection. *Hum Mol Genet,* 17, 1299–1305.
28. Yates, J. R., Sepp, T., Matharu, B. K., Khan, J. C., et al. 2007. Complement C3 variant and the risk of age-related macular degeneration. *N Engl J Med,* 357, 553–61.
29. Chen, W., Stambolian, D., Edwards, A. O., Branham, K. E., et al. 2010a. Genetic variants near TIMP3 and high-density lipoprotein-associated loci influence susceptibility to age-related macular degeneration. *Proc Natl Acad Sci U S A,* 107, 7401–6.
30. Udar, N., Atilano, S. R., Memarzadeh, M., Boyer, D. S., et al. 2009. Mitochondrial DNA haplogroups associated with age-related macular degeneration. *Invest Ophthalmol Vis Sci,* 50, 2966–74.
31. Seddon, J. M., Reynolds, R., Maller, J., Fagerness, J. A., et al. 2009. Prediction model for prevalence and incidence of advanced age-related macular degeneration based on genetic, demographic, and environmental variables. *Invest Ophthalmol Vis Sci,* 50, 2044–53.
32. Ho L., van Leeuwen R., Witteman J.C., van Duijn C.M., et al. Reducing the genetic risk of age-related macular degeneration with dietary antioxidants, zinc, and ω-3 fatty acids: the Rotterdam study. *Arch Ophthalmol,* 2011 Jun;129(6):758–66.
33. Seddon, J. M., George, S., and Rosner, B. 2006. Cigarette smoking, fish consumption, omega-3 fatty acid intake, and associations with age-related macular degeneration: The US Twin Study of Age-Related Macular Degeneration. *Arch Ophthalmol,* 124, 995–1001.
34. Thornton, J., Edwards, R., Mitchell, P., Harrison, R. A., et al. 2005. Smoking and age-related macular degeneration: A review of association. *Eye,* 19, 935–44.
35. Moeini, H. A., Masoudpour, H., and Ghanbari, H. 2005. A study of the relation between body mass index and the incidence of age related macular degeneration. *Br J Ophthalmol,* 89, 964–66.
36. Knudtson, M. D., Klein, R., and Klein, B. E. 2006. Physical activity and the 15-year cumulative incidence of age-related macular degeneration: The Beaver Dam Eye Study. *Br J Ophthalmol,* 90, 1461–63.
37. Zlateva, G. P., Javitt, J. C., Shah, S. N., Zhou, Z., and Murphy, J. G. 2007. Comparison of comorbid conditions between neovascular age-related macular degeneration patients and a control cohort in the medicare population. *Retina,* 27, 1292–99.
38. Schaumberg, D. A., Christen, W. G., Buring, J. E., Glynn, R. J., Rifai, N., and Ridker, P. M. 2007. High-sensitivity C-reactive protein, other markers of inflammation, and the incidence of macular degeneration in women. *Arch Ophthalmol,* 125, 300–305.
39. Glazer-Hockstein, C., and Dunaief, J. L. 2006. Could blue light-blocking lenses decrease the risk of age-related macular degeneration? *Retina,* 26, 1–4.
40. Ham, W. T., Jr., Mueller, H. A., and Sliney, D. H. 1976. Retinal sensitivity to damage from short wavelength light. *Nature,* 260, 153–55.
41. Delcourt, C., Carriere, I., Ponton-Sanchez, A., Fourrey, S., Lacroux, A., and Papoz, L. 2001. Light exposure and the risk of age-related macular degeneration: The Pathologies Oculaires Liees a l'Age (POLA) study. *Arch Ophthalmol,* 119, 1463–68.
42. Taylor, H. R., West, S., Munoz, B., Rosenthal, F. S., et al. 1992. The long-term effects of visible light on the eye. *Arch Ophthalmol,* 110, 99–104.
43. Bone, R. A., Landrum, J. T., and Tarsis, S. L. 1985. Preliminary identification of the human macular pigment. *Vision Res,* 25, 1531–35.

44. Connolly, E. E., Beatty, S., Thurnham, D. I., Loughman, J., et al. 2010. Augmentation of macular pigment following supplementation with all three macular carotenoids: An exploratory study. *Curr Eye Res*, 35, 335–51.

45. Khachik, F., Spangler, C. J., Smith, J. C., Jr., Canfield, et al. 1997. Identification, quantification, and relative concentrations of carotenoids and their metabolites in human milk and serum. *Anal Chem*, 69, 1873–81.

46. Bone, R. A., and Landrum, J. T. 2010. Dose-dependent response of serum lutein and macular pigment optical density to supplementation with lutein esters. *Arch Biochem Biophys*, 504, 50–55.

47. Snodderly, D. M., Handelman, G. J., and Adler, A. J. 1991. Distribution of individual macular pigment carotenoids in central retina of macaque and squirrel monkeys. *Invest Ophthalmol Vis Sci*, 32, 268–79.

48. Stringham, J. M., and Hammond, B. R., Jr. 2005. Dietary lutein and zeaxanthin: Possible effects on visual function. *Nutr Rev*, 63, 59–64.

49. Bernstein, P. S., Delori, F. C., Richer, S., Van Kuijk, F. J., and Wenzel, A. J. 2010. The value of measurement of macular carotenoid pigment optical densities and distributions in age-related macular degeneration and other retinal disorders. *Vision Res*, 50, 716–28.

50. Obana, A., Hiramitsu, T., Gohto, Y., Ohira, A., et al. 2008. Macular carotenoid levels of normal subjects and age-related maculopathy patients in a Japanese population. *Ophthalmology*, 115, 147–57.

51. Beatty, S., Murray, I. J., Henson, D. B., Carden, D., Koh, H., and Boulton, M. E. 2001. Macular pigment and risk for age-related macular degeneration in subjects from a Northern European population. *Invest Ophthalmol Vis Sci*, 42, 439–46.

52. Sangiovanni, J. P., Chew, E. Y., Clemons, T. E., Ferris, F. L., III, et al. 2007. The relationship of dietary carotenoid and vitamin A, E, and C intake with age-related macular degeneration in a case-control study: AREDS Report No. 22. *Arch Ophthalmol*, 125, 1225–32.

53. Mares, J. A., Larowe, T. L., Snodderly, D. M., Moeller, S. M., et al. 2006. Predictors of optical density of lutein and zeaxanthin in retinas of older women in the Carotenoids in Age-Related Eye Disease Study, an ancillary study of the Women's Health Initiative. *Am J Clin Nutr*, 84, 1107–22.

54. Bone, R. A., Landrum, J. T., Guerra, L. H., and Ruiz, C. A. 2003. Lutein and zeaxanthin dietary supplements raise macular pigment density and serum concentrations of these carotenoids in humans. *J Nutr*, 133, 992–98.

55. Hodge, W. G., Barnes, D., Schachter, H. M., Pan, Y. I., et al. 2007. Evidence for the effect of omega-3 fatty acids on progression of age-related macular degeneration: A systematic review. *Retina*, 27, 216–21.

56. Vu, H. T., Robman, L., Mccarty, C. A., Taylor, H. R., and Hodge, A. 2006. Does dietary lutein and zeaxanthin increase the risk of age related macular degeneration? The Melbourne Visual Impairment Project. *Br J Ophthalmol*, 90, 389–90.

57. Christen, W. G., Schaumberg, D. A., Glynn, R. J., and Buring, J. E. 2011. Dietary omega-3 fatty acid and fish intake and incident age-related macular degeneration in women. *Arch Ophthalmol*, 129, 921–29.

58. Salem, N., Jr., Litman, B., Kim, H. Y., and Gawrisch, K. 2001. Mechanisms of action of docosahexaenoic acid in the nervous system. *Lipids*, 36, 945–59.

59. Neuringer, M., Connor, W. E., Lin, D. S., Barstad, L., and Luck, S. 1986. Biochemical and functional effects of prenatal and postnatal omega 3 fatty acid deficiency on retina and brain in rhesus monkeys. *Proc Natl Acad Sci U S A*, 83, 4021–25.

60. Jump, D. B. 2002. The biochemistry of n-3 polyunsaturated fatty acids. *J Biol Chem*, 277, 8755–58.

61. Simopoulos, A. P. 2002. The importance of the ratio of omega-6/omega-3 essential fatty acids. *Biomed Pharmacother*, 56, 365–79.

62. Cordain, L., Eaton, S. B., Miller, J. B., Mann, N., and Hill, K. 2002. The paradoxical nature of hunter-gatherer diets: Meat-based, yet non-atherogenic. *Eur J Clin Nutr*, 56 Suppl 1, S42–52.

63. Parekh, N., Chappell, R. J., Millen, A. E., Albert, D. M., and Mares, J. A. 2007. Association between vitamin D and age-related macular degeneration in the Third National Health and Nutrition Examination Survey, 1988 through 1994. *Arch Ophthalmol*, 125, 661–69.

64. Millen, A. E., Voland, R., Sondel, S. A., Parekh, N., et al. 2011. Vitamin D status and early age-related macular degeneration in postmenopausal women. *Arch Ophthalmol*, 129, 481–89.

65. Crossland, M., and Rubin, G. 2007. The Amsler chart: Absence of evidence is not evidence of absence. *Br J Ophthalmol*, 91, 391–93.

66. Newsome, D. A., and Negreiro, M. 2009. Reproducible measurement of macular light flash recovery time using a novel device can indicate the presence and worsening of macular diseases. *Curr Eye Res*, 34, 162–70.

67. Jackson, G. R., and Edwards, J. G. 2008. A short-duration dark adaptation protocol for assessment of age-related maculopathy. *J Ocul Biol Dis Infor*, 1, 7–11.

68. Arup Laboratory Test Directory. *Carotenes, Fractionated, Plasma or Serum*: 0021021. http://www
    .aruplab.com/guides/ug/tests/0021021.jsp.
69. Gallaher, K. T., Mura, M., Todd, W. A., Harris, et al. 2007. Estimation of macular pigment optical density
    in the elderly: Test-retest variability and effect of optical blur in pseudophakic subjects. *Vision Res,* 47,
    1253–59.
70. Snellen, E. L., Verbeek, A. L., Van Den Hoogen, G. W., Cruysberg, J. R., and Hoyng, C. B. 2002.
    Neovascular age-related macular degeneration and its relationship to antioxidant intake. *Acta Ophthalmol
    Scand,* 80, 368–71.
71. Tanumihardjo, S. A., Li, J., and Dosti, M. P. 2005. Lutein absorption is facilitated with cosupplementa-
    tion of ascorbic acid in young adults. *J Am Diet Assoc,* 105, 114–18.
72. Seddon, J. M. 2007. Multivitamin-multimineral supplements and eye disease: Age-related macular
    degeneration and cataract. *Am J Clin Nutr,* 85, 304S–7S.
73. Goodman, G. E., Thornquist, M. D., Balmes, J., Cullen, M. R., et al. 2004. The Beta-Carotene and
    Retinol Efficacy Trial: Incidence of lung cancer and cardiovascular disease mortality during 6-year
    follow-up after stopping beta-carotene and retinol supplements. *J Natl Cancer Inst,* 96, 1743–50.
74. Siems, W., Wiswedel, I., Salerno, C., Crifo, C., et al. 2005. Beta-carotene breakdown products may
    impair mitochondrial functions—Potential side effects of high-dose beta-carotene supplementation.
    J Nutr Biochem, 16, 385–97.
75. *Archives of Opthalmology.* 2001. A randomized, placebo-controlled, clinical trial of high-dose supple-
    mentation with vitamins C and E, beta carotene, and zinc for age-related macular degeneration and vision
    loss: AREDS report no. 8. *Arch Ophthalmol,* 119, 1417–36.
76. Berger, A. 2002. What does zinc do? *BMJ,* 325, 1062.
77. Rowin, J., and Lewis, S. L. 2005. Copper deficiency myeloneuropathy and pancytopenia secondary to
    overuse of zinc supplementation. *J Neurol Neurosurg Psychiatry,* 76, 750–51.
78. Trumbo, P., Yates, A. A., Schlicker, S., and Poos, M. 2001. Dietary reference intakes: Vitamin A, vitamin
    K, arsenic, boron, chromium, copper, iodine, iron, manganese, molybdenum, nickel, silicon, vanadium,
    and zinc. *J Am Diet Assoc,* 101, 294–301.
79. Ellis, R., Kelsay, J. L., Reynolds, R. D., Morris, E. R., et al. 1987. Phytate:zinc and phytate X calcium:zinc
    millimolar ratios in self-selected diets of Americans, Asian Indians, and Nepalese. *J Am Diet Assoc,* 87,
    1043–47.
80. Menzano, E., and Carlen, P. L. 1994. Zinc deficiency and corticosteroids in the pathogenesis of alcoholic
    brain dysfunction—A review. *Alcohol Clin Exp Res,* 18, 895–901.
81. Naber, T. H., Van den Hamer, C. J., Baadenhuysen, H., and Jansen, J. B. 1998. The value of methods to
    determine zinc deficiency in patients with Crohn's disease. *Scand J Gastroenterol,* 33, 514–23.
82. Hoffman, H. N., II, Phyliky, R. L., and Fleming, C. R. 1988. Zinc-induced copper deficiency.
    Gastroenterology, 94, 508–12.
83. Tavani, A., Longoni, E., Bosetti, C., Maso, L. D., et al. 2006. Intake of selected micronutrients and the risk
    of surgically treated benign prostatic hyperplasia: A case-control study from Italy. *Eur Urol,* 50, 549–54.
84. Cuajungco, M. P., and Lees, G. J. 1997. Zinc and Alzheimer's disease: Is there a direct link? *Brain Res
    Brain Res Rev,* 23, 219–36.
85. Hooper, P. L., Visconti, L., Garry, P. J., and Johnson, G. E. 1980. Zinc lowers high-density lipoprotein-
    cholesterol levels. *JAMA,* 244, 1960–61.
86. Kowluru, R. A., and Odenbach, S. 2004. Effect of long-term administration of alpha-lipoic acid on retinal
    capillary cell death and the development of retinopathy in diabetic rats. *Diabetes,* 53, 3233–38.
87. Voloboueva, L. A., Liu, J., Suh, J. H., Ames, B. N., and Miller, S. S. 2005. (R)-alpha-lipoic acid protects
    retinal pigment epithelial cells from oxidative damage. *Invest Ophthalmol Vis Sci,* 46, 4302–10.
88. Tanito, M., Masutani, H., Kim, Y. C., Nishikawa, M., Ohira, A., and Yodoi, J. 2005. Sulforaphane induces
    thioredoxin through the antioxidant-responsive element and attenuates retinal light damage in mice.
    Invest Ophthalmol Vis Sci, 46, 979–87.
89. Hanneken, A., Lin, F. F., Johnson, J., and Maher, P. 2006. Flavonoids protect human retinal pigment
    epithelial cells from oxidative-stress-induced death. *Invest Ophthalmol Vis Sci,* 47, 3164–77.
90. Cremer, D. R., Rabeler, R., Roberts, A., and Lynch, B. 2006. Long-term safety of alpha-lipoic acid
    (ALA) consumption: A 2-year study. *Regul Toxicol Pharmacol,* 46, 193–201.
91. Johnson, E. J., Hammond, B. R., Yeum, K. J., Qin, J., et al. 2000. Relation among serum and tissue con-
    centrations of lutein and zeaxanthin and macular pigment density. *Am J Clin Nutr,* 71, 1555–62.
92. Berendschot, T. T., Goldbohm, R. A., Klopping, W. A., Van De Kraats, J., et al. 2000. Influence of lutein
    supplementation on macular pigment, assessed with two objective techniques. *Invest Ophthalmol Vis Sci,*
    41, 3322–26.

93. Feher, J., Kovacs, B., Kovacs, I., Schveoller, M., et al. 2005. Improvement of visual functions and fundus alterations in early age-related macular degeneration treated with a combination of acetyl-L-carnitine, n-3 fatty acids, and coenzyme Q10. *Ophthalmologica,* 219, 154–66.

94. Schalch, W., Cohn, W., Barker, F. M., Kopcke, W., et al. 2007. Xanthophyll accumulation in the human retina during supplementation with lutein or zeaxanthin—The LUXEA (LUtein Xanthophyll Eye Accumulation) study. *Arch Biochem Biophys,* 458, 128–35.

95. Trieschmann, M., Beatty, S., Nolan, J. M., Hense, H. W., et al. 2007. Changes in macular pigment optical density and serum concentrations of its constituent carotenoids following supplemental lutein and zeaxanthin: The LUNA study. *Exp Eye Res,* 84, 718–28.

96. Cangemi, F. E. 2007. TOZAL Study: An open case control study of an oral antioxidant and omega-3 supplement for dry AMD. *BMC Ophthalmol,* 7, 3.

97. Parisi, V., Tedeschi, M., Gallinaro, G., Varano, M., et al. 2008. Carotenoids and antioxidants in age-related maculopathy Italian study: Multifocal electroretinogram modifications after 1 year. *Ophthalmology,* 115, 324–33 e2.

98. Neelam, K., Hogg, R. E., Stevenson, M. R., Johnston, E., et al. 2008. Carotenoids and co-antioxidants in age-related maculopathy: Design and methods. *Ophthalmic Epidemiol,* 15, 389–401.

99. Richer, S., Stiles, W., Statkute, L., Pulido, J., et al. 2004. Double-masked, placebo-controlled, randomized trial of lutein and antioxidant supplementation in the intervention of atrophic age-related macular degeneration: The Veterans LAST study (Lutein Antioxidant Supplementation Trial). *Optometry,* 75, 216–30.

100. Richer, S., Devenport, J., and Lang, J. C. 2007. LAST II: Differential temporal responses of macular pigment optical density in patients with atrophic age-related macular degeneration to dietary supplementation with xanthophylls. *Optometry,* 78, 213–19.

101. Bartlett, H. E., and Eperjesi, F. 2007. Effect of lutein and antioxidant dietary supplementation on contrast sensitivity in age-related macular disease: A randomized controlled trial. *Eur J Clin Nutr,* 61, 1121–27.

102. Richer, S. P., Stiles, W., Graham-Hoffman, K., Levin, M., et al. 2011. Randomized, double-blind, placebo-controlled study of zeaxanthin and visual function in patients with atrophic age-related macular degeneration: The Zeaxanthin and Visual Function Study (ZVF) FDA IND #78, 973. *Optometry,* 82, 667–80 e6103. Droge, W. 2005. Oxidative stress and ageing: Is ageing a cysteine deficiency syndrome? *Philos Trans R Soc Lond B Biol Sci,* 360, 2355–72.

104. Breitkreutz, R., Holm, S., Pittack, N., Beichert, M., et al. 2000. Massive loss of sulfur in HIV infection. *AIDS Res Hum Retroviruses,* 16, 203–9.

105. Mcpherson, R. A., and Hardy, G. 2011. Clinical and nutritional benefits of cysteine-enriched protein supplements. *Curr Opin Clin Nutr Metab Care,* 14, 562–68.

106. Neuringer, M., and Sturman, J. 1987. Visual acuity loss in rhesus monkey infants fed a taurine-free human infant formula. *J Neurosci Res,* 18, 597–601.

107. Laidlaw, S. A., Shultz, T. D., Cecchino, J. T., and Kopple, J. D. 1988. Plasma and urine taurine levels in vegans. *Am J Clin Nutr,* 47, 660–63.

108. Christen, W. G., Glynn, R. J., Chew, E. Y., Albert, C. M., and Manson, J. E. 2009. Folic acid, pyridoxine, and cyanocobalamin combination treatment and age-related macular degeneration in women: The Women's Antioxidant and Folic Acid Cardiovascular Study. *Arch Intern Med,* 169, 335–41.

109. Morris, M. S., Jacques, P. F., Chylack, L. T., Hankinson, S. E., et al. 2007. Intake of zinc and antioxidant micronutrients and early age-related maculopathy lesions. *Ophthalmic Epidemiol,* 14, 288–98.

110. Chung, H. Y., Rasmussen, H. M., and Johnson, E. J. 2004. Lutein bioavailability is higher from lutein-enriched eggs than from supplements and spinach in men. *J Nutr,* 134, 1887–93.

111. Dionisio, A. P., Gomes, R. T., and Oetterer, M. 2009. Ionizing radiation effects on food vitamins—A review. *Brazilian Archives of Biology and Technology,* 52, 1267–78.

112. Cao, Y. and Cao, R. 1999. Angiogenesis inhibited by drinking tea. *Nature,* 398, 381.

113. Toi, M., Bando, H., Ramachandran, C., Melnick, S. J., et al. 2003. Preliminary studies on the anti-angiogenic potential of pomegranate fractions in vitro and in vivo. *Angiogenesis,* 6, 121–28.

114. Cao, Y., Cao, R., and Brakenhielm, E. 2002. Antiangiogenic mechanisms of diet-derived polyphenols. *J Nutr Biochem,* 13, 380–90.

115. Chiu, C. J., Milton, R. C., Klein, R., Gensler, G., and Taylor, A. 2007. Dietary carbohydrate and the progression of age-related macular degeneration: A prospective study from the Age-Related Eye Disease Study. *Am J Clin Nutr,* 86, 1210–18.

116. Goni, I., Serrano, J., and Saura-Calixto, F. 2006. Bioaccessibility of beta-carotene, lutein, and lycopene from fruits and vegetables. *J Agric Food Chem,* 54, 5382–87.

117. Yonekura, L., and Nagao, A. 2007. Intestinal absorption of dietary carotenoids. *Mol Nutr Food Res,* 51, 107–15.

118. Kostic, D., White, W. S., and Olson, J. A. 1995. Intestinal absorption, serum clearance, and interactions between lutein and beta-carotene when administered to human adults in separate or combined oral doses. *Am J Clin Nutr,* 62, 604–10.

119. Clevidence, B., Haynes, K., Rao, D., and Novotny, J. 2005. Effect of cooking method on xanthophyll content of yellow-fleshed potato. *United States Japan Natural Resources Protein Panel,* 34, 280–84.

120. Johnson, G. H., Keast, D. R., and Kris-Etherton, P. M. 2007. Dietary modeling shows that the substitution of canola oil for fats commonly used in the United States would increase compliance with dietary recommendations for fatty acids. *J Am Diet Assoc,* 107, 1726–34.

121. Cashman, K. D. 2007. Calcium and vitamin D. *Novartis Found Symp,* 282, 123–38; discussion 138–42, 212–18.

122. Bischoff-Ferrari, H. A., Giovannucci, E., Willett, W. C., Dietrich, T., and Dawson-Hughes, B. 2006. Estimation of optimal serum concentrations of 25-hydroxyvitamin D for multiple health outcomes. *Am J Clin Nutr,* 84, 18–28.

123. Marcason, W. 2007. Vitamin K: What are the current dietary recommendations for patients taking coumadin? *J Am Diet Assoc,* 107, 2022.

124. Vioque, J., Weinbrenner, T., Asensio, L., Castello, A., et al. 2007. Plasma concentrations of carotenoids and vitamin C are better correlated with dietary intake in normal weight than overweight and obese elderly subjects. *Br J Nutr,* 97, 977–86.

125. Madan, A. K., Orth, W. S., Tichansky, D. S., and Ternovits, C. A. 2006. Vitamin and trace mineral levels after laparoscopic gastric bypass. *Obes Surg,* 16, 603–6.

126. Vahlquist, A., Carlson, K., Hallberg, D., and Rossner, S. 1982. Serum carotene, vitamin A, retinol-binding protein and lipoproteins before and after jejunoileal bypass surgery. *Int J Obes,* 6, 491–97.

127. Alvarez-Leite, J. I. 2004. Nutrient deficiencies secondary to bariatric surgery. *Curr Opin Clin Nutr Metab Care,* 7, 569–75.

128. Kastin, D. A., and Buchman, A. L. 2002. Malnutrition and gastrointestinal disease. *Curr Opin Gastroenterol,* 18, 221–28.

129. Davidson, M. H., Hauptman, J., Digirolamo, M., Foreyt, J. P., et al. 1999. Weight control and risk factor reduction in obese subjects treated for 2 years with orlistat: A randomized controlled trial. *JAMA,* 281, 235–42.

130. Peters, J. C., Lawson, K. D., Middleton, S. J., and Triebwasser, K. C. 1997. Assessment of the nutritional effects of olestra, a nonabsorbed fat replacement: Introduction and overview. *J Nutr,* 127, 1539S–46S.

131. Rosell, M. S., Lloyd-Wright, Z., Appleby, P. N., Sanders, T. A., et al. 2005. Long-chain n-3 polyunsaturated fatty acids in plasma in British meat-eating, vegetarian, and vegan men. *Am J Clin Nutr,* 82, 327–34.

132. Plourde, M., And Cunnane, S. C. 2007. Extremely limited synthesis of long chain polyunsaturates in adults: Implications for their dietary essentiality and use as supplements. *Appl Physiol Nutr Metab,* 32, 619–34.

133. Gerster, H. 1998. Can adults adequately convert alpha-linolenic acid (18:3n–3) to eicosapentaenoic acid (20:5n–3) and docosahexaenoic acid (22:6n–3)? *Int J Vitam Nutr Res,* 68, 159–73.

134. Holden, J. M., Eldridge, A. L., Beecher, G. R., Buzzard, I. M., et al. 1999. Carotenoid content of U.S. foods: An update of the database. *J. Food Comp. Anal.,* 12, 169–96.

2 Chemosensory Disorders

Emerging Roles in Food Selection, Nutrient Inadequacies, and Digestive Dysfunction

Alan R. Hirsch, M.D., and Bradley W. Whitman, M.D., M.S.

INTRODUCTION

Nutrition regulates the chemosenses and reciprocally, taste and smell greatly influence food selection, satiety, dietary patterns, digestion, and nutrient intake. While the name "gustation" suggests the link between the sense of taste and food, the sense of olfaction is linked in a variety of complex ways. Approximately 90% of taste or flavor is actually smell [1]. It is a nonpathological form of synesthesia, wherein orthonasal smell is perceived as aroma and retronasal smell, from the posterior of the mouth, through the oropharnyx, is construed as taste [2,3]. Olfaction begins exerting its effects when stimuli are afar and its potential roles in nutritional assessments are an area of ongoing research [4]. Attributes of nutritional metabolism and physiology are both enmeshed in this nexus and serve as a powerful milieu regulating disparate chemosensory forces that powerfully come together and impact one another, to yield relevant changes in the human sensory response, behavioral outcomes, and finally in the results of human health. This chapter explores how diminution and alteration in taste and smell influence food selection and nutrient needs.

EPIDEMIOLOGY

Chemosensory dysfunction is endemic. Approximately 15 million Americans 55 years of age or older have olfactory abnormalities, and more than 200,000 individuals seek the medical advice of general practitioners and specialists each year because of complaints regarding smell or taste [5]. Causes of chemosensory dysfunction are many, and the underlying disorders are often associated with nutritional dysfunction [6].

ANATOMY AND PATHOPHYSIOLOGY

Smell is the only sensation to reach the cortex before reaching the thalamus. Furthermore, it is the only sensory system that is primarily ipsilateral in its projection to the cortex. In the future, neuroimaging techniques will be able to expand the understanding of this evolutionarily, precortical limbic system sense.

31

ANATOMY OF SMELL

Dirhinous inhalation occurs asymmetrically due to the olfactory cycle, which alternates open nostrils every four to eight hours. Parenthetically, olfaction demonstrates greatest sensitivity ipsilateral to the restricted nostril, as a result of eddy currents that are created by the smaller aperture. These tumultuous gusts of odorant, like rhinal tornadoes, stochastically distribute the odorants with greater concentration reaching the olfactory epithelium at the top of the nose, as opposed to bypassing this area in favor of the bronchi and lungs [7]. For a putative olfactory substrate to be processed, it needs to be solubilized in mucous. If through suboptimal alterations in nutritional metabolism, a disturbance in mucous production arises, it is possible that subsequent olfaction might be adversely affected. Increased nasal mucous production in the setting of the biology of a hyperimmune state might yield a disturbance in olfaction. Features of these conditions such as asthma and nasal polyps may also separately include problems with taste and smell.

Once an odor passes through the olfactory epithelium, it must stimulate the olfactory nerve, which consists of unmyelinated olfactory fila. The olfactory nerve has the slowest conduction rate of any nerve in the body. The olfactory fila pass through the cribiform plate of the ethmoid bone and enter the olfactory bulb. During trauma, much damage occurs in this bulb [8]. Different odors localize in different areas of the olfactory bulb. See Figure 2.1.

Inside the olfactory bulb is a conglomeration of neuropil called glomeruli. Approximately 2,000 glomeruli reside in the olfactory bulb. Four different cell types make up the glomeruli: processes of receptor cell axons, mitral cells, tufted cells, and second-order neurons that give off collaterals to the granule cells and to cells in the periglomerular and external plexiform layers. The mitral and tufted cells form the lateral olfactory tract and establish a reverberating circuit with the granule cells. The mitral cells stimulate firing of the granule cells, which in turn inhibit firing of the mitral cells [9].

A reciprocal inhibition exists between the mitral and tufted cells, which results in a sharpening of olfactory acuity. The olfactory bulb receives several efferent projections, including the primary olfactory fibers, the contralateral olfactory bulb and the anterior nucleus, the inhibitory prepiriform cortex, the diagonal band of Broca with neurotransmitters acetylcholine and gamma-aminobutryric acid (GABA), the locus coeruleus, the dorsal raphe, and the tuberomammillary nucleus of the hypothalamus.

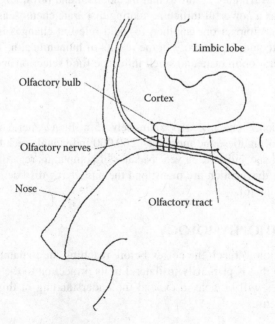

FIGURE 2.1 Cross-sectional anatomy of the nose and cranial nerve I.

The olfactory bulb's efferent fibers project into the olfactory tract, which divides at the olfactory trigona into the medial and lateral olfactory striae. The striae project to the anterior olfactory nucleus, the olfactory tubercle, the amygdaloid nucleus (which in turn projects to the ventral medial nucleus of the hypothalamus, a feeding center), the cortex of the piriform lobe, the septal nuclei, and the hypothalamus, especially the anterolateral regions of the hypothalamus, which are involved in reproduction.

The anterior olfactory nucleus receives afferent fibers from the olfactory tract and projects efferent fibers, which decussate in the anterior commissure and synapse in the contralateral olfactory bulb. Some of the efferent projections from the anterior olfactory nucleus remain ipsilateral, and synapse on internal granular cells of the ipsilateral olfactory bulb.

The olfactory tubercle receives afferent fibers from the olfactory bulb and the anterior olfactory nucleus. Efferent fibers from the olfactory tubercle project to the nucleus accumbens as well as the striatum. Neurotransmitters of the olfactory tubercle include acetylcholine and dopamine.

The area on the cortex where olfaction is localized, that is, the primary olfactory cortex, includes the prepiriform area, the periamygdaloid area, and the entorhinal area. The piriform cortex and the amygdala are the primary olfactory cortex, while the insula and orbitofrontal cortex are secondary olfactory cortex association areas [10]. Afferent projections to the primary olfactory cortex include the mitral cells, which enter the lateral olfactory tract and synapse in the prepiriform cortex (lateral olfactory gyrus) and the corticomedial part of the amygdala. Efferent projections from the primary olfactory cortex extend to the entorhinal cortex, the basal and lateral amygdaloid nuclei, the lateral preoptic area of the hypothalamus, the nucleus of the diagonal band of Broca, the medial forebrain bundle, the dorsal medial nucleus and submedial nucleus of the thalamus, and the nucleus accumbens.

It should be noted that the entorhinal cortex is both a primary and a secondary olfactory cortical area. Efferent fibers project via the uncinate fasciculus to the hippocampus, the anterior insular cortex next to the gustatory cortical area, and the frontal cortex. This may explain why temporal lobe epilepsy that involves the uncinate often produces parageusias of burning rubber, sometimes referred to as uncinate fits [11].

Some of the efferent projections of the mitral and tufted cells decussate in the anterior commissure and form the medial olfactory tract. They then synapse in the contralateral paraolfactory area and the contralateral subcallosal gyrus. The exact function of the medial olfactory stria and tract is not clear. The accessory olfactory bulb receives afferent fibers from the bed nucleus of the accessory olfactory tract and the medial and posterior corticoamygdaloid nuclei. Efferent fibers from the accessory olfactory bulb project through the accessory olfactory tract to the same afferent areas. The medial and posterior corticoamygdaloid nuclei project secondary fibers to the anterior and medial hypothalamus, the areas associated with reproduction. Therefore the accessory olfactory bulb in humans may be a mediator for human pheromones [12]. As well, the microneuroanatomy of these structures and other cortical projections may be adversely impacted by certain forms of poor nutrition.

NEUROTRANSMITTERS THAT MEDIATE SMELL

Neurotransmitters of the olfactory cortex are many, including glutamate, aspartate, cholcystekinin, luteinizing hormone-releasing hormone, and somatastatin. Furthermore, perception of odors causes modulation of olfactory neurotransmitters within the olfactory bulb and the limbic system. Virtually all known neurotransmitters are present in the olfactory bulb. Thus odorant modulation of neurotransmitter levels in the olfactory bulb, tract, and limbic system intended for transmission of sensory information may have unintended secondary effects on a variety of different behaviors and disease states that are regulated by the same neurotransmitters. For instance, odorant modulation of dopamine in the olfactory bulb/limbic system may affect manifestations of Parkinson's disease. This may act through mesolimbic override of aspects of Parkinson's disease with a mechanism similar to that which has been documented in response to motoric activation associated with emotional distress and fear of injury in a fire.

THE PHYSIOLOGY OF TASTE

True tastes—salt, sweet, sour, bitter, unami, and possibly lipids—are mediated through taste receptors on taste buds located primarily in the fungiform, but also circumvallate papillae. The fungiform papillae have the lowest threshold to salt and sweet, whereas the circumvallate are more sensitive to sweet stimuli [13,14]. Cranial nerves VII, IX, and X, mediating the gustatory stimuli, enter the pons and pontomedullary junction, ascending and descending through the tractus solitarius finally terminating topographically on the ipsilateral nucleus of the tractus solitarius with cranial nerve VII chorda tympani fibers synapsing rostrally and glossopharyngeal fibers caudally. Second order taste neurons progress through the parabrachial pontine nuclei where they diverge. Some synapse in the thalamus with tertiary order neurons progressing to the primary gustatory cortex in the insula. The others bypass the thalamus and project diffusely to the ventral forebrain with widespread limbic system connections.

Gustatory perception fluctuates between individuals and such variability is partially genetically determined. Such differences influence consumption patterns and gastrointestinal physiology, thereby influencing metabolic and health outcomes more broadly. Chemosenses promote gastric acid production and influence nutrient absorption, food allergenicity, and autonomic responses to food [15].

ETIOLOGIES OF CHEMOSENSORY DISORDERS

Nasal Obstruction

Decreased ability to detect odors can occur secondary to nasal obstruction from adenoid hypertrophy. Adenoidectomy causes a recovery of the threshold of odor detection. Steroid-dependent anosmia is a syndrome whose triad includes inhalant allergy, nasal polyps, and steroid reversal anosmia [16]. Its pathology is that of polyps, which cause a mechanical obstruction preventing odorants from reaching the olfactory epithelium.

Unknown Etiology

Acute viral hepatitis causes a reduction in olfactory sensitivity with dysgeusia and associated anorexia, which improve as the illness improves. Olfactory sensitivity in acute viral hepatitis is inversely proportional to the plasma bilirubin and directly proportional to the plasma retinal binding protein level. The function of these and other signaling molecules in connection with food choice–related chemosensory variability will become increasingly pertinent in the epidemiology of obesity and metabolic disturbance.

Endocrine Disorders

Several endocrine disorders are associated with anosmia. In hypothyroidism, 39% of afflicted individuals are aware of an alteration of sense of taste, 17% have dysosmia or distortion in sense of smell, and 39% have dysgeusia. Thyroid replacement reverses these problems. Individuals with both olfactory or gustatory problems and hypothyroidism have low parotid zinc levels.

Pseudohypoparathyroidism is a syndrome that includes short stature, rounded face, mental retardation, brachymetacarpia, brachymetatarsia, hypocalcemia, hyperphosphatemia, and resistance to parathyroid hormone. Hyposmia and hypogeusia are also seen in pseudohypoparathyroidism. Patients are usually unaware of their hyposmia and are unresponsive to hormones. The hyposmia has been well described as due to the X-linked dominant chromosome. Its onset is at birth.

Turner's syndrome, or chromatin-negative gonadal dysgenesis, is characterized by short stature, cubitus valgus, webbed neck, shield-like thorax, and XO-chromosome pattern. Though patients are unaware of olfactory defects, they are found to have both hyposmia and hypogeusia [17].

Olfactory sensitivity of patients with adrenocortical insufficiency is increased approximately 100,000 fold over that of unaffected individuals. Treatment with carbohydrate-active steroids such as prednisone 20 mg qd reduces olfactory sensitivity toward normal in one day. Since the olfactory response occurs prior to any change in electrolytes or body weight, one can postulate that endogenous central nervous system (CNS) carbohydrate-active steroids normally inhibit olfaction.

Congenital adrenal hyperplasia is a virilizing illness which presents in different subtypes. Congenital adrenal hyperplasia can cause hypertension. 11β-hydroxylase deficiency is an uncommon form of congenital adrenal hyperplasia. Treatment with steroids reduces the sometimes associated olfactory and gustatory hypersensitivity to normal in 8 to 14 days. Since 17-ketosteroids and pregnanetriol return to normal before the normalization of olfactory and gustatory sensitivity, it is unlikely that the reduction in olfactory sensitivity is due to carbohydrate-active steroids alone.

Kallmann's syndrome involves gonadotrophin-deficient hypogonadism associated with impaired olfactory acuity. Clomiphene induces luteinizing hormone and follicle-stimulating hormone release, which causes an increase in both gonadotrophin and testosterone. The olfactory deficit does not respond to clomiphene.

Meningiomas

Olfactory meningiomas are classically described as causing loss of ability to detect odors. These meningiomas, which occur along the olfactory groove, account for less than 10% of all intracranial meningiomas. They usually develop in middle-aged patients, with hyposmia as the first and only symptom, years before the meningioma would enlarge, causing dementia and impaired vision.

Temporal Lobe Lesions

The temporal lobe also has an important influence on olfaction. One patient, H.M., was studied for his olfactory sensitivity after undergoing bilateral resection of the medial temporal lobe that involved the amygdala, uncus, anterior two-thirds of the hippocampus, and parahippocampal gyrus. Although he could detect odors, he could not identify them, and when given two odors, he could not distinguish whether they were the same or different. This suggests that the medial temporal lobe is critical for perception of odor quality [18]. Temporal lobectomy patients demonstrate a mild, bilateral reduction in absolute olfactory sensitivity. In the ipsilateral nostril, odor perception is reduced, as is odor identification. Patients with temporal lobe epilepsy who have had no surgery display a bilateral reduction in odor identification. Of patients with temporal lobe tumors, 20% have an olfactory disturbance [19]. Speculated to be secondary to temporal lobe infarction [20], coronary artery bypass surgery can cause both dysosmia and cacosmia, whereby odors are distorted and previously hedonically pleasant aromas are now perceived as unpleasant.

Thalamic and Hypothalamic Lesions

Patients with estrogen-receptor-positive breast cancer have been found to have hyposmia, possibly secondary to hypothalamic lesions [21]. Significantly, hypothalamic lesions produce an increase in incidence of spontaneous mammary tumors in female rats. This suggests that a hypothalamic lesion may be the primary defect in both estrogen receptor positive breast carcinoma and associated hyposmia.

Korsakoff's psychosis is associated with an anatomic lesion of the dorsal medial nucleus of the thalamus, and is associated with impairment in odor perception corresponding to reduction in cerebrospinal fluid 3-methoxy-4-hydroxy-phenylethylene glycol (MHPG), a norephinephrine metabolite [22]. MHPG is reduced in Parkinson's disease and in senile dementia of the Alzheimer's type as well, and these patients also display an impaired ability to identify odors [23,24]. Related studies suggest that norephinephrine is important for olfaction, and that a drug to increase norephinephrine could potentially restore olfactory ability in some patients.

One such drug is d-amphetamine. This d-2 dopamine-receptor agonist increased olfactory detection in rats given 0.2 mg/kg body weight. With much higher doses (i.e., 1.6 mg/kg), the rats' ability to detect odors was reduced [25,26]. The mechanism whereby it increases odor detection ability is unknown. D-amphetamine may act as a reticular activating system stimulator. It may also act by increasing catecholamine levels in the olfactory tubercle, anterior olfactory nucleus, amygdala, and entorhinal cortex. It may stimulate the locus coeruleus to release norephinephrine, which projects to the lateral olfactory tract. The lateral olfactory tract then would act to inhibit granule cell discharge, causing a reduction in the inhibition of mitral cell discharge. The mitral cells would thus be allowed to fire, causing an increase in olfactory acuity. The latter mechanism is probably not applicable to d-amphetamine, however, because in experiments with rats, norephinephrine depletion of the olfactory bulb had no effect on odor detection ability, implying that d-amphetamine operates on a central basis.

Parkinsonism

Parkinsonism is associated with a decrease in odor sensitivity in 75% of cases and a reduced ability to identify odors in 90% of cases. These olfactory deficits occur independently of age, gender, stage, and duration of the disease. Before they were tested, 72% of Parkinson's disease patients were unaware of their deficits in olfaction, which tend to occur early in the disease process in both demented and nondemented patients, and do not worsen with time [27]. In monozygotic twins with Parkinson's disease, olfactory impairment has a low concordance rate, indicating that this aspect of the disease is probably not inherited [28]. Phantosmia has also been described [29].

Many mechanisms have been postulated for the olfactory defects associated with Parkinson's disease: 1. The same environmental agent that caused the Parkinson's disease damaged the olfactory pathway. 2. The olfactory receptor cells may actively transport viruses, proteins, and environmental toxins, bypassing the blood-brain barrier directly infiltrating the CNS. The substance so transported could damage the olfactory epithelium and olfactory system before invading the substantia nigra to cause the Parkinson's disease. 3. The underlying Parkinson's disease could reduce the olfactory system's resistance to viral or environmental toxins, which then could destroy olfactory pathways. 4. The degenerative process of Parkinson's disease may favor destruction of the olfactory pathways as it affects the substantia nigra. 5. A reduction in CNS neurotransmitters can impair olfaction. The absence of effect of levodopa/carbidopa on olfaction in Parkinson's disease argues against this hypothesis. In its favor is that d-2 dopamine-receptor agonist d-amphetamine increases olfaction in rats, as mentioned.

Aging

Olfactory deficit begins to be demonstrated at age 35 [30,31]. Olfaction in aging individuals has been extensively studied [32]. Odor sensitivity, in regards to both absolute threshold and odor identification is reduced with age. Over 50% of the people between 65 and 80 years of age have major impairments in olfaction. For those over 80 years old, the proportion with major impairments rises to 75%. Over the age of 75 years, 25% are anosmic. These effects of aging parallel those found in other senses.

Many possible mechanisms have been postulated for age-induced olfactory defects. One theory holds that degenerative processes caused by toxins and viruses produce a cumulative effect on the olfactory epithelium. A second theory suggests that age-related immunocompromise predisposes people to upper respiratory infections, which may be followed by postviral upper respiratory infection–induced anosmia. A third hypothesis suggests that in the elderly, the central olfactory neural pathway degenerates, or that neurotransmitters, for instance, norepinephrine, are reduced. A fourth theory postulates ossification of the foramina of the cribiform plate with secondary occlusion and compression of the olfactory fila. None of these theories excludes any of the others.

The implications of olfactory deficits among the aged are important, particularly regarding the detection of gas used for heating and cooking. Elderly persons succumb to accidental poisonings from leaking gas at a much higher rate than do younger people; 75% of such deaths were among persons over 60 years of age. Among persons over 65 years old, 30% could not smell natural gas in concentrations below 50 parts per 10,000, if they could smell it at all. Among those under age 65, in comparison, 95% could smell natural gas in concentrations below 20 parts per 10,000. Half of the people over age 60 could not detect the odor of gas at the maximum concentration allowed by the Department of Transportation. One-seventh of persons 70 to 85 years of age could not detect the odor of gas at explosive concentrations.

In reference to ethyl mercaptan, the agent that is added to propane gas to give it a noxious odor, persons 70 to 85 years of age have a threshold 10 times higher than that of persons under age 70.

The impaired olfactory abilities among the elderly imply impaired gustatory abilities since odor forms a large component of the sense of taste. This may factor in to the elderly consuming an unbalanced diet, such as one lacking in vegetables. Green peppers, for instance, have a bitter taste and a pleasant odor, but to the elderly, they merely taste bitter, making it unlikely that elderly people would eat them.

Among the aged, retronasal odor perception, odor perceived while chewing and swallowing, is also reduced. Despite this, elderly persons rarely complain of food lacking taste, possibly because of the slow, gradual loss of smell. Cooks preparing food for the elderly should use higher concentrations of odorants compared with those preparing food for the young. The elderly, because of their deficits, prefer foods with enhanced flavor.

Alzheimer's Disease (AD)

Patients with AD are usually unaware of their olfactory deficits [33]. Serby et al. postulated that the reduced odor threshold and identification ability found in this disorder are secondary to reduced acetylcholine in the olfactory system [34]. Acetylcholine has been found to be low in the olfactory tubercle in patients with AD. Arguing in favor of this hypothesis is the effect of the application of nasal acetylcholine producing an increase in olfactory sensitivity.

Koss et al. postulate that the decrease in olfactory sensitivity in Alzheimer's disease is secondary to temporal lobe dysfunction [35,36]. As mentioned, olfactory defects are found in individuals with temporal lobectomies and the same mechanism may operate in AD. Pearson et al. suggests that the olfactory pathway is the initial site of involvement both in AD and in Pick's disease [37]. In Alzheimer's disease, neuritic plaque and neurofibrillary tangles form in the olfactory bulb, olfactory tract, anterior olfactory nucleus, prepyriform cortex, uncus, and corticomedial part of the amygdaloid nucleus. Interestingly, the anterior olfactory nucleus, the uncus, and the corticomedial part of the amygdaloid nucleus all receive afferent input from the olfactory bulb. In the entorhinal cortex, layer II stellate cells, which are the end point for the lateral olfactory tract, are lost. Secondary connections of the olfactory cortex are involved with memory and cognition, including the amygdala, the dorsal medial nucleus of the thalamus, and the hippocampus.

A unified theory that could possibly explain the occurrence of both olfactory deficits and AD is a variant of that described for Parkinson's disease: viruses may enter the olfactory pathway via the olfactory epithelium, thereby bypassing the blood-brain barrier [38]. Once inside the olfactory pathway, the viruses could spread into the secondary connections of the limbic system. This route of infection is known to operate in St. Louis encephalitis and amebiasis.

Roberts' theory is that Alzheimer's disease begins in the nose and is caused by aluminosilicates [39]. Labeled glucose placed into the oropharynx is rapidly transported transneuronally to the glomeruli in the olfactory bulb. From there it spreads into the olfactory projections (i.e., the nucleus of Meynert), the locus ceruleus, and the brainstem raphe nuclei. Aluminum and silicon are found to increase in the brain with aging [40]. Widely dispersed in the environment, aluminosilicates can be found in diverse products including talc, deionizers, antacids, underarm spray, dental powder, cat litter, cigar ash, and cigarette ash. Roberts strongly recommends reducing exposure to these aerosolized toxins.

Toxic Agents

In addition to aluminum and silicon mentioned earlier as possible causes of Alzheimer's disease, other, more classic toxic agents, notably lead and arsenic, are well known to affect olfaction.

Perfume workers, varnish workers, and those exposed to cadmium dust also experience a marked reduction in olfactory abilities.

In a Texas petrochemical plant, workers who smoked cigarettes showed reduced olfactory sensitivity; the diminished acuity directly correlated with the amount they smoked [41]. Another aspect of cigarette smoking concerns its effect on the trigeminally-mediated reflex of transitory apnea (the "took-my-breath-away" reflex). Cigarette smoking raised the threshold of the reflex by 67% [42]. The mechanism is probably secondary to smoke-induced ciliastasis, which causes a mucostasis that induces viscid, static mucus. The viscid mucus impairs the transfer of odor molecules from the air to free nerve endings. Second-hand smoke may act through a similar mechanism to raise both olfactory and trigeminal thresholds.

Trauma

Subfrontal exploration of the anterior fossa can stretch or tear the olfactory nerves. Surgical repair of a dural tear with grafts covering the cribiform plate can block regenerating stem cells.

Head injury is a common cause of olfactory defects. Many possible mechanisms have been suggested. One is that acceleration injury produces shearing forces on the olfactory nerves as they pass through the cribiform plate of the ethmoid bone. Fracture of the cribiform plate may compress the olfactory nerves or a hematoma may compress them, thereby impairing olfaction. Another theory suggests that the primary insult in trauma is the destruction of pathways of central connection of olfaction [43].

Averaging the results of many studies of olfaction in head injury victims, we find that roughly 5% of them have olfactory disorders. No correlation has been observed between the loss of olfaction and the age of the victim at the time of the accident, or the category of the accident.

The incidence of olfactory disorder is proportional to the severity of the injury, but even a trivial injury can induce anosmia. In trauma severe enough to induce amnesia, occipital trauma is five times as likely to produce anosmia as is trauma to the forehead.

Usually any olfactory loss occurs shortly after the trauma, but sometimes it may not occur until several months later. Recovery from olfactory defects usually begins during the first few weeks after head trauma, but it can be delayed until as long as five years later.

Half of the individuals with anosmia secondary to head trauma experience distorted smell in response to odorants. Costanzo and Becker reported on 77 persons with anosmia due to head injury: 33% recovered, 27% worsened, and 40% remained unchanged [44]. Costanzo and Becker also reported on a sample of 1167 patients: 50% recovered, except for cases where injury was so severe as to cause amnesia of more than 24 hours. In these cases, fewer than 10% recovered [44].

Temporary anosmia of short duration, often found after trauma, could be due to mechanical blockage of airways, nasal hemorrhaging, inflammation, CSF rhinorrhea, or an increase in intracranial pressure. Increased intracranial pressure may reduce circulation of the olfactory bulbs causing secondary infarctions therein with associated anosmia.

Nutritional Deficiencies

Some primary nutritional deficiency states have also been associated with chemosensory pathology. Hypovitaminosis A induces both hyposmia and hypogeusia [45] that usually resolves within two months with vitamin A replacement. The mechanism of the deficit may be a result of epithelial proliferation and drying, which forms a physical barrier, preventing odorants and tastants from reaching their respective receptors [46].

Chemosensory dysfunction has been reported in those deficient in B complex vitamins [47]. Wernicke-Korsakoff syndrome associated with thiamine deficiency is linked to hyposmia [22]. Dysosmia and dysgeusia are seen in those with reduced vitamin B12 levels and pernicious anemia [47,48].

Zinc status has also been implicated. Hypocupria causes a reversible hypogeusia and is responsive to both copper sulfate and zinc sulfate [49,50]. Patients with anosmia induced by head trauma have been found to have reduced total serum zinc and increased total serum copper. This same chemical imbalance is found in the syndrome of idiopathic hypogeusia with dysgeusia, hyposmia, and dysosmia. The importance of zinc is further demonstrated in patients treated with L-histidine, which induces zincuria, causing a secondary hypozincemia and reduced total body zinc. This, in turn, causes hypogeusia, hyposmia, anorexia, dysgeusia, and dysosmia. All these symptoms are corrected by treating the patient with zinc. Improvement occurs even when the patient is still receiving L-histidine [51]. Excess zinc losses due to hemopyrrollactamuria associated with trauma and certain infections and autism may be a factor here.

PATIENT EVALUATION

When chemosensory disorders are associated with some of the aforementioned underlying conditions, it is important to diagnose the treatable medical conditions. This assessment is particularly relevant among hospitalized persons where the incidence of olfactory impairment is probably greater than among the general population [52,53].

Standard medical [54] and neurological texts [55,56,57] indicate that assessment of the olfactory nerve, cranial nerve I (CNI), is an essential part of a complete neurological examination. Given the likelihood of olfactory dysfunction among hospitalized patients, particularly those with neurological disorders, olfactory testing should be routine.

DIAGNOSES ASSOCIATED WITH OLFACTORY IMPAIRMENT

Lack of olfactory data may impair diagnostic accuracy. For example, Post's pseudodementia, which does not involve olfactory impairment, is sometimes misdiagnosed as Alzheimer's disease [58], which does involve olfactory impairment. Solomon et al. demonstrated that olfactory testing can aid in distinguishing these disorders [59]. Similarly, olfactory deficits are seen in idiopathic Parkinson's disease but not 1-methyl-4-phenyl-1,2,3,6-tetrahydropyridine (MPTP)-induced Parkinson's disease [60], progressive supranuclear palsy [61], or essential tremor [62]. Olfactory deficits are seen in a substantial proportion of those with sinusitis or migraines, but not in those with cluster headaches [63,64,65].

Olfactory deficits may be the first manifestation of an underlying disease state. Without olfactory data, vitamin B12 deficiency [6,66], and olfactory groove meningiomas [67], which display olfactory dysfunction early on, may remain undetected until more serious neurological deficits occur. General anxiety disorder [68] and sexual dysfunction [69] are associated with olfactory dysfunction, thus detection of olfactory deficits may facilitate diagnosis and treatment of these disorders.

Assessment of CNI allows detection of hyposmia and anosmia regardless of the origin. Patients may then receive medications, vitamins, food supplements [70], or special treatment to correct the underlying pathology, such as polypectomy for nasal polyps [71] and steroids for allergic rhinitis [72]. Appropriate counseling can be lifesaving prevention. Risks to personal safety such as inadvertent consumption of spoiled or over-salted food or fire injury can be averted with use of food tasters and gas detectors [73,74].

ASSESSING OLFACTION

Limiting testing to those who complain of chemosensory problems would leave many cases of smell-loss undetected. Self-recognition of olfactory deficits is poor across groups affected. Half of anosmic workers exposed to cadmium [75], and 100% of hyposmic chefs [76] were unaware of any deficits. Moreover, 87.5% of hyposmic or anosmic firefighters were unaware of their deficits [77]. Geriatric patients and those with neurodegenerative disorders tend to be unaware of their olfactory losses [78]. Of those with Parkinson's disease, fewer than 15% recognize their olfactory deficits [27].

In clinical practice, CNI is rarely tested [57]. To evaluate, we reviewed histories and physical examinations in 90 patient charts at a Chicago teaching hospital. Charts were selected from all adult patients admitted to this hospital from April through September 1988 who met the following criteria: a neurologic diagnosis upon discharge, ability to follow directions and respond verbally and not intubated, comatose, or admitted to an intensive care unit. None of the 94 physical exams performed by attending-level internists and neurologists indicated that CNI was tested. While four charts (4.2%) note "cranial nerves intact" or "neuro exam grossly normal," thereby implying that olfactory testing may have been performed, it appears to have been an overgeneralization.

Resources for testing have historically been limited and may therefore account for part of the olfactory-testing lacuna. There is a lack of standardization among the traditional test of asking patients to identify readily available fragrant substances such as coffee, almond, lemon, tobacco, anise, oil of clove, toothpaste, eucalyptus, vanilla, peppermint, camphor, rosewater, and soap [54,55,56,57,79]. Difficulties with standardized tests prevent their widespread use. The Chicago Smell Test [80,81] is not widely available. Individual odor olfactory threshold tests from Olfacto-Labs require several bulky bottles and hence, are not practical for the clinician [82,83]. The University of Pennsylvania Smell Identification Test (UPSIT) [84] is a 40-question scratch-and-sniff test, adjusted for age and sex, that requires a substantial amount of time to administer; patients with cognitive dysfunction may have difficulty completing it.

A simple, standardized test is available. The Alcohol Sniff Test (AST) [85,86,87] is standardized and can easily be performed at the bedside, even with children [88] and those with cognitive impairment [89]. The AST is rapid, cost-effective, and requires only a tape measure and an alcohol pad (see Figure 2.2). Olfactory ability is quantitatively determined by placing the centimeter (cm) marker of the tape measure at the philtrum (the medial cleft extending from the upper lip to the nose). With the patient's eyes closed, an alcohol pad, one-quarter exposed, is place at the 40 cm marker and gradually moved inward on inhalation at 1 cm/second until detected. This is repeated four times, waiting 45 seconds between each test, and the results are averaged. If detection is greater than or equal to 17 cm, it indicates normosmia; detection between 8 and 17 cm indicates hyposmia; and detection at less than 8 cm suggests anosmia.

The AST has been validated in comparison to threshold testing [85], and threshold testing correlates with the UPSIT [90]. A statistically significant correlation exists between the UPSIT and AST. UPSIT scores, in addition, are used to discriminate among anosmic, hyposmic, normosmic, and malingering patients.

In time-sensitive situations, the AST can grossly be interpreted such that if alcohol can be detected beyond the chin, olfaction is normal. Number of centimeters on AST can thus be recorded sequentially in office visits, analogous to office testing of visual acuity on the Snellen Acuity Test.

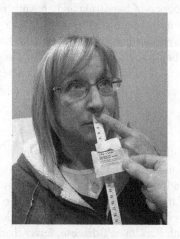

FIGURE 2.2   Demonstrating the Alcohol Sniff Test (AST), a standardized bedside clinical exam of olfaction.

More detailed testing such as the UPSIT and a functional MRI can then be performed on those with an abnormal AST.

TREATMENT

There are currently no FDA approved medications specifically for the treatment of chemosensory dysfunction. However, chemosensory disorders have been shown to be responsive to several nutritional approaches. Individual nutrient repletion is presented here.

PHOSPHATIDYLCHOLINE

Acetylcholine is important in olfaction as evidenced by the fact that normal persons' olfactory sense is impaired by taking scopolamine, which decreases the effect of acetylcholine. We cannot ascribe this impairment to drying of the nasal mucus since drying actually improves olfaction [91]. So we ascribe it to a decrease in acetylcholine. As further evidence of the importance of acetylcholine in olfaction, patients with senile dementia of the Alzheimer's type lose their ability to detect and identify odors relatively early; in this disease, reduced choline acetyltransferase causes a reduction of acetylcholine in the basal nucleus of Meynert [92]. Phosphatidylcholine is converted via choline acetyltransferase into acetylcholine. Thus, choline provides the essential precursor [93]. The amount of choline circulating in the body affects its content in the brain and affects release of acetylcholine in the CNS. Insufficient choline impairs nerve cells' ability to transmit messages across synapses. By supplementing choline, it is possible to amplify these messages in some forms of chemosensory disorders [94]. Phosphatidylcholine has been used to increase blood choline, brain choline, and brain acetylcholine levels in patients with brain diseases associated with impaired acetylcholine neurotransmission, such as tardive dyskinesia [95]. Due to its central role in the composition and function of neuronal membranes, phosphatidylcholine has been used for patients with brain diseases associated with dissolution of neuronal membranes such as Alzheimer's disease [96].

In an open label, followed by a double-blind trial of phosphatidylcholine at 9 grams a day for three months, mixed results were seen. A 40% improvement on the open-label study was followed by a negative result on the double-blind study. The double-blind study design is noteworthy to the conclusions. Experimental subjects dropped out of the double-blind trial with phosphatidylcholine saying that they disliked the taste of licorice. Since none of the patients voiced this complaint initially, it seems possible that their sense of smell, and therefore of taste, improved during treatment, making them more aware of the licorice taste. None of the control subjects who dropped out mentioned the licorice taste as a reason [97]. Given the aforementioned, in those with idiopathic hyposmia or anosmia, a three-month trial of phosphatidylcholine (Phoschol) at 9 grams per day in three divided doses may be beneficial.

THIAMINE

While a pilot trial of thiamine at 100 mg a day showed no effect, anecdotally, some anosmic and hyposmic patients showed remarkable improvement with this treatment. [98].

VITAMIN A

Since vitamin A exists in the olfactory epithelium and could be involved in olfactory neuron regeneration, it theoretically could improve hyposmia or anosmia [99].

Of 56 studied, 89% of anosmic patients who underwent intramuscular vitamin A injections, regained full or partial olfactory ability. Oral retinoid treatment (Etretinate) has also been reported to be effective [100]. Patients with cirrhosis and hypovitaminosis A display improvement in both taste and smell thresholds in response to vitamin A treatment [101].

CAFFEINE

Caffeine inhibits adenosine receptors and thus, may facilitate taste sensitivity. Although study results are mixed, there is a suggestion that topical caffeine enhances taste to sweet and bitter [102,103].

ZINC

Zinc has undergone the peripatetic course as the standard-bearer for treatment of smell and taste disorders. The zeitgeist of zinc was in the 1960s and 1970s when a series of articles suggested its efficacy in a wide range of chemosensory disorders [50,104,105]. Zinc was originally used during the polio epidemic in an attempt to prevent spread of the disease to victims' families. Family members were treated intranasally to destroy the receptor neuroepithelium. The stratagem was effective only for several months, since stem cells proliferated and underwent transformation into fully developed bipolar olfactory receptor cells, thus allowing the treated persons again to be exposed to the polio virus. This effect of zinc was the basis for the idea of using zinc on the stem cells of patients with anosmia to stimulate the development of bipolar olfactory receptor cells.

The frequent association between olfactory impairment and exposure to trace metals suggests another rationale for using zinc. Mercury, lead, cadmium, and gold have been associated with olfactory dysfunction. Iron deficiency alters taste and food selection. Zinc metabolism is abnormal in such altered physiologic states, with hyposmia, as liver disease, and first trimester pregnancy. Hypothyroid patients with hyposmia and hypogeusia have low parotid zinc levels. Treatment with Synthroid improves olfaction and taste as it returns parotid zinc levels to normal. Patients with post-influenza hypogeusia and hyposmia have low parotid zinc and low serum zinc.

Clinical trials have not produced the results one might anticipate from the observations noted here. A study of 106 patients with hypogeusia following influenza revealed that although zinc treatment corrected their low serum levels, it did not improve hypogeusia and hyposmia. A double-blind, crossover trial did not demonstrate efficacy of zinc and treatment of hypogeusia [106]. Another paper, comparing zinc treated versus non-zinc treated patients found no difference in taste ability [107]. Moreover, zinc is not necessarily benign: toxicity may occur. At 100 mg of zinc a day, a level at or below suggested therapeutic doses, inhibition of immune function, anemia, and neutropenia have been reported [108].

We have anecdotally found zinc to be remarkably effective in post-cardiac transplantation dysosmia and hyposmia, despite the presence of normal zinc levels [109]. Zinc at concentrations beyond those in a multivitamin may wisely be limited to use with laboratory evidence of hypozincemia or specific states where zinc has demonstrated efficacy including cirrhosis, dialysis, D-penicillimine treatment, hemopyrrollactamuria, and age-related macular degeneration.

Increasing Patients' Awareness of Altered Eating Habits

Chemosensory disorders in general are linked to changes in food selection. Most notably there is an aversion of foods that are bitter in taste and sweet in smell, as in dark chocolate, coffee, green peppers, and other green leafy vegetables. Also, a predilection develops toward more textured and trigeminally-mediated foods, as sensory compensation for loss and in an attempt to recreate a sapid experience, with such foods as sushi or hot chili peppers.

Table 2.1 presents the different types of chemosensory impairments and the resulting impacts on food selection and body weight:

- For congenital chemosensory dysfunction, no significant difference in weight, eating patterns, or food preferences exists compared to normosmics.
- People with acquired, noncongenital chemosensory dysfunction experience changes in food preferences and a compensatory increase in salt and sugar intake.

TABLE 2.1

Change in Nutrition with Chemosensory Disorders (1-A, 1-B, 1-C, 1-D, 1-E)

Chemosensory Disorders	Food Complaints	Increased Appetite	Decreased Appetite	Decreased Enjoyment	Increased Use of Sugar, Salt, and Spices	Mean Energy Intake Compared to Normosmics	Mean Micronutrient Intake Compared to Normosmics	Mean Body Weight Compared to Normosmics	% Who Gained 10% or More Body Weight Prior to Chemosensory Dysfunction	% Who Lost 10% or More Body Weight Prior to Chemosensory Dysfunction
Anosmia (noncongenital)	50% to 60%	20%	31%	88%	20% to 40% 4% decreased	No change	No change	No change	14%	6.50%
Anosmia (congenital)	20%									
Hyposmia	31% to 80%	30%	10% to 20%	50%	20% to 50% 20% decreased				1.50%	10.60%
Dysosmia & Phantosmia	75% to 85%		24%	83%	50%			113%		
Ageusia	100%		100%	100%						
Hypogeusia	75%		67%	33%			No change		Reported	Reported
Dysgeusia & Phantageusia	72% to 85%	24%	30% to 67%	42% to 70%	40% to 60% 18% decreased	No change			15% to 20%	15% to 20%

References

1-A. Mattes RD, Cowart BJ. Dietary assessment of patients with chemosensory disorders. J Am Dietet Assoc, 1994; 94:50–56.

1-B. Ferris AM, Schlitzer JL, Schierberl MJ, Catalanotta FA, Gent J, Peterson MG, Bartoshuk LM, Cain WS, Goodspeed RB, Leonard G, Donaldson JO. Anosmia and nutritional status. Nutr Res, 1985; 5:149–156.

1-C. Ferris AM, Schlitzer JL, Schierberl MJ. Nutrition and taste and smell deficits: A risk factor or an adjustment? In: Clinical Measurement of Taste and Smell. New York: MacMillan, 1986, 264–278.

1-D. Mattes-Kulig DA, Henkin RI. Energy and nutrient consumption of patients with dysgeusia. J Am Dietet Assoc, 1985; 85:822–826.

1-E. Mattes RD, Coward BJ, Schiavo MA, Arnold C, Garrison B, Kare MR, Lowry LD. Dietary evaluation of patients with smell and/or taste disorders. Am J Clin Nutr, 1990; 51:233–240.

- People with dysgeusia tend to ingest intense trigeminal stimuli, like mint, in an attempt to overcome the unpleasant sensation.
- In those with chemosensory loss, about 10% gain a substantial amount of weight, possibly increasing eating due to the narcissistic drive for the sensory experience or a lack of sensory-specific satiety. An approximately equal number lose weight, possibly secondary to lack of interest in food or an associated depression, or due to the hedonically unpleasant distortion in the taste of foods.
- Dysgeusia triggers most noted and avoided include meats, fresh fruits, coffee, eggs, carbonated beverages, and vegetables [110].
- Among patients with anorexia there is an elevation in sour and bitter recognition thresholds, but there is no abnormality in sweet or salt taste detection thresholds. Neither are there abnormal sweet superthreshold intensity judgments or detection threshold in anorexic or bulimic patients [111,112,113]. Furthermore, anorexics patients demonstrated an aversion to high fat foods, but this may have been due to texture rather than taste [114].
- In obesity there are normal sweet taste thresholds and normal sweet superthreshold intensity judgments [115,116,117,118]. In regards to sweet hedonics, studies are inconclusive with results suggesting more, same, or less sweet preference [116,117,119,120]. While high fat, low sugar mixtures appear to be preferred in the obese [121], not all studies confirm this preference [122,123]. Diverse results from studies suggest that presently unidentified subgroups of taste response exist among those with obesity and chemosensory disorders.

Increasing awareness to the predispositions of food selection may help some patients moderate their food selection [124,125].

SUMMARY

An anfractuous invisible universe at the tip of the nose is ripe for exploration. Compromised senses of smell and taste influence food selection, food preparation, dietary patterns, and digestion. Chemosensory impairments tend to have insidious onset and many patients are therefore unaware these sensations are diminished or altered. Physicians can diagnose chemosensory disorders using a simple screening test, the AST. Familiarity with the medical conditions and iatrogenic risk factors can increase clinical suspicion of smell and taste impairment. Diagnosis can bring awareness to patients for altered food habits and issues pertaining to home safety and food preparation. These can assist clinicians in identifying and managing both underlying nutrient disturbances and gustatory dysfunction to foster optimized eating education for improved overall human health.

REFERENCES

1. Hirsch AR. Scentsation, olfactory demographic and abnormalities. *Intl J Aromatherap*, 1992; 4:1:16–17.
2. Bingham AF, Birch GG, deGraaf C, Behan JM, Perring KD. Sensory studies with sucrose maltol mixtures. *Chem Sen*, 1990; 15:447–456.
3. Murphy C, Cain WS. Taste and olfaction: Independence vs. interaction. *Physiol Behav*, 1980; 24:601–605.
4. Griep MI, Mets TF, Collys K, Verté D, Verleye G, Ponjaert-Kristoffersen I, Massart DL. MNA and odor perception. VUB Free University of Brussels, Faculty of Medicine and Pharmacy, Belgium. (MNA is nutritional assessment), 1999; 1:41–59; discussion 59–60.
5. Murphy C, Schubert CR, Cruickshanks KJ, Klein BEK, Klein R, Nondahl DM. Prevalence of olfactory impairment in older adults. *JAMA*, 2002; 288:2307–2312.
6. Estrem SA, Renner G. Disorders of smell and taste. *Otolaryngol Clin North Am*, 1987; 20:1:133–147.
7. Frye RE. Nasal patency and the aerodynamics of nasal airflow: Measurement by rhinomanometry and acoustic rhinometry, and the influence of pharmacological agents. In: Doty RL (Ed). *Handbook of Olfaction and Gustation*, 2nd Ed., Revised and Expanded. New York: Marcel Dekker, Inc., 2003, 439–459.

8. Hirsch AR, Wyse JP. Posttraumatic dysosmia: Central vs peripheral. *J Neurol Orthop Med Surg,* 1993; 14:152–155.

9. Brodal A. *Neurological anatomy in relation to clinical medicine,* Ed. 3, Vol. 10, New York: Oxford University Press, 1969.

10. Doty RL, Bromley SM, Moberg PJ, Hummel T. Laterality in human nasal chemoreception. In: Christman S (Ed.). *Cerebral in Sensory and Perceptual Processing.* Amsterdam: Elsiever, 1997, 492–542.

11. Acharya V, Acharya J, Luders H. Olfactory epileptic auras. *Neurology,* 1996; 46:A446.

12. Hirsch AR. *Scentsational Sex.* Boston: Element Books, 1998.

13. Jeppson P. Studies on the structure and innervation of taste buds. *Acta Otolaryngol,* 1969; 259:1–95.

14. Smith DV. Taste, smell and psychophysical measurement. In: Meiselman HL, Rivlin RS (Eds.). *Clinical Measurement of Taste and Smell.* New York: Macmillan Co., 1986, 1–18.

15. Rolls ET. Taste, olfactory and food texture reward processing in the brain and obesity. *Intl J Obes,* 2010; 35:550–561.

16. Jefek BW, Moran DT, Eller PM. Steroid-dependent anosmia. *Arch Otolaryngol,* 1987; 113:547–549.

17. Heinkin R. Abnormalities of taste and olfaction in patients with chromatin negative gonadal dysgenesis. Taste and olfaction in Turner's syndrome. *J Clin Endocrin,* 1967; 27:1437.

18. Eichenbaum H, Morton T, Potter H, Corkin S. Selective olfactory deficits in case H.M. *Brain,* 1983; 106(2):459–472.

19. Eskenazi B, Cain W, Novelly R, Mattson R. Odor perception in temporal lobe epilepsy patients with and without temporal lobectomy. *Neuropsychologia,* 1986; 24:553–562.

20. Mohr PD. Early neurological complications of coronary artery bypass surgery. *BMJ,* 1986; 292:60–61.

21. Lehrer S, Levine E, Bloomer W. Abnormally diminished sense of smell in women with estrogen receptor positive breast cancer. *Lancet,* 1985; 2:333.

22. Mair RG, Doty RL, Kelly KM, Wilson CS, Langlais PJ, McEntree WJ, Vollmecke TA. Multimodal sensory deficits in Korsakoff's psychosis. *Neuropsychologia,* 1986; 24:831–839.

23. Potter H, Butters N. An assessment of olfactory deficits in patients with damage to prefrontal cortex. *Neuropsychologia,* 1980; 18:621–628.

24. Ward CD, Hess WA, Calne DB. Olfactory impairment in Parkinson's disease. *Neurology,* 1983; 33:943–946.

25. Doty RL, Ferguson-Segall M. Odor detection performance of rats following d-amphetamine treatment: A signal detection analysis. *Psychopharmacology (Berl),* 1987; 93:87–93.

26. Doty RL, Ferguson-Segall M, Lucki I, Kreider M. Effects of intrabulbar injections of 6-hydroxydopamine on ethyl acetate odor detection in castrate and non-castrate male rats. *Brain Res,* 1988; 44:95–103.

27. Doty RL, Deems DA, Stellar S. Olfactory dysfunction in Parkinsonism: A general deficit unrelated to neurologic signs, disease stage, or disease duration. *Neurology,* 1988; 38:1237.

28. Doty RL, Riklan M, Deems D, Reynolds C, Stellar S. The olfactory and cognitive deficits of Parkinson's disease: Evidence for independence. *Ann Neurol,* 1989; 25:166–171.

29. Hirsch, AR. Parkinsonism: The hyposmia and phantosmia connection. *Archives of Neurology,* 2009; 66:4:538–539.

30. Delahunty CM. Changing sensitivity of odour, taste, texture and mouth-feel with ageing. (Workshop summary). How do age-related changes in sensory physiology influence food liking and food intake? *Food Qual Pref,* 2004; 15:907–911.

31. Hawkes C, Fogo A, Shah M. Smell identification declines from age 36 years and mainly affects pleasant odors. *Chem Sen,* 2005; 30:A152–A153.

32. Stevens J, Cain W, Weinstein D. Aging impairs the ability to detect gas odors. *Fire Technol,* 1987; 23:198–204.

33. Doty R, Reys P, Gregor T. Presence of both odor identification and detection deficits in Alzheimer's disease. *Brain Res Bull,* 1987; 18:598.

34. Serby M, Corwin J, Novatt A, Conrad P, Rotrosen J. Olfaction in dementia. *Neurosurg Psychiat,* 1985; 14:848–849.

35. Koss E, Weiffenbach J, Haxby J, Friedland R. Olfactory detection and identification performance are dissociated in early Alzheimer's disease. *Neurology,* 1988; 38:1228.

36. Koss E, Weiffenbach J, Haxby J, Friedland R. Olfactory detection and identification performance are dissociated in early Alzheimer's disease. *Lancet,* 1987; 1:622.

37. Pearson R, Esiri M, Hiorns R, Wilcock G, Powell T. Anatomical correlates of the distribution of the pathological changes in the neocortex in Alzheimer's disease. *Proc Natl Acad Sci, USA,* 1985; 82:4531–4534.

38. Monath T, Cropp B, Harrison A. Mode of entry of a neurotropic arbovirus into the central nervous system. *Lab Invest,* 1983; 48:399.

39. Roberts R. Alzheimer's disease may begin in the nose and may be caused by aluminosilicates. *Neurbiol Aging,* 1986; 7:561–567.
40. Schwartz A, Frey J, Lukas R. Risk factors in Alzheimer's disease: Is aluminum hazardous to your health? *BNI Quarterly,* 1988; 4:2.
41. Frye R, Schwartz B, Doty R. Dose-related effects of cigarette smoking on olfactory function. *JAMA,* 1990; 263:1233.
42. Cain W, Cometto-Muniz JE. Perception of nasal pungency in smokers and nonsmokers. *Psychol Behav,* 1982; 29:727–732.
43. Levin H, High W, Eisenberg H. Impairment of olfactory recognition after closed head injury. *Brain,* 1985; 108:579–591.
44. Costanzo R, Becker D. Smell and taste disorders in head injury and neurosurgery patients. In: Meiselman HL, Rivlin RS (Eds.). *Clinical Measurement of Taste and Smell.* New York: Macmillan, 1986, 565–568.
45. Sauberlich HE. Vitamin metabolism and requirements. *S Afr Med J,* 1975; 49:2235–2244.
46. Friedman MI, Mattes RD. Chemical senses and nutrition. In: Getchell TV, Doty RL, Bartoshuk LM, Snow, Jr. JB (Eds.). *Smell and Taste in Health and Disease.* Chapter 21. New York: Raven Press, 1991, 392.
47. Green RF. Subclinical pellagra and idiopathic hypogeusia. (Letter). *JAMA,* 1971; 218:8:1303.
48. Smith AD. Legaloblastic anemias. In: Williams WJ, Beutler E, Erslev AJ, Lichtman MA (Eds.). *Hematology,* 3rd Ed. New York: McGraw-Hill, 1983, 434–465.
49. Smith DV, Seiden AM. Olfactory dysfunction. In: Laing DG, Doty RL, Briepohl W (Eds.). *The Human Sense of Smell.* Chapter 14. New York: Springer-Verlag, 1995, 298.
50. Schechter PJ, Friedewald WT, Bronzert DA, Raff MS, Henkin RI. Idiopathic hypogeusia: A description of the syndrome and a single blind study with zinc sulfate. *Int Rev Neurobiol Suppl,* 1972; 1:125–140.
51. Weismann K, Christensen E, Dreyer V. Zinc supplementation in alcoholic cirrhosis. *Acta Med Scand,* 1979; 205:361–366.
52. Public Health Service. *Report of the Panel on Communicative Disorders to the National Advisory Neurological and Communicative Disorders and Stroke Council.* (NIH Publication No. 79–1914). Washington, DC: National Institutes of Health, 1979, 319.
53. Ackerman BH, Kasbekar N. Disturbances of taste and smell induced by drugs. *Pharmacother,* 1997; 17:482–496.
54. Bates B. *Guide to Physical Examination.* Philadelphia: JB Lippincott, 1974, 272.
55. Haerer AF. *DeJong's The Neurological Examination.* 5th Ed. Philadelphia: Lippincott, 1992, 89.
56. Parsons M. *Color Atlas of Clinical Neurology.* Chicago: Year Book Medical, 1983, 18.
57. Fuller G. *Neurological Examination Made Easy.* Edinburgh, Scotland: Churchille Livingstone, 1993, 47.
58. Post F. Dementia, depression, and pseudodementia. In: Benson DV, Blumer D (Eds.). *Psychiatric Aspects of Neurologic Disease.* New York: Grune and Stratton, 1975, 99–120.
59. Solomon GS, Petrie WM, Hart JR, Brackin, Jr., HB. Olfactory dysfunction discriminates Alzheimer's dementia from major depression. *J Neuropsychiat Clin Neurosci,* 1998; 10:1:64–67.
60. Doty RL, Singh A, Tetrude J, Langston JW. Lack of olfactory dysfunction in MPTP-induced Parkinsonism. *Ann Neurol,* 1992; 32:97–100.
61. Sajjadian A, Doty RL, Gutnick DN, Chirurgi RJ, Sivak M, Perl D. Olfactory dysfunction in amyotrophic lateral sclerosis. *Neurodegener,* 1994; 3:153–157.
62. Busenbark KL, Huber ST, Greer G, Pahwa R, Koller WC. Olfactory function in essential tremor. *Neurol,* 1992; 42:1631–1632.
63. Hirsch AR. Olfaction in migraineurs. *Headache,* 1992; 32:233–236.
64. Loury MC, Kennedy DN. Chronic sinusitis and nasal polyposis. In: Getchell TV et al. (Eds.), *Smell and Taste in Health and Disease.* New York: Raven, 1991, 517–528.
65. Hirsch AR, Thakkar N, Olfaction in a patient with unclassifiable cluster headache-like disorder. *Headache Quarterly,* 1995; 6:113–122.
66. Hirsch AR. Neurotoxicity as a result of ambient chemicals: Denham Springs, La. *International Congress on Hazardous Waste: Impact on Human and Ecological Health.* U.S. Department of Health and Human Services. Atlanta: Public Health Agency for Toxic Substances and Disease Registry, 1995, 229.
67. Bakay L, Cares HL. Olfactory meningiomas. *Acta Neurochirurgia Fasc,* 1973; 26:1–12.
68. Hirsch AR, Trannel TH. Chemosensory disorders and psychiatric diagnoses. *J Neurol Ortho Med Surg,* 1996; 17:25–30.
69. Hirsch AR. Concurrence of chemosensory and sexual dysfunction. *Bio Psychiat,* 1998; 43:52S.
70. Davidson TM, Jalowayski A, Murphy C, Jacobs RJ. Evaluation and treatment of smell dysfunction. *West J Med,* 1987; 146:434–438.

71. Scott AE, Cain WS, Leonard G. Nasal/sinus disease and olfactory loss at the Connecticut Chemosensory Clinical Research Center. *Chem Senses,* 1989; 14:745.

72. Scott AE, Cain WS, Clavet G. Topical corticosteroids can alleviate olfactory dysfunction. *Chem Senses,* 1988; 13:735.

73. Chalke HD, Dewhurst JR. Accidental coal-gas poisoning. *Brit Med J,* 1957; 2:915–917.

74. Costanzo RM, Zasler ND. Head trauma. In: Getchell TV (Ed.). *Smell and Taste in Health and Disease.* New York: Raven, 1991, 711–730.

75. Adams RG, Crabtree N. Anosmia in alkaline battery workers. *Br J Industr Med,* 1961; 18:216–221.

76. Hirsch AR. Smell and taste: How the culinary experts compare to the rest of us. *Food Technol,* 1987; 23:198–204.

77. Hirsch AR, Colavincenzo ML. Olfactory deficits among Chicago firefighters. *Chgo Med,* 2000; 103:11: 18–19.

78. Nordin S, Monsoh AU, Murphy C. Unawareness of smell loss in normal aging and Alzheimer's disease: Discrepancy between self-reporting and diagnosed smell sensitivity. *J Gerentol,* 1995; 50:187–192.

79. Adams R, Victor M. *Principles of Neurology.* New York: McGraw-Hill, 1989, 482–496.

80. Hirsch AR, Gotway MB. Validation of the Chicago Smell Test (CST) in subjective normosmic neurologic patients. *Chem Senses,* 1993; 18:570–571.

81. Hirsch AR, Gotway MB, Harris AT. Validation of the Chicago Smell Test (CST) in patients with subjective olfactory loss. *Chem Senses,* 1993; 18:571.

82. Amoore JE, Ollman BG. Practical test kits for quantitatively evaluating sense of smell. *Rhinol,* 1983; 21:49–54.

83. Gent JP, Cain WS, Bartoshuk LM. Taste and smell management in a clinical setting. In: Meiselman HL, Rivlin RS (Eds.). *Clinical Measurement of Taste and Smell.* New York: Macmillan, 1986, 107–111.

84. Doty RL, Newhouse MG, Azzalina JD. Internal consistency and short-term test-retest reliability of the University of Pennsylvania Smell Identification Test. *Chem Sen,* 1985; 10:297–300.

85. Davidson TM, Murphy C. Rapid clinical evaluation of anosmia: The alcohol sniff test. *Arch Otolaryngol Head Neck Surg,* 1997; 123:591–594.

86. Schlotfeld CR, Geisler MW, Davidson TM, Murphy C. Clinical application of the alcohol sniff test on HIV positive and HIV negative patients with nasal sinus disease. *Chemical Sen,* 1998; 23:610.

87. Middleton CB, Geisler MW, Davidson TM, Murphy C. Relationship between the alcohol sniff test and sensory olfactory event-related potentials: Validation of a psychophysical test. *Chemical Sen,* 1998; 23:610.

88. Davidson TM, Freed C, Healy MP, Murphy C. Rapid clinical evaluation of anosmia in children: The Alcohol Sniff Test. *Ann NY Acad Sci,* 1998; 855:787–792.

89. Freed CL, Dalve-Endres AM, Davidson TM, Murphy C. Rapid screening of olfactory function in Down's syndrome. *Chemical Sen,* 1998; 23:610.

90. Doty RL, Shaman P, Applebaum SL, Gilberson R, Sikorsky L, Rosenberg L. Smell identification ability: Changes with age. *Sci,* 1984; 226:1441–1443.

91. Serby M. Olfaction and neuropsychiatry [Abstr.]. Distributed at Dr. Serby's lecture at the Institute for Research and Behavioral Neurosciences, New York, December 12, 1987.

92. Adams RB, Victor M. *Principles of Neurology.* New York: McGraw-Hill, 1989, 927.

93. Wurtman RJ. Sources of choline and lecithin in the diet. In: Barbeau JH, Growden JH, Wurtman RJ (Eds.). *Nutrition and the Brain,* Vol. 5. New York: Raven Press, 1979, 73–81.

94. Wurtman RJ, Hefti F, Melamed E. Precusor control of neurotransmitter synthesis. *Pharmacol Rev,* 1981; 32:315–335.

95. Jackson IV, Nuttal EA, Ibe IO, et al. Treatment of tardive dyskinesia with lecithin. *Am J Psychiat,* 1979; 136:1458–1460.

96. Little A, Levy R. Chuaqui-Kidd P, et al. Double blind placebo control trial of high dose lecithin in Alzheimer's disease. *J Neurol Nursury Psychiat,* 1985; 48:736–742.

97. Hirsch AR, Dougherty DD, Aranda JG, Vanderbilt JG, Weclaw GC. Medications for olfactory loss: Pilot studies. *J Neurol Orthop Med Surg,* 1996; 17:108–114.

98. Hirsch AR, Baker J. Lack of efficacy of thiamine treatment for chemosensory disorder. *J Psychiat Clin Neurosci,* 2001; 13:1:151.

99. Duncan RB, Briggs M. Treatment of uncomplicated anosmia by vitamin A. *Arch Otolaryngol,* 1962; 75:116–124.

100. Roydhouse N. Retinoid therapy and anosmia. *New Zealand Med J,* 1988; 101:465.

101. Garrett-Laster M, Russell RM, Jacques PF. Impairment of taste and olfaction in patients with cirrhosis: The role of vitamin A. *Human Nutr,* 1984; 38C:203–214.

102. Schiffman SS, Diaz C, Beeker TG. Caffeine intensifies taste of certain sweeteners: Role of adenosine receptor. *Pharm Biochem Behav*, 1986; 24:429–432.

103. DeMet E, Stein MK, Tran C, Chicz-DeMet A, Sangdahl C, Nelson J. Caffeine taste test for panic disorder: Adenosine receptor supersensitivity. *Psychiatr Res,* 1989; 30:231–242.

104. Henkin RI, Keiser HR, Jaffee IA, Sternlieb I, Scheinberg IH. Decreased taste sensitivity after D-penicillamine reversed by copper administration. *Lancet,* 1967; 2:1268–1271.

105. Henkin RI, Bradley DF. Regulation of taste acuity by thiols and metal ions. *Proc Natl Acad Sci, USA,* 1969; 62:30–37.

106. Henkin RI, Schechter PJ, Friedewald WT, Demets DL, Raff M. A double blind study of the effects of zinc sulfate on taste and smell dysfunction. *Am J Med Sci,* 1976; 272:285–299.

107. Deems DA, Doty RL, Settle RG, Moore-Gillon V, Shaman P, Mester AF, Kimmelman CP, Brightman VJ, Snow, Jr., JB. Smell and taste disorders. A study of 750 patients from the University of Pennsylvania Smell and Taste Center. *Arch Otolaryngol Head Neck Surg,* 1991; 117:519–528.

108. Fosmire GJ. Zinc toxicity. *Am J Clin Nutr,* 1990; 51:225–227.

109. Hirsch AR. Unpublished.

110. Markley EJ, Mattes-Kulig DA, Henkin RI. A classification of dysgeusia. *J Am Dietet Assoc,* 1983; 83:578–580.

111. Casper RC, Kirschner B, Sandstead HH, Jacob RA, Davis JM. An evaluation of trace metals, vitamins, and taste function in anorexia nervosa. *Am J Clin Nutr,* 1980; 33:1801–1808.

112. Lacey JH, Stanley PA, Crutchfield SM. Sucrose sensitivity in anorexia nervosa. *J Psychosom Res,* 1977; 21:17–21.

113. Sunday SR, Halmi KA. Taste perceptions and hedonics in eating disorders. *Psychol Behav,* 1990; 48:587–594.

114. Mela DJ. Sensory assessment of fat content in fluid dairy products. *Appetite,* 1988; 10:37–44.

115. Grinker J. Obesity and sweet taste. *Am J Clin Nutr,* 1978; 31:1078–1087.

116. Drewnowski A. Sweetness and obesity. In: Dobbing J (Ed.). *Sweetness.* New York: Springer-Verlag, 1987, 177–201.

117. Fritjers JER, Rasmussen-Conrad EL. Sensory discrimination, intensity perception, affective judgment of sucrose-sweetness in the overweight. *J Gen Psychol,* 1982; 107:233–247.

118. Witherly SA, Pangborn RM, Stern JS. Gustatory responses and eating duration of obese and lean adults. *Appetite,* 1980; 1:53–63.

119. Rodin J, Moskowitz HR, Bray GA. Relationship between obesity, weight loss, and taste responsiveness. *Physiol Behav,* 1976; 17:591–597.

120. Spitzer L, Rodin J. Human eating behavior: A critical review of studies in normal weight and overweight individuals. *Appetite,* 1981; 2:293–329.

121. Drewnowski A. Fat and sugar: Sensory and hedonic aspects of sweet, high-fat foods. In Friedman MI, Tordoff MG, Kare MR (Eds.). *Chemical Senses: Appetite and Nutrition,* New York: Marcel Dekker, 1991, 69–83.

122. Pangborn RM, Bos KEO, Stern J. Dietary fat intake and taste responses to fat in milk by under-, normal, and overweight women. *Appetite,* 1985; 6:25–40.

123. Warwick ZS, Schiffman SS, Anderson JJB. Relationship of dietary fat content to preferences in young rats. *Physiol Behav,* 1990; 48:581–586.

124. Hirsch AR, Gomez R. Weight reduction through inhalation of odorants. *J Neurol Orthop Med Surg,* 1995; 16:28–31.

125. Hirsch, AR. "Use of gustatory stimuli to facilitate weight loss." ATTD Abstracts, 2008, p. 39.

3 Periodontal Disease

Treatable, Nutrition-Related, and with Systemic Repercussions

David Kennedy, D.D.S.

INTRODUCTION

Periodontal disease (PD) is an encompassing term for gingivitis and periodontitis. PD is the predominant underlying pathology of adult tooth loss. It is caused by various microorganisms and parasites. Host susceptibility, moderated by nutritional deficiencies, plays a significant role in the progress of the disease. Among the risk factors are diabetes, smoking, a diet characterized by refined carbohydrates, and inadequate vitamin C.

PD has been called cyclical because it seems to come and go for reasons that are not totally clear. For example, when a woman is pregnant her periodontal problems seem to accelerate. This is commonly called pregnancy gingivitis and patients are often not counseled that PD is linked to the pregnancy outcome. The more severe the mother's periodontal condition, the more likely she is to have a low birth weight baby. In fact, periodontal pathogens have been isolated from the amniotic fluid [1,2]. In addition, periodontal disease has been linked to systemic illness including cancers, pneumonia, diabetes, and cardiovascular disease [3,4,5].

EPIDEMIOLOGY

Research has confirmed through DNA testing a number of vectors for this infectious disease. The most common transmission pattern is from mother to child or caregiver to child, the pattern by which the gut microbiome is obtained [6]. Unlike the intestinal tract, which is colonized during the birth process, the organisms associated with periodontal disease need teeth to colonize so they are typically not transferred until after the first teeth arrive.

Periodontal infections can also be transmitted to children from a father, siblings, or playmates. In addition, a surprising development uncovered with DNA testing found transfer from dogs to humans.

Nutritional factors in the population can abate the infectious microorganisms. Nutrition can also influence individual susceptibility; changes in nutrient status and dietary patterns are thought to contribute to the cyclical pattern of PD progression. Other factors include mercury/silver filling implants, smoking, and stress [7]. Both fluoride containing dentifrice and dental fluorosis have been linked to periodontal disease probably through the mechanism of direct bone injury and/or increased inflammation [8].

49

PATHOPHYSIOLOGY

The pathophysiology of PD is the result of an inflammatory response resulting from the interaction between the pathogenic bacteria, host's immune response, polymorph nuclear leukocytes (PMN), and heavy metal reactive oxygen species (ROS) production with depletion of glutathione [9,10,11]. The inflammation is induced by either direct action from bacterial invasion like most infections or by exotoxins released from colonizing bacteria.

Once the infection becomes established, amoebas that are secondary invaders play a significant role in the inflammatory process, producing large numbers of PMNs. Amoebas were identified in 1915 by the famous physician C. C. Bass as strongly implicated in periodontal disease [12]. He identified their presence by using a light microscope. They cannot be cultured and as a result are not picked up in most microbiological tests. Recently, the presence of amoebas in PD sites and their absence where PD-related inflammation is not present has been confirmed by polymerase chain reaction diagnostic techniques [13].

On microscopy, amoebas can be seen visibly attacking and consuming white blood cells—usually PMNs [14]. The damaged white blood cells then release histamine, which calls more PMNs to the area. The cycle produces enormous inflammation and accelerates the bone loss that is characteristic of the progressive destruction of the periodontal supporting structures. As the disease process advances, pockets form and eventually tooth mobility and abscess formation occurs.

Oral antibiotics such as metronidozole (Flagyl) for these parasites alone ultimately will fail to eradicate the oral infections as the gingival crevicular fluid (GCF) generally carries very little antibiotic. A direct application of antiseptics to the sulcus, followed by direct application of metronidozole in ophthalmic solution to the sulcus at the same time while simultaneously giving systemic metronidozole, provides oral and systemic antibiotic coverage that has proven effective in eliminating this kind of infection. This method essentially treats all areas of infection simultaneously; this way, the amoeba is eradicated.

HEAVY METAL MERCURY IN PERIDONTAL DISEASE PATHOPHYSIOLOGY

The dental profession has traditionally referred to a mixture of 50% elemental mercury and varying amounts of silver, copper, zinc, and tin as a "silver" amalgam filling. As a result, most of the general public in a recent Zogby poll did not realize that mercury was even a component of a "silver" filling, much less the principal ingredient. A more appropriate term for such a filling, in consideration of the patient's right to adequate informed consent, would be mercury/silver tooth filling.

Some dental organizations have claimed that the mercury forms a covalent bond with silver, a physical impossibility. It forms weak intermetallic bonds that are easily broken with heat or pressure, and forms micro-currents between the metals. Consequently, such fillings are now known to be a predominant source of human exposure to mercury [15].

In a series of elegant experiments at the University of Calgary School of Medicine, radioactively labeled mercury[203] fillings were installed in sheep and monkeys and the released mercury was imaged. In four weeks, the mercury had exited the fillings and accumulated in many distant organs including the kidney, liver, and heart [16]. The deposits in the gut are likely particulate forms of amalgam that abrade during normal mastication. Human studies of stool have found high levels of mercury in amalgam bearers [17]. Although the absorption rate of inorganic mercury is low, the sheer volume of material was quite large. The mercury deposited in the kidneys is thought to be derived from the blood stream because elemental mercury vapor absorbs rapidly from the lungs. The experiment with sheep was criticized by the American Dental Association as not reliable because sheep are ruminants, chewing more than humans. The authors of the research reported that a sheep was chosen precisely because the sheep is an exacerbated chewing model. However, the study was repeated a few months later in monkeys with similar results [18].

The sheep and monkey studies both revealed jawbone saturation with mercury. The mercury had rapidly migrated from the filling directly through the dental tissues into the bone. This appears to explain older research in humans that found bone loss surrounding teeth that have received "silver" fillings [19,20]. Taken together, "silver" fillings are implicated in periodontal destruction. This is likely due to the production of reactive oxygen species, depletion of GCF, glutathione, and inflammation.

In an interesting adaptation, exotoxin-producing bacteria, which inhabit the oral cavity, are able to couple mercury with their biological toxin to produce an even more toxic substance. This is particularly important in the case of root canals where dead roots are partially filled and retained in the jawbone. Research has confirmed that these root-filled teeth accumulate anaerobic bacteria in large numbers [21]. Wu reports that "histologic observation of root apices with surrounding bone removed from either patients or human cadavers has demonstrated that post-treatment apical periodontitis is associated with 50–90% of root filled human teeth" [22]. Apical periodontitis confirms that many root-filled teeth remain infected. The reaction of oral mercury with anaerobic toxicants can produce super-toxicants such as CH_3S-Hg^+ and $CH_3-S-Hg-S-CH_3$. Also, the excretion of mercury is variable, influenced by a diet containing milk or following an antibiotic by as much as thirtyfold [23]. Since no dental research evaluates the systemic impact of root canal therapy, this task falls upon the medical profession to identify and rectify any injury from such misinformed dental treatments.

PATIENT EVALUATION: REASONS TO NOTE PERIDONTAL DISEASE IN A PHYSICAL EXAM

The classic method of diagnosing periodontal disease is based upon measurement of the gingival sulcus with a measuring probe and noting the presence of pus and bleeding. Primarily, anaerobic motile bacteria create inflammation and denude the crevicular epithelium to cause pocket formation.

Anaerobic culture is difficult to do in a clinical practice; pocket measurement is easy but a very flawed approach. Even after the bacteria are eradicated, the pockets will remain as an artifact of the prior damage. Pus is not a consistently reliable feature of periodontal disease. Bleeding will occur in a healthy sulcus when sufficient pressure is applied to the probe. An undesirable consequence of probing an infected sulcus prior to disinfection is that the pathogenic organisms are seeded into deeper tissues. A much more accurate method of diagnosis is to visually assess the biological life in the gingival sulcus. Although this method is very easy in an office equipped with the necessary microscope, it is not typically found in most dental practices. The International Academy of Oral Medicine and Toxicology (IAOMT) strongly recommends this approach, but not all of its members provide the recommended level of examination. Less than 15% of the fees charged by dentists relate to periodontal disease, although an estimated 90% of adults have PD—pointing to a large disconnect between the problem and the treatment.

However, a physician during a routine exam may quickly screen for the presence of PD by assessing mouth odor, noting gingival color, and asking pertinent questions regarding the stability of the teeth. A sure sign of advancing inflammation is seen when teeth begin to drift out of place and food impacts interproximally. Like most things in medicine, a careful diagnosis is going to lead to an appropriate treatment; but in the absence of a microscopic examination, there are steps that can easily be taken to avoid advancing disease.

Based on the pathophysiologic research presented here, noting "silver" fillings as a PD risk factor may not only be helpful for prevention and treatment of PD but can inform other systemic conditions associated with overburdened biopathways for toxin removal.

Noting the presence of PD in the chart is an inexpensive biomarker, described in the medical literature to be as strong a predictor of cardiovascular disease as is cholesterol [2]. PD can therefore contribute to clinical acumen in a diagnostic work-up.

PD can further guide clinical decision making regarding compromised nutrient status and impaired digestion. Choice of antibiotics for a systemic illness may be appropriately influenced by the presence of PD, since responsive treatment regiments are better established than for some other conditions.

PD prevention is aligned with lifestyle medicine counseling. One of the most important steps in prevention is to promote healthful nutrition, optimum hydration, and the absence of negative oral habits like smoking or chewing tobacco.

PREVENTION

By far the simplest and most cost-effective approach to any dental disorder is prevention. Since almost all of the periodontal pathogens are anaerobic and highly motile organisms, the most efficacious approach in my opinion is daily application of antiseptics by oral irrigation. In the nineteenth century, physicians traditionally painted iodine on infected gums with a cotton swab. Applying a dilute solution with a pulsating water irrigator is the modern method, although some recent research into the prevention of baby bottle tooth decay found the cotton swab is still an effective way to prevent decay [24].

Adequate saliva is vital to both preventing periodontal infections from advancing and to arresting tooth decay. Therefore, careful attention to the side effects of drugs is needed.

Many medications can cause dry mouth. The most common ones are for blood pressure and psychiatric conditions. When such a medication is indicated, it should be accompanied with specific instructions on hydrating the mouth with sialogogue or another non-sugary method. Unfortunately, many people—when faced with this condition—reach for a sugary lozenge or sugary beverage that will greatly accelerate the problem of tooth decay.

Various solutions have been proposed including colloidal silver and even salt water. Early research found that water alone was more effective than nothing and antimicrobial solutions enhanced the results [25]. Therefore, the actual solution is likely one of availability and preference rather than any hard dictates. It remains clear that the outer layers of plaque need to be disturbed mechanically first, in order for the solution to penetrate sufficiently to flush out the periodontal pathogens. Simply put, stir it up and flush it out.

Fluoride irrigation solutions have been shown to promote destruction of bone in the presence of preexisting PD [26]. The mouth has a thin mucosa—especially the floor of the mouth—and superb circulation; therefore, it can be used to supply nutrients such as vitamin B12 directly to the bloodstream. By the same logic, a dentifrice that contains fluoride will give an unwanted systemic dose and impact the integrity of the jawbone. Inflammation is a known result of exposing soft tissues to fluoride. The patent application of a pharmaceutical company discloses that concentrations of fluorides from fluoridated toothpastes and mouthwashes activate G proteins in the oral cavity, thereby promoting PD and oral cancer. This is not surprising considering research has linked fluoride to G-protein activation [27].

In addition to the concerns about fluoride, there are two additional ingredients found in some toothpastes that have raised concerns about potential exacerbation of PD. Sodium laurel sulfate is a soap derivative that will disrupt the oral mucosa and dramatically increase the frequency of oral aphthous or herpes outbreaks [28]. Triclosan (2,4,4′ –trichloro-2′-hydroxydiphenyl ether) is a synthetic, broad-spectrum antimicrobial agent first registered as a pesticide in 1969 and now linked to chloroform production and thus certain cancers at the FDA [29,30]. This is not unreasonable considering that it may form dioxins in surface water and its active ingredient is a polychlorophenoxyphenol [31].

Prevention is especially important during pregnancy. The hormone shift and immunosuppression during pregnancy can exacerbate existing periodontal conditions. Research has confirmed that a woman's oral health plays a significant role in her pregnancy outcome [32,33]. Periodontal disease is associated with elevated risk of undesirable pregnancy outcomes such as preterm birth and low birth weight infants [34]. Treatment of PD and tooth decay during pregnancy is difficult. For example, placing a mercury/silver filling during pregnancy will significantly increase the cord blood mercury. And while disinfection is beneficial, even the trauma incurred during routine cleaning when PD is present may be sufficient to spread the organisms to the bloodstream.

Bacteria living in the sulcus or in nonvital teeth exude short molecular weight proteins that are more toxic than botulism. These short proteins migrate to distant locations and this is apparently how a septic sight can exert its biotoxin in a remote area such as a heart or joint. Or they can exert their effects more directly by getting into the placenta or inside the blood brain barrier [35].

TREATMENT

Surgical periodontal therapy has been the standard of care for more than half a century, but more modern considerations now dictate an anti-infectious approach while enhancing host immunity to achieve a more predictable outcome. Some evidence now suggests that surgery can accelerate tooth loss [36]. This is because the target for such therapy was pocket reduction by excision of pocket tissue and bone remodeling and occasionally tissue grafts. Since periodontal disease begins in children with apparently healthy gingival sulci and minimal depth the process is doomed to fail unless the underlying cause of host susceptibility and microorganism are addressed.

The IAOMT, after an extensive review of the literature and consultation with experts, concluded that the appropriate therapy for any periodontal condition starts with a careful analysis of the oral flora followed by nonsurgical disinfection both in office and at home [37]. Frequent follow-up evaluations, with a strong bias toward microbiological analysis, provided the best avenue toward health. Mercury/silver fillings often play a significant role in the pathogenesis of PD, adding to the reasons to support the ban of mercury/silver fillings as the IAOMT first recommended in 1985. Daily irrigation with an antimicrobial agent is the most effective way to remove this common infection.

CLINICAL SUMMARY

PD is not limited to the oral cavity: It is systemically influenced and has systemic repercussions such as cardiovascular disease, low birth weight babies, and cancers. It is an infectious process involving numerous forms of anaerobic bacteria and one-celled animals. Control of this condition is achieved by a combined approach of targeted oral hygiene with irrigation and antiseptics, mercury removal, optimizing nutrition, and frequent monitoring of the oral flora to guard against recurrent infection.

REFERENCES

1. León, R., et al. Detection of Porphyromonas gingivalis in the amniotic fluid in pregnant women with a diagnosis of threatened premature labor. *Journal of Periodontology* 2007, 78(7):1249–1255. (doi:10.1902/jop.2007.060368)
2. Xiaojing, L. I., et al. Systemic diseases caused by oral infections. *Clinical Microbiology Reviews* 2000, Oct. 13(4):547–558.
3. Marques da Silva, R. Human atherosclerotic plaque contains viable invasive Actinobacillus actinomycetemcomitans and Porphyromonas gingivalis. *J Vasc Surg* 2006, Nov. 44(5):1055–60.
4. Beck J. D., et al. Periodontal disease and cardiovascular disease. *J. Periodontology* 1996, 67:1123–1137.
5. Paju, S., and Scannapieco, F. A. Oral biofilms, periodontitis, and pulmonary infections. *Oral Dis* 2007, Nov. 13(6):508–512.
6. Li, Y., and Caufield, P. W. The fidelity of initial acquisition of mutans streptococci by infants from their mothers. *J Dental Res* 1995, Feb. 74(2):681–685.
7. Chapple, I. Potential mechanisms underpinning the nutritional modulation of periodontal inflammation. *JADA* 2009, 140(2):178–184.
8. Vandana, K. L., and Sesha Reddy, M. Assessment of periodontal status in dental fluorosis subjects using community periodontal index of treatment needs. *Indiana Journal of Dental Research* 2007, 18(2):67–71.
9. Iwamoto, Y., et al. Antimicrobial periodontal treatment decreases serum C-reactive protein, tumor necrosis factor-alpha, but not adiponectin levels in patients with chronic periodontitis. *J Periodontol* 2003, Aug. 74(8):1231–1236.

10. Salzberg, T. N., Overstreet, B. T., Rogers, J. D., Califano, J. V., Best, A. M., and Schenkein, H. A. C-reactive protein levels in patients with aggressive periodontitis. *J Periodontol* 2006, June 77(6):933–939.
11. Chapple, I. L. C. Role of free radicals and antioxidants in the pathogenesis of inflammatory periodontal diseases. *Clinical Molecular Pathology* 1996, 49:247–255.
12. Bass, C. C., and Johns, F. M. *Alveolodental Pyorrhea*. Philadelphia: WB Saunders, 1915.
13. Trim, Robert D., et al. Use of PCR to detect Entamoeba gingivalis in diseased gingival pockets and demonstrate its absence in healthy gingival sites. *Parasitol Res* 2011, Mar, 109(3):857–864.
14. Author's personal observation.
15. WHO Environmental Health Criteria 118 (1991), section 5.1. General population exposure, Table 2, http://www.inchem.org/documents/ehc/ehc/ehc118.htm.
16. Hahn, L. J., Kloiber, R., Vimy, M. J., Takahashi, Y., and Lorscheider, F. Dental "silver" tooth fillings: A source of mercury exposure revealed by whole-body image scan and tissue analysis. *FASEB J* 1989, 3:2641–2646.
17. Skare, I., and Engqvist, A. Amalgam restorations—An important source of human exposure of mercury and silver. *LÄKARTIDNINGEN* 1992, 15:1299–1301.
18. Hahn, L. J., Kloiber, R., Leininger, R. W., Vimy, M. J., and Lorscheider, F. L. Whole-body imaging of the distribution of mercury released from dental fillings into monkey tissues. *FASEB* 1990, 4:3256–3260.
19. Fisher, D., et al. NIDR/ADA Workshop. *J Oral Rehab* 1984, 11:399–405.
20. Ziff, M. F. Documented clinical side-effects to dental amalgam. 1992, *Adv Dent Res* 6:131–134.
21. Nagaoka S., et al. Bacterial invasion into dentinal tubules of human vital and nonvital teeth. *Journal of Endodontics* 1995, 21(2):70-73.
22. Wu, M. K., et al. Consequences of and strategies to deal with residual post-treatment root canal infections. *International Endodontic Journal* 2006, 39:343–356.
23. Rowland, I. R., Effects of diet on mercury metabolism and excretion in mice given methylmercury: Role of gut flora. *Archives of Environmental Health* 1984 39(6):401–408.
24. Lopez, L., Berkowitz, R., Spiekerman, C., and Weinstein, P. Topical antimicrobial therapy in the prevention of early childhood caries: A follow-up report. *Pediatr Dent* 2002, May-Jun 24(3):204–206.
25. Macaulay, W. J. Roy, and Newman, H. N. The effect on the composition of subgingival plaque of a simplified oral hygiene system including pulsating jet subgingival irrigation. *Journal of Periodontal Research* 1986, July, 21(4), 375–385.
26. Sjostrom, S., and Kalfas, S. Tissue necrosis after subgingival irrigation with fluoride solution. *J Clinical Periodontology* 1999, Apr 26(4):257–260.
27. Strunecká, A., and Patočkab, J. Pharmacological and toxicological effects of aminofluoride complexes. Research report 1999, *J Fluoride* 32:4.
28. Herlofson, B. B., and Barkvoll, P. Sodium lauryl sulfate and recurrent aphthous ulcers. A preliminary study. *Acta Odontol Scand* 1994, 52:257–259.
29. Layton, L. FDA says studies on triclosan, used in sanitizers and soaps, raise concerns. *Washington Post* April 8, 2010.
30. http://www.epa.gov/oppsrrd1/REDs/factsheets/triclosan_fs.htm#summary.
31. Rule, K. L., Ebbett, V. R., and Vikesland, P. J. Formation of chloroform and chlorinated organics by free-chlorine-mediated oxidation of triclosan. *Environ Sci Technol* 2005, 39(9):3176–3185.
32. Offenbacher, S., Jared, H. L., O'Reilly, P. G., Wells, S. R., Salvi, G. E., Lawrence, H. P., Socransky, S. S. and Beck, J. D. Potential pathogenic mechanisms of periodontitis associated pregnancy complications. *Ann Periodontol* 1998, 3:233–250.
33. Rubén, L., et al. Detection of orphyromonas gingivalis in the amniotic fluid in pregnant women with a diagnosis of threatened premature labor. *Journal of Periodontology* 2007, 78:7.
34. Offenbacher, S., Beck, J. D., Lieff, S. and Slade, G. Role of periodontitis in systemic health: Spontaneous preterm birth. *J Dent Educ* 1998, 62: 852–858.
35. Nicolson, G. Chronic bacterial and viral infections in neurodegenerative and neurobehavioral diseases. *LABMEDICINE* 2008, 39(5):291–299.
36. Ramfjord, S. P., Knowles, J. W., and Nissle, R. R. Longitudinal study of periodontal therapy. *J Periodontol* 1973, 44:66.
37. Biocompatible Perio. www.iaomt.org/articles/files/files188/biocompatible%20perio.pdf.

Section II

Cardiovascular, Hematologic, and Pulmonary Conditions

4 Dyslipidemia

How Diet, Food, and Nutrients Augment Treatment

Mark Houston, M.D., M.S., and Ruth DeBusk, Ph.D., R.D.

INTRODUCTION

The combination of a lipid lowering diet and scientifically proven nutraceutical supplements has the ability to significantly reduce low-density lipoprotein (LDL) cholesterol, increase LDL particle size, decrease LDL particle number, lower triglycerides (TG) and very low-density lipoprotein (VLDL), and increase total and type 2b high-density lipoprotein (HDL). In addition, inflammation, oxidative stress, and immune responses are decreased. In several prospective clinical trials, coronary heart disease (CHD) and cardiovascular disease (CVD) have been reduced with many of the nutraceutical supplements. This chapter uses food and nutrients to address the multitude of steps involved in lipid-induced vascular damage.

PATHOPHYSIOLOGY

Dyslipidemia is considered one of the top five risk factors for cardiovascular disease along with hypertension, diabetes mellitus (DM), smoking, and obesity [1]. The mechanisms by which certain lipids induce vascular damage are complex, but from a pathophysiologic and functional medicine viewpoint, these include inflammation, oxidative stress, and autoimmune dysfunction [2,3,4]. These pathophysiologic mechanisms lead to endothelial dysfunction and vascular smooth muscle dysfunction. The vascular consequences are CVD, coronary heart disease, myocardial infarction (MI), and cerebrovascular accidents (CVA) [4].

Genetics, poor nutrition, visceral obesity, some pharmacological agents such as select beta blockers and diuretics, tobacco products, DM, and lack of exercise contribute to dyslipidemia [5]. For example, several genetic phenotypes, such as apolipoprotein E (APO E), result in variable serum lipid responses to diet, as well as CHD and MI risk [6,7]. In addition, HDL proteomics such as paroxonase-1 (PON1) and scavenger receptor B-1 (SR–B1) increase CVD [8] and sortilin I allele variants on chromosome 1p13 increases LDL and CHD risk by 29% [9].

However, recent studies suggest that dietary cholesterol intake will not alter serum cholesterol levels or CHD significantly and that saturated fats have a minimal influence on serum lipids and CHD risk, whereas monounsaturated and polyunsaturated fats have a favorable influence on serum lipids and CHD risk. Increased refined carbohydrate intake may be more important in changing serum lipids and lipid subfractions than saturated fats and cholesterol through the effects on insulin resistance, atherogenic LDL, LDL particle number, VLDL, triglycerides, and total HDL

57

and HDL sub-fractions of cholesterol, and thus contribute more to CHD risk than saturated fats [5,10,11,12,13,14,15,16].

The validity of the diet-heart hypothesis that implies that dietary saturated fats, dietary cholesterol, and eggs increase the risk of CHD has been questioned [11,12,13]. Trans-fatty acids have definite adverse lipid effects and increase CVD and CHD risk but omega-3 fatty acids and mono-unsaturated fats improve serum lipids and reduce CVD risk [5,10,12,14,15,16]. Trans fats suppress TGF-B responsiveness, which increases the deposition of cholesterol into cellular plasma membranes in vascular tissue [15].

Expanded lipid profiles that measure lipids, lipid sub-fractions, particle size and number, and apolipoprotein B (APO B) are preferred to standard obsolete lipid profiles that measure only the total cholesterol, LDL, TG, or HDL. Expanded lipid profiles include: lipoprotein particles (Spectracell Labs), nuclear magnetic resonance testing (Liposcience), Berkley Heart Labs test (Berkley Heart Labs), and vertical auto profile (Atherotec). Each has been shown to improve CHD risk profiling and more readily reflect the serum lipid changes that occur with exercise, nutrition, and weight loss or gain, lifestyle changes, use of nutritional supplements, and initiation of pharmacotherapy [17,18]. Proper diagnosis, CHD risk assessment, and evaluation of nondrug or drug treatment is more accurate using the new expanded lipid profiles [17,18]. New concepts in dysfunctional or inflammatory HDL [19] and ability to evaluate it directly or indirectly measuring reverse cholesterol transport [20] or myeloperoxidase (MPO) [21] will allow even better assessment of serum lipids, CHD risk, and treatment.

An understanding of the pathophysiological steps in dyslipidemia-induced vascular damage is mandatory to properly treat this disease in a more logical and advanced manner. Table 4.1 displays nutrients for the treatment of dyslipidemia-induced vascular disease, organized by mechanism of action in descending order of research supporting each mechanism. The ability to interrupt all of the various steps in this pathway will allow more specific functional and metabolic medicine treatments to reduce vascular injury, improve vascular repair systems, and maintain or restore vascular health. Native LDL, especially large type A LDL, is not usually atherogenic until modified. However, there may exist an alternate pinocytosis mechanism that allows macrophage ingestion of native LDL and accounts for up to 30% of the foam cell formation in the subendothelium [22,23]. For example, decreasing LDL modification, the atherogenic form of LDL cholesterol—through decreases in oxidized (oxLDL), glycated (glyLDL), glyco-oxidized LDL (gly-oxLDL), and acetylated LDL (acLDL)—decreasing the uptake of modified LDL into macrophages by the scavenger receptors (CD 36 SR), and decreasing the inflammatory, oxidative stress, and autoimmune responses will reduce vascular damage beyond just treating the LDL cholesterol level [24–30]. There are at least 38 potential mechanisms that can be treated in the pathways that involve dyslipidemia-induced vascular damage and disease. Reductions in high-sensitivity C-reactive protein (HS-CRP), an inflammatory marker, lead to fewer vascular events independent of reductions in LDL cholesterol [29].

TREATMENT

Overview

Many patients cannot or will not use pharmacologic treatments such as statins, fibrates, bile acid resin binders, or ezetimibe to treat dyslipidemia [5]. Statin-induced or fibrate-induced muscle disease, abnormal liver function tests, neuropathy, memory loss, mental status changes, gastrointestinal disturbances, glucose intolerance, or diabetes mellitus are some of the medical contraindications [31–34]. With prolonged or high-dose usage of statin medications, patients may experience other clinical symptoms or lab abnormalities such as chronic fatigue, exercise-induced fatigue, myalgias, muscle weakness, memory loss, loss of lean muscle mass, reduced exercise tolerance, and reductions in coenzyme Q10, carnitine, vitamin E, Vitamin D, omega-3 fatty acids, selenium, and free T3 levels [5,31,35–42].

TABLE 4.1
Nutrients for the Treatment of Dyslipidemia-Induced Vascular Disease

Mechanism	Food or Nutrient Therapy (Alphabetically by Mechanism)
Inhibit LDL Oxidation	Citrus Bergamot
	Curcumin
	Epigallocatechin Gallate
	Garlic
	Glutathione
	Lycopene
	Monounsaturated Fatty Acids
	Niacin
	Oleic Acid
	Pantethine
	Polyphenols
	Pomegranate
	Resevertrol
	Sesame
	Tocotrienols (γ and δ)
Inhibit LDL Glycation	Carnosine
	Histidine
	Kaempferol
	Morin
	Myricetin
	Organosulfur Compounds Pomegranate
	Rutin
Reduce LDL	Citrus Bergamot
	Curcumin
	Epigallocatechin Gallate
	Flax Seed
	Garlic
	Monounsaturated Fatty Acids
	Niacin
	Omega-3 Fatty Acids
	Orange Juice
	Pantethine
	Plant Sterols
	Red Yeast Rice
	Resveratrol
	Sesame
	Soluble Fiber
	Tocotrienols
Convert Dense LDL B to Large LDL A	Niacin
	Omega-3 Fatty Acids
	Plant Sterols
Reduce Intestinal Cholesterol Absorption	Epigallocatechin Gallate
	Fiber
	Flax Seeds
	Garlic
	Plant Sterols
	Sesame
	Soy

continued

TABLE 4.1 (*continued*)

Nutrients for the Treatment of Dyslipidemia-Induced Vascular Disease

Mechanism	Food or Nutrient Therapy (Alphabetically by Mechanism)
Inhibit HMG CoA Reductase	Citrus Bergamot
	Curcumin
	Epigallocatechin Gallate
	Gamma-Linolenic Acid
	Garlic
	Omega-3 Fatty Acids
	Pantethine
	Plant Sterols
	Red Yeast Rice
	Sesame
	Tocotrienols (γ)
Reduce Lipoprotein (a)	Coenzyme Q10
	Flax Seed
	L-Arginine
	L-Carnitine
	L-Lysine
	N-Acetyl Cysteine
	Niacin
	Omega-3 Fatty acids
	Tocotrienols (γ and δ)
	Vitamin C
Reduce Triglycerides	Citrus Bergamot
	Flax Seed
	Krill Oil
	Monounsaturated Fatty Acids
	Niacin
	Omega-3 Fatty Acids
	Orange Juice
	Pantethine
	Red Yeast Rice
	Resveratrol
Increase Total HDL and HDL 2b Levels and Convert HDL 3 to HDL 2 and 2b	Citrus Bergamot
	Curcumin
	Krill Oil
	Monounsaturated Fatty Acids
	Niacin
	Omega-3 Fatty Acids
	Orange Juice
	Pantethine
	Pomegranate
	Red Yeast Rice
	Resveratrol
Alter Scavenger Receptor NADPH Oxidase and oxLDL Uptake into Macrophages	N-Acetyl Cysteine
	Resveratrol
Increase Reverse Cholesterol Transport	Glutathione
	Lycopene

TABLE 4.1 *(continued)*

Nutrients for the Treatment of Dyslipidemia-Induced Vascular Disease

Mechanism	Food or Nutrient Therapy (Alphabetically by Mechanism)
	Plant Sterols
Decrease LDL Particle	Niacin
Number	Omega-3 Fatty Acids
Reduce Inflammation	Flax Seed
	Glutathione
	Monounsaturated Fatty Acids
	Niacin
	Omega-3 Fatty Acids
	Plant Sterols
	Resveratrol
Lower Apolipoprotein B	Epigallocatechin Gallate
	Niacin
	Omega-3 Fatty Acids
	Plant Sterols
Increase Apolipoprotein A-1	Niacin
Decrease LDL Particle	Niacin
Number	Omega-3 Fatty Acids
Upregulate the LDL Receptor	Curcumin
	Epigallocatechin Gallate
	Plant Sterols
	Sesame
	Tocotrienols (γ and δ)
Increase PON1 and PON2	Epigallocatechin Gallate
	Glutathione
	Quercetin
	Pomegranate
	Resveratrol
Increase Bile Acid Excretion	Citrus Bergamot
	Fiber
	Probiotics
	Plant Sterols
	Resveratrol
	Sesame

HDL = High-Density Lipoprotein; LDL = Low-Density Lipoprotein;
NADPH = Nicotinamide Adenine Dinucleotide PHosphate;
PON = ParaxONase

New treatment approaches that combine weight loss, reduction in visceral and total body fat, increases in lean muscle mass, optimal aerobic and resistance exercise, scientifically proven nutrition, and use of nutraceutical supplements offer not only improvement in serum lipids but also reductions in inflammation, oxidative stress, immune dysfunction, and endothelial and vascular smooth muscle dysfunction. In addition, surrogate markers for vascular disease or clinical vascular target organ damage such as CHD are reduced in many clinical trials [5]. This chapter will review diet and nutraceutical supplements in the treatment of dyslipidemia. The reader is referred to an extensive body of literature on the role of exercise, weight loss, and other lifestyle treatments for dyslipidemia.

DIET

Diet therapy has long been recognized as an important modality for managing and preventing dyslipidemia and other risk factors for cardiovascular disease (reviewed by Van Horn et al., 2008) [43]. Studies such as the Framingham Heart Study and Seven Countries Study were instrumental in establishing the link between the dietary habits of Western civilizations and their association with cardiovascular disease [44–46]. These landmark studies laid the groundwork for experimental and intervention studies that focused on dietary approaches that could minimize cardiovascular risk, with particular emphasis on dietary fat and dyslipidemia.

The Framingham Heart Study formally began in 1950 with an initial cohort of 5209 healthy residents of Framingham, Massachusetts, aged 30–60 years. In 1971, a second cohort of 5124 offspring of the original cohort was added and formed the Framingham Offspring Study. More recently, 500 minorities have been recruited for the OmniHeart Trial, a third cohort of the Framingham study [47].

The Seven Countries Study was also a large prospective study but focused on investigating the diet and lifestyle habits of over 12,000 middle-aged men in four regions of the world: Asia, northern Europe, southern Europe, and North America. The countries participating were Finland, Greece, Italy, Japan, the Netherlands, Yugoslavia (Croatia, Serbia), and the United States. Among the primary diet/lifestyle-cardiovascular associations identified were the link between a high-fat diet and increased prevalence of cardiovascular disease and the finding that subjects in the United States and northern Europe had a much higher prevalence than those in southern Europe.

The Framingham and Seven Countries studies detected important associations between elevated serum levels of low-density lipoprotein-cholesterol (LDL-C) and total cholesterol with increased risk of cardiovascular disease, between elevated levels of high-density lipoprotein-cholesterol (HDL-C) and decreased risk of cardiovascular disease, and the association of diet and other lifestyle choices with cardiovascular risk, particularly dietary fat consumption. These studies laid the groundwork for subsequent intervention studies that sought to devise dietary approaches that would minimize the risk of developing cardiovascular disease.

Pritikin Principle Diet

Pritikin and colleagues were among the first to investigate whether adjusting the dietary fat content of the diet could improve cardiovascular health outcomes. The Pritikin Principle Diet was a low-fat diet based primarily on vegetables, grains, and fruits, with total fat supplying 10% of energy needs [48,49]. The outcomes from a small intervention study of this diet coupled with regular exercise undertaken with participants with type-2 diabetes suggested that this approach would be beneficial for improving dyslipidemia, specifically hypercholesterolemia [50].

Intensive Diet-and-Lifestyle Intervention

Ornish et al. [51] developed an intensive therapeutic approach that combined diet, exercise, and other lifestyle changes. This approach was initially tested in the Lifestyle Heart Trial, a randomized controlled trial that had as its one-year and five-year endpoints low-density lipoprotein-cholesterol (LDL-C) level, number of anginal episodes, and regression of coronary stenosis [52,53]. The low-fat, whole foods vegetarian diet contained 10% of total energy as fat, 10 mg of cholesterol per day, complex carbohydrates, and minimal simple sugars. Lifestyle modifications included moderate aerobic exercise, stress reduction, smoking cessation, and group psychosocial support. Compared with the control group that did not make intensive diet-and-lifestyle changes, the experimental group had statistically significant changes in LDL-C reduction, decreased frequency of angina episodes, and regression in coronary artery stenosis at years one and five. In contrast, the control group had minimal reduction in LDL-C, significant increase in frequency of angina episodes, and an increase in coronary artery stenosis. In spite of the small study population, these differences in the intensive lifestyle group were statistically significant after one year and five years, and the Ornish work was an important landmark in the use of diet therapy in the management and prevention of cardiovascular disease. The group has continued its exploration of the efficacy of an intensive diet-and-lifestyle intervention for minimizing the risk of developing cardiovascular disease as well as reversing existing disease [54].

Therapeutic Lifestyle Changes Diet

On behalf of the National Heart, Lung, and Blood Institute (NHLBI, U.S. National Institutes of Health), the Adult Treatment Panel III of the National Cholesterol Education Program recommends a therapeutic lifestyle changes (TLC) diet that reduces dietary saturated fat (SFA) to < 7% of total energy and dietary cholesterol to < 200 mg/day [55,56] The TLC diet also contains 10–25 g/day of viscous fiber and 2 g/day of plant sterols/stanols. In a small study of 36 moderately hypercholesterolemic subjects, a randomized crossover design was used to compare the TLC diet (28% total fat, < 7% SFA, 66 mg cholesterol/1000 kcal) with a Western diet (38% total fat, 15% SFA, 164 mg cholesterol/1000 kcal). Participants consumed each diet for 32 days. Compared to the Western diet, the TLC diet significantly reduced plasma LDL-C by 11% and HDL-C levels by 7%, with no significant effect on triglyceride or total cholesterol HDL-C levels [57].

A more recent NHLBI-sponsored study has been interpreted by many to suggest that a low-fat diet may not improve cardiovascular risk. The Women's Health Initiative (WHI) study of 48,835 postmenopausal women included the dietary modification trial, a multi-center randomized clinical trial. This trial was designed to evaluate the effect of a diet low in fat (20% of total calories), high in fruits and vegetables (five or more servings/day), and high in grains (six or more servings/day) on cardiovascular risk. Participants in the control group followed their usual diet. At the end of the 15-year study, neither a significant reduction in cardiovascular risk nor improvement in lipid profile was observed [58]. However, limitations in diet compliance and study design may have influenced the outcomes and precluded an appropriate testing of whether dietary fat modification could reduce cardiovascular risk and improve lipid profiles. The participants did not achieve the low-fat target of 20% total fat; average fat consumption was 23% at year one and 29% at year 15. Further, the diet focused on reducing total fat rather than modifying the types of fats consumed. Researchers are now addressing the benefits of reduced saturated and trans fats and increased levels of monounsaturated fat (MUFA) and polyunsaturated fat (PUFA).

OmniHeart Trial

The Optimal Macronutrient Intake for Heart Health Trial (OmniHeart Trial) investigated the effect of a Mediterranean-style diet on plasma lipids and blood pressure [47]. In this randomized controlled intervention trial of generally healthy adults, a crossover study design was used to test the effects of three diets: a carbohydrate-rich diet, a protein-rich diet, and a diet rich in monounsaturated fat (similar to the TLC diet). Among the significant outcomes were the findings that the monounsaturated fat-rich diet did not influence LDL-cholesterol levels but raised HDL-C levels, the protein-rich diet decreased LDL-C and HDL-C, and all three diets lowered triglycerides.

Portfolio Diet

Jenkins and colleagues have developed the Portfolio Diet for its ability to improve dyslipidemia compared with a low-saturated fat diet [59–60]. This diet is a vegetarian version of the low-fat TLC diet, with the addition of soluble fiber, nuts, soy protein, and plant sterols, all of which had been shown individually to lower plasma LDL-C [61]. In a randomized controlled feeding trial, 13 hyperlipidemic adults followed the Portfolio Diet and 12 followed the TLC control diet [59]. After four weeks, participants on the Portfolio Diet experienced an average 35.0% reduction in LDL-C compared with 12.1% on the control diet. Also in a four-week study, the Portfolio Diet reduced LDL-C at a level comparable to that achieved with statin medication [62]. In a subsequent study in which 66 hyperlipidemic adults followed the Portfolio Diet for one year, 31 participants had reductions in LDL-C > 20% [60]. LDL-C levels were inversely correlated with dietary adherence.

Increasing the monounsaturated fat content further enhanced the Portfolio Diet benefits for dys-lipidemia by raising HDL-C levels without altering the diet's ability to reduce LDL-C [63]. No effect on triglycerides was seen. In the largest randomized controlled trial of the Portfolio Diet to date, LDL-C levels in those following this diet were significantly lower than in those following a low-saturated fat diet [64].

Mediterranean Diet

The finding in the Seven Countries Study of a lower prevalence of cardiovascular disease in south-ern Europe suggested that the diet common to this Mediterranean region might be an impor-tant contributor to the observed outcomes. The diet of this region is typically referred to as a Mediterranean-style diet because the multiple countries that make up the geographical region bor-dering the Mediterranean Sea have diverse cultural, religious, economic, and agricultural practices [65]. In general, this dietary pattern is characterized by a high intake of vegetables and fruits, bread and other cereal grains, potatoes, legumes, nuts, and seeds. Monounsaturated fat is the primary fat consumed and is typically 15–20% of total calories, with olive oil being the most common source. Animal products (meat, poultry, fish, dairy, eggs) are included in the diet at a low-to-moderate level. Red wine is also frequently consumed in moderation. There have been several trials of a Mediterranean-style diet for lowering cardiovascular risk.

Lyon Diet Heart Study

The Lyon Diet Heart Study was the first intervention trial to investigate the effect of a Mediterranean-style diet on cardiovascular disease (CVD) risk. This randomized, single-blind, secondary preven-tion trial was conducted in the Lyon region of France and included more than 600 participants with a prior initial myocardial infarction (MI) [66–68]. The primary outcome measurement (fatal or nonfatal MI) was significantly reduced over the four-year study period. The Lyon Diet Heart Study contributed significantly to demonstrating that diet modification could improve CVD risk even fol-lowing an initial MI. Because it introduced sufficient changes to the usual Mediterranean-style diet consumed in southern Europe, it is not generally considered to be an appropriate test of the efficacy of that diet on CVD risk parameters. For example, the total fat in the experimental diet was 30.5%, with 12.5% as MUFA rather than the more typical 15–20% MUFA content of this diet as consumed in southern Europe. Further, the diet was enriched in alpha-linolenic acid, an omega-3 polyunsatu-rated fat, rather than the usual MUFA olive oil.

Indian Heart Study

In a case-control study of ischemic heart disease patients in India, the Indian Heart Study also used a Mediterranean-style diet that was enriched in alpha-linolenic acid for the experimental group [69]. The control group was advised on smoking cessation, stress management, and regular exercise and on reducing intake of dietary fat and alcohol. Compared to the control group at the one-year follow-up, the experimental group had a 38% reduction in nonfatal MI and a 32% reduction in fatal MI.

Prevención con Dieta Mediterránea (PREDIMED) Study

Additional studies in Europe and the United States found associations between a Mediterranean-style diet and a reduction in cardiovascular risk. However, none compared a Mediterranean-style diet with the standard low-fat TLC diet using a randomized controlled trial for primary prevention of cardiovascular disease. Further, several of the studies introduced modifications to the Mediterranean diet that were distinct from the diet typically consumed in southern Europe. In 2003, PREDIMED randomized cross-sectional study was initiated with the goal of addressing these limitations [70]. A cohort of 772 asymptomatic Spanish adults at high risk for cardiovascular disease participated in a three-month trial on one of three diets. The control group was instructed in the use of the TLC diet. The two experimental arms of the study used Mediterranean-style diets that differed only in their primary fat source: extra virgin olive oil (EVOO) or mixed nuts, both of which were supplied to participants. Compared with the low-fat control diet, lipid parameters improved with both the Mediterranean/EVOO and the Mediterranean/nuts diets. The most noteworthy improvement was in the total cholesterol:HDL-C ratio, with a mean change of –0.38 (95% CI, –0.55 to –0.22) for those on the Mediterranean/EVOO diet and of –0.26 (95% CI, –0.42 to –0.10) for those on the Mediterranean/nuts diet [71].

The PREDIMED study was also helpful in expanding the emphasis of diet associations to include inflammation as a key process underlying CVD risk. Four inflammatory markers were measured: high-sensitivity C-reactive protein (CRP), the proinflammatory cytokine interleukin-6 (IL-6), intracellular adhesion molecule-1 (ICAM-1), and vascular cell adhesion molecule-1 (VCAM-1). In the Estruch report [71], both Mediterranean diets lowered circulating levels of IL-6, ICAM-1, and VCAM-1 compared with the low-fat diet. Only the Mediterranean diet with EVOO reduced CRP levels significantly.

Salas-Salvadó and colleagues [72] further analyzed these data as to food groupings, arranging participants into tertiles of consumption within each food group and as to degree of adherence to a Mediterranean-style diet. Those who adhered more closely to the Mediterranean diets had lower but nonsignificant serum levels of the various inflammatory marker levels. When individual components of the diet were examined, all four markers were reduced. Those in the highest tertile for consumption of cereals and fruits had the lowest concentrations of IL-6. Those with a higher consumption of olive oil and nuts had lower CRP, IL-6, ICAM-1, and VCAM-1 levels. A higher intake of dairy products was associated with lower circulating levels of CRP and ICAM-1. However, statistical significance was attained only for VCAM-1 among participants with the highest consumption of EVOO and for ICAM-1 among those with the highest consumption of nuts.

Although the Mediterranean-style diet appears to be beneficial for managing and preventing dyslipidemia, many questions remain. One category of questions pertains to the macronutrient composition of the diet. In a diet modified for fat content, which macronutrient (or combination of macronutrients) should replace saturated and trans fats? Is it the amount of a macronutrient that influences the lipid profile, the type of dietary fat, or both? When protein replaces some or all of the saturated and trans fats, should only plant protein be used or is lean animal protein appropriate? Is there a different influence on the lipid profile between these two categories of lean protein? Why does increasing carbohydrate content reduce heart-protective HDL-C levels? Is the quality of the carbohydrate component (i.e., the glycemic load of the diet) important? Why is modification of the dietary carbohydrate component, rather than the dietary fat component, more effective for lowering elevated triglyceride levels? What is the balance among the amount and composition of the macronutrients that prevents dyslipidemia? Limited understanding of these important considerations hampers development of effective therapeutic diets for dyslipidemia.

Along this line of questioning, is it specific food components of a Mediterranean-style diet that influences the lipid profile or might it be the combination of whole foods that are beneficial to cardiovascular health? Further, might it be the diet within the context of the lifestyle that characterizes the approach to eating in this geographic region?

Dietary Approaches in the Genomics Era

Another category of questions relating to the use of a Mediterranean-style diet for reducing the risk for CVD in general and dyslipidemia in particular pertains to the genetic makeup (genotype) of the populations studied. Specifically, given the genetic heterogeneity among human populations, is it logical to anticipate that a diet that benefits the populations in the Mediterranean region is appropriate for Asian populations or African populations? In determining the suitability of a Mediterranean-style diet to be extrapolated to human beings in general, it is essential to know whether this approach is effective in other ethnic populations or might the genetic makeup of the Mediterranean population be particularly well adapted to this diet pattern?

This line of questioning hints at much broader issues that beg to be considered. An organism's functional capacity is directly tied to interactions between environmental factors and the organism's genomic and epigenomic makeup. How much of the inconsistencies that have been reported from otherwise well-designed and controlled studies are due to failure to stratify study populations by genotype? Are there significant outcomes within subpopulations that are hidden when the data are analyzed as if the participants belonged to a single, genetically homogeneous population? Further, chronic diseases such as dyslipidemia seldom result from alteration in a single gene. Instead, multiple genes are typically involved in the development of complex conditions. Further, it appears that the majority of these genes provide a susceptibility to disease but their influence is not sufficient to manifest the disease state. Instead, such genes require interaction with one or more environmental factors that in turn trigger cascading events that culminate in the development of the disease state. Studies are demonstrating that altering the environmental influence, such as changing specific characteristics of the diet, can affect gene expression and, thereby, functional outcomes. Key studies follow.

The FUNGENUT Study

Kallio and coworkers [73] were among the first to show that modifying the diet can influence both phenotypic outcomes and gene expression. A subset of 47 Finnish subjects with metabolic syndrome who participated in the Functional Genomics and Nutrition (FUNGENUT) Study were randomly assigned to one of two diets for 12 weeks. The diets differed in their carbohydrate composition: a low glycemic load rye-pasta diet that promoted a low postprandial insulin response and a high glycemic load oat-wheat-potato diet that promoted a high postprandial insulin response.

The metabolic syndrome is typically accompanied by abdominal obesity and insulin resistance. Using microarray technology to monitor gene expression, the researchers investigated whether diet influenced gene expression in subcutaneous adipose tissue (SAT). In the low glycemic load rye-pasta group, 71 genes were down-regulated (decreased in their expression), including genes involved in insulin signaling and apoptosis. In the high glycemic load oat-wheat-potato diet group, 62 genes were up-regulated and were related to oxidative stress and inflammation, including increased production of interleukin cytokines. Further, the insulinogenic index had improved by 12 weeks in the rye-pasta group but not in the oat-wheat-potato group. This measurement is informative because early insulin response is important to insulin appropriate glucose disposal. Deterioration of this early response typically accompanies the progression from insulin sensitivity to insulin resistance. In both groups, these changes occurred in the absence of changes in body weight.

The GEMINAL Study

In the Gene Expression Modulation by Intervention with Nutrition and Lifestyle (GEMINAL) pilot study, Ornish and coworkers [74] reported that gene expression in 30 men with low-risk prostate cancer could be modified by a three-month intensive diet-and-lifestyle intervention. The intervention consisted of a low-fat, whole-foods, plant-based diet; moderate exercise; stress management; and psychosocial group support. Microarray analysis of gene expression in prostate biopsies taken before and after the intervention detected 453 down-regulated genes, which were associated with tumorigenesis, as a result of the intensive diet-lifestyle intervention.

Mediterranean Diet and Gene Expression

In a cohort from the PREDIMED study, Llorente-Cortés et al. [75] studied the effect of three diet modifications on gene expression. The control diet was a low-fat TLC diet; the experimental diets were a Mediterranean-style diet enhanced with either extra-virgin olive oil (EVOO) or mixed nuts. The genes selected were involved in inflammation, foam cell formation, or thrombosis. Using microarray analysis, at the three-month point the researchers found that the Mediterranean-style diets, particularly the one enhanced with EVOO, decreased expression of key genes in each of the categories examined.

Also studying a cohort from the PREDIMED study, Razquin and colleagues [76] investigated whether following one of the aforementioned three diets for three years influenced the effects on body weight parameters of a variant of *IL6 (IL6–174G > C* [rs1800795]) that overproduces the proinflammatory cytokine IL-6. The variant is associated with increased body weight and waist circumference, with G being the usual allele and C being the variant allele. This study illustrates the importance of stratifying study populations by genotype. When the results from the total population were analyzed by diet group, the change in weight was greatest in the EVOO group, but not statistically significant in any group. When the population was stratified by genotype (GG + GC vs CC), a clear difference was evident, with the CC group experiencing greater weight loss (without consideration of diet type). Further, it was the contribution of the CC genotype individuals that was responsible for the decreased weight observed with the EVOO diet. Interestingly, these individuals had greater adiposity at baseline and yet lost significantly more weight than those with one or two copies of the G allele (p = 0.002). An additional finding was that, in the CC group, the nut diet actually led to weight gain.

Key Points to Consider

Information that is critical to the design of effective disease management and prevention can be lost if genotype is not factored into study design and, ultimately, into the clinician's thinking when developing the diet intervention. In the aforementioned Razquin study [76], the distinction between genetically different subpopulations would not have been detected had the study participants not been stratified by genotype. In the Razquin study [76], the data would have been interpreted as the EVOO diet being more beneficial for everyone, when in fact it had no effect on weight unless subjects had the CC genotype. Further, it could have been concluded that a Mediterranean-style diet enhanced in nuts was neutral, being neither helpful nor harmful for weight loss. This interpretation is likely to find its way into general recommendations for public health, when in fact for those with the CC genotype this diet appears to cause weight gain. These individuals, by virtue of being homozygous for a key proinflammatory gene variant, are already at increased risk for inflammatory disorders and, thus, chronic disease and should not be advised to follow a dietary intervention that will further exacerbate that risk.

These types of studies that incorporate genomics into their design are significant in that they demonstrate that diet modification influences key mechanisms that underlie cardiovascular disease and other chronic disorders. Further, such appropriately designed studies can provide direction for diet interventions that can be specifically targeted to root causes of cardiovascular risk. The studies highlighted here are examples of the types of studies being conducted now and illustrate the importance of integrating genomics into clinical decision making concerning chronic disease management and prevention. Space precludes our doing justice to the extensive body of work of José Ordovás and colleagues in reference to diet-gene-cardiovascular disease interactions. Instead we direct the reader to the scientific literature for exploration of the many hundreds of publications reporting on specific gene variants and their influence on cardiovascular risk factors.

The Hunter-Gatherer (Paleolithic) Diet

With the growing awareness of the key role of genes and gene expression in influencing the functional abilities of an organism, if one were designing a diet for human beings a logical place to start would be to come as close as possible to the food pattern on which our ancestors evolved. The human genome is thought to have evolved little in the past 40,000–50,000 years [77], yet the food supply in Western countries has changed substantially during that time and bears little resemblance to that on which the human species evolved. The hunter-gatherer diet (also called the Paleolithic diet) is considered to be close to Man's ancestral diet [78,79]. Early information of our ancestral diet dating back to the Miocene and early Pleistocene eras suggests a diet high in foliage, leafy vegetables, fruits, seeds, nuts, plant sterols, vegetable protein, fiber and omega-3 fatty acids [80]. Animal protein was added in the form of lean meat and fish during the Paleolithic period. The agricultural period began during the Neolithic era approximately 10,000 years ago and led to an introduction of starchy grains and legumes and, later, to the introduction of dairy products and vegetable oils. Subsequently, the Industrial Revolution of the twentieth century had a particularly dramatic impact on our ancestral diet. It was during this time that refined grains and convenience foods were introduced, which led to the modern diet of refined carbohydrates, animal products high in saturated fat, refined oils, high-sodium foods, and energy-dense foods. These changes were accompanied by a decrease in vegetables, fruits, nuts and seeds, omega-3-rich foods, dietary fiber, and numerous vitamins and minerals. A number of researchers are beginning to consider the value of the hunter-gatherer diet now that genetic considerations are being integrated into our thinking about the most appropriate diet for the human species and how to modify that core diet for genetically distinct human subpopulations.

SPECIFIC FOODS

Fats

Omega-3 Fatty Acids

Observational, epidemiologic, and controlled clinical trials have shown significant reductions in serum TG, VLDL-decreased LDL particle number, and increased LDL and HDL particle size as well as major reductions in all CVD events [5,81–88]. The DART trial demonstrated a decrease in mortality of 29% in men post MI; and the GISSI prevention trial found a decrease in total mortality of 20%, CV deaths of 30%, and sudden death of 45%. The Kuppio Heart Study demonstrated a 44% reduction in fatal and nonfatal CHD in subjects in the highest quintile of omega-3 intake compared to the lowest quintile [5,81,82]. Omega-3 fatty acids reduce CHD progression, stabilize plaque, reduce coronary artery stent restenosis, and reduce CABG occlusion [5,83]. In the Japan eicosapentaenoic acid (EPA) lipid intervention study (JELIS), the addition of 1.8 grams of omega-3 fatty acids to a statin resulted in an additional 19% relative risk reduction (RRR) in major coronary events and nonfatal MI and a 20% decrease in CVA [5,84].

There is a dose-related reduction in VLDL of up to 50%, TG of up to 50%, with little to no change or decrease in total cholesterol (TC), LDL, and APO B, and no change to a slight increase in HDL [5,85,86,87,88]. However, the number of LDL particles decrease and LDL particle size increases from small type B to large type A (an increase of .25 nm). The anti-atherogenic HDL2b also increases by up to 29%. The rate of entry of VLDL particles into the circulation is decreased and APOCIII is reduced, which allows lipoprotein lipase to be more active. There is a decrease in remnant chylomicrons and remnant lipoproteins [5,86]. Patients with LDL over 100 mg% usually have reductions in total LDL and those that are below 80 mg% have mild increases [87]. However, in both cases the LDL particle number decreases, the dense LDL B increases in size to the less atherogenic LDL A particle and APO B levels decrease. There is a net decrease in the concentration of cholesterol carried by all atherogenic particles and decreases in non-HDL cholesterol. Omega-3 fatty acids are anti-inflammatory and anti-thrombotic, lower blood pressure (BP) and heart rate, and improve heart rate variability [5,81]. There is a decrease in fatty acid synthesis and an increase in fatty acid oxidation with consistent weight loss [5].

Insulin resistance is improved and there are no significant changes in fasting glucose or hemoglobin A1C with long term treatment [89]. Doses of 3 grams per day of combined EPA and DHA at a 3:2 ratio with GLA at 50% of the total EPA and DHA content and 700 mg of gamma, delta, and alpha tocopherol at 80% gamma/delta and 20% alpha tocopherol per 3 grams of DHA and EPA are recommended (5). DHA and EPA may have variable, but favorable, effects on the various lipid levels [5,85,86,89]. The combination of plant sterols and omega-3 fatty acids are synergistic in improving lipids and inflammation [88].

Monounsaturated Fats

Monounsaturated fats (MUFA) such as olives, olive oil, and nuts reduce LDL by 5–10%, lower TG 10–15%, increase HDL 5%, decrease oxLDL, reduce oxidation and inflammation, improve endothelial dysfunction (ED), lower BP, decrease thrombosis, and reduce the incidence of CHD (Mediterranean diet) [5,90–93]. MUFA are among the most potent agents to reduce oxLDL. The equivalent of three to four tablespoons (30–40 grams) per day of extra virgin olive oil in MUFA content is recommended for the maximum effect in conjunction with omega-3 fatty acids. However, the caloric intake of this amount of MUFA must be balanced with the other beneficial effects.

Flax

Flax seeds and flax lignan complex with secoisolariciresinol diglucoside (SDG) and increased intake of ALA from other sources such as walnuts have been shown in several meta-analyses to reduce TC and LDL by 5–15%, Lp(a) by 14%, TG by up to 36%, with either no change or a slight reduction in HDL [5,93–95]. These properties do not apply to flax seed oil. In the Seven Countries Study CHD was reduced with increased consumption of ALA and, in the Lyon diet trial at four years, intake of flax reduced CHD and total deaths by 50–70% [5]. Flax seeds contain fiber and lignans and reduce the levels for 7 alpha hydrolyase and acyl CoA cholesterol transferase [5,93–95]. Flax seeds and ALA are anti-inflammatory, increase eNOS, improve endothelial dysfunction, contain phytoestrogens and decrease vascular smooth muscle hypertrophy, reduce oxidative stress, and retard development of atherosclerosis [5,93–95]. The dose required for these effects is from 14 to 40 grams of flax seed per day [5,93–95].

Garlic

Numerous placebo-controlled clinical trials in humans indicate reductions in TC and LDL of about 9–12% at doses of 600 to 900 mg per day of a standardized extract of allicin and ajoene [5,96]. However, many studies have been poorly controlled and use variable types and doses of garlic, which have given inconsistent results [5,96]. Garlic reduces intestinal cholesterol absorption, inhibits enzymes involved in cholesterol synthesis, and deactivates HMG CoA reductase [5,96]. In addition, garlic lowers BP, has fibrinolytic activity, anti-platelet activity, reduces oxLDL, and decreases coronary artery calcification by EBT [5,96,97].

Green Tea

Catechins, especially epigallocatechin gallate (EGCG) or green tea extract, may improve the lipid profile by interfering with micellar solubilization of cholesterol in the GI tract and reduce absorption [5]. In addition, EGCG reduces the fatty acid gene expression, inhibits HMG CoA reductase, increases mitochondrial energy expenditure, reduces oxLDL, increases PON1, up-regulates the LDL receptor, decreases APO B lipoprotein secretion from cells, mimics the action of insulin, improves endothelial dysfunction, and decreases body fat [5,98,99,100]. A meta-analysis of human studies of 14 trials shows that EGCG at 224–674 mg per day or 60 oz of green tea per day reduced TC 7.2 mg/dL and LDL 2.19 mg/dL (p < 0.001 for both). There was no significant change in HDL or TG levels [101]. The recommended dose is a standardized EGCG extract 500 to 700 mg per day.

Orange Juice

In one human study, 750 ml of concentrated orange juice per day over two months decreased LDL 11% with reductions in APO B and TG, and increased HDL by 21% [102]. The effects are due to polymethoxylated flavones, hesperitin, naringin, pectin, and essential oils [102]. Additional studies are needed to verify this data.

Pomegranate Juice

Pomegranate increases PON1 binding to HDL and increases PON2 in macrophages. It is a potent antioxidant, increases total antioxidant status, lowers oxLDL, decreases antibodies to oxLDL, inhibits platelet function, reduces glycosylated LDL, decreases macrophage LDL uptake, reduces lipid deposition in the arterial wall, decreases progression of carotid artery *intima-media thickness* (IMT), and lowers blood pressure especially in subjects with the highest oxidative stress, known carotid artery plaque, and the greatest abnormalities in TG and HDL levels [103–108]. Consuming about eight ounces of pomegranate juice per day is recommended.

Sesame Seeds

Sesame at 40 grams per day reduces LDL by 9% through inhibition of intestinal absorption, increasing biliary secretion, decreasing HMG CoA reductase activity, up-regulating the LDL receptor gene, up-regulating 7-alpha hydroxylase gene expression, and up-regulating the SREBP 2 genes [109,110]. A randomized placebo-controlled crossover study of 26 postmenopausal women who consumed 50 grams of sesame powder daily for five weeks had a 5% decrease in total cholesterol and a 10% decrease in LDL-C [109].

Soy

Numerous studies have shown mild improvements in serum lipids with soy at doses of about 30–50 grams per day [5,111,112]. Total cholesterol fell 2–9.3%, LDL decreased 4–12.9%, TG fell up to 10.5%, and HDL increased up to 2.4%. However, the studies are conflicting due to differences in the type and dose of soy used in the studies, as well as nonstandardized methodology [5,111,112]. Soy decreases the micellar content and absorption of lipids though a combination of fiber, isoflavones (genistin, glycitin, diadzin), and phytoestrogens [5,111,112]. The most reduction is seen with soy-enriched isoflavones with soy protein. Fermented soy is preferred.

NUTRIENTS AND DIETARY SUPPLEMENTS

Nutraceutical supplement management of dyslipidemia has been infrequently reviewed [5]. New important scientific information and clinical studies are required to understand the present role of these natural agents in the management of dyslipidemia [5,80]. These studies include clinical trials that show excellent reductions in both serum lipids and CHD (niacin, omega-3 fatty acids, red yeast rice, fiber, and alpha-linolenic acid [ALA]), and smaller studies with reductions in surrogate vascular markers with numerous other nutraceutical supplements (carotid intimal medial thickness and obstruction, plaque progression, coronary artery calcium score by electron beam tomography [EBT], generalized atherosclerosis, and endothelial function) [5,80,97,113]. The proposed mechanisms of action of some of the nutraceutical supplements on the mammalian cholesterol pathway are shown in Figure 4.1.

Citrus Bergamot

Citrus bergamot has been evaluated in several clinical prospective trials in humans. In doses of 1000 mg per day this compound lowers LDL up to 36%, TG 39%, increases HDL 40% by inhibiting HMG CoA reductase, increases cholesterol and bile acid excretion, and reduces ROS and oxLDL. The active ingredients include naringin, neroeriocitrin, neohesperidin, poncerin, rutin, neodesmin, rhoifolin, melitidine, and brutelidine [114,115].

Curcumin

Curcumin is a phenolic compound in turmeric and curry [5,116]. It induces changes in the expression of genes involved in cholesterol synthesis such as the LDL receptor mRNA, HMG CoA reductase, SREBP, cholesterol 7 alpha hydrolyze, PPAR, and LXR [5,116]. In one human study of 10 patients

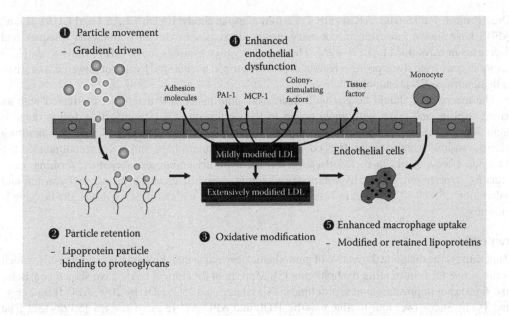

FIGURE 4.1 Proposed mechanisms of actions of nutraceuticals and statins in the cholesterol pathway. Diagrammed here are the various steps in the uptake of LDL cholesterol, modification, macrophage ingestion with scavenger receptors, foam cell formation, oxidative stress, inflammation, autoimmune cytokines, and chemokine production.

consuming 500 mg per day of curcumin, the HDL increased 29% and total cholesterol fell 12% [5,116]. This needs confirmation in larger randomized clinical trials.

Guggulipids (Not Recommended)

Guggulipids (*Commiphora mukul*) are resins from the mukul myrrh tree that contain active lipid-lowering compounds called guggulsterones [5,117–119]. These increase hepatic LDL receptors and bile acid secretion, and decrease cholesterol synthesis in animal experiments [5,117]. However, controlled human clinical trials have not shown these agents to be effective in improving serum lipids [117,118,119]. One study of 103 subjects on 50–75 mg of guggulsterones per day for eight weeks actually had a 5% increase in LDL; no change in TC, TG, or HDL; and insignificant reductions in Lp(a) and HS-CRP [117]. Guggulipids are not recommended at this time.

Lycopene

Lycopene has been shown in tissue culture to inhibit HMG CoA reductase, induce Rho inactivation, increase PPAR gamma and LXR receptor activities, and increase reverse cholesterol transport and efflux with ABCA1 and Caveolin 1 expression [120].

Niacin (Vitamin B3)

Niacin has a dose-related effect (1–4 grams per day) in reducing total cholesterol (TC), low-density lipoprotein (LDL), APO B, LDL particle number and triglycerides (TG) VLDL, increasing LDL size from small type B to large type A, and increasing high-density lipoprotein (HDL), especially the protective and larger HDL 2b particle and apolipoprotein (APO A1) [5]. The changes are dose-related and vary from about 10 to 30 percent for each lipid level as noted here [5,121,122]. Niacin inhibits LDL oxidation, increases TG lipolysis in adipose tissue, increases APO B degradation, reduces the fractional catabolic rate of HDL-APOA-1, inhibits platelet function, induces fibrinolysis, decreases cytokines and cell adhesion molecules (CAMs), lowers Lp(a), increases adiponectin, and is a potent antioxidant [5,121,122]. Randomized controlled clinical trials such as the Coronary

Drug Project, HATS trial, ARBITOR 2, Oxford Niaspan Study, FATS, CLAS I and CLAS II, and AFRS have shown reduction in coronary events, decreases in coronary atheroma (plaque), and decreases in carotid IMT [5,121–126]. The recent negative findings in the AIM HIGH study [127] do not detract from these positive results in previous trials, as this study was not powered to statistically determine CVD endpoints.

The niacin dose should be gradually increased, administered at mealtime, pretreated with an 81-mg aspirin, and taken with apple pectin to reduce flushing [5]. The effective dosing range is from 500 to 4000 mg per day. Only vitamin B3 niacin is effective in dyslipidemia. The nonflush niacin (inositol hexanicotinate, IHN) does not improve lipid profiles, and is not recommended [5]. The side effects of niacin include hyperglycemia, hyperuricemia, gout, hepatitis, flushing, rash, pruritus, hyperpigmentation, hyperhomocysteinemia, gastritis, ulcers, bruising, tachycardia, and palpitations [5,121–122]. If niacin is taken on a regular basis without missing doses, the flushing is minimized.

Pantethine

Pantethine is the disulfide derivative of pantothenic acid and is metabolized to cystamine-SH, which is the active form in treating dyslipidemia [5]. More than 28 clinical trials have shown consistent and significant improvement in serum lipids. TC is decreased 15%, LDL by 20%, APO B by 27.6%, and TG by 36.5% over four to nine months. HDL and APO A1 are increased 8% [5,128–132]. The effects on lipids are slow, with peak effects at four months but may take up to six to nine months. In addition, pantethine reduces lipid peroxidation of LDL, and decreases lipid deposition, intimal thickening, and fatty streak formation in the aorta and coronary arteries [5,128–132]. Pantethine inhibits cholesterol synthesis and accelerates fatty acid metabolism in the mitochondria by inhibiting hepatic acetyl-CoA carboxylase, increases CoA in the cytoplasm, which stimulates the oxidation of acetate at the expense of fatty acid and cholesterol synthesis, and increases the Krebs cycle activity [5,128–132]. In addition, cholesterol esterase activity increases and HMG-CoA reductase activity is decreased. There is 50% inhibition of FA synthesis and 80% inhibition of cholesterol synthesis [5]. The recommended effective dose is 300 mg three times per day or 450 mg twice per day with or without food [5,128–132].

Plant Sterols (Phytosterols)

The plant sterols are naturally occurring sterols of plant origin that include B-sitosterol (the most abundant), campesterol, stigmasterol (4-desmethyl sterols of the cholestane series), and the stanols, which are saturated [5,133–136]. The plant sterols are much better absorbed than the plant stanols. The daily intake of plant sterols in the United States is about 150–400 mg per day mostly from soybean oil, various nuts, and tall pine tree oil [136]. These have a dose dependent reduction in serum lipids [134]. Total cholesterol is decreased 8%, and LDL is decreased 10% (range 6–15%) with no change in TG and HDL on doses of 2 to 3 g/day in divided doses with meals [5,133,134,136]. A recent meta-analysis of 84 trials showed that an average intake of 2.15 g/day reduced LDL by 8.8% with no improvement with higher doses [134].The mechanism of action is primarily to decrease the incorporation of dietary and biliary cholesterol into micelles due to lowered micellar solubility of cholesterol, which reduces cholesterol absorption and increases bile acid secretion. In addition, there is an interaction with enterocyte ATP-binding cassette transport proteins (ABCG 8 and ABCG 5) that directs cholesterol back into the intestinal lumen [5,133]. The only difference between cholesterol and sitosterol consists of an additional ethyl group at position C-24 in sitosterol, which is responsible for its poor absorption. The plant sterols have a higher affinity than cholesterol for the micelles. Patients that have the rare homozygote mutations of the ATP-binding cassette are hyperabsorbers of sitosterol (they absorb 15–60% instead of the normal 5%) and will develop premature atherosclerosis [136]. This is a rare, autosomal recessive disorder termed sitosterolemia. The plant sterols are also anti-inflammatory and decrease the levels of proinflammatory cytokines such as hsCRP, IL-6, IL-1b, TNF alpha, PLA 2, and fibrinogen, but these effects vary among the various phytosterols [135,137]. Other potential mechanisms include modulation of signaling pathways, activation of cellular stress responses, growth arrest, reduction of APO B 48 secretion from intestinal and hepatic cells, reduction of cholesterol synthesis with suppression of HMG CoA reductase and CYP7A1, interference with SREBP, and promotion of reverse cholesterol transport via ABCA 1 and ABCG 1 [137]. The biological activity of phytosterols is both cell-type and sterol specific [137].

The plant sterols can interfere with absorption of lipid-soluble compounds such as fat-soluble vitamins and carotenoids such as vitamin D, E, and K, and alpha carotene [5,136]. Some studies have shown reduction in atherosclerosis progression, reduced carotid IMT, and decreased plaque progression, but the results have been conflicting [5,136]. There are no studies on CHD or other CVD outcomes. The recommended dose is about 2 to 2.5 grams per day (average 2.15 grams per day).

Policosanol (Not Recommended)

Policosanol is a sugarcane extract of eight aliphatic alcohols that has undergone extensive clinical studies with variable results [5]. Most of the earlier studies that showed positive results were performed in Cuba and these have been questioned as to their validity [5,136,138]. The more recent double–blind, placebo-controlled clinical trials have not shown any significant improvement in any measured lipids including TC, LDL, TG, or HDL. Policosanol is not recommended at this time for the treatment of any form of dyslipidemia [5,136,138,139].

Red Yeast Rice

Red yeast rice (RYR), *Monascus purpureus*, is a fermented product of rice that contains monocolins that inhibit cholesterol synthesis via HMG CoA reductase and thus has statin-like properties [5,136,140,141]. RYR also contains sterols, isoflavones, and monounsaturated fatty acids. At 2400 mg per day, LDL is reduced 22% (p < 0.001), TG falls 12% with little change in HDL [5,136,140]. In a recent placebo-controlled Chinese study of 5000 subjects over 4.5 years, an extract of RYR reduced LDL 17.6% (p < 0.001) and increased HDL 4.2% (p < 0.001) [141]. CV mortality fell 30% (p < 0.005) and total mortality fell 33% (p < 0.0003) in the treated subjects. The overall primary endpoint for MI and death was reduced by 45% (p < 0.001). A highly purified and certified RYR must be used to avoid potential renal damage induced by a mycotoxin, citrinin [5,136,141]. The recommended dose is 2400 to 4800 mg of a standardized RYR. No adverse clinical effects have been reported with long-term use. Although reductions in coenzyme Q10 may occur in predisposed patients and those on prolonged high-dose RYR due to its weaker statin-like effect. RYR provides an alternative to patients with statin-induced myopathy [5,136,140–141].

Resveratrol

Resveratrol reduces oxLDL, inhibits ACAT activity and cholesterol ester formation, increases bile acid excretion, reduces TC, TG, and LDL, increases PON1 activity and HDL, inhibits NADPH oxidase in macrophages, and blocks the uptake of modified LDL by CD36 scavenger receptors (SR) [135]. N-acetyl cysteine (NAC) has this same effect on CD 36 DR and should be used in conjunction with resveratrol [135]. The dose of *trans* resveratrol is 250 mg per day and NAC is 1000 mg twice per day.

Tocotrienols

Tocotrienols are a family of unsaturated forms of vitamin E termed alpha, beta, gamma, and delta [5]. The gamma and delta tocotrienols lower TC up to 17%, LDL 24%, APO B 15%, and Lp(a) 17% with minimal changes in HDL or APO A1 in 50% of subjects at doses of 200 mg per day given at night with food [5,142,143]. The gamma/delta form of tocotrienols inhibits cholesterol synthesis by suppression of HMG-CoA reductase activity by two posttranscriptional actions [5,142–144]. These include increased controlled degradation of the reductase protein and decreased efficiency of translation of HMG CoA reductase mRNA. These effects are mediated by sterol binding of the reductase enzyme to the endoplasmic reticulum membrane proteins called INSIGs [143]. The toco-trienols have natural farnesylated analogues of tocopherols that give them their effects on HMG CoA reductase [143]. In addition, the LDL receptor is augmented and they exhibit antioxidant activity.

The tocotrienol dose is very important because increased dosing will induce its own metabolism and reduce effectiveness, whereas lower doses are not as effective [5]. Also, concomitant intake (less than 12 hours) of alpha tocopherol reduces tocotrienol absorption. Increased intake of alpha tocoph-erol over 20% of total tocopherols may interfere with the lipid lowering effect [5,142]. Tocotrienols are metabolized by successive beta oxidation then catalyzed by the CYP P450 enzymes 3A4 and CYP 4F2 [5]. The combination of a statin with gamma/delta tocotrienols further reduces LDL cho-lesterol by 10% [142]. The tocotrienols block the adaptive response of up-regulation of HMG-CoA reductase secondary to competitive inhibition by the statins [5,142]. Carotid artery stenosis regres-sion has been reported in about 30% of subjects given tocotrienols over 18 months. They also slow progression of generalized atherosclerosis [5,144]. The recommended dose is 200 mg of gamma delta tocotrienol at night with food.

Vitamin C

Vitamin C supplementation lowers serum low-density lipoprotein cholesterol and triglycerides [145]. A meta-analysis of 13 randomized controlled trials in subjects given at least 500 mg of vita-min C daily for 3 to 24 weeks found a reduction in LDL cholesterol of 7.9 mg/dL (p < 0.0001) and TG fell 20.1 mg/dL (p < 0.003). HDL did not change. The reductions in LDL and TG were greatest in those with the highest initial lipid levels and the lowest serum vitamin C levels [146].

COMBINATION THERAPIES

A recent prospective, open-label human clinical trial of 30 patients for two months showed signifi-cant improvement in serum lipids using a proprietary product with a combination of pantethine, plant sterols, EGCG, and gamma/delta tocotrienols [147]. The TC fell 14%, LDL decreased 14%, VLDL dropped 20%, and small dense LDL particles fell 25% (type III and IV) [147]. In another study using the same proprietary product with RYR 2400–4800 mg per day and niacin 500 mg per day, the TC fell 34%, LDL decreased by 34%, LDL particle number fell 35%, VLDL dropped 27%, and HDL increased 10% [148]. Studies indicate a relative risk reduction of CVD mortality with omega-3 fatty acids of 0.68, with resins of 0.70 and with statins of 0.78 [149]. Combining statins with omega-3 fatty acids further decreases CHD by 19% [84]. The combination of gamma/delta tocotri-enols with a statin reduces LDL cholesterol an additional 10% [142]. Plant sterols with omega-3 fatty acids have synergistic lipid-lowering and anti-inflammatory effects [88]. Future studies are needed to evaluate various other combinations on serum lipids, surrogate vascular endpoints, and CHD and CVD morbidity and mortality.

SUMMARY AND CONCLUSIONS

The combination of a lipid-lowering diet and select food and nutrients has the ability to reduce LDL-C by up to 50%, increase LDL particle size, decrease LDL particle number, lower TG and VLDL, and increase total and type 2b HDL. In addition, inflammation, oxidative stress, and immune responses are decreased, and vascular target organ damage, atherosclerosis, and CVD are reduced. In several prospective clinical trials, CHD and CVD have been reduced with many of the interventions discussed in this chapter and summarized in Table 4.2. Our approach broadens treatment options by levering the effects of diet, food, and nutrients on the underlying, complex pathophysiology of lipid-induced vascular damage.

TABLE 4.2

Recommended Doses of Nutraceutical Supplements for Treatment of Dyslipidemia

Food or Nutrient (Alphabetical Listing)	Daily Recommended Dose
Citrus Bergamot	1000 mg
Curcumin	2000 mg in divided doses
Epigallocatechin Gallate	500–700 mg
Flax Seed	40 g
Monounsaturated Fats	20–40 g
N-Acetyl Cysteine	2000 mg in divided doses
Niacin (Vitamin B3)	500–4000 mg in divided doses
Omega-3 Fatty Acids	3000–5000 mg
Pantethine	900 mg in divided doses
Phytosterols	2.15 g
Pomegranate Juice	8 oz
Resveratrol (Trans Form)	250 mg
Sesame Seeds	40 g
Soy (Fermented)	30–50 g
Tocotrienols (γ and δ)	200 mg
Vitamin C	500 mg

REFERENCES

1. Kannel WB, Castelli WD, Gordon T., et al. Serum cholesterol, lipoproteins and risk of coronary artery disease. The Framingham Study. *Ann Intern Med* 1971; 74: 1–12.
2. Houston MC. Nutrition and nutraceutical supplements in the treatment of hypertension. *Expert Rev Cardiovasc Ther*. 2010; 8: 821–33.
3. Tian N, Penman AD, Mawson AR, Manning RD, Jr., and Flessner MF. Association between circulating specific leukocyte types and blood pressure: The atherosclerosis risk in communities (ARIC) study. *J Am Soc Hypertension* 2010; 4(6): 272–83.
4. Ungvari Z, Kaley G, de Cabo R, Sonntag WE, and Csiszar A. Mechanisms of vascular aging: New perspectives. *J Gerontol A Biol Sci Med Sci* 2010; 65(10): 1028–41.
5. Houston MC, Fazio S, Chilton FH, Wise DE, Jones KB, Barringer TA, and Bramlet DA. Non pharmacologic treatment of dyslipidemia. *Prog Cardiovasc Dis* 2009; 52: 61–94.
6. Plourde M, Vohl MC, Vandal M, Couture P, Lemieux S, and Cunnane SC. Plasma n-3 fatty acid supplement is modulated by apoE epsilon 4 but not by the common PPAR-alpha L162 polymorphism in men. *Br. J Nutr* 2009; 102: 1121–4.
7. Neiminen T, Kahonen M, Viiri LE, Gronroos P, and Lehtimaki T. Pharmacogenetics of apolipoprotein E gene during lipid-lowering therapy: Lipid levels and prevention of coronary heart disease. *Pharmacogenomics* 2008; 9(10): 1475–86.
8. Shih DM and Lusis AJ. The roles of PON1 and PON2 in cardiovascular disease and innate immunity. *Curr Opin Lipidol* 2009; 20(4): 288–92.
9. Calkin AC and Tontonoz P. Genome-wide association studies identify new targets in cardiovascular disease. *Sci Transl Med* 2010; 2(48): 48.
10. Djousse L and Caziano JM. Dietary cholesterol and coronary artery disease: A systematic review. *Curr Atheroscler Rep* 2009; 11(6): 418–22.
11. Werko L. End of the road for the diet-heart theory? *Scand Cardiovasc J* 2008; 42(4): 250–55.
12. Erkkila A, de Mello VD, Riserus U, and Laaksonen DE. Dietary fatty acids and cardiovascular disease: An epidemiological approach. *Prog Lipid Res* 2008; 47(3):172–87.
13. Weinberg SL. The diet-heart hypothesis: A critique. *J Am Coll Cardiol* 2004; 43(5):731–33.
14. Mozaffarian D and Willet WC. Trans fatty acids and cardiovascular risk: A unique cardiometabolic imprint. *Curr Atheroscler Rep* 2007; 9(6): 486–93.

15. Chen CL, Tetri LH, Neuschwander-Tetri BA, Huang SS, and Huang JS. A mechanism by which dietary trans fats cause atherosclerosis. *J of Nutrition Biochemistry* 2011; 22: 649–55.

16. Siri-Tarino PW, Sun Q, Hu FB and Krauss RM. Saturated fat, carbohydrate and cardiovascular disease. *Am J Clin Nutr.* 2010; 91(3): 502–9.

17. Otvos JD, Mora S, Shalaurova I, Greenland P, Mackey RH, and Goff DC Jr. *J Clin Lipidol* 2011; 5(2): 105–13.

18. Hodge AM, Jenkins AJ, English DR, O'Dea K, and Giles GG. NMR Determined lipoprotein subclass profile is associated with dietary composition and body size. *Nutr Metab Cardiovasc Dis* 2011; 21(8): 603–09.

19. Asztalos BF, Tani M, and Schaefer E. Metabolic and functional of HDL subspecies. *Curr Opin Lipidol* 2011; 22: 176–85.

20. Khera AV, Cuchel M, de la Llera-Moya M, Rodriguez A, Burke MF, Jafri K, French BC, et al. Cholesterol efflux capacity, high-density lipoprotein function, and atherosclerosis. *N Engl J Med* 2011; 64: 127–35.

21. Karakas M, Koenig W, Zierer A, Herder C, Rottbauer W, Meisinger C, and Thorand B. Myeloperoxidase is associated with incident coronary heart disease independently of traditional risk factors: Results form the MONICA/KORA Augsburg study. *J Intern Med* 2011; May 2, E PUB.

22. Lamarche B, Tchernof A, Mooriani S, Cantin B, Dagenais GR, Lupien PJ, and Despres JP. Small, dense low-density lipoprotein particles as a predictor of the risk of ischemic heart disease in men. Prospective results from the Quebec Cardiovascular Study. *Circulation* 1997; 95(1): 69–75.

23. Kruth HS. Receptor-independent fluid-phase pinocytosis mechanisms for induction of foam cell formation with native low density lipoprotein particles. *Current Opinion in Lipidology* 2011; 22(5): 386–93.

24. Zhao ZW, Zhu XL, Luo YK, Lin CG, and Chen LL. Circulating Soluble lectin-like oxidized low-density lipoprotein redeptor-1 levels are associated with angiographic coronary lesion complexity in patients with coronary artery disease. *Clin Cardiol* 2011; 34(3): 172–77.

25. Ehara S, Ueda M, Naruko T, et al. Elevated levels of oxidized low density lipoprotein show a positive relationship with the severity of acute coronary syndromes. *Circulation* 2001; 103(15): 1955–60.

26. Hansson GK. Inflammation, atherosclerosis, and coronary artery disease. *N Engl J Med.* 2005; 352(16): 1685–95.

27. Harper CR and Jacobson TA. Using apolipoprotein B to manage dyslipidemic patients: Time for a change? *Mayo Clin Proc.* 2010; 85(5): 440–45.

28. Curtiss LK. Reversing atherosclerosis? *N Engl J Med* 2009; 360(11): 1144–46.

29. Ridker PM, Danielson E, Fonseca FA, et al. Jupiter Study Group. Rosuvastatin to prevent vascular events in men and women with elevated C-eactive protein. *N Engl J Med* 2008; 359(21): 2195–207.

30. Shen GX. Impact and mechanism for oxidized and glycated lipoproteins on generation of fibrinolytic regulators from vascular endothelial cells. *Mol Cell Biochem* 2003; 246(1–2): 69–74.

31. Krishnan GM and Thompson PD. The effects of statins on skeletal muscle strength and exercise performance. *Curr Opin Lipidol* 2010;21(4): 324–28.

32. Mills EJ, Wu P, Chong G, Ghement K, Singh S, Aki EA, Eyawo O, Guyatt G, Berwanger O, and Briel M. Efficacy and safety of statin treatment for cardiovascular disease: A network meta-analysis of 170,255 patients from 76 randomized trials. *QJM* 2011; 104(2):109–24.

33. Mammen AL and Amato AA. Statin myopathy: A review of recent progress. *Curr Opin Rheumatol* 2010; 22(6): 544–50.

34. Russo MW, Scobev M and Bonkovsky HL. Drug-induced liver injury associated with statins. *Semin Liver Dis* 2009; 29(4): 412–22.

35. Moosmann B and Behl C. Selenoproteins, cholesterol-lowering durgs, and the consequences: Revisiting of the mevalonate pathway. *Trends Cardiovasc Med* 2004; 14(7): 273–81.

36. Liu CS, Lii CK, Chang LL, Kuo CL, Cheng WL, Su SL, Tsai CW, and Chen HW. Atorvastatin increases blood ratios of vitamin E/low-density lipoprotein cholesterol and coenzyme Q10/low-density lipoprotein cholesterol in hypercholesterolemic patients. *Nutr Res* 2010; 30(2): 118–24.

37. Wyman M, Leonard M, and Morledge T. Coenzyme Q 10: A therapy for hypertension and statin-induced myalgia? *Clev Clin J Med* 2010; 77(7): 435–42.

38. Mortensen SA. Low coenzyme Q levels and the outcome of statin treatment in heart failure. *J Am Coll Cardiol* 2011; 57(14): 1569.

39. Shojaei M, Djalali M, Khatami M, Siassi F, and Eshraghian M. Effects of carnitine and coenzyme Q 10 on lipid profile and serum levels of lipoprotein(a) in maintenance hemodialysis patients on statin therapy. *Iran J Kidney Dis* 2011; 5(20): 114–18.

40. Gupta A and Thompson PD. The relationship of vitamin D deficiency to statin myopathy. *Atherosclerosis* 2011; 215(1): 23–29.

41. Avis HJ, Hargreaves IP, Ruiter JP, Land JM, Wanders RJ, and Wijburg FA. Rosuvastatin lowers coenzyme Q 10 levels, but not mitochondrial adenosine triphosphate synthesis, in children with familial hypercholesterolemia. *J Pediatr* 2011; 158(3): 458–62.

42. Kiernan TJ, Rochford M, and McDermott. Simvastatin induced rhapdomyloysis and an important clinical link with hypothyroidism. *Int J Cardiol* 2007; 119(3): 374–76.

43. Van Horn L, McCoin, M, Kris-Etherton PM, et al. The evidence for dietary prevention and treatment of cardiovascular disease. *J Am Diet Assoc* 2008; 108: 287–331.

44. Dawber TR, Meadors GF, and Moore FE. Epidemiological approaches to heart disease: The Framingham Study. *Am J Public Health* 1951; 41: 279–86.

45. Keys A. 1970. Coronary heart disease in seven countries. *Circulation* 41(suppl 1): 1–21.

46. Keys A, Menotti A, Karvonen MJ, et al. The diet and 15-year death rate in the Seven Countries Study. *Am J Epidemiol* 1986; 124: 903–15.

47. Appel LJ, Sacks FM, Carey VJ, et al. Effects of protein, monounsaturated fat, and carbohydrate intake on blood pressure and serum lipids: Results of the OmniHeart randomized trial. *JAMA* 2005; 294: 2455–64.

48. Pritikin N. Dietary factors and hyperlipidemia. *Diabetes Care* 1982; 5: 647–48.

49. Pritikin N. The Pritikin diet. *JAMA* 2005; 1984; 251: 1160–61.

50. Barnard RJ, Lattimore L, Holly RG, et al. Response of non-insulin-dependent diabetic patients to an intensive program of diet and exercise. *Diabetes Care* 1982; 5: 370–74.

51. Ornish D, Scherwitz LW, Doody RS, et al. Effects of stress management training and dietary changes in treating ischemic heart disease. *JAMA* 1983; 249: 54–59.

52. Ornish D, Brown SE, Scherwitz LW, et al. Can lifestyle changes reverse coronary heart disease? The Lifestyle Heart Trial. *Lancet* 1990; 336: 129–33.

53. Ornish D, Scherwitz LW, Billings JH, et al. Intensive lifestyle changes for reversal of coronary heart disease. *JAMA* 1998; 280: 2001–7. Erratum in: *JAMA* 1999; 281: 1380.

54. Chainani-Wu N, Weidner G, Purnell DM, et al. Changes in emerging cardiac biomarkers after an intensive lifestyle intervention. *Am J Cardiol* 2011; 108: 498–507.

55. Expert Panel on Detection, Evaluation, and Treatment of High Blood Cholesterol in Adults. Executive summary of the third report of the National Cholesterol Education Program (NCEP) Expert Panel on Detection, Evaluation, and Treatment of High Blood Cholesterol in Adults (Adult Treatment Panel III). *JAMA* 2001; 16(285): 2486–97. 2004 update available at http://www.nhlbi.nih.gov/guidelines/cholesterol/atp3upd04.htm. Accessed November 27, 2011.

56. Lichtenstein AH, Appel LJ, Brands M, et al. Summary of American Heart Association Diet and Lifestyle Recommendations revision 2006. *Arterioscler Thromb Vasc Biol* 2006; 26: 2186–91.

57. Lichtenstein AH, Ausman LM, Jalbert SM, et al. Efficacy of a therapeutic lifestyle change/Step 2 diet in moderately hypercholesterolemic middle-aged and elderly female and male subjects. *J Lipid Res* 2002; 43: 264–73.

58. Howard BV, Van Horn L, and Hsia J. Low-fat dietary pattern and risk of cardiovascular disease: The Women's Health Initiative Randomized Controlled Dietary Modification Trial. *JAMA* 2006; 8; 295: 655–66.

59. Jenkins DJ, Kendall CW, Marchie, A, et al. The effect of combining plant sterols, soy protein, viscous fibers, and almonds in treating hypercholesterolemia. *Metabolism* 2003; 52: 1478–83.

60. Jenkins DJ, Kendal CW, Faulkner DA, et al. Assessment of the longer-term effects of a dietary portfolio of cholesterol-lowering foods in hypercholesterolemia. *Am J Clin Nutr* 2006; 83: 582–91.

61. Jenkins DJ, Kendall CW, Faulkner D, et al. A dietary portfolio approach to cholesterol reduction: Combined effects of plant sterols, vegetable proteins, and viscous fibers in hypercholesterolemia. *Metabolism* 2002; 51: 1596–604.

62. Jenkins DJ, Kendall CW, Marchie A, et al. Effects of a dietary portfolio of cholesterol-lowering foods vs lovastatin on serum lipids and C-reactive protein. *JAMA* 2003; 290: 502–10.

63. Jenkins DJ, Chiavaroli L, Wong JM, et al. Adding monounsaturated fatty acids to a dietary portfolio of cholesterol-lowering foods in hypercholesterolemia. *CMAJ* 2010; 182: 1961–67.

64. Jenkins DJ, Jones PJ, Lamarche B, et al. Effect of a dietary portfolio of cholesterol-lowering foods given at 2 levels of intensity of dietary advice on serum lipids in hyperlipidemia: A randomized controlled trial. *JAMA* 2011; 306: 831–39.

65. Kris-Etherton P, Eckel RH, Howard BV, et al. AHA Science Advisory: Lyon Diet Heart Study. Benefits of a Mediterranean-style, National Cholesterol Education Program/American Heart Association Step I dietary pattern on cardiovascular disease. *Circulation* 2001; 103: 1823–25.

66. de Lorgeril M, Renaud S, Mamelle N, et al. Mediterranean alpha-linolenic acid-rich diet in secondary prevention of coronary heart disease. *Lancet* 1994; 343: 1454–59. Erratum in: *Lancet* 1994; 345: 738.

67. de Lorgeril M, Salen P, Martin JL, et al. Mediterranean diet, traditional risk factors, and the rate of cardiovascular complications after myocardial infarction: Final report of the Lyon Diet Heart Study. *Circulation* 1999; 99: 779–85.

68. de Lorgeril M and Salen P. The Mediterranean diet: Rationale and evidence for its benefit. *Curr Atheroscler Rep* 2008; 10: 518–22.

69. Rastogi T, Reddy KS, Vaz M, et al. Diet and risk of ischemic heart disease in India. *Am J Clin Nutr* 2004; 79: 582–92.

70. PREDIMED Investigators. PREDIMED Study (protocol), available at: http://predimed.onmedic.net/LinkClick.aspx?fileticket=PPjQkaJqs20%3D&tabid=574. Accessed November 26, 2011.

71. Estruch R, Martínez-González MA, Corella D, et al. Effects of a Mediterranean-style diet on cardiovascular risk factors: A randomized trial. *Ann Intern Med* 2006; 145: 1–11.

72. Salas-Salvadó J, Garcia-Arellano A, Estruch R, et al. Components of the Mediterranean-type food pattern and serum inflammatory markers among patients at high risk for cardiovascular disease. *Eur J Clin Nutr* 2008; 62: 651–59.

73. Kallio P, Kolehmainen M, Laaksonen DE, et al. Dietary carbohydrate modification induces alterations in gene expression in abdominal subcutaneous adipose tissue in persons with the metabolic syndrome: the FUNGENUT Study. *Am J Clin Nutr* 2007; 85: 1417–27.

74. Ornish D, Magbanua MJ, Weidner G, et al. Changes in prostate gene expression in men undergoing an intensive nutrition and lifestyle intervention. *Proc Natl Acad Sci USA* 2008; 105: 8369–74.

75. Llorente-Cortés V, Estruch R, Mena MP, et al. Effect of Mediterranean diet on the expression of proatherogenic genes in a population at high cardiovascular risk. *Atherosclerosis* 2010; 208: 442–50.

76. Razquin C, Martinez JA, Martinez-Gonzalez MA, et al. A Mediterranean diet rich in virgin olive oil may reverse the effects of the -174G/C IL6 gene variant on 3-year body weight change. *Mol Nutr Food Res* 2010; 54(Suppl 1): S75–82.

77. Konner M and Eaton SB. Paleolithic nutrition: Twenty-five years later. *Nutr Clin Pract* 2010; 25: 594–602.

78. Eaton SB, Konner MJ, and Cordain L. Diet-dependent acid load, Paleolithic [corrected] nutrition, and evolutionary health promotion. *Am J Clin Nutr* 2010; 91: 295–97. Erratum in: *Am J Clin Nutr* 2010; 91: 1072.

79. O'Keefe, Jr., JH and Cordain L. Cardiovascular disease resulting from a diet and lifestyle at odds with our Paleolithic genome: How to become a 21st-century hunter-gatherer. *Mayo Clin Proc* 2004; 79: 101–8.

80. Jew S, AbuMweis SS, and Jones PJ. Evolution of the human diet: Linking our ancestral diet to modern functional foods as a means of chronic disease prevention. *J Med Food* 2009; 12: 925–34.

81. Saremi A and Arora R. The utility of omega-3 fatty acids in cardiovascular disease. *Am J Ther* 2009;16(5): 421–36.

82. Rissanen T, Voutilainen S, NyyssonenK, Lakka TA, and Salonen JT. Fish oil-derived fatty acids, docosahexaenoic acid and docosapentaenoic acid and the risk of acute coronary events: The Kuopio ischaemic heart disease risk factor study. *Circulation* 2000; 102(22): 2677–79.

83. Davis W, Rockway S, and Kwasny M. Effect of a combined therapeutic approach of intensive lipid management, omega 3 fatty acid supplementation, and increased serum 25(OH) D on coronary calcium scores in asymptomatic adults. *Am J Ther*. 2009; 16(4): 326–32.

84. Yokoyama M, Origasa H, Matsuzaki M, et al. Japan EPA lipid intervention study (JELIS) investigators. *Lancet*. 2007; 369(9567): 1090–98.

85. Ryan AS, Keske MA, Hoffman JP, and Nelson EB. Clinical overview of algal-docosahexaenoic acid: Effects on triglyceride levels and other cardiovascular risk factors. *Am J Ther* 2009; 16(2): 183–92.

86. Kelley DS, Siegal D, Vemuri M, Chung GH, and Mackey BE. Docosahexaenoic acid supplementation decreases remnant-like particle cholesterol and increases the (n-3) index in hypertriglyceridemic men. *J Nutr*. 2008; 138(1): 30–35.

87. Maki KC, Dicklin MR, Davidson MH, Doyle RT, and Ballantyne CM. Combination of prescription omega-3 with simvastatin (COMBOS) investigators. *Am J Cardiol* 2010; 105(10): 1409–12.

88. Micallef MA and Garg ML. The lipid-lowering effects of phytosterols and (n-3) polyunsaturated fatty acids are synergistic and complementary in hyperlipidemic men and women. *J Nutr* 2008; 138(6): 1085–90.

89. Mori TA, Burke V, Puddey IB, Watts GF, O'Neal DN, Best JD, and Beilin LJ. Purified eicosapentaenoic and docosahexaenoic acids have differential effects on serum lipids and lipoproteins, LDL particle size, glucose and insulin in mildly hyperlipidemic men. *Am J Clin Nutr* 2000; 71(5): 1085–94.

90. Bester D, Esterhuyse AJ, Truter EJ, and van Rooyen J. Cardiovascular effects of edible oils: A comparison between four popular edible oils. *Nutr Res Rev* 2010; 23(2): 334–48.

91. Brown JM, Shelness GS, and Rudel LL. Monounsaturated fatty acids and atherosclerosis: Opposing views from epidemiology and experimental animal models. *Curr Atherosclero Rpe* 2007; 9(6): 494–500.

92. Bogani P, Gali C, Villa M and Visioli F. Postprandial anti-inflammatory and antioxidant effects of extra virgin olive oil. *Atherosclerosis* 2007; 190(1): 181–86.

93. Prasad K. Flaxseed and cardiovascular health. *J Cardiovasc Pharmacol* 2009; 54(5): 369–77.

94. Bioedon LT, Balkai S, Chittams J, Cunnane SC, Berlin JA, Rader DJ, and Szapary PO. Flaxseed and cardiovascular risk factors: Results from a double-blind, randomized controlled clinical trial. *J Am Coll Nutr* 2008; 27(1): 65–74.

95. Mandasescu S, Mocanu V, Dascalita AM, Haliga R, Nestian I, Stitt PA, and Luca V. Flaxseed supplementation in hyperlipidemic patients. *Rev Med Chir Soc Med Nat Lasi* 2005; 109(3): 502–6.

96. Gardner CD, Lawson LD, Block E, Chatterjee LM, Kiazand A, Balise RR, and Kraemer HC. Effect of raw garlic vs commercial garlic supplements on plasma lipid concentration in adults with moderate hypercholesterolemia: A randomized clinical trial. *Arch Intern Med* 2007; 167 (4): 346–53.

97. Budoff MJ, Ahmadi N, Gul KM, Liu ST, Flores FR, Tiano J, Takasu J, Miller E, and Tsimikas S. Aged garlic extract supplemented with B vitamins, folic acid and L-arginine retards progression of subclinical atherosclerosis: A randomized clinical trial. *Prev Med* 2009; 49(2–3): 101–7.

98. Singh DK, Banerjee S, and Porter TD. Green and black tea extracts inhibit HMG-CoA reductase and activate AMP kinase to decrease cholesterol synthesis in hepatoma cells. *J Nutr Biochem* 2009; 20(10): 816–22.

99. Tinahones FJ, Rubio MA, Garrido-Sanchez L, Ruiz C, Cordillo E, Cabrerizo L, and Cardona F. Green tea reduces LDL oxidability and improves vascular function. *J Am Coll Nutr* 2008; 27(2): 209–13.

100. Brown AL, Lane J, Holyoak C, Nicol B, Mayes AE, and Dadd T. Health effects of green tea catechins in overweight and obese men: A randomized controlled cross-over trial. *Br J Nut* 2011; 7: 1–10.

101. Zheng XX, Xu YL, Li SH, Liu XX, Hui R, and Huang XH. Green tea intake lowers fasting serum total and LDL cholesterol in adults: A meta-analysis of 14 randomized controlled trials. *Am J Clin Nutr* 2011; 94: 601–10.

102. Cesar TB, Aptekman NP, Araujo MP, Vinagre CC, and Maranhao RC. *Nutr Res* 2010; 30(10): 689–94.

103. Aviram M. Atherosclerosis: Cell biology and lipoproteins-oxidative stress and paraoxonases regulate atherogenesis. *Curr Opin Lipidol* 2010; 21(2): 163–64.

104. Fuhrman B, Volkova N, Aviram M. Pomegranate juice polyphenols increase recombinant paroxonase-1 binding to high density lipoprotein: Studies in vitro and in diabetic patients. *Nutrition* 2010; 26(4): 359–66.

105. Avairam M, Rosenblat M, Gaitine D, et al. Pomegranate juice consumption for 3 years by patients with carotid artery stenosis reduces common carotid intima-media thickness, blood pressure and LDL oxidation. *Clin Nutr* 2004; 23(3): 423–33.

106. Mattiello T, Trifiro E, Jotti GS, and Pulcinelli FM. Effects of pomegranate juice and extract polypyenols on platelet function. *J Med Food* 2009; 12(2): 334–39.

107. Aviram M, Dornfeld L, Rosenblat M, Volkova N, Kaplan M, Coleman R, Hayek T, Presser D, and Fuhrman B. Pomegranate juice consumption reduces oxidative stress, atherogenic modifications to LDL, and platelet aggregation: Studies in humans and in atherosclerotic apolipoprotein E-deficient mice. *Am J Clin Nutr* 2000; 71(5): 1062–76.

108. Davidson MH, Maki KC, Dicklin MR, Feinstein SB, Witcher M. Bell M, McGuire DK, Provost JC, Liker H, and Aviram M. Effects of consumption of pomegranate juice on carotid intima-media thickness in men and women at moderate risk for coronary heart disease. *Am J Cardiol* 2009; 104(7): 936–42.

109. Wu WH., Kang YP, Wang NH, Jou HJ, and Want TA. Sesame ingestion affects sex hormones, antioxidant status and blood lipids in postmenopausal women. *J Nutr* 2006; 136(5): 1270–75.

110. Namiki M. Nutraceutical functions of sesame: A review. *Crit Rev Food Sci Nutr* 2007; 47(7): 651–73

111. Sacks FM, Lichtenstein A, Van Horn L, Harris W, Kris-Etherton P, and Winston M. *American Heart Association Nutrition Committee* Circulation 2006; 113(7): 1034–44.

112. Harland JI and Haffner TA. Systemic review, meta-analysis and regression of randomized controlled trials reporting an association between an intake of circa 25 g soya protein per day and blood cholesterol. *Atherosclerosis* 2008; 200(1): 13–27.

113. Houston MC. Juice powder concentrate and systemic blood pressure, progression of coronary artery calcium and antioxidant status in hypertensive subjects: A pilot study. *Evid Based Complementary Alternat Med.* 2007; 4(4): 455–62.

114. Di Donna L, De Luca G, Mazzotti F, Napoli A, Salerno R, Taverna D, and Sindona G. Statin-like principles of bergamot fruit (*Citrus bergamia*): Isolation of 3 hydroxymethylglutaryl flavonoid glycosides. *J Nat Prod* 2009; 72(7): 1352–54.

115. Mollace V, Sacco I, Janda E, et al. Hypolipidemic and hypoglycaemic activity of bergamot polyphenols: From animal modles to human studies. *Fitotherapia* 2011; 82(3): 309–16.
116. Soni KB and Kuttan R. Effect of oral curcumin administration on serum peroxides and cholesterol levels in human volunteers. *Indian J Physiol Pharmacol* 1992; 36(4): 273–75.
117. Szapary PO, Wolfe ML, BLoedon LT, Cucchiara AJ, DerMarderosian AH, Cirigliano MD, and Rader DJ. Guggulipid for the treatment of hypercholesterolemia: A randomized controlled trial. *JAMA* 2003; 290(6): 765–72.
118. Ulbricht C, Basch E, Szapary P, Hammerness, P, Axentsev S, Boon H, Kroll D, Garraway L, Vora M, and Woods J. Natural Standard Research Collaboration. Guggul for hyperlipidemia: A review by the Natural Standard Research Collaboration. *Complement Ther Med* 2005; 13(4): 279–90.
119. Nohr LA, Rasmussen LB, and Straand J. Resin from the Mukul Myrrh tree, guggul, can it be used for treating hypercholesterolemia: A randomized, controlled study. *Complement Ther Med* 2009; 17(1): 16–22.
120. Palozza P, Simone R, Gatalano A, Parrone N, Monego G, and Ranelletti F. Lycopene regulation of cholesterol synthesis and efflux in human macrophages. *J of Nutritional Biochemistry* 2011; 22: 971–78.
121. Ruparelia N, Digby JE, and Choudhury RP. Effects of niacin on atherosclerosis and vascular function. *Current Opinion in Cardiology* 2011; 26(1): 66–70.
122. Al-Mohissen MA, Pun SC, and Frohlich JJ. Niacin: From mechanisms of action to therapeutic uses. *Mini Rev Med Chem* 2010; 10(3): 204–17.
123. The Coronary Drug Project Group. Clofibrate and niacin in coronary heart disease. *JAMA* 1975; 231: 360–81.
124. Taylor AJ, Lee HJ, and Sullenberger LE. The effect of 24 months of combination statin and extended-release niacin on carotid intima-media thickness: ARBITER 3. *Curr Med Res Opin* 2006; 22(11): 2243–50.
125. Lee JM, Robson MD, Yu LM, et al. Effects of high dose modified release nicotinic acid on atherosclerosis and vascular function: A randomized, placebo controlled, magnetic resonance imaging study. *J Am Coll Cardiol* 2009; 54(19): 1787–94.
126. Taylor AJ, Villines TC, Stanek EJ, Devine PJ, Griffen L, Miller M, Weissman NJ, and Turco M. Extended release niacin or ezetimibe and carotid intima media thickness. *N Engl J Med* 2009; 361(22): 2113–22.
127. AIM HIGH Investigators. The role of niacin in raising high density lipoprotein cholesterols to reduce cardiovascular events in patients with atherosclerotic cardiovascular disease and optimally treated low density lipoprotein cholesterol: Baseline characteristics of study participants. The Atherothrombosis Intervention in Metabolic syndrome with low HDL/high triglycerides: Impact on Global Health outcomes (AIM-HIGH) trial. *Am Heart J* 2011; 161(3): 538–43.
128. McRae MP. Treatment of hyperlipoproteinemia with pantethine: A review and analysis of efficacy and tolerability. *Nutr Res* 2005; 25: 319–33.
129. Kelly G. Pantethine: A review of its biochemistry and therapeutic applications. *Altern Med Rev* 1997; 2: 365–77.
130. Horvath Z and Vecsei L. Current medical aspects of pantethine. *Ideggyogy Sz* 2009; 62(7–8): 220–29.
131. Pins LL and Keenan JM. Dietary and nutraceutical options for managing the hypertriglyceridemic patient. *Prog Cardiovasc Nurs* 2006; 21(2): 89–93.
132. No authors listed. Pantethine monograph. *Altern Med Rev* 2010; 15(3): 279–82.
133. Patch CS, Tapsell LC, Williams PG, and Gordon M. Plant sterols as dietary adjuvants in the reduction of cardiovascular risk: Theory and evidence. *Vasc Health Risk Manag* 2006; 2(2): 157–62.
134. Demonty I, Ras RT, van der Knaap HC, Duchateau GS, Meijer L, Zock PL, Geleijnse JM, and Trautwein EA. Continuous dose response relationship of the LDL cholesterol lowering effect of phytosterol intake. *J Nutr* 2009; 139(2): 271–84.
135. Othman RA and Moghadasian MH. Beyond cholesterol lowering effects of plant sterols: Clinical and experimental evidence of anti-inflammatory properties. *Nutrition Reviews* 2011; 69(7): 371–82.
136. Nijjar PS, Burke FM, Bioesch A, and Rader DJ. Role of dietary supplements in lowering low-density lipoprotein cholesterol: A review. *J of Clinical Lipidology* 2010; 4: 248–58.
137. Sabeva NS, McPhaul CM, Li, X, Cory, TJ, Feola DJ, and Graf GA. Phytosterols differiently influence ABC transporter expression, cholesterol efflux and inflammatory cytokine Secretion in macrophage foam cells. *J of Nutritional Biochemistry* 2011; 22: 777–83.
138. Berthold HK, Unverdorben S, Degenhardt R, Bulitta M, and Gourni Berthold I. Effect of policosanol on lipid levels among patients with hypercholesterolemia or combined hyperlipidemia: A randomized controlled trial. *JAMA* 2006; 295(19): 2262–69.
139. Greyling A, De Witt C, Oosthuizen W, and Jerling JC. Effects of a policosanol supplement on serum lipid concentrations in hypercholesterolemic and heterozygous familial hypercholesterolaemic subjects. *Br J Nutr* 2006; 95(5): 968–75.

140. Liu J, Zhang J, Shi Y, Grimsgaard S, Alraek T, and Fonnebo V. Chinese red yeast rice *(Monascus purpureus)* for primary hyperlipidemia: A meta-analysis of randomized controlled trials. *Chin Med* 2006; 1: 4.

141. Lu Z, Kou W, Du B, Wu, Y, Zhao S, Brusco OA, Morgan JM, Capuzzi DM, Chinese Coronary Secondary Prevention Study Group, and Li S. Effect of xuezhikang, an extract from red yeast Chinese rice, on coronary events in a Chinese population with previous myocardial infarction. *Am J Cardiol* 2008; 101(12) : 1689–93.

142. Qureshi AA, Sami SA, Salser WA, and Khan FA. Synergistic effect of tocotrienol-rich fraction (TRF 25) of rice bran and lovastatin on lipid parameters in hypercholesterolemic humans. *J Nutr Biochem* 2001; 12(6): 318–29.

143. Song BL and DeBose-Boyd RA. Insig-dependent ubiquitination and degradation of 3-hydroxy-3 methylglutaryl coenzyme a reductase stimulated by delta-and gamma-tocotrienols. *J Biol Chem* 2006; 281(35): 54–61.

144. Prasad K. Tocotrienols and cardiovascular health. *Curr Pharm Des* 2011; July 21, E PUB.

145. McRae MP. Vitamin C supplementation lowers serum low-density cholesterol and triglycerides: A meta-analysis of 13 randomized controlled trials. *J Chiropr Med* 2008; 7(2): 48–58.

146. McRae MP. The efficacy of vitamin C supplementation on reducing total serum cholesterol in human subjects: A review of 51 experimental trials. *J Chiropr Med* 2006; 5(1): 2–12.

147. Houston M and Sparks W. Effect of combination pantethine, plant sterols, green tea extract, delta-tocotrienol and phytolens on lipid profiles in patients with hyperlipidemia. *JANA* 2010; 13(1): 15–20.

148. Houston MC. Unpublished data. Personal communication 2011.

149. Studer M, Briel M, Leimenstoll B, Glass TR, and Bucher HC. Effect of different anti-lipidemic agents and diets on mortality: A systemic review. *Arch Int Med* 2005; 165(7): 725–30.

5 Hyperviscosity Syndrome

A Nutritionally Modifiable Cardiovascular Risk Factor

Ralph E. Holsworth, Jr., D.O., and Young I. Cho, Ph.D.

INTRODUCTION

Blood viscosity (BV) is a biomarker comparable to atherosclerosis and hypertension in the assessment of cardiovascular risk. Diet choices associated with dehydration, choline deficiency, and fatty acid imbalances predispose to unfavorable, high BV. Conversely, dietary changes that support hydration, digestion, and optimal nutrient status reduce BV. In this way, what someone eats affects not only the biochemical parameters measured in conventional laboratory tests, but also biophysical parameters such as pressure and flow.

Blood viscosity is defined as the resistance of blood to flow vis-à-vis the vessel wall; viscosity is the thickness and stickiness of blood. The cardiovascular system seeks to optimize blood flow, which in the vast majority of human cases means to increase or maximize oxygen delivery to local tissues. Since oxygen is bound to hemoglobin molecules that reside in erythrocytes, biochemically the greater the number of erythrocytes the more oxygen that can be delivered. However, biophysically this is not always the case because flow resistance increases nearly exponentially as a function of hematocrit. This chapter provides an overview on the hyperviscosity syndrome, its role in the pathophysiology of cardiovascular disease, a synopsis of relevant epidemiologic studies, and information on patient evaluation and treatment modalities.

HISTORICAL PERSPECTIVE

After the initial clinical description of angina by Heberden in 1772, more than a century elapsed before pathologists centered their attention on the coronary arteries and developed an understanding of thrombotic occlusions and ossification [1]. The initial discussions of angina pectoris were presented by John Warren, MD, in 1812 in the very first article of the first issue of the *New England Journal of Medicine and Surgery* [2].

The initial description of angina pectoris (from the Latin *angina*, "infection of the throat," the Greek *ankhon*, "strangling," and Latin *pectus,* "chest") mirrors the same presentation in patients for physicians today. The pathogenesis remained unknown until 1799, when Caleb H. Parry proposed that angina pectoris was related to coronary-artery ossification or calcification observed predominantly in men, 50 years of age, and seldom seen in women or children [3]. In 1879, the pathologist Ludvig Hektoen advanced our understanding of myocardial infarction as being caused by coronary thrombosis "secondary to sclerotic changes in the coronaries" [4].

From then on, our understanding and management of acute myocardial infarct remained virtually static until the 1960s when initial results of the Framingham Heart Study (which had started in 1948) were presented in "Factors of Risk in the Development of Coronary Heart Disease" [5]. Coronary risk factors such as elevations in blood pressure and cholesterol levels were associated with a higher incidence of ischemic heart disease and acute myocardial infarction (AMI). Large multicenter clinical trials provided primary intervention and secondary prevention facilitated by aggressive steps in controlling blood pressure and serum total cholesterol. Modern therapy continued to be refined in the 1970s, with cardiologists opening occluded coronary arteries by infusion of the fibrinolytic agent streptokinase, thereby reducing early mortality in patients with acute myocardial infarction [6]. The Second International Study of Infarct Survival (ISIS-2) indicated aspirin (an antiplatelet drug) could reduce AMI mortality [7]. Coronary angioplasty and stenting aided by more potent platelet inhibitors (e.g., $P2Y_{12}$ and glycoprotein IIb/IIIa platelet-receptor blockers) further reduced hospital mortality to 7%.

The 1998 Nobel Prize research of Furchgott, Ignarro, and Murad transformed our understanding of vascular biology by identifying nitric oxide as a physiological dilator of blood vessels intricately involved in thrombotic occlusion of a ruptured or eroded atherosclerotic plaque [8]. On the basis of these studies and others, we understand atherosclerosis is a chronic inflammation of arteries that develops slowly over decades in response to biologic effects of cardiac risk factors. Atherogenesis starts as a qualitative change in the intact endothelium cells after subjection to oxidative, hemodynamic, or biochemical stimuli (from smoking, hypertension, or dyslipidemia) and inflammatory factors summarized in the 1998 monograph *The Vulnerable Atherosclerotic Plaque: Understanding, Identification and Modification* by Fuster [9]. Approximately 300 independent risk factors for coronary heart disease were identified and prioritized in importance by Hopkins and Williams [10,11].

But a constant enigma in the historical development of the three major manifestations of atherosclerosis—coronary heart disease, cerebrovascular disease, and peripheral arterial disease—was to identify the initiating event or nidus of atherogenesis (see Figure 5.1). Blood viscosity is a parameter that can unify the risk factors for cardiovascular disease. In other words,

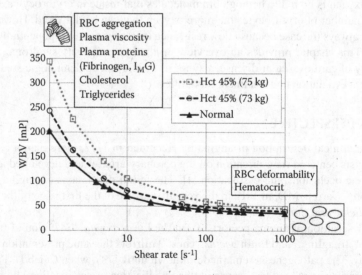

FIGURE 5.1 Typical profiles for whole blood viscosity. Factors affecting whole blood viscosity (WBV) at both low and high shear rates are shown. In addition, two men of comparable age and weight with identical hematocrit may have significantly different WBV particularly at low shear rates. At low shear rates, erythrocytes tend to produce Rouleaux formation, increasing blood viscosity, whereas at high shear rates the erythrocytes are dispersed due to high-flow velocity, resulting in minimal blood viscosity.

viscosity may be the reason why the biochemical, metabolic, and demographic factors proved important. Under this biophysical paradigm, increased blood viscosity acts as a biophysical stimulus and mechanism of action by which the other risk factors convey the preinflammatory insult to the patient's arterial walls [12]. Further development of this paradigm shift from biochemistry to biophysics was provided in *The Origin of Atherosclerosis—What Really Initiates the Inflammatory Process* by the late cardiologist Kensey and co-author of this chapter, fluid dynamist Cho [13].

PATHOPHYSIOLOGY AND EPIDEMIOLOGY: ROLE OF HYPERVISCOSITY SYNDROME IN CARDIOVASCULAR DISEASES

The hyperviscosity syndromes are a group of symptoms triggered by an increase in the viscosity of the blood [14]. Hyperviscosity can occur from pathologic elevations of either the cellular or acellular (protein) fractions of the circulating blood such as is found in the well-established examples of polycythemias, dysproteinemias, Waldenström macroglobulinemia, multiple myeloma, leukemia, sickle cell anemia, and sepsis [15–18]. Hyperviscosity typically presents with visual disturbances and neurologic signs of headache and vertigo. Categorically speaking, types of hyperviscosity syndromes include the syndromes of serum hyperviscosity where patients may experience neurologic or ocular disorders; syndromes of polycythemic hyperviscosity that result in reduced blood flow or capillary perfusion and increased organ congestion; and syndromes of hyperviscosity caused by reduced deformability of red blood cells as in sickle cell anemia [14].

Blood viscosity is the inherent resistance of blood to flow and represents the thickness and stickiness of blood. The blood becomes stickier when it moves slowly in small vessels, whereas it becomes thinner when blood moves quickly in large vessels. The phenomenon of the velocity-dependent blood viscosity can be described as the shear-thinning, non-Newtonian behavior of whole blood [19–21]. When blood moves quickly through large arteries, blood becomes thinner as erythrocytes are fully dispersed due to higher flow velocity in large arteries. When blood moves through small vessels whose diameter is less than 50 microns (as in microcirculation), the flow velocity is often less than 0.1 cm/s. Without the dispersing force of high velocity, serum proteins such as fibrinogen and LDL cholesterol molecules promote erythrocyte aggregation known as Rouleaux formation [20,22,23]. As erythrocytes at these small vessels cluster and crowd together, the flow resistance dramatically increases, resulting in hyperviscosity of whole blood.

Blood viscosity is affected by a number of variables that include blood cells (i.e., erythrocytes, white cells, platelets, etc.), plasma proteins (i.e., fibrinogen, immunoglobulins, and albumin), lipids (i.e., HDL, LDL, and TG), osmolality, and levels of inflammation and stress (i.e., emotional and oxidative). Hence, any abnormality in one of these variables could alter blood viscosity. Among these variables, the two most important parameters that influence the blood viscosity profile are hematocrit and plasma proteins, especially fibrinogen [20]. Hematocrit is the volume fraction of erythrocytes in whole blood. As hematocrit increases, flow resistance increases between the moving blood and the arterial wall, resulting in hyperviscosity as can be experienced in polycythemia vera, where hematocrit can be 60–65% or greater [20]. At such high levels of cellular content, blood viscosity increases exponentially with hematocrit.

An involvement of blood viscosity in the pathogenesis of various diseases has long been recognized. An understanding of the role of viscosity in cardiovascular diseases, specifically, is based on the epidemiologic evidence as well as key pathophysiologic insights relating to the site-specificity of lesions. It is worthwhile to note that blood viscosity has been independently correlated with the major risk factors for cardiovascular disease [24–35]. The epidemiologic research on the link between blood viscosity and major cardiovascular disease events, such as acute myocardial infarction and cardiovascular death, demonstrates that the risk of such events increases with increases in blood viscosity [36,37]. Elevated blood viscosity is at least as predictive of ischemic vascular diseases as several conventional major cardiac risk factors [38,39]. Strong evidence for a link between viscosity and cardiovascular events was provided by the Edinburgh Artery Study in a random population sample of 1592 men and women aged 55 to 74 years [39]. Over a period of five years, age and gender-adjusted mean rheological variables including blood viscosity, hematocrit, hematocrit-corrected blood viscosity, plasma viscosity, and fibrinogen were all significantly higher in patients who experienced cardiovascular events (ischemic heart disease and stroke) than in those who did not. The difference in mean high-shear blood viscosity between the two groups of patients was statistically very significant ($p = 0.0003$), and the relationship of blood viscosity to the occurrence of cardiovascular events was at least as strong as for diastolic blood pressure and LDL cholesterol and stronger than that of smoking. These results suggest that blood viscosity is an important predictor of cardiovascular events in the adult population [39].

Atherosclerosis, the established cause of cardiovascular diseases, is observed to develop at localized sites, such as at outer walls of arterial branches, which are regions of lower vascular shear stress and sites of blood recirculation and stasis [40]. The site specificity of lesions has provided pathological support for the critical involvement of hemodynamic forces in the initiation and progression of atherosclerotic lesions that evolve to a rupture-prone lesion [13]. For decades, hemodynamic forces have been implicated as important factors in the development of atherosclerosis, rupture of vulnerable atherosclerotic lesions, and thrombosis that are established pathological determinants responsible for the vast majority of acute ischemic events [41–43].

The key hemodynamic force is vascular shear stress, or wall shear stress, which is defined as the tangential frictional force per unit area applied by blood flow upon the endothelial wall. While normal physiological shear stress (> 15 dyne/cm^2) permits endothelial quiescence and atheroprotective gene expression, oscillatory low shear stresses ($< \pm 4$ dyne/cm^2) stimulate atherogenic phenotypes [42]. Wall shear stress applied by the blood against the vessel wall is defined as viscosity multiplied by the wall shear rate and expressed as

$$\tau_w = \mu \dot{\gamma}_w \cong \mu \left[8 \frac{V}{d} \right]$$

where τ_w = wall shear stress; μ = blood viscosity; $\dot{\gamma}_w$ = shear rate; V = blood flow velocity (spatially averaged mean velocity); and d = lumen diameter.

The proportionality μ that relates wall shear stress and wall shear rate is blood viscosity. Therefore, at any given moment and in a given vessel segment, if flow velocity and lumen diameter could be assumed to be fixed quantities, then wall shear stress depends primarily on blood viscosity. Blood viscosity is the biological parameter that adversely modulates vascular shear stress, particularly at bifurcation and inner wall of curved vessels. When endothelial cells are exposed to oscillatory low vascular shear stress, they lose their healthy elongated shape and adopt a pathological rounder profile associated with augmented expression of inflammatory genes responsible for increased synthesis of endothelial-localized adhesion molecules, transmigration of mononuclear cells into subendothelial space, and intrusion and incorporation of lipoproteins into tissue macrophages [44–51]. Through a process called mechanotransduction [52], hyperviscosity of the blood is the root cause of the preinflammatory injury that triggers endothelial dysfunction and sets in motion a cascade of events that results in the atherosclerosis and eventual atherothrombosis. Blood viscosity in the pathogenesis of atherosclerosis has been explored and substantiated [42,53,54]. The clinical relevance of whole blood viscosity was recognized at the beginning of the twentieth century, when Russell Burton-Opitz, in his long-recognized medical textbook, suggested that elevated whole blood viscosity affects the heart and other organs—proposing that cardiac hypertrophy would result from increased peripheral resistance caused by the greater thickness of blood [55,56]. From then to now, clinical researchers have continued to find significant associations between hyperviscosity and congestive heart failure as well as, importantly, atherosclerosis, myocardial infarction, peripheral artery disease, and stroke [57–59].

PATIENT EVALUATION

From a pure physiologic view, the instantaneous work of the heart is determined by pulse pressure, left ventricular contractility, heart rate, and whole blood viscosity. If the circulatory system is considered as a closed loop system, any excursions of these variables will necessarily increase the mechanical or biophysical nidus initiating atherogenesis. Within this context, elevated whole blood viscosity is the key mechanism by which the conventional risk factors influence the development of atherosclerosis.

In contrast to hypertension and atherosclerosis, which have well-established clinical biomarkers, viscosity is a parameter where direct clinical assessment is currently limited to research and specialty settings. However, elevated blood viscosity is associated with well-defined clinical conditions, lifestyle choices, and nonmodifiable risk factors. These risk factors are summarized in the following section.

The first 11 risk factors presented here are modifiable, some to a greater extent than others. By treating any of the modifiable risk factors, blood viscosity improves as the predisposing condition improves. In addition to the treatment of concurrent factors, direct treatments are detailed in the treatment section.

SIXTEEN RED FLAGS FOR ELEVATED WHOLE BLOOD VISCOSITY

Modifiable Factors

1. Cardiovascular and Cerebrovascular Diseases

Clinical and epidemiological studies provide compelling evidence that elevated blood viscosity is a significant causal determination of atherosclerosis. As part of the Edinburgh Artery Study, 1106 men and women 60 to 80 years of age were followed over an average duration of five years. The results of this study found that whole blood viscosity, plasma viscosity, fibrinogen, and hematocrit were linearly related to carotid intima-media thickness in men. The study concluded that, in men, whole blood viscosity and its major determinants were associated not only with incident cardiovascular events but also with the early stages of atherosclerosis [54].

Resch et al. investigated the prognostic relevance of blood rheological variables in patients with arteriosclerotic diseases. These findings indicated that patients who suffered a second stroke or myocardial infarction or cardiovascular death within two years of their first examination, compared with those who had not, had significantly higher whole blood viscosity, red blood cell aggregation, serum viscosity, fibrinogen, and cholesterol [54,60].

2. Smoking

A comparison between smokers and nonsmokers indicated that those who smoked more than 21 cigarettes per day had significantly higher whole blood viscosity and plasma viscosity, and higher hematocrit and fibrinogen than nonsmokers [61]. Supporting research confirms that smokers have significant increases in whole blood viscosity, hematocrit, red blood cell aggregation, plasma viscosity, and fibrinogen [62]. Additional effects of smoking include the increase in total white blood cell count and modifications of leukocyte function. Collectively, these changes cause a deterioration in the flow properties of blood and precipitous increases of whole blood viscosity by 10–20%. The demonstrated clinical effect of reduced blood flow and impaired microcirculatory function suggests that smoking increases the risk of vascular diseases by changing blood rheology [63]. From the clinician's perspective, the positive attributes of smoking cessation are quickly reflected in "substantial and persistent reductions in blood viscosity" within two days of stopping smoking and provides an additional educational tool to encourage a patient's smoking cessation [64].

3. Essential Hypertension

The relationship between blood pressure and viscosity is such that, given a constant systolic blood pressure, if blood viscosity increases, then the total peripheral resistance will necessarily increase, thereby reducing blood flow. Conversely, when viscosity decreases, blood flow and perfusion will increase. Because of the dependence of systemic arterial blood pressure on cardiac output and total peripheral resistance, if blood viscosity and total peripheral resistance rise, systolic blood pressure must then increase for cardiac output to be maintained. Consequently, blood viscosity has been established as a major determinant of the work of the heart and tissue perfusion [65]. Since increased viscosity requires a higher blood pressure to ensure the same circulating volume of blood, both the burden on the heart and the forces acting on the vessel wall are directly modulated by changes in blood viscosity.

4. Elevated Hematocrit

Hematocrit, the percent volume of red blood cells, is the most influential determinant of whole blood viscosity. Red blood cells (RBCs) contribute the vast majority of the cellular content in blood and as much as 50% of the total blood volume in normal male adults. A clinician's review of complete blood count and, specifically, mild-to-moderate elevations in hematocrit are a necessary diagnostic aspect in detecting a patient's increased risk for hyperviscosity. Whole blood viscosity increases by about 26% for every 10% increase in hematocrit [66]. In polycythemia, hematocrit increases to 60 to 70%, with corresponding increases in whole blood viscosity at high shear rates 10 times greater than the viscosity of water. The resultant flow of blood through blood vessels is greatly diminished.

As a clinician, maintaining patients' hematocrit levels below median values, of 40% for females and 45% for men, can be a helpful rule of thumb for sustaining healthy perfusion. Patients with hematocrit levels beyond median values may be viewed as prime candidates for evaluating blood viscosity. Elevated hematocrit may also indicate clinical hypovolemia secondary to dehydration. The combination of decreased thirst drive, loss of arterial compliance, and commonly prescribed diuretics in elderly populations may contribute to increased subclinical states of dehydration.

5. Inactivity (Sedentary Lifestyle)

The long-term benefit of exercise is an improved whole blood viscosity, specifically related to the decrease in both coronary and peripheral vascular morbidity. In a 1998 review of exercise rheology, Brun et al. demonstrated that exercise improved blood lipids and fibrinogen profiles and, additionally, modified the metabolic and rheologic properties of red blood cells. The research concluded that the hemorheological effects of exercise could be a marker of the risk reversal and that whole blood viscosity was a physiologic determinant of fitness [67].

In a study of standardized treadmill exercise for the treatment of intermittent claudication, 42 patients with claudication were assigned to two groups. Group I (n = 22) conducted regular standardized treadmill exercise for two months. This group's maximal and pain-free walking distances increased significantly, more than 100%. Group II (n = 20) patients did not receive exercise over the same two-month period and their pain-free walking distances remained unchanged [68].

The "fluidification" of blood initiated by regular exercise was qualitatively and quantitatively similar to that in patients administered hemorheologically active medications. The study suggests that physical training may be a form of hemorheologic therapy appropriate for decreasing whole blood viscosity in patients with ischemic diseases.

6. Dyslipidemia

The most widely recognized risk factor for cardiovascular disease is dyslipidemia. Whole blood viscosity is directly related to total blood cholesterol and LDL-C and inversely related to HDL-C [69]. Other studies reporting correlations between blood viscosity and lipids have been discussed elsewhere in this chapter [23,27,28]. Interestingly, in a large prospective study in more than 5000 middle-aged British men with no evidence of ischemic heart disease, a positive association between hematocrit and cholesterol was shown along with a negative association between hematocrit and HDL-C [70].

7. Age-related Macular Degeneration

Whole blood viscosity is a factor in the pathogenesis of visual field defects. The role of whole blood viscosity in 292 patients with branch retinal vein occlusion was studied by Remsky et al. in 1996. Hematocrit and plasma viscosity were significantly elevated in these patients relative to healthy controls, but red blood cell deformability and aggregation did not differ, indicating that whole blood viscosity may be important in the pathogenesis of retinal vein occlusion [71]. In addition, whole blood viscosity, plasma viscosity, and packed red blood cell volume were shown to be significantly higher in patients with glaucoma than in healthy controls [72].

8. Diabetes, Insulin Resistance, and Obesity

Adults with diabetes have more atherosclerosis in their arteries and microperfusion problems than those without diabetes. Most of the deaths in this population, upward to 80% of diabetics, are from the coronary diseases and associated micro- and macrovascular diseases [73]. In diabetics, whole blood viscosity, plasma viscosity, and hematocrit are elevated, and red blood cell deformability is consistently decreased. Specific increases in low-shear blood viscosity have been attributed to increased fibrinogen and globulin [74].

The Framingham Heart Study identified obesity as an independent risk factor for cardiovascular disease. A study of the relationship between excess weight and whole blood viscosity demonstrated elevations in whole blood viscosity, plasma viscosity, and red blood cell aggregation in a group of 14 obese adults relative to nonobese controls [75]. A litany of recent studies have reported relationships between obesity, body mass index, and whole blood viscosity [76].

9. Autoimmune Diseases (only some of which may be modifiable)

Tietjen et al. (1975) studied the blood rheology of 20 patients with Raynaud's syndrome. Whole blood viscosity and plasma viscosity were significantly elevated over normal controls as were fibrinogen and globulins [77]. The results suggest such circulatory complications may in part be the result of increased whole blood viscosity and red blood cell aggregation in hindrance of blood flow.

10. Systemic Inflammation and Endothelial Dysfunction

The levels of acute-phase proteins such as high sensitivity C-reactive protein and several soluble markers of inflammation, such as interleukin-6, are associated with the acute coronary syndromes. Fluid dynamics, secondary to hyperviscosity conditions, affect the interface between blood and the vascular wall in a process called mechanotransduction. This mechanism couples mechanical shear stress and shear rate imparted by blood flow to induce endothelial cells' modulation of vasoactive and antithrombotic substances. Flow-induced vasoadaptation is mediated by the release of prostacyclin PGI_2 and endothelium-derived relaxing factor (EDRF/NO), from shear-exposed endothelial cells [78].

11. Alzheimer's Disease

Age-related changes in hemorheological properties and cerebral blood flow are probable factors in the development of Alzheimer's disease. Proposed structural models for the pathogenesis of this disease consider structural abnormalities and subsequent disturbed blood flow to the brain to be a unifying factor for the multiple manifestations of the disease [79,80,81]. The overall effect of chronic blood flow disruption on the brain impairs the perfusion of oxygen and glucose to cerebral neurons.

In 2000, Solerte et al. found an association between mild Alzheimer's disease, whole blood and plasma hyperviscosities, decreased red blood cell deformability, increased red blood cell aggregation, hyperfibrinogenemia, and increased acute-phase protein levels [82]. Also in 2000, Wen et al. measured high-shear and low-shear whole blood viscosity, plasma viscosity, and hematocrit in 31 patients with probable early Alzheimer's disease. The results led them to suggest that hemorheological indices could be useful in the earlier diagnosis of Alzheimer's disease [83], potentially forestalling disease progression with the emergence of treatment options.

Non-modifiable Risks

12. Men Age 50 and Older

A study of the relative importance of cardiovascular risk factors states that age is the strongest risk factor for cardiovascular disease [10]. Reduced microvascular blood flow resulted from blood rheology abnormalities contributes to age-associated increases in the incidence of ischemic vascular disease [84]. Similarly, studies indicate older age groups trended with higher plasma viscosity and significantly higher plasma fibrinogen levels [85].

Women of reproductive age are less likely to develop heart disease than men of the same age. In alignment with other cardiovascular risk factors, including whole blood viscosity, hematocrit, fibrinogen, and red blood cell aggregation, risks are significantly higher in men than women [65,86].

13. Heritable Hematologic Disorders

Polycythemia is an increased concentration of red blood cells. As previously mentioned, mild-to-moderate polythemia, which may result from any cause of dehydration, such as deprivation of water, prolonged vomiting, diarrhea, or mismanagement of diuretics, is modifiable. Absolute or primary polycythemia results from an intrinsic abnormality of myeloid stem cells. Milligan et al. investigated the influence of iron-deficiency indices in 18 patients suffering from polycythemia. The study indicated that the reduced number of iron-deficient cells resulted in increased cell-to-cell interaction, causing an increase in the whole blood viscosity [87].

Lichtman and Rowe provided a review of data for whole blood viscosity in patients with acute or chronic leukemia who had significantly elevated white blood cell counts. Despite a higher fractional volume of white blood cells, whole blood viscosity was not increased because reductions in the fractional volume of red blood cells were associated with the increase in leukocytes. Nevertheless, the excessive number of leukocytes seriously altered the circulation at the lung, brain, and other organs by obstructing microvasculature or by forming aggregates [88].

Whole blood is able to move through small capillaries because red blood cells are extremely deformable. When the deformability of red blood cells is reduced as in sickle cell anemia, the abnormal red blood cells disturb perfusion and create congestion in the capillaries. This difficulty causes whole blood viscosity to increase and results in subsequent clinical complications in patients. The relationship between reduced red blood cell deformability and hyperviscosity has long been established in a number of studies [89,90]. Sickle cell disease is the most striking example of a disorder in which the loss of red blood cell deformability causes ischemia [20].

14. Plasma Protein Disorders

The tendency of red blood cells to form Rouleaux at low shear rates mainly results from plasma proteins: fibrinogen and immunoglobulins [20]. The hyperviscosity syndrome of Waldenstrom's macroglobulinemia is associated with retinopathy, loss of vision, bleeding of mucous membranes, and neurological disorders. A clinical study of 35 patients with Waldenstrom's macroglobulinemia examined the relationship of this disease state with whole blood viscosity. Most symptomatic patients had high shear whole blood viscosity from 8 to 15 cP, whereas asymptomatic patients had whole blood viscosity from 3 to 6 cP [91]. The study indicated that when plasma concentration of total proteins was greater than 9 g/100dL, the increase of whole blood viscosity was particularly pronounced in the presence of low-molecular weight IgG and IgA paraproteins [20,92].

15. History of Preeclampsia

Elevated whole blood viscosity is a prominent feature of preeclampsia, and monitoring whole blood viscosity may have clinical applicability in managing patients with this condition [93].

To examine the hypothesis that changes in whole blood viscosity were related to fetal or maternal complications, a study of 228 pregnant women assigned subjects to one of four groups, according to maximum diastolic pressure. The study found significantly higher whole blood viscosity values in the groups with higher blood pressure. Low-shear whole blood viscosity, independent of elevated blood pressure, was significantly associated with unfavorable fetal outcomes [94].

16. Postmenopause

In results from the Framingham study, the risk of cardiovascular disease increased in postmenopausal women. In contrast, among the group of 2873 women who were followed over a period of 24 years, none of the premenopausal women had a heart attack or died from coronary heart disease. Other research has shown that compared to premenopausal women, postmenopausal women had higher whole blood viscosity, plasma viscosity, hematocrit, and fibrinogen as well as lower red blood cell deformability. Additional cardiovascular risk factors such as total cholesterol, triglycerides, uric acid, fasting glucose, and fibrinogen were higher, but HDL-C lower, after menopause.

Regarding the nature of this phenomenon, Kameneva hypothesized that the regular monthly bleeding of premenopausal females improved the blood flow properties of their blood and was responsible for the fact that their risk for cardiovascular diseases was lower than that of men at any age [95]—specifically, the reduced concentration of red blood cells in premenopausal women, the higher proportion of younger red blood cells, and a lower proportion of older red blood cells in the premenopausal women [95]. The increased ratio of younger to older red blood cells is responsible for the differences in the mechanical properties of blood [95]. By extension of this hypothesis, the loss of menses, either surgical or hormonal, may explain the drastic alterations in risk factors.

HEMORHEOLOGIC THERAPIES

Phlebotomy

Therapeutic phlebotomy is one of medicine's oldest remedies and has been practiced by almost every culture in the world. It was still being used as recently as the nineteenth century for hypervolemic conditions such as acute congestive heart failure and preeclampsia [96]. Although it remains an integral component of the management of certain conditions such as polycythemia vera and hereditary hemochromatosis [97–99], in recent times, many have come to regard therapeutic phlebotomy as an outmoded concept belonging to a bygone era. Blood viscosity increases with hematocrit at all levels of hematocrit. However, blood viscosity increases almost exponentially with hematocrit and faster when Hct is greater than 50%, particularly the low-shear blood viscosity. Thus, when one removes 450 mL of blood, the benefit of phlebotomy will be greater in terms of the percentage of reduced blood viscosity if the initial, pretreatment hematocrit is relatively high. For example, one would expect a greater fall in blood viscosity in polycythemic subjects [100].

Phlebotomy reduces hematocrit, which has been shown to be a risk factor for atherosclerosis in the Framingham study [101]. However, the effect of bloodletting on hematocrit lasts only for days to a maximum of a few weeks [102]. Since phlebotomy reduces hematocrit, it also reduces whole blood viscosity because hematocrit is a primary determinant of blood viscosity. However, while the hematocrit reduction induced by a phlebotomy is relatively short lived, the reduction in blood viscosity as a result of phlebotomy tends to last much longer [103]. That is due to the fact that the phlebotomy replaces a part of old erythrocytes with new ones, and the life of the new erythrocytes is about 120 days. Red blood cells grow stiffer and less deformable with age, and reduced erythrocyte deformability is another major factor contributing to changes in blood viscosity [104]. In essence, younger red blood cells are softer and make blood thinner for an extended period of time [105]. Evidence that blood loss has a marked influence on the rheological properties of blood was demonstrated in a study comparing rheological variables in men and age-matched premenopausal women [95]. Compared with men, age-matched premenopausal women had significantly lower blood viscosity, hematocrit, and red blood cell aggregation and rigidity, which, as the study authors postulated, was a result of menstrual blood loss of approximately 50–100 mL per cycle. There was no significant difference in plasma viscosity between the genders in this study. Similarly, a study in healthy blood donors reported significantly lower blood viscosity values measured across a range of shear rates in females in comparison with age-matched males [106].

It is important to identify that phlebotomy is a process that does not hemoconcentrate the blood. Blood donations of 450 mL were observed to lead to immediate and significant reductions in both hematocrit and plasma viscosity in a study involving 42 elderly blood donors, a phenomenon that was attributed to rapid fluid shifts taking place during the bloodletting process [107]. The reduced total blood volume during bloodletting decreases intravascular hydrostatic pressure at the microvessels, while the osmotic pressure remains relatively unchanged. Thus, the balance between the two pressures is disrupted, forcing water influx to the intravascular space until fluid shift restores the balance between the two forces. Accordingly, plasma viscosity has been reported to decrease after phlebotomy [107].

There exists a widespread conviction that the more iron in the diet the better. This general premise is informed by centuries of physician experience with treatment malnutrition and iron-deficiency anemia; this point of view is still found in most medical textbooks [108]. However, in the context of the chronic inflammatory diseases that trend in industrialized countries, excess iron is known to be one of the major contributing causes of ischemic heart disease [109]. Since cardiovascular mortality was correlated with liver iron using published data from 11 countries, Yuan and Li proposed that redox-active iron in tissue was the atherogenic portion of total iron stores [110]. Separately, the effect of phlebotomy on the oxidation resistance of serum lipoprotein was also investigated in 14 Finnish men with raised serum ferritin concentrations [111]. After phlebotomy of 500 ml of blood three times in 14 weeks, serum ferritin concentration was reduced from 209 to 74 micro g/L with no change in serum iron.

Despite the prevailing view that therapeutic phlebotomy is largely an outmoded form of treatment belonging to a past era, interest in this approach as a practical and safe method of accomplishing hypovolemic hemodilution has been rekindled by reports of its benefits in improving blood rheological parameters and studies linking bloodletting with a reduction in the risk of cardiovascular disease. Phlebotomy has been shown to have a marked influence on the rheological properties of blood by significantly lowering blood viscosity, plasma viscosity, hematocrit, and fibrinogen, and there is a relationship between elevated blood viscosity and the occurrence of major cardiovascular events, underscoring the therapeutic potential phlebotomy in lowering the risk of cardiovascular disease. The Kuopio (Finland) Ischaemic Heart Disease Risk Factor study of 2682 men aged 42–60 years found that those who had donated blood showed a significantly reduced risk of myocardial infarction over a follow-up period of 5.5 years compared with nondonors ($p < 0.001$) [112]. Although the findings of this study have been questioned on the basis of their statistical significance and possible selection bias [113], a follow-up report by the investigators confirmed the association between a reduced risk of myocardial infarction and blood donation in middle-aged men (relative hazard = 0.12, 95% CI 0.02–0.86; $p = 0.035$) [102]. Frequent blood loss through voluntary donation has been highlighted for its important protective effect against the occurrence of myocardial infarction in this population.

This perspective is supported by the finding of a reduced incidence of cardiovascular events such as myocardial infarction, angina, and stroke and a reduced requirement for procedures such as percutaneous transluminal coronary angioplasty (PTCA) and coronary artery bypass surgery (CABG) in blood donors in comparison with nondonors, principally in men. Thus far, women have not been shown to benefit significantly from blood donation in terms of a decreased incidence of cardiovascular events, although in a key study [114] reporting the absence of a significant benefit in females, regular menstrual blood loss may have been an important factor. Nevertheless, the available data suggest that regular withdrawal of relatively small amounts of blood (i.e., < 250 ml) will lead to positive benefits in reducing the risk of cardiovascular disease, and that this safe and effective procedure can be considered alongside other risk-modifying measures such as treatment of high blood pressure or elevated plasma lipids in at-risk individuals.

The availability of technology capable of measuring blood viscosity across a range of shear rates is a valuable aid to cardiovascular risk profiling, as viscosity monitoring has the potential to provide early warning of an increased risk of atherosclerosis, and permits an assessment of the risk of plaque rupture and erosion. Rheological profiling of patients may help to identify those who can benefit from regular therapeutic phlebotomy.

Hemodilution

While related to therapeutic phlebotomy, hemodilution is a separate treatment modality that has been shown to reduce risk profiles in cardiovascular disease, subsequently improving or preventing ischemia. The three principal forms of hemodilution are as follows: hypovolemic hemodilution, isovolumic hemodilution, and hypervolemic hemodilution [115]. A critical consideration that the clinician must take into account in performing hemodilution is the patient's volume balance in order to determine which type of hemodilution should be utilized. Hypovolemic hemodilution, secondary to therapeutic phlebotomy, can be used to treat patients with overt hypervolemia. Typical candidates for this type of hemodilution would be patients with congestive heart failure, secondary parathyroidism, obstructive lung disease, polycythemia, early cirrhosis, and early dementia (if not anemic). Isovolumic hemodilution maintains a fairly constant blood volume balance through a combination of therapeutic phlebotomy and volume-repletion infusion therapy. Typical plasma substitute and repletion consist of albumin, amino acids, Dextran 40 (40,000 Daltons) and Dextran 70 (70,000 Daltons), and hydroxyethylstarch (HES) 200,000 and 450,000 Daltons. Hypervolemic hemodilution is primarily used during bypass surgery. Postbypass patients typically leave the hospital with hematocrit at or near 29, which translates to a one-third reduction in the work of the heart compared with the time when the patient's preoperative hematocrit of > 40. Autologous blood donation is routinely performed prior to surgery.

PHARMACOLOGIC TREATMENT

Hyperviscosity syndromes can be treated using active pharmaceutical agents. This section provides an overview of several different molecules and drug classes that have been reported to have anti-viscogenic effects.

Pentoxifylline (oxpentifylline)

This xanthine derivative is indicated for claudication, and although it has been reported to reduce blood viscosity, there are conflicting reports on this effect. Because it is the most widely recognized and broadly cited in the pharmaceutical community as a viscosity-lowering drug, it is helpful to provide a detailed review of the literature herein. Pentoxifylline has been shown in six different peer-reviewed studies to reduce blood viscosity [116–121]. In six other peer-reviewed studies, pentoxifylline was demonstrated to increase blood viscosity or have no effect on blood viscosity [122–127]. In three other publications, the compound was shown to have a mixed effect or an unclear rheological effect.

The increase of erythrocyte deformability is pentoxifylline's proposed mechanism of action, which has not yet been clearly validated and continues to be subject to debate. Pentoxifylline has been demonstrated to increase the filterability of the red blood cell, and this effect was thought to be a function of increased deformability of the red blood cells [119]. This increase would be expected to cause a resultant reduction in viscosity, most notably at systole—or at high shear rate. Other studies have demonstrated a decrease in viscosity at low shear rates, leading to the hypothesis that fibrinogen levels may also be reduced. Data have been generated in some studies supporting this hypothesis, but in others, no change in fibrinogen levels was detected [116,119]. Length of observation period, dosage, and the means of administration were widely different amongst these cited studies and were therefore likely to have played a role in the differing conclusions. Equally important, these studies focused their investigations on subjects in a variety of differing disease states, and this would also be expected to have played a role in the outcomes.

Statins

The correlations between blood viscosity and LDL cholesterol have been discussed previously in this chapter. Various lipid-lowering agents have, in turn, been shown to be antiviscogenic. The statin drugs in particular have been reported to lower blood viscosity. In subjects with familiar hypercholesterolemia, pravastatin has been demonstrated to have a significant blood viscosity lowering effect [128]. In addition, lovastatin was also shown to reduce blood viscosity after three months of treatment [129]. A separate clinical study found that after three months of treatment, lovastatin reduced both plasma viscosity and erythrocyte aggregation [130]. Neither of these studies observed any significant effect of statin on fibrinogen levels.

A 2003 study of patients with hypercholesterolemia showed that low-dose administration of atorvastatin for four weeks reduced low-shear blood viscosity by a mean of 16%. Atorvastatin at the administered dose reduced total cholesterol levels and LDL levels by 25% and 24%, respectively. It is reasonable to surmise that these changes were connected to the 16% mean reduction in low-shear blood viscosity observed in this study [131]. Lowering the LDL cholesterol concentration in the blood works to reduce blood viscosity by individually altering its major determinants, namely plasma viscosity, red cell rigidity, and aggregation. Therefore, certain statin medications may be acting to reduce the risk of atherosclerotic disease and acute cardiovascular events through their positive effects on LDL by improving blood rheology. The antiviscogenic effect would, by definition, improve microcirculation and tissue-level perfusion, attenuating systemic and focal ischemia.

Antiplatelet Agents

Various studies have examined the effect of aspirin on blood viscosity and suggested that aspirin may have a viscosity-lowering effect [132,133]. However, the most authoritative study on the effect of aspirin on blood viscosity was a randomized, double-blind, placebo-controlled study of 100 healthy, nonsmoking, normolipidemic adult males, using an automated scanning capillary viscometer. This instrument measured blood viscosity values at 10,000 different shear rates in increments of $0.1s^{-1}$ for each blood sample. The study showed that aspirin had no significant effect on blood viscosity [134]. Using the same automated scanning capillary viscometer, aspirin plus dipyridamole (Aggrenox) was shown to be more effective than aspirin alone in reducing low-shear blood viscosity in patients with hyperhomocystemia and stable cardiovascular disease [135]. The dipyridamole study was performed as a mechanistic follow-up study to the European/Australasian Stroke Prevention in Reversible Ischemia Trial (ESPRIT), a randomized controlled trial that reported combination aspirin/dipyridamole reduced composite vascular events including mortality after ischemic stroke as compared with aspirin monotherapy [136].

Separately, clopidogrel has been demonstrated to reduce low-shear blood viscosity values by 12%, 12%, and 18% on average from baseline levels one, two, and three weeks after administration, respectively [137]. High-shear blood viscosity values were also reduced 10% from baseline after the third week (all p values < 0.01). These findings were based on a double-blind, placebo-controlled study of 30 age- and gender-matched individuals with impaired blood viscosity and instrumental evidence of carotid and/or femoral atherosclerosis. Fibrinogen levels did not change from baseline at any of the time points in this study.

Other Pharmaceutical Agents

Streptokinase and recombinant tissue plasminogen activator were both shown to lower blood viscosity in patients with acute myocardial infarction [138]. Acipimox, a niacin analogue, was previously shown to reduce blood viscosity at both high and low shear rates in 21 subjects with hypertriglyceridemia (p < 0.05 and p < 0.01, respectively). The range of reduction in viscosity was 6–20% and was not related to changes in plasma triglycerides [139].

Because fibrinogen concentration is another major determinant of blood viscosity, defibrinating agents have long held some promise as a pharmaceutical target mechanism for lower blood viscosity. Ancrod, batroxobin, and crotalase are defibrinating enzymes extracted from three different venomous snakes, which have been shown to have powerful antiviscogenic effects [140]. Their mechanism of action involves stimulating phospholipase A2.

NUTRITIONAL INTERVENTIONS

Hydration

Dehydration has been underappreciated as a cause of hospitalization and increased hospital-associated mortality in older people. In 1991, 6.7% (731,695) of Medicare hospitalizations had dehydration listed as one of the five reported diagnoses, a rate of 236.2 per 10,000 elderly Medicare beneficiaries. Medicare reimbursed over $446 million for hospitalizations with dehydration as the principal diagnosis. Older people, men, and African Americans had elevated risks for hospitalization with dehydration. About 50% of elderly Medicare beneficiaries hospitalized with dehydration died within a year of admission [141]. Dehydration can increase whole blood viscosity as well as plasma viscosity, fibrinogen, and hematocrit, all of which are risk factors for coronary heart disease, as previously discussed. By definition, blood viscosity is a measure of hemoconcentration and can serve as an effective index for hydration status. In a six-year study of 8,280 men and 12,017 women who were without heart disease, stroke, or diabetes at baseline found five or more glasses of water per day were associated with a lower risk of fatal coronary heart disease than two or fewer glasses of water per day [142].

Oral Rehydration Solutions

Research published in 2004 showed that dehydration increases high-shear blood viscosity by 9.3% and low-shear blood viscosity by 12.5% [143]. The results are from a study of 12 healthy men who sat for four hours in a room with a dry-bulb temperature of 23.0–23.5°C and a relative humidity of 18–36%. The purpose of the study was to assess the effects of prehydration with water and an electrolyte-glucose beverage in comparison with control subjects who did not ingest either fluid prior to the study. Blood viscosity and plasma volume were measured every hour (including baseline prior to hydration), and routine laboratory hematological tests, urine volume, and body weight were recorded at two and four hours. At time points one, two, three, and four hours from baseline, control subjects had high-shear blood viscosity increases of 3.3, 9.3, 6.8, and 9.3% and low-shear blood viscosity increases of 3.0, 10.9, 6.8, and 12.5%. These increases were slightly attenuated in the subjects given water, demonstrating high-shear blood viscosity increases of 1.9, 4.6, 4.7, and 3.0% and low-shear blood viscosity increases of 4.6, 4.9, 7.3, and 5.4%. The electrolyte beverage was more effective than water in mitigating the harmful effects of dehydration, almost negating any viscosity increases at all. These subjects had high-shear blood viscosity increases of -0.7, 1.1, -1.1, and 3.1% and low-shear blood viscosity increases of 4.2, 1.4, 1.0, and 5.6% from baseline. The study is of interest because dehydration is a common condition that can exacerbate the potential for developing deep vein thrombosis and/or pulmonary embolism. Factors that can cause dehydration during air travel include consumption of diuretic beverages containing alcohol or caffeine, mild hypoxia, and increased evaporative water loss due to low humidity of the air in the cabin.

Eicosapentaenoic Acid

Fish oil supplements have been shown in a double-blind, randomized study to lower high-shear blood viscosity and low-shear blood viscosity, both by 15%. Five capsules were given twice daily for seven weeks (1.8 g/day), and blood viscosity tests were performed at the beginning of the study and at the end of seven weeks of supplementation [144].

No significant changes were observed in hematocrit or plasma viscosity despite the blood viscosity reductions of 15%, suggesting that the benefit of fish oil supplements to circulatory health may be due, at least in part, to increases of eicosapentaenoic acid (EPA) content in red cell membranes, which in turn reduce blood viscosity. Dietary supplementation with omega-3 fatty acids or fish oil has been previously shown to be effective in prevention of cardiovascular events. One major study of 11,324 patients following a recent heart attack showed that fish oil supplements reduced the incidence of death, cardiovascular death, and sudden cardiac death by 20%, 30%, and 45%, respectively [145].

Although the omega-3 fatty acid EPA may be the primary fat in fish oil to reduce blood viscosity, EPA should only be supplemented in conjunction with docosahexaenoic acid (DHA), also found in fish oil. In some clinical situations, the omega-6 fatty acid precursor of the prostaglandin 1 series gamma-linolenic acid (GLA) may also need to be supplemented. Algae such as chlorella species are a nonanimal derived source of both EPA/DHA and vitamin B12.

Proteolytic Enzymes

Therapies with applied proteolyitc enzymes are among the oldest methods of therapy known to humans. The application of masticated plant material has been mentioned in ancient descriptions and documents. Natives of Middle and South America used the leaves and fruits of the papaya tree (*Carica papaya*) or parts of the pineapple (*Bromeliaceae*) for cleaning poorly healing wounds. Even today, the local application of enzymatic preparations remains one of the most tried and tested treatment modalities in various areas of medicine. Topical application and oral ingestion of active ingredients supports the natural enzymatic degradation and subsequent absorption of cellular material that has become necrotic, and thereby promotes the healing of the ulcerated tissue. In today's industrialized food industry, enzyme activity is not preserved and devitalized foods are more commonplace in comparison to the traditional and native diets of our ancestors.

The introduction of oral substitution of pancreatic enzymes to treat disturbed endocrine activities began around 1900. The predecessors of our modern day endocrinology called organotherapy, implemented intravenous, peritumoral, and oral application of pancreatic enzymes such as pancreatin, trypsin, chymotrypsin, lipase, and amylase, to obtain an arrest or retrogression of cancerous growth. The intestinal efficacy of orally applied digestive enzymes, especially in regards to preservation in the environment of the gastric secretions and optimal release in the small intestine, has been refined by the development of modern galenic methods.

The influence of proteolytic enzymes or systemic enzyme therapy on coagulation and on the improvement of blood rheology is well documented [146–149]. Systemic enzyme therapy improves the circulation and supply of oxygen to tissues by (1) degrading fibrinogen, soluble fibrin monomers, and other globular serum proteins such as alpha-2 macroglobulin; and (2) improving red blood deformability. The use of oral administration in the treatment of venous disorders, arterial occlusive disease, and deep vein thrombosis as a prophylactic agent has been proven in clinical studies.

Patients with malignancy or chronic inflammatory diseases are at an increased incidence of thromboembolic complications. In these incidences, concentrations of fibrinogen and fibrin and fibrinolytic serum activity are elevated [150,151]. Oral and rectal applications of Wobenzym combinations increase proteolytic serum activity and reduce the risk of complications in thrombophilic patients [152]. In vitro results of nattokinase, a serine endopeptidase, showed a significant, dose-dependent decrease of erythrocyte aggregation and low-shear viscosity, with these beneficial effects evident at concentrations similar to those achieved in previous in vivo animal trials [153]. The preliminary data thus indicate positive in vitro hemorheological effects of nattokinase [154], suggesting its potential value as a therapeutic agent and the need for additional studies and clinical trials [155]. In a double-blind, crossover study comparing preparations of Wobenzym with placebo, the application of Wobenzym resulted in a substantial reduction of the blood viscosity, plasma viscosity, and the red blood cell aggregation. The overall ability of the blood to flow was improved with the administration of Wobenzym [156].

In a recent human clinical trial, supplemental nattokinase was found to reduce levels of fibrinogen by 7–10%, factor VII by 7–14%, and factor VIII by 17–19% within two months. The researchers noted the potential of nattokinase for improving circulation and reducing the risk of cardiovascular disease [157,158,159].

Dietary sources of proteolytic enzymes are primarily from fresh and fermented foods. Bromelain is a proteolytic enzyme found in fresh but not processed pineapple, mango, and papaya. As a way of illustrating this point, note that it is the bromelain that breaks down gelatin, the reason why only processed pineapple is used in gelatin salads. Fermented foods high in proteolytic enzymes include soy sauce, tempura, natto (source of nattokinase), and fermented fish. Supplemental enzymes and glandular dietary supplements derived from organ meats also are sources considered beneficial in certain disease states and with diets lacking fresh and fermented foods. Nattokinase and lumbroki-nase are available as dietary supplements and clinical trials described here support their use in some patients with cardiovascular disease.

Phospholipids

A highly purified fraction of soybean phosphatidyl choline sometimes called essential phospholip-ids (EPL) has been tested in vitro, to decrease platelet sensitivity to promoting aggregation. As refer-enced in *Phosphatidylcholine: Biochemical and Clinical Aspects of Essential Phospholipids* [160], the therapeutic application of EPL demonstrated enhanced blood flow properties and improved microcirculation [161,162]. Whether these results are directly and/or indirectly determinant upon EPL's favorable influences on increasing HDL and lowering LDL-C is not readily apparent. One ref-erence suggests increased red blood cell deformability secondary to use of EPL and citing over 60 various types of phosphatidyl choline within the RBC membrane [163]. Researchers have suggested the possible exchange of membrane phospholipids containing saturated fatty acids and facilitated filtration of RBCs and improved deformability [164].

The essential component, that which is dependent on dietary intake, is choline. Dietary sources of choline include egg yolks, nuts, seeds, and organ meats. Cholecystectomy and some gastrointestinal conditions require increased dietary intake to compensate for decreased absorption of this nutrient. Deficiency states are likely given the U.S. national statistics that choline intake has declined [165].

CLINICAL SUMMARY

Blood viscosity is a biophysical parameter that unifies the risk factors for cardiovascular disease, insofar as blood viscosity has been shown to correlate with all of the conventional cardiovascular risk factors and, at the same time, is able to clearly elucidate the site and region specificity of ath-erosclerotic lesions. Because blood is shear thinning, its viscosity is not a static quantity. Rather, the viscosity of blood is changing within the human body depending on blood flow velocity and vessel diameter— a characteristic that underscores the large dynamic range of clinical blood viscosity data as well as its utility as a means for patient stratification.

Clinicians may be able to refer their patients for assessment of blood viscosity in the future. Currently this testing is limited to research. However, a clinical suspicion of elevated blood viscos-ity can be made based on the presence of risk factors.

Some risk factors such as atherosclerosis, insulin resistance and diabetes, obesity, macular degeneration, hypertension, and physical inactivity can be modified with nutrition and lifestyle interventions. In so doing, blood viscosity improves commensurately.

In addition to the treatment of risk factors, antiviscogenic therapies are available. These include hematologic, pharmacologic, and nutritional interventions. Nutritional interventions are several:

- Hydration with water, electrolyte, or oral rehydration solutions, specifically those that do not pose a significant increase in caloric intake.
- Fish oil supplementation at 1 gram a day. Dietary and algal sources of EPA/DHA are also available.
- Proteolytic enzymes can be derived from increased dietary intake of fresh tropical fruits containing bromelain and fermented soy products. For some patients, supplementation with nattokinase or lumbrokinase may be indicated and can be initiated as follows: nattokinase,

6,000 fibrinolytic degradation units (FUs) daily divided into three to four doses for optimal serum activity.

- Increased dietary intake of choline-rich foods is merited. In 1998, the U.S. Institute of Medicine's Food and Nutrition Board established an adequate intake (AI) and a tolerable upper limit (UL) for choline. The AI is 425 and 550 mg/d for women and men, respectively, with more recommended during pregnancy and lactation [166]. Supplemental phosphatidyl choline may be of added benefit, and it is of note that a common gene polymorphism makes choline biosynthesis unresponsive to estrogen, suggesting women's dietary choline intake be comparable to men's requirements [167,168]. Therapeutic doses of phosphatidyl choline > 55% liposomal form (not triple lecithin) are 10 grams daily.

Future clinical applications for blood viscosity are many, for example:

- The treatment and monitoring of whole blood viscosity opens a new horizon of pharmaceutical agents acting as antiviscogenic agents that prevent or reverse elevated whole blood viscosity in the earliest stages of the disease.
- Presurgical screening of elective surgical patients for elevated whole blood viscosity may apprise the surgeon of high-risk patients for postsurgical deep vein thrombosis.
- Hydration status of surgical patients could be monitored by the anesthesiologist during prolonged surgeries and volume replacement could be adjusted and titrated to minimize renal insufficiencies, cerebrovascular and cardiac complications, and management of hypertension.
- Monitoring of whole blood viscosity in diabetic and dialysis patients may direct treatment to minimize the expansion of microvascular disease.

REFERENCES

1. Heberden, W., *Some account of a disorder of breast.* Medical Transactions, 1772. **2**: p. 59–67.
2. Warren, J., *Remarks on angina pectoris.* New England Journal of Medicine, Surgery and Collateral Branches of Science, 1812. **1**(1): p. 1–11.
3. Parry, C. H., *An Inquiry Into the Symptoms and Causes of the Syncope Anginosa: Commonly Called Angina Pectoris.* 1799, London: R. Cruttwell.
4. Hektoen, L., *Embolism of left coronary artery; sudden death.* Med Newsl (Lond), 1892. **61**: p. 210.
5. Kannel, W. B., et al., *Factors of risk in the development of coronary heart disease—Six-year follow-up experience.* Annals of Internal Medicine, 1961. **55**(1): p. 33.
6. GISSI, *Effectiveness of intravenous thrombolytic treatment in acute myocardial infarction.* Lancet, 1986. **1**: p. 397–402.
7. Grines, C. L., et al., *A comparison of immediate angioplasty with thrombolytic therapy for acute myocardial infarction.* New England Journal of Medicine, 1993. **328**(10): p. 673–79.
8. Furchgott, R. F., and J. V. Zawadzki, *The obligatory role of endothelial cells in the relaxation of arterial smooth muscle by acetylcholine.* Nature, 1980. **288**(5789): p. 373–76.
9. Fuster, V., *The Vulnerable Atherosclerotic Plaque: Understanding, Identification, and Modification.* American Heart Association, Monograph Series, ed. V. Fuster. 1998, Armonk, NY: Futura Publishing Company, Inc.
10. Hopkins, P. N., *A survey of 246 suggested coronary risk factors.* Atherosclerosis, 1981. **40**: p. 1–52.
11. Hopkins, P., and R. Williams, *Identification and relative weight of cardiovascular risk factors.* Cardiology Clinics, 1986. **4**(1): p. 3.
12. Sloop, G. D., *A unifying theory of atherogenesis.* Med Hypotheses, 1996. **47**(4): p. 321–25.
13. Kensey K. R., and Y. I. Cho. *The Origin of Atherosclerosis: What Really Initiates the Inflammatory Process.* 2nd Ed. 2007, Lewiston, NY: EPP Medica.
14. Kwaan, H. C., and A. Bongu, *The hyperviscosity syndromes.* Semin Thromb Hemost, 1999. **25**(2): p. 199–208.
15. Krol, T. C., and W. S. Wood, *Hyperviscosity syndrome in Waldenstrom's macroglobulinemia.* Am Fam Physician, 1981. **24**(2): p. 187–89.

16. Kwaan, H. C., and J. Wang, *Hyperviscosity in polycythemia vera and other red cell abnormalities.* Semin Thromb Hemost, 2003. **29**(5): p. 451–58.

17. Proctor, S., et al., *Hyperviscosity syndrome in IgE myeloma.* British Medical Journal (Clinical research ed.), 1984. **289**(6452): p. 1112.

18. Baer, M. R., R. S. Stein, and E. N. Dessypris, *Chronic lymphocytic leukemia with hyperleukocytosis. The hyperviscosity syndrome.* Cancer, 1985. **56**(12): p. 2865–69.

19. Cocklet, G. R., and H. J. Meiselman, *Blood Rheology,* in *Handbook of Hemorheology and Hemodynamics,* ed. O. K. Baskurt, M. R. Hardeman, M. W. Rampling, H. J. Meiselman. 2007, Washington, DC: IOS Press, p. 45–71.

20. Stoltz, J. F., M. Singh, and P. Riha, *Hemorheology in Practice.* 1999, Washington, DC: IOS Press.

21. Baskurt, O. K., and H. J. Meiselman, *Blood rheology and hemodynamics.* Semin Thromb Hemost, 2003. **29**(5): p. 435–50.

22. Bachorik, P. S., R. I. Levy, and B. M. Rifkind, *Lipids and dyslipoproteinemia,* in *Clinical Diagnosis and Management by Laboratory Methods,* ed. J. B. Henry. 2001, Philadelphia: Saunders, p. 1–2.

23. Sloop, G. D., and D. E. Mercante, *Opposite effects of low-density and high-density lipoprotein on blood viscosity in fasting subjects.* Clin Hemorheol Microcirc, 1998. **19**(3): p. 197–203.

24. Jax, T. W., et al., *Cardiovascular diabetology.* Cardiovascular Diabetology, 2009. **8**: p. 48.

25. Cecchi, E., et al., *Hyperviscosity as a possible risk factor for cerebral ischemic complications in atrial fibrillation patients.* Am J Cardiol, 2006. **97**(12): p. 1745–48.

26. Devereux, R. B., et al., *Possible role of increased blood viscosity in the hemodynamics of systemic hypertension.* Am J Cardiol, 2000. **85**(10): p. 1265–68.

27. Sloop, G. D., and D.W. Garber, *The effects of low-density lipoprotein and high-density lipoprotein on blood viscosity correlate with their association with risk of atherosclerosis in humans.* Clin Sci (Lond), 1997. **92**(5): p. 473–79.

28. Rosenson, R. S., A. McCormick, and E. F. Uretz, *Distribution of blood viscosity values and biochemical correlates in healthy adults.* Clin Chem, 1996. **42**(8 Pt 1): p. 1189–95.

29. Fowkes, F. G., et al., *The relationship between blood viscosity and blood pressure in a random sample of the population aged 55 to 74 years.* Eur Heart J, 1993. **14**(5): p. 597–601.

30. Smith, W. C., et al., *Rheological determinants of blood pressure in a Scottish adult population.* J Hypertens, 1992. **10**(5): p. 467–72.

31. de Simone, G., et al., *Relation of blood viscosity to demographic and physiologic variables and to cardiovascular risk factors in apparently normal adults.* Circulation, 1990. **81**(1): p. 107–17.

32. Ernst, E., et al., *Blood rheology in healthy cigarette smokers. Results from the MONICA project, Augsburg.* Arteriosclerosis, 1988. **8**(4): p. 385–88.

33. Levenson, J., et al., *Cigarette smoking and hypertension. Factors independently associated with blood hyperviscosity and arterial rigidity.* Arteriosclerosis, 1987. **7**(6): p. 572–77.

34. Ernst, E., et al., *Cardiovascular risk factors and hemorheology. Physical fitness, stress and obesity.* Atherosclerosis, 1986. **59**(3): p. 263–69.

35. Letcher, R. L., et al., *Elevated blood viscosity in patients with borderline essential hypertension.* Hypertension, 1983. **5**(5): p. 757–62.

36. Danesh, J., et al., *Haematocrit, viscosity, erythrocyte sedimentation rate: Meta-analyses of prospective studies of coronary heart disease.* Eur Heart J, 2000. **21**(7): p. 515–20.

37. Ciuffetti, G., et al., *Prognostic impact of low-shear whole blood viscosity in hypertensive men.* Eur J Clin Invest, 2005. **35**(2): p. 93–98.

38. Koenig, W., et al., *Plasma viscosity and the risk of coronary heart disease: Results from the MONICA-Augsburg Cohort Study, 1984 to 1992.* Arteriosclerosis, Thrombosis, and Vascular Biology, 1998. **18**(5): p. 768–72.

39. Lowe, G. D., et al., *Blood viscosity and risk of cardiovascular events: The Edinburgh Artery Study.* Br J Haematol, 1997. **96**(1): p. 168–73.

40. Zarins, C. K., et al., *Carotid bifurcation atherosclerosis. Quantitative correlation of plaque localization with flow velocity profiles and wall shear stress.* Circulation Research, 1983. **53**(4): p. 502–14.

41. Davies, P. F., *Hemodynamic shear stress and the endothelium in cardiovascular pathophysiology.* Nature Clinical Practice Cardiovascular Medicine, 2008. **6**(1): p. 16–26.

42. Malek, A. M., S. L. Alper, and S. Izumo, *Hemodynamic shear stress and its role in atherosclerosis.* JAMA, 1999. **282**(21): p. 2035–42.

43. Langille, B. L., and F. O'Donnell, *Reductions in arterial diameter produced by chronic decreases in blood flow are endothelium-dependent.* Science, 1986. **231**(4736): p. 405.

44. White, C. R., and J. A. Frangos, *The shear stress of it all: The cell membrane and mechanochemical transduction.* Philos Trans R Soc Lond B Biol Sci, 2007. **362**(1484): p. 1459–67.

45. Chachisvilis, M., Y. L. Zhang, and J. A. Frangos, *G protein-coupled receptors sense fluid shear stress in endothelial cells.* Proceedings of the National Academy of Sciences, 2006. **103**(42): p. 15463–68.

46. Eng, E., and B. J. Ballermann, *Diminished NF-[kappa] B activation and PDGF-B expression in glomerular endothelial cells subjected to chronic shear stress.* Microvascular Research, 2003. **65**(3): p. 137–44.

47. Li, Y. S., J. H. Haga, and S. Chien, *Molecular basis of the effects of shear stress on vascular endothelial cells.* J Biomech, 2005. **38**(10): p. 1949–71.

48. Dardik, A., et al., *Shear stress-stimulated endothelial cells induce smooth muscle cell chemotaxis via platelet-derived growth factor-BB and interleukin-1 [alpha].* Journal of Vascular Surgery, 2005. **41**(2): p. 321–31.

49. Malek, A. M., et al., *Induction of nitric oxide synthase mRNA by shear stress requires intracellular calcium and G-protein signals and is modulated by PI 3 kinase.* Biochemical and Biophysical Research Communications, 1999. **254**(1): p. 231–42.

50. Dardik, A., et al., *Differential effects of orbital and laminar shear stress on endothelial cells.* Journal of Vascular Surgery, 2005. **41**(5): p. 869–80.

51. Glagov, S., et al., *Hemodynamics and atherosclerosis. Insights and perspectives gained from studies of human arteries.* Arch Pathol Lab Med, 1988. **112**(10): p. 1018–31.

52. Chien, S., *Mechanotransduction and endothelial cell homeostasis: The wisdom of the cell.* Am J Physiol Heart Circ Physiol, 2007. **292**(3): p. H1209–24.

53. Frangos, S. G., V. Gahtan, and B. Sumpio, *Localization of atherosclerosis: Role of hemodynamics.* Arch Surg, 1999. **134**(10): p. 1142–49.

54. Lee, A. J., et al., *Blood viscosity and elevated carotid intima-media thickness in men and women: The Edinburgh Artery Study.* Circulation, 1998. **97**(15): p. 1467–73.

55. Burton-Opitz, R., *A Textbook of Physiology for Students and Practitioners of Medicine.* 1920, Philadelphia, PA: WB Saunders.

56. Burton-Opitz, R., *The viscosity of the blood.* Journal of the American Medical Association, 1911. **57**(5): p. 353–58.

57. Zhu, W., et al., *Association of hyperviscosity and subclinical atherosclerosis in obese schoolchildren.* Eur J Pediatr, 2005. **164**(10): p. 639–45.

58. Ernst, E., et al., *Hyperviscosity. An independent risk factor after a survived stroke.* Acta Med Austriaca, 1991. **18 Suppl 1**: p. 32–36.

59. Coull, B. M., et al., *Chronic blood hyperviscosity in subjects with acute stroke, transient ischemic attack, and risk factors for stroke.* Stroke, 1991. **22**(2): p. 162–68.

60. Resch, K. L., et al., *Can rheologic variables be of prognostic relevance in arteriosclerotic diseases?* Angiology, 1991. **42**(12): p. 963–70.

61. Gudmundsson, M., and A. Bjelle, *Plasma, serum and whole-blood viscosity variations with age, sex, and smoking habits.* Angiology, 1993. **44**(5): p. 384–91.

62. Lowe, G. D., et al., *The effects of age and cigarette-smoking on blood and plasma viscosity in men.* Scott Med J, 1980. **25**(1): p. 13–17.

63. Ernst, E., et al., *Dose-effect relationship between smoking and blood rheology.* Br J Haematol, 1987. **65**(4): p. 485–87.

64. Rothwell, M., et al., *Haemorheological changes in the very short term after abstention from tobacco by cigarette smokers.* British Journal of Haematology, 1991. **79**(3): p. 500–503.

65. Levy, B. I., et al., *Impaired tissue perfusion: A pathology common to hypertension, obesity, and diabetes mellitus.* Circulation, 2008. **118**(9): p. 968–76.

66. Brun, J. F., et al., *The paradox of hematocrit in exercise physiology: Which is the "normal" range from an hemorheologist's viewpoint?* Clin Hemorheol Microcirc, 2000. **22**(4): p. 287–303.

67. Brun, J. F., Khaled, S., et al., *The triphasic effects of exercise on blood rheology: Which relevance to physiology and pathophysiology?* Clin Hemorheol Microcirc, 1998. **19**(2): p. 89–104.

68. Ernst, E. E., and A. Matrai, *Intermittent claudication, exercise, and blood rheology.* Circulation, 1987. **76**(5): p. 1110–14.

69. Crowley, J. P., et al., *Low density lipoprotein cholesterol and whole blood viscosity.* Ann Clin Lab Sci, 1994. **24**(6): p. 533–41.

70. Wannamethee, G., and A. Shaper, *Haematocrit: Rrelationships with blood lipids, blood pressure and other cardiovascular risk factors.* Thrombosis and Haemostasis, 1994. **72**(1): p. 58.

71. Remky, A., et al., *Haemorheology in patients with branch retinal vein occlusion with and without risk factors.* Graefes Arch Clin Exp Ophthalmol, 1996. **234 Suppl 1**: p. S8–12.

72. Klaver, J.H., et al., *Blood and plasma viscosity measurements in patients with glaucoma.* BJO, 1985. **69**(10): p. 765–70.

73. Ridker, P., J. Genest, and P. Libby, *Heart Diseases: Textbook of Cardiovascular Medicine.* 6th ed. *Risk Factors for Artherosclerosclerotic Disease*, ed. E. Braunwald, D. Zipes, and P. Libby. 2001, Philadelphia: W. B. Saunders.

74. Dintenfass, L., *Blood viscosity factors in severe non-diabetic and diabetic retinopathy.* Biorheology, 1977. **14**: p. 151–57.

75. Carroll, S., C. B. Cooke, and R. J. Butterly, *Plasma viscosity, fibrinogen and the metabolic syndrome: Effect of obesity and cardiorespiratory fitness.* Blood Coagulation & Fibrinolysis: An International Journal in Haemostasis and Thrombosis, 2000. **11**(1): p. 71.

76. Yarnell, J. W. G., et al., *Lifestyle and hemostatic risk factors for ischemic heart disease: The Caerphilly Study.* Arteriosclerosis, Thrombosis, and Vascular Biology, 2000. **20**(1): p. 271–79.

77. Tietjen, G. W., et al., *Blood viscosity, plasma proteins, and Raynaud syndrome.* Archives of Surgery, 1975. **110**(11): p. 1343.

78. Alshihabi, S. N., et al., *Shear stress-induced release of PGE2 and PGI2 by vascular smooth muscle cells.* Biochemical and Biophysical Research Communications, 1996. **224**(3): p. 808–14.

79. De la Torre, J. C., and T. Mussivand, *Can disturbed brain microcirculation cause Alzheimer's disease?* Neurological Research, 1993. **15**(3): p. 146.

80. De la Torre, J. C., *Critical threshold cerebral hypoperfusion causes Alzheimer's disease.* Acta Neuropathologica, 1999. **98**(1): p. 1–8.

81. De la Torre, J. C., *Cerebrovascular changes in the aging brain.* Advances in Cell Aging and Gerontology, 1997. **2**: p. 77–107.

82. Solerte, S. B., et al., *Hemorheological changes and overproduction of cytokines from immune cells in mild to moderate dementia of the Alzheimer's type: Adverse effects on cerebromicrovascular system.* Neurobiology of Aging, 2000. **21**(2): p. 271–81.

83. Wen, Z., et al., *A study of hemorheological behaviour for patients with Alzheimer's disease at the early stages.* Clinical Hemorheology and Microcirculation, 2000. **22**(4): p. 261–66.

84. Armani, U., et al., *Evaluation of various hemorheological parameters in nonagenarians: Evidence of an increase of fibrinogen.* Bollettino Della Società Italiana di Biologia Sperimentale, 1990. **66**(10): p. 961.

85. Coppola, L., et al., *Blood viscosity and aging.* Arch Gerontol Geriatr, 2000. **31**(1): p. 35–42.

86. de Simone, G., et al., *Gender differences in left ventricular anatomy, blood viscosity and volume regulatory hormones in normal adults.* Am J Cardiol, 1991. **68**(17): p. 1704–8.

87. Milligan, D.W., et al., *The influence of iron-deficient indices on whole blood viscosity in polycythaemia.* British Journal of Haematology, 1982. **50**(3): p. 467–73.

88. Lichtman, M. A., and J. M. Rowe, *Hyperleukocytic leukemias: Rheological, clinical, and therapeutic considerations.* Blood, 1982. **60**(2): p. 279–83.

89. Chien, S., Sung, K. L., et al., *Theoretical and experimental studies on viscoelastic properties of erythrocyte membrane.* Biophys J, 1978. **24**(2): p. 463–87.

90. Weed, R. I., *The importance of erythrocyte deformability.* American Journal of Medicine, 1970. **49**(2): p. 147–50.

91. MacKenzie, M. R., and T. K. Lee, *Blood viscosity in Waldenstrom macroglobulinemia.* Blood, 1977. **49**(4): p. 507–10.

92. Alexanian, R., *Blood volume in monoclonal gammopathy.* Blood, 1977. **49**(2): p. 301–7.

93. Hobbs, J. B., et al., *Whole blood viscosity in preeclampsia.* Am J Obstet Gynecol, 1982. **142**(3): p. 288–92.

94. Zondervan, H. A., et al., *Maternal whole blood viscosity in pregnancy hypertension.* Gynecol Obstet Invest, 1988. **25**(2): p. 83–88.

95. Kameneva, M. V., M. J. Watach, and H. S. Borovetz, *Gender difference in rheologic properties of blood and risk of cardiovascular diseases.* Clin Hemorheol Microcirc, 1999. **21**(3–4): p. 357–63.

96. Seigworth, G. R., *Bloodletting over the centuries.* New York State Journal of Medicine, 1980. **80**(13): p. 2022.

97. Antle, E. A., *Who needs a therapeutic phlebotomy?* Clin J Oncol Nurs, 2010. **14**(6): p. 694–96.

98. Tefferi, A., *A contemporary approach to the diagnosis and management of polycythemia vera.* Curr Hematol Rep, 2003. **2**(3): p. 237–41.

99. Vautier, G., M. Murray, and J. K. Olynyk, *Hereditary haemochromatosis: Detection and management.* Med J Aust, 2001. **175**(8): p. 418–21.

100. Dayton, L. M., et al., *Symptomatic and puomonary response to acute phlebotomy in secondary polycythemia.* Chest, 1975. **68**(6): p. 785–90.

101. Gagnon, D. R., et al., *Hematocrit and the risk of cardiovascular disease—The Framingham study: A 34-year follow-up.* Am Heart J, 1994. **127**(3): p. 674–82.

102. Salonen, J. T., et al., *Donation of blood is associated with reduced risk of myocardial infarction. The Kuopio Ischaemic Heart Disease Risk Factor Study.* Am J Epidemiol, 1998. **148**(5): p. 445–51.

103. Kim, D., Y. I. Cho, and K. Kensey, *Reduction of major amputation by therapeutic phlebotomy in patients with chronic critical limb ischemia*, in 6th International Conference on Clinical Hemorheology. College Park, PA: <add publisher>, 2008.

104. Chien, S., et al., *Blood viscosity: Iinfluence of erythrocyte deformation*. Science, 1967. **157**(3790): p. 827–29.

105. Waugh, R. E., et al., *Rheologic properties of senescent erythrocytes: Loss of surface area and volume with red blood cell age*. Blood, 1992. **79**(5): p. 1351.

106. Fossum, E., et al., *Whole blood viscosity, blood pressure and cardiovascular risk factors in healthy blood donors*. Blood Press, 1997. **6**(3): p. 161–65.

107. Janetzko, K., et al., *The effect of moderate hypovolaemia on microcirculation in healthy older blood donors*. Anaesthesia, 2001. **56**(2): p. 103–7.

108. Tuomainen, T. P., et al., *Author's reply to comments from Hemila et al.on blood donation, body iron stores, and risk*. Lancet, 1997. **314**: p. 1830–31.

109. Sullivan, J. L., *The iron paradigm of ischemic heart disease*. Am Heart J, 1989. **117**(5): p. 1177–88.

110. Yuan, X. M. and W. Li, *The iron hypothesis of atherosclerosis and its clinical impact*. Annals of Medicine, 2003. **35**(8): p. 578–91.

111. Salonen, J. T., et al., *Lowering of body iron stores by blood letting and oxidation resistance of serum lipoproteins:A randomized cross-over trial in male smokers*. J Intern Med, 1995. **237**(2): p. 161–68.

112. Tuomainen, T. P., et al., *Cohort study of relation between donating blood and risk of myocardial infarction in 2682 men in eastern Finland*. BMJ, 1997. **314**(7083): p. 793–94.

113. Hemila, H., and M. Paunio, *Blood donation, body iron stores, and risk of myocardial infarction. Confidence intervals and possible selection bias call study results into question*. BMJ, 1997. **314**(7097): p. 1830–31.

114. Meyers, D. G., et al., *Possible association of a reduction in cardiovascular events with blood donation*. Heart, 1997. **78**(2): p. 188–93.

115. Kreimeier, U., and K. Messmer, *Hemodilution in clinical surgery: State of the art 1996*. World Journal of Surgery, 1996. **20**(9): p. 1208–17.

116. Berman, W., et al., *Effects of pentoxifylline (Trental) on blood flow, viscosity, and oxygen transport in young adults with inoperable cyanotic congenital heart disease*. Pediatric Cardiology, 1994. **15**(2): p. 66–70.

117. Sonkin, P., S. Sinclair, and D. Hatchell, *The effect of pentoxifylline on retinal capillary blood flow velocity and whole blood viscosity*. American Journal of Ophthalmology, 1993. **115**(6): p. 775.

118. Perego, M., et al., *Haemorrheological improvement by pentoxifylline in patients with peripheral arterial occlusive disease*. Current Medical Research and Opinion, 1986. **10**(2): p. 135–38.

119. Solerte, S. B., et al., *Retrospective analysis of long-term hemorheologic effects of pentoxifylline in diabetic patients with angiopathic complications*. Acta Diabetol, 1997. **34**(2): p. 67–74.

120. Di Perri, T., et al., *Studies of the clinical pharmacology and therapeutic efficacy of pentoxifylline in peripheral obstructive arterial disease*. Angiology, 1984. **35**(7): p. 427.

121. Ott, E., H. Lechner, and F. Fazekas, *Hemorheological effects of pentoxifylline on disturbed flow behavior of blood in patients with cerebrovascular insufficiency*. Eur Neurol, 1983. **22** Suppl 1: p. 105–7.

122. Dawson, D. L., et al., *Failure of pentoxifylline or cilostazol to improve blood and plasma viscosity, fibrinogen, and erythrocyte deformability in claudication*. Angiology, 2002. **53**(5): p. 509–20.

123. Karandashov, V., E. Petukhov, and V. Zrodnikov, *Effects of pentoxyphyllin drugs and UV photohemotherapy on blood viscosity*. Bulletin of Experimental Biology and Medicine, 1998. **126**(5): p. 1155–56.

124. Brown, M. M., *Effect of oxpentifylline on blood viscosity and cerebral blood flow in man*. Br J Clin Pharmacol, 1989. **28**(4): p. 488–92.

125. Billett, H., et al., *Pentoxifylline (Trental) has no significant effect on laboratory parameters in sickle cell disease*. Nouvelle Revue Française d'Hématologie, 1989. **31**(6): p. 403–7.

126. Reilly, D., D. Quinton, and W. Barrie, *A controlled trial of pentoxifylline (Trental 400) in intermittent claudication: Clinical, haemostatic and rheological effects*. New Zealand Medical Journal, 1987. **100**(828): p. 445.

127. Perhoniemi, V., et al., *Effects of flunarizine and pentoxifylline on walking distance and blood rheology in claudication*. Angiology, 1984. **35**(6): p. 366.

128. Tsuda, Y., et al., *Effects of pravastatin sodium and simvastatin on plasma fibrinogen level and blood rheology in type II hyperlipoproteinemia*. Atherosclerosis, 1996. **122**(2): p. 225–33.

129. Koenig, W., et al., *Lovastatin alters blood rheology in primary hyperlipoproteinemia: Dependence on lipoprotein(a)*. J Clin Pharmacol, 1992. **32**(6): p. 539–45.

130. Koppensteiner, R., E. Minar, and H. Ehringer, *Effect of lovastatin on hemorheology in type II hyperlipoproteinemia*. Atherosclerosis, 1990. **83**(1): p. 53–58.

131. Empen, K., et al., *Effect of atorvastatin on lipid parameters, LDL subtype distribution, hemorrheological parameters and adhesion molecule concentrations in patients with hypertriglyceridemia.* Nutr Metab Cardiovasc Dis, 2003. **13**(2): p. 87–92.

132. Bozzo, J., M. R. Hernandez, and A. Ordinas, *Reduced red cell deformability associated with blood flow and platelet activation:Improved by dipyridamole alone or combined with aspirin.* Cardiovasc Res, 1995. **30**(5): p. 725–30.

133. Bozzo, J., et al., *Prohemorrhagic potential of dipyrone, ibuprofen, ketorolac, and aspirin: Mechanisms associated with blood flow and erythrocyte deformability.* Journal of Cardiovascular Pharmacology, 2001. **38**(2): p. 183–90.

134. Rosenson, R., et al., *Aspirin. Aspirin does not alter native blood viscosity.* Journal of Thrombosis and Haemostasis, 2004. **2**(2): p. 340–41.

135. Rosenson, R. S., *Treatment with aspirin and dipyridamole is more effective than aspirin in reducing low shear blood viscosity.* Microcirculation, 2008. **15**(7): p. 615–20.

136. Halkes, P., et al., *Aspirin plus dipyridamole versus aspirin alone after cerebral ischaemia of arterial origin (ESPRIT): Randomised controlled trial.* Lancet, 2006. **367**(9523): p. 1665–73.

137. Ciuffetti, G., et al., *Clopidogrel: Hemorheological effects in subjects with subclinical atherosclerosis.* Clin Hemorheol Microcirc, 2001. **25**(1): p. 31–39.

138. Jan, K. M., et al., *Altered rheological properties of blood following administrations of tissue plasminogen activator and streptokinase in patients with acute myocardial infarction.* Adv Exp Med Biol, 1990. **281**: p. 409–17.

139. Montefusco, S., et al., *Blood and plasma viscosity after acipimox treatment in hypertriglyceridemic patients.* International Journal of Clinical Pharmacology, Therapy, and Toxicology, 1988. **26**(10): p. 492.

140. Bell, W. R., Jr., *Defibrinogenating enzymes.* Drugs, 1997. **54** Suppl 3: p. 18–30; discussion 30–31.

141. Warren, J. L., et al., *The burden and outcomes associated with dehydration among US elderly, 1991.* American Journal of Public Health, 1994. **84**(8): p. 1265.

142. Chan, J., et al., *Water, other fluids, and fatal coronary heart disease: The Adventist Health Study.* Am J Epidemiol, 2002. **155**(9): p. 827–33.

143. Doi, T., et al., *Plasma volume and blood viscosity during 4 h sitting in a dry environment: Effect of pre-hydration.* Aviat Space Environ Med, 2004. **75**(6): p. 500–504.

144. Woodcock, B., et al., *Beneficial effect of fish oil on blood viscosity in peripheral vascular disease.* British Medical Journal (Clinical research ed.), 1984. **288**(6417): p. 592–94.

145. *Dietary supplementation with n-3 polyunsaturated fatty acids and vitamin E after myocardial infarction: Results of the GISSI-Prevenzione trial. Gruppo Italiano per lo Studio della Sopravvivenza nell'Infarto miocardico.* Lancet, 1999. **354**(9177): p. 447–55.

146. Leipner, J., and R. Saller, *Systemic enzyme therapy in oncology: Effect and mode of action.* Drugs, 2000. **59**(4): p. 769–80.

147. Nouza, K., *Outlooks of systemic enzyme therapy in rheumatoid arthritis and other immunopathological diseases.* Acta Universitatis Carolinae. Medica, 1994. **40**(1–4): p. 101.

148. Smith, R., et al., *Fibrinolysis with acyl-enzymes: A new approach to thrombolytic therapy.* 1981.

149. Neurath, H., *Evolution of proteolytic enzymes.* Science, 1984. **224**(4647): p. 350–57.

150. Kleine, M. W., G. M. Stauder, and E. W. Beese, *The intestinal absorption of orally administered hydro-lytic enzymes and their effects in the treatment of acute herpes zoster as compared with those of oral acyclovir therapy.* Phytomedicine, 1995. **2**(1): p. 7–15.

151. Kleine M. W., G. M. Stauder, et al., *Kinetics of proteolytic enzyme activity of serum in controlled randomized double blind study,* in *Second International Congress on Biological Response Modifiers.* San Diego, CA: <add publisher>, 1993.

152. Mudrák, J., L. Bobák, and I. Šebová, *Adjuvant therapy with hydrolytic enzymes in recurrent laryngeal papillomatosis.* Acta Oto-Laryngologica, 1997. **117**(S527): p. 128–30.

153. Cengiz, M., et al., *Effect of nattokinase supplementation on plasma fibrinogen levels, whole blood viscosity and mortality in experimental sepsis in rats.* Critical Care, 2009. **13**(Suppl 1): p. P337.

154. Hitosugi, M., H. Maeda, and K. Omura, *Blood-viscosity reducing agent, US 7972835*, 2011.

155. Pais, E., et al., *Effects of nattokinase, a pro-fibrinolytic enzyme, on red blood cell aggregation and whole blood viscosity.* Clin Hemorheol Microcirc, 2006. **35**(1–2): p. 139–42.

156. Ernst, E., and A. Matrai, *Orale Therapie mit proteolytischen Enzymen modifiziert die Blutrheologie.* Klin. Wschr, 1987. **65**: p. 994.

157. Hsia, C-H., et al. *Nattokinase decreases plasma levels of fibrinogen, factor VII, and factor VIII in human subjects.* Nutrition Research. 2009. **29**: p. 190–96.

158. Yatagai, C., M. Maruyama, and H. Sumi. *Nattokinase-promoted tissue plasminogen activator release from human cells.* Pathophysiology of Haemmostasis and Thrombosis. 2008. **36**(5): p. 227–32.

159. Pais, E., et al. *Effects of nattokinase, a pro-fibrinolytic enzyme, on red blood cell aggregation and whole blood viscocity.* Clinical Hemorheology and Microcirculation. 2006. **35**(1–2): p. 139–42.

160. Peeters, H., *Phosphatidylcholine: Biochemical and Clinical Aspects of Essential Phospholipids. Proceedings of a Symposium Held at the Simon Stevin Institute November 15–18, 1975, Brugge, Belgium.* New York, NY: Springer, 1976.

161. Ehrly, A. M., and R. Blendin, *Influence of essential phospholipids on the flow properties of the blood,* in *Phosphatidylcholine—Biochemical and Clinical Aspects of Essential Phospholipids,* ed. H. Peeters. New York: Springer Press, 1976, p. 228–36.

162. Merchan, R., and G. Dona, *Microcirculation and haemorheology studies on polyunsaturated phosphatidyicholine (EPL; Lipostabil) in the aged.* Clin Trials J, 1984. **21**: p. 517–25.

163. Op den Kamp, J. A. F., B. Roelofsen, and L. L. M. van Deenen, *Structural and dynamic aspects of phosphatidylcholine in the human erythrocyte membrane.* Trends in Biochemical Sciences, 1985. **10**(8): p. 320–23.

164. Blagosklonov, A., et al., *Value of hemosorption and essential phospholipids in the complex treatment of patients with ischemic heart disease.* Kardiologiya, 1986. **26**: p. 112–15.

165. Zeisel, S. H., M-H Mar, J. C. Howe, and J. M. Holden. *Concentrations of choline-containing compounds and betaine in common foods.* J. Nutr. 2003. **133**: p. 1302–07. Erratum in: J Nutr. 2003. **133**: p. 2918–19.

166. Institute of Medicine, National Academy of Sciences. *Choline. Dietary reference intakes for folate, thiamin, riboflavin, niacin, vitamin B12, pantothenic acid, biotin, and choline.* Washington, DC: National Academies Press. 1998. p. 390–422.

167. Fischer, L.M., K. daCosta, L. Kwock, P. Stewart, T-S Lu, S. Stabler, R. Allen, and S. Zeisel. *Sex and menopausal status influence human dietary requirements for the nutrient choline.* Am J Clin Nutr. 2007. **85**: p. 1275–85.

168. Resseguie, M., J. Song, M. D. Niculescu, K. A. da Costa, T. A. Randall, and S. H. Zeisel. *Phosphatidylethanolamine N-methyltransferase (PEMT) gene expression is induced by estrogen in human and mouse primary hepatocytes.* FASEB J. 2007. **21**: p. 2622–32.

6 Hypertension

Nutrition, Nutraceuticals, Vitamins, Antioxidants, and Minerals in Prevention and Treatment

Mark C. Houston, M.D., M.S.

INTRODUCTION

Hypertension is a consequence of the interaction of genetics and environment. Macronutrients and micronutrients are crucial in the regulation of blood pressure (BP) and subsequent target organ damage (TOD). Nutrient-gene interactions, subsequent gene expression, oxidative stress, inflammation, and autoimmune vascular dysfunction have positive or negative influences on vascular biology in humans. Endothelial activation with endothelial dysfunction (ED) and vascular smooth muscle dysfunction (VSMD) initiate and perpetuate essential hypertension.

Macronutrient and micronutrient deficiencies are very common in the general population and may be even more common in patients with hypertension and cardiovascular disease due to genetics, environmental causes, and prescription drug use. These deficiencies will have an enormous impact on present and future cardiovascular health and outcomes such as hypertension, myocardial infarction, stroke, and renal disease. The diagnosis and treatment of these nutrient deficiencies will reduce blood pressure and improve vascular health, endothelial dysfunction, vascular biology, and cardiovascular events.

EPIDEMIOLOGY

The epidemiology underscores the etiologic role of diet and associated nutrient intake in hypertension. The transition from the Paleolithic diet to our modern diet has produced an epidemic of nutritionally related diseases (Table 6.1). Hypertension, atherosclerosis, coronary heart disease (CHD), myocardial infarction (MI), congestive heart failure (CHF), cerebrovascular accidents (CVA), renal disease, type 2 diabetes mellitus (DM), metabolic syndrome (MS), and obesity are some of these diseases [1,2]. Table 6.1 contrasts intake of nutrients involved in blood pressure regulation during the Paleolithic era and modern time. Evolution from a preagricultural, hunter-gatherer milieu to an agricultural, refrigeration society has imposed an unnatural and unhealthful nutritional selection process. In sum, diet has changed more than genetics can adapt.

TABLE 6.1

Dietary Intake of Nutrients Involved in Vascular Biology: Comparing and Contrasting the Diet of Paleolithic and Contemporary Humans

Nutrients and Dietary Characteristics	Paleolithic Intake	Modern Intake
Sodium	< 50 mmol/day (1.2 grams)	175 mmol/day (4 grams)
Potassium	> 10,000 meq/day (256 grams)	150 meq/day (6 grams)
Sodium/potassium ratio	< 0.13/day	> 0.67/day
Protein	37%	20%
Carbohydrate	41%	40–50%
Fat	22%	30–40%
Polyunsaturated/saturated fat ratio	1.4	0.4
Fiber	> 100 grams/day	9 grams/day

The human genetic makeup is 99.9% that of our Paleolithic ancestors, yet our nutritional, vitamin, and mineral intakes are vastly different [3]. The macronutrient and micronutrient variations, radical oxygen species (ROS), inflammatory mediators, cell adhesion molecules (CAMs), signaling molecules, and autoimmune dysfunction contribute to the higher incidence of hypertension and other cardiovascular diseases through complex nutrient-gene interactions and nutrient-caveolae interactions in the endothelium [4,5,6,7]. Reduction in nitric oxide bioavailability and endothelial activation initiate the vascular dysfunction and hypertension. Poor nutrition, coupled with obesity and a sedentary lifestyle have resulted in an exponential increase in nutritionally related diseases. In particular, the high Na^+/K^+ ratio of modern diets has contributed to hypertension, stroke, CHD, CHF, and renal disease [3,8] as have the relatively low intake of omega-3 PUFA, and increase in omega-6 PUFA saturated fat and trans fatty acids [9].

PATHOPHYSIOLOGY

Vascular biology assumes a pivotal role in the initiation and perpetuation of hypertension and target organ damage. Oxidative stress, inflammation, and autoimmune dysfunction of the vascular system are the primary pathophysiologic and functional mechanisms that induce vascular disease. All three of these are closely interrelated and establish a deadly combination that leads to endothelial dysfunction, vascular smooth muscle dysfunction, hypertension, vascular disease, atherosclerosis, and CVD.

OXIDATIVE STRESS

Oxidative stress, with an imbalance between ROS and the antioxidant defense mechanisms, contributes to the etiology of hypertension in animals [10] and humans [11,12]. Radical oxygen species are generated by multiple cellular sources, including NADPH oxidase, mitochondria, xanthine oxidase, uncoupled endothelium-derived NO synthase (U-eNOS), cyclo-oxygenase, and lipo-oxygenase [11]. Superoxide anion is the predominant ROS species produced by these tissues. Hypertensive patients have impaired endogenous and exogenous antioxidant defense mechanisms [13], an increased plasma oxidative stress, and an exaggerated oxidative stress response to various stimuli [13,14]. Hypertensive subjects also have lower plasma ferric reducing ability of plasma (FRAP), lower vitamin C levels, and increased plasma 8-isoprostanes, which correlate with both systolic and diastolic blood pressure. Various single-nucleotide polymorphisms (SNPs) in genes that codify for antioxidant enzymes are directly related to hypertension [15]. These include NADPH oxidase, xanthine oxidase, superoxide dismutase (SOD 3), catalase, glutathione peroxidase (GPx 1), and thioredoxin. Antioxidant deficiency and excess free radical production have been implicated in human hypertension in numerous epidemiologic, observational, and interventional studies [13,14,16]. See Table 6.2. Radical oxygen species directly damage endothelial cells;

TABLE 6.2

The Cytotoxic Reactive Oxygen Species and the Natural Defense Mechanisms

Reactive Oxygen Species		Antioxidant Defense Mechanisms	
Free Radicals		*Enzymatic Scavengers*	
$O_2\bullet^-$	Superoxide anion radical	SOD	Superoxide dismutase
OH•	Hydroxyl radical		$2O_2\bullet^- + 2H^+ \rightarrow H_2O_2 + O_2$
ROO•	Lipid peroxide (peroxyl)	CAT	Catalase (peroxisomal-bound)
RO•	Alkoxyl		$2H_2O_2 \rightarrow O_2 + H_2O$
RS•	Thiyl	GTP	Glutathione peroxidase
NO•	Nitric oxide		$2GSH + H_2O_2 \rightarrow GSSG + 2H_2O$
$NO_2\bullet$	Nitrogen dioxide		$2GSH + ROOH \rightarrow GSSG + ROH + 2H_2O$
$ONOO^-$	Peroxynitrite		
$CCl_3\bullet$	Trichloromethyl	*Nonenzymatic scavengers*	
		Vitamin A	
Nonradicals		Vitamin C (ascorbic acid)	
H_2O_2	Hydrogen peroxide	Vitamin E (α-tocopherol)	
HOCl	Hypochlorous acid	β-carotene	
$ONOO^-$	Peroxynitrite	Cysteine	
$^1O_2$	Singlet oxygen	Coenzyme Q	
		Uric Acid	
		Flavonoids	
		Sulfhydryl group	
		Thioether compounds	

The superscripted bold dot indicates an unpaired electron and the negative charge indicates a gained electron. GSH, reduced glutathione; GSG, oxidized gltathione; R, lipid chain. Singlet oxygen is an unstable molecule due to the two electrons present in its outer orbit spinning in opposite directions.

degrade NO; influence eicosanoid metabolism; oxidize LDL, lipids, proteins, carbohydrates, DNA, and organic molecules; increase catecholamines; damage the genetic machinery; and influence gene expression and transcription factors (1,11,12,13,14). The interrelations of neurohormonal systems, oxidative stress, and cardiovascular disease are shown in Figure 6.1. The increased oxidative stress, inflammation, and autoimmune vascular dysfunction in human hypertension results from a combination of increased generation of ROS, an exacerbated response to ROS, and a decreased antioxidant reserve [13–18].

INFLAMMATION

The link between inflammation and hypertension has been suggested in both cross-sectional and longitudinal studies [19]. Increases in high-sensitivity C-reactive protein (HS-CRP) as well as other inflammatory cytokines occur in hypertension and hypertensive-related target organ damage, such as increased carotid IMT [20]. HS-CRP predicts future CV events [19,20]. Elevated HS-CRP is both a risk marker and risk factor for hypertension and CVD [21,22]. Increases in HS-CRP of over 3 ug/ml may increase BP in just a few days; this increase is directly proportional to the increase in HS-CRP [21,22]. Nitric oxide and eNOS are inhibited by high-sensitivity C-reactive protein (HS-CRP) [21,22]. The AT2R, which normally counterbalances AT1R, is down-regulated by HS-CRP [21,22]. Angiotensin II (A-II) up-regulates many of the cytokines, especially interleukin 6 (IL-6), cell adhesion molecules (CAMs), and chemokines by activating nuclear factor kappa B (NFkb) leading to vasoconstriction. These events, along with the increases in oxidative stress and endothelin-1, elevate BP [19].

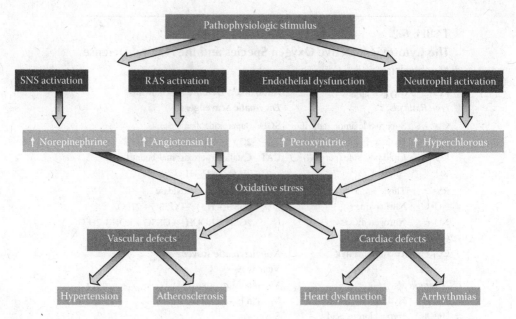

FIGURE 6.1. Interaction on the cardiovascular system. SNS = Sympathetic nervous system; RAAS = Renin angiotensin [aldosterone] system.

AUTOIMMUNE DYSFUNCTION

Innate and adaptive immune responses are linked to hypertension and hypertension-induced CVD through at least three mechanisms: cytokine production, central nervous system stimulation, and renal damage. This includes salt-sensitive hypertension with increased renal inflammation as a result of T-cell imbalance, dysregulation of CD+4 and CD+8 lymphocytes, and chronic leukocytosis with increased neutrophils and reduced lymphocytes [23,24]. Macrophages and various T-cell subtypes regulate blood pressure, invade the arterial wall, activate Toll-like receptors (TLRs), and induce autoimmune vascular damage [25,26]. Angiotensin II activates immune cells (T cells, macrophages, and dendritic cells) and promotes cell infiltration into target organs [26]. CD4 + T lymphocytes express AT1R and PPAR gamma receptors, when activated, release TNF alpha, interferon, and interleukins within the vascular wall [26]. Interleukin 17 (IL-17) produced by T cells may play a pivotal role in the genesis of hypertension caused by angiotensin II [26].

TREATMENT AND PREVENTION

Many of the natural compounds in food, certain nutraceutical supplements, vitamins, antioxidants, or minerals function in a similar fashion to a specific class of antihypertensive drugs. Although the potency of these natural compounds may be less than the antihypertensive drug, when used in combination with other nutrients and nutraceutical supplements, the antihypertensive effect is additive or synergistic. Table 6.3 summarizes these natural compounds into the major antihypertensive drug classes such as diuretics, beta blockers, central alpha agonists, CCB, ACEI, and ARBs.

SODIUM (NA±) REDUCTION

The average sodium intake in the United States is 5000 mg per day with some areas of the country consuming 15,000–20,000 mg per day [27]. However, the minimal requirement for sodium

TABLE 6.3

Natural Antihypertensive Compounds Categorized by Antihypertensive Class

Antihypertensive Therapeutic Class (Alphabetical Listing)	Foods and Ingredients Listed by Therapeutic Class	Nutrients and Other Supplements Listed by Therapeutic Class

Angiotensin converting enzyme inhibitors	Egg yolk
	Fish (specific):
	  Bonito
	  Dried salted fish
	  Fish sauce
	  Sardines
	  Tuna
	Garlic
	Gelatin
	Hawthorne berry
	Milk products (specific):
	  Casein
	  Sour milk
	  Whey (hydrolyzed)
	Sake
	Sea vegetables (kelp)
	Wheat germ (hydrolyzed)
	Zein (corn protein)
		Omega-3 fatty acids
		Pycnogenol
		Zinc

Angiotensin receptor blockers	Celery Fiber Garlic	Coenzyme Q10 Gamma-linolenic acid Potassium Resveratrol Vitamin C Vitamin B6 (pyridoxine)
Beta blockers	Hawthorne berry	
Calcium channel blockers	Celery Garlic Hawthorne berry	Alpha-lipoic acid Calcium Docosahexaenoic acid Eicosapentaenoic acid Magnesium N-acetyl cysteine Omega-3 fatty acids: Vitamin B6 Vitamin C Vitamin E
Central alpha agonists (reduce sympathetic nervous system activity)	Celery Fiber Garlic Protein	Coenzyme Q10 Gamma-linolenic acid Potassium Restriction of sodium Taurine Vitamin B6 Vitamin C Zinc

continued

TABLE 6.3 (*continued*)

Natural Antihypertensive Compounds Categorized by Antihypertensive Class

Antihypertensive Therapeutic Class (Alphabetical Listing)	Foods and Ingredients Listed by Therapeutic Class	Nutrients and Other Supplements Listed by Therapeutic Class
Direct vasodilators	Celery	Alpha-linolenic acid
	Cooking oils with monounsaturated fats	Arginine
		Calcium
	Fiber	Flavonoids
	Garlic	Magnesium
	Soy	Omega-3 fatty acids
		Potassium
		Taurine
		Vitamin C
		Vitamin E
Diuretics	Celery	Calcium
	Hawthorne berry	Coenzyme Q10
	Protein	Fiber
		Gamma-linolenic acid
		L-carnitine
		Magnesium
		Potassium
		Taurine
		Vitamin B6
		Vitamin C

is probably about 500 mg per day [27]. Epidemiologic, observational, and controlled clinical trials demonstrate that an increased sodium intake is associated with higher blood pressure [27]. A reduction in sodium intake in hypertensive patients, especially the salt sensitive patients, will significantly lower blood pressure by 4–6/2–3 mm Hg, which is proportional to the severity of sodium restriction and may prevent or delay hypertension in high-risk patients [28,29].

Salt sensitivity (≥ 10% increase in MAP with salt loading) occurs in about 51% of hypertensive patients and is a key factor in determining the cardiovascular, cerebrovascular, renal, and blood pressure response to dietary salt intake [30]. Cardiovascular events are more common in the salt-sensitive patients than in salt resistant ones, independent of BP [31].

Sodium intake per day in hypertensive patients should be between 1500 to 2000 mg. Sodium restriction improves blood pressure reduction in those patients that are on pharmacologic treatment [32,33]. Reducing dietary sodium intake may reduce damage to the brain, heart, kidney, and vasculature through mechanisms dependent on the small BP reduction as well as those independent of the decreased BP [34,35].

A balance of sodium with other nutrients, especially potassium and magnesium, is important not only in reducing and controlling BP, but also in decreasing cardiovascular and cerebrovascular events [3,32,33]. An increase in the sodium to potassium ratio is associated with significantly increased risk of CVD and all-cause mortality [34].

POTASSIUM

The average U.S. dietary intake of potassium (K^+) is 45 mmol per day with a potassium to sodium (K^+/Na^+) ratio of less than 1:2 [8,35]. The recommended intake of K^+ is 4700 mg day (120 mmol) with a K^+/Na^+ ratio of about 4–5 to 1 [8,35]. Numerous epidemiologic, observational, and clinical trials have demonstrated a significant reduction in BP with increased dietary K^+ intake in both normotensive and hypertensive patients [8,35,36]. The average BP reduction with a K^+ supplementation of 60 to120 mmol per day is 4.4/2.5 mm Hg in hypertensive patients but may be as much as 8/4.1 mm Hg with 120 mmol per day (4700 mg) [8,35,36]. The response depends on race (black > white), sodium, magnesium, and calcium intake [8]. Those on a higher sodium intake have a greater reduction in BP with potassium [8]. Alteration of the K^+/Na^+ ratio to a higher level is important for both antihypertensive as well as cardiovascular and cerebrovascular effects [37]. High potassium intake reduces the incidence of cardiovascular (CHD, MI) and cerebrovascular accidents independent of the BP reduction [8,35,36,37]. There are also reductions in CHF, LVH, diabetes mellitus, and cardiac arrhythmias [8]. If the serum potassium is less than 4.0 meq/dL, there is an increased risk of CVD mortality, ventricular tachycardia, ventricular fibrillation, and CHF [8]. Red blood cell potassium is a better indication of total body stores and thus CVD risk than is serum potassium [8]. Gu et al. [37] found that potassium supplementation at 60 mmol of KCl per day for 12 weeks significantly reduced SBP—5.0 mm Hg (range –2.13 mm Hg to –7.88 mm Hg) ($p < 0.001$) in 150 Chinese men and women aged 35 to 64 years.

Potassium increases natriuresis, modulates baroreflex sensitivity, vasodilates, decreases the sensitivity to catecholamines and Angiotensin II, and increases sodium potassium ATPase and DNA synthesis in the vascular smooth muscle cells and sympathetic nervous system cells resulting in improved function [8]. In addition, potassium increases bradykinin and urinary kallikrein, decreases NADPH oxidase, which lowers oxidative stress and inflammation, improves insulin sensitivity, decreases ADMA, reduces intracellular sodium, and lowers production of TGF-beta [8].

Each 1000 mg increase in potassium intake per day reduces all cause mortality by approximately 20%. Each 1000mg decrease in sodium intake per day will decrease all cause mortality by 20% [34]. The recommended daily dietary intake for patients with hypertension is 4.7 grams of potassium and less than 1500 mg of sodium [8]. Potassium in food or from supplementation should be reduced or used with caution in those patients with renal impairment or those on medications that increase renal potassium retention [8].

Magnesium (Mg$^{\pm\pm}$)

A high dietary intake of magnesium of at least 500–1000 mg per day reduces BP in most of the reported epidemiologic, observational, and clinical trials, but the results are less consistent than those seen with Na^+ and K^+ [35,38]. In most epidemiologic studies, there is an inverse relationship between dietary magnesium intake and BP [35,38,39]. A study of 60 essential hypertensive subjects given magnesium supplements showed a significant reduction in BP over an eight-week period documented by 24-hour ambulatory BP, and home and office blood BP [35,38,39]. The maximum reduction in clinical trials has been 5.6/2.8 mm Hg but some studies have shown no change in BP [40]. The combination of high potassium and low sodium intake with increased magnesium intake had additive antihypertensive effects [40]. Magnesium also increases the effectiveness of all antihypertensive drug classes [40].

Magnesium competes with Na^+ for binding sites on vascular smooth muscle and acts like a calcium channel blocker (CCB), increases PGE increase nitric oxide, improves endothelial function, binds in a necessary-cooperative manner with potassium, inducing (EDV) vasodilation and BP reduction [35,38–40].

Magnesium is an essential cofactor for the delta-6-desaturase enzyme that is the rate-limiting step for conversion of linoleic acid (LA) to gamma linolenic acid (GLA) [35,38,39] needed for synthesis of the vasodilator and platelet inhibitor prostaglandin E_1 (PGE$_1$).

Intracellular level of magnesium (RBC) is more indicative of total body stores and should be measured in conjunction with serum and urinary magnesium [40]. Magnesium may be supplemented in doses of 500 to 1000 mg per day. Magnesium formulations chelated to an amino acid may improve absorption and decrease the incidence of diarrhea [40]. Adding taurine at 1000 to 2000 mg per day will enhance the antihypertensive effects of magnesium [40]. Magnesium supplements should be avoided or used with caution in patients with known renal insufficiency or in those taking medications that induce magnesium retention [40].

CALCIUM (CA)

Population studies show a link between hypertension and calcium [41], but clinical trials that administer calcium supplements to patients have shown inconsistent effects on BP [35,41]. The heterogeneous responses to calcium supplementation have been explained by Resnick [42]. This is the ionic hypothesis [42] of hypertension, cardiovascular disease, and associated metabolic, functional, and structural disorders. Calcium supplementation is not recommended at this time as an effective means to reduce BP.

ZINC (ZN)

Low serum zinc levels in observational studies correlate with hypertension as well as CHD, type II DM, hyperlipidemia, elevated lipoprotein a (Lp[a]), two-hour postprandial plasma insulin levels, and insulin resistance [43]. Zinc is transported into cardiac and vascular muscle and other tissues by methothinein [44]. Genetic deficiencies of metallothionein with intramuscular zinc deficiencies may lead to increased oxidative stress, mitochondrial dysfunction, cardiomyocyte dysfunction, and apoptosis with subsequent myocardial fibrosis, abnormal cardiac remodeling, heart disease, heart failure, or hypertension [44]. Intracellular calcium increases oxidative stress, which is reduced by zinc [44].

Bergomi et al. [45] evaluated Zn status in 60 hypertensive subjects compared to 60 normotensive control subjects. An inverse correlation of BP and serum Zn was observed. The BP was also inversely correlated to a Zn dependent enzyme-lysyl oxidase activity. Zn inhibits gene expression and transcription through nuclear factor kappa-beta (NFK-B) and activated protein-1 (AP-1) [43,44]. These effects plus those on insulin resistance, membrane ion exchange, RAAS, and SNS effects may account for Zn antihypertensive effects [43,44]. Zinc intake should be 50 mg per day [1].

PROTEIN

Observational and epidemiologic studies demonstrate a consistent association between a high protein intake and a reduction in BP and incident BP [46,47]. The protein source is an important factor in the BP effect; animal protein being less effective than nonanimal or plant protein, especially almonds [46–49]. In the INTERSALT Study of over 10,000 subjects, those with a dietary protein intake 30% above the mean had a lower BP by 3.0/2.5 mm Hg compared to those that were 30% below the mean (81 grams versus 44 grams per day) [46]. However, lean or wild animal protein with less saturated fat and more essential omega-3 fatty acids may reduce BP, lipids, and CHD risk [46,49]. A meta-analysis confirmed these findings and also suggested that hypertensive patients and the elderly have THE greatest BP reduction with protein intake [47]. A randomized crossover study in 352 adults with prehypertension and stage I hypertension found a significant reduction in SBP of 2.0 mm Hg with soy protein and 2.3 mm Hg with milk protein compared to a high glycemic index diet over each of the eight-week treatment periods [50]. There was a nonsignificant reduction in DBP. The daily recommended intake of protein from all sources is 1.0 to 1.5 grams per kg body weight, varying with exercise level, age, renal function, and other factors [1,32,33].

Fermented milk supplemented with whey protein concentrate significantly reduces BP in human studies [51–55]. Administration of 20 grams per day of hydrolyzed whey protein supplement rich in bioactive peptides significantly reduced BP over six weeks by 8.0 +/– 3.2 mm Hg in systolic blood pressure and 5.5 +/– 2.1 mm in diastolic blood pressure [52]. Milk peptides that contain both caseins and whey proteins are a rich source of ACEI peptides. Val-Pro-Pro and Ile-Pro-Pro given at 5 to 60 mg per day have variable reductions in BP with an average decrease in pooled studies of about

4.8/2.2 mm Hg [33,50,53–55]. However, a recent meta-analysis did not show significant reductions in BP in humans [55]. Powdered fermented milk with *L. helveticus* given at 12 grams per day significantly lowered BP by 11.2/6.5 mm Hg in four weeks in one study. (53). The clinical response is attributed to fermented milk's two peptides, which inhibit ACE.

Pins and Keenan [56] administered 20 grams of hydrolyzed whey protein to 30 hypertensive subjects and noted a BP reduction of 11/7 mm Hg compared to controls at one week that were sustained throughout the study. These data indicate that the whey protein must be hydrolyzed in order to exhibit an antihypertensive effect, and the maximum BP response is dose dependent.

Bovine casein-derived peptides and whey protein-derived peptides exhibit ACEI activity [51–56]. These components include B-caseins, B-lg fractions, B2-microglobulin, and serum albumin [51–53,56]. The enzymatic hydrolysis of whey protein isolates releases ACEI peptides.

Marine collagen peptides (MCPs) from deep-sea fish have antihypertensive activity [57–59]. A double-blind, placebo-controlled trial in 100 hypertensive subjects with diabetes who received MCPs twice a day for three months had significant reductions in DBP and mean arterial pressure [57]. Bonito protein (*Sarda orientalis*) from the tuna and mackerel family has natural ACEI inhibitory peptides and reduces BP 10.2/7 mm Hg at 1.5 grams per day [58].

Sardine muscle protein, which contains valyl-tyrosine (VAL-TYR), significantly lowers BP in hypertensive subjects [60]. Kawasaki et al. treated 29 hypertensive subjects with 3 mg of valyl-tyrosine sardine muscle concentrated extract for four weeks and lowered BP 9.7 mm Hg/5.3 mm Hg (p < 0.05) [60]. Levels of A-I increased as serum A-II and aldosterone decreased indicating that valyl-tyrosine is a natural angiotensin converting enzyme inhibitor (ACEI). A similar study with a vegetable drink with sardine protein hydrolysates significantly lowered BP by 8/5 mm Hg in 13 weeks [61].

Soy protein intake was significantly and inversely associated with both SBP and DBP in 45,694 Chinese women consuming 25 grams per day or more of soy protein over three years and the association increased with age [62]. The SBP reduction was 1.9 to 4.9 mm lower and the DBP 0.9 to 2.2 mm Hg lower [62]. However, randomized clinical trials and meta-analysis have shown mixed results on BP with no change in BP to reductions of 7% to 10% for SBP and DBP [63–67]. Some studies suggest improvement in endothelial function, improved arterial compliance, reduction in HS-CRP and inflammation, ACEI activity, reduction in sympathetic tone, diuretic action, and reduction in both oxidative stress and aldosterone levels [66,68,69]. Fermented soy at about 25 grams per day is recommended.

In addition to ACEI effects, protein intake may also alter catecholamine responses and induce natriuresis [60,61]. Low protein intake coupled with low omega-3 fatty acid intake may contribute to hypertension in animal models [70]. The optimal protein intake, depending on level of activity, renal function, stress, and other factors, is about 1.0 to 1.5 grams/kg/day [1].

AMINO ACIDS AND RELATED COMPOUNDS

L-Arginine

L-arginine and endogenous methylarginines are the primary precursors for the production of nitric oxide (NO), which has numerous beneficial cardiovascular effects, mediated through conversion of L-arginine to NO by eNOS. Patients with hypertension, hyperlipidemia, diabetes mellitus, and atherosclerosis have increased levels of HS-CRP and inflammation, increased microalbumin, low levels of apelin (stimulates NO in the endothelium), increased levels of arginase (breaks down arginine), and elevated serum levels of ADMA, which inactivates NO [71–75].

Under normal physiological conditions, intracellular arginine levels far exceed the K(m) of eNOS. However, endogenous NO formation is dependent on extracellular arginine concentration. The NO production in endothelial cells is closely coupled to cellular arginine update indicating that arginine transport mechanisms play a major role in the regulation of NO-dependent function. Exogenous arginine can increase renal vascular and tubular NO bioavailability and influence renal perfusion, function, and BP (74).

Human studies in hypertensive and normotensive subjects of parenteral and oral administrations of L-arginine demonstrate an antihypertensive effect [71,76–80]. The BP decreased by 6.2/6.8 mm Hg on 10 grams per day of L-arginine when provided as a supplement or though natural foods to a group of hypertensive subjects [76]. Arginine produces a statistically and biologically significant decrease in BP and improved metabolic effect in normotensive and hypertensive humans that is similar in magnitude to that seen in the DASH-I diet [76]. Arginine given at 4 grams per day also significantly lowered BP in women with gestational hypertension without proteinuria, reduced the need for antihypertensive therapy, decreased maternal and neonatal complications, and prolonged the pregnancy [77,78]. The combination of arginine (1200 mg per day) and N-acetyl cysteine (600 mg bid) administered over six months to hypertensive patients with type 2 diabetes, lowered SBP and DBP (p < 0.05), increased HDL-C, decreased LDL-C and oxLDL, and reduced HS-CRP, ICAM, VCAM, PAI-I, fibrinogen, and IMT [79]. A study of 54 hypertensive subjects given arginine at 4 grams three times per day for four weeks had significant reductions in 24 hour ABM [80]. Although these doses of L-arginine appear to be safe, no long-term studies in humans have been published at this time; there are concerns of a pro-oxidative effect or even an increase in mortality in patients who may have severely dysfunctional endothelium, advanced atherosclerosis, CHD, or MI [81].

L-Carnitine

L-carnitine is a nitrogenous constituent of muscle primarily involved in the oxidation of fatty acids in mammals. Human studies on the effects of L-carnitine are small, limited to older studies in which there is minimal to no change in blood pressure [82–84]. Carnitine may be useful in the treatment of essential hypertension, type II DM with hypertension, hyperlipidemia, cardiac arrhythmias, CHF, and cardiac ischemic syndromes [1,82–84]. Doses of 2–3 grams twice per day are recommended.

Taurine

Taurine is a sulfonic beta-amino acid that is considered a conditionally essential amino acid that is not utilized in protein synthesis, but is found free or in simple peptides with its highest concentration in the brain, retina, and myocardium [85]. In cardiomyocytes, it represents about 50% of the free amino acids and has a role of an osmoregulator, inotropic factor, and antihypertensive agent [86].

Human studies have noted that essential hypertensive subjects have reduced urinary taurine as well as other sulfur amino acids [1,85,86]. Taurine lowers BP, SVR, and HR, decreases arrhythmias, CHF symptoms and SNS activity, increases urinary sodium and water excretion, increases atrial naturietic factor, improves insulin resistance, increases NO and improves endothelial function, and decreases A-II, PRA, aldosterone, plasma norepinephrine, plasma and urinary epinephrine [1,85,86,87]. A study of 31 Japanese males with essential hypertension placed on an exercise program for 10 weeks showed a 26% increase in taurine levels and a 287% increase in cysteine levels. The BP reduction of 14.8/6.6 mm Hg was proportional to increases in serum taurine and reductions in plasma norepinephrine [88]. Fujita et al.[86] demonstrated a reduction in BP of 9/4.1 mm Hg (p < 0.05) in 19 hypertension subjects given 6 grams of taurine for seven days. Taurine has numerous beneficial effects on the cardiovascular system and blood pressure [87]. The recommended dose of taurine is two to three grams per day at which no adverse effects are noted, but higher doses may be needed to reduce BP significantly [1,32,33,85–88].

Omega-3 Fats

The omega-3 fatty acids found in cold-water fish, fish oils, flax, flax seed, flax oil, and nuts lower BP in observational, epidemiologic, and in some small prospective clinical trials [89–93]. The findings are strengthened by a dose-related response in hypertension as well as a relationship to the specific concomitant diseases associated with hypertension [89–93].

Studies indicate that DHA reduces BP and heart rate [89]. The average reduction in BP is 8/5 mm Hg and heart rate falls about six beats per minute [1,32,33,89,94–96]. However, formation of EPA and ultimately DHA from ALA is decreased in the presence of high linoleic acid (the essential omega-6 fatty acid), saturated fats, trans fatty acids, alcohol, several nutrient deficiencies, and aging, all of which inhibit the desaturase enzymes [89]. Eating cold-water fish three times per week may be as effective as high-dose fish oil in reducing BP in hypertensive patients, and the protein in the fish may also have antihypertensive effects [1,89]. In patients with chronic kidney disease 4 grams of omega-3 fatty acids reduced BP measured with 24-hour ABM over eight weeks by 3.3/2.9 mm Hg compared to placebo (p < 0.0001) [97].

The ideal ratio of omega-6 FA to omega-3 FA is between 1:1 to 1:4 with a polyunsaturated to saturated (P/S) fat ratio greater than 1.5 to 2:0 [2]. The omega-6 FA family includes linoleic acid (LA), gamma-linolenic acid (GLA), dihomo-gamma linolenic acid (DGLA), and arachidonic acid (AA), which do not usually lower BP significantly, but may prevent increases in BP induced by saturated fats [99]. GLA may block stress-induced hypertension by increasing prostaglandin E 1 (PGE1) and PGI 2, reducing aldosterone levels, reducing adrenal AT1R density and affinity [95].

The omega-3 FA have a multitude of other cardiovascular consequences that modulate BP such as increases in eNOS and nitric oxide, improvement in endothelial dysfunction, reduction in plasma norepinephrine and increased parasympathetic nervous system tone, suppression of ACE activity, and improvement in insulin resistance [99]. The recommended daily dose is 3000 to 5000 mg per day of combined DHA and EPA in a ratio of three parts EPA to two parts DHA and about 50% of this dose as GLA combined with gamma/delta tocopherol at 100 mg per gram of DHA and EPA to get the omega-3 index of 8% or higher to reduce BP and provide optimal cardioprotection [100].

Omega-9 Fats

Olive oil is rich in the omega-9 monounsaturated fat (MUFA) oleic acid, which has been associated with BP and lipid reduction in Mediterranean and other diets [101,102]. Olive oil and monounsaturated fats have shown consistent reductions in BP in most clinical studies in humans [101,103–105]. In one study, the SBP fell 8 mm Hg (p ≤ 0.05) and the DBP fell 6 mm Hg (p ≤ 0.01) in both clinic and 24-hour ambulatory blood pressure monitoring in the MUFA-treated subjects compared to the PUFA-treated subjects [101]. In addition, the need for antihypertensive medications was reduced by 48% in the MUFA group versus 4% in the omega-6 PUFA group (p < 0.005). Extra virgin olive oil was more effective that sunflower oil in lowering SBP in a group of 31 elderly hypertensive patients in a double–blind, randomized crossover study [103]. The SBP was 136 mm Hg in the extra virgin olive oil treated subjects versus 150 mm Hg in the sunflower treated group (p < 0.01). Olive oil also reduces BP in hypertensive diabetic subjects [104].

Extra virgin olive oil also contains lipid-soluble phytonutrients such as polyphenol; approximately 5 mg of phenols are found in 10 grams of oil [101,102]. About four tablespoons of extra virgin olive oil is equal to 40 grams, which is the amount required to get significant reductions in BP.

Fiber

The clinical trials with various types of fiber to reduce BP have been inconsistent [106,107]. Soluble fiber, guar gum, guava, psyllium, and oat bran may reduce BP and reduce the need for antihypertensive medications in hypertensive subjects, diabetic subjects, and hypertensive-diabetic subjects [1,32,33,106,107]. The average reduction in BP is about 7.5/5.5 mm Hg on 40 to 50 grams per day of a mixed fiber. There is improvement in insulin sensitivity, endothelial function, reduction in sympathetic nervous system activity and increase in renal sodium loss [1,32,33,106].

Vitamin C

Vitamin C is a potent water-soluble electron-donor. At physiologic levels it is an antioxidant, although at supraphysiologic doses such as those achieved with intravenous vitamin C, it donates electrons to different enzymes, which results in pro-oxidative effects. At physiologic doses, vitamin C recycles vitamin E, improves endothelial dysfunction, and produces a diuresis [108]. Dietary intake of vitamin C and plasma ascorbate concentration in humans is inversely correlated to SBP, DBP, and heart rate [108–122].

An evaluation of published clinical trials indicates that vitamin C dosing at 250 mg twice daily will lower BP about 7/4 mm Hg [108–122]. Vitamin C will induce a sodium water diuresis, improve arterial compliance, improve endothelial function, increase nitric oxide and PGI2, decrease adrenal steroid production, improve sympathovagal balance, increase RBC Na/K ATPase, increase super-oxide dismutase, improve aortic elasticity and compliance, improve flow mediated vasodilation, decrease pulse wave velocity and augmentation index, increase cyclic GMP, activate potassium channels, reduce cytosolic calcium, and reduce serum aldehydes [120]. Vitamin C enhances the efficacy of amlodipine, decreases the binding affinity of the AT 1 receptor for angiotensin II by disrupting the ATR1 disulfide bridges, and enhances antihypertensive effects of medications in the elderly with refractory hypertension [1,32,33,112–117]. In elderly patients with refractory hypertension already on maximum pharmacologic therapy, 600 mg of vitamin C daily lowered the BP by 20/16 mm Hg [117]. The lower the initial ascorbate serum level, the better is the BP response. A serum level of 100 micromol/L is recommended [1,32,33]. The systolic BP and 24 ABM show the most significant reductions with chronic oral administration of Vitamin C [112–117]. Block et al. [118], in an elegant depletion-repletion study of vitamin C, demonstrated an inverse correlation of plasma ascorbate levels, SBP and DBP. In a meta-analysis of 13 clinical trials with 284 patients, vitamin C at 500 mg per day over six weeks reduced SBP 3.9 mm Hg and DBP 2.1 mm Hg [119]. Hypertensive subjects were found to have significantly lower plasma ascorbate levels compared to normotensive subjects (40 umol/liter versus 57 umol/liter respectively) [123], and plasma ascorbate is inversely correlated with BP even in healthy, normotensive individuals [118].

Vitamin E

Most studies have not shown reductions in blood pressure with most forms of tocopherols or toco-trienols [1,32,33]. Patients with type 2 diabetes mellitus and controlled hypertension (130/76 mm Hg) on prescription medications with an average BP of 136/76 mm Hg were administered mixed tocopherols containing 60% gamma, 25% delta, and 15% alpha tocopherols [124]. The BP actually increased by 6.8/3.6 mm Hg in the study patients ($p < 0.0001$) but was less compared to the increase with alpha tocopherol of 7/5.3 mm Hg ($p < 0.0001$). This may be a reflection of drug interactions with tocopherols via cytochrome P 450 (3A4 and 4F2) and reduction in the serum levels of the phar-macologic treatments that were simultaneously being given [124]. Gamma tocopherol may have natriuretic effects by inhibition of the 70pS potassium channel in the thick ascending limb of the loop of Henle and lower BP [125]. Both alpha and gamma tocopherol improve insulin sensitivity and enhance adiponectin expression via PPAR gamma dependent processes, which have the poten-tial to lower BP and serum glucose [126]. If vitamin E has an antihypertensive effect, it is probably small and may be limited to untreated hypertensive patients or those with known vascular disease or other concomitant problems such as diabetes or hyperlipidemia.

Vitamin D

Vitamin D3 may have an independent and direct role in the regulation of BP and insulin metabo-lism [127–133]. Vitamin D influences BP by its effects on calcium-phosphate metabolism, RAA system, immune system, control of endocrine glands, and endothelial dysfunction [128]. If the vita-min D level is below 30 ng/ml, the circulating PRA levels are higher, which increases angiotensin II, increases BP, and blunts plasma renal blood flow [133]. The lower the level of vitamin D, the greater the risk of hypertension, with the lowest quartile of serum vitamin D having a 52% inci-dence of hypertension and the highest quartile having a 20% incidence [133]. Vitamin D3 markedly suppresses renin transcription by a VDR-mediated mechanism via the JGA apparatus. Its role in electrolytes, volume, and blood pressure homeostasis indicates that vitamin D3 is important in amelioration of hypertension. Vitamin D lowers asymmetric dimethyl arginine (ADMA), suppresses pro-inflammatory cytokines such as TNF alpha, increases nitric oxide, improves endothelial function and arterial elasticity, decreases vascular smooth muscle hypertrophy, regulates electrolytes and blood volume, increases insulin sensitivity, reduces free fatty acid concentration, regulates the expression of the natriuretic peptide receptor, and lowers HS-CRP [129,130,132,133].

The hypotensive effect of vitamin D was inversely related to the pretreatment serum levels of $1_{,}25$ (OH)$_2$ D$_3$ and additive to antihypertensive medications. Pfeifer et al. showed that short-term supplementation with vitamin D3 and calcium is more effective in reducing SBP than calcium alone [134]. In a group of 148 women with low 25 (OH)$_2$ D$_3$ levels, the administration of 1200 mg calcium plus 800 IU of vitamin D3 reduced SBP 9.3% more (p < 0.02) compared to 1200 mg of calcium alone. The HR fell 5.4% (p = 0.02), but DBP was not changed. The range in BP reduction was 3.6/3.1 to 13.1/7.2 mm Hg. The reduction in BP is related to the pretreatment level of vitamin D3, the dose of vitamin D3, and serum level of vitamin D3, but BP is reduced only in hypertensive patients. A 25 hydroxyvitamin D level of 60 ng/ml is recommended.

Vitamin B6 (Pyridoxine)

Low serum vitamin B6 (pyridoxine) levels are associated with hypertension in humans [135]. One human study by Aybak et al. [136] proved that high-dose vitamin B6 significantly lowered BP. Pyridoxine (vitamin B6) is a cofactor in neurotransmitter and hormone synthesis in the central nervous system, increases cysteine synthesis to neutralize aldehydes, enhances the production of glutathione, blocks calcium channels, improves insulin resistance, decreases central sympathetic tone, and reduces end organ responsiveness to glucocorticoids and mineralocorticoids [1,32,33,137,138]. Vitamin B6 is reduced with chronic diuretic therapy and heme pyrollactams (HPU). Vitamin B6 thus has similar action to central alpha agonists, diuretics, and calcium channel blockers. The recommended dose is 200 mg per day orally.

Flavonoids

Over 4000 naturally occurring flavonoids have been identified in such diverse substances as fruits, vegetables, red wine, tea, soy, and licorice [139]. Flavonoids (flavonols, flavones, and isoflavones) are potent free-radical scavengers that inhibit lipid peroxidation, prevent atherosclerosis, promote vascular relaxation, and have antihypertensive properties [139]. In addition, they reduce stroke and provide cardioprotective effects that reduce CHD morbidity and mortality [140].

Resveratrol is a potent antioxidant and antihypertensive found in the skin of red grapes and in red wine. Resveratrol administration to humans reduces augmentation index, improves arterial compliance, and lowers central arterial pressure when administered as 250 ml of either regular or dealcoholized red wine [141]. There was a significant reduction in the aortic augmentation index of 6.1% with the dealcoholized red wine and 10.5% with regular red wine. The central arterial pressure was significantly reduced by dealcoholized red wine at 7.4 mm Hg and 5.4 mm Hg by regular red wine. Resveratrol increases flow-mediated vasodilation in a dose-related manner, improves endothelial dysfunction, prevents uncoupling of eNOS, increases adiponectin, lowers HS-CRP, and blocks the effects of angiotensin II [142–145]. The recommended dose is 250 mg per day of trans resveratrol [143].

Lycopene

Lycopene is a fat-soluble phytonutrient in the carotenoid family. Dietary sources include tomatoes, guava, pink grapefruit, watermelon, apricots, and papaya in high concentrations [146–150]. Lycopene has recently been shown to produce a significant reduction in BP, serum lipids, and oxidative stress markers [146–150]. Paran and Engelhard [150] evaluated 30 subjects with Grade I hypertension, ages 40–65, taking no antihypertensive or antilipid medications treated with a tomato lycopene extract (10 mg lycopene) for eight weeks. The SBP was reduced from 144 to 135 mm Hg (9 mm Hg reduction, $p < 0.01$) and DBP fell from 91 to 84 mm Hg (7 mm Hg reduction, $p < 0.01$). Another study of 35 subjects with Grade I hypertension showed similar results on SBP, but not DBP [146]. Englehard gave a tomato extract to 31 hypertensive subjects over 12 weeks demonstrating a significant BP reduction of 10/4 mm Hg [147]. Patients on various antihypertensive agents including ACEI, CCB, and diuretics had a significant BP reduction of 5.4/3 mm Hg over six weeks when administered a standardized tomato extract [148]. Other studies have not shown changes in blood pressure with lycopene [149]. The recommended daily intake of lycopene is 10–20 mg in food or supplement form.

Coenzyme Q10 (Ubiquinone)

Coenzyme Q10 has consistent and significant antihypertensive effects in patients with essential hypertension [151].

- Compared to normotensive patients, essential hypertensive patients have a higher incidence (sixfold) of coenzyme Q10 deficiency documented by serum levels.
- Doses of 120 to 225 mg per day of coenzyme Q10, depending on the delivery method or the concomitant ingestion with a fatty meal, are necessary to achieve a therapeutic level of 3 ug/ml. This dose is usually 3–5 mg/kg/day of coenzyme Q10. Oral dosing levels may become lower with nanoparticle and emulsion delivery systems intended to facilitate absorption. Adverse effects have not been characterized in the literature.
- Patients with the lowest coenzyme Q10 serum levels may have the best antihypertensive response to supplementation.
- The average reduction in BP is about 15/10 mm Hg based on reported studies.
- The antihypertensive effect takes time to reach its peak level at four weeks. Then the BP remains stable during long-term treatment. The antihypertensive effect is gone within two weeks after discontinuation of coenzyme Q10.
- Approximately 50% of patients on antihypertensive drugs may be able to stop between one and three agents. Both total dose and frequency of administration may be reduced.

Other favorable effects on cardiovascular risk factors include improvement in the serum lipid profile and carbohydrate metabolism with reduced glucose and improved insulin sensitivity, reduced oxidative stress, reduced heart rate, improved myocardial LV function and oxygen delivery, and decreased catecholamine levels.

Alpha Lipoic Acid

Alpha-lipoic acid (ALA) is known as thioctic acid in Europe where it is a prescription medication. It is a sulfur-containing compound with antioxidant activity both in water and lipid phases [1,32,33]. Its use is well established in the treatment of certain forms of liver disease and in the delay of onset of peripheral neuropathy in patients with diabetes. Recent research has evaluated its potential role in the treatment of hypertension, especially as part of the metabolic syndrome [152–154]. Lipoic acid reduces oxidative stress and inflammation, reduces atherosclerosis in animal models, decreases serum aldehydes and closes calcium channels (which improves vasodilation), improves endothelial function, and lowers BP. In addition, lipoic acid improves insulin sensitivity, which lowers glucose thereby improving BP control and lowering serum triglycerides. Morcos and others [155] showed stabilization of urinary albumin excretion in DM subjects given 600 mg of ALA compared to placebo for 18 months ($p < 0.05$).

The recommended dose is 100 to 200 mg per day of R-lipoic acid, with biotin 2–4 mg per day to prevent biotin depletion with long-term use of lipoic acid. R–lipoic acid is preferred to the L isomer because of its selected use by the mitochondria [1,32,33].

PYCNOGENOL

Pycnogenol, a bark extract from the French maritime pine, at doses of 200 mg/day resulted in a significant reduction in systolic BP from 139.9 mm Hg to 132.7 mmHg (p < 0.05) in 11 patients with mild hypertension over eight weeks in a double-blind, randomized placebo crossover trial. Diastolic BP fell from 93.8 mm Hg to 92.0 mm Hg. Pycnogenol acts as a natural ACEI, protects cell membranes from oxidative stress, increases NO and improves endothelial function, reduces serum thromboxane concentrations, decreases myelo-peroxidase activity, improves renal cortical blood flow, reduces urinary albumin excretion, and decreases HS-CRP [156–160]. Other studies have shown reductions in BP and a decreased need for ACEI and CCB, and reductions in Endothelin-1, HgA1C, fasting glucose, and LDL-C [157,158,160].

GARLIC

Clinical trials utilizing the correct dose, type of garlic, and well-absorbed, long-acting preparations have shown consistent reductions in BP in hypertensive patients with an average reduction in BP of 8.4/7.3 mm Hg [161,162]. Not all garlic preparations are processed similarly and are not comparable in antihypertensive potency [1]. In addition, cultivated garlic (*Allium sativum*), wild uncultivated garlic or bear garlic (*Allium urisinum*), and effects of aged, fresh, and long-acting garlic preparations differ [1,32–33,161–162]. Garlic is also effective in reducing BP in patients with uncontrolled hypertension already on antihypertensive medication [163]. In a double-blind, parallel, randomized placebo-controlled trial of 50 patients, 900 mg of aged garlic extract with 2.4 mg of S-allylcysteine was administered daily for 12 weeks and reduced SBP 10.2 mm Hg (p = 0.03) more than the control group in those with SBP over 140 mm Hg [163].

Approximately 10,000 mcg of allicin (one of the active ingredients in garlic) per day, the amount contained in four cloves of garlic (five grams) is required to achieve a significant BP lowering effect [1,32–33,162–163]. Garlic has ACEI activity, calcium channel blocking activity, reduces catecholamine sensitivity, improves arterial compliance, increases bradykinin and nitric oxide, and contains adenosine, magnesium, flavonoids, sulfur, allicin, phosphorous, and atoenes that reduce BP [1,32,33].

SEAWEED

Wakame seaweed (*Undaria pinnatifida*) is the most popular, edible seaweed in Japan [164]. In humans, 3.3 grams of dried wakame for four weeks significantly reduced both the SBP 14 ± 3 mm Hg and the DBP 5 ± 2 mm Hg (p < 0.01) [165]. In a study of 62 middle-aged, male subjects with mild hypertension given a potassium-loaded, ion-exchanging, sodium-adsorbing, potassium-releasing seaweed preparation, significant BP reductions occurred at four weeks on 12 and 24 grams/day of the seaweed preparation (p < 0.01) [166]. The MAP fell 11.2 mm Hg (p < 0.001) in the sodium-sensitive subjects and 5.7 mm Hg (p < 0.05) in the sodium-insensitive subjects, which correlated with plasma renin activity.

Seaweed and sea vegetables contain most all of the seawater's 771 minerals and rare earth elements, fiber, and alginate in a colloidal form [164–166]. The primary effect of wakame appears to be through its ACEI activity from at least four parent tetrapeptides and possibly their dipeptide and tripeptide metabolites, especially those containing the amino acid sequence Val-Tyr, Ile-Tyr, Phe-Tyr, and Ile-Try in some combination [164,167,168]. Its long-term use in Japan has demonstrated its safety. Other varieties of seaweed may reduce BP by reducing intestinal sodium absorption and increasing intestinal potassium absorption [166].

SESAME

Sesame has been shown to reduce BP in several small, randomized, placebo-controlled human studies over 30–60 days [169–174]. Sesame lowers BP alone [170–174] or in combination with nifedipine [169,173] and with diuretics and beta blockers [170,174]. In a group of 13 mild hypertensive subjects, 60 mg of sesamin for four weeks lowered SBP 3.5 mm Hg (p < 0.044) and DBP 1.9 mm Hg (p < 0.045) [171]. Black sesame meal at 2.52 grams per day over four weeks in 15 subjects reduced SBP by 8.3 mm Hg (p < 0.05) but there was a nonsignificant reduction in DBP of 4.2 mm Hg [172]. In addition, sesame lowers serum glucose, HgbAIC, and LDL-C; increases HDL; reduces oxidative stress markers; and increases glutathione, SOD, GPx, CAT, and vitamins C, E, and A [169–170,172–174]. The active ingredients are natural ACEIs, sesamin, sesamolin, sesaminol glucosides, furoufuran lignans, and suppressors of NF-kappa B [175,176]. All of these effects lower inflammation and oxidative stress, improve oxidative defense, and reduce BP [175,176].

BEVERAGES: TEA, COFFEE, AND COCOA

Green tea, black tea, and extracts of active components in both have demonstrated reduction in BP in humans [177–179].

Dark chocolate (100 grams) and cocoa with a high content of polyphenols (30 mg or more) have been shown to significantly reduce blood pressure in humans [180–189]. A meta-analysis of 173 hypertensive subjects given cocoa for a mean duration of two weeks had a significant reduction in BP 4.7/2.8 mm Hg (p = 0.002 for SBP and 0.006 for DBP) [180]. Fifteen subjects given 100 grams of dark chocolate with 500 mg of polyphenols for 15 days had a 6.4 mm Hg reduction in SBP (p < 0.05) with a nonsignificant change in DBP [181]. Cocoa at 30 mg of polyphenols reduced BP in prehypertensive and stage I hypertensive patients by 2.9/1.9 mm Hg at 18 weeks (p < 0.001) [182]. Two more recent meta-analysis of 13 trials and 10 trials with 297 patients found a significant reduction in BP of 3.2/2.0 mm Hg and 4.5/3.2 mm Hg respectively [184,187]. The BP reduction is the greatest in those with the highest baseline BP and those with a least 50–70% cocoa at doses of 6 to 100 grams per day [184,186]. Cocoa may also improve insulin resistance and endothelial function [181,188,189].

Polyphenols, chlorogenic acids (CGAs), the ferulic acid metabolite of CGAs, and di-hydro-caffeic acids decrease BP in a dose-dependent manner, increase eNOS, and improve endothelial function in humans [190–192]. CGAs in green coffee bean extract at doses of 140 mg per day significantly reduced SBP and DBP in 28 subjects in a placebo-controlled, randomized clinical trial. A study of 122 male subjects demonstrated a dose response in SBP and DBP with doses of CGA from 46 mg to 185 mg per day. The group that received the 185 mg dose had a significant reduction in BP of 5.6/3.9 mm Hg (p < 0.01) over 28 days. Hydroxyhydroquinone is another component of coffee beans that reduces the efficacy of CGAs in a dose-dependent manner, which partially explains the conflicting results of coffee ingestion on BP [190,192]. Furthermore, there is genetic variation in the enzyme responsible for the metabolism of caffeine that modifies the association between coffee intake, amount of coffee ingested, and the risk of hypertension, heart rate, myocardial infarction, arterial stiffness, arterial wave reflections, and urinary catecholamine levels [193]. Fifty-nine percent of the population has the IF/IA allele of the CYP1A2 genotype that confers slow metabolism of caffeine. Heavy coffee drinkers who are slow metabolizers had a 3.00 hazard ratio for developing hypertension. In contrast, fast metabolizers with the IA/IA allele had a 0.36 hazard ratio for incident hypertension [194].

ADDITIONAL COMPOUNDS

Melatonin demonstrates significant antihypertensive effects in humans in numerous double-blind, randomized, placebo-controlled clinical trials [195–205]. Beta blockers reduce melatonin secretion [206].

Hesperidin significantly lowered DBP 3–4 mm Hg (p < 0.02) and improved microvascular endo-thelial reactivity in 24 obese, hypertensive male subjects in a randomized, controlled crossover study over four weeks for each of three treatment groups consuming 500 ml of orange juice, hesperidin, or placebo [207].

Pomegranate juice reduces SBP 5–12%, reduces serum ACE activity by 36%, and has anti-atherogenic, antioxidant, and anti-inflammatory effects [208,209]. Pomegranate juice at 50 ml per day reduced carotid IMT by 30% over one year, increased PON 83%, decreased oxLDL by 59–90%, decreased antibodies to oxLDL by 19%, increased total antioxidant status by 130%, reduced TGF-b, and increased catalase, SOD, and GPx.

Grape seed extract (GSE) was administered to subjects in nine randomized trials, meta-analysis of 390 subjects, and demonstrated a significant reduction in SBP of 1.54 mm Hg (p < 0.02) [211]. Significant reduction in BP of 11/8 mm Hg (p < 0.05) was seen in another dose-response study with 150 to 300 mg per day of GSE over four weeks [212]. GSE has high phenolic content that activates the PI3K/Akt signaling pathway that phosphorylates eNOS and increases NO [212,213]. Hawthorn extract demonstrated borderline reductions on BP in patients not taking antihypertensive agents at 500 mg per day (p < 0.081), and significantly reduced DBP (p < 0.035) in diabetic patients taking antihypertensive drugs at doses of 1200 mg per day of hawthorn extract [214].

CLINICAL CONSIDERATIONS

COMPREHENSIVE APPROACH

Table 6.4 translates the basic science and clinical research into a comprehensive clinical approach. In the Hypertension Institute study [215], a comprehensive program using optimal nutrition with the DASH 2 diet, exercise, weight management, nutraceutical supplementation, renin profiling, and micronutrient analysis in lymphocytes, about 65% of patients were able to discontinue antihyper-tensive drug therapy over 12 months. The micronutrient analysis in lymphocytes gives a six-month picture of the patient's micronutrient deficiencies as well as their oxidative stress and defenses. This information allows for scientific administration of nutritional supplements to correct deficiencies as well as provide higher dose supplementation to reduce BP and improve vascular biology.

COMBINING FOOD AND NUTRIENTS WITH MEDICATIONS

Several of the strategic combinations of nutraceutical supplements with antihypertensive drugs mentioned in the previous section have been shown to lower blood pressure more than the medica-tion alone. These are:

- Sesame with beta blockers, diuretics, and nifedipine
- Pycnogenol with ACEI
- Lycopene with various antihypertensive medications
- Alpha-lipoic acid with ACEI
- Vitamin C with calcium channel blockers (CCB)
- N-acetyl cysteine with arginine
- Garlic with ACEI, diuretics and beta blockers
- Coenzyme Q10 with ACEI and CCB

Many antihypertensive drugs may cause nutrient depletions that can actually interfere with their antihypertensive action or cause other metabolic adverse effects manifest through the lab or with clinical symptoms [216,217]. Diuretics decrease potassium, magnesium, phosphorous, sodium, chloride, folate, vitamin B6, zinc, iodine, and coenzyme Q10; increase homocysteine, calcium, and creatinine; and elevate serum glucose by inducing insulin resistance. Beta blockers reduce coen-zyme Q10 and ACEI and ARB's reduce zinc.

TABLE 6.4

An Integrative Approach to the Treatment of Hypertension

Intervention Category	Therapeutic Intervention	Daily Intake
Diet characteristics	DASH I, DASH II-Na⁺, or PREMIER diet	Diet type
	Sodium restriction	1500 mg
	Potassium	4700 mg
	Potassium/sodium ratio	> 3:1
	Magnesium	1000 mg
	Zinc	50 mg
Macronutrients	Protein: Total intake from nonanimal sources, organic lean or wild animal protein, or cold-water fish	30% of total calories, which equals 1.5–1.8 gram/kg body weight
	Whey protein	30 grams
	Soy protein (fermented sources are preferred)	30 grams
	Sardine muscle concentrate extract	3 grams
	Milk peptides	30–60 mg
	Fat:	30% of total calories
	Omega-3 fatty acids	2–3 grams
	Omega-6 fatty acids	1 gram
	Omega-9 fatty acids	2–4 tablespoons of olive or nut oil or 10–20 olives
	Saturated fatty acids from wild game, bison, or other lean meat	< 10% total calories
	Polyunsaturated to saturated fat ratio	< 2:0
	Omega-3 to omega-6 ratio	1.1:1.2
	Synthetic trans fatty acids	None (completely remove from diet)
	Nuts in variety	Ad libidum
	Carbohydrates as primarily complex carbohydrates and fiber	40% of total calories
	Oatmeal or	60 grams
	Oatbran or	40 grams
	Beta-glucan or	3 grams
	Psyllium	7 grams
Specific foods	Garlic as fresh cloves or aged	4 fresh cloves (4 grams) or 600 mg aged garlic taken twice daily
	Sea vegetables, specifically dried wakame	3.0–3.5 grams
	Lycopene as tomato products, guava, watermelon, apricots, pink grapefruit, papaya, or supplements	10–20 mg
	Dark chocolate	100 grams
	Pomegranate juice	8 ounces
	Sesame	60 mg sesamin or 2.5 grams sesame meal
Exercise	Aerobic	20 minutes daily at 4200 KJ/week
	Resistance	40 minutes per day
Weight reduction	Body mass index < 25	Lose 1–2 pounds per week and increasing the proportion of lean muscle
	Waist circumference:	
	< 35 inches for women	
	< 40 inches for men	
	Total body fat:	
	< 22% for women	
	< 16% for men	

TABLE 6.4 (*continued*)

An Integrative Approach to the Treatment of Hypertension

Intervention Category	Therapeutic Intervention	Daily Intake
Other lifestyle recommendations	Alcohol restriction:	< 20 grams/day
	Among the choices of alcohol red wine is preferred due to its vasoactive phytonutrients	Wine < 10 ounces Beer < 24 ounces Liquor < 2 ounces
	Caffeine restriction or elimination depending on CYP 450 type	< 100 mg/day
	Tobacco and smoking	Stop
Medical considerations	Medications that may increase blood pressure	Minimize use when possible, such as by using disease-specific nutritional interventions
Supplemental foods and nutrients	Alpha-lipoic acid with biotin	100–200 mg twice daily
	Amino acids:	
	Arginine	5 grams twice daily
	Carnitine	1 to 2 grams twice daily
	Taurine	1 to 3 grams twice daily
	Chlorogenic acids	150–200 mg
	Coenzyme Q10	100 mg once to twice daily
	Grape seed extract	300 mg
	Melatonin	2.5 mg
	Resveratrol (trans)	250 mg
	Vitamin B6	100 mg once to twice daily
	Vitamin C	250–500 mg twice daily
	Vitamin D3	Dose to raise 25- hydroxyvitamin D serum level to 60 ng/ml
	Vitamin E as mixed tocopherols and delta and gamma tocotrienol	400 IU mixed tocopherols in the morning and 200 mg tocotrienols at bedtime

DIAGNOSTIC TESTING AND MONITORING DURING INTEGRATIVE THERAPY

Clinical monitoring of blood pressure is required in combination with patient awareness that dietary and supplemental interventions need to be taken as consistently as medication. Additional laboratory and diagnostic tests can inform clinical decision making. (See Table 6.5.) A test listed in Table 6.5 that particularly guides nutritional supplements for the management of hypertension is an assay of intracellular micronutrients in lymphocytes. From McCabe, 2003.

SUMMARY

Vascular biology such as endothelial and vascular smooth muscle dysfunction plays a primary role in the initiation and perpetuation of hypertension, CVD, and TOD.

- Nutrient-gene interactions are a predominant factor in promoting beneficial or detrimental effects in cardiovascular health and hypertension.
- Food and nutrients can prevent, control, and treat hypertension through numerous vascular biology mechanisms.
- Oxidative stress, inflammation, and autoimmune dysfunction initiate and propagate hypertension and cardiovascular disease.

TABLE 6.5

Clinical Monitoring and Laboratory Diagnostic Tests during Integrative Treatment of Hypertension

Category of Diagnostics Test	Test	Rationale and Other Notes	Interval for Repeating Tests
Blood	Electrolytes (serum) including magnesium	Low potassium can be clue to aldosteronism and low potassium increases BP. Giving potassium and magnesium reduces BP.	Every 2–3 months until normal, then once or twice per year
	Homocysteine	Indicates vitamins B6, B12, or folate deficiency and increases risk for CVA, CHD, and renal disease	Every 4 months until normal, then yearly
	Glucose and hemoglobin A1C	Evaluate insulin resistance, DM, and metabolic syndrome, which increase CVD; also helps in nutrient selection to lower glucose and BP	Every 4–6 months until normal then yearly
	Creatinine and blood urea nitrogen	Presence of renal insufficiency that will effect BP and CVD risk	Every 4–6 months
	High-sensitivity C-reactive protein	Indicates inflammation; increases CVD risk	Every 4–6 months
	Serum iron-, ferritin-, and total iron-binding capacity	Iron increases CHD risk and DM. Evaluate for hemochromatosis	Baseline, then every 4 months until normal, then yearly if elevated
	Advanced Lipid Profile	LDL and HDL particle number and size, Lp(a), Apo B, and A-1 that define CHD risk better than standard lipid profiles	Baseline, then every 4 months until normal with treatment then yearly
	Thyroid function	Hypothyroidism and hyperthyroidism increase BP and CHD risk.	Baseline, then every 4 months until normal with treatment then yearly
	Uric acid	Increases BP and CHD	Baseline, then every 4–6 months until normal, then yearly
	Vitamin D3	Low levels increase BP and CHD risk	Baseline, then every 4 months until normal, then yearly
	Micronutrient testing for intracellular nutrients	Measures 28 micronutrients with the average value for past 6 months in lymphocytes; allows for nutrient depletion analysis and replacement therapy as well as high-dose treatment	Baseline, then every 6 months until normal, then yearly
	Omega-3 index	Low levels increase risk for hypertension and CHD.	Baseline and every 6 months until normal, then yearly
	Plasma renin activity and serum aldosterone	Improves accuracy for nutrient and drug selection if not on therapy; helps define CHD risk	Baseline, and repeat in 4 months if resistant to treatment
	Male and female sex hormone levels	Low estrogen and testosterone increase BP and CHD risk	Baseline, and if abnormal, every 3–4 months while on treatment until normal, then every 6–12 months
Blood or cheek swab	CYP1A2 genotype	Hypertension responsive to caffeine restriction if IF/IA allele	Once if caffeine restriction is considered

TABLE 6.5 (*continued*)

Clinical Monitoring and Laboratory Diagnostic Tests during Integrative Treatment of Hypertension

Category of Diagnostics Test	Test	Rationale and Other Notes	Interval for Repeating Tests
Blood or urine	Heavy metals: lead mercury, cadmium, arsenic	Toxicity is associated with increased hypertension and nutritional strategies improve host defenses	Baseline
Urine	Urinalysis and microalbuminuria	Evaluates renal disease and CHD risk	Baseline, then every 4–6 months until normal, then yearly
Cardiac imaging and monitoring	Electrocardiogram	Evaluate for LAH, LVH, arrhythmias, electrical blocks	Baseline and then yearly
	Echocardiogram	Evaluate for LVH, valve function, ejection fraction	Yearly if abnormal
	Tests for endothelial dysfunction and arterial compliance such as ENDOPAT and HDI PROFILER	Endothelial dysfunction predicts BP, CHD risk and improves nutrient selection, drug selection, and response to treatment	Baseline, then yearly. If abnormal, every 6 months until normal
	Carotid IMT and Duplex	Risk for structural vascular disease with intimal medial thickening and plaque: predicts risk for CVA and correlates with other vascular diseases such as CHD and PAD	Baseline, then yearly
	Treadmill test	Evaluate for hypertensive response to exercise, arrhythmias, CHD	Baseline, then yearly
	24-hour ambulatory blood pressure monitor	Monitors BP more accurately than office and home readings; evaluates dipping status, BP load, average BP, lability, circadian rhythm, AM surges, adequate control	Baseline, then as needed to assess response to therapy every 4–6 months until all parameters are normal
Other	Body composition analysis	Visceral fat increases inflammation and HSCRP, increase BP and CHD risk	Baseline, then every 3 months until normal, then yearly
	Retinal scan	BP evaluation for target organ damage to retina; window to the brain	Baseline, then yearly

- There is a role for the selected use of single and component nutraceutical supplements, vitamins, antioxidants, and minerals in the treatment of hypertension based on scientifically controlled studies as a complement to optimal nutritional, dietary intake from food, and other lifestyle modifications [215].
- A clinical approach that incorporates diet, foods, nutrients, exercise, weight reduction, smoking cessation, alcohol and caffeine restriction, and other lifestyle strategies can be systematically and successfully incorporated into clinical practice. The protocol used by the author is outlined in Table 6.4.

REFERENCES

1. Houston, MC. Treatment of hypertension with nutraceuticals. Vitamins, antioxidants and minerals. Exper Rev Cardiovasc. Ther. 2007; 5(4): 681–91.
2. Eaton SB, Eaton SB, III, and Konner MJ. Paleolithic nutrition revisited: A twelve-year retrospective on its nature and implications. Eur J Clin Nutr 1997; 51:207–16.

3. Houston MC and Harper KJ. Potassium, magnesium, and calcium: Their role in both the cause and treatment of hypertension. J. Clin. Hypertens. 2008; 10 (7 supp 2): 3–11.

4. Layne J, Majkova Z, Smart EJ, Toborek M, and Hennig B. Caveolae: A regulatory platform for nutritional modulation of inflammatory diseases. J of Nutritional Biochemistry 2011; 22:807–11.

5. Dandona P, Ghanim H, Chaudhuri A, Dhindsa S, and Kim SS. Macronutrient intake induces oxidative and inflammatory stress: Potential relevance to atherosclerosis and insulin resistance. Exp Mol Med 2010; 42(4): 245–53.

6. Berdanier CD. Nutrient-gene interactions. In: Ziegler EE, Filer LJ, Jr, eds. *Present Knowledge in Nutrition*, 7th Ed. Washington, DC: ILSI Press, 1996, 574–80.

7. Talmud PJ and Waterworth DM. In-vivo and in-vitro nutrient-gene interactions. Curr Opin Lipidol 2000; 11:31–36.

8. Houston MC. The importance of potassium in managing hypertension. Curr Hypertens Rep 2011; 13(4): 309–17.

9. Broadhurst CL. Balanced intakes of natural triglycerides for optimum nutrition: An evolutionary and phytochemical perspective. Med Hypotheses 1997; 49:247–61.

10. Nayak DU, Karmen C, Frishman WH, and Vakili BA. Antioxidant vitamins and enzymatic and synthetic oxygen-derived free radical scavengers in the prevention and treatment of cardiovascular disease. Heart Disease 2001; 3:28–45.

11. Kizhakekuttu TJ and Widlansky ME. Natural antioxidants and hypertension: Promise and challenges. Cardiovasc Ther. 2010; 28(4): e20–e32.

12. Kitiyakara C and Wilcox C. Antioxidants for hypertension. Curr Opin Nephrol Hypertens 1998; 7:531–38.

13. Russo C, Olivieri O, Girelli D, Faccini G, Zenari ML, Lombardi S, and Corrocher R. Antioxidant status and lipid peroxidation in patients with essential hypertension. J Hypertens 1998; 16:1267–71.

14. Tse WY, Maxwell SR, Thomason H, Blann A, Thorpe GH, Waite M, and Holder R. Antioxidant status in controlled and uncontrolled hypertension and its relationship to endothelial damage. J Hum Hypertens 1994; 8:843–49.

15. Mansego ML, Solar Gde M, Alonso MP, Martinez F, Saez GT, Escudero JC, Redon J, and Chaves FJ. Polymorphisms of antioxidant enzymes, blood pressure and risk of hypertension. J Hypertens 2011; 29(3): 492–500.

16. Galley HF, Thornton J, Howdle PD, Walker BE, and Webster NR. Combination oral antioxidant supplementation reduces blood pressure. Clin Sci 1997; 92:361–365.

17. Dhalla NS, Temsah RM, and Netticadam T. The role of oxidative stress in cardiovascular diseases. J Hypertens 2000; 18:655–673.

18. Saez G, Tormos MC, Giner V, Lorano JV, and Chaves FJ. Oxidative stress and enzymatic antioxidant mechanisms in essential hypertension. Am J Hypertens 2001; 14:248A. Abstract P-653.

19. Ghanem FA and Movahed A. Inflammation in high blood pressure: A clinician's perspective. J Am. Soc Hypertens. 2007; 1(2): 113–19.

20. Amer MS, Elawam AE, Khater MS, Omar OH, Mabrouk RA, and Taha HM. Association of high–sensitivity C reactive protein with carotid artery intima-media thickness in hypertensive older adults. J Am Soc Hypertens. 2011; 5(5): 395–400.

21. Vongpatanasin W, Thomas GD, Schwartz R, Cassis LA, Osborne-Lawrence S, Hahner L, Gibson LL, Black S, Samois D, and Shaul PW. C-reactive protein causes downregulation of vascular angiotensin subtype 2 receptors and systolic hypertension in mice. Circulation 2007; 115(8): 1020–28.

22. Razzouk L, Munter P, Bansilal S, et al. C reactive protein predicts long-term mortality independently of low-density lipoprotein cholesterol in patients undergoing percutaneous coronary intervention. Am Heart J 2009; 158(2): 277–83.

23. Kvakan H, Luft FC, and Muller DN. Role of the immune system in hypertensive target organ damage. Trends Cardiovasc Med 2009; 19(7): 242–46.

24. Rodriquez-Iturbe B, Franco M, Tapia E, Quiroz Y, and Johnson RJ. Renal inflammation, autoimmunity and salt-sensitive hypertension. Clin Exp Pharmacol Physiol 2012; 39(1): 96–103.

25. Tian N, Penman AD, Mawson AR, Manning RD, Jr, and Flessner MF. Association between circulating specific leukocyte types and blood pressure. The Atherosclerosis Risk in Communities (ARIC) study. J Am Soc Hypertens 2010; 4(6): 272–83.

26. Muller DN, Kvakan H, and Luft FC. Immune-related effects in hypertension on and target-organ damage. Curr Opin Nephrol Hypertens. 2011; 20(2): 113–17.

27. Kotchen TA and McCarron DA. AHA Science Advisory. Dietary electrolytes and blood pressure. Circulation 1998; 98:613–17.

28. Cutler JA, Follmann D, and Allender PS. Randomized trials of sodium reduction: An overview. Am J Clin Nutr 1997; 65:643S–51S.
29. Svetkey LP, Sacks FM, Obarzanek E, et al. The DASH diet, sodium intake and blood pressure (the DASH-Sodium Study): Rationale and design. JADA 1999; 99:S96–S104.
30. Weinberger MH. Salt sensitivity of blood pressure in humans. Hypertension 1996; 27:481–90.
31. Morimoto A, Usu T, Fujii T, et al. Sodium sensitivity and cardiovascular events in patients with essential hypertension. Lancet 1997; 350:1734–37.
32. Houston MC. Nutraceuticals, vitamins, antioxidants and mineral in the prevention and treatment of hypertension. Prog Cardiovasc Dis. 2005; 47(6): 396–449.
33. Houston MC. Nutrition and nutraceutical supplements in the treatment of hypertension. Exper Rev Cardiovasc Ther 2010; 8(6): 821–33.
34. Messerli FH, Schmieder RE, and Weir MR. Salt: A perpetrator of hypertensive target organ disease? Arch Intern Med 1997; 157:2449–52.
35. Kawasaki T, Delea CS, Bartter FC, and Smith H. The effect of high-sodium and low-sodium intakes on blood pressure and other related variables in human subjects with idiopathic hypertension. Am J Med 1978; 64:193–98.
36. Whelton PK, He J. Potassium in preventing and treating high blood pressure. Semin Nephrol 1999; 19:494–99.
37. Gu D, He J, Xigui W, Duan X, and Whelton PK. Effect of potassium supplementation on blood pressure in Chinese: A randomized, placebo-controlled trial. J Hypertens 2001; 19:1325–31.
38. Widman L, Wester PO, Stegmayr BG, and Wirell MP. The dose dependent reduction in blood pressure through administration of magnesium: A double blind placebo controlled cross-over trial. Am J Hypertens 1993; 6:41–45.
39. Laurant P and Touyz RM. Physiological and pathophysiological role of magnesium in the cardiovascular system: Implications in hypertension. J Hypertens 2000; 18:1177–91.
40. Houston MC. The role of magnesium in hypertension and cardiovascular disease. J. Clinical Hypertension in press as of January 2012.
41. McCarron DA. Role of adequate dietary calcium intake in the prevention and management of salt sensitive hypertensive. Am J Clin Nutr 1997; 65:712S–16S.
42. Resnick LM. Calcium metabolism in hypertension and allied metabolic disorders. Diabetes Care 1991; 14:505–20.
43. Garcia Zozaya JL and Padilla Viloria M. Alterations of calcium, magnesium, and zinc in essential hypertension: Their relation to the renin-angiotensin-aldosterone system. Invest Clin 1997; 38:27–40.
44. Shahbaz AU, Sun Y, Bhattacharya SK, Ahokas RA, Gerling IC, McGee JE, and Weber KT. Fibrosis in hypertensive heart disease: Molecular pathways and cardioprotective strategies. J Hypetens 2010; 28: S25–32.
45. Bergomi M, Rovesti S, Vinceti M, Vivoli R, Caselgrandi E, and Vivoli G. Zinc and copper status and blood pressure. J Trace Elem Med Biol 1997; 11:166–69.
46. Stamler J, Elliott P, Kesteloot H, Nichols R, Claeys G, Dyer AR, and Stamler R. Inverse relation of dietary protein markers with blood pressure. Findings for 10,020 men and women in the Intersalt Study. Intersalt Cooperative Research Group. International study of salt and blood pressure. Circulation 1996; 94:1629–34.
47. Altorf-van der Kuil W, Engberink MF, Brink EJ, van Baak MA, Bakker SJ, Navis G, van t'Veer P, and Geleijnse JM. Dietary protein and blood pressure: A systematic review. PLoS One 2010; 5(8); e12102–17.
48. Jenkins DJ, Kendall CW, Faulkner DA, et al. Long-term effects of a plant-based dietary portfolio of cholesterol-lowering foods on blood pressure. Eur J Clin Nutr 2008; 62(6): 781–88.
49. Elliott P, Dennis B, Dyer AR, et al. Relation of dietary protein (total, vegetable, animal) to blood pressure: INTERMAP epidemiologic study. Presented at the 18th Scientific Meeting of the International Society of Hypertension, Chicago, IL, August 20–24, 2000.
50. He J, Wofford MR, Reynolds K, Chen J, Chen CS, Myers L, Minor DL, Elmer PJ, Jones DW, and Whelton PK. Effect of dietary protein supplementation on blood pressure: A randomized controlled trial. Circulation 2011; 124(5);589–95.
51. FitzGerald RJ, Murray BA, and Walsh DJ. Hypotensive peptides from milk proteins. J Nutr 2004: 134(4): 980S–88S.
52. Pins JJ and Keenan JM. Effects of whey peptides on cardiovascular disease risk factors. J Clin Hypertens 2006; 8(11): 775–82.
53. Aihara K, Kajimoto O, Takahashi R, and Nakamura Y. Effect of powdered fermented milk with lactobacillus helveticus on subjects with high-normal blood pressure or mild hypertension. J Am Coll Nutr. 2005; 24(4): 257–65.

54. Gemino FW, Neutel J, Nonaka M, and Hendler SS. The impact of lactotripeptides on blood pressure response in stage 1 and stage 2 hypertensives. J Clin Hypertens. 2010; 12(3): 153–59.

55. Geleijnse JM and Engberink MF. Lactopeptides and human blood pressure. Curr Opin Lipidol 2010; 21(1): 58–63.

56. Pins J and Keenan J. The antihypertensive effects of a hydrolyzed whey protein supplement. Cardiovasc Drugs Ther 2002; 16(Suppl): 68.

57. Zhu CF, Li GZ, Peng HB, Zhang F, Chen Y, and Li Y. Therapeutic effects of marine collagen peptides on Chinese patients with type 2 diabetes mellitus and primary hypertension. Am J Med Sci 2010; 340(5): 360–66.

58. De Leo F, Panarese S, Gallerani R, and Ceci LR. Angiotensin converting enzyme (ACE) inhibitory peptides: Production and implementation of functional food. Curr Pharm Des 2009; 15(31): 3622–43.

59. Lordan S, Ross P, and Stanton C. Marine bioactives as functional food ingredients: Potential to reduce the incidence of chronic disease. Mar Drugs 2011; 9(6): 1056–1100.

60. Kawasaki T, Seki E, Osajima K, Yoshida M, Asada K, Matsui T, and Osajima Y. Antihypertensive effect of valyl-tyrosine, a short chain peptide derived from sardine muscle hydrolyzate, on mild hypertensive subjects. J Hum Hypertens 2000; 14:519–23.

61. Kawasaki T, Jun CJ, Fukushima Y, and Seki E. Antihypertensive effect and safety evaluation of vegetable drink with peptides derived from sardine protein hydrolysates on mild hypertensive, high-normal and normal blood pressure subjects. Fukuoka Igaku Zasshi 2002; 93(10): 208–18.

62. Yang G, Shu XO, Jin F, Zhang X, Li HL, Li Q, Gao YT, and Zheng W. Longitudinal study of soy food intake and blood pressure among middle-aged and elderly Chinese women. Am J Clin Nutr 2005; 81(5): 1012–17.

63. Teede HJ, Giannopoulos D, Dalais FS, Hodgson J, and McGrath BP. Randomised, controlled, cross-over trial of soy protein with isoflavones on blood pressure and arterial function in hypertensive patients. J Am Coll Nutr 2006; 25(6): 533–40.

64. Welty FK, Lee KS, Lew NS, and Zhou JR. Effect of soy nuts on blood pressure and lipid levels in hypertensive, prehypertensive and normotensive postmenopausal women. Arch Inter Med 2007; 167(10): 1060–67.

65. Rosero Arenas MA, Roser Arenas E, Portaceli Arminana MA, and Garcia MA. Usefulness of phyto-oestrogens in reduction of blood pressure. Systematic review and meta-analysis. Aten Primaria 2008; 40(4): 177–86.

66. Nasca MM, Zhou JR, and Welty FK. Effect of soy nuts on adhesion molecules and markers of inflammation in hypertensive and normotensive postmenopausal women. Am J Cardiol 2008; 102(1): 84–86.

67. He J, Gu D, Wu X, Chen J, Duan X, Chen J, and Whelton PK. Effect of soybean protein on blood pressure: A randomized, controlled trial. Ann Intern Med 2005; 143(1): 1–9.

68. Hasler CM, Kundrat S, and Wool D. Functional foods and cardiovascular disease. Curr Atheroscler Rep 2000; 2(6): 467–75.

69. Tikkanen MJ and Adlercreutz H. Dietary soy-derived isoflavone phytoestrogens. Could they have a role in coronary heart disease prevention? Biochem Pharmacol 2000; 60(1): 1–5.

70. Begg DP, Sinclari AJ, Stahl LA, Garg ML, Jois M, and Weisinger RS. Dietary proteins level interacts with omega-3 polyunsaturated fatty acid deficiency to induce hypertension. Am. J. Hyperten. 2009; Nov 5 E pub. Ahead of Print.

71. Vallance P, Leone A, Calver A, Collier J, and Moncada S. Endogenous dimethyl-arginine as an inhibitor of nitric oxide synthesis. J Cardiovasc Pharmacol 1992; 20: S60–S62.

72. Sonmez A, Celebi G, Erdem G, et al. Plasma apelin and ADMA levels in patients with essential hypertension. Clin Exp Hypertens 2010; 32(3): 179–83.

73. Michell DL, Andrews KL and Chin-Dusting JP. Endothelial dysfunction in hypertension: The role of arginase. Front Biosci (Schol Ed) 2011; 3: 946–60.

74. Rajapakse NW and Mattson DL. Role of L-arginine in nitric oxide production in health and hypertension. Clin EWxp Pharmacol Physiol. 2009; 36(3): 249–55.

75. Tsioufis C, Dimitriadis K, Andrikou E, Thomopoulos C, Tsiachris D, Stefanadi E, Mihas C, Miliou A, Papademetriou V, and Stefanadis C. ADMA, C-reactive protein and albuminuria in untreated essential hypertension: A cross-sectional study. Am J Kidney Dis. 2010; 55(6): 1050–59.

76. Siani A, Pagano E, Iacone R, Iacoviell L, Scopacasa F, and Strazzullo P. Blood pressure and metabolic changes during dietary L-arginine supplementation in humans. Am J Hypertens 2000; 13: 547–51.

77. Facchinetti F, Saade GR, Neri I, Pizzi C, Longo M, and Volpe A. L-arginine supplementation in patients with gestational hypertension: A pilot study. Hypertens Pregnancy 2007; 26(1): 121–30.

78. Neri I, Monari F, Sqarbi L, Berardi A, Masellis G, and Facchinetti F. L-arginine supplementation in women with chronic hypertension: Impact on blood pressure and maternal and neonatal complications. J Matern Fetal Neonatal Med. 2010; 23(12): 1456–60.

79. Martina V, Masha A, Gigliardi VR, et al. Long-term N-acetylcysteine and L-arginine administration reduces endothelial activation and systolic blood pressure in hypertensive patients with type 2 diabetes. Diabetes Care. 2008; 31(5): 940–44.

80. Ast J, Jablecka A, Bogdanski I, Krauss H, and Chmara E. Evaluation of the antihypertensive effect of L-arginine supplementation in patients with mild hypertension assessed with ambulatory blood pressure monitoring. Med Sci Monit. 2010; 16(5): CR 266–71.

81. Schulman SP, Becker LC, Kass DA, et al. L arginine therapy in acute myocardial infarction: The vascular interaction with age in myocardial infarction (VINTAGE MI) randomized clinical trial. JAMA 2006; 295(1): 58–64.

82. Digiesi V, Cantini F, Bisi G, Guarino G, and Brodbeck B. L-carnitine adjuvant therapy in essential hypertension. Clin Ter 1994; 144:391–95.

83. Ghidini O, Azzurro M, Vita G, and Sartori G. Evaluation of the therapeutic efficacy of L-carnitine in congestive heart failure. Int J Clin Pharmacol Ther Toxicol. 1988; 26(4): 217–20.

84. Digiesi V, Palchetti R, and Cantini F. The benefits of L-carnitine therapy in essential arterial hypertension with diabetes mellitus type II. Minerva Med 1989; 80(3): 227–31.

85. Huxtable RJ. Physiologic actions of taurine. Physiol Rev 1992; 72:101–63.

86. Fujita T, Ando K, Noda H, Ito Y, and Sato Y. Effects of increased adrenomedullary activity and taurine in young patients with borderline hypertension. Circulation 1987; 75:525–32.

87. Huxtable RJ and Sebring LA. Cardiovascular actions of taurine. Prog Clin Biol Res 1983; 125:5–37.

88. Tanabe Y, Urata H, Kiyonaga A, Ikede M, Tanake H, Shindo M, and Arakawa K. Changes in serum concentrations of taurine and other amino acids in clinical antihypertensive exercise therapy. Clin Exp Hypertens 1989; 11:149–65.

89. Mori TA, Bao DQ, Burke V, Puddey IB, and Beilin LJ. Docosahexaenoic acid but not eicosapentaenoic acid lowers ambulatory blood pressure and heart rate in humans. Hypertension 1999; 34:253–60.

90. Bønaa KH, Bjerve KS, Straume B, Gram IT, and Thelle D. Effect of eicosapentaenoic and docosahexanoic acids on blood pressure in hypertension: A population-based intervention trial from the Tromso study. N Engl J Med 1990; 322:795–801.

91. Mori TA, Burke V, Puddey I, and Irish A. The effects of omega 3 fatty acids and coenzyme Q 10 on blood pressure and heart rate in chronic kidney disease: A randomized controlled trial. J Hypertens 2009; 27(9): 1863–72.

92. Ueshima H, Stamler J, Elliot B, and Brown, CQ. Food omega 3 fatty acid intake of individuals (total, linolenic acid, long chain) and their blood pressure: INTERMAP study. Hypertension 2007; 50(20): 313–19.

93. Mon TA. Omega 3 fatty acids and hypertension in humans. Clin Exp Pharmacol Physio 2006: 33(9): 842–46.

94. Liu JC, Conkin SM, Manuch SB, Yao JK, and Muldoon MF. Long-chain omega 3 fatty acids and blood pressure. Am J Hypertens. 2011: July 14 E PUB.

95. Engler MM, Schambelan M, Engler MB, and Goodfriend TL. Effects of dietary gamma-linolenic acid on blood pressure and adrenal angiotensin receptors in hypertensive rats. Proc Soc Exp Biol Med 1998; 218(3): 234–37.

96. Sagara M, Njelekela M, Teramoto T, Taquchi T, Mori M, Armitage L, Birt N, Birt C, and Yamori Y. Effects of docozhexaenoic acid supplementation on blood pressure, heart rate, and serum lipid in Scottish men with hypertension and hypercholesterolemia. Int J Hypertens. 2011; 8:8091–98.

97. Mori TA, Burke V, Puddey I, Irish A, Cowpland CA, Beilin L, Dogra G, and Watts GF. The effects of omega 3 fatty acids and coenzyme Q 10 on blood pressure and heart rate in chronic kidney disease: A randomized controlled trial. J Hypertens 2009; 27:1863–72.

99. Chin JP. Marine oils and cardiovascular reactivity. Prostaglandins Leukot Essent Fatty Acids 1994; 50:211–22.

100. Saravanan P, Davidson NC, Schmidt EB, and Calder PC. Cardiovascular effects of marine omega-3 fatty acids. Lancet 2010; 376(9740): 540–50.

101. Ferrara LA, Raimondi S, and d'Episcopa I. Olive oil and reduced need for antihypertensive medications. Arch Intern Med. 2000; 160:837–42.

102. Thomsen C, Rasmussen OW, Hansen KW, Vesterlund M, and Hermansen K. Comparison of the effects on the diurnal blood pressure, glucose, and lipid levels of a diet rich in monounsaturated fatty acids with a diet rich in polyunsaturated fatty acids in type 2 diabetic subjects. Diabet Med 1995; 12:600–606.

103. Perona JS, Canizares J, Montero E, Sanchez-Dominquez JM, Catala A, and Ruiz-Gutierrez V. Virgin olive oil reduces blood pressure in hypertensive elderly patients. Clin Nutr 2004; 23(5): 1113–21.

104. Perona JS, Montero E, Sanchez-Dominquez JM, Canizares J, Garcia M, and Ruiz-Gutierrez V. Evaluation of the effect of dietary virgin olive oil on blood pressure and lipid composition of serum and low-density lipoprotein in elderly type 2 subjects. J Agric Food Chem. 2009; 57(23): 11427–33.

105. Lopez-Miranda J, Perez-Jimenez F, Ros E, et al. Olive oil and health: Summary of the II international conference on olive oil and health consensus report, Jaen and Cordoba (Spain) 2008. Nutr Metab Cardiovasc Dis 2010; 20(4): 284–94.

106. He J and Whelton PK. Effect of dietary fiber and protein intake on blood pressure: A review of epidemiologic evidence. Clin Exp Hypertens 1999; 21:785–96.

107. Pruijm M, Wuerzer G, Forni V, Bochud M, Pechere-Bertschi A, and Burnier M. Nutrition and hypertension: More than table salt. Rev Med Suisse 2010; 6(282):1715–20.

108. Sherman DL, Keaney JF, Biegelsen ES, et al. Pharmacological concentrations of ascorbic acid are required for the beneficial effect on endothelial vasomotor function in hypertension. Hypertension 2000; 35:936–41.

109. Ness AR, Khaw K-T, Bingham S, and Day NE. Vitamin C status and blood pressure. J Hypertens 1996; 14:503–08.

110. Duffy SJ, Bokce N, and Holbrook M. Treatment of hypertension with ascorbic acid. Lancet 1999; 354: 2048–49.

111. Enstrom JE, Kanim LE, and Klein M. Vitamin C intake and mortality among a sample of the United States population. Epidemiology 1992; 3:194–202.

112. Block G, Jensen, CD, Norkus EP, Hudes M, and Crawford PB. Vitamin C in plasma is inversely related to blood pressure and change in blood pressure during the previous year in young black and white women. Nut J 2008; 17(7): 35–46.

113. Hatzitolios A, Iliadis F, Katsiki N, and Baltatzi M. Is the antihypertensive effect of dietary supplements via aldehydes reduction evidence based: A systemic review. Clin Exp Hypertens. 2008; 30(7): 628–39.

114. Mahajan AS, Babbar R, Kansai N, Agarwai, SK, and Ray PC. Antihypertensive and antioxidant action of amlodipine and vitamin C in patients of essential hypertension. J CLin Biochem Nutr. 2007; 40(2) 141–47.

115. Ledlerc PC, Proulx CD, Arquin G, and Belanger S. Ascorbic acid decreases the binding affinity of the AT! Receptor for angiotensin II. Am J Hypertens. 2008: 21(1): 67–71.

116. Plantinga Y, Ghiadone L, Magagna, A, and Biannarelli C. Supplementation with vitamins C and E improves arterial stiffness and endothelial function in essential hypertensive patients. Am J Hypertens. 2007; 20(4): 392–97.

117. Sato K, DohiY, Kojima, M, and Miyagawa K. Effects of ascorbic acid on ambulatory blood pressure in elderly patients with refractory hypertension. Arzneimittelforschung. 2006; 56(7): 535–40.

118. Block G, Mangels AR, Norkus EP, Patterson BH, Levander OA, and Taylor PR. Ascorbic acid status and subsequent diastolic and systolic blood pressure. Hypertension 2001; 37:261–67.

119. McRae MP. Is vitamin C an effective antihypertensive supplement? A review and analysis of the literature. J. Chiropr Med 2006; 5(2): 60–64.

120. Simon JA. Vitamin C and cardiovascular disease: A review. J Am Coll Nutr 1992; 11(2): 107–25.

121. Ness AR, Chee D, and Elliott P. Vitamin C and blood pressure—An overview. J Hum Hypertens 1997; 11(6): 343–50.

122. Trout DL. Vitamin C and cardiovascular risk factors. Am J Clin Nutr. 1991; 53(1 Suppl): 322S–25S.

123. National Center for Health Statistics, Fulwood R, Johnson CL, and Bryner JD. Hematological and nutritional biochemistry reference data for persons 6 months–74 years of age: United States, 1976–80. Washington, DC; US Public Health Service; 1982 Vital and Health Statistics series 11, No. 232, DHHS publication No. (PHS) 83–1682.

124. Ward NC, Wu JH, Clarke MW, and Buddy IB. Vitamin E effects on the treatment of hypertension in type 2 diabetics. J of Hypertension 2007; 227: 227–34.

125. Murray ED, Wechter WJ, Kantoci D, Wang WH, Pham T, Quiggle DD, Gibson KM, Leipold D, and Anner BM. Endogenous natriuretic factors 7: Biospecificity of a natriuetic gamma-tocopherol metabolite LLU alpha. J Pharmacol Exp Ther 1997; 282(2): 657–62.

126. Gray B, Swick J, and Ronnenberg AG. Vitamin E and adiponectin: Proposed mechanism for vitamin E-induced improvement in insulin sensitivity. Nutr Rev. 2011; 69(3): 155–61.

127. Hanni LL, Huarfner LH, Sorensen OH, and Ljunghall S. Vitamin D is related to blood pressure and other cardiovascular risk factors in middle-aged men. Am J Hypertens 1995; 8:894–901.

128. Bednarski R, Donderski R, and Manitius L. Role of vitamin D in arterial blood pressure control. Pol Merkur Lekarski 2007;136: 307–10.

129. Ngo DT, Sverdlov AL, McNeil JJ, and Horowitz JD. Does vitamin D modulate asymmetric dimethyl-argine and C-reactive protein concentrations? Am J Med 2010; 123(4): 335–41.

130. Rosen CJ. Clinical practice. Vitamin D insufficiency. N Engl J. Med 2011; 364(3): 248–54.

131. Pittas AG, Chung M, Trikalinos T, Mitri J, Brendel M, Patel K, Lichtenstein HA, Lau J, and Balk EM. Systematic review: Vitamin D and cardiometabolic outcomes. Ann Intern Med 2010; 152(5): 307–14.

132. Motiwala SR and Want TJ. Vitamin D and cardiovascular disease. Curr Opin Nephrol Hypertens 2011; 20(4): 345–53.

133. Bhandari SK, Pashayan S, Liu IL, Rasgon SA, Kujubu DA, Tom TY, and Sim JJ. 25–hydroxyvitamin D levels and hypertension rates. J Clin Hypertens 2011; 13(3): 170–77.

134. Pfeifer M, Begerow B, Minne HW, Nachtigall D, and Hansen C. Effects of a short-term vitamin D(3) and calcium supplementation on blood pressure and parathyroid hormone levels in elderly women. J Clin Endocrinol Metab 2001; 86: 1633–37.

135. Keniston R and Enriquez JI, Sr. Relationship between blood pressure and plasma vitamin B6 levels in healthy middle-aged adults. Ann N Y Acad Sci 1990; 585:499–501.

136. Aybak M, Sermet A, Ayyildiz MO, and Karakilcik AZ. Effect of oral pyridoxine hydrochloride supplementation on arterial blood pressure in patients with essential hypertension. Arzneimittelforschung 1995; 45:1271–73.

137. Paulose CS, Dakshinamurti K, Packer S, and Stephens NL. Sympathetic stimulation and hypertension in the pyridoxine-deficient adult rat. Hypertension 1988; 11(4): 387–91.

138. Dakshinamurti K, Lal KJ, and Ganguly PK. Hypertension, calcium channel and pyridoxine (vitamin B 6). Mol Cell Biochem 1998;188(1–2): 137–48.

139. Moline J, Bukharovich IF, Wolff MS, and Phillips R. Dietary flavonoids and hypertension: Is there a link? Med Hypotheses 2000; 55:306–9.

140. Knekt P, Reunanen A, Järvinen R, Seppänen R, Heliövaara M, and Aromaa A. Antioxidant vitamin intake and coronary mortality in a longitudinal population study. Am J Epidemiol 1994; 139:1180–89.

141. Karatzi KN, Papamichael CM, Karatizis EN, Papaioannou TG, Aznaouridis KA, Katsichti PP, and Stamatelopuolous KS. Red wine acutely induces favorable effects on wave reflections and central pressures in coronary artery disease patients. Am. J Hypertension 2005; 18(9): 1161–67.

142. Biala A, Tauriainen E, Siltanen A, Shi J, Merasto S, Louhelainen M, Martonen E, Finckenberg P, Muller DN, and Mervaala E. Resveratrol induces mitochondrial biogenesis and ameliorates Ang II- induced cardiac remodeling in transgenic rats harboring human renin and angiotensinogen genes. Blood Press 2010; 19(3): 196–205.

143. Wong RH, Howe PR, Buckley JD, Coates AM, Kunz L, and Berry NM. Acute resveratrol supplementation improves flow-mediated dilatation in overweight obese individuals with mildly elevated blood pressure. Nutr Metab Cardiovasc Dis. 2011 Nov; 21(11): 851–56.

144. Bhatt SR, Lokhandwala MF, and Banday AA. Resveratrol prevents endothelial nitric oxide synthase uncoupling and attenuates development of hypertension in spontaneously hypertensive rats. Eur J Pharmacol 2011; 667(1–3): 258–64.

145. Rivera L, Moron R, Zarzuelo A, and Galisteo M. Long-term resveratrol administration reduces metabolic disturbances and lowers blood pressure in obese Zucker rats. Biochem Pharmacol 2009; 77(6): 1053–63.

146. Paran E and Engelhard YN. Effect of lycopene, an oral natural antioxidant on blood pressure. J Hypertens 2001; 19:S74. Abstract P 1.204.

147. Engelhard YN, Gazer B, and Paran E. Natural antioxidants from tomato extract reduce blood pressure in patients with grade-1 hypertension: A double blind placebo controlled pilot study. Am Heart J 2006; 151(1):100.

148. Paran E, Novac C, Engelhard YN, and Hazan-Halevy I. The effects of natural antioxidants from tomato extract in treated but uncontrolled hypertensive patients. Cardiovasc Durgs Ther 2009; 23(2): 145–51.

149. Reid K, Frank OR, and Stocks NP. Dark chocolate or tomato extract for prehypertension: A randomized controlled trial. BMC Complement Altern Med 2009; 9:22.

150. Paran E and Engelhard Y. Effect of tomato's lycopene on blood pressure, serum lipoproteins, plasma homocysteine and oxidative stress markers in grade I hypertensive patients. Am J Hypertens 2001; 14:141A. Abstract P-333.

151. Rosenfeldt FL, Haas SJ, Krum H, and Hadu A. Coenzyme Q 10 in the treatment of hypertension: A meta-analysis of the clinical trials. J Hum Hypertens 2007; 21(4): 297–306.

152. McMackin CJ, Widlansky ME, Hambury NM, and Haung AL. Effect of combined treatment with alpha lipoic acid and acetyl carnitine on vascular function and blood pressure in patients with coronary artery disease. Journal of Clinical Hypertension 2007: 9: 249–55.

153. Salinthone S, Schillace RV, Tsang C, Regan JW, Burdette DN, and Carr DW. Lipoic acid stimulates cAMP production via G protein-coupled receptor-dependent and -independent mechanisms. J Nutr Biochem 2011; 22(7): 681–90.

154. Rahman ST, Merchant N, Hague T, Wahi J, Bhaheetharan S, Ferdinand KC, and Khan BV. The impact of lipoic acid on endothelial function and proteinuria in Quinapril-treated diabetic patients with stage I hypertension: Results from the QUALITY study. J Cardiovasc Pharmacol Ther 2012; 17(2): 139–45.

155. Morcos M, Borcea V, Isermann B, et al. Effect of alpha-lipoic acid on the progression of endothelial cell damage and albuminuria in patients with diabetes mellitus: An exploratory study. Diabetes Res Clin Prac 2001; 52(3): 175–83.

156. Hosseini S, Lee J, Sepulveda RT, et al. A randomized, double-blind, placebo-controlled, prospective 16 week crossover study to determine the role of pycnogenol in modifying blood pressure in mildly hypertensive patients. Nutr Res 2001; 21:1251–60.

157. Zibadi S, Rohdewald PJ, Park D, and Watson RR. Reduction of cardiovascular risk factors in subjects with type 2 diabetes by pycnogenol supplementation. Nutr Res 2008; 28(5): 315–20.

158. Liu X, Wei J, Tan F, Zhou S, Wurthwein G, and Rohdewald P. Pycnogenol French maritime pine bark extract improves endothelial function of hypertensive patients. Lif Sci 2004; 74(7): 855–62.

159. Van der Zwan LP, Scheffer PG, and Teerlink T. Reduction of myeloperoxidase activity by melatonin and pycnogenol may contribute to their blood pressure lowering effect. Hypertension 2010; 56(3): e35.

160. Cesarone MR, Belcaro G, Stuard S, et al. Kidney flow and function in hypertension: Protective effects of pycnogenol in hypertensive participants–a controlled study. J Cardiovasc Pharmacol Ther 2010; 15(1): 41–46.

161. Simons S, Wollersheim H, and Thien T. A systematic review on the influence of trial quality on the effects of garlic on blood pressure. Neth. J. Med 2009; 67(6): 212–19.

162. Reinhard KM, Coleman CI, Teevan C, and Vacchani P. Effects of garlic on blood pressure in patients with and without systolic hypertension: A meta-analysis. Ann Pharmacother 2008; 42(12): 1766–71.

163. Reid K, Frank OR, and Stocks NP. Aged garlic extract lowers blood pressure in patients with treated but uncontrolled hypertension: A randomized controlled trial. Maturitas 2010; 67(2): 144–50.

164. Suetsuna K and Nakano T. Identification of an antihypertensive peptide from peptic digest of wakame (undaria pinnatifida). J Nutr Biochem 2000; 11:450–54.

165. Nakano T, Hidaka H, Uchida J, Nakajima K, and Hata Y. Hypotensive effects of wakame. J Jpn Soc Clin Nutr 1998; 20: 92.

166. Krotkiewski M, Aurell M, Holm G, Grimby G, and Szckepanik J. Effects of a sodium-potassium ion-exchanging seaweed preparation in mild hypertension. Am J Hypertens 1991; 4:483–88.

167. Sato M, Oba T, Yamaguchi T, Nakano T, Kahara T, Funayama K, Kobayashi A, and Nakano T. Antihypertensive effects of hydrolysates of wakame (Undaria pinnatifida) and their angiotnesin-1-converting inhibitory activity. Ann Nutr Metab 2002; 46(6): 259–67.

168. Sato M, Hosokawa T, Yamaguchi T, Nakano T, Muramoto K, Kahara T, Funayama K, Kobayashi A, and Nakano T. Angiotensin I converting enzyme inhibitory peptide derived from wakame (Undaria pinnatifida) and their antihypertensive effect in spontaneously hypertensive rats. J Agric Food Chem 2002; 50(21): 6245–52.

169. Sankar D, Sambandam G, Ramskrishna Rao M, and Pugalendi KV. Modulation of blood pressure, lipid profiles and redox status in hypertensive patients taking different edible oils. Clin Chim Acta 2005; 355(1–2): 97–104.

170. Sankar D, Rao MR, Sambandam G, and Pugalendi KV. Effect of sesame oil on diuretics or beta-blockers in the modulation of blood pressure, athropometry, lipid profile and redox status. Yale J Biol Med. 2006; 79(1): 19–26.

171. Miyawaki T, Aono H, Toyoda-Ono Y, Maeda H, Kiso Y, and Moriyama K. Antihypertensive effects of sesamin in humans. J Nutr Sci Vitaminol (Tokyo) 2009; 55(1): 87–91.

172. Wichitsranoi J,Weerapreeyakui N, Boonsiri P, Settasatian N, Komanasin N, Sirjaichingkul S, Teerajetgul Y, Rangkadilok N, and Leelayuwat N. Antihypertensive and antioxidant effects of dietary black sesame meal in pre-hypertensive humans. Nutr J 2011; 10(1): 82–88.

173. Sudhakar B, Kalaiarasi P, Al-Numair KS, Chandramohan G, Rao RK, and Pugalendi KV. Effect of combination of edible oils on blood pressure, lipid profile, lipid peroxidative markers, antioxidant status, and electrolytes in patients with hypertension on nifedipine treatment. Saudi Med J 2011; 32(4): 379–85.

174. Sankar D, Rao MR, Sambandam G, and Pugalendi KV. A pilot study of open label sesame oil in hypertensive diabetics. J Med Food 2006; 9(3): 408–12.

175. Harikumar KB, Sung B, Tharakan ST, Pandey MK, Joy B, Guha S, Krishnan S, and Aggarwai BB. Sesamin manifests chemopreventive effects through the suppression of NF-kappa-B-regulated cell survival, proliferation, invasion and angiogenic gene products. Mol Cancer Res 2010; 8(5): 751–61.

176. Nakano D, Ogura K, Miyakoshi M, et al. Antihypertensive effect of angiotensin I-converting enzyme inhibitory peptides from a sesame protein hydrolysate in spontaneously hypertensive rats. Biosci Biotechnol Biochem 2006; 70(5): 1118–26.

177. Hodgson JM, Puddey IB, Burke V, Beilin LJ, and Jordan N. Effects on blood pressure of drinking green and black tea. J Hypertens 1999; 17:457–63.

178. Kurita I, Maeda-Yamamoto M, Tachibana H, and Kamei M. Antihypertensive effect of Benifuuki tea containing O-methylated EGCG. J Agric Food Chem 2010; 58(3): 1903–8.

179. McKay DL, Chen CY, Saltzman E, and Blumberg JB. Hibiscus sabdariffa L. tea (tisane) lowers blood pressure in pre-hypertensive and mildly hypertensive adults. J Nutr 2010; 140(2): 298–303.

180. Taubert D, Roesen R, and Schomig E. Effect of cocoa and tea intake on blood pressure: A meta-analysis. Arch Intern Med 2007; 167(7): 626–34.

181. Grassi D, Lippi C, Necozione S, Desideri G, and Ferri C. Short-term administration of dark chocolate is followed by a significant increase in insulin sensitivity and a decrease in blood pressure in health persons. Am J Clin Nutr 2005; 81(3): 611–14.

182. Taubert D, Roesen R, Lehmann C, Jung N, and Schomig E. Effects of low habitual cocoa intake on blood pressure and bioactive nitric oxide: A randomized controlled trial. JAMA 2007; 298(1): 49–60.

183. Cohen DL and Townsend RR. Cocoa ingestion and hypertension–another cup please? J Clin Hypertens 2007; 9(8): 647–48.

184. Reid I, Sullivan T, Fakler P, Frank OR, and Stocks NP. Does chocolate reduce blood pressure? A meta-analysis. BMC Med 2010; 8:39–46.

185. Egan BM, Laken MA, Donovan JL, and Woolson RF. Does dark chocolate have a role in the prevention and management of hypertension? Commentary on the evidence. Hypertension 2010; 55(6): 1289–95.

186. Desch S, Kobler D, Schmidt J, Sonnabend M, Adams V, Sareben M, Eitel I, Bluher M, Shuler G, and Thiele H. Low vs higher-dose dark chocolate and blood pressure in cardiovascular high-risk patients. Am J Hypertens 2010; 23(6): 694–700.

187. Desch S, Schmidt J, Sonnabend M, Eitel I, Sareban M, Rahimi K, Schuler G, and Thiele H. Effect of cocoa products on blood pressure: Systematic review and meta-analysis. Am J Hypertens 2010; 23(1): 97–103.

188. Grassi D, Desideri G, Necozione S, Lippi C, Casale R, Properzi G, Blumberg JB, and Ferri C. Blood pressure is reduced and insulin sensitivity increased in glucose intolerant hypertensive subjects after 15 days of consuming high-polyphenol dark chocolate. J Nutr 2008; 138(9): 1671–76.

189. Grassi D, Necozione S, Lippi C, Croce G, Valeri L, Pasqualetti P, Desideri G, Blumberg JB, and Ferri C. Cocoa reduces blood pressure and insulin resistance and improved endothelium-dependent vasodilation in hypertensives. Hypertension 2005; 46(2): 398–405.

190. Yamaguchi T, Chikama A, Mori K, Watanabe T, Shiova Y, Katsuraqi Y, and Tokimitsu I. Hydroxyhydroquinone-free coffee: A double-blind, randomized controlled dose-response study of blood pressure. Nutr Metab Cardiovasc Dis 2008; 18(6): 408–14.

191. Chen ZY, Peng C, Jiao R, Wong YM, Yang N, and Huang Y. Antihypertensive nutraceuticals and functional foods. J Agric Food Chem 2009; 57(11): 4485–99.

192. Ochiai R, Chikama A, Kataoka K, Tokimitsu I, Maekawa Y Ohsihi M, Rakugi H, and Mikmai H. Effects of hydroxyhydroquinone-reduced coffee on vasoreactivity and blood pressure. Hypertens Res 2009; 32(11): 969–74.

193. Kozuma K, Tsuchiya S, Kohori J, Hase T, and Tokimitsu I. Antihypertensive effect of green coffee bean extract on mildly hypertensive subjects. Hypertens Res 2005; 28(9): 711–18.

194. Palatini P, Ceolotto G, Ragazzo F, Donigatti F, Saladini F, Papparella I, Mos L, Zanata G, and Santonastaso M. CYP 1A2 genotype modifies the association between coffee intake and the risk of hypertension. J Hypertens 2008; 27(8): 1594–601.

195. Scheer FA, Van Montfrans GA, van Someren EJ, Mairuhu G, and Buijs RM. Daily nighttime melatonin reduces blood pressure in male patients with essential hypertension. Hypertension 2004; 43(2): 192–97.

196. Cavallo A, Daniels SR, Dolan LM, Khoury JC, and Bean JA. Blood pressure response to melatonin in type I diabetes. Pediatr Diabetes 2004; 5(1): 26–31.

197. Cavallo A, Daniels SR, Dolan LM, Bean JA, and Khoury JC. Blood pressure-lowering effect of melatonin in type 1 diabetes. J Pineal Res 2004; 36(4): 262–66.

198. Cagnacci A, Cannoletta M, Renzi A, Baldassari F, Arangino S, and Volpe A. Prolonged melatonin administration decreases nocturnal blood pressure in women. Am J Hypertens 2005; 18(12 Pt 1): 1614–18.

199. Grossman E, Laudon M, Yalcin R, Zengil H, Peleg E, Sharabi Y, Kamari Y, Shen-Orr Z, and Zisapel N. Melatonin reduces night blood pressure in patients with nocturnal hypertension. Am J Med 2006; 119 (10): 898–902.

200. Rechcinski T, Kurpese M, Trzoa E, and Krzeminska-Pakula M. The influence of melatonin supplementation on circadian pattern of blood pressure in patients with coronary artery disease-preliminary report. Pol Arch Med Wewn 2006; 115(6): 520–28.

201. Merkureva GA and Ryzhak GA. Effect of the pineal gland peptide preparation on the diurnal profile of arterial pressure in middle-aged and elderly women with ischemic heart disease and arterial hypertension. Adv Gerontol 2008; 21(1): 132–42.

202. Zaslavskaia RM, Scherban EA, and Logvinenki SI. Melatonin in combined therapy of patients with stable angina and arterial hypertension. Klin Med (Mosk) 2009; 86: 64–77.

203. Zamotaev IuN, Enikeev AKh, and Kolomets NM. The use of melaxen in combined therapy of arterial hypertension in subjects occupied in assembly line production. Klin Med (Mosk) 2009; 87(6): 46–49.

204. Rechcinski T, Trzos E, Wierzbowski-Drabik K, Krzeminska-Pakute M, and Kurpesea M. Melatonin for nondippers with coronary artery disease: Assessment of blood pressure profile and heart rate variability. Hypertens Res 2002; 33(1): 56–61.

205. Kozirog M, Poliwczak AR, Duchnowicz P, Koter-Michalak M, Sikora J, and Broncel M. Melatonin treatment improves blood pressure, lipid profile and parameters of oxidative stress in patients with metabolic syndrome. J Pineal Res 2011; 50(3): 261–66.

206. De-Leersnyder H, de Biois MC, Vekemans M, Sidi D, Villain E, Kindermans C, and Munnich A. Beta (1) adrenergic antagonists improve sleep and behavioural disturbances in a circadian disorder, Smith-Magenis syndrome. J Med Genet 2110; 38(9): 586–90.

207. Morand C, Dubray C, Milenkovic D, Lioger D, Martin JF, Scalber A, and Mazur A. Hesperidin contributes to the vascular protective effects of orange juice: A randomized crossover study in healthy volunteers. Am J Clin Nutr 2011; 93(1): 73–80.

208. Basu A and Penugonda K. Pomegranate juice: A heart-healthy fruit juice. Nutr Rev 2009; 67(1): 49–56.

209. Aviram M, Rosenblat M, Gaitine D, et al. Pomegranate juice consumption for 3 years by patients with carotid artery stenosis reduces common carotid intima-media thickness, blood pressure and LDL oxidation. Clin Nutr 2004; 23(3): 423–33.

210. Aviram M and Dornfeld L. Pomegranate juice inhibits serum angiotensin converting enzyme activity and reduces systolic blood pressure. Atherosclerosis 2001; 18(1): 195–98.

211. Feringa HH, Laskey DA, Dickson JE, and Coleman CI. The effect of grape seed extract on cardiovascular risk markers: A meta-analysis of randomized controlled trials. J Am Diet Associ 2011; 111(8): 1173–81.

212. Sivaprakasapillai B, Edirsinghe K, Randolph J, Steinberg F, and Kappagoda T. Effect of grape seed extract on blood pressure in subjects with the metabolic syndrome. Metabolism 2009: 58(12): 1743–46.

213. Edirisinghe I, Burton-Freeman B, and Tissa Kappagoda C. Mechanism of the endothelium-dependent relaxation evoked by grape seed extract. Clin Sci (Lond) 2008; 114(4): 331–37.

214. Walker AF, Marakis G, Simpson E, Hope JL, Robinson PA, Hassanein M, and Simpson HC. Hypotensive effects of hawthorn for patients with diabetes taking prescription drugs: A randomized controlled trial. Br J Gen Pract 2006; 56(527): 437–43.

215. Houston MC. The role of cellular micronutrient analysis and minerals in the prevention and treatment of hypertension and cardiovascular disease. Therapeutic Advances in Cardiovascular Disease 2010; 4:v165–83.

216. Trovato A, Nuhlicek DN, and Midtling JE. Drug-nutrient interactions. Am Fam Physician 1991; 44(5): 1651–58.

217. McCabe BJ, Frankel EH, and Wolfe JJ. Eds Handbook of Food-Drug Interactions. Boca Raton, FL: CRC Press, 2003.

7 Congestive Heart Failure and Cardiomyopathy

The Metabolic Cardiology Solution

Stephen T. Sinatra, M.D.

INTRODUCTION

The consensus opinion is that failing hearts are energy starved. Disruption in the metabolic processes controlling myocardial energy metabolism is characteristic in failing hearts, and this loss of energetic balance directly impacts heart function. Treatment options that include metabolic intervention with therapies shown to preserve energy substrates or accelerate energy turnover are indicated for at-risk populations or patients at any stage of disease.

EPIDEMIOLOGY

More than five million Americans suffer from chronic congestive heart failure (CHF) and 550,000 new cases are diagnosed annually, making CHF the most costly diagnosis in the Medicare population and the most common cause of hospitalization in patients over age 65. With an aging population, the number of CHF cases continues to grow annually, as evidenced by the growth in hospital discharges, which increased from 400,000 in 1979 to more than 1.08 million in 2005, or 171%.

Approximately 28% of men and women over the age of 45 have mild to moderate diastolic dysfunction with preserved ejection fraction [1]. Decline in diastolic heart function marks an early stage of disease that can progress in the absence of clinical and metabolic intervention.

The same study presented additional data that CHF is a growing medical concern, with the lifetime risk of developing CHF for those over the age of 40 years now at 20%, a level well in excess of many conditions commonly monitored with age [1].

PATHOPHYSIOLOGY

CHF is a clinical syndrome characterized by well-established symptoms, clinical findings, and standard of care pharmaceutical interventions. CHF occurs when the heart muscle weakens or the myocardial wall becomes stiff, resulting in an inability to meet the metabolic demands of the peripheral tissues. This chronic condition is predisposed by hypertension, cardiac insult such as myocardial infarction, ischemic heart disease, valvular disease, chronic alcohol abuse, or infection of the heart muscle, to mention a few. They all contribute to dysfunction or permanent loss of myocytes and decrease in contractility, cardiac output, and perfusion to vital organs of the body. Frequently, excess fluid accumulates in the liver, lungs, lining of the intestines, and the lower extremities.

Many cardiovascular diseases such as hypertension, coronary artery disease, and cardiomy-opathies can lead to the progressive onset of CHF that is accompanied by systolic and/or dia-stolic dysfunction. Most patients with systolic cardiac dysfunction exhibit some degree of diastolic involvement, but approximately half of the patients with CHF show marked impairment of dia-stolic function with well-preserved ejection fraction. Deficits in both systolic and diastolic dysfunc-tion frequently go undiagnosed until the onset of overt heart failure.

BASICS OF CARDIAC ENERGY METABOLISM

It is now widely accepted that one characteristic of the failing heart is the persistent and progressive loss of energy. The requirement for energy to support the systolic and diastolic work of the heart is absolute. Therefore, a disruption in cardiac energy metabolism, and the energy supply–demand mismatch that results, can be identified as the pivotal factor contributing to the inability of failing hearts to meet the hemodynamic requirements of the body. In her landmark book, *ATP and the Heart*, Joanne Ingwall [2] describes the metabolic maelstrom associated with the progression of CHF and identifies the mechanisms that lead to a persistent loss of cardiac energy reserves as the disease process unfolds.

The heart contains approximately 700 milligrams of adenosine triphosphate (ATP), enough to fuel about 10 heartbeats. At a rate of 60 beats per minute, the heart will beat 86,400 times in the average day, forcing the heart to produce and consume an amazing 6000 g of ATP daily and caus-ing it to recycle its ATP pool 10,000 times every day. This process of energy recycling occurs primarily in the mitochondria of the myocyte. These organelles produce more than 90% of the energy consumed in the healthy heart, and in the heart cell, the approximately 3500 mitochondria fill about 35% of the cell volume. Disruption in mitochondrial function significantly restricts the energy-producing processes of the heart, causing a clinically relevant impact on heart function that translates to peripheral tissue involvement.

The heart consumes more energy per gram than any other organ, and the chemical energy that fuels the heart comes primarily from ATP (Figure 7.1). The chemical energy held in ATP is resident in the phosphoryl bonds, with the greatest amount of energy residing in the outermost bond holding the ultimate phosphoryl group to the penultimate group. When energy is required to provide the chemical driving force to a cell, this ultimate phosphoryl bond is broken and chemical energy is released. The cell then converts this chemical energy to mechanical energy

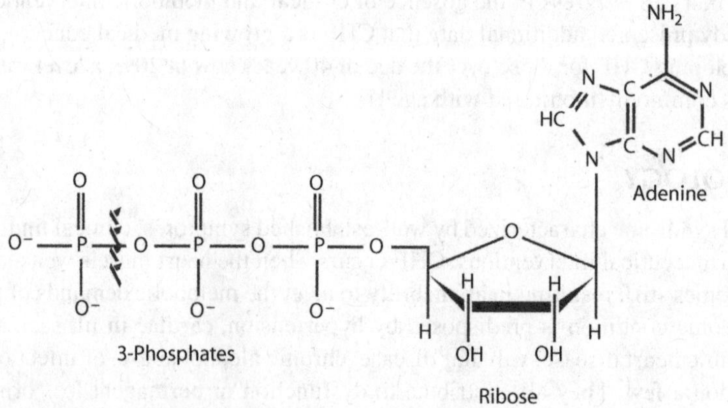

FIGURE 7.1 The ATP molecule.

to do work. In the case of the heart, this energy is used to sustain contraction, drive ion pump function, synthesize large and small molecules, and perform other necessary activities of the cell. The consumption of ATP in the supply of cellular energy yields the metabolic byproducts adenosine diphosphate (ADP) and inorganic phosphate (Pi). A variety of metabolic mechanisms have evolved within the cell to provide rapid rephosphorylation of ADP to restore ATP levels and maintain the cellular energy pool. In significant ways, these metabolic mechanisms are disrupted in CHF, tipping the balance in a manner that creates a chronic energy supply–demand mismatch.

The normal nonischemic heart is capable of maintaining a stable ATP concentration despite large fluctuations in workload and energy demand. In a normal heart, the rate of ATP synthesis via rephosphorylation of ADP closely matches ATP utilization. The primary site of ATP rephosphorylation is the mitochondria, where fatty acid and carbohydrate metabolic products flux down the oxidative phosphorylation pathways. ATP recycling can also occur in the cytosol via the glycolytic pathway of glucose metabolism, but in normal hearts this pathway accounts for only about 10% of ATP turnover. ATP levels are also maintained through the action of creatine kinase in a reaction that transfers a high-energy phosphate creatine phosphate (PCr) to ADP to yield ATP and free creatine. Because the creatine kinase reaction is approximately 10 times faster than ATP synthesis via oxidative phosphorylation, creatine phosphate acts as a buffer to assure a consistent availability of ATP in times of acute high metabolic demand. Although there is approximately twice as much creatine phosphate in the cell as ATP, there is still only enough to supply energy to drive about 10 heartbeats, making the maintenance of high levels of ATP availability critical to cardiac function.

The content of ATP in heart cells progressively falls in CHF, frequently reaching and then stabilizing at levels that are 25% to 30% lower than normal [3,4]. The fact that ATP falls in the failing heart means that the metabolic network responsible for maintaining the balance between energy supply and demand is no longer functioning normally in these hearts. It is well established that oxygen deprivation in ischemic hearts contributes to the depletion of myocardial energy pools [2,4], but the loss of energy substrates in the failing heart is a unique example of chronic metabolic failure in the well-oxygenated myocardium. The mechanism explaining energy depletion in heart failure is the loss of energy substrates and the delay in their resynthesis. In conditions where energy demand outstrips supply, ATP is consumed at a rate that is faster than it can be restored via oxidative phosphorylation or the alternative pathways of ADP rephosphorylation. The net result of this energy overconsumption is the loss of ATP catabolic products that leave the cell by passing across the cell membrane into the bloodstream. This loss of catabolic byproducts lowers the cellular concentration of energy substrates and depletes energy reserves. In diseased hearts, the energy pool depletion via this mechanism can be significant, reaching levels that exceed 40% in ischemic heart disease and 30% in heart failure.

Under high workload conditions, even normal hearts display a minimal loss of energy substrates. These substrates must be restored via the de novo pathway of ATP synthesis. This pathway is slow and energy costly, requiring consumption of six high-energy phosphates to yield one newly synthesized ATP molecule. The slow speed and high energy cost of de novo synthesis highlights the importance of cellular mechanisms designed to preserve energy pools. In normal hearts, the salvage pathways are the predominant means by which the ATP pool is maintained. While de novo synthesis of ATP proceeds at a rate of approximately 0.02 nM/min/g in the heart, the salvage pathways operate at a tenfold higher rate [5]. The function of both the de novo and salvage pathways of ATP synthesis is limited by the cellular availability of 5-phosphoribosyl-1-pyrophosphate, or PRPP (Figure 7.2). PRPP initiates these synthetic reactions and is the sole compound capable of donating the D-ribose-5-phosphate moiety required to re-form ATP and preserve the energy pool. In muscle tissue, including that of the heart, formation of PRPP is slow and rate limited, impacting the rate of ATP restoration via the de novo and salvage pathways.

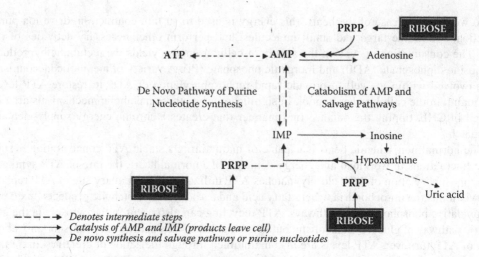

FIGURE 7.2 De novo synthesis and salvage of energy compounds.

ENERGY STARVATION IN THE FAILING HEART

The long-term mechanism explaining the loss of ATP in CHF is decreased capacity for ATP synthesis relative to ATP demand. In part, the disparity between energy supply and demand in hypertrophied and failing hearts is associated with a shift in relative contribution of fatty acid versus glucose oxidation to ATP synthesis. The major consequence of the complex readjustment toward carbohydrate metabolism is that the total capacity for ATP synthesis decreases, while the demand for ATP continually increases as hearts work harder to circulate blood in the face of increased filling pressures associated with CHF and hypertrophy. The net result of this energy supply–demand mismatch is a decrease in the absolute concentration of ATP in the failing heart; this decrease in absolute ATP level is reflected in a lower energy reserve in the failing and hypertrophied heart. A declining energy reserve is directly related to heart function, with diastolic function being first affected, followed by systolic function, and finally global performance (Figure 7.3).

LaPlace's law confirms that pressure overload increases energy consumption in the face of abnormalities in energy supply. In failing hearts, these energetic changes become more profound as left ventricle remodeling proceeds [6–8], but they are also evident in the early development of the disease [9]. It has also been found that similar adaptations occur in the atrium, with energetic abnormalities constituting a component of the substrate for atrial fibrillation in CHF [10]. Left ventricular hypertrophy is initially an adaptive response to chronic pressure overload, but it is

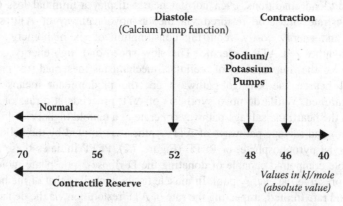

FIGURE 7.3 Free energy of hydrolysis of ATP required to fuel certain cell functions.

ultimately associated with a tenfold greater likelihood of subsequent chronic CHF. While metabolic abnormalities are persistent in CHF and left ventricular hypertrophy, at least half of all patients with left ventricular hypertrophy–associated heart failure have preserved systolic function, a condition referred to as diastolic heart failure.

Oxidative phosphorylation is directly related to oxygen consumption, which is not decreased in patients with pressure-overload left ventricular hypertrophy [11]. Metabolic energy defects, instead, relate to the absolute size of the energy pool and the kinetics of ATP turnover through oxidative phosphorylation and creatine kinase. The deficit in ATP kinetics is similar in both systolic and diastolic heart failure and may be both an initiating event and a consequence. Inadequate ATP availability would be expected to initiate and accentuate the adverse consequences of abnormalities in energy-dependent pathways. Factors that increase energy demand, such as adrenergic stimulation and biochemical remodeling, exaggerate the energetic deficit. Consequently, the hypertrophied heart is more metabolically susceptible to stressors such as increased chronotropic and inotropic demand and ischemia.

In humans, this metabolic deficit is shown to be greater in compensated left ventricular hypertrophy (with or without concomitant CHF) than in dilated cardiomyopathy [12,13]. Hypertensive heart disease alone was not shown to contribute to alterations in high-energy phosphate metabolism, but it can contribute to left ventricular hypertrophy and diastolic dysfunction that can later alter cardiac energetics [14,15]. Further, for a similar clinical degree of heart failure, volume overload hypertrophy does not, but pressure overload does, induce significant high-energy phosphate impairment [16]. Type 2 diabetes has also been shown to contribute to altering myocardial energy metabolism early in the onset of diabetes, and these alterations in cardiac energetics may contribute to left ventricular functional changes [17]. The effect of age on progression of energetic altering has also been reviewed, with results of both human [18] and animal [19] studies suggesting that increasing age plays a moderate role in the progressive changes in cardiac energy metabolism that correlates to diastolic dysfunction, left ventricular mass, and ejection fraction.

Cardiac energetics also provide important prognostic information in patients with heart failure, and determining the myocardial contractile reserve has been suggested as a method of differentiating which patients would most likely respond to cardiac resynchronization therapy (CRT) seeking to reverse LV remodeling [20]. Patients with a positive contractile reserve are more likely to respond to CRT and reverse remodeling of the left ventricle. Nonresponders show a negative contractile reserve, suggesting increased abnormality in cardiac energetics.

Studies confirm that energy metabolism in CHF and left ventricular hypertrophy are of vital clinical importance impacting both the heart and peripheral tissue. Loss of diastolic function associated with energy depletion can directly affect diastolic filling and stroke volume, limiting the delivery of oxygen-rich blood to the periphery. This chronic oxygen deprivation forces peripheral tissue, especially muscle, to adjust and down-regulate energy turnover mechanisms, a contributing cause of peripheral tissue involvement in CHF and a factor in the symptoms of fatigue, dyspnea, and muscle pain associated with the disease.

PATIENT EVALUATION

While the symptoms of CHF are well known and diagnostic procedures are defined, early diastolic dysfunction may be more difficult to diagnose. Clinical suspicion can be raised by the symptoms of shortness of breath and fatigue. While CHF can generally be determined by a careful physical examination and chest X-ray, more complex cases may require further assessment, such as that uncovered by increases in B-type natriuretic peptide (BNP) or by right heart catheterization. An echocardiogram with careful assessment of the mitral valve velocity and function will assist the clinician in making the diagnosis.

It should be noted that a presumption of energy deficiency in all patients presenting with CHF symptoms is warranted. While the absolute energy requirement for diastolic filling exceeds that of

TABLE 7.1

Nutrient-Drug Interactions for Energy Nutrients

Nutrient	Drugs Depleting Tissue Levels
D-Ribose	There are no known nutrient-drug interactions
CoQ10	Statins, beta blockers, oral hypoglycemic agents, certain antidepressants
L-Carnitine	Dilantin

systolic emptying, patients with systolic heart failure frequently present with diastolic and peripheral tissue involvement. Therefore, energy deficiency should be a paramount consideration.

Blood levels of certain of the nutrients involved in energy production can be assayed and have been shown to correlate with cardiomyocyte energy needs. Assays for free L-carnitine and CoQ10 are not routinely done by hospitals with the exception of the Mayo Clinic, but testing is routinely available and blood levels of CoQ10 and L-carnitine can be determined by qualified medical diagnostic laboratories, such as Quest Diagnostics or Metametrix Clinical Laboratory. The normal ranges show considerable variation. In my own clinical experience after testing hundreds of patients, I feel that the normal baseline levels of CoQ10 and L-carnitine approximate the plasma baseline levels of the Mayo Clinic, which are 0.43–1.53 µg/mL and 25–54 µmol/L for CoQ10 and free L-carnitine, respectively.

Although the medical literature generally supports the use of CoQ10 in CHF, the evaluated dose-response relationships for the nutrient have been confined to a narrow dose range, with the majority of clinical studies having been conducted in doses ranging from 90 to 200 mg daily. At such doses, some patients have responded, while others have not. In my patients with moderate to severe CHF or dilated cardiomyopathy, I generally use higher doses of CoQ10 in ranges of 300 to 600 mg in order to get a biosensitive result frequently requiring a blood level greater than 2.5 µg/mL and preferably up to 3.5 µg/mL [21,22]. Blood levels are particularly important and should be ordered, especially in patients who do not respond clinically when higher doses of CoQ10 and carnitine are utilized.

Some specialty laboratories provide both normal and optimal ranges. The slightly higher optimal range is clinically meaningful and more reflective of the range needed for patients with CHF. Since L-carnitine is predominantly made in the liver and kidney, additional consideration should be given to patients with renal failure or insufficiency because low levels of L-carnitine may adversely affect multiple organ systems. I suggest testing these patients more frequently to monitor L-carnitine levels in an attempt to move them into the optimum range. To maintain a blood level of L-carnitine sufficient to impact cardiac energy metabolism in CHF, I recommend 2000 to 2500 mg/day. Since L-carnitine is not well absorbed, smaller doses given multiple times a day on an empty stomach appear to be most effective. Most preparations of L-carnitine are offered in capsules. Patients on the medications listed in Table 7.1 are also at risk for low serum levels and priority should be placed on diagnostic testing in these patients.

D-ribose is produced by each cell individually and is not transported from one tissue to another. Therefore, a minimal blood level has not been established. In all energy-depleted patients, a lack of adequate D-ribose should be presumed, since the natural synthesis of D-ribose in tissue is generally inadequate to preserve or restore tissue energy levels in conditions of chronic energy deficiency. Blood levels of D-ribose range from 0.0 to 3.0 mg/dL and can be evaluated by laboratory evaluation, but results are of limited diagnostic value.

PHARMACOLOGIC TREATMENT

In large part, the objective of drug therapy is to inhibit certain of the compensatory mechanisms that may contribute to progression of CHF.

First-line pharmaceutical therapies for CHF include angiotensin-converting enzyme (ACE) inhibitors, diuretics, and digoxin. Angiotensin receptor blockers (ARBs) are also used as alternatives to ACE inhibitors in patients who are unable to tolerate the side effects of ACE inhibitors—cough being the most common and annoying symptom. Beta blockers have shown promising results in clinical trials designed to evaluate improvement in quality of life, exercise tolerance, and functional classification. Various types of diuretics are often utilized when fluid retention interferes with quality-of-life issues such as dyspnea and/or peripheral edema.

Digoxin, a natural constituent of the foxglove flowering plant, exerts a mild positive inotropic effect on cardiac contractility by inhibiting sodium-potassium pump function. Inhibiting this pump leads to accumulation of calcium within the cell, making it available to myosin to promote contraction. In general, however, while inotropic agents relieve symptoms in CHF patients, there is no evidence they prolong life and, in fact, may worsen the mortality rate. Inotropic agents such as Dobutamine increase contractility and cardiac output but may force the heart to work beyond its energetic reserve, further reducing the cardiac energy pool. Inotropic agents may increase the frequency of cardiac arrhythmias and the potential for sudden cardiac death, effects that may be exacerbated by depletion of the cardiac energy pool.

Although the pharmacological treatment of CHF improves symptoms, the options are often limited. An integrative approach with positive lifestyle considerations and nutraceutical support will improve quality of life and reduce human suffering. Nutraceutical support with energy-enhancing nutraceuticals has improved quality-of-life issues in patients awaiting heart transplant. In my personal experience, I have had several patients taken off transplant lists who improved so much while waiting for a transplant that they decided not to undergo the surgery.

FOOD AND NUTRIENT TREATMENT

One of the major issues associated with heart failure is fluid retention. Compensatory mechanisms in heart failure lead to fluid and sodium retention to maintain blood pressure. Processed foods further increase fluid retention, an effect that may lead to increased blood pressure that could aggravate the energy-depleted condition.

Conversely, CHF patients are frequently deficient in magnesium and potassium, which are depleted in heart failure often by the use of diuretic medications. Low potassium can increase blood pressure, while depleted magnesium can lead to a number of factors, including poor energy metabolism and insulin resistance. Similarly, thiamin levels can be low in CHF, and this can further sodium retention and disease progression. Finally, patients with CHF should limit fluid consumption to two quarts per day. Fluids are broadly defined as foods that are liquid at room temperature, and therefore include water, milk, juices, Jell-O or gelatins, popsicles, and ice cream (see Table 7.2).

TABLE 7.2
Nutrient Recommendations for Congestive Heart Failure

Nutrient	Recommendation
Salt	Avoid: processed salt in fast food, canned soups and sauces, lunch meats, frozen dinners, snack foods
Magnesium	Increase: wheat germ, navy beans, oatmeal, nuts, seeds, figs, tofu, low-fat dairy items, seafood
Potassium	Increase: fresh fruits and vegetables, beans, whole grains, low-fat dairy items, fish, potatoes
Thiamin	Increase: beans, peas, peanuts, whole grains, eggs, fish, poultry
Fats	Avoid: all trans fats; Restrict: saturated fats
Processed sugars	Avoid all
Fluids	Restrict to 2 quarts per day or less; Alternatives: hard candies or gum to stimulate saliva, ice chips to lessen thirst

---

TABLE 7.3
Foods High in Energy Nutrients

Energy Nutrient	Food Sources (Descending Order of Importance)
D-Ribose	Veal, beef
CoQ10	Beef heart, wild salmon, chicken liver
L-Carnitine	Mutton, lamb, beef, pork, poultry

Because the failing heart shows a shift in metabolism from fatty acids to carbohydrates, and since ischemic disease contributes to CHF progression by depleting ATP substrates, dyslipidemia resulting from consumption of fatty foods is problematic. Patients should be instructed to choose lower-fat dairy products, lean meats and fish, and to prepare foods with no added fat (see Table 7.3). This is a dilemma with diet alone because vegetarians generally have lower serum levels of CoQ10 and L-carnitine. Supplemental dosing can help avoid a diet high in saturated fats.

Energy metabolic deficit is additionally related to depletion of cellular compounds that contribute to energy metabolism, notably the pentose D-ribose, CoQ10, and L-carnitine. These nutrients are provided by foods that are metabolically active, such as red meat, heart, and liver. The normal diet is generally not adequate to provide sufficient levels of these nutrients and supplemental consumption is strongly recommended. Although one six-ounce portion of wild Alaskan salmon may well provide 10–15 mg of CoQ10, it would take the equivalent of 10 pounds of salmon to give the additional CoQ10 required to help make a difference in the compromised patient with CHF. This dietary scenario is not possible or practical.

D-ribose is a pentose carbohydrate that is found in every living tissue. Natural synthesis is via the oxidative pentose phosphate pathway of glucose metabolism, but the poor expression of gatekeeper enzymes glucose-6-phosphate dehydrogenase and 6-phosphogluconate dehydrogenase limit its natural production in heart and muscle tissue. The primary metabolic fate of D-ribose is the formation of 5-phosphoribosyl-1-pyrophosphate (PRPP) required for energy synthesis and salvage. The concentration of PRPP in tissue defines the rate of flux down the energy synthetic pathway and, in this way, ribose is rate limiting for preservation of the cellular energy pool. As a pentose, D-ribose is not consumed by cells as a primary energy fuel. Instead, ribose is preserved for the metabolic task of stimulating de novo energy synthesis and salvage.

CoQ10 resides in the electron transport chain of the mitochondria and is vital for progression of oxidative phosphorylation. In CHF, oxidative phosphorylation slows due to a loss of mitochondrial protein and lack of expression of key enzymes involved in the cycle. Disruption of mitochondrial activity may lead to a loss of CoQ10 that can further depress oxidative phosphorylation. In patients taking statin-like drugs, the mitochondrial loss of CoQ10 may be exacerbated by restricted CoQ10 synthesis resulting from HGM-CoA reductase inhibition. Such a decrease in CoQ10 occurring after years of statin therapy may be a major factor in the increase in CHF over the last decades. A small study reported in the *American Journal of Cardiology* demonstrates that diastolic dysfunction occurs in approximately two-thirds of previously normal patients given low-dose statin therapy. Supplemental CoQ10 helps to resurrect the previous vulnerable myocardium [23].

Carnitine is derived naturally in the body from the amino acids lysine and methionine. Its principal role is to facilitate the transport of fatty acids across the inner mitochondrial membrane to initiate beta oxidation and to remove metabolic waste products from the inner mitochondria for disposal. Carnitine also exhibits antioxidant and free-radical scavenger properties. Carnitine, like CoQ10, is found predominantly in animal flesh, and deficiencies in both of these nutrients are realized in those on vegetarian diets. The relationship between carnitine availability in heart tissue, carnitine metabolism in the heart, and left ventricular function is elucidated in Table 7.4.

TABLE 7.4

Clinical and Laboratory Evaluation of D-Ribose, CoQ10, and L-Carnitine in Congestive Heart Failure

Nutrient	Research Result	Reference
D-Ribose	NYHA Class II/III CHF. Administration resulted in significant improvement in all indices of diastolic heart function and led to significant improvement in patient quality of life score and exercise tolerance. No tested parameters were improved with glucose (placebo) treatment.	25
	NYHA Class II-IV CHF. Ribose improved ventilation efficiency, oxygen uptake efficiency, stroke volume, Doppler Tei Myocardial Performance Index (MPI), and ventilatory efficiency while preserving VO_{2max}. All are powerful predictors of heart failure survival. Ribose stimulates energy metabolism along the cardiopulmonary axis, thereby improving gas exchange.	25–27
	Lewis rat model. Remote myocardium exhibits a decrease in function within four weeks following myocardial infarction. To a significant degree, ribose administration prevents the dysfunction. Increased workload on the remote myocardium impacts cardiac energy metabolism resulting in lower myocardial energy levels. Elevating cardiac energy level improves function and may delay chronic changes in a variety of CHF conditions.	28
CoQ10	CHF with dilated cardiomyopathy and/or hypertensive heart disease. Therapy maintained blood levels of CoQ10 above 2.0 µg/mL and allowed 43% of the participants to discontinue one to three conventional drugs over the course of the study.	29
	Hypertensive heart disease with isolated diastolic dysfunction. Supplementation resulted in clinical improvement, lowered elevated blood pressure, enhanced diastolic cardiac function, and decreased myocardial wall thickness in 53% of study patients.	30
	Idiopathic dilated cardiomyopathy. Significant therapeutic effect of CoQ10. Affirmed the use of SPET-imaging as a way to measure the clinical impact of CoQ10 in hearts. Results are significant in that they show even small doses of coenzyme Q10 can have significant implications for some patients with dilated cardiomyopathy.	31
	End-stage CHF and cardiomyopathy. Designed to determine if CoQ10 could improve the pharmacological bridge to transplantation. Significant findings: (1) Following six weeks of therapy, the study group showed elevated blood levels of CoQ10 (0.22 mg/dL to 0.83 mg/dL, increase of 277%). Placebo group showed no increase (0.18 mg/dL to 0.178 mg/dL). (2) Study group showed improvement in six-minute walk test distance, shortness of breath, NYHA functional classification, fatigue, and episodes of waking for nocturnal urination with no changes in the placebo group. Results show that therapy may augment pharmaceutical treatment of patients with end-stage CHF and cardiomyopathy.	32
L-Carnitine	End-stage CHF and transplant. Compared to controls, concentration of carnitine in the heart muscle was significantly lower in patients; the level of carnitine in the tissue was directly related to ejection fraction. Study concluded that carnitine deficiency in heart tissue might be directly related to heart function.	33
	CHF and cardiomyopathy. Patients with CHF had higher plasma and urinary levels of carnitine, suggesting that carnitine was being released from the heart. Results showed that the level of plasma and urinary carnitine was related to the degree of left ventricular systolic dysfunction and ejection fraction, showing that plasma and urinary carnitine levels could serve as markers for myocardial damage and impaired left ventricular function.	34
	MI survivors. All-cause mortality significantly lower in the carnitine group than the placebo group (1.2% and 12.5%, respectively).	35
	MI survivors. Patients taking carnitine showed improvement in arrhythmia, angina, onset of heart failure, mean infarct size; reduction in total cardiac events. Significant reduction in cardiac death and nonfatal infarction versus placebo (15.6% vs. 26.0%, respectively).	36
	CHF. Improvement in ejection fraction and a reduction in left ventricular size in carnitine-treated patients. Combined incidence of CHF death after discharge was lower in the carnitine group than the placebo group (6.0% vs. 9.6%, respectively), a reduction of more than 30%.	37

The therapeutic advantage ribose provides in CHF suggests its value as an adjunct to traditional therapy for CHF [24]. Researchers and practitioners using ribose in cardiology practice recommend a dose range of 10 to 15 g/day as metabolic support for CHF or other heart disease. In my practice, patients are placed on the higher dose following a regimen of 5 g/dose three times per day. If patients respond favorably, the dose is adjusted to 5 g/dose two times per day. Individual doses of greater than 10 g are not recommended because high single doses of hygroscopic (water-retaining) carbohydrate may cause mild gastrointestinal discomfort or transient lightheadedness.

It is suggested that ribose be administered with meals or mixed in beverages containing a secondary carbohydrate source. In diabetic patients prone to hypoglycemia, I frequently recommend ribose in fruit juices. Ribose does have a negative glycemic impact and in diabetic patients taking insulin I have realized that bouts of hypoglycemia have occurred. This is why I have started with smaller doses and used a fruit juice to compensate for the reductions in blood sugar that I have clinically seen. Ribose has 20 calories per serving and does not necessarily have to be placed in a liquid. My patients have used a teaspoon of ribose in yogurt, protein shakes, as well as in oatmeal. Ribose can also be added to hot tea and is especially tasty in a green tea beverage. Ribose is a sugar and it tastes sweet.

HEART MUSCLE RENEWAL

For years, the consensus in medical science was that heart muscle cells could not regenerate. The theory was that these cells, or cardiomyocytes, grow bigger during childhood, but they do not divide and renew. Now, new evidence suggests otherwise, which may provide hope for people suffering with heart muscle damage or heart failure.

Swedish cellular biologists found that cardiomyocytes do indeed renew themselves, though at a very slow rate. Specifically, a 1% exchange occurs every year during early adulthood, and the rate decreases with age. At age 75 years, the annual renewal rate is 0.45%. During the course of a long life one will have approximately 40% cardiomyocyte turnover [38].

The Swedish researchers measured carbon-14, a radioactive isotope, present in proteins expressed exclusively by the DNA of cardiomyocytes. Carbon-14 levels in the environment soared during the nuclear bomb testing of the Cold War and then dropped when the testing stopped. By measuring the cardiomyocyte DNA carbon-14, the DNA within these cells reflects a mark as well as a time. Retrospectively, scientists can determine how old cells are and then infer how much turnover there must have been. Carbon-14 dating is also a widely used technique in archeology.

In a later review of the Swedish study, doctors at the University of Pennsylvania's Cardiovascular Institute wrote in the *New England Journal of Medicine* [39] that it was "ironic that the environmental devastation created by the testing of nuclear weapons . . . may have provided a glimpse into the future of regenerative medicine. This study provides the most definitive evidence to date that human cardiomyocytes are renewed during postnatal life."

What does this mean for patients suffering from severe congestive heart failure or end stage cardiomyopathy? In medical school, we physicians were taught that the chances of surviving heart failure are worse than many types of cancer, with a 50% mortality within five years. Despite that discouraging statistic, I have seen patients with initial ejection fractions of 10, 15, and 20% not just survive but thrive for decades after their initial diagnosis. After reading the article in *Science*, I often thought about my very ill patients with CHF and especially those who came off heart transplant lists. Did a metabolic approach facilitating the turnover and production of ATP give these patients time for the process of cardiomyocyte renewal? Could ATP support repair, rejuvenate, and restore vulnerable heart cells? Could a metabolic approach with ATP support be the missing ingredient? Based on my clinical experience, ATP support with lifestyle modification improves survival through mechanisms associated with cardiomyocyte regeneration.

SUMMARY

The complexity of cardiac energy metabolism is often misunderstood but is of vital clinical importance. One characteristic of the failing heart is a persistent and progressive loss of cellular energy substrates and abnormalities in cardiac bioenergetics that directly compromise diastolic performance, which has the capacity to impact global cardiac function. It took me 35 years of cardiology practice to learn that the heart is all about ATP, and the bottom line in the treatment of any form of cardiovascular disease, especially CHF and cardiomyopathy, is restoration of the heart's energy reserve. I have coined the term "metabolic cardiology" [40] to describe the biochemical interventions that can be employed to directly improve energy metabolism in heart cells. In simple terms, sick hearts leak out and lose vital ATP and when ATP levels drop, diastolic function deteriorates. The endogenous restoration of ATP cannot keep pace with this insidious deficit and relentless depletion. Treatment options that include metabolic intervention with therapies shown to preserve energy substrates or accelerate ATP turnover are indicated for at-risk populations or patients at any stage of disease.

In treating patients with mild CHF, I specifically recommend the following daily metabolic therapy:

- Multivitamin/mineral combination
- Fish oil: 1 g
- D-ribose: 10 to 15 g (two or three 5 g doses)
- CoQ10: 300 to 360 mg
- L-carnitine: 1500 to 2500 mg
- Magnesium: 400 to 800 mg

For severe CHF, dilated cardiomyopathy, and patients awaiting heart transplantation, I recommend daily:

- Multivitamin/mineral combination
- Fish oil: 1 g
- D-ribose: 15 g (three 5 g doses)
- CoQ10: 360 to 600 mg
- L-carnitine: 2500 to 3500 mg
- Magnesium: 400 to 800 mg

Metabolic cardiology may also be the supportive missing link in the new concept of cardiomyocyte renewal and offers great hope to patients with congestive heart failure and cardiomyopathy.

REFERENCES

1. Redfield MM, SJ Jacobson, JC Burnett, DW Mahoney, KR Bailey, RJ Rodenheffer. Burden of systolic and diastolic ventricular dysfunction in the community. Appreciating the scope of the heart failure epidemic. *JAMA*, 2003;289(2):194–202.
2. Ingwall JS. *ATP and the Heart.* Kluwer Academic Publishers, Boston, Massachusetts. 2002.
3. Ingwall JS. On the hypothesis that the failing heart is energy starved: Lessons learned from the metabolism of ATP and creatine. *Cur Hypertens Rep*, 2006;8:457–464.
4. Ingwall JS, RG Weiss. Is the failing heart energy starved? On using chemical energy to support cardiac function. *Circ Res*, 2004;95:135–145.
5. Manfredi JP, EW Holmes. Purine salvage pathways in myocardium. *Ann Rev Physiol*, 1985;47:691–705.
6. Gourine AV, Q Hu, PR Sander, AI Kuzmin, N Hanafy, SA Davydova, DV Zaretsky, J Zhang. Interstitial purine metabolites in hearts with LV remodeling. *Am J Physiol Heart Circ Physiol*, 2004; 286:H677–H684.

7. Hu Q, Q Wang, J Lee, et al. Profound bioenergetic abnormalities in peri-infarct myocardial regions. *Am J Physiol Heart Circ Physiol*, 2006;291:H648–H657.

8. Ye Y, G Gong, K Ochiai, J Liu, J Zhang. High-energy phosphate metabolism and creatine kinase in failing hearts: A new porcine model. *Circulation*, 2001;103:1570–1576.

9. Maslov MY, VP Chacko, M Stuber, AL Moens, DA Kass, HC Champion, RG Weiss. Altered high-energy phosphate metabolism predicts contractile dysfunction and subsequent ventricular remodeling in pressure-overload hypertrophy mice. *Am J Physiol Heart Circ Physiol*, 2007;292:H387–H391.

10. Cha Y-M, PP Dzeja, WK Shen, A Jahangir, CYT Hart, A Terzic, MM Redfield. Failing atrial myocardium: Energetic deficits accompany structural remodeling and electrical instability. *Am J Physiol Heart Circ Physiol*, 2003;284:H1313–H1320.

11. Bache RJ, J Zhang, Y Murakami, Y Zhang, YK Cho, H Merkle, G Gong, AH From, K Ugurbil. Myocardial oxygenation at high workstates in hearts with left ventricular hypertrophy. *Cardiovasc Res* 1999;42(3):567–570.

12. Smith CS, PA Bottomley, SP Schulman, G Gerstenblith, RG Weiss. Altered creatine kinase adenosine triphosphate kinetics in failing hypertrophied human myocardium. *Circulation*, 2006;114:1151–1158.

13. Weiss RG, G Gerstenblith, PA Bottomley. ATP flux through creatine kinase in the normal, stressed, and failing human heart. *Proc Nat Acad Sci*, 2005;102(3):808–813.

14. Beer M, T Seyfarth, J Sandstede, W Landschutz, C Lipke, H Kostler, M von Kienlin, K Harre, D Hahn, S Neubauer. Absolute concentrations of high-energy phosphate metabolites in normal, hypertrophied, and failing human myocardium measured noninvasively with (31)P-SLOOP magnetic resonance spectroscopy. *J Am Coll Cardiol*, 2002;40(7):1267–1274.

15. Lamb HJ, HP Beyerbacht, A van der Laarse, BC Stoel, J Doornbos, EE van der Wall, A de Roos. Diastolic dysfunction in hypertensive heart disease is associated with altered myocardial metabolism. *Circulation*, 1999;99(17):2261–2267.

16. Neubauer S, M Horn, T Pabst, K Harre, H Stromer, G Bertsch, J Sandstede, G Ertl, D Hahn, K Kochsiek. Cardiac high-energy phosphate metabolism in patients with aortic valve disease assessed by 31P-magnetic resonance spectroscopy. *J Investig Med*, 1997;45(8):453–462.

17. Diamant M, HJ Lamb, Y Groeneveld, EL Endert, JW Smith, JJ Bax, JA Romijn, A de Roos, JK Radder. Diastolic dysfunction is associated with altered myocardial metabolism in asymptomatic normotensive patients with well-controlled type 2 diabetes mellitus. *J Am Coll Cardiol*, 2003;41(2):328–335.

18. Schocke MF, B Metzler, C Wolf, P Steinboeck, C Kremser, O Pachinger, W Jaschike, P Lukas. Impact of aging on cardiac high-energy phosphate metabolism determined by phosphorous-31 2-dimensional chemical shift imaging (31P 2D CSI). *Magn Reson Imaging*, 2003;21(5):553–559.

19. Perings SM, K Schulze, U Decking, M Kelm, BE Strauer. Age-related decline of PCr/ATP-ratio in progressively hypertrophied hearts of spontaneously hypertensives rats. *Heart Vessels*, 2000;15(4):197–202.

20. Ypenburg C, A Sieders, GB Bleeker, ER Holman, EE van der Wall, MJ Schalij, JJ Bax. Myocardial contractile reserve predicts improvement in left ventricular function after cardiac resynchronization therapy. *Am Heart J*, 2007;154(6):1160–1165.

21. Sinatra ST. Coenzyme Q10 and congestive heart failure. Letter to the editor, *Annals of Int Med*, 2000;133(9).

22. Sinatra ST. Refractory congestive heart failure successfully managed with high doses of coenzyme Q10 administration. *Molec Aspects Med*, 1997;18:299–305.

23. Silver MA, PH Langsjoen, S Szabo, H Patil, A Zelinger. Effect of atorvastatin on left ventricular diastolic function and ability of coenzyme Q10 to reverse that dysfunction. *Am J Cardiol*, 2004;94(10):1306–1310.

24. Omran H, S Illien, D MacCarter, JA St. Cyr, B Luderitz. D-Ribose improves diastolic function and quality of life in congestive heart failure patients: A prospective feasibility study. *Eur J Heart Failure*, 2003;5:615–619.

25. Vijay N, D MacCarter, M Washam, J St. Cyr. Ventilatory efficiency improves with d-ribose in congestive heart failure patients. *J Mol Cell Cardiol*, 2005;38(5):820.

26. Carter O, D MacCarter, S Mannebach, J Biskupiak, G Stoddard, EM Gilbert, MA Munger. D-Ribose improves peak exercise capacity and ventilatory efficiency in heart failure patients. *JACC*, 2005;45(3 Suppl A):185A.

27. Sharma R, M Munger, S Litwin, O Vardeny, D MacCarter, JA St. Cyr. D-Ribose improves Doppler TEI myocardial performance index and maximal exercise capacity in stage C heart failure. *J Mol Cell Cardiol*, 2005;38(5):853.

28. Befera N, A Rivard, G Gatlin, S Black, J Zhang, JE Foker. Ribose treatment helps preserve function of the remote myocardium after myocardial infarction. *J Surg Res*, 2007;137(2):156.

29. Langsjoen PH, P Langsjoen, R Willis, et al. Usefulness of coenzyme Q10 in clinical cardiology: A long-term study. *Mol Aspects Med,* 1994;15:S165–175.
30. Burke BE, R Neuenschwander, RD Olson. Randomized, double-blind, placebo-controlled trial of coenzyme Q10 in isolated hypertension. *So Med J,* 2001;94(11):1112–1117.
31. Kim Y, Y Sawada, G Fujiwara, et al. Therapeutic effect of coenzyme Q10 on idiopathic dilated cardiomyopathy: Assessment by iodine-123 labelled 150(p-iodophenyl)-3(R,S)-methyl-pentadecanoic acid myocardial single-photon emission tomography. *Eur J Nuc Med,* 1997;24:629–634.
32. Berman M, A Erman, T Ben-Gal, et al. Coenzyme Q10 in patients with end-stage heart failure awaiting cardiac transplantation: A randomized, placebo-controlled study. *Clin Cardiol,* 2004;27:295–299.
33. El-Aroussy W, A Rizk, G Mayhoub, et al. Plasma carnitine levels as a marker of impaired left ventricular functions. *Mol Cell Biochem,* 2000;213(1–2):37–41.
34. Narin F, N Narin, H Andac, et al. Carnitine levels in patients with chronic rheumatic heart disease. *Clin Biochem,* 1997;30(8):643–645.
35. Davini P, A Bigalli, F Lamanna, A Boem. Controlled study on L-carnitine therapeutic efficacy in post-infarction. *Drugs Exp Clin Res,* 1992;18:355–365.
36. Singh RB, MA Niaz, P Agarwal, et al. A randomized, double-blind, placebo-controlled trial of L-carnitine in suspected acute myocardial infarction. *Postgrad Med,* 1996;72:45–50.
37. Iliceto S, D Scrutinio, P Bruzzi, et al. Effects of L-carnitine administration on left ventricular remodeling after acute anterior myocardial infarction: The L-Carnitine Ecocardiografia Digitalizzata Infarto Miocardioco (CEDIM) trial. *J Am Coll Cardiol,* 1995;26(2):380–387.
38. Bergmann O, RD Bhardwaj, S Bernard, et al. Evidence for caridomyocyte renewal in humans. *Science.* 2009 Apr3;324(5923):47–48.
39. Parmacek MS, JA Epstein. Cardiomyocyte renewal. *N. Engl J Med.* 2009;361(1):86–88.
40. Sinatra ST. *The Sinatra Solution/Metabolic Cardiology.* Laguna Beach, CA: Basic Health Publications, 2005.

8 Cardiac Arrhythmias

Fish Oil and Omega-3 Fatty Acids in Management

Stephen Olmstead, M.D., and Dennis Meiss, Ph.D.

INTRODUCTION

The accumulated evidence suggests that fish oil has heterogeneous antiarrhythmic properties. Its effects vary according to the type of arrhythmia, the underlying cardiac disorder, amount and type of dietary fish consumption, and other factors. This chapter reviews the basic biochemistry of polyunsaturated fatty acids (PUFA) and electrophysiologic effects of omega-3 long-chain polyunsaturated fatty acids (LCPUFA), examines the antiarrhythmic properties of fish oil, and critically evaluates the available clinical evidence as to which patients may benefit and who may not benefit from fish oil supplementation.

OVERVIEW OF THE IMPACT OF FISH AND FISH OIL ON CARDIOVASCULAR DISEASE

In 1976, Bang and coworkers insightfully proposed that the low mortality from coronary heart disease (CHD) observed in Greenland Inuit people despite a high dietary fat intake was due to the consumption of abundant amounts of omega-3 LCPUFA from fish and other seafoods [1]. The Greenland Inuit hypothesis came concurrently with publication of research by Gudbjarnason and his group showing that increased dietary availability of omega-3 LCPUFA supplied by cod liver oil paradoxically lowered isoproterenol stress tolerance in rats leading to greater cardiac necrosis and death [2]. Over the ensuing decades, a considerable body of evidence from tissue culture and animal model studies has been developed showing that omega-3 LCPUFA favorably alter myocardial excitability and reduce the risk of ventricular arrhythmias [3–10]. Observational studies have disclosed that one to two fatty fish meals weekly and higher omega-3 LCPUFA blood levels are associated with a lower risk of sudden cardiac death (SCD) [11–14]. Two large meta-analyses were published in 2004 that examined the effect of fish consumption on fatal CHD [15,16]. Wharton and coworkers analyzed 19 observational studies comprising approximately 220,000 subjects followed for about 12 years [15]. Regular weekly fish intake reduced the incidence of fatal CHD by 17%. He and coworkers evaluated 13 cohort studies also consisting of over 220,000 participants followed for nearly 12 years [16]. They also found that one meal of fish weekly reduced fatal CHD incidence by 15%. His group also demonstrated a dose-response association between fish intake and CHD death rates. Participants consuming fish five or more times a week had a 38% reduction in the risk of fatal CHD. The evidence for a favorable impact of low amounts of fish intake on nonfatal myocardial infarction (MI) was flimsy although weekly

149

consumption of high amounts of fish appeared to protect against nonfatal MI. Three randomized, controlled trials have demonstrated that fish consumption and fish oil supplementation decrease total and cardiovascular mortalities primarily by reducing the risk of SCD [17–19]. However, one large study found that men with angina pectoris and no prior myocardial infarction (MI) who regularly consumed fish or fish oil experienced an excess incidence of SCD [20]. The results of two randomized prospective trials were published in 2010 that evaluated the effects of omega-3 LCPUFA on outcomes following MI [21,22]. Doses of 400 mg and 1 g of omega-3 LCPUFA, respectively, were administered to patients after MI who were followed for 41 and 12 months. Neither study found any reduction in the occurrence of SCD or major cardiovascular (CV) events. A study of fish oil and B vitamins in a heterogeneous group of patients with coronary artery and cerebrovascular disease found no reduction in major vascular events with a daily dose of 600 mg of fish oil [23]. In contrast, a large Japanese study of 1800 mg of eicosapentaenoic acid (EPA) together with a statin in patients with hypercholesterolemia found that in the subgroup with a history of CAD, EPA significantly reduced aggregate major coronary events by 19%. In the only study thus far of omega-3 LCPUFA in people with heart failure (HF), ingestion of 1 g per day significantly reduced death rates and first hospitalizations for ventricular arrhythmias, but had no significant effect on SCD [24]. Three studies of fish oil in patients with implantable cardiac defibrillators (ICD) at high risk for recurrent ventricular arrhythmias have yielded conflicting results ranging from protective benefit to proarrhythmic adverse effects [25–27].

PATHOPHYSIOLOGY

POLYUNSATURATED FATTY ACID BIOCHEMISTRY

PUFA are carboxylic acids with hydrocarbon (acyl) tails of varying length containing two or more C = C double bonds. There are two families of PUFA: omega-3 and omega-6 [28]. (See Figure 8.1.) In omega-3 PUFA, the first C = C double bond is located at carbon 3 counting from the terminal or omega methyl group of the acyl tail. In omega-6 PUFA, the first C = C double bond is located at carbon 6 from the omega methyl group. Omega-3 and -6 PUFA are also called n-3 and n-6 fatty acids respectively. Eukaryotes normally make and metabolize *cis* fatty acids; the C = C double bonds in both monounsaturated and PUFA are in the *cis* conformation, meaning the substituent groups are on the same side of the double bond. Both PUFA families are essential for human health. Following intake, omega-3 and omega-6 PUFA are ubiquitously disseminated throughout the body and mediate or regulate a host of physiological processes that include cardiovascular, immunological, hormonal, metabolic, neural, and visual functions. At the cellular level, these effects are brought about by changes in membrane lipid structure, alterations of membrane physical properties, interactions with membrane receptors and ion channels, modulation of eicosanoid signaling, and control of gene transcription [29].

POLYUNSATURATED FATTY ACID METABOLISM

Although omega-3 and -6 PUFA are necessary for normal cellular function, humans and other mammals lack the ability to insert a C = C double bond at the omega-3 and -6 positions making dietary intake of these fatty acids essential. The omega-3 alpha-linolenic acid (18:3n-3) and the omega-6 linoleic acid (18:3n-6) are the primary essential fatty acids because they cannot be synthesized by mammalian cells. These essential fatty acids may be transformed in the liver into longer chain PUFA. (See Figure 8.2.) Alpha-linolenic acid is the precursor of the omega-3 LCPUFA eicosapentaenoic acid (EPA; 20:5n-3) and docosahexaenoic acid (DHA; 22:6n-3). Linoleic acid is the precursor of the omega-6 arachidonic acid (AA; 20:4n-6). The conversion of alpha-linolenic acid to EPA and DHA is very inefficient [30,31]. EPA and DHA synthesis is further compromised by high dietary intake of omega-6 PUFA because alpha-linolenic acid and linoleic acid compete for entry into metabolic pathways [31]. Excessive consumption of omega-6 PUFA relative to omega-3 PUFA predisposes to a proinflammatory, prothrombotic, and vasoconstrictive physiology [29]. This

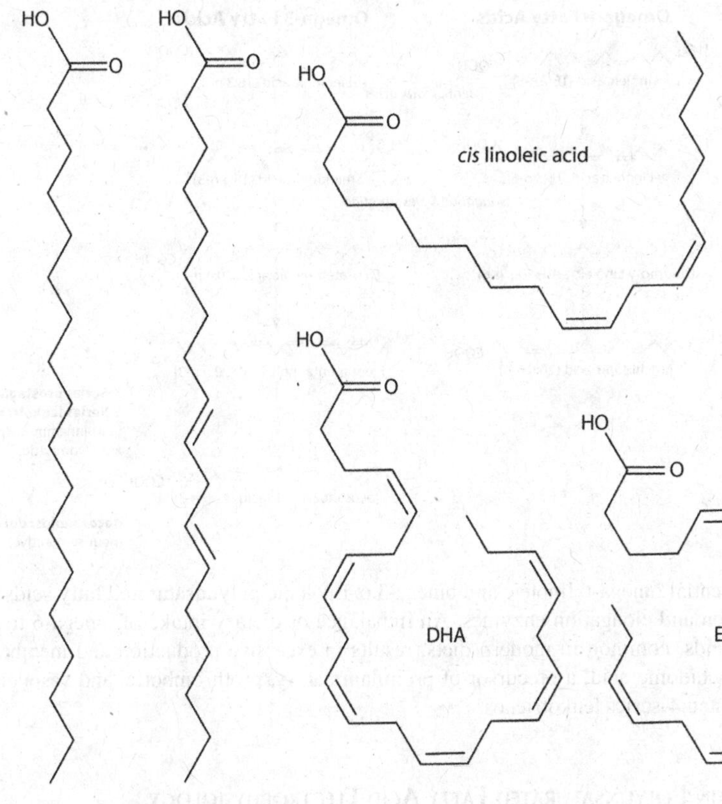

FIGURE 8.1 The structures of the long chain polyunsaturated fatty acids eicosapentaenoic acid (EPA) and docosahexaenoic acid (DHA) are compared to the *cis* isomer of the omega-6 polyunsaturated fatty acid linoleic acid, the *trans* isomer of linoleic acid, and stearic acid, a common dietary saturated fatty acid. Note how the acyl tail of the *cis* isomers folds back on itself. This results in less dense lipid packing within cell membranes. The *trans* conformation makes a polyunsaturated fatty acid structurally equivalent to a saturated fatty acid leading to greater lipid packing and reduced cell membrane fluidity.

makes dietary intake of EPA and DHA, commonly found in oily fish and other marine sources, vital to meet the body's need for omega-3 LCPUFA.

POLYUNSATURATED FATTY ACID MEMBRANE PHYSIOLOGY

Omega-3 LCPUFA have profound effects on cell membrane physiology. These effects are believed to be due to the multiple *cis* C = C double bonds that cause the acyl tail to fold back upon itself [32]. (See Figure 8.1.) This highly flexible three-dimensional conformation results in significantly less lipid packing within the membrane than is permitted by saturated or *trans* unsaturated fatty acids. In general, cell membranes with excessive concentrations of saturated or *trans* unsaturated fatty acids are stiff and inflexible while membranes containing higher amounts of LCPUFA are more fluid and dynamic [33]. DHA in particular has profound effects on membrane function [34]. These include increased membrane permeability [35], enhanced membrane fusion [36], more efficient vesicle formation [37], greater membrane inplane plasticity [38], increased phospholipid "flip-flops" [39], and promotion of intramembrane lipid domain formation [40]. It is also becoming increasingly clear that membrane physical properties significantly influence the function of membrane proteins such as cell signaling receptors and ion channels [41,42].

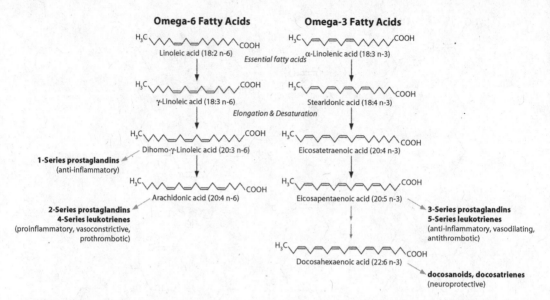

FIGURE 8.2. The essential omega-6 linoleic and omega-3 α-linolenic polyunsaturated fatty acids compete for the same desaturation and elongation enzymes. An imbalance of dietary intake of omega-6 to omega-3 polyunsaturated fatty acids, common in modern diets, results in excessive production and membrane content of the omega-6 arachidonic acid, a precursor of proinflammatory, prothrombotic, and vasoconstrictive 2-series prostaglandins and 4-series leukotrienes.

OMEGA-3 LONG CHAIN POLYUNSATURATED FATTY ACID ELECTROPHYSIOLOGY

A series of in vitro and animal experiments have elucidated the basic electrophysiology of omega-3 LCPUFA. In a perfused isolated rabbit heart, LCPUFA antagonize hypoxia-mediated ventricular arrhythmias [3]. In rats, dietary LCPUFA reduced the risk of ventricular fibrillation (VF) during coronary occlusion and reperfusion [4]. In marmoset monkeys, dietary LCPUFA reduced vulnerability to ventricular arrhythmias during coronary occlusion and reperfusion [6]. Omega-3 LCPUFA have been found to be more effective than omega-6 LCPUFA at increasing the VF threshold [43]. Exercise studies of dogs have shown that intravenous infusions of fish oil can prevent ischemia-induced VF [7]. In the dog model, EPA, DHA, and alpha-linolenic acid possessed similar anti-arrhythmic effects [44]. Elegant experiments involving cultured neonatal rat cardiomyocytes have provided extensive insights into the antiarrhythmic mechanisms of omega-3 LCPUFA at the transmembrane ion channel level [9,45–48]. The electrophysiologic effects of omega-3 LCPUFA are summarized in Table 8.1.

CURRENT HYPOTHESIS OF ANTI-ARRHYTHMIC EFFECTS OF FISH OIL

Experimental data primarily by Leaf and coworkers show that free omega-3 LCPUFA must partition into or enter the lipophilic acyl chains of membrane phospholipids to exert antiarrhythmic effect [47–49]. Only the free omega-3 LCPUFA are antiarrhythmic. They do not become incorporated into membrane phospholipids or form other covalent bonds to exert their antiarrhythmic effects because when the free omega-3 LCPUFA are extracted from myocytes, the antiarrhythmic effects cease. Free omega-3 LCPUFA concentrations in the nM to mcM range have been found to be antiarrhythmic. These molar concentrations and resultant free omega-3 LCPUFA to phospholipid ratios are considered too low for omega-3 LCPUFA to cause a generalized increase in membrane fluidity due to reduced lipid packing. Current thinking hypothesizes that free omega-3 LCPUFA enhance the fluidity of membrane microdomains surrounding channel proteins. Theoretically, small localized increases in free omega-3 LCPUFA concentrations in perichannel microdomains could

TABLE 8.1

Electrophysiologic Effects of Omega-3 Long-Chain Polyunsaturated Fatty Acids

Increase action potential duration (QT interval) [8]

Increase atrioventricular conduction (PR interval) [8]

Decrease rate of contraction [45]

Maintain steady myocyte resting potential [46]

Increase effective refractory period [46]

Inhibit the fast-voltage-dependent sodium current (INA) [9,47,48]

Accelerate INA channel transition from resting to inactive state [9,47,48]

Stabilize the INA channel inactive state [9,47,48]

Inhibit voltage-gated L-type calcium current [9,47,48]

Inhibit sarcoplasmic reticulum calcium release [9,47,48]

Inhibit repolarizing outward potassium current (I_{to1}) [9,47,48]

Inhibit fast outward potassium current (I_{Kr}) [9,47,48]

Inhibit delayed-rectifier potassium current (I_{KS}) [9,47,48]

Activate inward potassium current (I_{ir}) [9,47,48]

correct membrane protein hydrophobic mismatches in which the size of the hydrophobic portion of the transmembrane portion of the channel protein is less than the hydrophobic portion of the lipid bilayer. Omega-3 LCPUFA, by virtue of the folding of their double-bonded acyl tails, will reduce the size of hydrophobic portion of the lipid bilayer [42]. This may alter the resting conformation of the ion channels and modify their conductance. Further research remains to be done to test this hypothesis for the antiarrhythmic mechanism of action of omega-3 LCPUFA.

TREATMENT CONSIDERATIONS

PREVENTION OF ARRHYTHMIAS AFTER MYOCARDIAL INFARCTION

The Diet and Reinfarction Trial (DART) [17] randomized 2033 Welsh men under age 70 who had suffered an acute MI into four groups to receive no dietary advice or dietary advice on reduced fat intake, increased fish intake, or increased fiber intake. Subjects who received dietary advice to increase fish intake and could not tolerate fish were asked to take 3 MaxEPA® capsules delivering 500 mg daily of EPA. The portion of fish intake advised was relatively small, providing around 300 grams of fatty fish, or about 2.5 g of EPA, per week. Follow-up was obtained at six months and two years.

The risk of death at two years was reduced by 29% in subjects advised to increase fish intake or consume EPA supplements compared to those given no dietary fish advice (p < 0.05). The absolute risk reduction was 3.5%. The reduction in total mortality was due almost entirely to a 32.5% decrease in the risk of death from CHD (p < 0.01). The absolute reduction in ischemic heart disease death rate was 3.7%. There was no significant difference in the incidence of nonfatal MI between patients randomized to receive advice to increase fish consumption and those receiving no such advice. Dietary advice on reduced fat and increased fiber consumption also had no significant effect on mortality and reinfarction. The reduction in total mortality and ischemic heart disease mortality without an effect on the rate of recurrent MI was interpreted to mean fish oil reduces mortality by decreasing the incidence of arrhythmia-mediated SCD.

The Indian Experiment of Infarct Survival–4 (IEIS–4) study randomized 360 patients admitted with suspicion of acute myocardial infarction to receive fish oil containing 1.08 grams of EPA and 0.72 grams of DHA daily, 20 grams daily of mustard oil containing 2.9 grams of alpha-linolenic acid, or placebo [18]. The trial was double-blind. Over 90% of subjects received aspirin and approximately 30% were on beta blockers. No information was provided on the use of lipid-lowering agents. Follow-up of all outcomes took place over 12 months.

The total of cardiac events after one year was significantly less in subjects randomized to fish oil and mustard oil compared to the placebo group (24.5% and 28% versus 34.7%). Relative to placebo, patients receiving fish oil had a 48.2% reduction in cardiac mortality (10.6% absolute risk reduction) while mustard oil reduced cardiac mortality by 40% (6.7% absolute risk reduction). Both fish oil and mustard oil significantly reduced the incidence of nonfatal reinfarction (13% and 15% versus 25.4%). Fish oil was also found to reduce the incidence of left ventricular dilatation and ventricular arrhythmias.

The Gruppo Italiano per lo Studio della Sopravvivenza nell'Infarto Miocardico Prevenzione (GISSI-Prevenzione) is the largest trial to date on the effect of omega-3 LCPUFA on outcomes following acute MI [19]. This open-label trial randomized 11,324 recently discharged patients to 1 gram fish oil, 300 milligrams vitamin E (synthetic dl-alpha-tocopherol), both, or neither. The fish oil contained 570–588 mg of DHA and 280–294 mg of EPA as ethyl esters. All subjects consumed a Mediterranean-type diet that included moderate fish consumption. Most patients were on a secondary CHD risk reduction program consisting of an antiplatelet agent (82.8%), a lipid-lowering agent (45.5%), an ACE inhibitor (39%), and/or a beta blocker (38.5%).

After 3.5 years of follow-up, four-way analysis found patients randomized to fish oil had a significant 15% reduction in the relative risk of the aggregate endpoint of cardiovascular death, recurrent nonfatal MI, and stroke. The relative risk reduction in incidence of the aggregate endpoint was due to a decrease in death and nonfatal MI. Fish oil had no effect on the incidence of fatal or nonfatal stroke. All cause mortality was reduced by 20.2% (2.1% absolute risk reduction). Cardiovascular death was reduced by 30% (2% absolute risk reduction). SCD was decreased by 45% (1.6% absolute risk reduction). Fish oil supplementation had no effect on the incidence of nonfatal cardiovascular events such as recurrent MI. Vitamin E supplementation alone had no effect on the aggregate endpoint, but in four-way analysis reduced cardiovascular deaths by 20% and sudden death by 35%. There was no increased benefit to combining fish oil with synthetic vitamin E. Of interest is that neither fish oil nor vitamin E were associated with any reported increased bleeding risk to revascularization procedures calling into question the often repeated advice to discontinue these agents prior to surgery—advice that has no basis in clinical studies.

A time-course reanalysis of the original data reaffirmed the GISSI-Prevenzione trial results [50]. The survival curves of subjects randomized to fish oil significantly diverged early from those of patients randomized to vitamin E or no treatment. Total mortality was 41% lower by three months. The risk of SCD was reduced by 53% by four months. Significant reductions in other cardiovascular deaths were observed six to eight months after randomization. As with the DART findings, the early improvements in total mortality rate and reduced incidence of SCD provide support for the hypothesis that the omega-3 LCPUFA in fish oil exert their benefit through antiarrhythmic effects.

The Danish High-Dose n-3 Fatty Acid versus Corn Oil after Myocardial Infarction study details 300 subjects recruited following acute MI. The double-blind trial was designed to assess the effect of high-dose fish oil on serum lipid levels and outcomes [51]. Patients were randomized to receive 4 grams daily of fish oil (2.28–2.36 grams daily DHA and 1.12–1.16 grams daily EPA) or corn oil. Approximately 85% of subjects received aspirin, about 60% were on beta blockers, about 10% were using ACE inhibitors, and 68% were prescribed statins. Prior to study entry, 30% of those randomized to fish oil and 25% of subjects randomized to corn oil were regularly consuming fish oil. The median follow-up period was 18 months.

The cardiac death rate was identical in both groups (5.3%) as was total mortality (7.3%). Recurrent nonfatal MI occurred more frequently in patients receiving fish oil (14%) than in patients receiving corn oil (10%), but the difference was not significant. Patients receiving high-dose fish oil had significant reductions in serum triacylglycerol levels especially in conjunction with statin therapy.

While the Danish failed to find that fish oil reduced adverse outcomes following MI, a number of factors must be considered when evaluating the results of this trial. The first is the low rate of mortality and recurrent infarction. The observed mortality rate is about half that seen in DART and the GISSI-Prevenzione study. This means the study lacked the statistical power to observe a real benefit for fish oil. The low adverse events rate may have been related to a high rate of revascularization. In the GISSI-Prevenzione study, 24% of subjects had undergone revascularization after 42 months. In contrast, in the Danish trial, 31% of patients had undergone revascularization after a median time of 18 months. Recurrent adverse events were uncommon in revascularized patients. Another factor biasing this study against finding a benefit for fish oil is the high number of subjects using fish oil prior to study entry. Patients already consuming and benefiting from fish oil would be unlikely to accrue significant additional benefits from recommended fish oil intake. The low mortality in both groups may have been related to the high consumption of fish oil and fish in the Danish population.

The OMEGA trial randomized 3851 German patients three to 14 days after an acute MI to 1 g of omega-3 LCPUFA containing 460 mg of EPA and 380 mg of DHA or placebo [52]. The primary endpoint was SCD and subjects were followed for 12 months. All patients received aggressive, current guideline-adjusted treatment. Acute coronary arteriography was performed in 93.8% of all subjects and 77.8% underwent percutaneous coronary revascularization. Medical therapy was extensive with 83.7% of all subjects receiving beta blockers, 79.7% statins, 94.4% aspirin, and 86.2% clopidogrel. Most subjects were treated with angiotensin-converting enzyme inhibitors and heparin. Glycoprotein IIb/IIIa inhibitors were commonly used. Prior to study entry, 65.3% of subjects consumed fish occasionally while 27.7% ate fish several times a week. Significantly more participants randomized to receive omega-3 LCPUFA regularly consumed fish multiple times a week. Fish consumption significantly increased in both study groups during the trial. After one year, the incidence of SCD was 1.5% in both groups. Total mortality was 4.6% in subjects receiving omega-3 LCPUFA and 3.7% in those receiving placebo. Omega-3 LCPUFA had no effect on the incidence of major adverse cardiovascular and cerebrovascular events. There was no significant difference between the study groups in the number of survivors undergoing revascularization during follow-up.

The principal conclusion from the OMEGA study is that aggressive interventional and medical guideline-adjusted therapy during and following acute MI results in low rates of SCD and other adverse cardiovascular events. While supplementation with omega-3 LCPUFA was not shown to provide additional risk reduction, the study was seriously underpowered and unable to detect a benefit for fish oil in the setting of low rates of adverse events. The high level of fish consumption at study entry as well as the increased consumption of fish in both the omega-3 LCPUFA and placebo groups serve to further confound the OMEGA findings.

The Alpha-Omega trial recruited 4837 subjects with a history of prior MI and randomized them into 4 groups to receive margarine supplemented with DHA and EPA; margarine supplemented with ALA; margarine supplemented with DHA, EPA, and ALA; and margarine alone [53]. Participants consumed an average of 18.8 g of margarine daily. The average daily intake of DHA was 150 mg, of EPA 226 mg, and of ALA 1.9 g in the respective treatment groups. The mean time since MI was 4.3 years. Subjects received state-of-the-art therapy with antihypertensives, antithrombotics, and hypolipemic agents. The primary end point was the aggregate incidence of major CV events defined as fatal and nonfatal CV events and cardiac interventions. The median follow-up time was 40.8 months (interquartile range, 37.2 to 41.5 months). All analyses were by intention-to-treat.

During the Alpha-Omega trial follow-up period, a major CV event occurred in 13.9% of participants. DHA/EPA, ALA, and DHA/EPA together with ALA did not significantly reduce the risk of adverse CV events. There were 27% fewer adverse CV events among women receiving ALA compared to DHA/EPA and placebo. This difference did not attain statistical significance.

The Alpha-Omega trial has numerous limitations. The combination of omega-3 PUFA with margarine is problematic. Margarine contains *trans* fatty acids (TFA) and there is epidemiologic evidence that margarine intake may increase the risk of coronary artery disease [54,55]. It is possible margarine intake negated possible benefits of omega-3 PUFA. The division of subjects into four research groups rendered the study significantly underpowered to detect a risk reduction if present. Finally, omega-3 PUFA may have limited benefit in a population of patients more than four years post MI who are well treated medically and are at low risk of adverse effects.

To summarize the effects of fish, fish oil, and omega-3 LCPUFA following MI, five interventional trials have assessed the effect on adverse outcomes in patients following acute MI. Two relatively small trials yielded conflicting results. The Danish trial failed to show a reduction in mortality or nonfatal myocardial infarction rates. However, the high number of subjects consuming fish oil prior to study entry, the high revascularization rate, and the low adverse event rate bias this study against finding a benefit for fish oil. IEIS–4 found that fish oil substantially reduced cardiac mortality and nonfatal reinfarction. However, the mortality and nonfatal reinfarction rates in the placebo group were approximately twice the rate reported by DART as well as by the GISSI-Prevenzione trial summarized later in this chapter. While the benefit of fish oil is apparent, the magnitude of any benefit may have been exaggerated. A more unfortunate and troubling worry is that the validity of a prior study by the IEIS–4 leading author has been questioned and fabrication of data has been alleged [56,57]. While the validity or integrity of the IEIS–4 data has not been questioned, the results of IEIS–4 are regrettably tainted by this unrelated allegation.

The two larger and older trials found significant benefit for fish oil following acute MI. These studies unequivocally show that fish oil or fish intake reduces total and cardiovascular mortality following myocardial infarction. The magnitude of the reduction of mortality rate post MI is comparable to that obtained with statins, aspirin, ACE inhibitors, and beta blockers [58]. Fish oil supplementation following MI offers additive benefits to those provided by standard therapies. Both studies demonstrate a reduction in the incidence of sudden death, but no significant effect on recurrent MI. An antiarrhythmic mechanism appears to be the likely means by which the risk of death is reduced in this population. Based on the available clinical evidence of concordant, large, randomized, controlled trials, the recommendation of 1 gram of fish oil daily in patients following acute MI is warranted. In contrast, the more recent OMEGA study failed to show a benefit for omega-3 LCPUFA following acute MI. This may primarily be a function of low adverse event rates in an aggressively guideline-adjusted treated population. This hypothesis receives confirmation from subgroup analysis of the Alpha-Omega participants. The absolute incidence of CAD death in Alpha-Omega subjects with diabetes was 17.1/1000 person-years, which is the same order of magnitude as fatal CAD rates in the control group of the GISSI-Prevenzione study. In this Alpha-Omega subgroup, supplemental DHA/EPA significantly reduced fatal CAD at a level comparable to that found in the GISSI-Prevenzione. Fish and fish oil may offer the greatest benefit to patients with the highest risk of fatal CAD, but may offer little incremental benefit to optimized medically treated and revascularized people at low risk for subsequent SCD and other adverse events.

MORTALITY IN PATIENTS WITH ANGINA PECTORIS

A single study conducted by the DART principal investigator and coworkers assessed the long-term effect of increased dietary fish or fish oil intake on outcomes in men with chronic stable angina pectoris [20]. After three to nine years of follow-up, all-cause mortality was 26% greater in people assigned to increased fish intake. The risk of SCD was increased by 54%. The excess risk was largely among subjects given fish oil. The increase in mortality was confined to the second phase of the trial. An analysis of the data to evaluate the possibility of an interaction between fish oil and medications found that fish oil interacted favorably with beta blockers to reduce the risk of sudden death. No adverse fish oil–medication interactions were apparent. The authors speculate that fish oil intake may have been associated with an increase in risk-taking behavior, although the reasons for the observed increase in mortality with fish oil in this population are entirely unclear. The results provide a caveat against blanket recommendations for fish oil consumption and highlight the fact that patients with CHD are a heterogeneous population.

HEART FAILURE MORTALITY

The Gruppo Italiano per lo Studio della Sopravvivenza nell'Infarto Miocardico-Heart Failure (GISSI-HF) study randomized 6975 patients with chronic heart failure (HF) from any cause to 1 g daily of omega-3 LCPUFA containing 850–882 mg of EPA and DHA ethyl esters in a 1:1.2 ratio or placebo [59]. The co-primary endpoints were time to death and the aggregate of time to death and hospitalization for cardiovascular indications. The average age of participants was 67 years and 42% were older than 70 years. Subjects received standard medical therapy for HF. The median follow-up was 3.9 years. GISSI-HF found that omega-3 LCPUFA supplementation significantly reduced the risk of death by 9% and the risk of death or hospitalization for cardiovascular indications by 8%. The number needed to treat to prevent one death was 56 and to avoid death or hospitalization for cardiovascular reasons was 44. First hospital admissions for ventricular arrhythmias were significantly reduced by 28%. The incidence of sudden death was remarkably low and not impacted by omega-3 LCPUFA. Benefits were observed irrespective of whether HF was ischemic or nonischemic in etiology or whether left ventricular systolic function was impaired or preserved. The GISSI-HF results provide strong support for fish oil as an adjunctive measure to standard medications in the treatment of HF.

PREVENTION OF CARDIOVASCULAR EVENTS IN PATIENTS WITH HYPERCHOLESTEROLEMIA

The Japan EPA Lipid Intervention Study (JELIS) tested the hypothesis that EPA reduces the incidence of major coronary events in people with hypercholesterolemia in an open-label trial [60]. The amount of EPA administered was 600 mg three times daily. All participants received either pravastatin or simvastatin. The study randomized 18,645 patients, 69% of who were postmenopausal women. A primary prevention subgroup had 14,981 subjects, while 3664 patients with a history of CAD were in a secondary prevention subgroup. The follow-up period was five years. A major coronary event was defined as sudden cardiac death, fatal and nonfatal myocardial infarction, unstable angina pectoris, and coronary angioplasty, stenting, or surgical bypass grafting. Compared with placebo, EPA reduced major coronary events by 19%. The risk reduction was due to a decrease in the incidence of fatal and nonfatal myocardial infarction, unstable angina, and revascularization. The risk of sudden death was not affected. When subgroup analysis was performed, the risk reduction was statistically significant in subjects with preexisting CAD, but did not attain significance in the primary prevention subgroup. Although moderate doses of EPA did not reduce the risk of lethal arrhythmias in hypercholesterolemic Japanese consuming high amounts of fish, it did lower the risk of nonfatal major coronary events offering significant potential as a preventive intervention.

RISK OF SUDDEN CARDIAC DEATH

Siscovik and coworkers in Seattle first reported that dietary intake and blood levels of omega-3 LCPUFA were inversely associated with the risk of SCD [11]. In a population-based, case-control study, they compared 334 patients with primary cardiac arrest attended by paramedics and 493 randomly identified, population-based community controls, matched for age and sex. All cases and controls had no history of clinical heart disease or fish oil supplement use. The spouses of case patients and control subjects were interviewed to determine dietary omega-3 LCPUFA intake from seafood during the preceding month. Blood specimens from 82 cases and 108 controls were analyzed to determine red blood cell membrane fatty acid composition. The investigators found that compared with no consumption of EPA and DHA, an intake of 5.5 g of omega-3 LCPUFA per month, approximately one fatty-fish meal per week, and the mean of the third quartile, was associated with a 50% reduction in the risk of primary cardiac arrest. A red blood cell omega-3 LCPUFA level of 5.0% of total fatty acids, the third quartile mean, was associated with a 70% reduction in the risk of primary cardiac arrest compared with a red blood cell membrane omega-3 LCPUFA level of 3.3% of total fatty acids, the lowest quartile mean.

These convincing data were subsequently confirmed by two prospective cohort studies among healthcare professionals. In the Physicians' Health Study, which followed apparently healthy male physicians for up to 17 years, the incidence of SCD was related to fish consumption [12]. The risk of SCD was significantly reduced by 52% in men consuming fish at least once a week compared with the risk in men who ate fish less than once a month. The authors went on to explore the relation between baseline blood levels of omega-3 LCPUFA and the incidence of SCD in a nested, case-control study within the Physicians' Health Study [13]. Higher baseline blood omega-3 LCPUFA levels were significantly associated with a reduction in the risk of SCD. After adjusting for confounding factors, compared to the lowest quartile blood levels, omega-3 LCPUFA levels in the third quartile were associated with a 72% reduction and levels in the fourth quartile were associated with an 81% reduction in SCD risk (p for trend = 0.007). Red blood cell fatty acid analyses are not routinely available as clinical tests, but plasma fatty acid panels are available from integrative medicine clinical laboratories. Such testing may assist clinicians in risk assessment and assessment of dietary or supplemental fish oil interventions.

In the second prospective cohort study, the Health Professional Follow-Up Study, involving 45,722 men free of apparent heart disease, the relation of dietary intake of omega-6 PUFA and omega-3 PUFA from both seafood and plant sources to CHD risk was assessed [61]. Intake of both long-chain and intermediate-chain omega-3 PUFA was associated with lower CHD risk without any modification by omega-6 PUFA intake. Men with a median omega-3 LCPUFA intake of 250 mg/d or more had a reduced risk of SCD regardless of the amount of daily omega-6 PUFA intake. Plant-based intermediate-chain omega-3 PUFA appeared to reduce CHD risk when omega-3 LCPUFA intake from seafood is low, which has health implications for populations with low availability or consumption of fatty fish.

In another study, 5201 men and women over 65 were selected in four US communities from Medicare rolls [14]. The consumption of tuna and other broiled or baked fish consumption was associated with higher plasma EPA and DHA phospholipid levels while intake of fried fish and fish sandwiches was not. The clinical correlates of this association were that tuna and other broiled or baked fish intake were related to a lower rate of ischemic heart disease (IHD) death and arrhythmias, but not nonfatal myocardial infarction. Consumption of fried fish and fish sandwiches had no protective effect. This study highlights the importance of the type of fish, rich in omega-3 LCPUFA, and the method of preparation, baked or broiled, in conferring protection from SCD. These observational studies provide strong support for advising apparently healthy people to consume modest amounts of baked or broiled fatty fish one to two times per week or to consume fish oil supplements in a dose of 250 mg per day.

A growing body of evidence implicates dietary *trans* fatty acids (TFA) in an increased risk of SCD. TFA are unsaturated fatty acids in which at least one C = C double bond is in the *trans* configuration with the substituent groups oriented in the opposite directions [62]. In nature, TFA have only been found in a few bacteria and are not normally made by eukaryotic cells [63]. TFA are produced in large amounts when PUFA in vegetable oils are partially hydrogenated for use in commercial food production and cooking [64]. TFA are also found in beef and dairy products due to the metabolic activities of gut bacteria in ruminants [65]. Dietary TFA consist chiefly of *trans* oleic acid with one C = C double bond, *trans* linoleic acid with two C = C double bonds, and *trans* palmitoleic acid with one C = C double bond [66]. The *trans* configuration causes the acyl tail of TFA to resemble the linear structure of saturated fatty acids and facilitates greater lipid packing both within foodstuffs and within cell membranes (Figure 8.1). Diets rich in saturated fats are known to increase the risk of VF and SCD in primates [6,67]. In a case-control study from investigators in Seattle, increased levels of red cell TFA were associated with a moderate increase in the risk of primary cardiac arrest [65]. Levels of *trans* isomers of oleic acid with its single C = C double bond were not associated with an increased risk, but levels of the *trans* isomer of linoleic acid with its two C = C double bonds were linked to a threefold increase in the risk of SCD. It is conceivable that production of TFA during high-heat frying contributed to the lack of protective effect of fried fish on IHD death and arrhythmias observed in the previously described trial on Medicare recipients [14]. While further research is clearly warranted, dietary restrictions of TFA coupled with increased intakes of omega-3 LCPUFA seem prudent.

HIGH-RISK PATIENTS WITH IMPLANTABLE CARDIAC DEFIBRILLATORS

SCD is almost always caused by ventricular arrhythmias. SCD is the leading cause of death in Western countries and its incidence may be increasing [68]. Patients who have survived SCD are generally treated by placement of an implantable cardiac defibrillator (ICD). These patients are at high risk of recurrent arrhythmias and the ICD makes it possible to determine the nature and frequency of such arrhythmias and treat them by electrical shock or antitachycardia pacing.

Christensen and coworkers in Denmark evaluated the relation between serum omega-3 LCPUFA levels and the incidence of recurrent ventricular arrhythmias over a 12-month period in patients with an ICD [69]. They found that patients with more than one recurrent arrhythmic event had significantly lower serum omega-3 LCPUFA levels compared to patients without arrhythmias. When patients were divided into quintiles based on serum omega-3 LCPUFA levels, those in the lowest quintile had significantly more ventricular arrhythmic events than did those in the highest quintile (mean 1.3 event versus 0.2 event, $p < 0.05$).

The Fatty Acid Antiarrhythmia Trial (FAAT) randomized 402 patients with ICDs to either 4 grams daily of fish oil (2.6 grams EPA plus DHA) or olive oil [25]. The primary end point was time to first ICD event for ventricular tachycardia or fibrillation (VT or VF). As would be expected in patients with serious ventricular arrhythmias, 79% had coronary artery disease (CAD) and approximately half had severe left ventricular dysfunction with ejection fractions less than 0.30. Fish oil prolonged the time to first ICD event by 28%, but this failed to reach significance ($p = 0.057$). When probable episodes of VT and VF were included in the analysis, the beneficial effect of fish oil became statistically significant. A high proportion (35%) of subjects did not comply with consuming either the fish oil or olive oil. When on-treatment analysis was confined to subjects compliant for at least 11 months, fish oil significantly prolonged the time to first ICD event by 38%. Multivariate analysis found that fish oil reduced the risk of an ICD event for VT or VF by a highly significant 48%. The study authors suggest that regular consumption of fish oil may reduce the risk of potentially fatal ventricular arrhythmias in a high-risk population with a high proportion of patients suffering from CAD and severe left ventricular systolic dysfunction.

In contrast, a trial by Raitt and collaborators from Oregon found that omega-3 LCPUFA in fish oil may be proarrhythmic in certain patients with an ICD [26]. These investigators randomized 200 patients (73% with CAD) to either 1.8 grams daily of fish oil or olive oil. The primary end point was time to first ICD treatment for VT or VF. At 6, 12, and 24 months, more patients receiving fish oil had ICD therapy for VT or VF than did patients randomized to olive oil. The difference was not statistically significant. Multivariate analysis revealed that VT as the ICD qualifying arrhythmia and low ejection fraction were independent predictors of time to ICD treatment for VT or VF— suggesting that omega-3 LCPUFA may have proarrhythmic properties in these patients, especially the subset of patients with VT as the qualifying arrhythmia.

The Study on Omega-3 Fatty Acids and Ventricular Arrhythmia (SOFA) was a double-blind, placebo-controlled trial carried out by Brouwer and colleagues at cardiology clinics across Europe [27]. The study enrolled 546 subjects with an ICD and a history of VT or VF. Patients were randomized to 2 g/d of fish oil (containing 464 mg EPA/335 mg DHA) or 2 g/d of high-oleic sunflower oil. The primary end point was appropriate ICD treatment (shock or antitachycardia pacing) for VT or VF or death. Fish oil did not improve event-free survival. Among subjects receiving fish oil, 27% received appropriate ICD therapy compared to 30% of patients receiving placebo. In the fish oil group, eight patients (3%) died, six (2%) from cardiac causes, compared to 14 (5%) deaths, 13

(5%) from cardiac causes, in the placebo group. The differences were not significant. Overall, fish oil conferred no survival or event-free benefit in these patients, but was also not associated with any proarrhythmic effects. In the subset of patients with a prior myocardial infarction, there was a nonsignificant trend toward longer event-free survival (28% reaching the primary endpoint in the fish oil group versus 35% in the sunflower oil group; p = 0.13).

A meta-analysis of the three trials of fish oil in people with an ICD has been performed [70]. The analysis confirmed what is readily apparent in any close reading of the three studies: there is considerable heterogeneity in the response of this patient population to fish oil. Heterogeneity was particularly high between the Raitt study and the Leaf study (p = 0.01). In contrast, no significant heterogeneity was found between the Leaf study and the Brouwer study (p = 0.30) or between the Raitt study and the Brouwer study (p = 0.10). When the Leaf and Brouwer studies are analyzed together using a fixed-effects model, fish oil significantly reduced ICD discharge for recurrent ventricular arrhythmias. The current data prompt caution in the use of fish oil in patients with an ICD and suggest that high-dose (> 1 g/d) fish oil should be avoided in patients with primary VT, especially in the absence of CHD.

Atrial Dysrhythmias

Atrial fibrillation (AF) is an increasingly common and complex atrial dysrhythmia [71]. AF is characterized by a process of electrical remodeling that perpetuates the arrhythmia and may be facilitated by inflammation and oxidative stress [72]. Omega-3 LCPUFA have been hypothesized to have benefit in the prevention of AF through antiarrhythmic and anti-inflammatory mechanisms of action [73,74]. Limited animal studies suggest that fish oil may reduce susceptibility to AF. In a rabbit model of increased vulnerability to rapid pacing-induced AF due to left atrial stretch, dietary supplementation with tuna oil significantly reduced the pressure and pacing thresholds for stretch-induced AF [75]. In a dog model, fish oil limited heart failure–induced structural remodeling and prevented associated AF but had no effect on atrial pacing remodeling and associated AF [76]. The benefit was thought to be related to omega-3 LCPUFA-mediated reductions in protein kinase activation.

Prospective cohort studies have yielded conflicting data. A population-based study of 4815 elderly people by Mozaffarian and colleagues found that consumption of tuna or other broiled or baked fish was associated with a reduced risk of AF [77]. The much larger Danish Diet, Cancer, and Health Study involving 47,949 people found that consumption of fish was not associated with a lower risk of AF [78]. However, this study was not designed to assess the effect of fish intake on risk of atrial arrhythmias and did not elicit any information on the use of fish oil supplements, an important potential confounding factor. Patients with heart disease were excluded from the study and this may be the population that benefits most.

Clinical trials of fish oil and atrial dysrhythmias are sparse. In a small Italian study of 40 patients with dual-chamber pacemakers, omega-3 LCPUFA supplements (1 g/d) significantly reduced the incidence of atrial tachycardias [79]. When fish oil supplements were withdrawn, the incidence of recurrent atrial tachycardias reverted to baseline levels. The number of subjects was small and the population highly selected. Two larger studies have provided contradictory findings.

Kowey and coworkers randomized 663 US outpatients with symptomatic paroxysmal (n = 542) or persistent (n = 121) AF and no substantial structural heart disease to high dose omega-3 LCPUFA or placebo [80]. Paroxysmal AF was defined as a previous AF episode, but no long-term medical or electrical therapy to maintain sinus rhythm. Persistent AF was defined as previous medical or electrical treatment of AF. All subjects were in normal sinus rhythm at baseline. Participants randomized to omega-3 LCPUFA received 8 g per day for one week followed by 4 g per day. Each 1 g omega-3 LCPUFA contained approximately 465 mg of EPA and 375 mg of DHA. Treatment was for 24 weeks and follow-up was for six months. After 24 weeks, in subjects with paroxysmal AF, 129 of 269 (48%) receiving placebo and 135 of 258 participants (52%) receiving omega-3 LCPUFA had recurrent symptomatic AF or atrial flutter. In subjects with persistent AF, 18 participants (33%) in the placebo group and 32 (50%) in the omega-3 LCPUFA group had documented symptomatic AF or flutter events. Omega-3 LCPUFA had no effect on recurrent AF or atrial flutter over the six-month follow-up period.

Omega-3 LCPUFA supplements have been studied by Nodari and colleagues in the clinically challenging population of patients with persistent AF with at least one relapse following cardioversion [81]. Of 254 screened subjects, 199 were randomized to either 2 g per day of omega-3 LCPUFA containing 850–882 mg of EPA and DHA in a ratio ranging from 0.9 to 1.5 or placebo. All patients were treated with amiodarone and a renin-angiotensin-aldosterone system inhibitor. Four weeks after randomization, participants underwent direct current cardioversion. After a one-year follow-up, subjects receiving omega-3 LCPUFA were significantly more likely to remain in normal sinus rhythm (hazard ratio 0.62 vs. 0.36). Fifty-six of 103 patients receiving placebo experienced recurrent AF compared with 37 of 102 receiving omega-3 LCPUFA. Fish oil also prolonged the time to the onset of recurrent AF.

The conflicting findings of the Kowey and Nodari studies may be explained by variations in subject methodologies and subject populations. The Kowey study had a younger population, people with structural heart disease were excluded, and only a minority of subjects had persistent AF, which was really misdefined and not truly persistent but rather was medically or electrically treated paroxysmal AF. Nodari and coworkers recruited an older population of whom approximately 90% had structural heart disease. All subjects in the Nodari trial truly had persistent AF. A further difference is that subjects in the Nodari study were all treated with amiodarone. Finally, nearly half of all episodes of recurrent AF in the Kowey study occurred early during follow-up while omega-3 LCPUFA were started four weeks prior to cardioversion in the Nodari after which follow-up began. Animal studies show that maximal incorporation of omega-3 LCPUFA requires up to 28 days [82]. Rather than showing lack of efficacy, the Kowey findings may merely be a function of a poor study design that failed to allow sufficient time for omega-3 LCPUFA to exert their full antiarrhythmic effects. It is reasonable to conclude from currently available data that fish oil may be a useful adjunct to amiodarone and possibly other antiarrhythmics in the treatment of persistent AF in patients with structural heart disease, while the possible benefit to young patients with paroxysmal AF and no significant structural heart disease is presently uncertain.

Calò and coworkers were the first investigators to show that administration of omega-3 LCPUFA significantly reduced the incidence of postoperative AF in patients undergoing coronary bypass surgery [83]. They studied 160 patients undergoing coronary bypass surgery and found significantly fewer subjects randomized to 2 g/d of fish oil experienced postoperative AF compared to patients receiving placebo (15.2% versus 33.3%; p = 0.013). The benefits of perioperative fish oil with cardiac surgery appeared subsequently confirmed by Heidt and colleagues who randomized 102 patients undergoing coronary bypass surgery to fish oil 100 mg/kg body weight/d or soya oil 100 mg/kgd given intravenously beginning on hospital admission and continued until discharge from the intensive care unit (ICU) [84]. Postoperative AF occurred in nine (17.3%) in the fish oil group and in 15 patients (30.6%) in the control group (p < 0.05). Patients receiving fish oil required shorter times in the ICU than the control patients. In contrast, two randomized, double-blind, placebo-controlled trials have failed to show that perioperative fish oil reduces the incidence of AF following surgery. Heidarsdottir and coworkers studied randomized 168 patients undergoing coronary bypass surgery or heart valve repair to omega-3 LCPUFA supplying 1240 mg of EPA and 1000 mg DHA per day or olive oil. The study intervention began five to seven days before surgery. Fish oil had no effect on the incidence of postoperative AF, which occurred in 54.2% of patients receiving omega-3 LCPUFA and 54.1% of controls. Saravanan and colleagues randomized 108 patients undergoing coronary bypass surgery to 2 g/d of fish oil or olive oil initiated 12 to 21 days before surgery [86]. Omega-3 LCPUFA did reduce the risk of post operative AF. However, Saravanan and coworkers used a cutoff of 15 seconds to define an episode of AF, which overestimates the incidence of clinically significant AF making their data difficult to compare to those of the other trials. In all of these clinical studies, fish oil was not associated with significant adverse effects. Fish oil in conjunction with cardiac surgery was not associated with any increase in bleeding risk. A meta-analysis of the four studies of fish oil to reduce the incidence of postoperative AF following heart surgery concluded that there is insufficient evidence to recommend the use of fish oil in this clinical setting.

The clinical data on fish oil and atrial arrhythmias are intriguing and certainly justify larger prospective clinical trials. Study design should consider clinically relevant definitions of arrhythmia episodes or outcomes and strive to include homogeneous populations to minimize confounding factors. Fish oil should be initiated at least four weeks before the assessment of endpoints.

CLINICAL SUMMARY

- Omega-3 LCPUFA are antiarrhythmic.
- Omega-3 LCPUFA reduce lipid packing in cells membranes affecting ion channels.
- *Trans* fatty acids with two or more double bonds are proarrhythmic.
- One g/d of fish oil appears to lower mortality following MI.
- Doses in excess of 1 g/d of fish oil may increase risk of arrhythmia in patients with primary VT and idiopathic dilated cardiomyopathy.
- One g/d of fish oil may be a useful adjunction to antiarrhythmic medications to maintain sinus rhythm following cardioversion in patients with structural heart disease.
- Fish oil in addition to standard medical therapy may reduce mortality in HF.
- No data support discontinuing fish oil perioperatively at customary doses.

REFERENCES

1. Bang HO, Dyeberg J, Hjorne N. The composition of food consumed by Greenland Eskimos. Acta Med Scand 1976;200:69–73.
2. Gudbjarnason S, Óskarsdóttir G, Hallgrímsson J, Doell B. Role of myocardial lipids in development of cardiac necrosis. Recent Adv Stud Cardiac Struct Metab 1976;11:571–82.
3. Murnaghan MF. Effect of fatty acids on the ventricular arrhythmia threshold in the isolated heart of the rabbit. Br J Pharmacol 1981;73:909–15.
4. McLennan PL, Abeywardena MY, Charnock JS. Dietary fish oil prevents ventricular fibrillation following coronary artery occlusion and reperfusion. Am Heart J 1988;116:709–17.
5. McLennan PL. Relative effects of dietary saturated, monounsaturated, and polyunsaturated fatty acids on cardiac arrhythmias in rats. Am J Clin Nutr 1993;57:207–12.
6. McLennan PL, Bridle TM, Abeywardena MY, Charnock JS. Dietary lipid modulation of ventricular fibrillation threshold in the marmoset monkey. Am Heart J 1992;123:1555–61.
7. Billman GE, Hallaq H, Leaf A. Prevention of ischemia-induced ventricular fibrillation by omega 3 fatty acids. Proc Natl Acad Sci USA 1994;91:4427–30.
8. Billman GE, Kang JX, Leaf A. Prevention of ischemia-induced cardiac sudden death by n-3 polyunsaturated fatty acids in dogs. Lipids 1997;32:1161–8.
9. Leaf A, Xiao YF. The modulation of ionic currents in excitable tissues by n-3 polyunsaturated fatty acids. J Membr Biol 2001;184:263–71.
10. Leaf A, Xiao YF, Kang JX, Billman GE. Membrane effects of the n-3 fish oil fatty acids, which prevent fatal ventricular arrhythmias. J Membr Biol 2005;206:129–39.
11. Siscovick DS, Raghunathan TE, King I, et al. Dietary intake and cell membrane levels of long-chain n-3 polyunsaturated fatty acids and the risk of primary cardiac arrest. JAMA 1995;274:1363–7.
12. Albert CM, Hennekens CH, O'Donnell CJ, et al. Fish consumption and decreased risk of sudden cardiac death. JAMA 1998;279:23–8.
13. Albert CM, Campos H, Stampfer MJ, et al. Blood long-chain n-3 fatty acids and risk of sudden death. N Engl J Med 2002;346:1113–8.
14. Mozaffarian D, Lemaitre RN, Kuller LH, et al. Cardiac benefits of fish consumption may depend on the type of fish meal consumed. The Cardiovascular Health Study. Circulation 2003;107:1372–7.
15. Whelton SP, He J, Whelton PK, Muntner P. Meta-analysis of observational studies on fish intake and coronary heart disease. Am J Cardiol 2004;93:1119–23.

16. He K, Song Y, Daviglus ML, et al. Accumulated evidence on fish consumption and coronary heart disease mortality: A meta-analysis of cohort studies. Circulation 2004;109:2705–11.
17. Burr ML, Fehily AM, Gilbert JF, et al. Effects of changes in fat, fish, and fibre intakes on death and myocardial reinfarction: Diet and reinfarction trial (DART). Lancet 1989;2:757–61.
18. Singh RB, Niaz MA, Sharma JP, et al. Randomized, double-blind, placebo-controlled trial of fish oil and mustard oil in patients with suspected acute myocardial infarction: The Indian Experiment of Infarct Survival–4. Cardiovasc Drugs Ther 1997;11:485–91.
19. GISSI-Prevenzione Investigators. Dietary supplementation with n-3 polyunsaturated fatty acids and vitamin E after myocardial infarction: Results of the GISSI-Prevenzione trial. Lancet 1999;354:447–55.
20. Burr ML, Ashfield-Watt PA, Dunstan FD, et al. Lack of benefit of dietary advice to men with angina: Results of a controlled trial. Eur J Clin Nutr 2003;57:193–200.
21. Kromhout D, Giltay EJ, Geleijnse JM. N-3 fatty acids and cardiovascular events after myocardial infarction. N Engl J Med 2010;363:2015–26.
22. Rauch B, Schiele R, Schneider S, et al. OMEGA, a randomized, placebo-controlled trial to test the effect of highly purified omega-3 fatty acids on top of modern guideline-adjusted therapy after myocardial infarction. Circulation 2010;122:2152–9.
23. Yokoyama M, Origasa H, Matsuzaki M, et al. Effects of eicosapentaenoic acid on major coronary events in hypercholesterolaemic patients (JELIS): A randomized open-label, blinded endpoint analysis. Lancet 2007;369:1090–8.
24. Tavazzi L, Maggioni AP, Marchioli R, et al. Effect of n-3 polyunsaturated fatty acids in patients with chronic heart failure (the GISSI-HF trial): A randomized, double-blind, placebo-controlled trial. Lancet 2008;372:1223–30.
25. Leaf A, Albert CM, Josephson M, et al. Prevention of fatal arrhythmias in high-risk subject subjects by fish oil n-3 fatty acid intake. Circulation 2005;112:2762–8.
26. Raitt MH, Conner WE, Morris C, et al. Fish oil supplementation and risk of ventricular tachycardia and ventricular fibrillation in patients with implantable defibrillators. A randomized controlled trial. JAMA 2005;293:2884–91.
27. Brouwer IA, Zock PL, Camm AJ, et al. Effect of fish oil on ventricular tachyarrhythmia and death in patients with implantable cardioverter defibrillators: The Study on Omega-3 Fatty Acids and Ventricular Arrhythmia (SOFA) randomized trial. JAMA 2006;295:2613–9.
28. Jump DB. The biochemistry of n-3 polyunsaturated fatty acids. J Biol Chem 2002;277:8755–8.
29. Colussi G, Catena C, Baroselli S, et al. Omega-3 fatty acids: From biochemistry to their clinical use in the prevention of cardiovascular disease. Recent Patents Cardiovasc Drug Discov 2007;2:13–21.
30. Burdge GC. Metabolism of alpha-linolenic acid in humans. Prostaglandins Leukot Essent Fatty Acids 2006;75:161–8.
31. Burdge GC, Calder PC. Conversion of alpha-linolenic acid to longer-chain polyunsaturated fatty acids in human adults. Reprod Nutr Dev 2005;45:581–97.
32. Onuki Y, Morishita, M, Chiba Y, Tokiwa S, Takayama K. Docosahexaenoic acid and eicosapentaenoic acid induce changes in the physical properties of a lipid bilayer model membrane. Chem Pharm Bull 2006;54:68–71.
33. Valentine RC, Valentine DL. Omega-3 fatty acids in cellular membranes: A unified concept. Prog Lipid Res 2004;43:383–402.
34. Wassall SR, Brzustowicz MR, Shaikh SR, Cherezov V, Caffrey M, Stillwell W. Order from disorder, corralling cholesterol with chaotic lipids. The role of polyunsaturated lipids in membrane raft formation. Chem Phys Lipids 2004;132:79–88.
35. Huster D, Albert JJ, Arnold K, Gawrisch K. Water permeability of polyunsaturated lipid membranes measured by 17O NMR. Biophys J 1997;73:856–64.
36. Kafrawy O, Zerouga M, Stillwell W, Jenski LJ. Docosahexaenoic acid in phosphatidylcholine mediates cytotoxicity more effectively than other omega-3 and omega-6 fatty acids. Cancer Lett 1998;132:23–9.
37. Williams EE, Jenski LJ, Stillwell W. Docosahexaenoic acid (DHA) alters the structure and composition of membranous vesicles exfoliated from the surface of a murine leukemia cell line. Biochim Biophys Acta 1998;1371:351–62.
38. Smaby JM, Momsen MM, Brockman HL, Brown RE. Phosphatidylcholine acyl unsaturation modulates the decrease in interfacial elasticity induced by cholesterol. Biophys J 1997;73:1492–505.
39. Armstrong VT, Brzustowicz MR, Wassall SR, Jenski LJ, Stillwell W. Rapid flip-flop in polyunsaturated (docosahexaenoate) phospholipid membranes. Arch Biochem Biophys 2003;414:74–82.
40. Stillwell W, Wassall SR. Docosahexaenoic acid: Membrane properties of a unique fatty acid. Chem Phys Lipids 2003;126:1–27.

41. Lundbaek JA, Birn P, Hansen AJ, et al. Regulation of sodium channel function by bilayer elasticity: The importance of hydrophobic coupling. Effects of Micelle-forming amphiphiles and cholesterol. J Gen Physiol 2004;123:599–621.

42. Bruno MJ, Koeppe RE II, Andersen OS. Docosahexaenoic acid alters bilayer elastic properties. Proc Natl Acad Sci U S A 2007;104:9638–43.

43. McLennan PL, Bridle TM, Abeywardena MY, Charnock JS. Comparative efficacy of n-3 and n-6 poly-unsaturated fatty acids in modulating ventricular fibrillation threshold in marmoset monkeys. Am J Clin Nutr 1993;58:666–9.

44. Billman GE, Kang JX, Leaf A. Prevention of sudden cardiac death by dietary pure omega-3 polyunsatu-rated fatty acids in dogs. Circulation 1999;99:2452–7.

45. Kang JX, Leaf A. Effects of long-chain polyunsaturated fatty acids on the contraction of neonatal rat cardiac myocytes. Proc Natl Acad Sci USA 1994;91:9886–90.

46. Kang JX, Xiao YF, Leaf A. Free long-chain polyunsaturated fatty acids reduce membrane electrical excit-ability in neonatal rat cardiac myocytes. Proc Natl Acad Sci USA 1995;92:3997–4001.

47. Leaf A. The electrophysiologic basis for the antiarrhythmic and anticonvulsant effects of n-3 polyunsatu-rated fatty acids: Heart and brain. Lipids 2001;36 Suppl:S107–10.

48. Leaf A, Kang JX, Xiao YF. Fish oil fatty acids as cardiovascular drugs. Curr Vasc Pharmacol 2008;6:1–12.

49. Leaf A. Electrophysiologic basis for the antiarrhythmic and anticonvulsant effects of omega 3 polyun-saturated fatty acids. World Rev Nutr Diet 2001;88:72–8.

50. Marchioli R, Barzi F, Bomba E, et al. Early protection against sudden death by n-3 polyunsaturated fatty acids after myocardial infarction. Time-course analysis of the results of the Gruppo Italiano per lo Studio della Sopravvivenza nell'Infarto Miocardico (GISSI)-Prevenzione. Circulation 2002;105:1897–1903.

51. Nilsen DW, Albrektsen G, Landmark K, et al. Effects of high-dose concentrate of n-3 fatty acids or corn oil introduced early after acute myocardial infarction on serum triacylglycerol and HDL cholesterol. Am J Clin Nutr 2001;74:50–6.

52. Rauch B, Schiele R, Schneider S, et al. OMEGA, a randomized, placebo-controlled trial to test the effect of highly purified omega-3 fatty acids on top of modern guideline-adjusted therapy after myocardial infarction. Circulation 2010;122:2152–9.

53. Kromhout D, Giltay EJ, Geleijnse JM. N-3 Fatty acids and cardiovascular events after myocardial infarc-tion. N Engl J Med 2010;363:2015–26.

54. Micha R, King IB, Lemaitre RN, et al. Food sources of individual plasma phospholipid *trans* fatty acid isomers: The Cardiovascular Health Study. Am J Clin Nutr 2010;91;8855.

55. Clifton PM, Keogh JB, Noakes M. *Trans* fatty acids in adipose tissue and the food supply are associated with myocardial infarction. J Nutr 2004;134:874–9.

56. Expression of concern. BMJ 2005;331:266.

57. Al-Marzouki S, Evens S, Marshall T, Roberts I. Are these data real? Statistical methods for the detection of data fabrication in clinical trials. BMJ 2005;331:267–70.

58. Lee KW, Lip GYH. The role of omega-3 fatty acids in the secondary prevention of cardiovascular dis-ease. Q J Med 2003;96:465–80.

59. Tavazzi L, Maggioni AP, Marchioli R, et al. Effect of n-3 polyunsaturated fatty acids in patients with chronic heart failure (the GISSI-HF trial): A randomized, double-blind, placebo-controlled trial. Lancet 2008;372:1223–30.

60. Yokoyama M, Origasa H, Matsuzaki M, et al. Effects of eicosapentaenoic acid on major coronary events in hypercholesterolaemic patients (JELIS): A randomized open-label, blinded endpoint analysis. Lancet 2007;369:1090–8.

61. Mozaffarian D, Ascherio A, Hu FB, et al. Interplay between different polyunsaturated fatty acids and risk of coronary heart disease in men. Circulation 2005;111:157–64.

62. Emken EA. Nutrition and biochemistry of *trans* and positional fatty acid isomers in hydrogenated oils. Annu Rev Nutr 1984;4:339–76.

63. Ferreri C, Panagiotaki M, Chatgilialoglu C. *Trans* fatty acids in membranes: The free radical path. Mol Biotechnol 2007;37:19–25.

64. Mozaffarian D. *Trans* fatty acids—effects on systemic inflammation and endothelial function. Atheroscler Suppl 2006;7:29–32.

65. Lemaitre RN, King IB, Raghunathan TE, et al. Cell membrane *trans*-fatty acids and the risk of primary cardiac arrest. Circulation 2002;105:697–701.

66. Lemaitre RN, King IB, Mozaffarian D, Sootodehnia N, Siscovick DS. *Trans*-fatty acids and sudden car-diac death. Atheroscler Suppl 2006;7:13–5.

67. Charnock JS. Dietary fats and cardiac arrhythmia in primates. Nutrition 1994;10:161–9.

68. Zheng ZJ, Croft JB, Giles WH, et al. Sudden cardiac death in the United States, 1989 to 1998. Circulation 2001;104:2158–63.
69. Christensen JH, Riahi S, Schmidt EB, et al. N-3 Fatty acids and ventricular arrhythmias in patients with ischaemic heart disease and implantable cardioverter defibrillators. Europace 2005;7:338–44.
70. Jenkins DJ, Josse AR, Beyene J, et al. Fish-oil supplementation in patients with implantable cardioverter defibrillators: A meta-analysis. CMAJ 2008;178:157–64.
71. Gersh BJ, Tsang TS, Seward BJ. The changing epidemiology and natural history of nonvalvular atrial fibrillation: Clinical implications. *Trans* Am Clin Climatol Assoc 2004;115:149–60.
72. Korantzopoulos P, Kolettis T, Siogas K, Goudevenos J. Atrial fibrillation and electrical remodeling: The potential role of inflammation and oxidative stress. Med Sci Monit 2003;9:RA225–9.
73. Harrison RA, Elton PJ. Is there a role for long-chain omega3 or oil-rich fish in the treatment of atrial fibrillation? Med Hypotheses 2005;64:59–63.
74. Liu T, Li G. Anti-inflammatory effects of long-chain omega 3 fatty acids: Potential benefits for atrial fibrillation. Med Hypotheses 2005;65:200–1.
75. Ninio DM, Murphy KJ, Howe PR, Saint DA. Dietary fish oil protects against stretch-induced vulnerability to atrial fibrillation in a rabbit model. J Cardiovasc Electrophysiol 2005;16:1189–94.
76. Sakabe M, Shiroshita-Takeshita A, Maguy A, et al. Omega-3 polyunsaturated fatty acids prevent atrial fibrillation associated with heart failure but not atrial tachycardia remodeling. Circulation 2007;116:2101–9.
77. Mozaffarian D, Psaty BM, Rimm EB, et al. Fish intake and risk of incident atrial fibrillation. Circulation 2004;110:368–73.
78. Frost L, Vestergaard P. N-3 fatty acids consumed from fish and risk of atrial fibrillation or flutter: The Danish Diet, Cancer, and Health Study. Am J Clin Nutr 2005;81:50–4.
79. Biscione F, Totteri A, De Vita A, Lo Bianco F, Altamura G. Effect of omega-3 fatty acids on the prevention of atrial arrhythmias. Ital Heart J Suppl 2005;6:53–9 (abstract in English; article in Italian).
80. Kowey PR, Reiffel JA, Ellenbogen KA, et al. Efficacy and safety of prescription omega-3 fatty acids for the prevention of recurrent symptomatic atrial fibrillation: A randomized controlled trial. JAMA 2010;304:2363–72.
81. Nodari S, Triggiani M, Campia U, et al. N-3 polyunsaturated fatty acids in the prevention of atrial fibrillation recurrences after electrical cardioversion: A prospective, randomized study. Circulation 2011;124:1100–6.
82. Owen AJ, Peter-Przyborowska BA, Hoy AJ, McLennan PL. Dietary fish oil dose- and time-response effects on cardiac phospholipid fatty acid composition. Lipids 2004;39:955–61.
83. Calò L, Bianconi L, Colivicchi F, et al. N-3 Fatty acids for the prevention of atrial fibrillation after coronary artery bypass surgery: A randomized, controlled trial. J Am Coll Cardiol 2005;45:1723–8.
84. Heidt MC, Vician M, Stracke SK, et al. Beneficial effects of intravenously administered N-3 fatty acids for the prevention of atrial fibrillation after coronary artery bypass surgery: A prospective randomized study. Thorac Cardiovasc Surg 2009;57:276–80.
85. Heidarsdottir R, Arnar DO, Skuladottir GV, et al. Does treatment with n-3 polyunsaturated fatty acids prevent atrial fibrillation after open heart surgery? Europace 2010;12:356–63.
86. Saravanan P, Bridgewater B, West AL, et al. Omega-3 fatty acid supplementation does not reduce risk of atrial fibrillation after coronary artery bypass surgery: A randomized, double-blind, placebo-controlled clinical trial. Circ Arrhythm Electrophysiol 2010;3:46–53.
87. Armaganijan L, Lopes RD, Healey JS, et al. Do omega-3 fatty acids prevent atrial fibrillation after open heart surgery? A meta-analysis of randomized controlled trials. Clinics (São Paolo) 2011;66:1923–8.

9 Anemia

Which Patients Benefit from Nutritional Therapies?

Nicole M. Farmer, M.D.

INTRODUCTION

"It is more important to know what patient has the disease than what disease the patient has." The esteemed Dr. William Osler addresses how knowledge about a patient can outweigh knowledge of the disease process in this quote. Dr. Osler's words ring especially true for patients with anemia.

Derived from a French medical term first used in 1761, anemia is most often linked to a deficiency of iron status, to the extent that other modifiable underlying causes may go under recognized. Causes of anemia vary from genetic, infectious, trauma related, to nutritional deficiencies.

The goal of this chapter is twofold. One, to evaluate anemia through a lens focused on the central and important role of iron homeostasis and regulation in the most common types of anemia. Two, to explore the management of anemia as a patient-centered process driven by the need for a balanced review of an individual's physiologic, environmental, and nutritional states.

EPIDEMIOLOGY

Anemia is defined as a decrease in the number of red blood cells or less than the normal quantity of hemoglobin in the blood. Today it is regarded as one of the most common diseases in the world. In 2002, anemia was considered as one of the most important factors contributing to the global burden of disease [1].

Anemia can occur as a result of a variety of etiologic factors—genetic, dietary and nutritional, environmental, or from acute or chronic blood loss. Iron deficiency anemia occurs in 50% of cases of diagnosed anemia, and the presence of anemia is often used as a proxy for iron deficiency anemia [1]. Anemia of inflammation, formerly called anemia of chronic disease, is the second most prevalent type of anemia and is the most common type of anemia present when chronic illness occurs in a patient [2]. Anemia of inflammation often causes a less severe level of anemia than iron deficiency.

In many instances, iron deficiency plays an important role in anemia, either causally or as a downstream effect from the initial anemic disease process. Globally, iron deficiency anemia remains a significant problem due to either decreased dietary access to iron or as a result of infections, such as helminthes or malaria.

In developed countries, there may be a role for poor intake of foods and supplements that enhance iron absorption or of foods and supplements that are involved in red blood cell production. A study of data from the National Health and Nutrition Examination Survey (NHANES) from 2003 to

2006 found that the usual total intake of iron was 15.8 mg/day from natural and fortified sources [3]. The recommended daily intake range is 8–15 mg/day. Furthermore, other studies have shown the important role of iron bioavailability in determining iron deficiency in Western type diets [4]. To further showcase the impact dietary factors may have on iron bioavailability, a study of elderly patients from the Framingham Heart Study found that if a low intake of inhibitory foods occurred in a 2000 kcal/day diet then 1.8 mg of iron was absorbed. But, when dietary iron inhibitors were consumed, the amount of iron absorption declined to less than 1 mg a day [5].

As dietary choices in developed countries become varied and shifted towards vegan, vegetarian, or convenience based foods, it is conceivable that a continued decrease in the intake of foods that are highly iron bioavailable may have an impact on the degree of iron deficiency and anemia seen. Inadequate dietary intake may be combined with poor absorption due to rising prevalence of gluten-related digestive disorders.

PATHOPHYSIOLOGY

Iron is an important micronutrient for the body and is required for many vital cellular functions, including cellular oxidation and metabolism. When coupled with the protoporphyrin-based protein, heme, iron plays an important physiologic role in several cellular functions: carrying oxygen to tissues in hemoglobin, oxygen storage in muscles in myoglobin, and making oxygen available for cellular oxidation reaction needs to form ATP in cytochromes a, b, and c. In fact, iron's contribution to vital cellular and oxidation reactions is heralded before anemia manifests, by the finding of decreased oxygen consumption on vital capacity studies [6]. Iron is also the major element in the cytochrome P450 enzyme system that is responsible for the hepatic clearance of toxins and medications. Iron compounds, not united with heme, also have important functions in immune defense reactions involving cell-mediated immunity. Given iron's involvement in many vital cellular and immune functions, it is not surprising that iron deficiency may place a high burden on a society and greatly affect quality of life. Several studies have shown impairments in cognition, mood, and even restless leg syndrome in nonanemic iron deficiency [7]. Interventions where iron stores are repleted successfully have shown varied benefits, such as improved work capacity and improved childhood behavior [8].

As vital as iron is to cellular function, excess or free iron can be harmful. Unless bound or chelated, iron can play a key role in the formation of oxygen radicals through the Fenton reaction—leading to free-radical creation and possibly programmed cell death [9]. Iron is also an important factor needed for pathogenic microbial growth. Therefore, restriction of iron from bacteria is thought to be an evolutionary-based defense mechanism. Lastly, excess iron levels can be otherwise deleterious to organ function, such as occurs in hemochromatosis. Free iron is taken up by proteins that are responsible for iron storage, acquisition, and transport (Table 9.1).

Iron homeostasis is closely linked with the primary system that uses iron, red blood cell production. When needed, iron is released from senescent red blood cells through phagocytosis by macrophages involved in the reticuloendothelial system. The inherent interrelationship between red blood cell production and iron homeostasis creates a relationship where the effects on one system affect the other. Functioning as interdependent systems, specific contributors to both iron homeostasis and erythropoiesis, such as vitamins, co factors, trace element concentrations, and the immune system may also interface at times.

ERYTHROPOIESIS

Erythropoiesis involves the production of new hemoglobin containing red blood cells that deliver oxygen to tissues (Figures 9.1 and 9.2). Because the synthesis of hemoglobin is dependent on available iron concentrations, signals for production are closely linked to the replacement of old red blood cells destroyed through the reticuloendothelial system daily.

TABLE 9.1
Proteins Involved in Iron Homeostasis

Protein	Function
Divalent metal transporter 1	Transports divalent metal ions such as iron, zinc, copper, and cobalt by a proton-coupled mechanism
Ferrireductase	Reduction of Fe^{3+} to Fe^{2+}
Heme carrier protein 1	Traffics heme across the membrane
	Intestinal uptake of heme iron
Heme oxygenase	Dissembles heme to liberate iron
Ferroportin 1 (Iron regulatory protein 1)	Fe^{2+} transporter (exporter)
	Hepcidin receptor
Hephaestin	Multicopper ferroxidase, similar to plasma ceruloplasmin, oxidizes Fe^{2+} to Fe^{3+} to load it onto transferrin
Transferrin	Maintenance of cell-surface ferroportin
	Plasma Fe^{3+} binding protein
Transferrin receptor 1	Cellular uptake of transferrin bound iron
Transferrin receptor 2	Diferric transferrin; regulates hepcidin expression
Mitoferrin	Mitochondrial iron importer that supplies iron to ferrochelatase for insertion into protoporphyrin IX
Ferritin	Iron-storage protein (H and L chains); ferroxidase activity (H chain)
Iron regulatory proteins	Cytoplasmic proteins that bind and regulate iron-response elements of ferritin mRNAs
Hemosiderin	Iron-storage protein; breakdown product of ferritin that occurs when iron levels are high
Heme exporters	ATP-independent heme exporter
HFE	Interacts with TRF2 to induce hepatic hepcidin expression
Hemojuvelin	Acts as a bone morphogenic protein co receptor to stimulate hepcidin transcription
Hepcidin	Iron-regulatory protein, binds ferroportin to cause its internalization and degradation
Erythropoietin	Upregulates the expression of iron-transport and export proteins: ferroportin, TfR1, intestinal DMT1, and hephaestin
	Downregulates hepcidin expression in hepatocytes and macrophage DMT1

Adapted from Munoz, 2009.

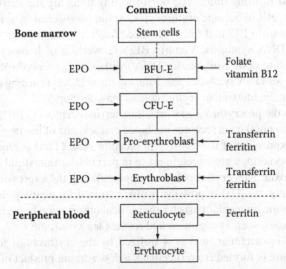

FIGURE 9.1 Erythropoiesis stages with involvement of erythropoietin, folate, vitamin B12, transferrin, and ferritin receptors at different stages of erythrocyte development. (From Munoz, 2009.)

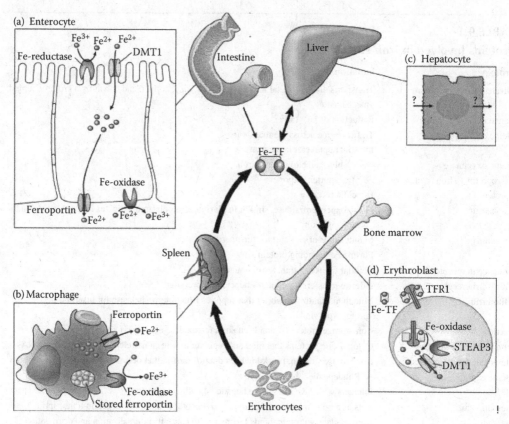

FIGURE 9.2 Iron homeostasis overview. Sites involved in absorption, utilization, and storage of iron. Detailed pictures show transporters and enzymes involved in iron absorption, cellular storage, and export. (From NC Andrews, 2008.)

The process of erythropoiesis occurs first in the bone marrow where progenitor stem cells transition to erythroid burst forming units. The burst-forming units are the earliest stage of commitment for the progenitor cells to become erythrocytes. At the burst-forming unit phase, erythroblasts express receptors for vitamin B12 and folate. Reduced folate availability can lead to a reduction in thymidine needed for DNA synthesis. Vitamin B12's conversion of homocysteine to methionine helps keep an active folate pool available for DNA synthesis in the erythroblast. A deficiency of either may lead to a longer DNA synthesis phase during the cell cycle causing enlarged megaloblastic erythrocytes; ultimately, ineffective erythropoiesis may develop.

As development into the proerythroblast starts, transferrin receptors (TFR1) are expressed on the cell surface to allow iron uptake via receptor mediated endocytosis of the iron and diferric transferrin protein complex. Expression of the transferrin receptor gene (Tfr1) is required for erythrocyte differentiation. Erythropoietin, a glycoprotein made in peritubular interstitial cells of the renal cortex in response to hypoxia, aids erythropoiesis by upregulating the expression of the Tfr1 on the erythroblast. Interestingly, the Tfr1 expression is also required for neuroepithelial cell differentiation [10]. Perhaps this is the molecular basis for the clinical observation between iron deficiency and various neurological issues, such as cognition and restless leg syndrome.

Once iron becomes intracellular, it is now utilized by the erythroblast for incorporation into heme. The heme structure is formed from succinate, a downstream product of the Kreb Cycle. The use of succinate therefore links red blood cell production with manganese and pyroxidine (vitamin B6) levels, which are important in the Krebs cycle [11].

Heme formation occurs mostly in the cytoplasm of the red blood cell and leads to the formation of a protoporphyrin ring. The site of heme production fluctuates between the mitochondria and cytoplasm of the red blood cell. Incorporation of iron into the protoporphyrin ring occurs in the mitochondria. Iron is transported to the mitochondria through the iron importer, mitoferrin. The synthesis of heme is closely linked with the transcription of globin chains in the nucleus of the proerythroblast. The pyknotic nucleus of the proerythroblast is ultimately removed once globin mRNA is amplified. The hemoglobin molecule is continually made in the cytoplasm and mitochondria of the reticulocyte cell from the globin mRNA and heme protoporphyrin ring and accounts for approximately 98% of the cytoplasm mass at the reticulocyte stage [11]. The reticulocyte stays in the bone marrow for two to three days before entering the peripheral circulation. The mitochondria and ribosomes from the reticulocyte are lost. A mature red cell starts to form and becomes dependent on the hemoglobin already produced to determine its oxygen carrying capacity. The erythrocyte expresses a heme exporter, feline leukemia virus subgroup C receptor (FLVCR), which prevents excess hemoglobin concentrations [12].

The normal life span of a mature red blood cell is approximately 120 days. Under periods of oxidative stress or during certain infections, such as malaria, the life span of an erythrocyte may be shortened. Eryptosis, the programmed cell death of erythrocytes, is characterized by cell shrinkage and cell membrane scrambling with phosphatidylserine exposure at the erythrocyte surface. Lead, gold, and bismuth are proeryptotic, as may be the phytonutrient curcumin. Lipid therapies for heavy metal toxin–related anemia may be effective through altering cell membrane lipids, and thus decreasing the membrane signaling response needed for induction of eryptosis.

From development to the end of the cellular life cycle, erythrocytes are sensitive to numerous factors surrounding oxidation, the presence of eryptotic factors, and erythropoietic promoting factors. Vitamin A, ascorbic acid, and vitamin E interact with a variety of the mechanisms needed to maintain a circulating pool of erythrocytes (Figure 9.3).

Iron Homeostasis

The iron requirements for erythropoiesis are 20–30 mg per day. Each red blood cell contains about 10^9 atoms of iron [9]. Dietary iron contributes 12–20 mg of iron to the body's stores. From that amount, the body absorbs 1–2 mg of iron a day [13]. Because there is no regulated excretion of iron through the liver or kidneys, iron balance is primarily controlled at the level of intestinal absorption [14]. The regulation of iron levels via the intestinal system acts in response to three factors: bioavailability of dietary iron for absorption, erythropoietic system demands, and immune system response [15].

Dietary iron occurs in two main forms: heme iron and nonheme iron. Heme iron is united with the protoporphyrin ring in either myoglobin or hemoglobin. Nonheme iron occurs mostly as ferric salts found in dairy products, animal source products, vegetables, legumes, grains, and iron fortified cereals [15]. Heme iron accounts for only 10–20% of dietary iron, but accounts for up to 50% of the iron absorbed [16]. Heme iron likely has increased bioavailability due to the iron-protein complex that protects the iron molecule from inhibitory absorption factors that may be present in a meal. An important factor in determining heme iron absorption includes the presence of transport proteins on the enterocyte microvilli surface [17]. Calcium can also affect heme iron absorption possibly at the gastrointestinal mucosa level [18].

Nonheme iron absorption is determined by the ability to keep iron in a soluble form in the intestinal lumen, transport proteins on the enterocyte, and by the presence of inhibitory or complementary dietary factors.

Most of nonheme iron is in the ferric form (Fe^{3+}). Ferric iron preciptiates at pH > 3 if it is not kept in solution by chelators [18]. Dietary forticants such as ethylenediaminetetraacetic acid (EDTA), organic acids, or amino acids from meats can serve as weak chealtors that keep ferric iron from precipitating. Vitamin C and vitamin A also help to increase iron absorption through chealtion of ferric iron.

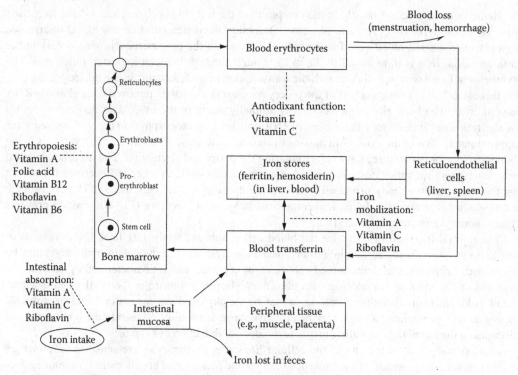

FIGURE 9.3 Role of vitamins in erythropoiesis and iron homeostasis. (From Fishman, 2000.)

At the surface of the enterocyte, the nonheme iron molecule moves through a layer of secreted mucus before reaching the microvilli for uptake [18]. Next, a reduction from ferric (Fe^{3+}) to ferrous (Fe^{2+}) iron occurs by the brush border ferrireductase, duodenal cytochrome b, before the transport protein divalent metal transporter 1 (DMT-1) cotransports the iron molecule with a proton. The reduction of ferric to ferrous iron is heavily dependent on the presence of an acidic gastric pH and the presence of the reducing agent, ascorbic acid. Calcium is a low-affinity, noncompetitive inhibitor of DMTI-1 explaining in part the effect of high dietary calcium on iron bioavailability [19]. Inflammation may also play a role in nonheme absorption, as injection of lipopolysaccharide leads to a decreased expression of the nonheme absorption proteins in the small intestine [20].

Once absorption through the apical and mucosal surface of the enterocyte occurs, nonheme and heme iron follow a common pathway. Iron either remains in the enterocyte for use or leaves the enterocyte to become absorbed into plasma. Iron that remains in the enterocyte is sloughed off into the gut lumen during enterocyte senescence. Once exported out of the basolateral layer of the cell by the export protein, ferroportin iron is oxidized by hephaestin, an oxidase protein, and then becomes bound to plasma transferrin [13]. Transferrin receptors on the surface of cells uptake the iron-transferrin complex by receptor mediated endocytosis. After the intracellular endosomes release iron, it is now available for cellular processes or becomes a complex with the protein ferritin for intracellular storage.

Lastly, iron homeostasis can be affected by the presence or absence of antagonistic or synergistic vitamins or trace elements. DMT-1 also transports manganese, zinc, copper, and lead. Lead toxicity can directly inhibit iron absorption and cause iron deficiency anemia. Copper and iron have a synergistic relationship. Copper is needed for activity of the ferrioxidases, ceruloplasmin and hephaestin, which aid in binding iron to transferrin. There are emerging studies that the copper ferrioxidases are involved in cellular iron efflux, especially from enterocytes [21]. Significant copper deficiency can lead to an increase in iron tissue stores and a decrease in iron availability. Chromium, an important element in glucose and insulin regulation, binds to transferrin in competition with iron during times of iron or chromium excess [22]. However, since iron concentrations are greater than chromium concentrations, iron is more likely to inhibit chromium absorption. During states of glucose dysregulation such as gestational diabetes, the potential for supplemental iron to reduce chromium stores may merit clinical consideration [23]. Cobalt, a major component of vitamin B12, can also compete with iron for absorption [24].

Iron Regulation in Anemia of Inflammation

Anemia frequently occurs in both acute (sepsis) and chronic inflammatory disease (congestive heart failure, kidney disease, rheumatoid arthritis, and inflammatory bowel disease). Iron and red blood cell production are both intimately regulated by the immune system through proinflammatory cytokines (Figure 9.4): 1) impaired responsiveness of erythroid cells to erythropoietin; 2) decreased red blood cell half-life from dyserythropoiesis and inhibited proliferation and differentiation; 3) inhibited erythropoietin response; 4) inhibited iron absorption from intestine, inhibited iron recirculation, and increased iron storage.

Initially reported in the 1930s and then fully described by Cartwright and Wintrobe in the 1960s, the decrease in available serum iron and the presence of anemia in response to injections of lipopolysaccharide were the first experiments to suggest a causative role of cytokines and inflammation in anemia. The synthesis of both transferrin and ferritin by iron regulatory proteins is also regulated by a nitric oxide–based mechanism in the presence of inflammation.

Protection from excess iron could be advantageous even in noninfectious conditions. In addition to hemochromatosis, increased serum iron is linked to carcinogenesis, atherosclerosis [25,26,27], and osteoporosis [25]. Furthermore, since some neutrophil-based reactions may be involved in oxidative stress generation, there may be instances where limiting iron availability in order to prevent iron-driven cell-mediated immune reactions would be advantageous.

The body regulates iron levels through the gastrointestinal tract, where absorption occurs, and by controlling the release of iron from the body's stores in the reticuloendothelial system. The protein hepcidin is now known to be the orchestrating protein involved in centrally regulating iron homeostasis. Elevated levels of hepcidin are now considered the cause of anemia of inflammation.

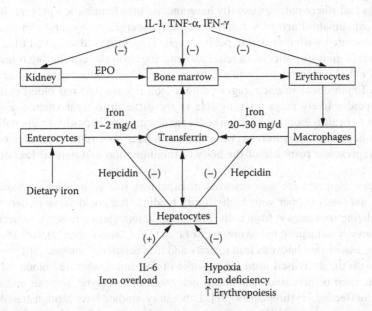

FIGURE 9.4 Role of cytokines in erythropoiesis and iron metabolism regulation, including regulation of hepcidin. (From Munoz, 2009.)

Hepcidin was first uncovered as an antimicrobial protein. Initial analysis of hepcidin (named from hepatic bactericidal protein) demonstrated significant antibacterial and antifungal activities [28]. Hepcidin is able to decrease the release of cellular iron through the induction and degradation of its receptor, ferroportin, the only known cellular iron exporter. Decrease in ferroportin leads to hepcidin-induced restriction of cellular iron from enterocytes, macrophages, and hepatocytes [29]. Direct injection of hepcidin into mice can result in a dramatic drop in serum iron within one hour, similar to the response induced in prior studies with lipopolysaccharide injection. Even though hepcidin is rapidly cleared from the plasma by the kidneys, the effect of a single dose can be apparent for up to 72 hours, due to the time required to resynthesize ferroportin [30].

Hepcidin is detected in biologic fluids as a 20 or 25 amino acid isoform, hepcidin-20 or hepcidin-25. Hepcidin-20 appears to behold antibacterial and antifungal properties. Hepcidin-25 contains an important five N-terminal amino acids and is the isoform involved in regulating iron homeostasis. Hepcidin levels are indirectly influenced by hypoxia and erythroid demand. The immune system, iron levels, and the action of the TGF-beta growth factor, bone morphogenic protein, are among the most influential direct hepcidin regulators. Within hours after an inflammatory stimulus (such as lipopolysaccrahide [LPS]), hepcidin levels greatly increase [31]. Interleukin 6 (IL-6), a cytokine of the innate immune system, plays a large role in the induction of hepcidin via the signal transducer and activator of transcription 3 (STAT3) pathway [32]. Other cytokines and factors in the innate immune system, independent of IL-6, are also involved in hepcidin production, such as Interleukin 22 (IL-22) and toll-like receptor proteins. In addition, endoplasmic reticulum (ER) stress can induce hepcidin expression. ER stress occurs from the accumulation of improperly folded proteins and may occur from inflammation mediated by IL-6 [33]. Bone morphogenetic protein-6 (BMP6) and its coreceptor hemojevulin play a key role in inducing hepcidin production. BMP6's positive effect on hepcidin is increased in response to chronic iron loading and decreased through the serine protease, TMPRSS6. Possibly the reason for BMP6's role in hepcidin expression is related to the finding that increased iron stores in bones can lead to osteoclastic activity [34] and a decrease in bone morphogenetic protein-2 induced osteoblastogenesis.

Elevated hepcidin levels are found in diseases where inflammation plays a critical role in the disease process and where patients usually have anemia of inflammation present. Inflammatory bowel disease, rheumatoid arthritis–related anemia, visceral obesity, and end-stage renal disease are all associated with elevated hepcidin levels. Hepcidin is also linked to erythropoietin resistant anemia in dialysis patients. In renal patients, the naturally conflicting roles of hepcidin, an inhibitor of cellular iron release, and erythropoietin, which encourages cellular iron release, are amplified. Erythropoietin encourages cellular iron release and red blood cell differentiation, while hepcidin likely plays a strong role in the difficult-to-treat anemia. Erythropoietin administration to healthy humans can markedly reduce urinary hepcidin levels within 48 hours [33]. The high hepcidin levels in renal patients may reflect poor renal clearance of the protein but may also represent a response of the body to inflammation and natural loss of erythropoietin levels.

Essential trace elements are also involved in hepcidin's role in iron homeostasis. Hepcidin's N-terminal region binds copper with high-affinity binding that could serve to decrease copper's effect on mobilizing iron release from cells. Endoplasmic reticulum stress, an inducer of hepcidin expression, is heavily influenced by the presence of lead [35]. Consequently, elevated hepcidin levels may explain the association between lead toxicity and iron deficiency anemia [36].

Consistent with the decreased need for hepcidin during times when red blood cell destruction or eythropoietic need is increased, hepcidin is decreased in hemolytic anemias and in hereditary anemias with ineffective erythropoiesis [37]. Laboratory studies have demonstrated that altered hepcidin expression is responsible for the increased iron absorption often observed in β-thalassemia [30]. Also, hepcidin levels are decreased in sickle cell anemia, where ongoing hemolysis can lead to increased organ iron storage, especially of hepatocytes and macrophages [38]. There appears to be an ongoing incongruously low hepcidin level present, despite the degree of tissue iron loading that occurs.

PATIENT EVALUATION

Based on current knowledge, hepcidin's role in iron homeostasis leads to an increase in tissue and cellular stores of iron that effectively decreases ability for iron utilization in the hematopoietic system. The end result is a potential functional iron deficient state where a tug-of-war relationship exists between the benefits and costs of restricting available iron versus the needs of the body for iron.

Categories for anemia involving iron imbalance are: true iron deficiency anemia, anemia of inflammation, and anemia of inflammation that has evolved into iron deficiency. Differentiation between the three categories depends on measurement of serum ferritin, a measure of iron stores, in conjunction with serum transferrin receptor levels, a measure of tissue iron needs (Figure 9.5). Primary dependence on ferritin is avoided due to significant intra individual variation [39]. Also ferritin is an acute phase reactant and elevated levels may occur with inflammatory mediated hepcidin expression.

In pure iron deficient states, hepcidin levels are reduced, due to the body's need to increase iron absorption and utilization. Recently, investigators have started to employ this finding in order to develop hepcidin as a lab test for iron deficiency anemia [40]. A marker of iron deficiency, serum zinc protoporphyrin is elevated in patients that have true iron deficiency and in patients with anemia of inflammation and iron deficiency [37].

Mechanisms that determine the progression from anemia of inflammation to anemia of inflammation with iron deficiency have not been fully elucidated. Morphologically, iron restriction related to hepcidin does not usually lead to a microcytic red blood cell, as in conventional iron deficiency.

For the clinician, it is important to utilize available lab studies with a clinical picture of symptoms to help determine the extent that a subclinical cause for the patient's anemia could be present (Table 9.2). Evaluating anemic patients first through use of functional iron categories may be beneficial in developing treatment plans to determine which patients benefit from a) an increase of iron intake and absorption or b) promoting the mobilization of iron stores when elevated hepcidin expression occurs.

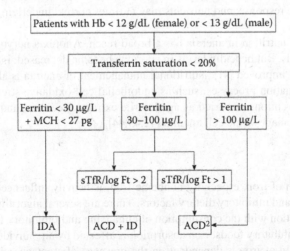

FIGURE 9.5 Classification of anemia based on iron functional status. ACD + ID anemia of chronic disease (or anemia of inflammation) with iron deficiency. IDA iron deficiency anemia. ACD2 anemia of chronic inflammation only. (From Munoz, 2009.)

TABLE 9.2

Classification of Anemia Based on Functional Iron Status: Iron Deficiency, Anemia of Inflammation, and Anemia of Inflammation with Iron Restriction

Anemia Type	Diseases	Hepcidin	Laboratory Values
Iron deficiency	GI blood loss Poor dietary intake Poor bioavailability	Decreased	Moderate to severe low Hgb Low to normal MCV Decreased ferritin with MCH < 27 Decreased transferrin saturation
Anemia of inflammation	Inflammatory bowel disease Rheumatoid arthritis Obesity	Increased	Mild to moderate Hgb Normal MCV Normal or increased ferritin Decreased transferring saturation Transferrin receptor level < 1
Anemia of chronic disease with iron restriction and deficiency	Chronic kidney disease* Congestive heart failure*	Increased	Mild to moderate Hgb Normal MCV Normal ferritin Decreased transferring saturation Transferrin receptor level > 2

*Signifies disease conditions with decreased erythropoietin production and resulting in very low iron stores in the setting of inflammatory conditions. MCV = Mean Cell Volume; Hgb = Hemoglobin

TREATMENT

When determining clinical management options for anemia, the best course of action is to treat the underlying condition causing the anemia. However, anemia may involve complex interactions of physiologic, pathologic, and dietary factors—making the treatment of a sole cause, outside of acute blood loss, difficult.

Treatment of anemia using nutritional interventions is effective due to nutrition's engagement of multiple etiologic factors that contribute to anemia: regulation of iron homeostasis occurs mostly at the level of intestinal absorption; iron absorption promotion and inhibition is influenced by the intake of vitamin and trace metals in supplements or food; the intestinal tract serves as a location of regulation for immune response; and nutrients may at times correct underlying metabolic dysfunction (Table 9.3).

The importance of nutrition in anemia has a broad reach. Anorexia nervosa is associated with elevated hepcidin levels. But hepcidin levels in anorexia become decreased, independent of inflammation, as nutrition is improved [41]. Nutritional management of anemia is also beneficial to help cell-mediated inflammation processes, such as endothelial cell oxidative stress in sickle cell anemia. Nutritional interventions as varied as aged garlic extract, green tea, and essential fatty acids are reported to help manage sickle cell anemia [42,43,44].

Iron

The overall absorption of iron, especially nonheme iron, is heavily influenced by the presence of absorption enhancing and inhibitory dietary factors. There are several algorithms developed to help determine iron absorption with the consumption of enhancing and inhibitory factors [45].

Besides intake of inhibitory foods, iron absorption is affected by an individual's intestinal physiologic state. Absorption of iron is dependent on the presence of stomach acid in order to form a soluble complex with proteins, such as uptake receptor proteins in small intestinal enterocytes. In an alkaline stomach, iron forms into insoluble complexes that lead to decreased absorption.

TABLE 9.3
Enhancing and Inhibitory Nutrients on Iron Absorption
and Erythropoiesis

	Enhancing	Inhibitory
Iron absorption	Ascorbic acid	Calcium
	Vitamin A	Vitamin D
	Vitamin B6 and B2	Phytate
	Copper	Flavonoids, specifically
	Organic acids	polyphenol tannins
	Fermented foods	
	Ascorbic acid	
Anti oxidation	Vitamin A	Phytate
	Riboflavin	
	Folate and B12	
	Vitamin E	
Mobilization of iron	Ascorbic acid	
stores	Copper	
Erythropoiesis	Folate and B12	
Inflammation related	Omega-3 fatty acids	
Detoxification of	Folate and B12	Mercury
heavy metals	Vitamin B6	Lead
		Cadmium

Therefore, the induction of gastric juices from smelling food during the cephalic phase of digestion, or the intake of meat proteins that produce gastric juice are important for iron absorption.
Hypochlorhydia, from a variety of causes such as gastric surgery, gastric atrophy, and pharmacotherapy such as proton pump inhibitor and histamine-2 blockers, may impair iron absorption.
Pancreatic enzyme replacement may also decrease iron absorption; intestinal iron absorption is
increased in patients that have deficiency of pancreatic enzyme excretion [24].

Culinary methods to increase dietary iron content from foods include use of unsalted water for
cooking vegetables and steaming or boiling [46]. Cooking with iron-rich herbs such as peppermint
leaves, comfrey root, and goldenseal root can improve iron status [24]. Use of cast iron or stainless
steel pans can lead to increased iron intake through the process of mineral migration [47]. Patients
familiar with the use of iron skillets may be advised to season iron pans with heated cooking oil [48].

Traditional cultures and diets have used foods containing iron for centuries to treat anemia.
Intake of iron from foods may be preferential as a replacement source compared to supplementation.
Dietary iron does not have the side effect profile of oral supplements. However, changes in modern
dietary selections along with shifts away from traditional foods may be responsible for the shift
away from use of dietary iron.

Supplementation with iron should not to be considered a low-risk intervention by clinicians.
In addition to the side-effect profile, excessive amounts of iron supplements can lead to further
decreased intestinal absorption due to oversaturation at the mucosa surface [49]. That residual
iron not absorbed into the lumen could also mediate the gastrointestinal side effects. Excessive
iron intake can cause perturbations in absorption of other trace elements, such as zinc, cobalt, and
chromium. The U.S. Institute of Medicine has established a lowest observed adverse effect level
(LOAEL) for iron of 60 mg/day [50]. One study has even reported 15 mg/day in an elderly population as still being effective in correcting iron deficiency [51].

For oral iron therapy, ferrous iron salts are often used. Ferrous fumerate, lactate, succinate,
glutamate, and sulfate all have similar bioavailability [15]. Due to accessibility and cost, ferrous

sulfate is the most commonly used supplement, but it is associated with more gastrointestinal side effects compared to some of the other ferrous salts. Ferrous glycinate has the least reported risk of gastrointestinal side effects, such as constipation.

Oral iron therapy can increase reticulocytes within 4 to 7 days. And a dose of 200–300 mg a day will result in absorption of 50 mg a day [11]. The ultimate goal of iron therapy is to provide stores of 500 mg to 1 gram to prepare for decreased absorption. Sustained treatment of iron for several months is recommended because as hemoglobin values increase, erythropoietin levels decrease and so does iron absorption. However, the sustained treatment recommended may ultimately lead to decreased compliance due to the risk of increased side effects with prolonged iron use.

Research into optimal iron supplement dosing frequency is desirable to help decrease side effects and help improve compliance. A Cochrane meta-analysis review of intermittent oral supplementation showed no overall difference between intermittent and daily supplementation in menstruating women. An explanation for the effectiveness of intermittent iron supplementation may rest in the increased ability of new enterocytes made in the intestinal lumen every 5 to 6 days to uptake iron. In addition to dosing frequency, the meta-analysis evaluated dosing and found the provision of supplements once a week with 60 to 120 mg of iron was enough to produce a positive hematological response [52].

When an expected increase in hemoglobin does not occur in a compliant patient, it is important to determine three factors before considering increase in dosing or frequency: 1) If the patient is eating a diet or taking supplements that promote iron absorption, for example ascorbic acid or vitamin A. In addition, copper can help to increase serum iron levels through promotion of tissue utilization of iron stores. Studies have also shown the addition of micronutrient supplements containing trace elements and vitamins to iron supplements can increase hemoglobin levels more than iron alone [53,54,55,56]. 2) If a medication taken by the patient is interfering with iron absorption. 3) If normal absorption of oral iron is occurring. Adequate absorption of supplemental oral iron can be determined through use of an iron absorption test. Two iron tablets are given to the patient on an empty stomach, and the serum iron is measured serially over the subsequent two hours. Normal absorption will result in an increase in the serum iron of at least 100 μg/dL. If an iron deficiency persists despite adequate treatment, it may be necessary to switch to parenteral iron therapy.

When iron supplementation is needed in the setting of blood loss, oral iron therapy should not be expected to correct iron stores if there is more than 20–30 ml of blood loss daily [57]. There are also clinical instances in which iron deficiency can occur from a gastrointestinal source and not involve any blood loss. Conventional gastrointestinal diagnostic workups fail to establish a cause of iron deficiency in about one-third of patients [58].

In *Helicobacter pylori*–related iron deficiency, blood loss may not be the prominent cause for iron loss due to the loss of parietal cell gastric proton secretion. In addition, *H. pylori* injection adversely affects gastrointestinal ascorbate levels [58].

For patient populations with noncompliance to oral therapy or who have absorption impairment, such as in celiac disease, post bariatric surgery, or inflammatory bowel disease, parenteral iron can be used. In parenteral formulations, iron is joined with a carbohydrate molecule. With older formulations of parenteral iron, such as iron dextran, the iron-carbohydrate complex is less stable allowing iron to become free at a faster rate. Labile iron may then lead to leaky capillary syndrome. In addition, anaphylaxis may occur to the carbohydrate molecule. Newer formulations of parenteral iron, such as ferric gluconate or carboxymaltose, that have a stronger iron-carbohydrate complex are available, and thus have lower side-effect risk profile.

VITAMIN C AND ANTIOXIDANTS

Ascorbic acid is an important antioxidant and enhancer of iron absorption. Physiologically, ascorbic acid is involved in reducing the chemical state of metal components in enzymatic reactions. Ascorbic acid leads to increased iron absorption through various mechanisms:

- Promotes an acidic environment in the stomach and intestine that helps to keep iron in a soluble form [59]
- Chelates ferric iron, which also helps to maintain iron's stability, even in high pH conditions [59]
- Reduces ferric iron to the ferrous form and helps to prevent iron from precipitating into ferric hydroxide [59]
- Antioxidant effect of ascorbic acid on iron absorption involves the duodenal cytochrome b enzyme located in the mucosal surface of enterocytes [60]

Foods in the citrus fruit group, peppers, and leafy green vegetables have the highest amounts of vitamin C. Biochemically alkalizing foods, such as citrus foods, that have an acidic pH level but still donate bicarbonate contain the highest amounts of vitamin C. For example, lemons are an alkalizing source of ascorbic acid and are acidic by pH, which can additionally enhance iron absorption. Canned fruit juices retain most of the vitamin C content from fresh fruit, but their ascorbic acid content decreases rapidly with exposure to air. Regarding infant intake of ascorbic acid, human breast milk contains four to six times as much vitamin C as cow's milk.

Both food sources and ascorbic acid supplements can improve iron absorption [61,62]. When eating a meal, complementary to iron absorption, ascorbic acid should be taken at the same time as iron tablets. Meals containing low to medium levels of iron inhibitors require the addition of ascorbic acid at a molar ratio of 2:1 (for example 20 mg ascorbic acid:3 mg iron). When a large amount of iron inhibitors are present in a meal, the effective molar ratio increases to 4:1.

In addition to absorption, ascorbic acid mobilizes iron tissue stores. Ascorbic acid is used in iron refractory iron deficiency anemia (IRIDA), a recessive genetic condition with excessively elevated hepcidin levels. Patients with IRIDA do not respond to oral iron pills, and only partially respond to parenteral iron therapy [63] due to restriction of iron into tissues. End-stage renal disease patients with hyperferratinemia and increased tissue iron also benefit from ascobic acid with increased hemoglobin levels after intravenous treatment [64,65]. A safe intravenous regimen of ascorbic acid for dialysis patients is 500 mg of ascorbic acid twice a week for eight weeks [66]. One possible side effect of intravenous ascorbic acid is extravascular deposition of oxalate, a concern for patients with a history of recurring calcium oxalate stones. To avoid oxalate deposition, treatment may be restricted to patients with serum vitamin C of less than 10 mcg/min [66].

Clinical situations in which decreased ascorbic acid absorption may occur are: an excessive intake of supplemental ascorbic acid, the presence of pectin or zinc in foods, or a high iron concentration in the intestinal tract [67]. In addition, *H. pylori* infections can decrease the gastrointestinal levels of ascorbate and therefore decrease iron absorption. Culinary factors that may decrease nutritional ascorbic acid levels are cooking with baking soda or with copper pans. Keeping foods away from sunlight and from refrigeration can help to maintain vitamin C levels. Also, an alkalizing diet enhances vitamin C status in part by decreasing the utilization of ascorbic acid.

Since eryptosis is responsive to the presence of oxidative stress, the antioxidant activity of ascorbic acid may also help to preserve the number of circulating erythrocytes. Other antioxidants, such as vitamin E, have also shown potential to help manage anemia through reduction in oxidative stress [68,69].

FOLATE

Folate, named from the Latin word for leaf (*folium*), is a water-soluble vitamin found in limited amounts in the body. Short periods of even one month of no folate intake or absorption can lead to significant deficiencies. Folate is involved in RNA and DNA synthesis in erythropoiesis. Folate functions as a carbon source in the formation of heme [70]. And, it is involved in the conversion of the byproduct, homocysteine, into the amino acid methionine intimately linking folate with vitamin B12.

Folate can be found in the natural form as a pteroylpolyglutamate and in the synthetic form as pteroylmonoglutamate. In its natural state, folate has to be hydrolyzed by an enzyme in the small intestinal brush border before it can be absorbed. This enzyme, folate hydrolase, can be inhibited by yeast, beans, and acidic pH levels. The synthetic form of folate, folic acid, does not require extensive digestion prior to absorption. In fact, due to bioavailability, folic acid supplements are preferred over folate food sources. When taken on an empty stomach or with food, folic acid is more bioavailable for absorption than folate from food [71].

Food sources of folate include legumes, leafy greens, citrus, broccoli, sprouts, sea vegetables, liver, and fermented dairy products. Many commercial fermented dairy products contain significant folate levels, especially if the cows are grass fed. Fermented yogurt has on average 100 μg/L of folate, while milk contains 20 μg/L [71]. During winter months, seasonal sources of folate include dried herbs such as spearmint, rosemary, basil, parsley, or chervil. Other dried sources include peanuts and sunflower seeds.

An important disadvantage with dietary folate is decreased bioavailability compared to folate in supplements. Dietary folate is also often lost during cooking as a result of thermal degradation and leaching into cooking water. One study assessing folate levels in broccoli and spinach after cooking found boiling significantly reduced levels [72], while steaming preserved precooking levels. Alternatively, there are concerns regarding use of supplemental folate of more than 1 mg/day due to increased risk of cancer, especially prostate cancer [73].

VITAMIN B12

Vitamin B12, also known as cobalamin, is a vital cofactor in many cellular functions, including providing available folate stores for DNA synthesis. Vitamin B12 is produced as a byproduct of bacterial metabolism. When obtained through meat sources, it is found in high quantities in liver, kidney, fish, and eggs. An alternative to meat sources for vitamin B12 is algae. The algae species, *Chlorella vulgaris* and *Anabaena cylindrical* contain 10–50 μgm of vitamin B12 per 100 g of dry weight. Some algae sources of vitamin B12 are contaminated with vitamin B12–producing bacteria or may have cobalamin analogues that may not be biologically active. Dietary supplements contain cobalamin in different forms: cyanocobalamin, hydroxycobalamin, adenosylcobalamin, and methylcobalamin. Cyanocobalamin is the most common oral form and requires activation to an active form. Methylcobalamin is the active form that is involved in the conversion of homocysteine to methionine.

Because vitamin B12, like folate, can be easily destroyed by heat and cooking processes, fortification of grains and flour with vitamin B12 has become a topic of interest. However, the effectiveness of food fortification with vitamin B12 needs to be determined since vitamin B12 deficiency can arise not only from a decreased amount but also from individual absorption problems [74]. Vitamin B12 deficiency can occur from the effects of the loss of the intrinsic factor needed for absorption (i.e., pernicious anemia), medications that interfere with absorption (i.e., metformin and orlistat), gastric bypass surgery, and inflammatory ileal disease (inflammatory bowel disease).

Hypochlorhydria from either pernicious anemia or medications is a clinical scenario that links both vitamin B12 deficiency and iron deficiency in some patients. Iron deficiency may occur in patients with pernicious anemia, and a low serum B12 level may also occur in iron deficiency anemia. The presence of a concomitant iron deficiency may retard the hematological response to B12 or folate therapy. Furthermore, vitamin B12 levels may also rise to normal on iron therapy alone [75].

PYROXIDINE (B6) AND RIBOFLAVIN (B2)

Vitamin B6 is involved in the synthesis of the heme molecule, making it an important vitamin for erythropoiesis. Deficiency of pyroxidine can occur in microcytic, normocytic, and sideroblastic anemia. Studies with acquired sideroblastic anemia have not shown marked improvements in ane-mia with pyroxidine supplementation; however, they have with inherited forms. In iron deficiency anemia, supplementation with vitamin B6 can lead to increased hemoglobin concentration com-pared to patients treated with iron alone [76]. In pregnant women, supplements of vitamin B6 were shown to improve anemia in women otherwise not responsive to iron supplementation [77]. Foods high in pyroxidine include brewer's yeast, sunflower seeds, and beef liver.

Like folate, vitamin B6 is needed for critical methylation required for the body's innate detoxi-fication pathway. Therefore, pyroxidine is involved in heavy metal detoxification that can help pre-vent anemia related to heavy metal exposure.

Riboflavin may help in the management of anemia through the ability to increase erythro-cyte B6 levels [78]. Iron levels may also increase in response to a riboflavin oxidase that aids in release of iron from ferritin stores [79]. Foods high in riboflavin include brewer's yeast, liver, and almonds. As a dietary source, riboflavin is best absorbed with food and in the presence of bile salts. Dietary sources exposed to excessive light may, however, lose significant riboflavin content.

VITAMIN A

Vitamin A is an important fat soluble vitamin. Also known as the metabolite form, retinoic acid, vitamin A acts as a hormone growth factor needed by epithelial and many other cells. It is known to stimulate erythropoietin expression [80]. It may also lead to increased iron mobilization from intracellular stores and increased bioavailability of dietary nonheme iron [81]. Vitamin A can also reverse the effect of iron absorption inhibitors such as polyphenols and phytates.

Supplementary vitamin A occurs in the form of palmitate, vitamin A acetate, or retinol palma-late in oral supplements. In dietary sources, vitamin A occurs either as retinol when absorbed from animal products or as carotene when absorbed from fruits and vegetables. Carotene is changed into the biologically active retinol. Of note, diabetes is a metabolic state where this conversion is impaired.

The carotenes are part of the carotenoid bioflavonoid family. Carotenes that function as vitamin A include alpha-carotene, beta-carotene, gamma-carotene, and xanthophyll beta-cryptoxanthin. Retinol absorbed from animal products occurs as a yellow fat-containing substance. However, vita-min A carotenes do not inherently contain fat and thus must be taken with 3–5 grams of fat for absorption. Foods that have been traditionally recommended for prevention or treatment of anemia, such as liver and spinach, are rich in both iron and vitamin A.

As a daily dose supplement, intermittent use dosing, or as a fortified food, vitamin A can increase iron and hemoglobin concentrations. Multiple studies in both children and pregnant women show vitamin A as effective in managing anemia. Some studies even suggest a synergystic relationship between iron and vitamin A when used in a micronutrient biscuit supplement [82]. The dietary use of red palm oil, which is rich in vitamin A, was also shown to significantly improve vitamin A levels and reduce prevalence of anemia in pregnant women [83].

COPPER

Copper is a trace element essential for iron utilization. Copper deficiency can lead to decreased iron available for erythropoiesis and to increased iron stores. Intake of copper through dietary sources and avoidance of dietary and environmental causes of copper deficiency is therefore important to help prevent iron deficiency. Apricots are a dietary source with high levels of copper, and tradition-ally they are used as a food to treat anemia. Other dietary sources of copper include liver, cauli-flower, kale, sesame seeds, and oysters. Excessive amounts of copper can compete with iron for absorption [24]. To help keep the system in balance, ascorbic acid, another iron enhancer, can help prevent excess copper levels by inhibiting copper absorption.

FERMENTED FOODS

Traditional cultures often use fermented foods as vehicles for important nutrients and minerals. Use of fermented foods may also be beneficial in the management of anemia for several reasons. Fermented foods contain high levels of organic acids that may enhance iron absorption through a weak chelating effect [59]. Fermentation methods and other traditional food processing methods, such as soaking and germinating, may also decrease phytate levels in foods and increase microbial production of B vitamins, such as folate [84]. In addition, fermented foods like kimchee or sauerkraut are rich, bioavailable sources of glutamine, an amino acid needed for healthy small intestine cell turnover. The presence of glutamine also helps to reduce gastrointestinal (GI) tract inflammation and cytokine response during digestion. Thus, glutamine from foods may be especially beneficial to anemic patients in order to avoid a cytokine response that may cause inappropriate or elevated hepcidin levels.

FATTY ACIDS AND LIPIDS

The essential fatty acids, omega-3 (linoelic acid) and omega-6 (linoic acid) are polyunsaturated fatty acids (PUFAs) needed for normal growth and development. Both omega-3 and omega-6 fatty acids use the same enzymes, desaturases (delta 5 and delta 6), to create their respective downstream elongated fatty acid derivatives. The desaturases are dependent on iron for enzymatic activity. This implies that there may be a deficiency in the higher order omega-3 fatty acid derivatives (EPA and DHA) and omega-6 derivatives (GLA). Experimental rat studies have shown a connection between iron deficiency and altered fatty acid metabolism. A strong connection between iron deficiency and the role of higher order PUFAs is still lacking. A cross-sectional study conducted of the Inuits, an indigenous population with iron deficiency, suggests the presence of a nutritional interaction between reduced iron intake and reduced omega-3 fatty acid synthesis. It could be reasoned that since desaturase activity relies on iron, omega-3 PUFAs would function best when iron is optimally available and hepcidin expression is lowest, such as at times of reduced inflammation.

Omega-3 intake may be important in the management of anemia in end-stage kidney disease. A study of dialysis patients using daily omega-3 acids with 1050 mg EPA and 690 mg DHA showed increased hemoglobin and decreased need for injection erythropoietin after eight weeks [85]. Omega-3 fatty acids may also decrease the number of crises and increase hemoglobin concentrations in sickle cell patients [86].

Omega-6 fats are the precursors of the proinflammatory eicosanoids. However, the omega-6 fatty acid gamma linolenic acid (GLA) is required in the synthesis of antiinflammatory prostaglandins. GLA synthesis is impaired by elevated blood glucose, excess omega-3 fatty acid intake, consumption of trans fats, and the depletion of metabolic cofactors. Hepcidin and eicosanoid production are both positively regulated by interleukin-6. However, to date there are no published studies on the interactions between eicosanoid levels and hepcidin levels or regulation of iron homeostasis.

Recommendations to maximize a patient's use of omega-3 for anemia include taking EPA and DHA sources that are independent of destaturase activity, avoiding possible vitamin A toxicity by excluding halibut or shark liver oils, and choosing brands with 1 to 2 mg of vitamin E to help prevent fatty acid oxidation [87]. Evening primrose oil, borage, and black currant oils are dietary sources of GLA, providing a source of this antiinflammatory fatty acid not affected by impaired destaurase activity in iron deficienct patients.

DIETARY AND SUPPLEMENT FACTORS CONTRIBUTING TO IRON DEFICIENCY

Calcium

Primarily, calcium decreases iron absorption by inhibiting the transfer of both heme and nonheme iron into mucosal cells. Calcium also can cause a decrease in iron absorption by interfering with the degradation of phytic acid [88]. When the amount of calcium in human milk was increased to that in cow's milk, iron absorption decreased to the same degree in both [89,90]. However, there may be a calcium interpendent inhibition of iron absorption in dairy, as milk proteins alone are inhibitory [91]. Studies of whole diets and studies conducted over several weeks tend to show no effect of increased calcium intake on iron absorption. In addition, experimental studies of calcium and iron status measures such as serum ferritin show no long-term effect of calcium supplementation on iron status [92]. Therefore, it is proposed that the inhibitory effect may be of short duration; there also may be compensatory mechanisms to circumvent calcium's inhibition on iron absorption [93].

Phytates and Flavonoids

As the primary storage compound of phosphorus in seeds, phytic acid provides a negatively charged phosphate that binds metallic cations such as calcium, iron, magnesium, potassium, manganese, and zinc. These elements are then rendered relatively unavailable for absorption. Iron absorption is inhibited when the phytic acid:metal ratio is increased above 10:1 [94].

It is possible to decrease phytic acid effects on iron. The inhibition on iron absorption can be overridden by foods such as oily fish [95] and fermented oats [96]. Phytates are found primarily in grains. Soaking and rinsing grains that contain phytic acid also plays a part in reducing the final

---

TABLE 9.4

A Treatment Approach for Patients with Anemia

Evaluate patient:
- Diagnose any potentially inherited, acute, or easily reversible causes of anemia (i.e., gastrointestinal blood loss)

If true iron deficiency present:
- Determine if related to decreased dietary intake, poor bioavailability from dietary inhibitors through complete dietary assessment
- Determine if oral versus parenteral iron replacement is needed
- Advise patient of important complementary foods to add to diet such as ascorbic acid, vitamin A, pyroxidine, riboflavin
- Encourage regular intake of foods that contain both iron and also enhancers of iron absorption, such as brewer's yeast, liver, and parsley

If anemia of inflammation (i.e., chronic disease related):
- Determine the role of chronic disease state and inflammation in determining the functional iron state
- Determine if oral versus parenteral iron replacement is needed. Advise patient of important complementary foods to add to diet
- Evaluate ferritin and transferrin receptor levels to determine functional iron status
- Recommend anti-inflammatory foods that may decrease gastrointestinal immune response and also complement iron absorption (i.e., traditional, fermented foods) and anti-inflammatory supplements (i.e., omega-3 fatty acids)

Evaluate for other deficient nutrients:
- Physical examination for clinical signs of vitamin deficiencies
- Check red blood cell folate, serum vitamin B12, methylmalonic acid levels
- Assess for medication and disease conditions affecting vitamin B12 absorption
- Encourage dietary sources of folate repletion including fermented foods; supplemental folate may be needed. For some patients, consider genetic testing for methylenetetrahydrofolate reductase (MTHFR) mutations before encouraging folate supplementation
- Advise patient of important complementary vitamins to add to diet or to take as supplements—ascorbic acid, vitamin A, pyroxidine, riboflavin
- Remember vitamin C to help absorption, mobilization of iron stores in presence of elevated hepcidin, end-stage renal disease; can help overcome inhibitory effect of phytates and flavonoids on iron absorption

Evaluate for foods and nutrients that can decrease inflammation and cellular toxicity:
- Recommend anti-inflammatory foods (i.e., traditional, fermented foods) and supplements (i.e. omega-3 fatty acids)
- Recommend algae, which contain vital nutrients to help with iron absorption, vitamin A carotenoids, ascorbic acid, vitamin B12, and detoxification support due to methyl content that can help with toxin-related anemia

amount of phytate present. In addition to a strong chelating effect on iron, phytic acid also can cause anemia through the ability to promote eryptosis [97].

Flavonoid polyphenols such as tannins in tea and coffee can also decrease iron bioavailability. The effect of tea tannins on iron absorption can be reduced by consuming tea between meals and by consuming iron absorptive enhancers when drinking tea [98]. Red wine and some legumes also contain iron-inhibiting tannin polyphenols that inhibit iron absorption [99,100]. The herbal medications and supplements saw palmetto, feverfew, nettle, and green tea contain tannins that inhibit iron absorption [100]. Nonpolyphenol flavonoids, such as rosemary extract, have also shown the ability to decrease nonheme iron bioavailability [101].

Flavonoids can lead to an increase in enterocyte uptake of iron and also inhibition of iron release from the enterocyte, resulting in increased enterocyte intracellular iron [102,103]. The inhibitory effect of flavonoids on enterocyte release of iron is offset, however, by the addition of ascorbic acid [104]. Ascorbic acid and flavonoids are usually found in the same foods. Limiting supplemental use of flavonoids among patients with anemia may therefore be prudent [99].

CLINICAL SUMMARY

During times of infection, or inflammatory or oxidative stress, iron regulation is downregulated, sometimes leading to anemia. Distinguishing between primary iron deficiency and anemia of inflammation is a clinical assessment that can guide not only iron supplementation but a broader range of food and nutrient approaches that can augment the management of anemia. One clinical approach is represented in Table 9.4.

REFERENCES

1. DeBenoist B, McLean E, Egli I, and Cogswell, M. "Worldwide prevalence of anemia in 1993–2005." WHO Global Database of Anemia, WHO, 2008.
2. Zarychanski R., Houston DS. "Anemia of chronic disease: A harmful disorder or an adaptive, beneficial response?" *CMAJ* 2008: 333–337.
3. Fulgoni VL III, Keast DR, Bailey Rl, Dweyer J. "Foods, forticants and supplements: Where do Americans get their nutrients?" *J Nutr*, 2011: 1847–1854.
4. Hallberg L. "Does calcium interfere with iron absorption?" *Am J Clin Nutr*, 1998: 3–4.
5. Fleming DJ. "Dietary determinants of iron stores in a free living elderly population." *Am J Clin Nutr*, 1998: 722–733.
6. Hinton PS, Giordano C, Brownlie T, Haas JD. "Iron supplementation improves endurance after training in iron-depleted non-anemic women." *J Appl Physiol*, 2000: 1103–1111.
7. Garrison R, Somer E. *Nutrition Desk Reference*. 3rd ed. New Canaan, CT: Keats Publishing, 1995, 204.
8. Stoltzfus RJ. "Iron deficiency anemia: Reexamining the nature and magnitude of the public health problem." *J Nutr*, 2001: 697S–700S.
9. Templeton, M. *Molecular and Cellular Iron Transport*. New York, NY: CRC Press, 2002.
10. Levy JE, Jin O, Fujiwara Y, Kuo F, Andrews NC. "Transferrin receptor is necessary for development of erythrocytes and the nervous system." *Nat Genet*, 1999: 396–399.
11. Kasper DL, Braunwald E, Fauci AS, Hauser SL, Longo DL, Jameson JL, Loscalzo J. *Harrison's Principles of Internal Medicine*. New York, NY: McGraw-Hill, 2008.
12. Quiqley, JG. "Identification of a heme exporter." *Cell*, 2004: 757–766.
13. Munoz M, Villar I, Garcia-Erce JA. "An update on iron physiology." *World J Gastroenterol*, 2009: 4617–4626.
14. Andrews, N. "Forging a field: The golden age of iron biology." *Blood*, 2008: 219–230.
15. Aspuru, K. "Optimal management of iron deficiency anemia due to poor dietary intake." *Int J of Gen Med*, 2011: 741–750.
16. Carpenter CE, Mahoney AW. "Contributions of heme and nonheme iron to human nutrition." *Critical Reviews in Food Science and Nutrition*, 1992: 333–367.
17. Krishnamurthy P, Xie T, Schuetz JD. "The role of transporters in cellular heme and porphyrin homeostasis." *Pharmacology and Therapeutics*, 2007: 345–358.

18. Bohn L, Meyer AS, Rasmussen SK. "Phytate: Impact on environment and human nutrition. A challenge for molecular breeding." *Journal of Zhejiang University,* 2008: 165–191.

19. Shawki A, Mackenzie B. "Interaction of calcium with the human divalent metal-ion transporter-1." *Biochem Biophys Res Commun,* 2010: 471–475.

20. Krijt J, Vokurka M, Sefc L, Duricová D, Necas E. "Effect of lipopolysaccharide and bleeding on the expression of intestinal proteins involved in iron and haem transport." *Folia Biol,* 2006: 1–5.

21. Tselepis C. "Characterization of the transition-metal binding properties of hepcidin." *Biochem J,* 2010: 289–296.

22. Quarles CD, Marcus RK, Brumaghim JL. "Competitive binding of Fe^{3+}, Cr^{3+}, and Ni^{2+} to transferrrin." *J Biol Inorg Chem,* 2011: 913–921.

23. Anderson RA. "Chromium in the prevention and control of diabetes." *Diabetes Metab,* 2000: 22–27.

24. Watts DL. "The nutritional relationships of iron." *Journal of Orthomolecular Medicine,* 1988: 110–116.

25. Weinberg, ED. "Iron depletion: A defense against intracellular infection and neoplasia." *Life Sci,* 1992: 50:1289–1297.

26. Sengoelge G, et al. "Potential risk for infection and atherosclerosis due to iron therapy." *J Ren Nutr,* 2005: 105–110.

27. Sullivan JL. "Iron and the sex difference in heart disease risk." *The Lancet,* 1981: 1293.

28. Fleming RE, Sly WS. "Hepcidin: A putative iron-regulatory hormone relevant to hereditary hemochromatosis and the anemia of chronic disease." *Proc Natl Acad Sci USA,* 2001: 8160–8162.

29. Ganz, T. "Hepcidin, a key regulator of iron metabolism and mediator of anemia of inflammation." *Blood,* 2003: 783–788.

30. Nemeth E, Ganz T. "The role of hepcidin in iron metabolism." *Acta Haematol,* 2009: 78–86.

31. Nemeth E, Valore EV, Territo M, Schiller G, et al. "Hepcidin, a putative mediator of anemia of inflammation, is a type II acute phase protein." *Blood,* 2003: 24613.

32. Wrighting DM, Andrews NC. "Interleukin-6 induces hepcidin expression through STAT3." 2006.

33. Finberg KE. "Unraveling mechanisms regulating systemic iron homeostasis." *Hematology Am Soc Hematol Educ Program,* 2011: 532–537.

34. Weinberg ED. "Iron loading: A risk factor for osteoporosis." *Biometals,* 2006: 633–635.

35. Allen LH, Rosenberg IH, Oakley GP, Omenn GS. "Considering the case for vitamin B12 fortification of flour." *Food Nutr Bull,* 2010: S36–46.

36. Arnold J, Busbridge M, Sangwaiya A, Bhatkal B, et al. "Prohepcidin levels in refractory anemia caused by lead poisoning." *Case Rep Gastroenterol,* 2008: 49–54.

37. Ganz T, Nemeth E. "Hepcidin and disorders of iron metabolism." *Annu Rev Med,* 2011: 347–360.

38. Kroot JJ, Laarakkers CM, Kemna EH, Biemond BJ, Swinkels DW. "Regulation of serum hepcidin levels in sickle cell anemia." *Haematologica,* 2009: 885–887.

39. Cooper SH, Zlotkin MJ. "Day-to-day variation of transferrin receptor and ferritin in healthy men and women." *Am J Clin Nutr,* 1996: 738–742.

40. Parischa SR, McQuitten Z, Westerman M, Keller A, et al. "Serum hepcidin as a diagnostic test of iron deficiency in premenopausal female blood donors." *Haematologica,* 2011: 1099–1105.

41. Papillard-Marechal S, Sznajder M, Hurtado-Nedelec M, Alibay Y, et al. "Iron metabolism in patients with anorexia nervosa: Elevated serum hepcidin concentrations in absence of inflammation." *Am J Clin Nutr,* 2012: 548–554.

42. Takasu J, Uykimpang R, Sunga MA, Amagase H, et al. "Aged garlic extract is a potential therapy for sickle-cell anemia." *J Nutr,* 2006: 803S–805S.

43. Ohnishi ST, Ohnishi T. "In vitro effects of aged garlic extract and other nutritional supplements on sickle erythrocytes." *J Nutr,* 2001: 1085S–92S.

44. Reed JD, Redding-Lallinger R, Orringer EP. Nutrition and sickle cell disease. *Am J Hematol,* 1987: 441–455.

45. Fairweather-Tait S, Lynch S, Hotz C, Hurrell R, et al. "The usefulness of in vitro models to predict the bioavailability of iron and zinc: A consensus statement from the HarvestPlus expert consultation." *Int J Vitam Nutr Res,* 2005: 371–374.

46. Lowe, B. *Experimental Cookery.* New York, NY: Wiley & Sons, 1937.

47. Adish AA, Esrey SA, Gyorkos TW, Jean-Baptiste J, Rojhani A. "Effect of consumption of food cooked in iron pots on iron status and growth of young children: A randomised trial." *Lancet,* 1999: 712–716.

48. McGee, H. *On Food and Cooking.* New York, NY: Scribner, 2004.

49. Roughead ZK, Hunt JR. "Adaptation in iron absorption: Iron supplementation reduces nonheme-iron but not heme-iron absorption from food." *Am J Clin Nutr,* 2000: 982–989.

50. Allen, LH. "Iron supplements: Scientific issues concerning efficacy and implications for research and programs." *J Nutr,* 2002: 813S–819S.

51. Rimon E, Kagansky N, Kagansky M, Mechnick L, Mashiah T, Namir M, Levy S. "Are we giving too much iron? Low-dose iron therapy is effective in octogenarians." *Am J Med*, 2005: 1142–1147.

52. Fernández-Gaxiola AC, De-Regil LM. "Intermittent iron supplementation for reducing anemia and its associated impairments in menstruating women." *Cochrane Database Syst Rev*, 2011: CD009218.

53. Bilenko N, Belmaker I, Vardi H, Fraser D. "Efficacy of multiple micronutrient supplementations on child health: Study design and baseline characteristics." *Israel Medical Assoc Journal*, 2010: 342–347.

54. Lung'aho MG, Glahn RP. "Micronutrient sprinkles add more bioavailable iron to some Kenyan complementary foods: Studies using an in vitro digestion/Caco-2 cell culture model." *Matern Child Nutr*, 2009: 151–158.

55. Adu-Afarwuah S, Lartey A, Brown KH, Zlotkin S, Briend A, Dewey KG. "Home fortification of complementary foods with micronutrient supplements is well accepted and has positive effects on infant iron status in Ghana." *AM J Clin Nutr*, 2008: 929–938.

56. Menon P, Ruel MT, Loechl CU, Arimond M, Habicht JP, Pelto G, Michaud L. "Micronutrient sprinkles reduce anemia among 9- to 24-mo-old children when delivered through an integrated health and nutrition program in rural Haiti." *J Nutr*, 2007: 1023–1030.

57. Bayraktar UD, Bayraktar S. "Treatment of iron deficiency anemia associated with gastrointestinal tract diseases." *World J Gastro*, 2010: 2720–2725.

58. Hershko C, Skikne B. "Pathogenesis and management of iron deficiency anemia: Emerging role of celiac disease, helicobacter pylori, and autoimmune gastritis." *Semin Hematol*, 2009: 339–350.

59. Teucher B, Olivares M, Cori H. "Enhancers of iron absorption: Ascorbic acid and other organic acids." *Int J Vit Nutr Res*, 2004: 403–419.

60. Lane DJ, Lawen A. "Ascorbate and plasma membrane electron transport—enzymes vs efflux." *Free Rad Biol Med*, 2009: 485–495.

61. Balay KS, Hawthorne KM, Hicks PD, Griffin IJ, Chen Z, Westerman M, Abrams SA. "Orange but not apple juice enhances ferrous fumarate absorption in small children." *J Ped Gastroenterol Nutr*, 2010: 545–550.

62. Lundqvist H, Sjöberg F. "Food interaction of oral uptake of iron/a clinical trial using 59Fe." *Arzneimittelforschung*, 2007: 401–416.

63. Cau M, Galanello R, Giagu N, Melis MA. "Responsiveness to oral iron and ascorbic acid in a patient with IRIDA." *Blood Cells Mol Dis*, 2012: 121–123.

64. Einerson B, Nathorn C, Kitiyakara C, Sirada M, Thamlikitkul V. "The efficacy of ascorbic acid in suboptimal responsive anemic hemodialysis patients receiving erythropoietin: A meta-analysis." *J Med Assoc Thai*, 2011: S134–S146.

65. Deved V, Poyah P, James MT, Tonelli M, Manns BJ, Walsh M, Hemmelgarn BR, Alberta Kidney Disease Network. "Ascorbic acid for anemia management in hemodialysis patients: A systematic review and meta-analysis." *Am J Kid Dis*, 2009: 1089–1097.

66. Sezer S, Ozdemir FN, Yakupoglu U, Arat Z, Turan M, Haberal M. "Intravenous ascorbic acid administration for erythropoietin-hyporesponsive anemia in iron loaded hemodialysis patients." *Artif Organs*, 2002: 366–370.

67. Gropper SA, Smith JL, Groff JL. *Advanced Nutrition and Human Metabolism*, 2005: 268–269.

68. Tesoriere L, D'Arpa D, Butera D, Allegra M, Renda D, Maggio A, Bongiorno A, Livrea MA. "Oral supplements of vitamin E improve measures of oxidative stress in plasma and reduce oxidative damage to LDL and erythrocytes." *Free Rad Res*, 2001: 529–540.

69. Winklhofer-Roob BM, Rock E, Ribalta J, Shmerling DH, Roob JM. "Effects of vitamin E and carotenoid status on oxidative stress in health and disease." *Mol Aspects Med*, 2003: 391–402.

70. Hoffbrand AV, Herbert V. Nutritional anemias. *Semin Hematol*, 1999: 13–23.

71. Iyer R, Tomar SK. "Folate: A functional food constituent." *J Food Sci*, 2009: R114–122.

72. McKillop DJ, Pentieva K, Daly D, McPartlin JM, Hughes J, Strain JJ, Scott JM, McNulty H. "The effect of different cooking methods on folate retention in various foods that are amongst the major contributors to folate intake in the UK diet." *Br J Nutr*, 2002: 681–688.

73. Wien TN, Pike E, Wisløff T, Staff A, et al. "Cancer risk with folic acid supplements: A systematic review and meta-analysis." *BMJ Open*, 2012: e000653.

74. Green R. "Is it time for vitamin B-12 fortification? What are the questions?" *Am J Clin Nutr*, 2009: 712S–716S.

75. Chanarin I. *The Megalobastic Anemias*. Oxford: Blackwell Sciences, 1979.

76. Reinken L, Kurz R. "Activity studies of an iron-vitamin B6 preparation for euteral treatment of iron deficiency anemia." *Int J Vitam Nutr Res*, 1975: 411–418.

77. Hisano M, Suzuki R, Sago H, Murashima A, Yamaguchi K. "Vitamin B6 deficiency and anemia in pregnancy." *Eur J Clin Nutr*, 2010: 221–223.

78. Perry GM. "The effect of riboflavin on red cell vitamin B6 metabolism and globin synthesis." *Biomedicine*, 1980: 36–38.

79. Fishman SM, Christian P, West KP. "The role of vitamins in the prevention and control of anemia." *Pub Health Nutr*, 2000: 125–150.

80. Evans T. "Regulation of hematopoiesis by retinoid signaling." *Exp Hematol*, 2005: 1055–1061.

81. Zimmermann MB, Biebinger R, Rohner F, Dib A, Zeder C, Hurrell RF, Chaouki N. "Vitamin A supplementation in children with poor vitamin A and iron status increases erythropoietin and hemoglobin concentrations without changing total body iron." *Am J Clin Nutr*, 2006: 580–586.

82. Hieu NT, Sandalinas F, de Sesmaisons A, Laillou A, Tam NP, Khan NC, Bruyeron O, Wieringa FT, Berger J. "Multi-micronutrient-fortified biscuits decreased the prevalence of anaemia and improved iron status, whereas weekly iron supplementation only improved iron status in Vietnamese school children." *Br J Nutr*, 2012: 109.

83. Radhika MS, Bhaskaram P, Balakrishna N, Ramalakshmi BA. "Red palm oil supplementation: A feasible diet-based approach to improve the vitamin A status of pregnant women and their infants." *Food Nutr Bull*, 2003: 208–217.

84. Sandberg AS. "Bioavailability of minerals in legumes." *Br J Nutr*, 2002: S281–285.

85. Jones WL, Kaiser SP. "Pilot study: An emulsified fish oil supplement significantly improved C-reactive protein, hemoglobin, albumin and urine output in chronic hemodialysis volunteers." *J Am Nutr Assoc*, 2010: 45–50.

86. Okpala I, Ibegbulam O, Duru A, Ocheni S, et al. "Pilot study of omega-3 fatty acid supplements in sickle cell disease." *APMIS*, 2011: 442–448.

87. Vergili-Nelsen JM. "Benefits of fish oil supplementation for hemodialysis patients." *J Am Diet Assoc*, 2003: 1174–1177.

88. Food and Nutrition Board, Institute of Medicine. *Dietary Reference Intakes for Vitamin A, Vitamin K, Arsenic, Boron, Chromium, Copper, Iodine, Iron, Manganese, Molybdenum, Nickel, Silicon, Vanadium, and Zinc in Iron.* Washington, DC: National Academies Press, 2000.

89. Hallberg L, Hulthén L, Garby L. "Iron stores in man in relation to diet and iron requirements." *Eur J Clin Nutr*, 1998: 623–631.

90. Hallberg L, Rossander-Hultén L, Brune M, Gleerup A. "Bioavailability in man of iron in human milk and cow's milk in relation to their calcium contents." *Pediatr Res*, 1992: 524–527.

91. Hurrell RF, Lynch SR, Trinidad TP, Dassenko SA, Cook JD. "Iron absorption in humans as influenced by bovine milk proteins." *Am J Clin Nutr*, 1989: 546–552.

92. Harris SS. "The effect of calcium consumption on iron absorption and iron status." *Nutr Clin Care*, 2002: 231–235.

93. Lönnerdal B. "Calcium and iron absorption—Mechanisms and public health relevance." *Int J Vitam Nutr Res.*, 2010: 293–299.

94. Gharib AG, Mohseni SG, Mohajer M, Gharib M. "Bioavailability of essential trace elements in the presence of phytate, fiber and calcium." *J Rad Nucl Chem*, 2006: 209–215.

95. Navas-Carretero S, Pérez-Granados AM, Sarriá B, Carbajal A, et al. "Oily fish increases iron bioavailability of a phytate rich meal in young iron deficient women." *J Am Coll Nutr*, 2008: 96–101.

96. Bering S, Suchdev S, Sjøltov L, Berggren A, et al. "A lactic acid-fermented oat gruel increases nonheme iron absorption from a phytate rich meal in healthy women of childbearing age." *Br J Nutr*, 2006: 80–85.

97. Eberhard M, Foller M, Lang F. "Effect of phytic acid on suicidal erythrocyte death." *J Agric Food Chem*, 2010: 2028–2033.

98. Zijp IM, Korver O, Tijburg LB. "Effect of tea and other dietary factors on iron absorption." *Crit Rev Food Sci Nutr*, 2000: 371–398.

99. Egert S, Rimbach G. "Which sources of flavonoids: complex diets or dietary supplements?" *Adv Nutr*, 2011: 8–14.

100. De Smet PA. "Herbal remedies." *N Engl J Med*, 2002: 2046–2056.

101. Samman S, Sandström B, Toft MB, Bukhave K, Jensen M, Sørensen SS, Hansen M. "Green tea or rosemary extract added to foods reduces nonheme-iron absorption." *Am J Clin Nutr*, 2001: 607–612.

102. Ma Q, Kim EY, Han O. "Bioactive dietary polyphenols decrease heme iron absorption by decreasing basolateral iron release in human intestinal Caco-2 cells." *J Nutr*, 2010: 1117–1121.

103. Vlachodimitropoulou E, Naftalin RJ, Sharp PA. "Quercetin is a substrate for the transmembrane oxidoreductase Dcytb." *Free Radic Biol Med*, 2010: 1366–1369.

104. Kim EY, Ham SK, Bradke D, Ma Q, Han O. "Ascorbic acid offsets the inhibitory effect of bioactive dietary polyphenolic compounds on transepithelial iron transport in Caco-2 intestinal cells." *J Nutr*, 2011: 828–834.

10 Asthma

Nutrient Strategies in Improving Management

Kenneth Bock, M.D., and Michael Compain, M.D.

INTRODUCTION

Asthma is a well-characterized immune response that targets the lung. Our understanding of the condition has evolved from the simple manifestations of airway reactivity with cough, wheezing, and shortness of breath to the present awareness of asthma as one of a growing number of inflammatory conditions that are at the interface of genetics and environmental influences.

Although primary care physicians have a full array of pharmacological therapies available in a classic step-care structure, these treatments of course have their attendant side effects. Fortunately, there is now a solid body of basic and clinical research showing how nutritional and environmental factors can either trigger asthma or be used to modify and treat it. This chapter presents nonpharmacological interventions that can be both preventive and therapeutic.

EPIDEMIOLOGY

There are an estimated 300 million people with asthma, and the geographic distribution is not uniform [1]. As with other immune and allergic disorders, asthma is on the rise. Between 1981 and 2002, asthma prevalence in US children increased from 3% to approximately 6% [2]. Over the past several decades, an association has been found between the increase in allergy and asthma and the spread of a Western lifestyle [3]. This has often been attributed to environmental pollution, but there may be other factors involved, such as the degradation of nutritional quality in the food supply of industrialized nations [4], or diminished vitamin D levels due to decreased sun exposure. Furthermore, there are questions being raised about the effect of early life environmental influences such as exposure to microorganisms on immune development in industrialized societies.

Air quality is a major contributing factor. In addition to the known inhalant allergens such as dust mites, mold, and cockroach antigens, there are well-established associations with indoor pollutants such as cigarette smoke [5–7]. Although there is not clear evidence that outdoor pollution is causing an increase in prevalence, it is documented that compounds such as sulfur dioxide [8], ozone [9], and particulates exacerbate asthma. This certainly suggests that these pollutants are at least partly responsible for the increased prevalence in urban areas [10–11]. The effect of pollutants also raises the issue of oxidative stress in genetically susceptible individuals, which may have therapeutic implications [12]. Investigation is also taking place regarding other genetic factors that may play a role in the way people with asthma respond to pollutants [13]. Furthermore, there is speculation as to whether environmental immunotoxins such as heavy metals might contribute to the increased prevalence of atopic disease [14].

PATHOPHYSIOLOGY

The rapid expansion of our understanding of immunology has revealed insights into the genesis of allergic phenomena in general and asthma in particular. This is particularly relevant to issues regarding immune tolerance.

The pathophysiology of airway inflammation has been known for many years, with the role of IgE, eosinophils and mast cells established. These effectors are in turn known to be directed by proinflammatory cytokines such as IL-4, IL-5, IL-9, and IL-13, which are elaborated by TH_2 lymphocytes.

Until recently it was felt that the TH_2 lymphocytes were involved in a dance of mutual regulation/inhibition with TH_1 lymphocytes [15]. It now appears more likely that some other group of T cells, called regulatory T (Treg) cells, elaborate cytokines such as IL-10 and transforming growth factor beta (TGFB) to modulate the activity of effector T cells. Regulatory T cells themselves are subject to many influences. Vitamin D, for example, has been shown to promote Treg cells [16,17], and vitamin D deficiency has been proposed as one of the causes of the increased prevalence of asthma [18]. Allergy and asthma appear to represent situations where Treg control of TH_2 cells is loosened [19,20].

But what messages do the regulatory T cells receive that cause them to direct a response of immune tolerance versus one of reactivity? This is the central question that underpins the development of allergic responses such as asthma.

The hygiene hypothesis was proposed to explain a body of epidemiologic evidence [3] that indicates that atopic and autoimmune conditions are more common in industrialized societies. It was found that the presence of older siblings and early daycare were associated with reduced incidence of later wheezing and atopy [21,22]. Furthermore, there are studies showing that children who live on farms or have early exposure to animals have reduced risk of developing allergy [23]. The increased exposure to antibiotics in industrialized societies, both therapeutically and in the food supply, has a negative effect on intestinal flora. In fact, a variety of studies have demonstrated that childhood use of antibiotics is indeed associated with increased risk of later development of asthma and allergy [24–26]. These data are consistent with our growing appreciation of how early exposure to commensal organisms is essential for developing immune tolerance.

Species of healthful bacteria that inoculate the intestinal tract early in life secrete lipopolysaccharides, which interact with toll-like receptors on dendritic and epithelial cells at the GI mucosa. This leads to cell signaling, which stimulates regulatory T cells to elaborate IL-10 and TGFB, keeping the effector T cells (TH_1 and TH_2) in check. The result is an immune response of either tolerance or appropriate inflammation when the gut-associated lymphoid tissue (GALT) is exposed to other antigens. The GALT is estimated to represent 65% of our immune tissue and therefore holds sway over immune responses throughout the body. In sum, the intestinal immune system not only tolerates healthful bacteria but requires them for its early education and long-term immune regulation. There is even evidence that gastric presence of *Helicobacter pylori* is associated with a 30% to 50% reduction of asthma incidence [27,28]. Therefore, when these toll-receptor ligands are absent or depleted by antibiotics early in life, the result is immune dysregulation and inflammatory disorders such as asthma and allergy. Recent evidence suggests an increased incidence of genetic polymorphisms involving the function of toll receptors themselves in individuals with asthma [29].

The gut flora has a significant effect on intestinal permeability. Increased intestinal permeability is commonly present in atopic diseases [30] and may cause sensitization to a larger number of antigens that then have access to the GALT. Therapeutic agents such as steroids can increase permeability further [31], so that short-term benefit may come at the price of further sensitization.

Nonsteroidal anti-inflammatory drugs (NSAIDs) also increase intestinal permeability. The use of probiotics has been shown to reduce permeability in atopic individuals [32].

Oxidative stress is another aspect of the inflammatory process that may offer therapeutic opportunities in asthma. In addition to environmental oxidants, which may trigger lung injury, the inflammatory process itself generates free radicals. A number of studies have shown that people with asthma have a higher incidence of genetic polymorphisms for glutathione S-transferase activity, which would make them more susceptible to oxidative stress [33,34]. Levels of antioxidants such as vitamin C, carotenoids, and selenium have also been found to be lower in people with asthma than in controls [35–37].

NUTRITIONAL THERAPIES

There have been numerous epidemiological and interventional studies to explore the use of diet and nutrients in the treatment of asthma, although the studies are generally smaller and have less statistical power than those in the literature supporting conventional pharmacological therapies.

One area of investigation has been the role of foods as triggers. Although the incidence of classic IgE food allergy is relatively low [38], there is evidence of IgG-mediated food sensitivity and food intolerances leading to increased airway reactivity in a higher percentage of patients [39–41]. Given the fact that food allergies are poorly understood and frequently undiagnosed, an elimination diet can be used for both diagnosis and treatment [38,42,43]. Food allergies may be especially important in asthma that flares randomly and seems unrelated to inhaled triggers.

Another potential source of dietary impact on asthma is that of food additives [44–46]. This has been reviewed extensively in the case of wine reactions in asthma. Although it was formerly felt that sulfites were largely responsible, there is now more controversy regarding the incidence as well as the cause of this phenomenon [47,48]. In either case, wine sensitivity is frequently reported by people with asthma. A diet trial without additives may be of benefit in some patients, and commercially available food and wine products are now offered sulfite free.

There is evidence that increased fish consumption has been associated with lowered risk [49,50], which may be due to the anti-inflammatory effect of omega-3 oils or a relative decrease in the intake of proinflammatory arachidonic acid from meat and poultry. Increased seafood consumption might also provide more vitamin D or micronutrients, such as selenium or iodine. Due to their high mercury content, however, large fish such as tuna, shark, and swordfish should generally be avoided. Although mercury has not been directly tied to asthma, it promotes oxidative stress and TH_2 skewing of immune function, which one would expect to be deleterious in those with asthma.

There is also an association between asthma and obesity. Obese individuals and those with asthma seem to have polymorphisms for receptors that are significant in both inflammation and asthma [51]. Leptin has been shown to increase airway reactivity in animal studies [52], and adipokines from fat cells are known to foster inflammation. Obesity has an obvious restrictive effect on lung function, and conversely, asthma can often impede an exercise and conditioning program. Furthermore, the frequent use of corticosteroids will promote obesity. Together, these factors can generate a number of vicious cycles in those with severe asthma.

The role of micronutrients in the diet has been studied more extensively. As noted earlier, there is strong epidemiologic literature showing the inverse association between antioxidant levels and asthma activity [53–55]. This has led to the proposition that the decline in antioxidant content in the highly processed Western diet is partly responsible for the prevalence trends. Therefore it would seem prudent to advise people with asthma to increase their intake of colored fruits and vegetables in order to raise antioxidant capacity.

Other micronutrient and trace elements such as selenium [56] and manganese [57] have also been found to be at reduced levels in people with asthma. The data on magnesium are mixed. In addition to the extensive literature on the therapeutic use of magnesium, there remains the question of whether there is an actual magnesium deficiency in patients with asthma, and the studies point in both directions [58–62]. A diet high in nuts, seeds, and leafy green vegetables to provide magnesium seems prudent.

Magnesium has been shown to be a bronchodilator in vitro [63] and in vivo [64]. Interventional studies with magnesium deal extensively with the use of intravenous magnesium in the acute setting, and they have shown it to be effective [65,66]. There is less clarity about the use of oral magnesium in the treatment of chronic asthma, with some studies supporting its use [67,68] and others not [69]. Since this cation is very safe in those with adequate renal function, one practical approach might be to check a red blood cell magnesium level and supplement those who are deficient or low normal. Measuring serum selenium levels and supplementing in doses up to 200 μg might also be considered. Zinc is another nutrient found to be at reduced levels in asthmatics, and there is evidence that zinc deficiency creates a cytokine environment conducive to asthma [70]. Zinc deficiency may decrease the activity of delta-6-desaturase, which is an important enzyme in the metabolism of essential fatty acids.

Vitamin B6 has been shown to have an inhibitory effect on inflammatory mediators such as thromboxanes and leukotrienes [71]. Among its many physiologic functions, vitamin B6 is important in trytophan metabolism, which may be abnormal in patients with asthma [72], a population found to be low in vitamin B6 [73]. Small studies have shown clinical improvement with vitamin B6 supplementation in the dosage range of 100 to 200 mg/day [74].

Vitamin E has been less well studied as a therapeutic agent, but there has been an association noted between reduced intake history and increased presence of asthma [75]. In addition, one prospective diet study showed reduced asthma incidence with higher dietary vitamin E consumption [76]. Vitamin E obtained from the diet is a mixture of alpha-, beta-, delta-, and gamma-tocopherols and the corresponding tocotrienols. Vitamin E from supplements tends to be only alpha-tocopherol. Clinical trials should be evaluated for the type of vitamin E used. Presently there are select vitamin E supplements that contain the full spectrum of tocopherols and tocotrienols, similar to the vitamin E obtained from diet. Additionally, antioxidant nutrients work well in groups, so using vitamin E in conjunction with vitamin C, selenium, carotenoids, and flavonoids might offer further benefit. Vitamin C alone has been studied with some positive results [77].

Diverse dietary polyphenolic compounds can mediate antioxidant reactions. One recently studied compound is an extract of pine bark called pycnogenol. Two controlled trials [78,79] of this agent have shown significant benefit with a dose of about 2 mg/kg body weight per day up to 200 mg. Lycopene, an antioxidant that confers the red color to tomatoes, guava, and pink grapefruit, has also been found beneficial [80]. Another class of nutrients that has been used in supplemental form is flavonoids such as quercetin [81]. This compound has been shown to down regulate the inflammatory contribution of mast cells [82,83], as well as the expression of cytokines in bronchial epithelium [84]. It has also been shown in vitro to induce gene expression of TH_1 cytokines in monocytes and to inhibit the TH_2 cytokine IL-4 [85]. Quercetin has been employed therapeutically in a dose range of 1 to 2 g/day, but well-controlled studies have not been performed. The herb *Euphorbia stenoclada* has been used traditionally in the treatment of asthma, and it appears that quercetin may be the major active ingredient [86,87].

The role of prostanoids and leukotrienes in the inflammatory response of asthma is well documented [88,89] and was exploited in the development of drugs such as the montelukasts. Because essential fatty acids are integral in the genesis of leukotrienes, they present logical therapeutic options. Eicosapentaenoic acid (EPA), an omega-3 fatty acid from fish oil, produces the anti-inflammatory series 3 prostanoids (PGE3), and gamma-linoleic acid (GLA) from borage and primrose oil generates the anti-inflammatory series 1 prostanoids (PGE1). Although GLA is an omega-6 essential fatty acid (EFA), the anti-inflammatory series 1 compounds are distinct from the proinflammatory series 2 (PGE2) that arise from arachadonic acid. The literature in the therapeutic use of supplemental EFAs is not as rich or convincing in asthma as it is in other inflammatory conditions, such as rheumatoid arthritis and inflammatory bowel disease. Epidemiologic dietary exposure studies have been positive [90–92], and a number of supplementation trials with

EPA have been positive as well [93–96], but negative results have also been obtained [97–99]. It is important to note that compared to the micronutrients and antioxidants discussed earlier, EFAs have to be supplemented with some caution. In the dose range of 1 to 3 g, which was used in the clinical trials, one must consider the mild negative effect on coagulation as well as occasional gastrointestinal tolerability issues. Clinical benefit has also been shown in a small study using 10 to 20 g/day of perilla seed oil, which is high in the precursor compound alpha-linolenic acid [100].

Adequate hydration is essential in asthma management. Water intake is important as is the adequacy of intracellular cations.

Propolis from bees has been studied in asthma [101]. In addition to the herbal extract of *Euphorbia stenoclada*, *Gnaphalium liebmannii* [102], gingko [103], and *Tylopohera indica* have also been studied as potential adjunct treatments for asthma [104].

Results of nutritional therapies can be augmented with relaxation techniques shown to improve lung function and reduce medication use [105,106]. Studies of acupuncture have shown some improvement but not in measures of lung function [107–109].

PATIENT EVALUATION

The concept of asthma as a completely reversible condition has long been supplanted by the knowledge that active airway inflammation leads to tissue damage and chronic changes. Early and aggressive treatment is therefore essential.

The diagnosis of asthma is usually straightforward and easily established by the primary care physician on clinical grounds and pulmonary function testing. One caveat is that the contribution of factors such as GERD may be more difficult to determine. Findings on history and physical exam may also, however, indicate the presence of coexisting nutritional factors that may influence the development and severity of a patient's asthma. The elements of a medical history suggesting common inhalant triggers such as dust, mold, and pollens should of course be obtained, but the discussion here focuses on the nutritional aspects.

A dietary history can be very revealing and can be obtained with a food diary. Foods that are eaten most frequently may in fact cause sensitization and are usually removed in elimination diets. In our clinical experience, removal of food triggers can be every bit as effective in treatment as environmental controls for dust and mold. In addition, a dietary history can reveal the degree of additives, preservatives, and sulfites consumed as well as the sufficiency of micronutrients discussed earlier.

Certain symptoms are often considered by nutritionally oriented practitioners to reflect possible food sensitivity. This especially includes postprandial symptoms such as dermal or oral pruritis, fatigue, gas, or bloating. Urticaria and recurrent apthous ulcers may raise the suspicion of food triggers. Certainly any symptom that the patient connects to a particular food should be considered.

Regarding micronutrients, one may also get clues from the history. Magnesium deficiency should be suspected in those with symptoms such as muscle cramps or twitches or a tendency toward constipation. Poor wound healing and frequent infections might suggest zinc deficiency.

Physical examination may reveal infra-orbital darkening sometimes referred to as allergic shiners. Oral thrush may indicate an imbalance of gastrointestinal flora and apthous ulcers may be present. Eczema in an atopic distribution of antecubital and popliteal regions might cause one to suspect food triggers. Dry skin or follicular hyperkeratosis identified as roughness over the triceps region can represent an imbalance of essential fatty acids.

Laboratory evaluation may be helpful as well. Most commercial labs can run assays for erythrocyte magnesium, serum selenium, and plasma zinc. Measuring 25-hydroxyvitamin D is becoming common practice for a variety of reasons and should be checked in those with asthma. Several diagnostic techniques are available to assay food reactivities and they can buttress diagnostic use of an elimination diet.

DRUG–NUTRIENT INTERACTIONS

The nutritional agents used in asthma therapy do not seem to adversely impact pharmacologic agents, outside of the concern that imbalances from higher dosing of essential fatty acids can influence coagulation. Nutritional agents can have a medication-sparing effect. Asthma medications as well as medications for other conditions discussed in this text may need to be adjusted downward.

The major conventional agents used in asthma treatment that can impact nutritional and immune function adversely are corticosteroids. This is becoming more important given the increasing emphasis on these anti-inflammatory, "asthma controller" medications from clinical guidelines. The FDA issued a clear warning against using long-acting beta agonists (LABAs) without concurrent use of steroid medications [110].

As discussed earlier, steroids can cause negative physiologic effects by virtue of weight gain and increased intestinal permeability. These agents often have a deleterious effect on gut flora, which might lead to immune dysregulation. This effect could presumably be mitigated by use of probiotics, and permeability can improve with gut healing agents such as glutamine and zinc.

There are certain classes of medications that are not used to treat asthma per se but negatively impact some of the nutrient levels discussed here:

- Diuretics: magnesium depletion, dehydration
- Oral contraceptives: diminished vitamin B6
- NSAIDs: increased intestinal permeability
- Antibiotics: disturbance of gut flora (dysbiosis)

SPECIAL CONSIDERATIONS

In light of the previous discussion regarding pathophysiology, a word should be said about the concept of asthma prevention. Since primary care physicians are obviously caring for women of child-bearing age as well as for young children, they might consider the implications of the hygiene hypothesis, especially when treating individuals with a family history of atopy.

The use of antibiotics should be minimized in order to maintain normal intestinal flora. Consuming antibiotic-free meat and poultry products may also be helpful, as well as the regular consumption of probiotic supplements. In the perinatal period, one should weigh the theoretically beneficial effects of vaginal delivery and breastfeeding on the establishment of intestinal flora as well. Given the results of some of the prospective studies [111,112] and the extreme safety of these agents, it might be reasonable to consider probiotic supplementation in infants with a family history of allergy.

Another preventive strategy has been proposed to reduce the development of asthma, possibly by impacting the known role of oxidative stress on lung dysfunction. The use of whey protein has been studied and found to be associated with a decreased incidence of asthma in children [113–115]. This is likely due to its role as a cysteine donor that may augment lung glutathione levels. Furthermore, it may help explain the epidemiologic data indicating diminished asthma in children raised on farms [23]. There is even some evidence that the nutritional factors such as flavonoids used therapeutically may have a role in prevention as well [116].

SUMMARY

There are many patients for whom nutritional interventions can effectively treat asthma, requiring either no other treatment or only occasional beta-agonist use instead of the chronic anti-inflammatory agents that they would otherwise require. For others, one can achieve a significant medication-sparing effect with decreased costs and side effects. Especially in children, one can create a more normal life and possibly avoid some of the vicious cycles that medications can create related to obesity, intestinal permeability, and gut flora disturbances.

These are the major diagnostic and therapeutic points to consider in using a nutritional approach to asthma treatment:

- Investigate for food triggers by diet history, elimination diet, and if necessary, additional food allergy testing.
- Avoid preservatives and sulfites, which may function as triggers.
- Consider measurement of RBC magnesium, serum selenium, and plasma zinc.
- Increase flavonoids and micronutrients in diet by enhanced consumption of colored fruits and vegetables, whole grains, nuts, and seeds, as well as weekly fish consumption, avoiding large fish that may be high in mercury.
- Maintain ideal body weight.
- Consider supplementing the following minerals: magnesium 250 to 500 mg, selenium 200 µg, zinc 20 to 40 mg. Daily dosage refers to amount of elemental mineral, which can be bound to a variety of salts or amino acid chelates.
- Consider supplementing the following antioxidants: vitamin C at least 500 to 1000 mg, vitamin E 100 to 400 IU (high gamma-tocopherol), pycnogenol 2 mg/kg body weight/day up to 200 mg, lycopene 30 mg for exercise-induced asthma, and quercetin 1 to 2 g/day in divided doses.
- Balance essential fatty acids, which can frequently be achieved with supplemental dosing of fish oil 1 to 3 g/day (use caution due to coagulation effect in patients on anticoagulants, NSAIDS, etc.) and gamma-linolenic acid 240 to 960 mg.
- Supplement vitamin B6 at 100 to 200 mg/day.
- Dose vitamin D to normalize blood levels.
- Use relaxation techniques and yoga training as an adjunct to dietary recommendations.
- Practice primary prevention strategies for pregnant women and infants by encouraging breast feeding (and/or whey supplementation), minimizing antibiotics, and using probiotics.

REFERENCES

1. Masoli M, Fabian D, et al. The global burden of asthma: Executive summary of the GINA Dissemination Committee Report. *Allergy*, 2004; 59: 469–478.
2. National Health Interview Survey 1981–2004, National Center for Health Statistics. US Dept. of Health and Human Services.
3. Asher M, Innes I. Worldwide time trends in the prevalence of asthma, allergic rhinoconjunctivitis, and eczema in childhood: ISAAC phase one and three report multicountry cross-sectional surveys. *Lancet*, 368: 733–743.
4. Magkos F, Arvaniti F, Zampelas A. Organic food: Nutritious food or food for thought? A review of the evidence. *Int J Food Sci Nutr*, 2003 Sep; 54(5): 357–371.
5. Guidelines for the Diagnosis and Management of Asthma, NAEP Expert Panel Report II. *NIH Publ* 97-4051, Bethesda, MD, National Heart, Lung and Blood Inst, 1997.
6. Evans R, Mellins R, et al. Improving care for minority children with asthma: Professional education in public health clinics. *Pediatrics*, 1997; 99: 157–164.
7. Sarnat JA, Asthma and air quality. *Curr Opin Pulm Med*, 2007 Jan; 13(1): 63–66.
8. Sole D, Camelo-Nunes IC, et al. Prevalence of asthma, rhinitis and atopic eczema in Brazilian adolescents related to exposure to gaseous air pollutants and socioeconomic status. *J Investig Allergol Clin Immunol*, 2007; 17(1): 6–13.
9. Villeneuve PJ, Chen L, et al. Outdoor pollution and emergency department visits for asthma among children and adults: A case-crossover study in northern Alberta, Canada. *Eviron Health*, 2007 Dec 24; 6(1): 40.
10. Hock G, Brunekreef B. Effect of photochemical air pollution on acute respiratory symptoms in children. *Am J Respir Crit Care Med*, 1995; 151: 27–32.
11. Byrd RS, Joad JP. Urban asthma. *Curr Opin Pulm Med*, 2006; 12(1): 68–74.

12. Imboden M, Downs S, et al. Glutathione S-transferase genotypes modify lung function decline in the general population: SAPALDIA cohort study. *Resp Res*, 2007; 8: 2.
13. London SJ. Gene-air pollution interactions in asthma. *Proc Am Ther Soc*, 2007 Jul; 4(3): 217–220.
14. Gurrie MJ. Exogenous Type I cytokines modulate mercury-induced hyper-IgE in the rat. *Clin Exp Immunol*, 2000; 121: 17–22.
15. Massarella G, Bianco A, et al. The Th_1/Th_2 lymphocyte polarization in asthma. *Allergy*, 2000; 55: suppl. 61: 6–9.
16. Gregori S, Giarratana N, et al. A 1 alpha, 25-dihydroxyD(3) analog enhances regulatory T-cells and arrests autoimmune diabetes in NOD mice. *Diabetes*, 2002; 51: 1367–1374.
17. Xystrakis E, Kusumakar S, et al. Reversing the defective induction of IL-10-secreting regulatory T-cells in glucocorticosteroid-resistant asthma patients. *J Clin Invest*, 2006; 116: 146–155.
18. Litonjua A, Weiss S. Is vitamin D deficiency to blame for asthma epidemic? *J Allerg Clin Immunol*, 2007 Nov; 120(5): 1031–1035.
19. Umetsu D, Akbar O, DeKruyff. Regulatory T cells control the development of allergic disease and asthma. *J Allerg Clin Immunol*, 112(3): 480–487.
20. Romagna S. Regulatory T Cells: Which role in the pathogenesis and treatment of allergic disorders? *Allergy*, 2006; 61: 3–14.
21. von Mutius E. The influence of birth order on the expression of atopy in families: A gene-environment interaction? *Clin Exp Allergy*, 1998; 28: 1454–1456.
22. Ball T, Castro-Rodriguez J, et al. Siblings, day-care attendance, and the risk of asthma and wheezing during childhood. *N Engl J Med*, 2000; 343: 538–543.
23. Braun-Fahrlander C, Riedler J, et al. Environmental exposures to endotoxin and its relation to asthma in school age children. *NEJM*, 2002; 347: 869–877.
24. Wickens K, Pearce N, et al. Antibiotic use in early childhood and the development of asthma. *Clin Exp Aller*, 1999; 29: 766–771.
25. Yan F, Polk DB. Commensal bacteria in the gut: Learning who our friends are. *Curr Opin Gastroenterol*, 2004; 20: 565–571.
26. Kozyrskyj A, Ernst P, Becker A. Increased risk of childhood asthma from antibiotic use in early life. *Chest*, 2007; 31: 1753–1759.
27. Matysiak-Budnik T, Heyman M. Food allergy and H. Pylori. *J Ped Gastro Nutr*, 2002; 34: 5–12.
28. H. Pylori may protect against asthma, other respiratory conditions. *Int Med World Report*, 2007; (1): 15.
29. Yang IA, et al. The role of TLR's and…. *Curr Opin Allerg Clin Immunol*, 2006 Feb; 6(1): 23–28.
30. Bernard A. Increased intestinal permeability in bronchial asthma. *J Allerg Clin Immunol*, 1996; 97: 1173–1178.
31. Kiziltas S, Imeryuz N, et al. Corticosteroid therapy augments gastroduodenol permeability to sucrose. *Am J Gastroenterol*, 1998 Dec; 93(12): 2420–2425.
32. Rosenfeldt V, Benfeldt B. Effect of probiotics on gastrointestinal symptoms and small intestinal permeability in children with atop dermatitis. *J Pediatrics*, 2004: 612–616.
33. Romieu, GSTM1 and GSTP1 and respiratory health. *Eur Resp J*, 2006 Nov; 28(5): 953–959.
34. Tamer L, et al. GST gene polymorphisms. *Respirology*, 2004 Nov; 9(4): 493–498.
35. Suguira H, Ichinose M, et al. Oxidative and nitrative stress in bronchila asthma. *Antiox Redox Signal*, 2008 April; 10(4): 785–798.
36. Misso NL, et al. Plasma concentration of dietary and non-dietary antioxidants….*Eur Respir J*, 2005 Aug; 9(4): 493–498.
37. Ford ES, et al. Serum antioxidant concentrations among U.S. adults with self-reported asthma. *J Asthma*, 2004; 41(2): 179–187.
38. Bousquet J, Michel F. Food allergy and asthma. *Ann Allerg*, 1998 Dec; Part II; 61: 70–74.
39. Anthony HM et al. Food intolerance. *Lancet*, 1994 July 9; 344: 136–137.
40. Watson W, et al. Food hypersensitivity and changes in airway function. *J Allerg and Clin Immunol*, 1992; (I/Part II): 184/159.
41. Wilson N, et al. Bronchial hyperactivity in food and drink intolerance. *Ann Allerg*, 1988 Dec; 61: 75–79.
42. Hoj L, et al. A double blind controlled trial of elemental diet in severe, perennial asthma. *Allergy* 1981; 36: 257–262.
43. Borok G, et al. Childhood asthma—food the trigger? *South Afr Med Journ*, 1990 March 3; 77: 269.
44. Weber R, Col MC, et al. Food additives and allergy. *Ann Allerg*, 70: 183–191.
45. Lessof MH, et al. Reactions to food additives. *Clin and Exp Allergy*, 1995; 25 (suppl): 27–28.

46. Hodge L, Yank Y, et al. Assessment of food chemical intolerance in adult asthmatic subjects. *Thorax*, 1996 Aug; 51(8): 805–809.

47. Valley H, et al. Changes in hyperresponsiveness following high- and low-sulfite wine challenge in wine-sensitive asthma patients. *Clin Exp Allerg*, 2007 July; 37(7): 1062–1066.

48. Vally H, Thompson PJ. Role of sulfite additives in wine-induced asthma: Single dose and cumulative dose studies. *Thorax*, 2001 Oct; 56(10): 763–769.

49. Hodge L. Consumption of oily fish and asthma risk. *Med J Australia*, 1996; 164: 137–140.

50. Thien F, et al. Oily fish and asthma—a fish story? *Med J Australia*, 1996 Feb 5; 164: 135–136.

51. Beuther DA. Obesity and asthma. *Am J Resp Crit Care Med*, 2006 Jul 15; 174(2): 112–119.

52. Lu FL, Johnston RA, et al. Increased pulmonary responses to ozone exposure in obese db/db mice. *Am J Physiol Cell Mol Physiol*, 2006 May; 290(5): L856–865.

53. Kelly J, et al. Altered lung antioxidant status in patients with mild asthma. *Lancet*, 1999; 354: 482–483.

54. Ochs-Balcom HM, Grant BJ, et al. Antioxidants, oxidative stress and pulmonary function in individuals diagnosed with asthma or COPD. *Eur J Clin Nutr*, 2006 Aug; 60(8): 991–999.

55. Misso NL, Brooks-Wildhaber J, et al. Plasma concentration of dietary and nondietary antioxidants are low in severe asthma. *Eur Resp J*, 2005 Aug; 26(2): 257–264.

56. Kadrabova J, et al. Selenium status is decreased in patients with intrinsic asthma. *Biol Trace Elem Res*, 1996; 52: 241–248.

57. Kocyigit A, Armutcu F, et al. Alterations in plasma essential trace elements … and the possible role of these elements on oxidative status in patients with childhood asthma. *Biol Trac Elem Res*, 2004 Jan; 97(1): 31–41.

58. Panaszek K, Barg W, Obojski A. The use of magnesium in bronchial asthma: A new approach to an old problem. *Arch Immunol Ther Exp*, 2007 Feb 5; 5(1): 354.

59. Sedighi M, Pourpak Z, et al. Low magnesium concentrations in erthrocytes of children with acute asthma. *Iran J Aller*, 2006 Dec; 5(4): 183–186.

60. Kazaks AG, Uriu-Adams JY, et al. Multiple measures of magnesium status are comparable in mild asthma and control subjects. *J Asthma*, 2006 Dec; 43(10): 783–788.

61. Zerras E, Papatherdorou G, et al. Reduced intracellular magnesium concentration in patients with acute asthma. *Chest*, 2003 Jan; 123(1): 113–118.

62. Sinert R, Spektor M, et al. Ionized magnesium levels and the ratio of ionized calcium to magnesium in asthma patients before and after treatment with magnesium. *Scand J Clin Lab Invest*, 2005; 65(8): 659–670.

63. Spivy WH, Skobellof EM, Levin RM. Effect of magnesium chloride on rabbit bronchial smooth muscle. *Ann Emerg Med*, 1990; 19: 1107–1112.

64. Nuppen M, Vanmaele L, et al. Bronchodilating effect of intravenous magnesium sulfate in acute severe bronchial asthma. *Chest*, 1990; 97: 373–377.

65. Skobelloff EM, Spivy WH, et al. Intravenous magnesium sulfate for treatment of acute severe asthma in the emergency department. *JAMA*, 1989; 262: 1210–1213.

66. Ciarallo J, Sauer A, Shannon MW. Intravenous magnesium for moderate to severe asthma: Results of a randomized, placebo-controlled trial. *J Pediatr*, 1996; 129: 809–814.

67. Gantijo-Amaral E, Ribeiro MA, et al. Oral magnesium supplementation in asthmatic children: A double blind placebo-controlled trial. *Eur J Clin Nutr*, 2007 Jan; 61(1): 54–60.

68. Bede D, Suranyi A, et al. Urinary magnesium excretion in asthmatic children receiving magnesium supplementation: A randomized, placebo-controlled double blind study. *Manges Res*, 2003 Dec; 16(4): 1262–1270.

69. Fogarty A, Lewis SA, et al. Oral magnesium and vitamin C supplementation in asthma: A parallel group randomized placebo-controlled trial. *Clin Exp Allerg*, 2003 Oct; 33(10): 1355–1359.

70. Tudor R, Zalewski PD, et al. Zinc in health and chronic disease. *J Nutr Health Aging*, 2005; 9(1): 45–51.

71. Saaereks V, Ylatilo P, et al. Opposite effects of nicotinic acid and pyridoxine on systemic prostacycline, thromboxane and leukotriene production in man. *Pharmacol Toxicol*, 2002 June; 90(6): 338–342.

72. Collip PJ, Chen SY, et al. Tryptophan metabolism in bronchial asthma. *Ann Allerg*, 1975 Sep; 35(3): 153–158.

73. Reynolds RD, Natta CL. Depressed plasma pyridoxal phosphate concentration in adult asthmatics. *J Clin Nutr*, 1985 Apr; 41(4): 684–688.

74. Collipp PJ, Goldzier S, III, et al. Pyridoxine treatment of childhood bronchial asthma. *Annal Allerg*, 1975 Aug; 35(2): 93–97.

75. Fogarty A, Lewis S, et al. Dietary vitamin E, IgE concentration and atopy. *Lancet* 2000; 356: 1573–1574.

76. Troisi RJ, Willet WC, et al. A prospective study of diet and adult onset asthma. *Am J Resp Crit Care Med*, 1995; 151: 1401–1408.

77. Bielory L, Gandhi R. Asthma and vitamin C. *Ann Allerg*, 1994 Aug; 73(2): 89–96.

78. Lau BH, Riesen SK, et al. Pycnogenol as an adjunct in the management of childhood asthma. *J Asthma*, 2004; 41(8): 825–832.

79. Hosseini S, Pishnamazi S, et al. Pycnogenol in the management of asthma. *J Med Food*, 2001 Winter; 4(4): 201–209.

80. Neuman I, Nahum H. Reduction of exercise-induced asthma oxidative stress by lycopene, a natural antioxidant. *Allergy*, 2000; 55: 1184–1189.

81. Tanaka T, Higa S, et al. Flavanoids as potential anti-allergy substances. *Curr Med Chem—Antiinflamm and Anti-Allerg Ag*, 2003 (2): 57–65.

82. Min YD, Choi CH, et al. Quercetin inhibits expression of inflammatory cytokines through attenuation of NFkB and p38MAPk in the HMC-1 human mast cell line. *Inflamm Res*, 2007 May; 56(5): 210–215.

83. Kandere-Grzybowska K, Kempuraj D, et al. Regulation of IL1-induced selective IL6 release from human mast cells and inhibition by quercetin. *Br J Pharmacol*, 2006 May; 148(2): 208–215.

84. Nanua S, Zick SM, et al. Quercetin blocks airway epithelial cell chemokine expression. *Am J Resp Cell Mol Biol*, 2006 Nov; 35(5): 602–610.

85. Nair MP, Kandaswami C, et al. The flavonoid, quercetin, differentially regulates Th-1 (IFNgamma) and Th-2 (IL4) cytokine gene expression by normal peripheral blood mononuclear cells. *Biochem Biophys Acta*, 2002 Dec 16; 1593(1): 29–36.

86. Ekpo OE, Pretorius E. Asthma, Euphorbia hirta and its anti-inflammatory properties. *South Afr J Science*, 2007 May/June; 103: 201–203.

87. Chaabi M, Freund-Michel V, et al. Anti-proliferative effect of Euphorbia stenoclada in human airway smooth muscle cells in culture. *J Ethnopharm*, 2007; 109: 134–139.

88. Carey MA, Germolec DR, et al. Cyclogenase enzymes in allergic inflammation and asthma. *Leukot Essent Fatty Acids*, 2003; 69(2–3): 157–162.

89. Calabrses C, Triggliano M, et al. Arachadonic acid metabolism in inflammatory cells of patients with bronchial asthma. *Allergy*, 2000; 55(suppl 61): 27–30.

90. Oddy WH, deKler NH, et al. Ratio of omega 6 to omega 3 fatty acids and childhood asthma. *J Asthma*, 2004; 41(3): 319–326.

91. Schwarz J, Weiss ST. The relationship of dietary fish intake to level of pulmonary function in the first National Health and Nutrition Survey. *Eur Respir J*, 1994; 7: 1821–1824.

92. Hodge L, Salmoc CM, et al. Effect of dietary intake of omega 3 and omega 6 fatty acids on severity of asthma in children. *Eur Respir J*, 2008; 11: 361–365.

93. Mihrshahi S, Peat JK, et al. Effect of omega 3 fatty acid concentration in plasma on symptoms of asthma at 18 months of age. *Ped Allerg Immunol*, 2004 Dec; 15(6): 517–522.

94. Nagakkura T, Matsuda S, et al. Dietary supplementation with fish oil rich in omega 3 polyunsaturated fatty acids in children with bronchial asthma. *Eur Respir J*, 2000 Nov; 16(5): 861–865.

95. Peat J, Mihrsahi S, et al. Three year outcomes of dietary fatty acid modification and house dust mite reduction in the Childhood Asthma Prevention Study. *J Allerg Clin Immunol*, 114(4): 807–813.

96. Dry J, Vincent D. Effect of a fish oil diet on asthma: Results of a one year double blind trial. *Int Arch Allerg Appl Immunol*, 1991; 85: 156–157.

97. Reisman J, Schachter HM, et al. Treating asthma with omega 3 fatty acids: Where is the evidence? *BMC Compl Altern Med*, 2006 Jul 19; 6: 26.

98. Thien FC, et al. Dietary fish oil effects on seasonal hay fever and asthma in pollen-sensitive subjects. *Am J Resp Dis*, 1993; 147: 1138–1143.

99. Arm J, et al. The effect of dietary supplementation with fish oil lipids on the airway response to inhalant allergy and bronchial asthma. *Am Rev Resp Dis*, 1989; 139: 1395–1400.

100. Markham A, Wilkinson J. Complementary and alternative medicine in the management of asthma. An examination of the evidence. *J Asthma*, 2004; 41(2): 131–139.

101. Khayyall MT, El-Ghazaly MA, et al. A clinical study of the potential beneficial effects of a propolis food product as an adjuvant in asthmatic patients.

102. Sanchez-Mendoza ME, Torres G, et al. Mechanisms of relaxant of a crude hexane extract of Gnaphalium liebmannii in guinea pig tracheal smooth muscle. *J Ethnopoharmocol*, 2007; 111: 142–147.

103. Wilkins JH, et al. Effects of a platelet activating factor-antagonist (BN52063) on bronchoconstriction and platelet activation during exercise-induced asthma. *Br J Clin Pharmacol*, 1990; 29: 85–91.

104. Shivpuri DN, et al. Treatment of asthma with an alcoholic extract of tylophora indica: A crossover, double blind study. *Ann Allerg*, 1972 July; 30: 407–412.

105. Lowe TH. Efficacy of "functional relaxation" in comparison to terbutaline and a "placebo relaxant" method in patients with acute asthma. *Psychother Psychosom*, 2001; 70: 151–157.

106. Jain SC, Rai L, et al. Effect of yoga training on exercise tolerance in adolescents with childhood asthma. *J Asthma*, 1991; 28: 437–442.
107. Shapiro MY, Berkman N, et al. Short term acupuncture treatment is of no benefit in patients with moderate persistent asthma. *Chest*, 2002; 121(5): 1396–1400.
108. Biernacki WP, Acupuncture in the treatment of stable asthma. *Respir Med*, 1998; 92: 1143–1145.
109. Joo S, Schott C, et al. Immunological effects of acupuncture in the treatment of allergic asthma: A randomized, controlled trial. *J Altern Compl Med*, 2000; 6(6): 519–525.
110. FDA Drug Safety Advisory, 2-18-10.
111. Bjorksten B. Evidence of probiotics in prevention of allergy and asthma. *Curr Drug Targ–Inflam Allerg*, 2005; 4: 599–604.
112. Kalliomaki M, Salminen S, et al. Probiotics in primary prevention of atopic disease: A randomized, placebo-controlled trial. *Lancet*, 2001; 357: 1076–1079.
113. Loss G, et al. The protective effect of farm milk consumption on childhood asthma and atopy: The GABIRELA study. *J Allergy Clin Immunol*. 2011 Oct; 128(4): 766–773.
114. von Berg A, et al. Preventive effect of hydrolyzed infant formulas persists until age 6 years: Long-term results from the German Infant Nutritional Intervention Study (GINI). *J Allergy Clin Immunol*. 2008 Jun; 121(6): 1442–1447.
115. Chandra RK. Five-year follow-up of high-risk infants with family history of allergy who were exclusively breast-fed or fed partial whey hydrolysate, soy, and conventional cow's milk formulas. *J Pediatr Gastroenterol Nutr*. 1997 Apr; 24(4): 380–388.
116. Willers SM, Devereux G, et al. Maternal food consumption during pregnancy and asthma, respiratory and atopic symptoms in 5-year-old children. *Thorax*, 2007; 62: 773–779.

Section III

Gastrointestinal Disorders

11 Gastroesophageal Reflux Disease

Food and Nutrients as First-Line Therapy

Eileen Marie Wright, M.D., and Mark Hyman, M.D.

INTRODUCTION

Although humans have suffered from heartburn for millennia, gastroesophageal reflux disease, or GERD, has only been recently recognized as a disease. GERD is defined as chronic symptoms or mucosal damage resulting from the abnormal reflux of gastric or duodenal contents into the esophagus. The disease and its treatment have been the target of aggressive pharmaceutical marketing to both professionals and consumers. The proton-pump inhibitor (PPI) class of medications is the third best-selling pharmaceutical class of drugs worldwide, accounting for $24 billion in sales in 2010.

Symptoms related to GERD are among the most common presenting complaints to the primary care physician, affecting 20–30% of the population in Western countries. GERD is now recognized as an increased risk factor for erosive esophagitis, strictures, and Barrett's esophagus, a metaplastic change of the esophageal epithelium associated with an increased incidence of adenocarcinoma. Significant questions remain about the true risk of reflux and adenocarcinoma. Mounting evidence documents harm from long-term pharmacologic acid suppression, including osteoporosis, depression, vitamin B12 and mineral deficiencies, small intestinal bacterial overgrowth, irritable bowel syndrome, pneumonia, and increased susceptibility to enteric pathogens.

Clearly a new approach is needed to address the underlying causes of GERD. This approach would ideally limit the use of pharmacologic agents while simultaneously relying on dietary, nutritional, and other lifestyle therapies targeted toward removing the underlying causes and restoring normal intestinal function.

Conventional approaches to GERD include limiting dietary triggers, elevating the head of the bed, and pharmacologic treatments: antacids, H_2 blockers, proton-pump inhibitors, and motility agents are highly effective immediately upon use. However, their cessation can lead to rebound symptoms resulting in reliance and long-term use. Better solutions for clinical resolution require novel approaches that address the underlying causes of GERD.

EPIDEMIOLOGY

One in 10 American adults has daily episodes of heartburn; of those with heartburn, 10% to 20% have weekly symptoms, and 44% have occasional symptoms. GERD is a medical condition experienced by 25% to 35% of the U.S. population. Only 50% of patients with GERD present with typical symptoms of heartburn and regurgitation, while other patients may experience heartburn yet not have GERD. This makes an accurate diagnosis challenging [1]. Up to 70% of GERD patients have overlapping symptoms such as diarrhea, dyspepsia, and constipation. Extraesophageal manifestations of GERD are in some cases the only clinical symptom [2]. Only 30% of patients with GERD-related symptoms in Western countries show erosive changes (ERD) in the esophageal mucosa and 60% have no visible lesions (NERD); 10% of GERD patients have Barrett's esophagus, which is considered a precancerous lesion, and many of these have no symptoms of reflux. Studies in adults show that over five years, there is a low risk of progression from NERD to ERD or from NERD or ERD to Barrett's esophagus [3]. However, progression of GERD is more likely to occur in patients with metabolic syndrome, elevated cholesterol, low HDL-cholesterol, elevated triglycerides, elevated uric acid, hypertension, and enlarged waist circumference; these patients are less likely to demonstrate disease regression [4].

An important clinical question when evaluating and treating patients with chronic GERD involves how to measure their risk of esophageal adenocarcinoma (EAC). While the overall incidence of GERD has increased 300% to 500% over the last 30 to 40 years in developed countries, the number of individuals with adenocarcinoma of the esophagus remains low. However, it is the fastest rising cancer and the third most common digestive cancer. In 2002, only half of the 13,100 diagnosed esophageal cancers in the United States were adenocarcinomas. But, in 2011, 16,980 new cases of EAC were reported there. Even in those with Barrett's esophagus, new cohort data indicates that the increased risk of EAC is much lower than previously suspected. This risk, once thought to be 30–40 times greater than those in the general population, still remains substantial, however, at 11 times the average [5].

A study published in 2011 aimed to estimate the symptom-, age-, and sex-specific incidences of EAC and to place these incidences in perspective with other cancer-screening endorsements [6]. Although the absolute risk of EAC in those with GERD is not known, GERD symptoms are a relative risk factor for EAC. Male sex, white race, and advancing age are also factors that increase the risk of EAC. The incidence of EAC in women is likely extremely low and is similar to the incidence of breast cancer in men. In white men older than 60 years of age with weekly GERD, the incidence of EAC is substantial, but it is only one-third their incidence of colorectal cancer. The incidence of EAC in younger white men with GERD is lower. The study concluded that screening for EAC is indicated only in white men over 60 years of age with weekly GERD symptoms.

PATHOPHYSIOLOGY

The functional and structural abnormalities associated with GERD are caused by exposure of the esophagus to recurrent episodes of acidic and nonacidic gastric refluxate. Gastric contents may contain duodenal and intestinal proteases as well as bile, acid, and gastric pepsin. Studies have shown that a combination of acid and pepsin causes more esophageal mucosal damage, although pepsin (a proteinase) is thought to be the dominant player [7]. Some degree of reflux occurs normally in most people (Figure 11.1); a combination of conditions can increase the amount and frequency of refluxate to pathologic levels by overwhelming innate protective mechanisms including esophageal acid clearance and mucosal resistance (Figures 11.2, 11.3, 11.4). Well-established mechanisms for GERD include abnormal pressure of the lower esophageal sphincter (LES) and frequent episodes of transient lower esophageal sphincter relaxation (TLESR) leading to reflux of stomach contents into the distal esophagus. Although, the importance of TLESRs in generating reflux is established, the mechanism(s) by which these events are perceived is/are unclear. Mechanisms relating to reflux perception include the content, proximal extent, and volume of reflux, impairment of mucosal

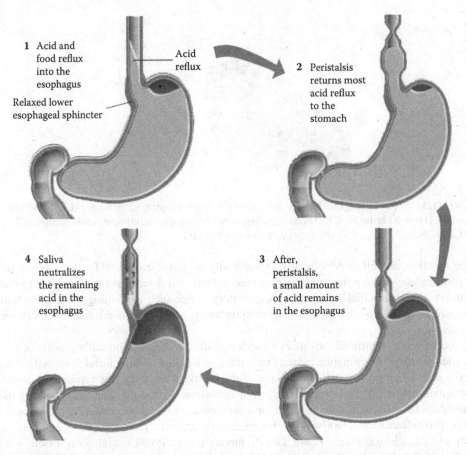

FIGURE 11.1 What happens during nonpathologic reflux. (From Kahrilas PJ. GERD pathogenesis, pathophysiology, and clinical manifestations. *Cleve Clin J Med.* 2003 Nov; 70 Suppl 5:S4–19. Reprinted with permission.)

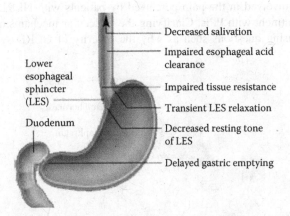

FIGURE 11.2 Potential etiologic factors involved in GERD. Acid clearance is particularly impaired in those with hiatal hernia. (From Kahrilas PJ. GERD pathogenesis, pathophysiology, and clinical manifestations. *Cleve Clin J Med.* 2003 Nov; 70 Suppl 5:S4–19. Reprinted with permission.)

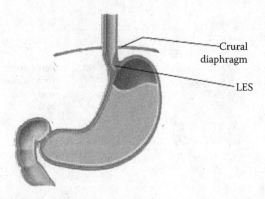

FIGURE 11.3   Normal antireflux barrier containing the lower esophageal sphincter (LES) and the crural diaphragm. (From Kahrilas PJ. GERD pathogenesis, pathophysiology, and clinical manifestations. *Cleve Clin J Med*. 2003 Nov; 70 Suppl 5:S4–19. Reprinted with permission.)

barrier function, as well as peripherally and centrally mediated esophageal sensitivity [8]. In specific patients, one or more mechanisms may predominate and determine their response to therapy. Secondary causes of GERD include hypersecretory states such as Zollinger-Ellison syndrome, gastroparesis, pyloric dysfunction, duodenal dysmotility, and connective tissue disorders such as scleroderma.

In recent years, significant advances in understanding the molecular pathogenesis of GERD-associated mucosal inflammation indicate an immune-mediated multifactorial process. Esophageal injury occurs when proteolytic components of the refluxate modulate the immune response and cause inflammation [2]. The molecular signs of inflammation and mucosal inflammatory mediators are detected even before microscopic or macroscopic changes become apparent in those with GERD. The molecular mechanisms involve proteinase-activated receptor 2 (PAR2), interleukin 8 (IL-8), and the acid-sensitive receptor TRVP1, among others. PAR2 is highly expressed on and in cells throughout all epithelial layers of the esophageal mucosa in patients with GERD. Acidic and even weakly acidic media can activate this receptor leading to the release of IL-8, a chemokine that recruits immune effector cells to infiltrate the area. In addition to its immune effects, PAR2 is also implicated in the modulation of visceral hypersensitivity and pain generation as well as increased epithelial permeability. PAR2 interacts with the acid-sensitive receptor TRVP1 in the mucosa of both ERD and NERD patients. TRVP1 activation induces the sensation of burning and produces inflammation and neuroinflammation. TRPV1 expression is higher in those with NERD than ERD and may be involved in the pain perceived by patients with NERD whose symptoms often persist despite treatment with PPIs. Clarifying the molecular mechanisms should gradually resolve clinically confusing questions such as why the severity of GERD symptoms correlates

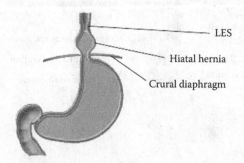

FIGURE 11.4   Hiatal hernia characterized by separation of the lower esophageal sphincter (LES) from the crural diaphragm. (From Kahrilas PJ. GERD pathogenesis, pathophysiology, and clinical manifestations. *Cleve Clin J Med*. 2003 Nov; 70 Suppl 5:S4–19. Reprinted with permission.)

poorly with the level of pathology seen on biopsy. Hopefully, a more thorough understanding of the molecular mechanisms of GERD will also lead to treatment options beyond the current first line acid-suppressive therapies.

In addition to the typical symptoms of GERD, which include heartburn, regurgitation, and dysphagia, atypical (extraesophageal) symptoms may include coughing, chest pain, and wheezing. Other consequences may result from abnormal reflux, including damage to the lungs (e.g., pneumonia, asthma, idiopathic pulmonary fibrosis), vocal cords (e.g., laryngitis, globus, cancer), ear (e.g., otitis media), and teeth (e.g., enamel decay).

A number of dietary and lifestyle recommendations are advised for patients with GERD. These recommendations fall into two broad categories: 1) avoidance of foods that, when ingested are associated with physiologic changes that can aggravate GERD, and 2) adoption of behaviors that may reduce esophageal acid exposure. A number of dietary and lifestyle factors have been demonstrated to trigger reflux, including portion size, late-night eating, fried foods, spicy foods, citrus, tomato-based foods, caffeine, alcohol, chocolate, mint, and smoking.

While there are physiologic reasons to advise against certain food choices, studies to support clinical efficacy in avoiding these triggers are lacking. Mint is known to reduce lower esophageal sphincter (LES) tone, which can aggravate GERD. However, mint also speeds gastric emptying time [9], which can improve GERD. Foods that potentially trigger or aggravate GERD include deep-fried, fatty foods, chocolate, carbonated beverages, acidic foods, and spicy foods. Deep-fried foods delay gastric emptying and reduce LES tone. Chocolate reduces LES tone. Carbonated beverages [10] cause gastric distention and reduce the resting pressure and length of the LES. Spicy foods enhance gastric-acid secretion by increasing parietal cell activity. Acidic food may aggravate mucosal damage and cause symptoms. Late-night eating increases the risk of GERD from subsequent supine positioning on a full stomach for sleep. There is also physiologic evidence that tobacco and alcohol reduce LES tone and smoking decreases salivation. However, the cessation of alcohol and tobacco use does not predictably improve esophageal pH profiles or symptoms [11]. The clinical improvement from following avoidance recommendations based on known physiology is highly variable from one patient to the next. A trial of removing these possible triggers certainly causes no harm, and some patients identify personal triggers and gain benefit.

There is a strong relationship between BMI and GERD. Obese patients who lose in the range of 20 pounds show symptomatic improvement [12–14]. Physiologically, GERD is caused by lower esophageal sphincter (LES) relaxation not related to swallowing but due to stimulation of mechanoreceptors programmed in the brainstem. Eating too fast and eating too much can cause gastric distension, which stimulates these mechanoreceptors, triggering GERD. Delayed gastric emptying after eating causes gastric distension, which is another risk factor for GERD. One or more mechanisms may be dominant in any given case and may influence their response to a chosen therapy.

In addition to obesity, pregnancy also increases the risk of reflux through direct compression of stomach contents and other mechanisms [15]. The multiple alterations in physiology and function caused by pregnancy, including elevation of progesterone, morning sickness, need for increased volume of food, and worsening of hiatal hernias, all increase the risk of reflux. Eating later as well as going to bed earlier makes lying down on a full stomach difficult to avoid during pregnancy. In addition, acidic foods are often selected during pregnancy partly because of the body's cues to absorb more minerals.

Hypothyroidism can cause hypotension of the LES. This has been shown to reverse with treatment of the hypothyroidism [16]. Head of bed elevation and left lateral decubitus position reduce the time that esophageal pH is less than 4.0 [11] and improves symptoms, at least in those with moderate to severe esophagitis [13,17]. Avoiding oral intake for two to three hours before going to bed is helpful in those with moderately severe esophagitis [13].

Many classes of medication can promote GERD. Medications that affect esophageal motility, decrease LES tone, or decrease salivation can induce or exacerbate reflux. These include anticholinergics, sedative/hypnotics (especially benzodiazepines), tricyclic antidepressants, theophylline, calcium channel blockers, alpha-adrenergic blockers, beta-adrenergic agonists, nitrates, and progesterone. NSAIDs, aspirin, steroids, sustained-release potassium tablets, and bisphosphonates such as alendronate can cause direct mucosal irritation and increase the risk of gastritis and GERD.

Dysfunction of the enteric nervous system from altered autonomic tone between the sympathetic and parasympathetic systems is implicated in reflux [18]. Physical or psychological stress increases sympathetic tone, increasing contraction of the pylorus and gastric outlet while relaxing the lower esophageal sphincter (LES), thereby setting the conditions for reflux. Autonomic dysfunction promotes an acquired gastroparesis leading to postprandial dyspepsia and bloating. Conversely, activation of the parasympathetic nervous system through the relaxation response or deep breathing relaxes the pylorus and increases LES tone, preventing reflux [19].

Nutritional deficiencies, intolerances, and sensitivities are also implicated. Zinc deficiency causes altered intestinal permeability triggering inflammation, food allergies, and increased sympathetic tone [20]. Zinc is necessary for proenzyme activation in the stomach and deficiency increases gastric acid, pepsin, and secretory volume. Pathologic changes in the stomach can be associated with zinc deficiency. Magnesium deficiency is associated with altered intestinal motility that may contribute to reflux [21]. Gluten intolerance and celiac disease can be associated with esophageal reflux, and a gluten-free diet frequently results in resolution symptoms [22–24]. These observations should prompt more research investigating the link between food allergies, sensitivities, and intolerances and GERD. A 2006 study in children demonstrated a cause-and-effect relationship between specific food allergens and GERD [25] suggesting this is indeed the case [25]. More controversial are the roles that IgG- and non-IgE-mediated food allergies play in GERD although clinical experience with elimination diets supports a trial for treatment.

While data is limited [26], clinical experience suggests that dysbiosis, the alteration of normal gut flora [27], and small intestinal bacterial overgrowth (SIBO) [28] lead to increased intestinal inflammation, disruption of the normal epithelial barrier function, and stimulation of the enteric nervous system. Such dysbiosis is commonly experienced as postprandial bloating and may also manifest as reflux. Small bowel yeast overgrowth secondary to the use of antibiotics, steroids, hormones, or a diet high in refined sugars and carbohydrates may also trigger upper intestinal symptoms. Changes in gut pH alter the microbial environment and may result in overgrowth of certain bacteria and yeast [29,30]. Reflux of alkaline bile and pancreatic secretions often go undiagnosed. Gastric pH is rarely measured in clinical practice, and empirical treatment with PPIs is recommended for conditions that may not be due to hyperacidity. This may lead to further small intestinal bacterial overgrowth and symptoms of irritable bowel syndrome (IBS). There is an overlap in prevalence of GERD and IBS. Together they form a continuous spectrum of functional gastrointestinal motility disorders. Most (> 50%) patients with GERD have delayed gastric emptying, which sets the stage not only for GERD but also bacterial overgrowth and IBS.

Food quality and composition have been shown to play a role in altered gastric and intestinal function. Calorie-dense, high-fat [31] foods contribute to reflux. High-glycemic-load foods with highly processed sugar content can also adversely influence gastric emptying and result in worsening reflux.

Helicobacter Pylori and Gastroesophageal Reflux Disease

The relationship between *Helicobacter pylori* (*H. pylori*) and gastroesophageal reflux disease (GERD) is controversial. Data from epidemiologic studies indicates an inverse relationship between the incidence of *H. pylori* infection and the prevalence of GERD, Barrett's esophagus, and esophageal adenocarcinoma (EAC). It is postulated that this relationship is due to *H. pylori*–induced gastric atrophy and hypochlorhydria, both of which reduce acid exposure in the lower esophagus. Recognizing the existence of three main gastric phenotypes resulting from *H. pylori* infection helps explain the controversy. These phenotypes are described as follows: (1) mild pangastritis does not affect gastric physiology, is not associated with significant human disease, and is the most common; (2) corpus-predominant gastritis (the gastric cancer [GC] phenotype) is associated with multifocal gastric atrophy, hypochlorhydria, and increased risk of gastric cancer; and (3) focal antral-predominant gastritis (the duodenal ulcer [DU] phenotype) is associated with high gastric acid secretion and increased risk of duodenal ulcer disease [32]. These three divergent phenotypes are due to a combination of host, bacterial, and environmental factors. Host and environmental factors relate to anatomy, physiology, and behavior discussed earlier as well as two proinflammatory genetic polymorphisms. The risk of gastric atrophy, hypochlorhydria, and gastric cancer are all increased by polymorphisms in the interleukin-1β (IL-1β) and tumor necrosis factor-α (TNF-α) genes [32]. IL-1β is more potent in its suppression of gastric acid from parietal cells and in its promotion of gastric atrophy, a precursor of gastric cancer. Bacterial factors involve the location of colonization and the strain of *H. pylori* [33]. When *H. pylori* is limited to the gastric antrum, the inflammatory reaction there causes destruction of somatostatin secreting D cells with loss of negative feedback on gastric acid secretion. This results in hyperchlorhydria, which may increase GERD severity. When *H. pylori* infection spreads to the corpus of the stomach, a condition apt to be associated with the more virulent CagA+ and VacAs1+ strains, inflammation causes progressive damage to the acid-secreting parietal cells leading to gastric atrophy and hypo- or achlorhydria. This may reduce the severity of GERD and its complications (Figure 11.5). It is important to remember that this subset of *H. pylori* patients may suffer all the nutritional consequences of hypo- or achlorhydria. Studies on eradication of *H. pylori* infection in GERD have been mixed, with some showing benefit and others not. Long-term acid suppression with PPIs facilitates the spread of *H. pylori* from the gastric antrum to the gastric corpus, which increases the risk of gastric carcinoma in those with *H. pylori* infection [34]. Diagnostic evaluation for *H. pylori* and its treatment are reasonable; however, *H. pylori* eradication may worsen GERD before it improves.

H. pylori infection has been linked to food allergy [35], rosacea, and B12 deficiency, all understandable given its potential for producing hypochlorhydria. Via molecular mimicry of host structures by its constituents, *H. pylori* infection is also implicated in a number of inflammatory and autoimmune diseases. These diseases include atherosclerosis [36], Raynaud's [23], Sjögren's [23,37], rheumatoid arthritis [38], Hashimoto's thyroiditis [38], and idiopathic thrombocytopenic purpura [38].

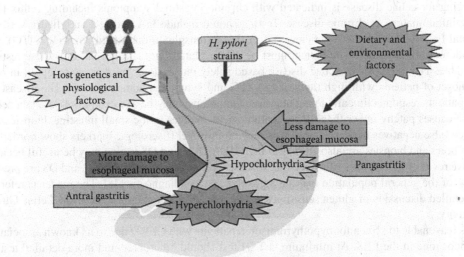

FIGURE 11.5 Possible role of various factors including *H. pylori* in pathogenesis of GERD. (From Ghoshal UC, Chourasia D. Gastroesophageal reflux disease and *Helicobacter pylori*: What may be the relationship? *J Neurogastroenterol Motil.* 2010 Jul; 16(3):243–50. Reprinted with permission.)

PATIENT EVALUATION

Esophagogastroduodenoscopy (EGD), ambulatory pH monitoring, and motility studies document the dysfunction but do little to uncover the etiology of reflux other than hiatal hernia. Their benefit and cost effectiveness as diagnostic or screening tools for Barrett's esophagus or adenocarcinoma are not supported by existing research [6]. Published data indicates that patients with GERD symptoms without alarm features may be treated empirically without endoscopic or motility evaluation. This approach avoids invasive procedures, reduces cost, and does not impact health-related quality of life [39]. Dysphagia, odynophagia, hematemesis, anemia, weight loss, hemoptysis, or respiratory distress are all possible alarm symptoms indicating the need for further investigation rather than empiric therapy alone [40].

Testing for *H. pylori* should be performed. Except for serology, PPIs should be discontinued for at least two weeks before testing. Serology or antibody testing, stool antigen, and urea breath testing (UBT) can all document infection. The diagnostic accuracy of UBT is > 95% in studies except in the presence of acute upper gastrointestinal (GI) bleeding where the test is not sensitive. Specimens for stool antigen tests must be properly stored and transported. The sensitivity of these tests may decrease to 69% after two to three days at room temperature unless the laboratory provides an appropriate fixative. When properly collected and performed, the sensitivity and specificity of stool antigen tests are 91% and 93%, respectively [41]. Serology is a widely available and inexpensive, noninvasive test, but the diagnostic accuracy is lower (80–84%). Breath and stool antigen testing should be used to confirm eradication of *H. pylori* four to eight weeks after treatment to reduce false negatives that might occur with earlier testing.

DIAGNOSTICS OF PHYSIOLOGY AND FUNCTION

Novel tests provide useful lenses for looking at the etiology and pattern of gut dysfunction that may contribute to GERD. IgG food testing, though problematic due to a high rate of false positives and some false negatives, may help identify trigger foods associated with gastrointestinal dysfunction, such as irritable bowel syndrome [42], GERD, obesity [43], and systemic inflammatory diseases. The results of IgG food testing serve as a starting point for dietary changes that may reduce symptoms and provide insight for both patient and practitioner.

Testing for celiac disease is indicated with chronic intestinal symptoms including reflux [44], or any inflammatory or chronic disease. Testing should include IgA and IgG antigliadin antibodies, total IgA (to check for IgA deficiency), IgA tissue transglutaminase antibodies (IgA tTG), and antiendomesial antibodies. The patient must be eating gluten on a regular basis for these tests to be reliable. The diagnosis of celiac disease based solely on serologic markers is accepted in only that subset of patients with high titers of IgA tTG and symptoms compatible with the disease. If these patients respond clinically to a gluten-free diet, biopsy may be avoided [45–47]. When celiac disease causes patchy rather than diffuse pathological changes in the small intestine, biopsies can produce false negatives but serological tests may be positive. If serologic markers show borderline or low titers and biopsies are also equivocal then HLA DQ2 and D8 testing may be useful because negative results on these tests rule out celiac disease 99% of the time. HLA DQ2 and D8 are present in 30% of the general population making a positive test nondiagnostic [48]. The reader is referred to a detailed discussion of gluten sensitivity in Chapter 16: Celiac Disease and Non-Celiac Gluten Sensitivity.

It is reasonable to screen for hypothyroidism in patients with GERD due to its known association with poor tone in the LES. At minimum, a TSH test should be ordered and more detailed testing added if other symptoms compatible with hypothyroidism are present.

Assessment of body weight and body mass index (BMI) contributes to understanding the etiology of reflux. Charting these values, along with waist circumference, at each visit allows patient and practitioner to observe changes in symptoms associated with decreases in size.

Urinary organic acid analysis, the analysis of nonhuman microbial metabolites that are absorbed through the intestinal epithelium and excreted in the urine, can identify markers of intestinal flora overgrowth including small bowel overgrowth [49] and yeast overgrowth [50].

Digestive stool analysis provides a broad picture of intestinal health, including information about digestion, absorption and assessment of beneficial flora, pathogenic bacteria, yeast, and parasites. In research circles, the race is on to define human enterotypes based on the genetic fingerprint of the gut microbiome. The information that is forthcoming is fascinating and proves that human beings are, indeed, superorganisms. We are, however, years away from enough data to make the information clinically relevant on a personal level.

Nutritional analyses should include plasma or red blood cell (RBC) zinc, RBC magnesium, vitamin D, serum iron, ferritin, and methylmalonic acid (vitamin B12 assessment). Magnesium deficiency can be seen even in those with normal stomach acid as a result of competitive absorption with calcium in those taking Tums for heartburn or calcium supplements for bone support, as well as from prescription or over-the-counter (OTC) medications for GERD.

PATIENT TREATMENT

PHARMACOLOGIC INTERVENTIONS AND RISKS

In the past, heartburn was traditionally treated with sodium bicarbonate and antacids such as calcium carbonate. H2 blockers followed by proton-pump inhibitors (PPIs) are now the main treatment modalities. They are among the mostly widely used and profitable pharmaceuticals in the market today.

Conventional reflux medications reduce acid and include:

- Calcium carbonate
- Antacid-alginic acid combinations
- H2 blockers (cimetidine, famotidine, nizatidine, ranitidine)
- Proton-pump inhibitors (esomeprazole, lansoprazole, omeprazole, pantoprazole, rabeprazole)

PPIs limit the final common pathway in gastric acid secretion. Therefore, they inhibit gastric acid secretion regardless of the biochemical pathway involved in its activation and are thus the most potent antacids. However, not all patients with GERD have normal gastric acidity or hyperacidity. A known subset have hypochlorhydria [51], and this may account for part of the up to 40% of GERD patients for whom PPIs do not provide adequate symptom relief [2]. Pharmacological suppression of gastric acid secretion with proton-pump inhibitors or H2 blockers is common practice for treating GERD symptoms because they often resolve the symptom(s) that brought the patient to the office. Moreover, the empirical use of these agents, based on symptoms alone, is supported by the literature. More detailed assessment looking for underlying causes such as hypochlorhydria and food allergy are seldom performed. The prolonged use of PPIs for symptoms that can often be managed with lifestyle modification and nutritional approaches as discussed in the following section is not without its downside. Mounting evidence documents the risks of long-term suppression of normal physiologic acid, which is required for the initiation of protein digestion in the stomach, mineral absorption, normal intrinsic factor function, suppression of pathogens, and the activation of pancreatic enzymes.

DRUG-FOOD INTERACTIONS, DRUG-NUTRIENT INTERACTIONS, AND DRUG-DRUG INTERACTIONS

A number of important considerations involving interactions between drugs and foods, drugs and nutrients, and one drug with another are delineated here.

1. Medication results in permissive behavior. Instead of losing weight, eating less, eating fewer fatty "rich" foods, or attempting to isolate food triggers, people use and depend upon a pill.

2. Choices such as vinegar, spices, and decaffeinated coffee, which increase stomach acid, improve diabetes. The mechanism of action for this effect is not established, but concern that prolonged pharmacological suppression of stomach acid may have an adverse effect on diabetes is valid.

3. Suppression of parietal cell acid function also impairs intrinsic factor function and B12 absorption [52]. Long-term used of PPIs is associated with B12 deficiency and all its associated complications including depression, neuropathy, fatigue, and dementia. Measuring serum B12 levels is an inadequate measure of functional B12 status; serum methylmalonic acid is a more sensitive indicator of B12 deficiency.

4. Stomach acid is required for protein digestion. When proteins are inadequately broken down to their constituent amino acids, they travel further down the GI tract where they are exposed to gut-associated lymphoid tissue (GALT). These partially digested proteins can trigger food intolerances and immune upregulation. A 2011 study documents that antacid medications—including PPIs, H_2 blockers, and sucralfate—act as risk factors for development of IgE-mediated food allergies [53]. In addition, PPIs may contribute to the development of IgG- or non-IgE-mediated food sensitivities.

5. Adequate gastric acid is necessary for proper mineral absorption. PPIs are linked to magnesium [54–57], zinc [58–60], calcium, and iron [61] deficiency. Plasma zinc levels increased by 37% in those taking long-term PPIs and zinc supplementation compared to a 126% increase in healthy controls [59]. On their normal diet without zinc supplementation, PPI-users had a 28% lower plasma zinc level than healthy controls ($p < 0.005$) [59]. Since 2006, there have been several publications documenting PPI-induced hypomagnesemia causing parathyroid dysfunction and significant hypokalemia, after as little as one year of use [55,57]. Data on the effects of PPIs on calcium absorption is conflicting. Although the mechanism is not clear, it is apparent that long-term use of PPIs can cause hypocalcemia and is associated with increased fracture risk [57,62–66].

6. Inadequate mineral status leads to greater uptake of heavy metal toxicants because zinc, for example, is a necessary cofactor for metallothionein, which complexes and removes intracellular metals. Selenium is a cofactor for glutathione peroxidase, necessary for detoxification and as part of the body's antioxidant system.

7. *H. pylori* can shift from cohabitation status to disease-causing concentrations in the presence of acid suppression. Profound acid suppression affects the pattern and distribution of *H. pylori* gastritis favoring corpus dominant gastritis and may accelerate progression to atrophic gastritis [41].

8. In patients being treated with thyroxine for hypothyroidism, PPIs decrease the absorption of thyroxine and cause a statistically significant increase in serum TSH [67]. Those taking thyroxine should be monitored for a rise in TSH and the need for an increased dose when placed on PPIs. The dosage increase needed in one study was 37% [68]. Likewise, those who have had their thyroxine dose stabilized while on PPIs may need a decrease in dose when PPIs are successfully withdrawn.

9. PPIs decrease the bioavailability of vitamin C and its serum concentration. *H. pylori* infection increases this effect [69].

10. Protein and food maldigestion are common side effects of pharmacological acid suppression, and may cause nausea, bloating, abdominal pain, and diarrhea.

11. Recent literature suggests that PPIs may affect the gut microflora in two different ways: a) PPIs may directly target the proton pumps of bacteria and fungi, and/or b) PPIs may indirectly affect the microenvironment of the flora via changes in pH. This can lead to small intestinal bacterial overgrowth and gut dysbiosis in general. PPIs are systemically

distributed and may affect the proton pumps of acid-producing host cells in areas of the body besides the stomach with unintended results [70].

12. PPIs increase susceptibility to multiple enteric pathogens including *Salmonella, Campylobacter jejuni*, invasive strains of *Escherichia coli, Clostridium difficile, Vibrio cholera*, and *Listeria* [71,72].

IMMUNE DYSREGULATION AND ACID BLOCKADE: CANCER AND ALLERGIES

PPIs may also increase the risk of gastric cancer [73]. Other consequences of long-term PPI use include an increase in gastric polyps [74], community-acquired pneumonia, pediatric pneumonia, and gastroenteritis [72,75].

In developing countries, allergic diseases such as asthma (30 million cases) and environmental allergies (50 million cases), particularly IgE type 1 hypersensitivity food allergy (9 million cases), are increasing at an alarming rate [76]. Adding autoimmunity (24 million cases), we are facing an epidemic of inflammatory and allergic disease. The prevailing hypothesis suggests that increased hygiene and reduced exposure to infectious agents in early childhood impedes normal development of tolerance and immunity [77].

However, another hypothesis merits consideration and is supported by the literature [78]. Food reactions including intolerances, allergies, and hypersensitivities can result from reduced gastric digestion of protein caused by acid-suppressing therapies, including PPIs and H2 blockers. In 152 patients medicated with acid-blocking medication, 25% developed IgE antibodies to regular food constituents as confirmed by oral provocation and skin testing. Allergenicity of potential food allergens is reduced 10,000-fold by gastric digestion. Although not yet adequately investigated, impaired or partial digestion of dietary proteins may also induce delayed hypersensitivity or IgG antibody formation to dietary constituents. This may be compounded in the setting of bacterial overgrowth in the small intestine induced by PPIs, which alters intestinal permeability leading to activation of the GALT and both local and systemic inflammation.

The collective influence of a processed, low-fiber, high-sugar, nutrient-deficient, low-phytonutrient-content diet combined with stress and the overuse of antibiotics, gastric acid-suppressing medication, nonsteroidal anti-inflammatory medications (NSAIDs), aspirin, steroids, and antihypertensive medications can trigger a vicious cycle of altered motility, autonomic dysfunction, nutrient malabsorption, maldigestion, altered intestinal flora, inflammation, and immune dysfunction.

The rationale for long-term treatment with PPIs is questionable. Years of use of powerful acid-suppressing medication alters normal digestion, leads to nutrient malabsorption and deficiency, disrupts normal intestinal flora and immunity, and increases the risk of cancer, allergic disease, and bone fractures. Long-term use of PPIs is also associated with pneumonia and colitis. These medications should be used with caution and only as a last resort for relatively benign conditions. Even in cases of Barrett's esophagus, PPIs are not proven to reduce progression to esophageal adenocarcinoma (EAC) [79,80].

SURGICAL INTERVENTIONS AND RISKS

GERD patients with troublesome symptoms despite PPI therapy or with complications of reflux such as recurrent or refractory esophagitis, stricture, Barrett's metaplasia, and asthma may be candidates for surgical intervention. Patients who are unable to tolerate medications or are unwilling to take long-term medication are also potential surgical candidates. Laparoscopic fundoplication is now the most common surgical approach to GERD. It can often remove the need for long-term PPI therapy in many patients thereby eliminating the known side effects [81]. Like any surgical intervention, the quality of the results depends upon the clinical acumen of the surgeon with respect to patient selection and to their surgical experience and skill [82]. Endoscopic surgical procedures including suturing and radiofrequency application remain in the research phase.

FOOD AND NUTRIENT TREATMENTS

Clinical tools can be useful in improving gut function and addressing GERD and NERD. A starting point is to remove what harms and provide what heals. The details may be different from person to person, but the concept will guide diagnosis and therapy. This is an area of medicine where the practical art has exceeded the clinical science. The positive clinical outcomes from this low-risk approach warrant its application because conventional approaches, even in the face of symptom control, are fraught with a myriad of consequences discussed earlier. Typical conventional approaches do not solve the problem except where obesity is causative and weight loss is sustained.

A careful dietary history noting responses to common triggers is essential. Assessing and modifying triggering factors or behaviors such as stress levels, use of medications that alter intestinal function and lead to altered motility or dysbiosis, smoking, late-night eating, poor sleep quality, and obesity are important.

TREATMENT OF POTENTIAL CAUSES

Elimination of Dietary Triggers

Elimination of typical dietary triggers can often be helpful. These may include caffeine, alcohol, chocolate, garlic, onions, mint, spicy foods, fried or fatty foods, citrus- or tomato-based foods, and highly processed or "junk foods." A whole-food, low-glycemic-load, phytonutrient-rich, plant-based, high-fiber diet often resolves reflux symptoms.

Modification of Medications

Medication begets medication. There is a slippery pharmaceutical slope, down which many patients begin to slide as they start that first long-term prescription. New symptoms appearing after the medication is started are often addressed by adding another drug, and so it goes until polypharmacy makes it impossible to determine if the next new symptoms represent new pathology or simply the result of drug interaction effects. Nutrient interventions described throughout this text can reduce the dose or eliminate the need for several medications known to worsen GERD. Cessation or substitution of medications that alter motility, reduce LES tone, or decrease salivation resolves symptoms in certain patients. Anticholinergics, sedative/hypnotics (especially benzodiazepines), tricyclic antidepressants, theophylline, prostaglandins, calcium channel blockers, alpha-adrenergic blockers, beta-adrenergic blockers, nitrates, and progesterone all have the potential to cause or aggravate GERD. Medications such as steroids, aspirin, NSAIDs, sustained release potassium tablets, and bisphosphonates, which alter intestinal permeability leading to intestinal inflammation and increased enteric sympathetic tone, can also cause/aggravate GERD.

Food Allergy Elimination Diet

Many patients with GERD are found to consume foods that trigger symptoms. Dietary changes, starting with foods having physiologic associations potentially causing GERD symptoms are a good place to start. For some, however, this does not produce success [83]—whereas a more broad-based elimination diet will. Such a diet can be empiric, starting with foods with known low allergenicity and progressively adding back foods with greater allergen potential, while keeping a diary of symptoms. On the other hand, a more personalized approach, supported by observation and clinical experience often gives a more rapid response and involves designing a customized diet after testing for food allergy/sensitivity. What is the best way to test for food reactions? This is a good question, but has no perfect answer; opinions are often conflicting and passionately debated. Most patients are aware of Type I, IgE-mediated food allergy because their symptoms, which are usually severe or even life-threatening, are hard to ignore. Milder Type I allergies can often be confirmed with serum IgE testing, or immediate-type skin prick testing. This type of food allergy testing generates little disagreement. IgE-mediated Type I allergies are not, however, the type most likely to plague those with GERD or functional GI complaints. It is the delayed type hypersensitivity responses (Type II, III, and IV) that need to be identified for these patients. Type II hypersensitivities can be determined by measuring the level of IgG antibodies to specific host proteins. Type III hypersensitivities can be detected with serum IgG antibody tests to specific antigens. When it comes to food testing, there is a great deal of debate over accuracy, pathologic significance, and clinical relevance of IgG testing [84,85]. Although largely based on empirical observation and clinical experience, an allergy elimination diet based on IgG testing may improve symptoms and is a benign intervention. A two- or three-week elimination diet removing common food allergens followed by careful reintroduction of each food class every three days may identify trigger foods without testing. The most common food allergens include gluten, dairy, eggs, yeast, corn, soy, citrus, nightshades, and nuts. Gluten elimination in celiac patients relieves reflux [24]. Type IV hypersensitivities are determined by delayed skin testing or in vitro tests based on effector and memory lymphocyte responses, but no blood tests of this type are yet proven for foods [86]. Delayed skin testing is invasive, time consuming, requires extensive training, and is not freely available.

The body's largest immune organ is the gut associated lymphoid tissue (GALT). The purpose of eliminating sensitizing foods is to reduce total antigenic load in the GALT, and thereby reduce local GI and systemic inflammatory drivers. Reintroduction of foods must be performed cautiously and slowly in order to identify any GI or systemic symptoms that occur as foods are added. This identification of trigger foods is an essential component of the elimination/challenge process. Depending on the severity of dysbiosis and altered intestinal permeability, this process can take anywhere from four to 12 weeks. Chapter 16 discusses diagnosis and treatment of food sensitivities in detail. Food trigger identification is an important part of a comprehensive gut repair program designed to return the enteric neuroendoimmune system to balance, restoring normal digestion, motility, mucosal integrity, and barrier function. Hypochlorhydria, whether primary or induced by a pathogen, toxin, drug, or nutrient deficiency, is a cause of food allergy due to increased antigenic load from partially digested food protein. Once the underlying cause of low stomach acid is addressed, the food allergies often gradually resolve.

Treatment of *Helicobacter Pylori*

Controversy remains not only because *H. pylori* has colonized human stomachs since Paleolithic times but also because its progressive eradication in the population as a whole has been linked to increases in asthma and allergic diseases via the hygiene hypothesis. Whether this is an epiphenomenon of increased hygiene or a causal relationship still remains to be proven [87].

While no consensus exists, and some experts propose that certain strains of *H. pylori* may protect against GERD [88], it is reasonable to attempt to identify and eradicate *H. pylori* in patients with GERD. A single course of treatment will often relieve symptoms while reducing the risk of peptic ulcer disease and gastric cancer. Eradication of *H. pylori* may increase the risk of adenocarcinoma of the esophagus (EAC). Over time, it may be found that this is true for only certain strains of *H. pylori* with specific anatomic distributions [32,41,89].

Certain foods inhibit or reduce *H. pylori* proliferation, including cruciferous vegetables and licorice, as does maintaining an appropriate pH. Combining foods that inhibit *H. pylori* provides greater effects than one food alone; in a 2010 publication, the combination of broccoli sprouts and black currant oil had the most potent results [90].

This bacterium has come into prominence over the last few years as the identified cause of stomach ulcers but also may be linked to reflux. It is found in 90% to 100% of people with duodenal ulcers, 70% of people with gastric ulcers, and about 50% of people over the age of 50. Benign cohabitation with *H. pylori* is common but may progress to symptomatic infection. It may be associated with stomach cancer as well as inflammation throughout the body and may even be linked to heart disease. It is often acquired in childhood and may be the cause of lifelong gastritis or stomach inflammation. Genetic and nutritional differences seem to determine whether or not *H. pylori* causes gut symptoms or cancer. Large-population studies may miss unique subpopulations with susceptibility to *H. pylori* for this reason. In patients with elevated C-reactive protein, inflammatory diseases, chronic digestive symptoms, or a family history of gastric cancer, treatment is logical. Currently, most physicians only treat documented ulcers. However, this may neglect many people who could benefit from treatment. A trial of a single course of treatment may be helpful in some patients with GERD.

Low stomach acid predisposes to development and proliferation of *H. pylori* as does a low antioxidant defense system. Low levels of vitamins C and E in gastric fluids promote the growth of *H. pylori* [91]. Natural therapies can sometimes be effective, but pharmacological triple therapy, comprised of two antibiotics and a proton-pump inhibitor, is often necessary for eradication of *H. pylori* [92]. Treatment of *H. pylori* infection is facing a challenge. Current treatment regimens are associated with more frequent treatment failure than in the past. Several new treatment strategies developed are now suggested with the intention of overcoming antibiotic resistance. Quadruple therapies are now considered first-line alternatives in areas of high clarithromycin resistance [93]. Natural agents may help with resolution. Expanding research with specific strains of probiotics and their effects on colonization with *H. pylori* alone and in combination with standard therapy may substantially enhance treatment options in the future. One recent meta-analysis concluded that adequate evidence exists to recommend the use of *Sacchromyces boulardii*, in addition to standard triple therapy, in patients with *H. pylori* infection. Adding *Sacchromyces boulardii* increased eradication rates and decreased overall therapy-related side effects, particularly diarrhea [94,95]. Zinc carnosine (prolaprezinc) also demonstrates the ability to enhance response to standard triple antibiotic therapy [96].

Food and Nutrient Treatment of Dysbiosis

Largely based on clinical experience and empirical observation, normalizing intestinal function through a comprehensive approach can resolve reflux symptoms. Restoring normal intestinal function takes two to three months or more and requires a methodical approach, often referred to as the 4R approach since it involves: 1) removing trigger foods, toxins, and pathogens; 2) replacing enzymes, hydrochloric acid, and fiber; 3) reinoculating the gut with beneficial bacteria; and 4) repairing the gut mucosa. Alterations of gut flora may not cause reflux. However, treatment with antibiotics for *H. pylori* and the long-term use of PPIs that further disrupt digestion by altering pH may lead to dysbiosis. In either case, to treat the cause of reflux or the side effects of medication, a gut repair protocol often results in significant clinical improvement.

Remove

The first step is removing any triggers for altered intestinal function, including food allergens, pathogens, and, when possible, offending medications as mentioned earlier. The most common microbial influences on the gut include small bowel bacterial overgrowth, yeast overgrowth, *H. pylori* infection, and parasites. The "remove" phase may also include detoxification therapy for environmental toxins including heavy metals.

Targeted antimicrobial therapies are often necessary. Small bowel bacterial overgrowth can be successfully treated with rifaximin (Xifaxan) [97]. Common antifungal therapies include both herbal and pharmacological treatments. Medications used include fluconazole, itraconazole, nystatin, terbinafine, and ketoconazole. Herbal and natural therapies include caprylic acid and lauric acid (both contained in coconut oil), undecylenic acid, oregano, garlic, berberine, grapefruit seed extract, and black walnut hull extract. Herbal combinations are often more effective than monotherapy. Pharmacologic treatments for parasites include metronidazole, iodoquinole (Yodoxin), paramomycin (Humatin), trimethoprim/sulfamethoxazole, and nitazoxanide (Alinia). Herbal therapies for parasites include artemesinin [98], oregano, quassia, garlic, and berberine. Again, combinations tend to have greater clinical efficacy than single herbs alone. Treatment of *H. pylori* can be accomplished with triple therapy [99], although resistance is becoming more widespread and sequential or quadruple therapy is necessary in areas where clarithromycin resistance is high [94]. In vitro studies show a number of natural substances and foods have the ability to inhibit or kill *H. pylori* including mastic gum [100] and zinc carnosine (prolaprezinc) [96,101] but in vivo studies are few and small. It is likely that natural products, much like conventional drugs, will need to be combined for the eradication of this tenacious organism, and more positive results will likely occur in concert with a comprehensive gut repair program.

It may be necessary to use natural agents to assist in weaning patients from their H2 blockers and PPIs as part of the "remove" step because withdrawal is often associated with rebound symptoms. This is especially true for PPIs. Three natural agents that can assist in the weaning of these potent acid blockers are neem (*Azadirachta indica*) [102,103], melatonin [104], and D-limonene [105]. The herb neem has a long history of traditional use in Ayurvedic medicine for many and varied conditions. One of its traditional applications is for peptic and duodenal ulcers. In human studies, neem decreases gastric acid secretion, volume of gastric secretion, and pepsin activity. Neem bark extract given at 30–60 mg b.i.d. for 10 weeks significantly improved or healed duodenal ulcers. Gastric and esophageal ulcer healing occurred at six weeks with a 30-mg b.i.d. dose. Results with neem for these conditions are comparable to results obtained with H2 blockers and PPIs. Neem did not show activity against *H. pylori*. Neem is a natural proton-pump inhibitor that blocks against stress and NSAID-induced depletion of protective gastric mucus and provides antioxidant protection preventing both lipid peroxidation and thiol depletion. Its anti-inflammatory activity is due to inhibition of neutrophil activation. One-quarter teaspoon of neem powder in hot water sipped as a tea before meals can relieve symptoms of GERD. Melatonin in doses of 3–6 mg per day, both alone and mixed with amino acids and vitamins, resolves symptoms of GERD and heals gastric ulcers [106]. Melatonin prevents esophageal injury in cases of both acid-pepsin and acid-pepsin-bile exposure. Melatonin can be considered a novel esophagoprotector that acts through cyclo-oxygenase, prostaglandins, and nitric oxide synthase in a dose- and duration-dependent manner [107]. D-limonene is a common terpene in nature and is a major constituent in several citrus oils. It is used for relief of heartburn because of its gastric acid neutralizing effects and its support of normal peristalsis. Any of these three natural agents may be started while a patient is still on their acid-blocking pharmaceuticals. While symptoms are monitored, the dose of prescription medication can be gradually withdrawn. Completion of a comprehensive gut repair program often also allows for discontinuation of the natural agent.

Replace

Replacing insufficient digestive enzymes and hydrochloric acid as indicated based on symptoms and testing follows the removal of triggers. Because the typical Western diet is often low in soluble and insoluble fiber, the use of prebiotic fibers is included in the "replace" category. Broad-spectrum digestive enzyme support can improve intestinal function and reduce symptoms of GERD and bloating. Plant- or animal-based enzymes may be used. Acid-stable formulas survive digestion in the stomach and often provide the best results. Proteases, lipases, cellulases, and saccharidases are all potential candidates for replacement. They are all normally secreted on demand by the pancreas or intestinal mucosa, but in the face of gut barrier compromise and inflammation, normal feedback signaling may be impaired. Dyspeptic symptoms can result from frank or functional hypochlorhydria and may be clinically indistinguishable from acid reflux. Measurement of gastric pH at baseline and after bicarbonate challenge is the ideal way to assess for the presence of hypochlorhydria. This testing reveals those patients with an elevated baseline gastric pH (hypochlorhydria), and also those whose baseline pH is normal but who do not reacidify appropriately after an alkaline challenge (functional hypochlorhydria). Testing must be done at least two weeks after discontinuation of PPIs and at least three days after stopping H2 blockers. Hypochlorhydria is most common in those over 60 years of age but can be seen at any age, especially in those with certain strains of *H. pylori*. Zinc is necessary for hydrochloric acid (HCl) production. When clinical evaluation and/or testing is consistent with zinc deficiency, a period of zinc replacement, balanced with appropriate doses of copper, is prudent before testing gastric acid status, or before starting HCl in those with proven hypochlorhydria. Otherwise, a trial of hydrochloric acid (betaine HCl/pepsin) should be given to those with acid deficiency. A starting dose of 500 to 600 mg per tablet or capsule is taken at the start of the meal and titrated up to five tablets or capsules until a warm feeling in the stomach area, nausea, or heartburn occurs. These sensations indicate the presence of excess acid and the dose producing symptoms should be reduced at the next meal. Acid challenges can be given empirically, but since the symptoms from acid reflux and hypochlorhydria are not easily distinguished clinically, it is preferable to test before treatment. When suggesting an empirical HCl challenge, it is wise to suggest that patients have sodium bicarbonate on hand to resolve heartburn should it occur as a result of the challenge. Often, after several months of a comprehensive gut repair program, treatment with HCl and enzymes is no longer necessary.

Reinoculate

The next step, done concurrently, is reinoculating the gut with beneficial bacteria or probiotics [108]. Mounting evidence links altered intestinal flora or dysbiosis to many chronic diseases of the twenty-first century, including obesity, allergies, atopy, irritable bowel syndrome, chronic inflammatory diseases, and certain cancers. A therapeutic effect often requires large doses ranging from 10 billion to 450 billion probiotic organisms daily. Cultured and fermented traditional foods such as sauerkraut, tempeh, miso, yogurt, and kefir contain live bacteria, but usually probiotic supplementation is necessary for therapeutic reinoculation. Live or freeze-dried bacteria packaged in powders, tablets, or capsules are available and contain a variety of *Lactobacillus* species, *Bifidobacteria, Streptococcus,* and *Saccharomyces boulardii*. Prebiotics such as fructans, inulin, arabinogalactans, and fructooliosaccharides provide substrates for colonization and growth of normal commensal flora. They can enhance results with probiotics although they can be associated with bloating especially when dysbiosis is severe.

The immune effects of probiotic species and even subspecies differ substantially one from another. It is important to understand the effects of the species used with respect to the patient's condition because certain probiotic bacteria can, for instance, upregulate the TH1 side of the immune system while others can downregulate TH1 or cellular immunity. Clinical response may depend on appropriate choices. These data are now available for many probiotic bacteria along with information about which cytokines they up- or downregulate. Choosing a species known to downregulate IL-8 is appropriate for GERD based on its known molecular pathophysiology. *L. acidophilus* Bar13 and *B. longum* Bar33 [109] and *Sacchromyces boulardii* can inhibit IL-8 [110]. Different species also have different effects on secretory IgA, the most abundant and crucial immunoglobulin in the gut. Low secretory IgA (sIgA) is often present in patients with GI symptoms. Studies of *Saccharomyces boulardii* and *Lactobacillus rhamnosus GG* demonstrate that both can enhance sIgA activity.

Repair

Certain nutrients, herbs, and foods can assist the gut in self-repair. In the 4R approach, the addition of these substances follows reinoculation. A whole-food, high-fiber, phytonutrient-rich diet appropriately supplemented with nutrients and herbs such as zinc, glutamine, omega-3 fatty acids, gamma-oryzanol, butyrate, antioxidants, vitamin A, turmeric, marshmallow, and ginger [111] can soothe and restore an inflamed gut.

The last step in normalization of digestive and intestinal function is to repair by providing nutritional support for regeneration and healing of damaged intestinal mucosa. Key nutrients involved in intestinal mucosal differentiation, growth, functioning, and repair include glutamine, zinc, pantothenic acid, and essential fatty acids such as eicosapentaenoic acid, docosahexaenoic acid, and gamma-linolenic acid.

Small bowel epithelial cells use glutamine as their main energy substrate. PPIs reduce glutamine availability, creating an iatrogenic glutamine insufficiency. Stress also reduces glutamine availability. The amino acid glutamine [112], which provides both a source of fuel and precursors for growth to the rapidly dividing cells of the intestinal lining, can aid in repair and healing of gut mucosal injury. Glutamine improves gut and systemic immune function, especially in patients on long-term parenteral nutrition. Glutamine improves repair of gut mucosa after damage from radiation or chemotherapy and reduces episodes of bacterial translocation and clinical sepsis in critically ill patients.

Zinc-carnosine reduces NSAID-induced epithelial injury, induces mucosal repair, and reduces intestinal permeability [101,113]. Chewable or powdered deglycyrrhizinated licorice root (DGL) is an herbal anti-inflammatory, which may reduce heartburn, reflux, and gastritis [114]. It provides a protective coating to the esophagus and the gastric mucosa. Aloe vera *(Aloe barbadensis)* reduces mucosal inflammation, reduces reflux, and improves gut healing [115]. Chapter 12 outlines the specific dosing of these and many other nutrient and herbal treatments related to gastrointestinal mucosal healing. Ultimately, gut repair results from removing insults such as inflammatory foods, toxins, allergens, and infections while replacing enzymes and hydrochloric acid, if needed, adding fiber and prebiotics, re-establishing a balanced intestinal flora, and finally adding nutrients capable of assisting the gut's mucosal healing.

Special Considerations

Patients with peptic ulcer disease should be tested and aggressively treated for *H. pylori*. Pregnant women can undertake a 4R approach but should carefully ensure adequate caloric intake and review the use of medications and herbs with their physician.

Additional Benefits of the 4R Approach

The GI tract is the key portal to the human mucosal immune system, the body's first line of protection and prevention. Aberrations in mucosal immunity can have profound systemic effects. Chronic inflammation secondary to dysfunction of the gut's complex neuroendoimmune physiology underlies many chronic diseases of the twenty-first century, including obesity and its complications [43]. The 4R approach can ameliorate or cure many chronic health problems. It should be used as a first step in addressing the underlying etiology of a chronic complex illness whenever possible. As a low-risk, high-yield therapeutic modality, it merits more aggressive clinical use and further study.

CLINICAL SUMMARY

GERD is a common, annoying, but mostly benign condition that limits the quality of life for millions of people around the world. Acid-suppressive therapies, prescription and OTC, may be effective in reducing symptoms but may lead to unnecessary and potentially life-threatening complications. Identifying and addressing food sensitivities, celiac disease, *Helicobacter pylori* infection, maldigestion, hypochlorhydria, small bowel bacterial and yeast overgrowth, as well as modifying more commonly recognized lifestyle and dietary factors that contribute to symptoms of GERD can often preclude the need for pharmacologic intervention. It takes time and effort to address symptoms at a fundamental level rather than just popping a pill. It is necessary to highlight for patients the long-term negative consequences of short-term symptom suppression. Knowledge is power. Awareness helps patients appreciate the benefit of approaching an illness or symptom complex in a manner that ultimately supports long-term health and well-being. Table 11.1 summarizes a therapeutic, functional medicine approach to GERD.

TABLE 11.1

Therapeutic Options for Gastroesophageal Reflux Disease

I. Lifestyle and Dietary Recommendations

A. Potential Dietary Triggers

Caffeine, alcohol, chocolate, garlic, onions, and peppermint; and spicy, fried or fatty, citrus- or tomato-based, and processed or "junk" foods

B. Lifestyle and Behavioral Factors

Avoid large meals

Finish eating three hours before bedtime

Practice active relaxation to increase parasympathetic tone

Eat slowly

Chew food completely

Ensure adequate quality sleep

Stop smoking

Elevate head of the bed six to eight inches

Lose weight if body mass index is elevated

C. Medications That May Induce or Aggravate Reflux

Calcium channel blockers

Beta-adrenergic agonists

Alpha-adrenergic blockers

Theophylline

Nitrates

Progesterone

Aspirin

Non-steroidal anti-inflammatory drugs

Anticholinergics

Sedative/hypnotics (especially benzodiazepines)

Tricyclic antidepressants

Antibiotics in the tetracycline and erythromycin classes

Potassium chloride (especially sustained release preparations)

Bisphosphonates

D. Food Allergy Elimination Diet

A two-week trial of an oligo-antigenic diet followed by food challenge:

Eliminate gluten, dairy, eggs, yeast, corn, soy, citrus, nightshades, and nuts

II. Treatment of Microbial Imbalances or Infections

A. Helicobacter Pylori Treatment

Select Natural Therapies

Bismuth subcitrate 240 mg twice daily before meals for two weeks

(temporary, harmless blackening of the tongue and stool may occur)

Deglycyrrhizinated licorice (DGL) can help eradicate the organism while relieving symptoms

Myrrh gum resin

Mastic gum (*Pistacia lentiscus*)

Zinc-carnosine (enhances response to antibiotic therapy)

    Saccharomyces boulardii (enhances response to antibiotic therapy)

Medications

Amoxicillin 1 g b.i.d., clarithromycin 500 mg b.i.d, omeprazole 20 mg b.i.d for 10 days

Prevpac: lansoprazole/amoxicillin/clarithromycin combination b.i.d for 14 days

Helidac (bismuth/metronidazole/tetracycline) q.i.d with meals for two weeks

Tritec (ranitidine bismuth citrate) 400 mg b.i.d for 28 days

TABLE 11.1 (*continued*)

Therapeutic Options for Gastroesophageal Reflux Disease

B. Treatment of Small Bowel Bacterial Overgrowth

Nonprescription Preparations

Oregano, citrus seed extract, *Isatis*, or berberine compounds

Spices that support healthy digestive function provided they do not trigger symptoms include garlic, onions, turmeric, ginger, cinnamon, sage, rosemary, oregano, and thyme; these may be freely added to the diet

Medications

Useful compounds when prescription medication is needed:

Rifamixin 200–400 mg t.i.d. (the preferred treatment and a nonabsorbed antibiotic)

Metronidazole 250 mg t.i.d. for seven days (for anaerobes such as Bacteroides or Clostridia species)

Tetracycline 500 mg b.i.d. for seven days (also for anaerobes)

Ciprofloxacin 500 mg b.i.d. for three days (for aerobes)

C. Treatment of Yeast Overgrowth

Test for yeast overgrowth: stool microbiology, urinary organic acid testing

Address predisposing factors (such as chronic use of antibiotics, steroids, hormones)

Address diet to eliminate refined carbohydrates, sugar, and yeast-fermented foods

Nonprescription antifungals: oregano, garlic, citrus seed extract, berberine, tannins, undecylenate, *Isatis tinctoria*, caprylic acid, monolaurin—combinations work best

Antifungal medications: nystatin, fluconazole, itraconazole, terbinafine, ketoconazole

Immunotherapy

Identify potential environmental toxic fungi (*Stachybotrys*, strains of *Aspergillus*, *Chaetomium*, and *Penicillium*); remove patient from contaminated environment if remediation is not possible

4R approach (remove triggers, replace nutrients, reinoculate probiotics, and repair intestinal mucosa)

Stress reduction

D. Treatment of Parasites

Nonprescription parasite treatments

Take digestive enzymes for a few months during and after treatment: parasites often cause malabsorption and maldigestion

Avoid vitamins during treatment because vitamins may help parasites flourish

Herbal therapies: *Artemesia annua*, oregano, clove and berberine containing plants (*Hydrastis canadensis*, *Berberis vulgaris*, *Berberis aquifolium* and *Coptis chinesis*); combinations work best

Prescription Medication for Parasites

Humatin (paramomycin) in adult doses of 250 mg t.i.d. X 14 days and Bactrim DS or Septra DS (trimethoprim and sulfamethoxazole) q12h X 14 days.

Yodoxin (iodoquinole) 650 mg t.i.d. X 14 days; Yodoxin is antifungal and antiparasitic.

Flagyl (metronidazole) 500 mg t.i.d. X 10 days with meals

Alinia (nitazoxanid) 500 mg t.i.d. X 10 days

III. Use of Digestive Enzymes and Hydrochloric Acid

Enhance digestion by replacing missing digestive enzymes and hydrochloric acid

Recommend consumption of soluble fiber (vegetables, fruits, beans, and whole, nongluten grains)

Most potent enzymes are from animals and are available by prescription.

Dose = two to three just before or at the beginning of a meal. They are generally well tolerated and without side effects. Look for a formula containing at least:

- Protease 100,000 USP units
- Lipase 20,000 USP units
- Amylase 100,000 USP units

continued

TABLE 11.1 (continued)

Therapeutic Options for Gastroesophageal Reflux Disease

Vegetarians can take a mixed plant-based form of digestive enzymes. Dose = two to three just before or at the beginning of a meal. These are grown from *Aspergillus oryzae* and an optimal formula contains about 500 mg/dose including:

- Amylase 100,000 USP units
- Protease 100,000 USP units
- Lipase 10,000 USP units
- Lactase 1600 Lactase Units (LacU)

Digestive bitters may also aid digestion. Swedish bitters or other aperitifs stimulate digestion function including enzymes and HCl. Herbal bitters formulas may contain gentian, artichoke, cardamom, fennel, ginger, and dandelion and are available in concentrated forms that should be diluted with water.

IV. Prebiotics

Prebiotics, nondigestible components of fibrous plants, serve as growth factors for healthy intestinal microflora, which metabolize the fiber to produce important short chain fatty acids (butyrate, propionate, acetate) necessary for normal large bowel function and colonocyte health.

In addition to supplementing with the healthy bacteria, studies show that providing food for the flora can improve outcomes.

Traditional dietary sources that are rich enough in fructooligosaccharides in their raw state to actually provide a prebiotic effect when eaten in reasonably small amounts (<2 oz) are chicory, jicama, Jerusalem artichoke, dandelion greens, garlic, and leek.

V. Probiotics

Preparations include freeze-dried bacteria packaged in powder, tablet, or capsule form; many preparations no longer require refrigeration for potency.

Average dosing: 5–10+ billion organisms per day on an empty stomach in two divided doses.

Higher doses may be necessary for certain conditions with doses of 50–450 billion organisms per day.

Look for reputable brands of mixed flora with organisms balanced for the type of immune response desired and guaranteed potency.

Not all strains are meant to colonize; some are used to provide a specific immune response only while being ingested. *Saccharomyces boulardii* is a good example of this type of probiotic; it is absent from stool within four to five days of being discontinued.

Some strains are particularly adapted to colonize such as *Lactobacillus* GG.

Strains backed by research provide the practitioner with information about their best application.

Saccharomyces boulardii, Lactobacillus GG, the DDS-1 strain of *Lactobacillus acidophilus,* and VSL#3 are some of the best researched with respect to human use.

Research in this field is rapidly advancing. Probiotic/prebiotic formulas and functional foods are expected to become progressively more condition specific.

VI. Nutrients for Gut Repair

Specialized gut support products and nutrients provide the necessary support for gut healing and repair. These are the final tools for correcting digestive problems, healing a leaky gut, and reducing relapse and recurrence of digestive and immune problems. These should be taken for at least one to three months depending on the severity of symptoms and response to treatment.

The compounds helpful for gut repair can be divided into four main categories:

A. Gut Food

Glutamine 1000–10,000 mg/day

This is a nonessential amino acid that is the preferred fuel for the lining of the small intestine and can greatly facilitate healing. It can be taken for one to two months. It generally comes in powder form, and is often combined with other compounds that facilitate gut repair.

B. Nutrients, Antioxidants, Demulcents (These can be taken separately or as part of a good high-potency multivitamin)

Zinc carnosine 75–150 mg b.i.d. between meals

TABLE 11.1 *(continued)*

Therapeutic Options for Gastroesophageal Reflux Disease

Zinc 20–50 mg qd (not needed in addition to zinc carnosine)

Vitamin A 5,000–10,000 IU/day

Vitamin B5 (pantothenic acid) 100–500 mg/day

Vitamin E 400 to 800 IU/day in the form of mixed tocopherols

Quercitin/Rutin 500mg twice a day and other bioflavonoids

N-acetyl-D-glucosamine

Vitamin *D*

Gingko biloba

Green tea polyphenols

Deglycyrrhizinated licorice

Althea officinalis (marshmallow)

C. Essential Fats and Oils

Gamma-linolenic acid 2–6 g/day (give with Omega-3 fatty acids)

Gamma-oryzanol (rice brain or rice brain oil) 100 mg t.i.d.

Omega-3 fatty acids 2 to 4 g/day of eicosapentaenoic acid and docosahexaenoic acid (give with long-chain Omega-6 fatty acids)

D. Anti-inflammatories and Gut/Liver Detoxifiers

N-acetylcysteine 500 mg twice a day

Reduced glutathione 300 mg twice a day

Andrographis paniculata

Phosphatidylcholine (> 45%, i.e., not lecithin or triple lecithin)

Silymarin

Curcumin (for gut application use brands without "enhanced" absorption)

Neem (*Azadirachta indica*) leaf powder ¼ tsp. in warm water taken as a bitter tea

REFERENCES

1. Scott M, Gelhot AR. Gastroesophageal reflux disease: Diagnosis and management. *Am Fam Physician.* 1999 Mar 1; 59(5):1161–9, 1199. Review.
2. Kandulski A, Malfertheiner P. Gastroesophageal reflux disease—from reflux episodes to mucosal inflammation. *Nature Reviews Gastroenterology and Hepatology.* 2012 Jan; 9:15–22.
3. Malfertheiner P, Nocon M, Vieth M, et al. Evolution of gastro-oesophageal reflux disease over 5 years under routine medical care—the ProGERD study. *Alimentary Pharmacology & Therapeutics.* 2012; 35(1):154–64.
4. Patrick L. Gastroesophageal reflux disease (GERD): A review of conventional and alternative treatments. *Altern Med Rev.* 2011; 16(2):116–33.
5. Hvid-Jensen F, Pedersen L, Drewes AM, Sørensen HT, Funch-Jensen P. Incidence of adenocarcinoma among patients with Barrett's esophagus. *N Engl J Med.* 2011 Oct 13; 365(15):1375–83.
6. Rubenstein JH, Scheiman JM, Sadeghi S, Whiteman D, Inadomi JM. Esophageal adenocarcinoma incidence in individuals with gastroesophageal reflux: Synthesis and estimates from population studies. *Am J Gastroenterol.* 2011 Feb; 106(2):254–60.
7. Kahrilas PJ. GERD pathogenesis, pathophysiology, and clinical manifestations. *Cleve Clin J Med.* 2003 Nov; 70 Suppl 5:S4–19.
8. Bredenoord AJ. Mechanisms of reflux perception in gastroesophageal reflux disease: A review. *Am J Gastroenterol.* 2012; 107:8–15.
9. Inamori M, Akiyama T, Akimoto K, et al. Early effects of peppermint oil on gastric emptying: A crossover study using a continuous real-time 13C breath test (BreathID system). *J Gastroenterol.* 2007 Jul; 42(7):539–42.
10. Hamoui N, Lord RV, Hagen JA, Theisen J, DeMeester TR, Crookes PF. Response of the lower esophageal sphincter to gastric distention by carbonated beverages. *J Gastrointestinal Surgery.* 2006; 10(6):870–77.

11. Kaltenbach T, Crockett S, Gerson LB. Are lifestyle measures effective in patients with esophageal reflux disease? *Arch Intern Med.* 2006; 166: 965–71.

12. Dore MP, Maragkoudakis E, Fraley K, et al. Diet, lifestyle and gender in gastro-esophageal reflux disease. *Dig Dis Sci.* 2008; 53(8):2027–32.

13. Kahrilas PJ, Shaheen NJ, Vaezi MF. American Gastroenterological Association I, Clinical Practice and Quality Management Committee. American Gastroenterological Association Institute, technical review on the management of gastroesophageal reflux disease. *Gastroenterology.* 1413; 135(4):1392–413.

14. De Groot NL, Burgerhart JS, Van De Meeberg PC, de Vries DR, Smout AJ, Siersema PD. Systematic review: The effects of conservative and surgical treatment for obesity on gastro-oesophageal reflux disease. *Aliment Pharmacol Ther.* 2009; 30(11–12):1091–102.

15. El-Serag HB, Graham DY, Satia JA, Rabeneck L. Obesity is an independent risk factor for GERD symptoms and erosive esophagitis. *Am J Gastroenterol.* 2005 Jun; 100(6):1243–50.

16. Eastwood GL, Braverman LE, White EM, Vander Salm TJ. Reversal of lower esophageal sphincter hypotension and esophageal aperistalsis after treatment for hypothyroidism. *J Clin Gastroenterol.* 1982 Aug; 4(4):307–10.

17. Bashir A. Khan DM, Jaswinder Singh Sodhi DM, Showkat Ali Zargar DM, Gul Javid DM, GN Yattoo DM, Altaf Shah DM, GM Gulzar DM, Mushtaq A, Khan DM. Effect of bed head elevation during sleep in symptomatic patients of nocturnal gastro esophageal reflux. *J Gastroenterol Hepatol.* 2011 Nov; 18:1440–1746.

18. Bhatia V, Tandon RK. Stress and the gastrointestinal tract. *J Gastroenterol Hepatol.* 2005 Mar; 20(3):332–9. Review.

19. Keohane J, Quigley EM. Functional dyspepsia: The role of visceral hypersensitivity in its pathogenesis. *World J Gastroenterol.* 2006 May 7; 12(17):2672–6. Review.

20. Davidson G, Kritas S, Butler R. Stressed mucosa. *Nestle Nutr Workshop Ser Pediatr Program.* 2007; 59:133–42; discussion 143–6. Review.

21. Landin WE, Kendall FM, Tansy MF. Metabolic performance and GI function in magnesium-deficient rats. *J Pharm Sci.* 1979 Aug; 68(8):978–83.

22. Cuomo A, Romano M, Rocco A, Budillon G, Del Vecchio Blanco C, Nardone G. Reflux oesophagitis in adult coeliac disease: Beneficial effect of a gluten free diet. *Gut.* 2003 Apr; 52(4):514–7.

23. Gasbarrini A, Franceschi F. Does *H. pylori* infection play a role in idiopathic thrombocytopenic purpura and in other autoimmune diseases? *Am J Gastroenterol.* 2005 Jun; 100(6):1271–3.

24. Nachman F, Vázquez H, González A, et al. Gastroesophageal reflux symptoms in patients with celiac disease and the effects of a gluten-free diet. *Clin Gastroenterol Hepatol.* 2011 Mar; 9(3):214–19.

25. Semeniuk J, Kaczmarski M. Gastroesophageal reflux (GER) in children and adolescents with regard to food intolerance. *Adv Med Sci.* 2006; 51:321–6.

26. Waldron B, Cullen PT, Kumar R, Smith D, Jankowski J, Hopwood D, Sutton D, Kennedy N, Campbell FC. Evidence for hypomotility in non-ulcer dyspepsia: A prospective multifactorial study. *Gut.* 1991 Mar; 32(3):246–51.

27. Othman M, Agüero R, Lin HC. Alterations in intestinal microbial flora and human disease. *Curr Opin Gastroenterol.* 2008 Jan; 24(1):11–6. Review.

28. Lin HC. Small intestinal bacterial overgrowth: A framework for understanding irritable bowel syndrome. *JAMA.* 2004 Aug 18; 292(7):852–8. Review.

29. O'May GA, Reynolds N, Macfarlane GT. Effect of pH on an in vitro model of gastric microbiota in enteral nutrition patients. *Appl Environ Microbiol.* 2005 Aug; 71(8):4777–83.

30. Gościmski A, Matras J, Wallner G. Microflora of gastric juice in patients after eradication of *Helicobacter pylori* and treatment with a proton pump inhibitor. *Wiad Lek.* 2002; 55(1–2):19–28. Polish.

31. Fox M, Barr C, Nolan S, Lomer M, Anggiansah A, Wong T. The effects of dietary fat and calorie density on esophageal acid exposure and reflux symptoms. *Clin Gastroenterol Hepatol.* 2007 Apr; 5(4):439–44.

32. McLean MH, El-Omar EM. Esophageal cancers and *Helicobacter pylori*: Do host genes matter? *Gastroenterology.* 2010 Jul; 139(1):17–9.

33. Ghoshal UC, Chourasia D. Gastroesophageal reflux disease and *Helicobacter pylori*: What may be the relationship? *J Neurogastroenterol Motil.* 2010 Jul; 16(3):243–50.

34. Suerbaum S, Michetti P. *Helicobacter pylori* infection. *N Engl J Med.* 2002 Oct 10; 347(15):1175–86. Review.

35. Matysiak-Budnik T, Heyman M. Food allergy and *Helicobacter pylori*. *J Pediatr Gastroenterol Nutr.* 2002 Jan; 34(1):5–12. Review.

36. Nazmi A, Diez-Poux AV, Jenny NS, Tsai MY, Szklo M, Aiello AE. The influence of persistent pathogens on circulating levels of inflammatory markers: A cross-sectional analysis from the Multi-Ethnic Study of Atherosclerosis. *BMC Public Health.* 2010; 10:706.

37. Aragona P, Magazzù G, Macchia G, Bartolone S, Di Pasquale G, Vitali C, Ferreri G. Presence of antibodies against *Helicobacter pylori* and its heat-shock protein 60 in the serum of patients with Sjögren's syndrome. *J Rheumatol.* 1999 Jun; 26(6):1306–11.

38. Emilia G, Longo G, Luppi M, Gandini G, Morselli M, Ferrara L, Amarri S, Cagossi K, Torelli G. *Helicobacter pylori* eradication can induce platelet recovery in idiopathic thrombocytopenic purpura. *Blood.* 2001 Feb 1; 97(3):812–4.

39. Giannini EG, Zentilin P, Dulbecco P, Vigneri S, Scarlata P, Savarino V. Management strategy for patients with gastroesophageal reflux disease: A comparison between empirical treatment with esomeprazole and endoscopy-oriented treatment. *Am J Gastroenterol.* 2008 Feb; 103(2):267–75.

40. Altmán KW, Prufer N, Vaezi MF. A review of clinical practice guidelines for reflux disease: Toward creating a clinical protocol for the otolaryngologist. *Laryngoscope* 2011 April; 121(4): 717–23.

41. Malfertheiner P, Megraud F, O'Morain C, Bazzoli F, El-Omar E, Graham D, Hunt R, Rokkas T, Vakil, N, Kuipers EJ. Current concepts in the management of *Helicobacter pylori* infection: The Maastricht III Consensus Report. *Gut* 2007; 56:772–81.

42. Atkinson W, Sheldon TA, Shaath N, Whorwell PJ. Food elimination based on IgG antibodies in irritable bowel syndrome: A randomized controlled trial. *Gut.* 2004 Oct; 53(10):1459–64.

43. Wilders-Truschnig M, Mangge H, Lieners C, Gruber HJ, Mayer C, März W. IgG antibodies against food antigens are correlated with inflammation and intima media thickness in obese juveniles. *Exp Clin Endocrinol Diabetes.* 2008, Apr; 16(4):241–45.

44. Lee SK, Green PH. Celiac sprue (the great modern-day imposter). *Curr Opin Rheumatol.* 2006 Jan; 18(1):101–7. Review.

45. Mubarak A, Wolters VM, Gerritsen SA, Gmelig-Meyling FH, Ten Kate FJ, Houwen RH. A biopsy is not always necessary to diagnose celiac disease. *J Pediatr Gastroenterol Nutr.* 2011 May; 52(5): 554–7.

46. Clouzeau-Girard H, Rebouissoux L, Taupin JL, et al. HLA-DQ genotyping combined with serological markers for the diagnosis of celiac disease: Is intestinal biopsy still mandatory? *J Pediatr Gastroenterol Nutr.* 2011 Jun; 52(6):729–33.

47. Hill PG, Holmes GK. Coeliac disease: A biopsy is not always necessary for diagnosis. *Aliment Pharmacol Ther.* 2008 Apr 1; 27(7):572–77.

48. Alaedini A, Green PH. Narrative review: Celiac disease: Understanding a complex autoimmune disorder. *Ann Intern Med.* 2005 Feb 15; 142(4):289–98. Review.

49. Elsden SR, Hilton MG, Waller JM. The end products of the metabolism of aromatic amino acids by Clostridia. *Arch Microbiol.* 1976 Apr 1; 107(3):283–88.

50. Shaw W, Kassen E, Chaves E. Increased urinary excretion of analogs of Krebs cycle metabolites and arabinose in two brothers with autistic features. *Clin Chem.* 1995 Aug; 41(8 Pt 1):1094–104.

51. Ayazi S, Leers JM, Oezcelik A, Abate E, et al. Measurement of gastric pH in ambulatory esophageal pH monitoring. *Surg Endosc.* 2009; 23:1968–73.

52. Ruscin JM, Page RL, II, Valuck RJ. Vitamin B(12) deficiency associated with histamine(2)-receptor antagonists and a proton-pump inhibitor. *Ann Pharmacother.* 2002 May; 36(5):812–16.

53. Pali-Scholl I, Jensen-Jarolim E. Review article: Anti-acid medication as a risk factor for food allergy. *Allergy.* 2011; 66:469–77.

54. Epstein M, McGrath S, Law F. Proton-pump inhibitors and hypomagnesemic hypoparathyroidism. *N Engl J Med.* 2006 Oct 26; 355(17):1834–6.

55. Cundy T, Mackay J. Proton pump inhibitors and severe hypomagnesaemia. *Curr Opin Gastroenterol.* 2011 Mar; 27(2):180–85.

56. MacKay JD, Blandon PT. Hypomagnesaemia due to proton-pump inhibitor therapy: A clinical case series. *Q J Med.* 2010; 103:387–95.

57. Hoorn EJ, van der Hoek J, de Man RA, Kuipers EJ, Bolwerk C, Zietse R. A case series of proton pump inhibitor-induced hypomagnesemia. *Am J Kidney Dis.* 2010 Jul; 56(1):112–6.

58. Ozutemiz AO, Aydin HH, Isler M, Celik HA, Batur Y. Effect of omeprazole on plasma zinc levels after oral zinc administration. *Indian J Gastroenterol.* 2002 Nov-Dec; 21(6):216–8.

59. Farrell CP, Morgan M, Rudolph DS, Hwang A, Albert NE, Valenzano MC, Wang X, Mercogliano G, Mullin JM. Proton pump inhibitors interfere with zinc absorption and zinc body stores. *Gastroenterology Research.* 2011; 4(6):243–51.

60. Sturniolo GC, Montino MC, Rossetto L, Martin A, D'Inca R, D'Odorico A, Naccarato R. Inhibition of gastric acid secretion reduces zinc absorption in man. *J Am Coll Nutr.* 1991 Aug; 10(4):372–75.

61. Hutchinson C, Geissler CA, Powell JJ, Bomford A. Proton pump inhibitors suppress absorption of dietary non-haem iron in hereditary haemochromatosis. *Gut.* 2007 Sep; 56(9):1291–95.

62. Yang YX, Lewis JD, Epstein S, Metz DC. Long-term proton pump inhibitor therapy and risk of hip fracture. *JAMA*. 2006 Dec 27; 296(24):2947–53.

63. Hansen KE, Jones AN, Lindstrom MJ, Davis LA, Ziegler TE, Penniston KL, Alvig AL, Shafer MM. Do proton pump inhibitors decrease calcium absorption? *J Bone Miner Res.* 2010 Dec; 25(12): 2786–95.

64. Targownik LE, Leslie WD. The relationship among proton pump inhibitors, bone disease and fracture. *Expert Opin Drug Saf.* 2011 Nov; 10(6):901–12.

65. Targownik LE, Lix LM, Leung S, Leslie WD. Proton-pump inhibitor use is not associated with osteoporosis or accelerated bone mineral density loss. *Gastroenterology*. 2010 Mar; 138(3):896–904.

66. Fournier MR, Targownik LE, Leslie WD. Proton pump inhibitors, osteoporosis, and osteoporosis-related fractures. *Maturitas*. 2009 Sep 20; 64(1):9–13.

67. Sachmechi I, Reich DM, Aninyei M, Wibowo F, Gupta G, Kim PJ. Effect of proton pump inhibitors on serum thyroid-stimulating hormone level in euthyroid patients treated with levothyroxine for hypothyroidism. *Endocr Pract.* 2007 Jul-Aug ;13(4):345–9.

68. Centanni M, Gargano L, Canettieri G, Viceconti N, Franchi A, Delle Fave G, Annibale B. Thyroxine in goiter, *Helicobacter pylori* infection, and chronic gastritis. *N Engl J Med.* 2006 Apr 27; 354(17): 1787–95.

69. McColl KEL. Effect of proton pump inhibitors on vitamins and minerals. *Am J Gastroenterol.* 2009; 104:S5–S9.

70. Vesper BJ, Jawdi A, Altman KW, Haines III GK, Tao L, Radosevich, JA. The effect of proton pump inhibitors on the human microbiota. *Current Drug Metabolism.* 2009; 10:84–9.

71. Dial S, Delaney JAC, Barkun AN, Suissa S. Use of gastric acid-suppressive agents and the risk of community acquired Clostrium difficile-associated disease. *JAMA*. 2005; 294(23):2989–95.

72. Bavishi C, DuPont HL. Systemic review: The use of proton pump inhibitors and increased susceptibility to enteric infection. *Aliment Pharmacol Ther.* 2011; 34:1269–81.

73. Waldum HL, Gustafsson B, Fossmark R, Qvigstad G. Antiulcer drugs and gastric cancer. *Dig Dis Sci.* 2005 Oct; 50 Suppl 1:S39–44. Review.

74. Jalving M, Koornstra JJ, Wesseling J, Boezen HM, DE Jong S, Kleibeuker JH. Increased risk of fundic gland polyps during long-term proton pump inhibitor therapy. *Aliment Pharmacol Ther.* 2006 Nov 1; 24(9):1341–8.

75. Hauben M, Horn S, Reich L, Younus M. Association between gastric acid suppressants and *Clostridium difficile* colitis and community-acquired pneumonia: Analysis using pharmacovigilance tools. *Int J Infect Dis.* 2007 Sep; 11(5):417–22.

76. Leonardi S, Miraglia del Giudice M, La Rosa M, Bellanti JA. Atopic disease, immune system, and the environment. *Allergy Asthma Proc.* 2007 Jul-Aug; 28(4):410–7. Review.

77. Guarner F. Hygiene, microbial diversity and immune regulation. *Curr Opin Gastroenterol.* 2007 Nov; 23(6):667–72. Review.

78. Untersmayr E, Jensen-Jarolim E. The effect of gastric digestion on food allergy. *Curr Opin Allergy Clin Immunol.* 2006 Jun; 6(3):214–9.

79. Reid BJ, Li X, Galipeau PC, Vaughan TL. Barrett's oesophagus and oesophageal adenocarcinoma: Time for a new synthesis. *Nat Rev Cancer.* 2010 Feb; 10(2):87–101.

80. Sharma P. Clinical practice. Barrett's esophagus. *N Engl J Med.* 2009 Dec 24; 361(26):2548–56.

81. Comparative Effectiveness Review Number 29: *Comparative Effectiveness of Management Strategies for Gastroesophageal Reflux Disease: Update of Comparative Effectiveness Review No. 1. Comparative Effectiveness of Management Strategies for Gastroesophageal Reflux Disease.* Prepared by: Tufts Medical Center Evidence-based Practice Center Boston, MA. September 2011.

82. Limongelli P, et al. Laparoscopic total fundoplication for refractory GERD: How to achieve optimal long-term outcomes. In *Gastroesophageal Reflux Disease*, Mauro Bortolotti, ed.

83. Cao Q, Kolasa KM. Gut check: Finding the effective dietary approach. *Nutrition Today.* 2011; 46 (4):171–77.

84. Ménard S, Cerf-Bensussan N, Heyman M. Multiple facets of intestinal permeability and epithelial handling of dietary antigens. *Mucosal Immunol.* 2010 May; 3(3):247–59.

85. Heyman M. Gut barrier dysfunction in food allergy. *Eur J Gastroenterol Hepatol.* 2005 Dec; 17(12):1279–85.

86. Mullin GE, Swift KM, Lipski L, Turnbull LK, Rampertab D. Testing for food reactions: The good, the bad, and the ugly. *Nutr Clin Pract.* 2010; (25):192.

87. Blaser MJ, Chen Y, Reibman J. Does *Helicobacter pylori* protect against asthma and allergy? *Gut.* 2008;57:561–67.

88. Loffeld RJ, Werdmuller BF, Kuster JG, Pérez-Pérez GI, Blaser MJ, Kuipers EJ. Colonization with cagA-positive *Helicobacter pylori* strains inversely associated with reflux esophagitis and Barrett's esophagus. *Digestion.* 2000; 62(2–3):95–9.

89. Bauer B, Meyer TF. Review article: The human gastric pathogen *Helicobacter pylori* and its association with gastric cancer and ulcer disease. *Ulcers.* 2011; Article ID 340157, 23 pages. doi:10.1155/2011/340157.

90. Keenan JI, Salm N, Hampton MB, Wallace AJ. Individual and combined effects of foods on *Helicobacter pylori* growth. *Phytother Res.* 2010 Aug; 24(8):1229–33.

91. Kim HJ, Kim MK, Chang WK, Choi HS, Choi BY, Lee SS. Effect of nutrient intake and *Helicobacter pylori* infection on gastric cancer in Korea: A case-control study. *Nutr Cancer.* 2005; 52(2):138–46.

92. Wolle K, Malfertheiner P. Treatment of *Helicobacter pylori*. *Best Pract Res Clin Gastroenterol.* 2007; 21(2):315–24. Review.

93. Selgrad M, Malfertheiner P. Treatment of *Helicobacter pylori*. *Current Opinion in Gastroenterology.* 2011; 27:565–70.

94. Szajewska H, Horvath A., Piwowarczyk A. Meta-analysis: The effects of *Saccharomyces boulardii* supplementation on *Helicobacter pylori* eradication rates and side effects during treatment. *Alimentary Pharmacology & Therapeutics.* 2010; 32(9):106.

95. Vitor JMB, Vale FF. Alternative therapies for *Helicobacter pylori*: Probiotics and phytomedicine. *FEMS Immunology & Medical Microbiology.* 2011 Nov; 63(2):153–64.

96. Kashimura H, Suzuki K, Hassan M, et al. Polaprezinc, a mucosal protective agent, in combination with lansoprazole. amoxycillin and clarithromycin increases the cure rate of Helicobacter pylori infection. *Aliment Pharmacol Ther.* 1999 Apr; 13(4):483–7.

97. Majewski M, McCallum RW. Results of small intestinal bacterial overgrowth testing in irritable bowel syndrome patients: Clinical profiles and effects of antibiotic trial. *Adv Med Sci.* 2007; 52:139–42.

98. Karunajeewa HA, Manning L, Mueller I, Ilett KF, Davis TM. Rectal administration of artemisinin derivatives for the treatment of malaria. *JAMA.* 2007 Jun 6; 297(21):2381–90. Review.

99. Bergamaschi A, Magrini A, Pietroiusti A. Recent advances in the treatment of *Helicobacter pylori* infection. *Recent Patents Anti-Infect Drug Disc.* 2007 Nov; 2(3):197–205. Review.

100. Paraschos S, Magiatis P, Mitakou S, Petraki K, Kalliaropoulos A, Maragkoudakis P, Mentis A, Sgouras D, Skaltsounis AL. In vitro and in vivo activities of chios mastic gum extracts and constituents against *Helicobacter pylori*. *Antimicrob Agents Chemother.* 2007 Feb; 51(2):551–9.

101. Matsukura T, Tanaka H. Applicability of zinc complex of L-carnosine for medical use. *Biochemistry (Mosc).* 2000 Jul; 65(7):817–23.

102. Maity P, Biswas K, Chattopadhyay I, Banerjee RK, Bandyopadhyay U. The use of neem for controlling gastric hyperacidity and ulcer. *Phytother Res.* 2009 Jun; 23(6):747–55.

103. Life Bandyopadhyay U, Biswas K, Sengupta A, Moitra P, Dutta P, Sarkar D, Debnath P, Ganguly CK, Banerjee RK. Clinical studies on the effect of neem (*Azadirachta indica*) bark extract on gastric secretion and gastroduodenal ulcer. *Sci.* 2004 Oct 29; 75(24):2867–78.

104. Kandil TS, Mousa AA, El-Gendy AA, Abbas AM. The potential therapeutic effect of melatonin in gastroesophageal reflux disease. BMC *Gastroenterol.* 2010 Jan 18; 10:7.

105. Sun J. D-Limonene: Safety and clinical applications. *Altern Med Rev.* 2007 Sep; 12(3):259–64.

106. de Souza Pereira R. Regression of gastroesophageal reflux disease symptoms using dietary supplementation with melatonin, vitamins and aminoacids: Comparison with omeprazole. *J Pineal Res.* 2006 Oct; 41(3):195–200.

107. de Oliveira Torres JD, de Souza Pereira R. Which is the best choice for gastroesophageal disorders: Melatonin or proton pump inhibitors? *World J Gastrointest Pharmacol Ther.* 2010 Oct 6; 1(5): 102–6.

108. Isolauri E. Probiotics in human disease. *Am J Clin Nutr.* 2001 Jun; 73(6):1142S–6S. Review.

109. Candela M, Perna F, Carnevali P, Vitali B, Ciati R, Gionchetti P, Rizzello F, Campieri M, Brigidi P. Interaction of probiotic *Lactobacillus* and *Bifidobacterium* strains with human intestinal epithelial cells: Adhesion properties, competition against enteropathogens and modulation of IL-8 production. *Int J Food Microbiol.* 2008 Jul 31; 125(3):286–92.

110. Sougioultzis S, Simeonidis S, Bhaskar KR, Chen X, Anton PM, Keates S, Pothoulakis C, Kelly CP. *Saccharomyces boulardii* produces a soluble anti-inflammatory factor that inhibits NF-kappaB-mediated IL-8 gene expression. *Biochem Biophys Res Commun.* 2006 Apr 28; 343(1):69–76.

111. Duggan C, Gannon J, Walker WA. Protective nutrients and functional foods for the gastrointestinal tract. *Am J Clin Nutr.* 2002 May; 75(5):789–808. Review.

112. Vicario M, Amat C, Rivero M, Moretó M, Pelegrí C. Dietary glutamine affects mucosal functions in rats with mild DSS-induced colitis. *J Nutr.* 2007 Aug; 137(8):1931–7.

113. Mahmood A, FitzGerald AJ, Marchbank T, Ntatsaki E, Murray D, Ghosh S, Playford RJ. Zinc carnosine, a health food supplement that stabilizes small bowel integrity and stimulates gut repair processes. *Gut.* 2007 Feb; 56(2):168–75.

114. Tarnawski A, Hollander D, Cergely H. Cytoprotective drugs. Focus on essential fatty acids and sucralfate. *Scand J Gastroenterol Suppl.* 1987; 127:39–43. Review.

115. Eamlamnam K, Patumraj S. Visedopas N, Thong-Ngam D. Effects of aloe vera and sucralfate on gastric microcirculatory changes, cytokine levels and gastric ulcer healing in rats. *World J Gastroenterol.* 2006 Apr 7; 12(13):2034–9.

12 Peptic Ulcer Disease and *Helicobacter Pylori*

Georges M. Halpern, M.D., Ph.D.

INTRODUCTION

Here are some facts and numbers [1]:

- 10% of Americans feel heartburn every day.
- 44% of Americans have heartburn monthly.
- 20 million Americans will suffer from an ulcer in their lifetime.
- The major cause of ulcers is *Helicobacter pylori*.
- The second one is nonsteroidal anti-inflammatory drugs (NSAIDs).
- Over-the-counter antacids account for > $1 billion in sales/year.
- > 60 million Americans experience acid indigestion once a month.
- > 15 million experience it daily.
- > 10 million are hospitalized each year for gastric problems at a cost of > $40 billion.
- 6,000 Americans die each year from ulcer-related complications.
- > 40,000 Americans have surgery (persistent symptoms, complications of ulcers).

Should the primary care provider be actively involved to change this course? Obviously, yes. Can foods or natural substances help? The answer is yes, but not necessarily how one may think and the choice may prove difficult. This chapter will help you select the appropriate strategy best suited for your specific patient.

EPIDEMIOLOGY

Peptic ulcer disease is common worldwide. The overall lifetime prevalence is about 12% for men and 9% for women. The lifetime risk of peptic ulcer disease is about 10%. At any given time, about 2% of the general population of the United States has symptomatic peptic ulcer disease, which translates into about four million people who have active peptic ulcers; about 350,000 new cases are diagnosed each year. Four times as many duodenal ulcers as gastric ulcers are diagnosed. Approximately 3000 deaths per year in the United States are due to duodenal ulcers and 3000 to gastric ulcers. There has been a marked decrease in reported hospitalization and mortality rates for peptic ulcers in the United States, but changes in criteria for selecting the underlying cause of death might account for some of the apparent decreases in ulcer mortality rates. Hospitalization rates for duodenal ulcers decreased nearly 50% from 1970 to 1978, but hospitalization rates for gastric ulcers did not decrease [2]. Physician office visits for peptic ulcer disease have decreased in the last few decades. The hospitalization rate is approximately 30 patients per 100,000 cases. Although this decrease in hospitalization rates may reflect a decrease in duodenal ulcer disease incidence, it appears that changes in coding practices, hospitalization criteria, and diagnostic procedures have contributed to the reported declines in peptic ulcer hospitalization and mortality rates; the mortality rate has decreased modestly in the last few decades and is approximately one death per 100,000 cases. In Peru, the prevalence of gastric ulcer and duodenal ulcer decreased from 3.15% and 5.05% respectively in 1985, to 1.62% and 2.00% respectively in 2002 [3]. There is no good evidence to support the popular belief that peptic ulcers are most common in the spring and autumn; the most consistent pattern appears to be low ulcer rates in the summer. There is strong evidence that cigarette smoking, regular use of aspirin or nonsteroidal anti-inflammatory drugs (NSAIDs including coxibs), and prolonged use of steroids are associated with the development of peptic ulcers. There is some evidence that coffee may affect ulcers, but most studies do not implicate alcohol, food, or psychological stress as causes of ulcer disease. Genetic factors play a role in both duodenal and gastric ulcers; the first-degree relatives of patients with duodenal ulcers have a two- to threefold increase in risk of getting duodenal ulcers and relatives of gastric ulcer patients have a similarly increased risk of getting a gastric ulcer. About half of the patients with duodenal ulcers have elevated plasma pepsinogen I; a small increase in risk of duodenal ulcers is found in persons with blood group O and in subjects who fail to secrete blood group antigens into the saliva. In most Western countries, morbidity from duodenal ulcers is more common than from gastric ulcers, even though deaths from gastric ulcers exceed or equal those from duodenal ulcers; in Japan, both morbidity and mortality are higher for gastric ulcers than for duodenal ulcers [2].

H. pylori is associated with peptic ulcers in adults (< 60), mostly males; while NSAIDs are the major cause of peptic ulcers in the elderly, more in women. The currently accepted knowledge is that *H. pylori* is transmitted by the fecal-oral route, which may or may not be water- or food-borne.

H pylori is so common as to seem ubiquitous in many areas of the world. In developing nations, four of five persons are infected by age 20 years [4]. However, in the United States, infection is unusual in children, and the likelihood of being infected is roughly correlated with age and ethnic background [4]. Today, the prevalence of *H. pylori* infection in the United States is about 30%, which represents a 50% decline from 30 years ago. Persons born before 1950 are much more likely to have the infection than those born after 1950. Twice as many black and Hispanic people are infected as white people [5]. This difference is not racial but reflects socioeconomic and educational factors, especially socioeconomic status during childhood. Although the prevalence of *H. pylori* infection is relatively low in the United States and other countries in which the standard of living is high, the prevalence exceeds 50% in industrialized areas of Asia and Europe. The EUROGAST Study Group [6] found that among asymptomatic persons 25 to 34 years of age, the prevalence of infection in Minneapolis–St. Paul (MN) was 15%, compared with 62% in Yokote, Japan, and 70% in parts of Poland. Because infection is typically acquired in childhood and is almost ubiquitous in Russia, Asia, Latin America, South America, and parts of Europe, patient age and country of origin may be important for detection. Mortality data (1971–2004) from eight different countries, including Argentina, Australia, Chile, Hong Kong, Japan, Mexico, Singapore, and Taiwan, were characterized by a decline in gastric and duodenal ulcer mortality [7]. Gastritis is almost always associated with *H. pylori* infection, but peptic ulcer disease develops in only about one in six infected persons. A number of studies [8] have shown that more than 90% of patients with duodenal ulcers and more than 70% of those who have a gastric ulcer are infected with *H. pylori*. However, recent reports [9,10] describe ulcer disease that is *H. pylori*–negative and apparently not associated with use of NSAIDs, suggesting there may be other rare causative factors.

PATHOPHYSIOLOGY

Peptic ulcers are defects in the gastric or duodenal mucosa that extend through the muscularis mucosa. *H. pylori* infection and NSAID use are the most common etiologic factors. *H. pylori* can elevate acid secretion in people who develop duodenal ulcers, decrease acid through gastric atrophy in those who develop gastric ulcers or cancer, and leave acid secretion largely unchanged in those who do not develop these diseases. Duodenal ulcers did not occur in achlorhydric people or in those secreting < 15 mmol/h of acid; duodenal ulcers can be healed, but not cured, by pharmacological suppression of acid secretion below this threshold. Areas of gastric metaplasia in the duodenum can be colonized by *H. pylori*, causing inflammation (duodenitis) and leading to further damage of the mucosa. The extent of gastric metaplasia is related to the amount of acid entering the duodenum— lowest in patients with pernicious anemia who secrete no acid and highest in patients with acid hypersecretion due to gastrin-secreting tumors (Zollinger-Ellison syndrome). Acid hypersecretion in duodenal ulcer disease is virtually always due to *H. pylori* infection because secretion returns to normal after the infection is eradicated. The predominantly antral gastritis in duodenal ulcer disease leads to acid hypersecretion by suppressing somatostatin cells and increasing gastrin release from the G cells in the gastric antrum. Other less common causes are mastocytosis, and basophilic leukemias. Under normal conditions, a physiologic balance exists between peptic acid secretion and gastroduodenal mucosal defense. Mucosal injury and, thus, peptic ulcers occur when the balance between the aggressive factors and the defensive mechanisms is disrupted. Aggressive factors, such as NSAIDs, *H. pylori*, alcohol (liquor), bile salts, acid, and pepsin, can alter the mucosal defense by allowing back diffusion of hydrogen ions and subsequent epithelial cell injury. The defensive mechanisms include tight intercellular junctions, mucus, mucosal blood flow, cellular restitution, and epithelial renewal. *H. pylori* infection predisposes the patient to distal gastric cancer, but patients who develop this complication have diminished acid secretion. Low acid secretion in gastric cancer was, until recently, thought to be predominantly due to gastric corpus gastritis, the associated gastric atrophy leading to loss of parietal cells. However, *H. pylori*–associated acid hyposecretion can in part be reversed by eradicating *H. pylori*, suggesting that hyposecretion is due to inflammation rather than to permanent loss of cells.

Most strains of *H. pylori* can be divided into two distinct phenotypes based on the presence or absence of a vacuolating toxin (Vac A toxin) and the products of the cag pathogenicity island (cagPI), a large chromosomal region that encodes virulence genes and is similar to that found in other enteric pathogens such as *Escherichia coli* and *Salmonella typhimurium*. People infected with strains of *H. pylori* with the cagPI have more severe mucosal damage and are more likely to have duodenal ulcers or gastric cancer. However, research has not so far identified *H. pylori* genes that predispose to either duodenal ulcers or gastric cancer. Furthermore, in developing countries, where *H. pylori* infects most of the population, cagPI strains of *H. pylori* are present in almost all infected people but only a few develop clinical disease [11].

TREATMENT RECOMMENDATIONS

FOOD

Since *H. pylori* infection is the leading cause of peptic ulcer disease (PUD) and it is transmitted through the gastrointestinal exposure, some patients and their practitioners are focused on risk of reinfection. Food and nutrient selection should instead be focused on what improves gastrointestinal linings and immune resistance.

A diet imposed by a physician or a dietician creates stress, will not be followed for more than a few days, and can exacerbate symptoms such as the recommending of large amounts of milk [1]. Furthermore, most people are wired to like—or dislike—foods, dishes, textures, smells, or carry prejudices they were infected with at a young age. A clinically measurable example is the "supertaster" who finds cruciferous vegetables intensely, and therefore avoidably, bitter. Rather than imposing a diet, certain foods should be recommended over others as detailed here:

Broccoli sprouts, brussels sprouts, and other leafy vegetables of the large cabbage family, preferably cooked to prevent infection. Lactic fermentation of cabbage (e.g., sauerkraut) is safe and provides the added benefits of a probiotic.

Yogurt, kefir, and other lactic fermented foods do help, and could cure a peptic ulcer. See Table 12.1 [12–66]. Conversely, large amounts of live probiotics, even 10^{10} live lactic bacteria, pale when compared to the $> 10^{14}$ bacteria that form our usual intestinal flora. Somewhere between 300 and 1000 different species live in the gut [67]. Probiotics alone might not make much difference at the usual available dosage; if absorbed during a treatment with antibiotics, they might be wiped out if not taken at least four hours before or after the medicine.

Foods rich in quercetin should be part of the diet: apples, tea, and red wine are the most acceptable. A regular consumption of onions and capers is recommended. Regular, moderate consumption of red wine (even de alcoholized) during meals could help control *H. pylori* proliferation [68] and toxicity [69].

To provide a supplemental, absorbable, iron supply, a diet rich in red meat, liver, and other entrails is recommended in patients with confirmed blood loss due to a bleeding ulcer. The only iron we can readily absorb comes from animal sources. These same foods are rich in vitamin B12, which can be absorbed less readily in a hypochlorhydric environment of acid-suppressing medication.

Beverages can increase stomach acid production. Patients must be aware of the acid-inducing properties of some beverages presented in Figure 12.1. Of particular note is that milk, but not fermented dairy products, induces acid production.

TABLE 12.1

Brief Review of Natural Products Proposed to Control/Eradicate *H. Pylori* or Cure Peptic Ulcers

Nutrient/Food/Herb	Proposed Mechanism of Action	Dosage/Precautions
Aloe Vera [12] gel *Aloe barbadensis*	Reduction of leukocyte adherence in postcapillary veinule. Increased level of IL-10; decreased level of TNF-α. Reduction of gastric inflammation. Elongated gastric glands. Healing of gastric ulcers.	1 teaspoon (5 g) of gel after meals **Caveat**: Use only the translucent gel without alloin, a cathartic purgative
Astragaloside IV [13] *Astragalus zahlbruckneri*	Participation of nitric oxide (NO), prostaglandins, and sulfhydryls	100 mg t.i.d.
Broccoli Sprouts, Brussels Sprouts [14–16] (sulforaphanes)	Antioxidant. Stimulate nrf-2 gene-dependent antioxidant enzyme activities. Protect and repair gastric mucosa during *H. pylori* infection [3], Bacteriostatic against three reference strains and 45 clinical isolates of *H. pylori* irrespective of their resistance to conventional antibiotics. Brief exposure to sulforaphane was bactericidal [4]. Consumption of broccoli sprouts twice daily for seven days resulted in normal urea breath tests that remained normal at day 35; 78% of patients became stool antigen-negative and 60% remained negative at day 35 [5].	50 g of cooked broccoli/brussels sprouts b.i.d. for seven days
Cat's Claw/Uña de Gato [17] *Uncaria tomentosa, Uncaria guianensis* (3% alkaloids [rhynchophylline]; 15% polyphenols)	Carboxyl-alkyl esters; pentacyclic oxindole alkaloids (POA). Proanthocyanidins. Antioxidants, anti-inflammatory. Cytoprotection with inhibition of TNF-α production (> 70%).	Inner bark of stems and leaves 1g of vine powder capsules t.i.d. (and up to 5 g daily) with lemon juice (one-half teaspoon/cup of water) **Caveat**: Potentiates coumadin/warfarin

TABLE 12.1 (*continued*)

Brief Review of Natural Products Proposed to Control/Eradicate *H. Pylori* or Cure Peptic Ulcers

Nutrient/Food/Herb	Proposed Mechanism of Action	Dosage/Precautions
Centella Asiatica, Gotu Kola [18]	Brahmi, bacosides A and B. Bacoside assists in release of NO. Asiaticosides are immuno-stimulants. Extract and asiaticosides reduced size of ulcers at day three and seven with concomitant attenuation of myeloperoxidase activity in ulcer tissue. Epithelial cell proliferation and angiogenesis were promoted, as well as expression of basic fibroblast growth factor in the ulcer tissues.	Eaten raw as salad leaf (Sri Lanka) Boil one-half teaspoon of dry leaves in one cup; drink three cups daily. **Caveat:** Potentiates sedative effects of diphenhydramine, barbiturates, tricyclic antidepressants, zolpidem, anticonvulsants. Interferes with oral antidiabetics and insulin.
Cranberry [19] *Vaccinium oxycoccus palustris*	Polyphenol antioxidants with antibacterial activity. Antiadhesion against *H. pylori* [13]. Urea breath test was negative after one week of treatment. Eradication was 82.5%; better in female patients (95.2%).	250 ml of juice b.i.d.
Cumin, Black [20] *Nigella sativa*	Albino rats with acetylsalicylic acid-induced stomach ulcers experienced the same cure rate with *N. sativa* extract as with cimetidine.	One 400 mg or 500 mg capsule of black cumin seed q.d or b.i.d.
Dangshen [21] *Conopsis pilosula*	Reduces gastric acid secretion and gastrointestinal movements and propulsion	Roots: 10–15 g daily in decoction
Dragon's Blood [22] *Dracaena cochinchinensis*	New flavonoids derivatives 6 and 7 and (2S)-4',7-dihydroxy-8-methylflavan were very active against *H. pylori* (ATC c45504) with MIC values of 29.5, 29.5, and 31.3 microM, respectively.	10 grains q.d., preferably in liquor **Caveat:** Cathartic (risk of diarrhea)
Ginger [23] *Zigimber officinale* rhizome	Sesquiterpenoids. Phenylpropanoloids (gingerols, shogaols). Zingerone (during cooking) Sialagogue (Stimulates production of saliva). Gastrokinetic. Ginger rhizome extract containing the gingerols inhibits the growth of *H. pylori* Cag+ strains in vitro.	1–5 g of fresh ginger daily **Caveat:** Interacts with warfarin Cholecystokinetic contra indicated if gallstones. Can cause heartburn if taken in large amounts or as powder
Guarana [24] *Paullinia cupana*	Tannins and other polyphenols. Pretreatment with guarana (50 and 100 mg/kg orally) provides gastroprotection against pure ethanol, similar to caffeine (2–30 mg/kg orally). But guarana protected against indomethacin-induced gastric ulceration while caffeine was ineffective.	Guarana extract: 500 mg q.d. with food **Caveat:** Risk of seizures at high doses (cf. caffeine). Do not mix with ephedrine!
Honey [20,25,26]	Honey eradicates *H. pylori*, and healed acetic acid 100% and acetylsalicylic acid-induced gastric ulcers in rats as well as cimetidine.	One to three tablespoons/day
Kamala or Red Kamala [27] *Mallotus philippensis*	*Mallotus phillipinesis* (Lam) Muell; 70% aqueous-ethanol extract completely killed *H. pylori* at concentration 15.6–31.2 µg/ml.	Red dye tea is popular in the Philippines, Afghanistan, and Australia (NSW). **Caveat:** Cathartic (risk of diarrhea).

continued

TABLE 12.1 (*continued*)
Brief Review of Natural Products Proposed to Control/Eradicate *H. Pylori* or Cure Peptic Ulcers

Nutrient/Food/Herb	Proposed Mechanism of Action	Dosage/Precautions
Deglycyrrhizinated licorice, DGL [28] Caved-S®	Equal to cimetidine; 44% healing vs. 6% with placebo.	> 760 mg chewed before each meal. Daily dosage: 4.5 g
Marigold [29,30] *Calendula officinalis*	Methanolic extract and its 1-butanol-soluble fraction show gastroprotective effects. The active constituents are saponin glycosides A, B, C, D, and F against indomethacin-induced lesions in rats [14]. In 90% of patients, spontaneous pain disappeared. Gastric acidity was statistically decreased post treatment [15].	Calendula extract (45% water): 1–5 ml b.i.d.
Mastic Gum [31–33] Resin from *Pistacia lenticus,* from the island of Chios, Greece	Decreases free acidity in six-hour pylorus-ligated rats and cytoprotective against 50% ethanol in rats [16]. Acid fraction of total mastic extract was very active (MBC = 0.139 mg/ml), as well as isomasticadienolic acid (MBC = 0.202 mg/ml) [17]. A double-blind study on 38 patients with 1 g daily for two weeks provided symptomatic relief in 80% of mastic patients (vs. 50% in the placebo group); endoscopically proven healing occurred in 70% mastic patients vs. 22% with placebo (p < 0.01). No side effects were reported [18].	1g daily
Melatonin [34–41]	Melatonin is released by the pineal gland and in large amounts by the digestive tract; it has major antioxidant properties. Average concentration of melatonin was lower in patients with GERD or recurrent gastroduodenal ulcers when compared to normal. Melatonin helps eliminate *H. pylori*. Melatonin is synthesized from L-tryptophan given orally from the gastrointestinal tract, after pinealectomy (500 X); it heals peptic ulcers. Melatonin (MT) and its precursor l-tryptophan (lTrpt) significantly attenuate gastric mucosal lesions induced by aspirin in human volunteers due to (a) direct gastroprotective action of exogenous melatonin or that generated from l-tryptophan and (b) gastrin released from the gastric mucosa by melatonin or l-tryptophan. The gastroprotective action of melatonin and lTrpt is independent of gastric mucosal PGE2 generation. Esophageal mucosal protection elicited by melatonin against experimental reflux esophagitis is not only dependent on its free-radical scavenging activity but also mediated in part through its effect on the associated inflammatory events in a receptor-independent manner.	L-tryptophan: 500–1000 mg q.d or b.i.d. Melatonin: 1–6 mg q.d. **Caveat**: L-tryptophan must be taken under strict medical supervision.

TABLE 12.1 (*continued*)

Brief Review of Natural Products Proposed to Control/Eradicate *H. Pylori* or Cure Peptic Ulcers

Nutrient/Food/Herb	Proposed Mechanism of Action	Dosage/Precautions
Optiberry® [42] Blend of wild blueberry, strawberry, cranberry, wild bilberry, edelberry, and raspberry seed extracts, with standardized levels of malvidin, cyanidin, delphinidin, and petunidin.	Anthocyanins: better bioavailability with antioxidant activity. *H. pylori* strain 49503 suspension in PBS was exposed for 18 hours to Optiberry 0.25–1% concentration that significantly inhibited ($p < 0.05$) *H. pylori* and increased its susceptibility to clarithromycin.	30 mg b.i.d. with meals
Parsley [43] *Petroselinum crispum* Tannins, flavonoids, sterols, triterpenes.	Inhibits gastric secretion, protects gastric mucosa against injuries caused by pyloric ligation, indomethacin, and cytodestructive agents at 1–2 g/kg in rats.	6 g daily **Caveat**: Emmenagogue and abortifaciens (apiol). Photosensitizer (furanocoumarins and psoralens). Rich in oxalic acid (urolithiasis).
Plantain [44–46] *Musa spp.* Extract from unripe plantain bananas. Effects may vary according to variety; *Hom* seems to be more active.	Stimulates growth of gastric mucosa [21]. Antiulcer caused by aspirin, indomethacin, phenylbutazone, prednisolone, and cysteamine in rats; caused by histamine in guinea pigs. Increased staining of alcian blue in apical cells with staining in deeper layers of mucosal glands [22]. Extract of *Hom* variety is both gastroprotective (vs. indomethacin) and ulcer healing [23].	5–10 g of powder daily, with food. **N.B.** Ripe fruit plantain and dessert bananas are inactive.
Primrose, Evening [47,48] *Oenothera biennis* The seeds contain 7–10% of gamma-linolenic acid (GLA), an omega-6 PUFA. The oil (EPO) is used in medicine (anti-inflammatory).	EPO (5–10 mg/kg) inhibits damage induced by pylorus ligation and NSAIDs; it demonstrates anti secretory and anti ulcerogenic effects in rats [24]. EPO inhibited growth of *H. pylori*, suppressed acid production, healed the ulcer, and protected gastric mucosa from aspirin- and steroid-induced damage in humans [28].	4–8 g of EPO daily, divided in small doses to be taken throughout the day **Caveat**: Seizures in some patients, notably if taking antipsychotic phenothiazines
Polyunsaturated Fatty Acids, PUFAs [49] Commonly found in seed and marine oils. GLA (omega-6), docosahexaenoic (DHA), and EPA (omega-3 C20:5) acids are most effective.	Linolenic acid is associated with membrane function (^{14}C studies) [25]	Diets rich in PUFAs protect against duodenal ulcers by inhibiting growth of *H. pylori*. Doses of $10(^{-3})$ M or $2.5 \times 10(^{-4})$ M are effective in killing most *H. pylori*.
Probiotics, Yogurt/Yoghurt [50,51] Live microorganisms that, when administered in adequate amounts, confer a health benefit on the host; mostly lactic bacteria.	Lactic bacteria inhibit growth of *H. pylori*. Regular intake of yogurt containing Bb12 and La5 (AB yogurt) decreased the urease activity (^{13}C breath test) after six weeks of therapy ($p < 0.0001$) and *H. pylori* infection in 59 adults vs. 11 in milk (placebo) control group [26]. Pretreatment with AB yogurt for four weeks improved the efficacy of quadruple one-week treatment of *H. pylori* infection despite microbial resistance [27].	Two to four, 6-oz. or 8-oz. yogurts with live active cultures/day. Brands associating *bifidobacteria* claim more efficacy.

continued

TABLE 12.1 (*continued*)

Brief Review of Natural Products Proposed to Control/Eradicate *H. Pylori* or Cure Peptic Ulcers

Nutrient/Food/Herb	Proposed Mechanism of Action	Dosage/Precautions
Propolis [26,52] A resinous substance that bees collect from tree buds or other botanical sources. The composition of propolis is variable, depending on season, bee species, and geographic location.	The composition of propolis will vary from hive to hive, district to district, and from season to season. Even propolis samples taken from within a single colony can vary, making controlled clinical tests virtually impossible. Propolis has been shown to target *H. pylori*, and is anti-inflammatory and antioxidant; it healed acetic acid-induced gastric ulcers in rats. Combination of propolis and clarithromycin improved inhibition of *H. pylori* synergistically.	Two 250-mg capsules t.i.d. for one week **Caveat:** Propolis may cause severe allergic reactions if the user is sensitive to bees or bee products.
Quercetin [53] 3,3',4',5,7-pentahydroxy-2-phenylchromen-4-one. The aglycone form of a number of other flavonoid glycosides, such as rutin and quercitrin.	Quercetin is the most active of the flavonoids with significant anti-inflammatory activity; it inhibits both the manufacture and release of histamine; it exerts potent antioxidant activity and vitamin C-sparing action. Pretreatment (120') with 200 mg/kg quercetin prevented gastric necrosis due to ethanol; all animals treated with quercetin showed increased gastric mucus production.	Foods rich in quercetin include capers (1800 mg/kg), lovage (1700 mg/kg), apples (440 mg/kg), tea (*Camellia sinensis*), onions (higher concentrations of quercetin occur in the outermost rings), red grapes (higher concentration in red wine), citrus fruits, broccoli, and other leafy green vegetables. Organic tomatoes have 79% more quercetin than conventionally grown ones. FRS soft chews are a commercial supplement: two soft chews t.i.d. **Caveat:** Quercetin is contraindicated with antibiotics; it may interact with fluoroquinolones. It is also a potent inhibitor of CYP3A4 (drug interaction).
Reishi, Lingzhi [54] *Ganoderma lucidum*	Reishi polysaccharide (GLPS) 250 and 500 mg/kg by intragastric administration healed ulcers in rats, with suppression of TNF-α gene expression and ornithine decarboxylase (ODC) activity. GLPS at 0.25–1mg/ml increased mucus synthesis. Besides suppression of TNF-α, GLPS induced c-Myc and ODC gene expression.	One to two capsules of 500 mg (with spores) of ReishiMax® b.i.d with vitamin C supplement (250 mg) or fruit juice
Sanogastril® [55] Extract of *Glycine maximus* with *Lactobacillus bulgaricus* LB51.	Active against gastric hyperacidity; 80% of gastric and duodenal ulcers improved after 10 days of treatment.	Chew one to three1.5- tablet(s) each day. Active within five minutes in 70% of cases
Sea-Buckthorn(56) *Hippophaerhamnoides*	Constituents of sea-buckthorn berries, particularly oils, have exceptional properties as antioxidants. In rats, oral administration of CO_2-extracted oil from seeds and pulp at dosage of 7 ml/kg/day significantly reduced ulcer formation by water immersion or reserpine in rats. At 3.5 ml/kg/day it also reduced gastric ulcer by pylorus ligation and sped up healing of acetic acid-induced gastric ulcer ($p < 0.01$).	Fresh juice, syrup, and berry or seed oils are used for stomach ulcers. The recommended dosage for esophagus and stomach disorders is one-half teaspoon two to three times a day of sea-buckthorn oil.

TABLE 12.1 (*continued*)

Brief Review of Natural Products Proposed to Control/Eradicate *H. Pylori* or Cure Peptic Ulcers

Nutrient/Food/Herb	Proposed Mechanism of Action	Dosage/Precautions
Swallowroot, Sariva [57] *Decalepis hamiltonii* Bioactive polysaccharide (SRPP)	Prevented (80–85%) stress-induced gastric ulcers in animal models. Normalized gastric mucin, antioxidants, and upregulated X 3 H(+),K(+)-ATPase. Protected gastric mucosa and epithelial glands. Inhibited *H. pylori* growth at 77mg/ml. SRPP is non toxic.	Decoction of root (India, Ayurvedic) t.i.d.
Tea, Green [58] *Camellia sinensis*	Inhibition of *H. pylori* urease with IC(50) of 13µg/ml. Active components are catechins. In Mongolian gerbils infected with *H. pylori*, 500, 1000, and 2000 ppm of green tea extract in water suppressed gastritis and *H. pylori* in six weeks, in dose-dependent manner.	Four to eight cups (2.25 grams of tea per six ounces of water) daily. Decaffeinated green tea is available.
Turmeric, Curcumin [59] *Curcuma longa* Its rhizomes are boiled for several hours and then dried in hot ovens, after which they are ground into a deep orange-yellow powder. Turmeric contains up to 5% essential oils and up to 3% curcumin, a polyphenol. It can exist at least in two tautomeric forms, keto and enol. The keto form is preferred in solid phase and the enol form in solution.	Anti-H2 histamine receptor. In pylorus-ligated rat stomachs, it reduced gastric secretion and prevented lesions. Pretreatment with *Curcuma longa* extract reduced Dimaprit® (H2 agonist)-induced cAMP production in a concentration-dependent manner. The ethanol and ethylacetate extracts are both active as H2 receptor competitive blockers.	Two 500-mg curcumin 95% capsules b.i.d.
Vitamin C [60,61] Ascorbic acid	Adding vitamin C (ascorbic acid) for one week to the triple treatment (omeprazole 20mg q.d. + clarithromycin 500mg q.d. + amoxicillin 1g q.d.) can reduce the dosage of clarithromycin from 500 to 250 mg and help eradicate *H. pylori* [37]. However, administration of 5g q.d. vitamin C during 28 days had no effect on *H. pylori* infection [38].	250 mg b.i.d.
Water hyssop, Brahmi [62] *Bacopa monniera* Contains two saponins (bacopaside I and II), betulinic acid, wogonin, oxeoxindin, apigenin, and luteolin.	In both normal and diabetic (NIDDM) rats, *B. monniera* extract (BME, 20–100 mg/kg) did not influence blood glucose levels. BME (50 mg/kg) showed significant anti ulcer and ulcer-healing activities. The ulcer-protective effects of BME were more pronounced in nondiabetic rats; BME affects various mucosal offensive and defensive factors.	One to two 225-mg tablet(s) b.i.d. Antioxidant. Treats epilepsy. Nootropic (enhances cognition); protects against memory deterioration due to phenytoin
Yarrow [63] *Achillea millefolium* Multiple antioxidants: isovaleric acid, salicylic acid, asparagin, sterols, flavonoids, bitters, tannins, and coumarins.	In rats, hydroalcoholic extract of yarrow (HE) protected the gastric mucosa vs. ethanol and 80% acetic acid and promoted complete regeneration at 10 mg/kg HE.	Yarrow herbal tea: one-half teaspoon to a cup of hot water t.i.d.

continued

TABLE 12.1 (*continued*)

Brief Review of Natural Products Proposed to Control/Eradicate *H. Pylori* or Cure Peptic Ulcers

Nutrient/Food/Herb	Proposed Mechanism of Action	Dosage/Precautions
Bolivian Medicinals [64] *Phoradendron crassifolium* and *Franseria artemisioides* Tannins, saponins, flavonoids, and coumarins.	Cytoprotective against ethanol-induced ulcer in rats. Cytoprotective activity is comparable to atropine.	As decoction, several times daily **Caveat**: *Phoradendron* is mistletoe, with poorly defined toxicity. *Franseria artemisioides* is a ragweed, with cross-allergenicity with all *Ambrosiae*.
Traditional Chinese Medicine (TCM) [65] 30 Chinese herbals divided into the following groups.	In vitro assessment of ethanol extracts against *H. Pylori*. Extracts of group #1 were active at a concentration of 40 µg/ml while extracts of groups #2 and #3 were active at 60 µg/ml. These 30 well-known plants require more studies for identification of active components and standardization, but offer great hope for eradication of *H. pylori*, possibly in combination.	As "tea" (decoction) t.i.d. **Caveat**: Sourcing, toxicology, standardization—and even proper identification—are poor, unknown, or ignored. Contamination with heavy metals, pathogens, pesticides, etc., is common.

TCM Treatment of Peptic Ulcer

Insufficiency-Cold Type: Modified Decoction of *Astragalus*

Astragalus root
Cinnamon twig bark
White peony root
Cuttlefish bone
Dahurian angelica root
Prepared licorice root

Stagnated-Heat Type: Modified Two-Old Herbs Decoction + Eliminating Pathogenic Heat from Liver

Coptis rhizome
Cape jasmine fruit
Scutellaria root
Anemarrhema rhizome
White peony root
Tangerine peel
Piniella Tuber
Poria
Finger citron
Dendrobium
Prepared licorice root
N.B. If presence of hematemesis or melena, add 6 g of natoginseng powder to be taken after decoction.

Advanced Stomach Support Formula, Standardized

Corydalis tuber
Astragalus root
San-qi root
Chekiang fritillary bulb
Chinese licorice root
Gambir leaf & stem
Bletilla striata (Thumb.) root
Sepia esculenta (Hoyle) shell

TABLE 12.1 (*continued*)

Brief Review of Natural Products Proposed to Control/Eradicate *H. Pylori* or Cure Peptic Ulcers

Nutrient/Food/Herb	Proposed Mechanism of Action	Dosage/Precautions
Qi-Stagnation Type: Modified Powder Against Cold Limbs + Sichuan Chinaberry Powder		
Bupleurum root		
Cyperus tuber		
White peony root		
Bitter orange		
Tangerine peel		
Sichuan Chinaberry		
Corydalis tuber		
Aucklandia root		
Perilla stem		
Ark shell		
Finger citron		
Prepared licorice root		
Zinc-Carnosine [66] Chelate of elemental zinc and carnosine in a 1:1 ratio.	Carnosine is a free-radical scavenger that prevents lipid peroxidation. Zinc-carnosine blocks the effects of TNF-α or IL-1β in MKN28 human gastric cells, and reduces IL-8 in supernatant. It prevents reduction of mucus production caused by ethanol and inhibits proliferation of *H. pylori* by inactivating urease. Many studies confirm 100% control of symptoms and > 80% endoscopic cure after eight weeks of treatment. Zinc-carnosine improved efficacy and shortens duration of treatment with antibiotics.	75 mg q.d. or b.i.d., preferably chewable, for eight weeks

NUTRIENT AND HERBAL SUPPLEMENTS

The marketing of "natural cures" is an exponentially growing business on the Internet, in magazines, health food stores, supermarkets, or large outlets (e.g., Costco, Walmart). Most claims are unsubstantiated, and most products are unreliable if not toxic.

Table 12.1 summarizes current acceptable knowledge based on extensive search on Medline/PubMed mid-2011. Even in this list, many products have not been submitted to the test of controlled clinical studies and base their claims on limited animal or lab results. Here, more than ever, caution is required.

Treatment of peptic ulcer disease can involve nutrient-drug interactions. Specifically, if proton-pump inhibitors have been used for a long period of time, the patient's vitamin B12 status must be checked, and oral supplementation or injection considered.

SUMMARY

Based on details shared by experienced practitioners in the United States and abroad, and screening of peer-reviewed publications, we feel that we can recommend the following, for their good record on safety and efficacy. Most foods can be consumed regularly together, in groups or individually; supplements' activity should be checked after eight weeks.

- Cooked broccoli sprouts: 50 g daily
- Cranberry juice (pure): 250 ml twice daily

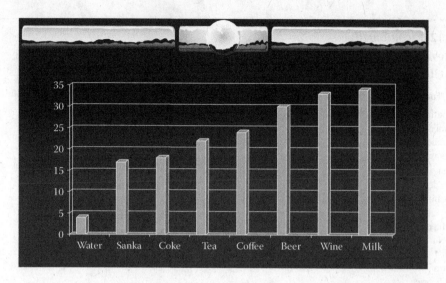

FIGURE 12.1 Stomach acid output 3.5 hours after consumption of beverage. The volume of each beverage consumed was 360 ml except for wine, which was 240 ml. The acid output was measured in mmol/3.5 hours.

- Deglycyrrhizinated licorice: 760 mg t.i.d.
- Mastic gum: 1 g daily
- Unripe plantain powder: 5–10 g daily
- Yogurt, natural, low fat, with live cultures (possibly *Bifidobacteria* spp.): two–four, six-ounce servings daily
- Diet high in vegetables rich in quercetin and moderate amounts of red wine (even de-alcoholized) with meals
- Sanogastril®: one–three tablets daily
- Green tea (eventually decaffeinated): ad libitum
- Zinc-carnosine: 75 mg q.d. or b.i.d. (preferably chewable).

REFERENCES

1. Yamada T, Alpers DH, Kaplowitz N, Laine L, Owyang C, Powell DW. *Textbook of Gastroenterology*, 4th ed. Philadelphia: Lippincott, Williams & Wilkins, 2003.
2. Kurata GH, Haile BM. Epidemiology of peptic ulcer disease. *Clin Gastroenterol* 1984;13:289–307.
3. Ramírez-Ramos A, Watanabe-Yamamoto J, Takano-Morón J, et al. Decrease in prevalence of peptic ulcer and gastric adenocarcinoma at the Policlínico Peruano Japones, Lima, Peru, between the years 1985 and 2002. Analysis of 31,446 patients. *Acta Gastroenterol Latinoam* 2006;36:139–46.
4. Breuer T, Malaty HM, Graham DY. The epidemiology of *H pylori*-associated gastroduodenal diseases. In: Ernst PB, Michetti P, Smith PD, eds. *The Immunobiology of H Pylori: From Pathogenesis to Prevention*. Philadelphia: Lippincott-Raven, 1997:1–14.
5. Graham DY, Malaty HM, Evans DG, et al. Epidemiology of *Helicobacter pylori* in an asymptomatic population in the United States: Effect of age, race, and socioeconomic status. *Gastroenterology* 1991;100(6):1495–501.
6. The EUROGAST Study Group. Epidemiology of, and risk factors for, *Helicobacter pylori* infection among 3194 asymptomatic subjects in 17 populations. *Gut* 1993;34(12):1672–6.
7. Sonnenberg A. Time trends of ulcer mortality in non-European countries. *Am J Gastroenterol* 2007;102:1101–7.
8. Isenberg JI, Soll AH. Epidemiology, clinical manifestations, and diagnosis of peptic ulcer. In: Bennett JC, Plum F, eds. *Cecil Textbook of Medicine*. 20th ed. Philadelphia: Saunders, 1996:664–6.
9. McColl KEL. How I manage *H. pylori*-negative, NSAID/aspirin-negative peptic ulcers. *Am J Gastroenterol* 2009;104:180–93.

10. Goenka MK, Majumber S, Sathy PK, Chakrborty M. *Helicobacter pylori*-negative, non-steroidal anti-inflammatory-negative peptic ulcers in India. *Indian J Gastroenterol* 2011;30:33–7.
11. Calam J, Baron JH. ABC of the upper gastrointestinal tract. *BMJ* 2001;323:980–2.
12. Eamlamnam K, Patumraj S, Visedopas N, Thong-Ngam D. Effects of Aloe vera and sucralfate on gastric microcirculatory changes, cytokine levels and gastric ulcer healing in rats. *World J Gastroenterol* 2006;12(13):2034–9.
13. Navarrete A, Arrieta J, Terrones L, Abou-Gazar H, Calis I. Gastroprotective effect of Astragaloside IV: Role of prostaglandins, sulfhydryls and nitric oxide. *J Pharm Pharmacol* 2005;57(8):1059–64.
14. Yanaka A, Zhang S, Tauchi M, Suzuki H, Shibahara T, Matsui H, Nakahara A, Tanaka N, Yamamoto M. Role of nrf-2 gene in protection and repair of gastric mucosa against oxidative stress. *Inflammopharmacology* 2005;13(1–3):83–90.
15. Fahey JW, Haristoy X, Dolan PM, Kensler TW, Scholtus I, Stephenson KK, Talalay P, Lozniewski A. Sulforaphane inhibits extracellular, intracellular, and antibiotic-resistant strains of *Helicobacter pylori* and prevents benzo[a]pyrene-induced stomach tumors. *Proc Natl Acad Sci USA* 2002;99(11): 7810–5.
16. Galan MV, Kishan AA, Silverman AL. Oral broccoli sprouts for the treatment of *Helicobacter pylori* infection: A preliminary report. *Dig Dis Sci* 2004;49(7–8):1088–90.
17. Gattuso M, Di Sapio O, Gattuso S, Pereyra EL. Morphoanatomical studies of *Uncaria tomentosa* and *Uncaria guianensis* bark and leaves. *Phytomedicine* 2004;11(2–3):213–23.
18. Cheng CL, Guo JS, Luk J, Koo MW. The healing effects of *Centella* extract and asiaticoside on acetic acid induced gastric ulcers in rats. *Life Sci* 2004;74(18):2237–49.
19. Shmuely H, Yahav J, Samra Z, Chodick G, Koren R, Niv Y, Ofek I. Effect of cranberry juice on eradication of *Helicobacter pylori* in patients treated with antibiotics and a proton pump inhibitor. *Mol Nutr Food Res* 2007;51(6):746–51.
20. Bukhari MH, Khalil J, Qamar S, Qamar Z, Zahid M, Ansari N, Bakhshi IM. Comparative gastroprotective effects of natural honey, *Nigella sativa* and cimetidine against acetylsalicylic acid induced gastric ulcer in albino rats. *J Coll Physicians Surg Pak* 2011 Mar;21(3):151–6.
21. Wang ZT, Du Q, Xu GJ, Wang RJ, Fu DZ, Ng TB. Investigations on the protective action of *Condonopsis pilosula* (Dangshen) extract on experimentally-induced gastric ulcer in rats. *Gen Pharmacol* 1997;28(3):469–73.
22. Zhu Y, Zhang P, Yu H, Li J, Wang MW, Zhao W. Anti-*Helicobacter pylori* and thrombin inhibitory components from Chinese Dragon's Blood, *Dracaena cochinchinensis*. *J Nat Prod* 2007;70(10):1570–7.
23. Mahady GB, Pendland SL, Yun GS, Lu ZZ, Stoia A. Ginger (*Zinzinber officinalis* Roscoe) and the gingerols inhibit the growth of Cag A+ strains of *Helicobacter pylori*. *Anticancer Res* 2003;23(SA): 3699–702.
24. Campos AR, Barros AI, Santos FA, Rao VS. Guarana (*Paullinia cupana* Mart.) offers protection against gastric lesions induced by ethanol and indomethacin in rats. *Phytother Res* 203;17(10):1199–202.
25. Tanih NF, Dube C, Green E, Mkwetshana N, Clarke AM, Ndip LM, Ndip RN. An African perspective on *Helicobacter pylori*: Prevalence of human infection, drug resistance, and alternative approaches to treatment. *Ann Trop Med Parasitol* 2009 Apr;103(3):189–204
26. Belostotskiĭ NI, Kasianenko VI, Dubtsova EA, Lazebnik LB. Influence of honey, royal jelly and propolis on accelerating acetate healing of experimental gastric ulcers in rats. *Eksp Klin Gastroenterol* 2009;(6):46–50.
27. Zaidi SF, Yamada K, Kadowaki M, Usmanghani K, Sugiyama T. Bactericidal activity of medicinal plants, employed for the treatment of gastrointestinal ailments, against *Helicobacter pylori*. *J Ethnopharmacol* 2009 Jan 21;121(2):286–91.
28. Glick L. Deglycyrrhizinated liquorice for peptic ulcer. *Lancet* 1982;2(8302):817.
29. Yoshikawa M, Murakami T, Kishi A, Kageura T, Matsuda H. Medicinal flowers. III. Marigold.(1): hypoglycemic, gastric emptying inhibitory, and gastroprotective principles and new oleanane-type triterpene oligoglycosides, calendasaponins A, B, C, and D, from Egyptian *Calendula officinalis*. *Chem Pharm Bull* (Tokyo) 2001;49(7):863–70.
30. Chakürski I, Matev M, Stefanov G, Koĭchev A, Angelova I. Treatment of duodenal ulcers and gastroduodenitis with a herbal combination of *Symphitum officinalis* and *Calendula officinalis* with and without antacids. *Vutr Boles* 1981;20(6):44–7.
31. Al-Said MS, Ageel AM, Parmar NS, Tariq M. Evaluation of mastic, a crude drug obtained from *Pistacia lentiscus* for gastric and duodenal anti-ulcer activity. *Ethnopharmacol* 1986;15(3):271–8.
32. Paraschos S, Magiatis P, Mitakou S, Petraki K, Kalliaropoulos A, Maragkoudakis P, Mentis A, Sgouras D, Skaltsounis AL. In vitro and in vivo activities of Chios mastic gum extracts and constituents against *Helicobacter pylori*. *Antimicrob Agents Chemother* 2007;51(2):551–9.

33. Al-Habbal MJ, Al-Habbal Z, Huwez FU. A double-blind controlled clinical trial of mastic and placebo in the treatment of duodenal ulcer. *Clin Exp Pharmacol Physiol* 1984;11(5):541–4.
34. Klupinska G, Wißßniewska-Jarosińska M, Harasiuk A, Chojnacki C, Stec-Michalska K, Błasiak J, Reiter RJ, Chojnacki J. Nocturnal secretion of melatonin in patients with upper digestive tract disorders. *J Physiol Pharmacol* 2006 Nov;57 Suppl 5:41–50.
35. Konturek SJ, Konturek PC, Brzozowski T. Melatonin in gastroprotection against stress-induced acute gastric lesions and in healing of chronic gastric ulcers. *J Physiol Pharmacol* 2006 Nov;57 Suppl 5:51–66.
36. Malinovskaia NK, Rapoport SI, Zhernakova NI, Rybnikova SN, Postnikova LI, Parkhomenko IE. Antihelicobacter effects of melatonin. *Klin Med (Mosk)* 2007;85(3):40–3.
37. Konturek SJ, Konturek PC, Brzozowska I, Pawlik M, Sliwowski Z, Cześnikiewicz-Guzik M, Kwiecień S, Brzozowski T, Bubenik GA, Pawlik WW. Localization and biological activities of melatonin in intact and diseased gastrointestinal tract (GIT). *J Physiol Pharmacol* 2007 Sep;58(3):381–405.
38. Konturek SJ, Konturek PC, Brzozowski T, Bubenik GA. Role of melatonin in upper gastrointestinal tract. *J Physiol Pharmacol* 2007 Dec;58 Suppl 6:23–52.
39. Konturek PC, Celinski K, Slomka M, Cichoz-Lach H, Burnat G, Naegel A, Bielanski W, Konturek JW, Konturek SJ. Melatonin and its precursor L-tryptophan prevent acute gastric mucosal damage induced by aspirin in humans. *J Physiol Pharmacol* 2008 Aug;59 Suppl 2:67–75.
40. Lahiri S, Singh P, Singh S, Rasheed N, Palit G, Pant KK. Melatonin protects against experimental reflux esophagitis. *Pineal Res* 2009 Mar;46(2):207–13.
41. Konturek PC, Konturek SJ, Celinski K, Slomka M, Cichoz-Lach H, Bielanski W, Reiter RJ. Role of melatonin in mucosal gastroprotection against aspirin-induced gastric lesions in humans. *J Pineal Res* 2010 May;48(4):318–23.
42. Chatterjee A, Yasmin T, Bagchi D, Stohs SJ. Inhibition of *Helicobacter pylori* in vitro by various berry extracts, with enhanced susceptibility to clarithromycin. *Mol Cell Biochem* 2004;265(1–2):19–26.
43. Al-Howiriny T, Al-Sohaibani M, El-Tahir K, Rafatullah S. Prevention of experimentally-induced gastric ulcers in rats by an ethanolic extract of Parsley *Petroselinum crispum. Am J Chin Med* 2003;31(5): 699–711.
44. Best R, Lewis DA, Nasser N. The anti-ulcerogenic activity of the unripe plantain banana (*Musa* species). *Br J Pharmacol* 1984;82(1):107–16.
45. Goel RK, Gupta S, Shankar R, Sanyal AK. Anti-ulcerogenic effect of banana powder (*Musa sapientum* var. *paradisiaca*) and its effect of mucosal resistance. *J Ethnopharmacol* 1986;18(1):33–44.
46. Pannangpetch P, Vuttivirojana A, Kularbkaew C, Tesana S, Kongyingyoes B, Kukongviriyapan V. The antiulcerative effect of Thai *Musa* species in rats. *Phytother Res* 2001;15(5):407–10.
47. al-Shabanah OA. Effect of evening primrose oil on gastric ulceration and secretion induced by various ulcerogens and necrotizing agents in rats. *Food Chem Toxicol* 1997;35(8):769–75.
48. Das UN. Hypothesis: Cis-unsaturated fatty acids as potential anti-peptic ulcer drugs. *Prostaglandins Leukot Essent Fatty Acids* 1998;58(5):377–80.
49. Thompson L, Cockayne A, Spiller RC. Inhibitory effect of polyunsaturated fatty acids on the growth of *Helicobacter pylori*: A possible explanation of the effect of diet on peptic ulceration. *Gut* 1994;35(11):1557–61.
50. Wang KY, Li SN, Liu CS, Perng DS, Su YC, Wu DC, Lai CH, Wang TN, Wang WM. Effects of ingesting *Lactobacillus*- and *Bifidobacterium*-containing yogurt in subjects with colonized *Helicobacter pylori. Am J Clin Nutr* 2004;80(3):737–41.
51. Sheu BS, Cheng HC, Kao AW, Wang ST, Yang YJ, Yang HB, Wu JJ. Pretreatment with *Lactobacillus*- and *Bifidobacterium*-containing yogurt can improve the efficacy of quadruple therapy in eradicating residual *Helicobacter pylori* infection after failed triple therapy. *Am J Clin Nutr* 2006;83(4):864–9.
52. Nostro A, Cellini L, Di Bartolomeo S, Canatelli MA, Di Campli E, Procopio F, Grande R, Marzio L, Alonzo V. Effects of combining extracts from propolis or *Zigiber officinalis* with clarithromycin on *Helicobacter pylori. Phytother Res* 2006;20(3):187–90.
53. Alarcon de la Lastra C, Martin MJ, Motilva V. Antiulcer and gastroprotective effects of quercetin: A gross and histologic study. *Pharmacology* 1994;48(1):56–62.
54. Gao Y, Zhou S, Wen J, Huang M, Xu A. Mechanism of the antiulcerogenic effect of *Ganoderma lucidum* polysaccharides on indomethacin-induced lesions in the rat. *Life Sci* 2002;72(6):731–45.
55. http://www.yalacta.com/public/index.php?a=sano-gastril&yalacta=b05753a2c79ecc5517a3554ea87df2de.
56. Xing J, Yang B, Dong Y, Wang B, Wang J, Kallio HP. Effects of sea buckhorn (*Hippophae rhamnoides* L.) seed and pulp oil on experimental models of gastric ulcer in rats. *Fitoterapia* 2002;73(7–8):644–50.
57. Srikanta BM, Siddaraju MN, Dharmesh SM. A novel phenol-bound pectic polysaccharide from *Decalepis hamiltonii* with multi-step ulcer preventive activity. *World J Gastroenterol* 2007;13(39):5196–207.

58. Matsubara S, Shibata H, Ishikawa F, Yokokura T, Takahashi M, Sugimura T, Wakabayashi K. Suppression of *Helicobacter pylori*-induced gastritis by green tea extract in Mongoian gerbils. *Biochem Biophys Res Commun* 2003;310(3):715–9.

59. Kim DC, Kim SH, Choi BH, Baek NI, Kim D, Kim MJ, Kim KT. *Curcuma longa* extract protects against gastric ulcers by blocking H2 histamine receptors. *Biol Pharm Bull* 2005;28(12):2220–4.

60. Chuang CH, Sheu BS, Kao AW, Cheng HC, Huang AH, Yang HB, Wu JJ. Adjuvant effect of vitamin C on omeprazole-amoxicillin-clarithromycin triple therapy for *Helicobacter pylori* eradication. *Hepatogastroenterology* 2007;54(73):320–6.

61. Kamiji MM, Oliveira RB. Effect of vitamin C administration on gastric colonization by *Helicobacter pylori*. *Arch Gastroenterol* 2005;42(3):167–72.

62. Darababu M, Prabha T, Pryambada S, Agrawal VK, Aryya NC, Goel RK. Effect of *Bacopa monnieri* and *Azadirachta indica* on gastric ulceration and healing in NIDDM rats. *Indian J Exp Biol* 2004;42(4):389–97.

63. Potrich FB, Allemand A, daSilva LM, Dos Santos AC, Baggio CH, Freitas CS, Mendes DA, Andre E, Werner MF, Marques MC. Antiulcerogenic activity of hydroalcoholic extract of *Achillea millefolium* L.: Involvement of the antioxidant system. *J Ethnopharmacol* 2010 Jul 6;130(1):85–92.

64. Gonzales E, Iglesias I, Carretero E, Villar A. Gastric cytoprotection of Bolivian medicinal plants. *J Ethnopharmacol* 2000;70(3):329–33.

65. Li Y, Xu C, Zhang Q, Liu JY, Tan RX. In vitro anti-*Helicobacter pylori* action of 30 Chinese medicines used to treat ulcer diseases. *J Ethnopharmacol* 2005;98(3):329–33.

66. Halpern GM. *Zinc-Carnosine: Nature's Safe and Effective Remedy for Ulcers*. Garden City Park, NY; SquareOne Publishers. 2005:42.

67. Steinhoff U. Who controls the crowd? New findings and old questions about the intestinal microflora. *Immunol Lett* 2005;99(1):12–16.

68. Daroch F, Hoeneisen M, Gonzalez CL, et al. In vitro antibacterial activity of Chilean red wines against *Helicobacter pylori*. *Microbios* 2001;104:79–85.

69. Tombola F, Campello S, De Luca L, Ruggiero P et al. Plant polyphenols inhibit VacA, a toxin secreted by the gastric pathogen *Helicobacter pylori*. *FEBS Lett* 2003;543:184–89.

13 Viral Hepatitis and Nonalcoholic Steatohepatitis

Nutrient Interventions in Management

Trent W. Nichols, Jr., M.D.

INTRODUCTION

A liver detoxifies potentially harmful foreign substances and endogenous metabolic by-products. Failure to detoxify harms the liver and human host. Historically, the focus on liver disease management has been reducing the toxic burden where possible. More recent research points to biochemical individuality in response to the same toxin burden.

Hepatitis can be thought of as a genetotrophic disease for which genetic uniqueness creates demands for specific nutrients beyond the average and for which unmet nutrient demands are associated with disease [1]. This chapter focuses on dietary patterns, food, and nutrients that can augment the liver's detoxifying system and metabolism in the face of liver disease and, if practiced before disease presents, lessen or prevent tissue and organ damage.

EPIDEMIOLOGY

Hepatitis A, hepatitis B (HBV), hepatitis C, and hepatitis E cause 95% of cases of acute viral hepatitis in the United States. (Hepatitis D requires coexisting HBV infection.) Hepatitis C is the most common cause of chronic hepatitis [2].

Viral hepatitis epidemiology is changing with immigrants and adoptees from areas where HBV is endemic. In these areas, hepatitis B is often acquired transplacentally with a chronic carriage rate of 90% without medical intervention. Due to improved viral testing, blood transfusions have decreased as a cause of transferring hepatitis B and C. Intravenous drug use, unsafe sex, and tattoos are now the leading means of acquiring hepatitis B and C. There are 1.4 million deaths annually in the United States from hepatocellular carcinoma and cirrhosis as a complication of hepatitis B [3]. Hepatitis C infects an estimated three to four million people in the United States and is only self-limiting in 15% of the cases. Of the 85% who have chronic hepatitis C, the majority will have elevated or fluctuating serum alanine aminotransferase (ALT) and one-third will have persistently normal ALT. The latter group is now eligible for peginterferon and ribavirin therapy to prevent continued liver injury and detectable viremia [4]. Triple therapy using a protease inhibitor, either boceprevir or telaprevir, in addition to pegintron and ribavirin, is available now for hepatitis C therapy with increased viral clearing in patients in 24 weeks instead of the previous 48-week course.

Nonalcoholic steatohepatitis (NASH) has recently become the third cause for liver transplantation. It is projected to be the leading cause sometime in the future as obesity and diabetes prevalence increases. The spectrum of fatty liver ranges from nonalcoholic fatty liver disease (NAFLD) with normal enzymes to NASH as the leading cause of transaminasemia. By proton magnetic resonance (MR) spectroscopy, the Dallas Heart study (a population-based cohort study performed in an ethnically diverse community in the United States) reported that one in three adult Americans have hepatic steatosis. The findings indicate that more than 70 million Americans have NAFLD [5].

Preliminary genetic data for NASH suggest that polymorphisms in genes encoding microsomal triglyceride transfer protein, superoxide dismutase 2, the CD14 endotoxin receptor, tumor necrosis factor a, transforming growth factor b, and angiotensinogen may be associated with steatohepatitis or hepatic fibrosis or both [6].

In summary, inheritance, gender, lifestyle habits, nutrition, and health status influence the activities of various detoxification enzymes. Polymorphism of liver detoxification enzymes have been associated with increased prevalence of many degenerative diseases [7].

PATHOPHYSIOLOGY

Hepatic steatosis arises from an imbalance between triglyceride accumulation and removal as outlined in Figure 13.1 [8]. Genetic defects have been discovered that prevent the removal of triglycerides from the liver, which cause steatosis. Additionally, defects in the enzymes required for oxidation of free fatty acids in mitochondria (the hydroxyacyl-CoA transferase) also cause hepatic steatosis [9], Recent insight into the pathophysiology of fatty liver now suggest deficits in oxidative phosphorylation, glucose, and fatty acid disposal in various stages of insulin resistance with a common pathway of impairments in mitochondrial function [10].

Adipose tissue IL-6 expression is increased in obesity and is a strong predictor of abnormalities in adipocyte and systemic metabolism. A study demonstrated that IL-6 impairs insulin signaling in both the 3T3-L1 model of adipocyte model system and human adipocytes [11].

Magnetic resonance spectroscopy studies in humans suggest that a defect in insulin-stimulated glucose transport occurs by inhibiting insulin-stimulated tyrosine phosphorylation of insulin receptor substrate-1 (IRS-1) and IRS-1–associated phosphatidylinositol 3 kinase activity. A number of different metabolic abnormalities may increase fat delivery to muscle and liver as a consequence of either excess energy intake or defects in adipocyte fat metabolism, and acquired or inherited defects in mitochondrial fatty acid oxidation [12].

Liver detoxification is a two-phase process where each phase requires nutrients. If those nutrients are inadequately present, the liver's ability to manage the oxidative by-products is compromised. Phase I detoxification is conducted by the specialized members of the cytochrome P450 mixed-function oxidase family of enzymes resulting in production of a new class of compounds called biotransformed intermediates. These are converted into a form that can be easily excreted. Many toxins are fat soluble and tend to accumulate in fatty tissues. Phase II detoxification involves the combination of these newly biotransformed intermediates with substances in the liver to make them water soluble for excretion as nontoxic substances in the urine and bile [13].

In order for phase I and the eight separate phase II processes to function properly, specific nutrients are required: vitamins C, E, and B complex, bioflavonoids, glutathione, and the sulfur-containing amino acid cysteine [14]. The amino acids glycine, taurine, methionine, and vitamins and minerals are additionally needed to activate the conjugation phase II pathways [15].

Viral hepatitis and NASH both exert inflammatory stress on the liver. The liver in turn requires more detoxifying nutrients to manage inflammation, mitochondrial stress, and other processes

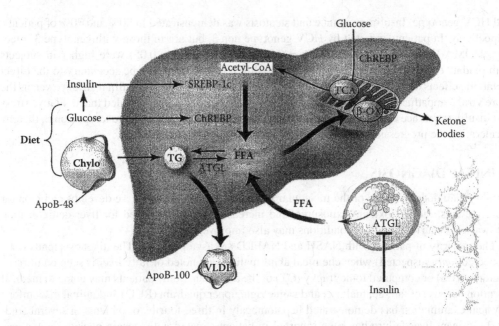

FIGURE 13.1 Metabolism of TG in the liver. The three major sources of free fatty acids (FFA) are diet, endogenous synthesis, and peripheral tissues. FFA have four possible fates. They can be metabolized by B oxidation (B-ox) in mitochondria, esterified and stored as TG in lipid droplets, used to form other lipids (not shown), or packed with apoB into VLDL and secreted into blood. Processes that increase FFA and triglyceride (TG) input or reduce FFA and TG output cause hepatic steatosis. Carbohydrate intake increases glucose and insulin levels, which activate two transcription factors in the liver that promote de novo lipogensis: ChREBP and SREBP-1c. Insulin inhibits lipolysis in adipose tissue by suppressing ATGL, chylo, chylomicron, TCA, and tricarboxylic acid. (Reproduced with permission from Cohen JC, Horton JD, Hobs HH; *Science*, vol 332, p. 1519–23, June 24, 2011.)

occurring at the molecular and cellular levels. When the molecular insults are not fully neutralized, inflammation results. Free radicals overwhelm the antioxidant reserve of the mitochondria of the cell. Repeated and ongoing inflammation results in liver damage visible at the tissue level. Fibrosis from the stellate cells is an overzealous attempt to wall off the inflammation to keep it from spreading. This process may result in altered architecture of the liver lobule reducing access to the arterial and portal blood flow and bile removal leading to cirrhosis and portal hypertension [16]. When the liver is inflamed, insulin resistance and abdominal fat increase the steatosis in the liver and predispose the gallbladder to stone formations.

In chronic hepatitis, hepatic hypoxia and oxidative stress may occur during the inflammatory and fibrotic processes that characterize these chronic liver diseases of viral origin. As a consequence, new vascular structures are formed to provide oxygen and nutrients and to repair cellular damage from oxidative stress. Angiogenesis with growth factors and molecules involved in matrix remodeling, cell migration, and vessel maturation–related factors are involved with liver diseases and liver regeneration [17].

A study published in the *Journal of Hepatology* confirmed the aforementioned hypothesis on the pathophysiology of hepatitis C. This study investigated the relationship among oxidative stress, insulin resistance, steatosis, and fibrosis in patients with chronic hepatitis C (CHC). IgG against malondialdehyde-albumin adducts and homeostasis model assessment derived from fasting plasma glucose and insulin level (HOMA-IR) were measured as markers of oxidative stress and insulin resistance in 107 consecutive CHC patients. Oxidative stress was present in 61% of the patients, irrespective of age, gender, viral load, BMI, aminotransferase level, histology activity index (HAI), and HCV genotype. Insulin resistance and steatosis was demonstrated in 80% and 70% of patients, respectively. In patients infected by HCV genotype non-3, but not in those with genotype 3 infection, HOMA-IR ($p < 0.03$), steatosis ($p = 0.02$), and fibrosis ($p < 0.05$) were higher in subjects with oxidative stress than in those without. The difference is thought to be secondary to the direct metabolic effects of genotype 1 infection that result in hepatic steatosis/insulin resistance versus the more viral cytopathic effect of genotype 3 infection. The researchers concluded that oxidative stress and insulin resistance contribute to steatosis in patients infected with HCV genotype non-3, thereby accelerating the progression of fibrosis [18].

CLINICAL DIAGNOSIS

Primary care doctors aware of the molecular process by which liver disease develops can monitor these patients, reduce toxicant exposures, and increase nutrients required for liver detoxification pathways. Concurrent medical conditions may also improve.

The majority of patients with NASH and NAFLD are asymptomatic. The diagnosis tends to be suspected (*only* suspected) when chemical abnormalities are noted or fatty liver is seen on ultrasonography (US) or computed tomography (CT) of the abdomen. Some patients may come to medical attention because of fatigue, malaise, and vague right upper quadrant (RUQ) abdominal discomfort. Physical examination has demonstrated hepatomegaly in three-fourths of patients in several studies. Fulminant liver failure has been reported in patients treated with certain nucleoside analogs, antimiotic agents, and tetracycline. In other patients with inborn errors of metabolism, such as tyrosinemia, fatty liver or steatosis appear to progress rapidly to cirrhosis and commonly lead to death from various liver-related complications including hepatocellular carcinoma. Liver biopsy is seldom necessary to diagnose NAFLD, and is currently made to exclude other causes of chronic hepatitis [19].

However, many patients with chronic illnesses have some impairment of liver detoxification of which they and many of their doctors are unaware. They do not have elevated aspartate aminotransferase (AST), ALT, or gamma-glutamyl transferase (GGT) but are often on a number of pharmaceuticals and often have drug interactions and sensitivities. Symptoms often demonstrate sensitivities to perfumes, car exhaust, fumes from gasoline or paint, and common household cleansing agents and chemicals. Physical examination often reveals palmar erythema, which hepatologists would say indicates that they have cirrhosis, but they do not. These patients are experiencing liver disease at the molecular and cellular level, which is not yet visible on a tissue level.

Hypertrigyleridemia is associated with fatty liver (NASH and NAFLD). A ratio of the triglycerides divided by the HDL of 3.0 or greater and triglycerides of 130 mg/dl or greater can be used in the absence of standardized insulin assays to screen patients for insulin resistance [20]. However, this ratio is not a reliable marker of insulin resistance in African American or Hispanic [21] populations in the United States with higher rates of diabetes. Another calculation is the *homeostatic model assessment for insulin* resistance (HOMA-IR) that multiples the fasting insulin by the fasting glucose divided by 405 if glucose is expressed as mg/dL and insulin expressed as μU/ml. Insulin resistance is usually diagnosed with a HOMA of 3.0 or greater [22]. A number of online calculators are available; if glucose is measured in mmol/l, the constant 22.5 is used.

Presently, the only laboratory offering a liver detox profile is Doctors Data. Accordingly, a reliable biomarker for exposure to toxic chemicals is urinary D-glucaric acid. Elevated levels of D-glucaric acid indicate induction of cytochrome P-450 enzymes (phase 1) as a result of exposure to xenobiotics. Urinary levels of mercapturic acids indicate quantitatively the degree of activity of phase 2 detoxification. Mercapturic acids are the final excretory products of detoxification and include a spectrum of xenobiotics that have been conjugated with glutathione of L-cysteine prior to excretion. Low levels of mercapturic acids are consistent with insufficient levels of glutathione and or L-cysteine [23].

VIRAL HEPATITIS

Antioxidants protect the liver from oxidative damage to the mitochondria, and their effects in the regulation of angiogenesis and fibrosis are also highly protective [24].

Researchers at Shandong University in China investigated the impacts of interferon alpha-2b (IFN alpha-2b) on the oxidative stress states in the treatment of chronic hepatitis B (CHB) with different genotypes. Thirty-five patients with chronic hepatitis B and 18 healthy volunteers as a control were enrolled in the study. In control and patient groups, the serum alanine aminotransferase (ALT), aspartate aminotransferase (AST), malondialdehyde (MDA), and total antioxidative stress capacity (TAC) were measured spectrophotometrically. After the therapy with interferon alpha-2b via intramuscular injection thrice a week for 12 weeks, these parameters were measured again in the patient group. The serum levels of MDA after the treatment with IFN alpha-2b were significantly lower than the pretreatment levels ($p < 0.05$), which even returned to the normal concentration ($p > 0.05$) in the responsive group. There were also significant increases in the TAC after the IFN alpha-2b therapy in this group. However, the significant differences in the TAC levels before and after the INF alpha-2b treatment were not observed in the nonresponsive group. They concluded that oxidative stress could be improved with IFN alpha-2b treatment of chronic hepatitis B patients. The results suggested that antioxidant treatment for chronic hepatitis B patients may help improve the effect of antivirus therapy [25].

The good news is that there are several promising treatment options for completely eradicating the hepatitis B virus. Currently, there are seven FDA-approved drugs in the United States to treat chronic HBV: Intron A (Interferon Alpha), Pegasys (Pegylated Interferon), Epivir HBV (Lamivudine), Hepsera (Adefovir), Baraclude (Entecavir), Tyzeka (Telbivudine), and Viread (Tenofovir). There is still viral resistance that develops in some of the older drugs, such as Lamivudine. As a result, the newer drugs are now used to avoid viral relapse on therapy.

A review of the effects of silymarin on viral hepatitis by studying 148 papers elucidated its actions as follows: Silymarin is reported to have antioxidant properties, by increasing superoxide dismutase activity in erythrocytes and lymphocytes. It is also reported to stabilize hepatocyte membrane structure, thereby preventing toxins from entering the cell through enterohepatic recirculation, and to promote liver regeneration by stimulating nucleolar polymerase A and increasing ribosomal protein synthesis. Silybin selectively inhibits leukotriene formation by Kupffer cells and is a mild chelator of iron. It also prevents gluthatione depletion in human hepatocyte cultures, protecting cells from methotrexate and ethanol induced damage in vitro. Studies concluded that the silymarin—when used to treat viral hepatitis, decreased serum transaminases in patients with chronic viral hepatitis, but did not appear to affect viral load or liver histology. Nevertheless, it may be worthwhile to determine its effects in conjunction with standard antiviral treatment [26].

The aim of another study was to determine oxidant/antioxidant status of patients with chronic hepatitis C (CHC), and the effect of pegylated interferon alfa-2b plus ribavirin combination therapy on oxidative stress. Nineteen patients with chronic HCV infection and 28 healthy controls were included in the research. In control and patient groups, serum alanine aminotransferase (ALT), aspartate aminotransferase (AST), erythrocyte malondialdehyde (MDA), erythrocyte CuZn-superoxide dismutase (SOD), and erythrocyte glutathione peroxidase (GSH-Px) activities were measured. After pegylated interferon alfa-2b and ribavirin combination therapy for 48 weeks, these parameters were measured again in the patient group. Serum MDA levels increased significantly in CHC patients ($n = 19$) before the treatment when compared with healthy subjects ($n = 28$), 9.28 +/– 1.61, 4.20 +/– 1.47 mmol/ml, $p < 0.001$, respectively. MDA concentration decreased significantly ($p < 0.001$) after the treatment as did ALT and AST activity in erythrocytes of these patients. Superoxide dismutase and glutathione peroxidase were significantly lower in erythrocytes of patients with CHC before treatment compared with the control group (both, $p < 0.001$). These results show that patients with chronic HCV infection are under the influence of oxidative stress associated with lower levels of antioxidant enzymes. These impairments return to the levels of healthy controls after pegylated interferon alfa-2b plus ribavirin combination therapy of CHC patients. The study concluded that although interferon and ribavirin are not antioxidants, their antiviral capacity might reduce viral load and inflammation, and perhaps through this mechanism might reduce virus-induced oxidative stress [27].

In another study, 100 chronic HCV infection patients who failed interferon treatment were enrolled and randomly assigned to receive combined intravenous and oral antioxidants or placebo or oral treatment alone. Primary end points were liver enzymes, HCV-RNA levels, and histology. The investigators found that combined oral and intravenous antioxidant therapy was associated with a significant decline in ALT levels in 52% of patients who received antioxidant therapy versus 20% of patients who received placebo (P = 0.05). Histology activity index (HAI) scores at the end of treatment were reduced in 48% of patients who received antioxidant therapy versus 26% of patients who received placebo (P = 0.21). HCV-RNA levels decreased by 1-log or more in 28% of patients who received antioxidant therapy versus 12% who received placebo (P = NS). In part II of the trial, oral administration of antioxidants was not associated with significant alterations in any of the end points. The authors concluded that antioxidant therapy has a mild beneficial effect on the inflammatory response of chronic HCV infection patients who are nonresponders to interferon. Combined antiviral and antioxidant therapy may be beneficial for these patients [28].

Dr. Burt Berkson at New Mexico State University's Integrative Medical Center described a low-cost and efficacious treatment program in three patients with cirrhosis, portal hypertension, and esophageal varices secondary to chronic hepatitis C infection. This regimen combined alpha-lipoic acid 300 mg twice daily, silymarin 300 mg daily, and selenium 200 mcg twice a day. (Berkson used what was available then. Alpha-lipoic acid was only available from Germany as a mixture of dextro and levo forms.) Each substance protects the liver from free-radical damage, increases the levels of other fundamental antioxidants, and interferes with viral proliferation. The three patients presented in this paper followed the triple antioxidant program, recovered quickly, and their laboratory values remarkably improved. Furthermore, liver transplantation was avoided and the patients were back at work, carrying out their normal activities, and feeling healthy. The author concluded that the conservative triple antioxidant treatment approach should be considered prior to liver transplant surgery evaluation or during the transplant evaluation process. If these is a significant betterment in the patient's condition, liver transplant surgery may be avoided [29]. Because alpha-lipoic acid increases the liver cells' ability to make glutathione, it has been used to treat other forms of hepatitis [30,31].

NONALCOHOLIC STEATOHEPATITIS (FATTY LIVER)

Nonalcoholic fatty liver disease (NAFLD) is the leading cause of abnormal liver enzymes in the United States. Nonalcoholic steatohepatitis (NASH), a more serious form of NAFLD, can proceed to cirrhosis and even hepatocellular carcinoma. These liver diseases represent the hepatic component of the metabolic syndrome, and this spectrum of liver disease represents a major health problem both in the United States and worldwide with NASH projected to be the leading reason for liver transplantation in the near future.

Unfortunately, from a strictly clinical medicine perspective, NASH is a disease in search of an effective therapy. Most of the current regimens have been tested in open label, uncontrolled trials that have been carried out over a relatively short period of time; most of these studies did not adhere to a strict histologic end point [32]. None have been convincingly effective. However, understanding how liver disease at the tissue level is the result of aberrant molecular and cellular processes that generally began years beforehand presents broader possibilities for treatment interventions and is therefore a reason to diagnose disease early.

Diet and Weight Reduction

Hepatic steatosis is closely linked to diet. Lifestyle choices and altered genetic signaling are intertwined in a vicious cycle that produces abnormalities in lipid and glucose metabolism. Dr. Joseph L Goldstein, Nobel laureate, professor of medicine and genetics at the Southwestern School of Medicine, University of Texas, said that although many assume the process requires years of poor diet, inadequate exercise, and less than optimal lifestyle, it could be accelerated enormously. He cited the 2004 documentary *Super Size Me* in which Morgan Spurlock monitored his metabolic function while consuming all his meals at a fast food restaurant over a 30-day period. "Morgan Spurlock was able to develop metabolic syndrome in less than a month and it took him six months to reverse it." Goldstein stated the major physiological change in Spurlock as well as others with metabolic syndrome is a fatty liver. "One of the most important mediators of metabolic function in the liver is (SREBP) sterol regulatory element binding protein. A high glucose intake in the diet triggers the pancreas to produce increased amounts of insulin. The liver continues to produce glucose despite the high glucose intake. Ultimately, the downstream effects of sustained hyperglycemia leads to type 2 diabetes mellitus and the abnormally elevated SREPB-1c activity leads to increased synthesis of fatty acids and triglyceride in the liver, resulting in a fatty liver" [33].

Refined carbohydrates can increase inflammation and triglyceride levels. A study of 74 obese patients undergoing bariatric surgery at Johns Hopkins was conducted by Dr. Steve Solga and Dr. Anna Mae Diehl. All patients underwent a preoperative dietary evaluation using a standardized 24-hour food recall. Food intake was evaluated for total calories and macronutrients and compared to liver histopathology from biopsies routinely obtained during surgery. The authors found there were no significant associations between total caloric intake or protein intake and steatosis, fibrosis, or inflammation. However, higher carbohydrate intake was associated with significantly higher odds of inflammation, while higher fat intake was associated with significantly lower odds of inflammation [34]. This contradicted previous recommendation of fat restriction and the increase therefore of carbohydrates.

It has also been demonstrated that rapid weight loss may actually elevate liver enzymes. It can also spasm the gallbladder and theoretically cause more oxidative stress by release of toxins that have been stored in fat. Therefore, most experts recommend that the reduction of weight in obese patients with NAFLD should be gradual (< 1.6 kg per week) [35]. Sibutramine (Meridia)—which now has been removed from the market, and orlistat (Xenical) used in weight reduction have shown improved results of liver function tests and decreased sonographic evidence of steatosis in NASH patients [36].

Bariatric surgery has also been studied in NASH. Roux-en-Y gastric bypass surgery was retrospectively studied in 29 patients undergoing surgery. At that time, patients had achieved a mean weight loss of 116.9 lbs, with a significant decrease in body mass index (28.9 ± 5.8 kg/m^2 vs. 47.8 ± 6.6 kg/m^2), relative to presurgery baseline. Mean scores revealed that liver histology other than portal fibrosis improved after gastric bypass. The author concluded that fibrosis or scarring may be permanent. "Liver function tests showed some improvement in test results after gastric bypass, but even at baseline the values were within the normal range," noted Dr. R. H. Clements, a noted gastric bypass surgeon, emphasizing the role of biopsy in diagnosing NASH [37].

Toxin Avoidance

The most studied toxins that can be avoided are smoking tobacco products. Smoking increases the fibrosis and progression to cirrhosis in both chronic viral hepatitis and NASH. Cigarette smoking induces three major adverse effects on the liver: direct or indirect toxic effects, immunological effects, and oncogenic effects. Smoking yields chemical substances with cytotoxic potential that increase necroinflammation and fibrosis. In addition, smoking increases the production of proinflammatory cytokines (IL-1, IL-6, and TNF- alpha) that would be involved in liver cell injury.

Smoking affects both cell-mediated and humoral immune responses by blocking lymphocyte proliferation and inducing apoptosis of lymphocytes. Smoking also increases serum and hepatic iron that
induce oxidative stress and lipid peroxidation and lead to activation of stellate cells and development
of fibrosis. Smoking yields oncogenic chemicals that increase the risk of hepatocellular carcinoma
(HCC) in patients with viral hepatitis and are independent of viral infection as well. Tobacco smoking has been associated with suppression of p53 (tumor suppressor gene). Heavy smoking affects
the sustained virological response to interferon (IFN) therapy in hepatitis C patients, which can be
improved by repeated phlebotomy to alleviate the secondary polycythemia caused by it [38].

Food, water, and air exposure to toxins play a role in NASH. There is increasing interest in the
potential interaction of toxins and liver detoxification and their interactions with nutrients [39]. Is
that because some exposures can be avoided or mitigated through nutrient optimization? All genes
are epigenetic and avoidance of exposure and nutrient optimization modify gene expression.

Low doses of bisphenol A induce gene expression related to lipid synthesis and trigger triglyceride accumulation in adult mouse liver [40]. Rubratoxin B is a mycotoxin that causes hypoglycemia
and fatty liver. It induces signs of fatty acid oxidation disorders (FAODs) in mice by depleting
hepatic glycogen stores by inhibiting PEPCK gene transcription [41]. Fumanisin, a mycotoxin from
fungi, and aflatoxins also are well established to cause fatty liver disease [42].

The majority of research published in studies of NASH excludes any patients who consume alcohol because the pathology is virtually identical with steatosis, including Mallory bodies (alcoholic
hyaline) in both entities. Alcohol consumption is considered a risk factor in NAFLD progressing to
NASH [43].

Specific Foods

Sulfur-containing foods include onions, cabbages, some water sources, and cruciferous vegetables
that include broccoli, brussels sprouts, and cauliflower. Sulfation couples toxins with sulfur containing compounds, important in detoxifying drugs, food additives, environmental toxins, and toxins
from gut bacteria. This is also the main pathway for detoxifying steroid and thyroid hormones.

Citrus fruits contain glucuronic acid, which provides the process of glucuronidation with toxins. This detoxification is important because many commonly used OTC medications are handled
through this pathway, including aspirin, and food additives such as benzoates and menthol [44].

Nutrients

A number of nutrients or naturally occurring substances have also been tried for NASH. Historically
nutrients have been used, some like silymarin—since Roman times—and others like vitamin E,
since the discovery of antioxidants, have found a place in NASH armentarium.

Recently, n-3 polyunsaturated fatty acid (n-3 PUVA)–enriched diets have been shown in animal
studies to reduce hepatic triglyceride content and the development of steatohepatitis [44]. A clinical
trial studying the role of n-3 PUVA in NAFLD was conducted in 2005. ALT, GGT, and ultrasound
improvement in NAFLD were shown in the 42 patients who received 1 gm n-3 PUVA daily over a
period of 12 months. A larger study evaluating 134 patients randomized to a control group (calorie
restricted diet and placebo) and the study group who received 2 g thrice daily of n-3 PUVA demonstrated a 53% reduction in fatty liver compared to 35% reduction in those on diet and placebo
[45]. Similar improvements in imaging and biochemical markers in NAFLD was seen in another
study [46].

Betaine

Betaine (which is N-trimethylglycine), a methyl donor initially found in sugar beets, has been
used in a number of clinical trials along with folate and vitamin B12 to reduce homocysteine, a
toxic amino acid implicated in cardiovascular and neurodegenerative disease [47]. A small clinical

trial conducted at the Mayo Clinic and published in the *American Journal of Gastroenterology* in 2001 demonstrated that betaine, a naturally occurring metabolite of choline had been shown to raise S-adenosylmethionine (SAMe) levels that may decrease hepatic steatosis. Ten adult patients with NASH were enrolled and received betaine in two daily doses for 12 months. A significant improvement in serum levels of AST (p = 0.002) and ALT (p = 0.007) occurred during treatment. Aminotransferase normalized in three of seven patients that completed the year-long trial. Similarly, a marked improvement in the degree of steatosis, necroinflammatory grade, and stage of fibrosis was also noted at one year [48].

The effect of betaine on steatohepatitis has been elucidated. In this study, the effects of betaine on fat accumulation in the liver induced by high-sucrose diet and mechanisms by which betaine could attenuate or prevent hepatic steatosis were examined. Male C57BL/6 mice were divided into four groups (eight mice per group) and started on one of four treatments: standard diet (SD), SD + betaine, high-sucrose diet (HS), and HS + betaine. Betaine was supplemented in the drinking water at a concentration of 1% (anhydrous). Long-term feeding of a high-sucrose diet to mice caused significant hepatic steatosis accompanied by markedly increased lipogenic activity. Betaine significantly attenuated hepatic steatosis in this animal model, and this change was associated with increased activation of hepatic AMP-activated protein kinase (AMPK) and attenuated lipogenic capability (enzyme activities and gene expression) in the liver [49].

Ursodeoxycholic Acid

Ursodeoxycholic acid, a bile salt that has been approved by the FDA for primary biliary cirrhosis (PBC), is marketed as URSO Forte™ and URSO 250. URSO has, in more than 10 years of clinical studies, proven its effectiveness and safety to delay the progression of PBC, normalize liver function tests and decrease the incidence of esophageal varices by 60%.

In pilot studies, it was found by itself not to be effective in NASH and therefore was used in combination with antioxidants and other agents. Patients with elevated aminotransferase levels with biopsy-proven NASH were randomly assigned to receive UDCA 12-15 mg/kg-1/day-1 with vitamin E 400 IU twice a day (UDCA/Vit E), UDCA with placebo (UDCA/P), or placebo/placebo (P/P). After two years, they underwent a second liver biopsy. Forty-eight patients were included, 15 in the UDCA/Vit E group, 18 in the UDCA/P group, and 15 in the P/P group; 8 patients dropped out, none because of side effects. Baseline parameters were not significantly different among the three groups. Body mass index remained unchanged during the study. AST and ALT levels diminished significantly in the UDCA/Vit E group. Neither the AST nor the ALT levels improved in the P/P group and only the ALT levels in the UDCA/P group. Histologically, the activity index was unchanged at the end of the study in the P/P and UDCA/P groups, but it was significantly better in the UDCA/Vit E group, mostly as a result of regression of steatosis. The authors concluded that two years of treatment with UDCA in combination with vitamin E improved laboratory values and hepatic steatosis of patients with NASH. Larger trials are warranted [50]. Ursodeoxycholic acid (UDCA) is marketed as Actigall and Urso.

N-Acetylcysteine

N-acetylcysteine (NAC) has been used to increase glutathione in the liver, which is one of the detoxifying enzymes used for liver conjugation of toxins. Its use in NASH follows the logic that abnormalities in liver detoxification may be in part important in pathogenesis of fatty liver and transaminasemia. N-acetylcysteine was studied in models of NASH in a research project with male Sprague-Dawley rats with three groups of diets. Group 1 (control, n = 8) had free access to regular dry rat chow (RC) for six weeks. Group 2 (NASH, n = 8) was fed with a 100% fat diet for six weeks. Group 3 (NASH+NAC (20), n = 9) was fed with a 100% fat diet plus 20 mg/kg per day of NAC orally for six weeks. All rats were sacrificed to collect blood and liver samples at the end of the study. The study found the levels of total glutathione (GSH) and hepatic malondialdehyde (MDA) were increased significantly in the NASH group as compared with the control group (P < 0.05).

Livers from group 2 showed moderate to severe macrovesicular steatosis, hepatocyte ballooning, and necroinflammation. NAC treatment improved the level of GSH (P < 0.05), and led to a decrease in fat deposition and necroinflammation. The authors concluded that NAC treatment could attenuate oxidative stress and improve liver histology in rats with NASH [51].

S-Adenosylmethionine

In another model, rats were fed a methionine-choline deficient (MCD) diet and given S-adenosylmethionine (SAMe), or 2(RS)-n-propylthiazolidine-4(R)-carboxylic acid (PTCA), two agents that stimulate glutathione (GSH) biosynthesis on the development of experimental steato-hepatitis. These two agents suppressed abnormal enzyme activities in the treated rats, whereas the control rats developed elevated transaminasemia. MCD rats developed severe liver pathology manifested by fatty degeneration, inflammation, and necrosis, which significantly improved with therapy. Blood levels of GSH were significantly depleted in MCD rats but normalized in the treated groups. The researchers found a significant upregulation of genes involved in tissue remodeling and fibrosis (matrix metalloproteinases, collagen-alpha1), suppressors of cytokines signaling, and the inflammatory cytokines in the livers of rats fed MCD. The authors concluded that GSH-enhancing therapies significantly attenuated the expression of deleterious proinflammatory and fibrogenic genes in this dietary model [52].

Phosphatidycholine

Suboptimal amounts of the nutrient choline have been measured in the US population. A study of two-month inpatient diets of 15 female subjects controlled for choline level was conducted. Using pyrosequencing of 16s ribosomal RNA bacterial genes, the authors characterized the microbiota in stool samples collected over the course of the study. They identified bacterial biomarkers of fatty liver that resulted from choline deficiency [53]. Phosphatidylcholine (PC) is a phosphorylated fatty acid incorporated into cell membranes where it influences membrane movement and the function of transmembrane proteins [54].

Phosphatidylcholine became of interest in NAFLD research when it was demonstrated to be reduced in a mouse model of starvation-induced hepatic steatosis. After 24 hours of fasting, it appears that starvation reduced the phospholipids (PL). Phosphatidylcholine was used in another animal model of NASH. Rats were fed orotic acid (OA) containing triglyceride (TG) or PC (20% of dietary lipid, PC + OA group) for 10 days. Rats fed the TG diet without OA supplementation served as the control group. Administering OA significantly increased the weights and TG accumulation in livers of the TG + OA group compared with the control group. The researchers found that the PC + OA group did not show TG accumulation and OA-induced increases of these enzyme activities; a significant increase in the activity of carnitine palmityl transferase, a rate-limiting enzyme of fatty acid beta-oxidation, was found in the PC + OA group. The researchers concluded that dietary PC appears to alleviate the OA-induced hepatic steatosis and hepatomegaly, mainly through the attenuation of hepatic TG synthesis and enhancement of fatty acid beta-oxidation in Sprague-Dawley rats [55].

Silymarin

Silymarin or milk thistle has been used in a number of clinical trials of NASH. Silybin is the main component of silymarin, which is absorbed when linked with a phytosome. In rats, this substance reduces the lipid-peroxidation and the activation of hepatic stellate cells. In humans, some non-controlled studies show that silybin is able to reduce insulin resistance, liver steatosis, and plasma markers of liver fibrosis [56].

The regulatory action of silymarin on cellular and mitochondrial permeability associated with increased membrane stability against xenobiotics injury is supported by a number of studies [57]. In a rat model of ischemia reperfusion injury, silymarin reversed the severity of mitochondrial bio-energetics including increasing ATP levels, decreasing susceptibility to mitochondrial permeability transition (MPT), and improving defects in mitochondrial respiration [58].

Silymarin has direct effects on fibrinogenesis-inhibiting collagen accumulation, even when administered late, inhibiting increases in serum aminoterminal propetide of type III procollagen [59].

Silybin in combination with vitamin E and phospholipids to improve its antioxidant activity was used in the following study. Eighty-five patients were divided into two groups: those affected by nonalcoholic fatty liver disease (group A) and those with HCV-related chronic hepatitis associated with nonalcoholic fatty liver disease (group B). After treatment, group A showed a significant reduction in ultrasonographic scores for liver steatosis. Liver enzyme levels, hyperinsulinemia, and indexes of liver fibrosis showed an improvement in treated individuals. A significant correlation among indexes of fibrosis, body mass index, insulinemia, plasma levels of cytokines, degree of steatosis, and gamma-glutamyl transpeptidase was observed. The author's data suggest that silybin conjugated with vitamin E and phospholipids could be used as a complementary approach to the treatment of patients with chronic liver damage [60].

A clinical trial sponsored by Madaus, Inc., at the University of Pennsylvania, University of North Carolina, Thomas Jefferson University, Beth Israel Deaconess Medical Center, Brooke Army Medical Center, and University of Pittsburgh is currently recruiting patients with NASH using silymarin: "A Multicenter, Randomized, Double Masked, Placebo Controlled Phase II Study to Assess the Safety and Efficacy of a Standardized Orally Administered Silymarin Preparation (Legalon®) for the Treatment of Non-Cirrhotic Patients With Nonalcoholic Steatohepatitis" [61].

Unfortunately, silymarin—and even more—silybin have poor intestinal absorption that limits their bioavailability. Therefore, many studies on liver-protectant flavolignans have used phospholipid-complexed ingredients made through Phytosomes technology such as Silymarin Phytosome®, Siliphos®, or Silipide®, or the equivalent of the latter for health food applications [62].

Probiotics

Beneficial bacteria have been demonstrated to have protective effects exerted directly by specific bacterial species, control of epithelial cell proliferation and differentiation, production of essential mucosal nutrients—such as short-chain fatty acids and amino acids, prevention of overgrowth of pathogenic organisms, and stimulation of intestinal immunity. Oral probiotics are living microorganisms that upon ingestion in specific numbers exert health benefits beyond those of inherent basic nutrition. The accumulation of fat in hepatocytes with a necroinflammatory component—steatohepatitis—that may or may not have associated fibrosis is becoming a frequent lesion, as discussed earlier. Probiotics have therefore attracted attention for their inclusion in the therapeutics for NASH after being used in inflammatory bowel disease and irritable bowel. Although steatohepatitis is currently recognized to be a leading cause of cryptogenic cirrhosis, the pathogenesis has not been fully elucidated. Among the various factors implicated, intestinal bacterial overgrowth may play a role. In fact, various rat models of intestinal bacterial overgrowth have been associated with liver lesions similar to NASH, and bacterial overgrowth has been observed significantly more often in patients with NASH compared with control subjects. The authors of this paper discuss the relationship among intestinal bacterial overgrowth, steatohepatitis development, and probiotic treatment [63].

Carnitine

The lipid-lowering effects of carnitine and its precursors, lysine and methionine, were studied in an animal model of alcoholic steatosis where Sprague-Dawley rats were fed ethanol as 36% of total calories. The ethanol caused hepatic steatosis. Supplementation of the ethanol diet with 1% DL-carnitine, 0.5%L-lysine, and 0.2% L-methionine significantly lowered ethanol-induced lipid fractions. It was concluded that dietary carnitine more effectively prevented alcohol-induced hyperlipemia and accumulation of fat in livers. A deficiency of functional carnitine may indeed exist in chronic alcoholic cases [64]. A deficiency in nutrients such as carnitine, choline, and other amino acids may result from total parental nutrition (TPN) due to formulation, poor delivery, and degradation of TPN. Carnitine deficiency has been documented on long-term TPN resulting in fatty liver. Mobilization of long chain fatty acids into the mitochondria cannot occur without fatty acid shuttling, resulting from an increase in free fatty acids and the development of hepatic steatosis. However, human studies with carnitine supplementation have failed to confirm previously mentioned effects on fatty liver [65,66]. In an experimental model of insulin resistance using fructose-fed rats, L-carnitine reduced skeletal muscle lipid including triglycerides and reduced oxidative stress [67].

Glutathione

Glutathione in the form of glutathione-sulfate transferase (GSH) helps to process a large number of xenobiotics. The availability of GSH depends upon the sufficient amounts of its amino acid precursors (cysteine, glycine, and glutamic acid). Magnesium is an essential cofactor in GSH synthesis and B vitamins for methionine recycling and reducing agents. S-adenosylmethionine (SAMe) is a methyl donor and precursor of GSH. Low SAMe levels have been seen in experimental liver injury, and impaired methylation is associated with elevated homocysteine, Vitamins B2, B6, and B12, folic acid, and serine. B6 and magnesium support amino acid coupling, which is another process in which nutrients combine with drug toxins and detoxify them [68]. Hyperhomocysteinemia causes steatosis; the methylenetetrahydrofolate reductase (MTHFR) gene polymorphism (A1298) has been described in 57 well-diagnosed NASH patients and thus is a risk factor for this disease [69]. Vitamins B6 and B12, folic acid, and a methyl donor all exist at critical biochemical interactions in the methionine cycle between SAMe, and high levels of homocysteine signal a breakdown of this vital process [70].

Chlorella

Chlorella has been found to have a protective effect on liver toxicity. In a rat experiment, when chlorella was fed to the animals that were exposed to cadmium they were protected against the heavy metal by induction of metallothioneins in their livers, as compared to a control group who were not treated [71].

Branched Chained Aminoacids

Branched chain amino acids have been used in severe hepatic encephalopathy mainly by administration via total parental hyperalimentation. A study of 19 patients with grade 3–4 hepatic encephalopathy was conducted in which the patients treated regained consciousness in a mean of 27.6 and 31.5 hours of the oral lactulose group. However, the therapeutic affect was not significant between the control group and the treated group [72].

On the other hand, a Cochrane review of the literature in 2009 of clinical trials using branched chain amino acids concluded that when including trials of higher quality, the modest effect seen was not convincing enough to support the use for patients with hepatic encephalopathy [73].

SUMMARY

Patients in my practice often have established illness. This generally means that the nutrients involved in liver detoxification are in high demand, perhaps higher than they could easily obtain by select foods and diet alone. For this reason, I have expanded on my dietary, food, and lifestyle interventions to optimize the nutrients needed for liver detoxification.

In my gastroenterology and nutritional practice, I presently have many patients on nutrient powders that can be consumed as foods or beverages at usually two scoops daily [15] (Ultra Clear™ and Medi-Clear™ from Metagenics and Thorne, respectively). Powders may be better tolerated than a handful of pills and may work more effectively in the gastrointestinal lumen.

In addition, viral hepatitis patients are advised nutritionally to reduce saturated fats in their diets and cease any alcohol ingestion. They are also encouraged to use one of the previously mentioned medical food liver detoxification products and in many cases to add silymarin, standardized extract 300 mg b.i.d. A trial at the National Institutes of Health (NIH) is now ongoing involving patients with hepatitis C with silymarin at this concentration. The trial is expected to close in the near future (2012).

If a patient declines medication or is not a candidate for them, then I strongly encourage them to follow the Berkson protocol (alpha-lipoic acid 300 mg twice daily, silymarin 300 mg daily, and selenium 200 mcg twice a day).

In addition to nutrient powders, I advise NAFLD patients to lose weight with a restricted carbohydrate diet after consultation with a registered dietician, exercise with weight resistance training, and to do daily liver detoxification with one of the aforementioned medical food detoxification products. NASH patients are advised the same plus silymarin, standardized extract of silybin 300 mg, and vitamin E 400 mg (E-Thistle™) once or twice a day depending on the degree of ALT elevation. If no transaminases reduction is seen, then medical therapy with metformin is started before trying any other additional nutritional therapy.

REFERENCES

1. Wolf DC. Viral hepatitis, in *Medscape: emedicine.medscape.com/article/775507-treatment,* ed. Katz, J. Updated Oct 20, 2011.
2. Williams R. *Biochemical Individuality.* New York: John Wiley and Sons, 1956.
3. Carey WD. The prevalence and natural history of hepatitis B in the 21st century. *CCJM* 2009; 76. Suppl 3:S2–S5.
4. Berenguer M, Wright T. Viral hepatitis, in *Sleisinger and Fordtran's Gastrointestinal and Liver Disease,* ed. M. Feldman, L.S. Friedman, and M. H. Sleisinger, Vol. 2., Philadelphia: Saunders, 2002; 2385.
5. Angulo P. GI epidemiology: Nonalcoholic fatty liver disease. *Medscape: Alim Pharm Therp* 2007; 25(8):883–89.
6. de Alwis MW, Day CP. Genetics of alcoholic liver disease and nonalcoholic fatty liver disease. *Semin Liver Dis* 2007; 27(1):44–54.
7. Hyman M et al. Detoxification and biotransformational imbalances, in *Textbook of Functional Medicine,* ed. D. Jones. Gig Harbor, WA: Institute of Functional Medicine, 2006; 275–99.
8. Cohen JC. Human fatty liver disease: Old questions and new insights. *Science* 2011; 322(24):1519–23.
9. Hooper AJ et al. Genetic determinants of hepatic steatosis in man. *J. Lipid Res* 2011; 52(4):593–617.
10. Lowell BB, Shulman GI. Mitochondrial dysfunction and type 2 diabetes. *Science* 2005; 307:384–87.
11. Trujillo ME et al. Interleukin-6 regulates human adipose tissue lipid metabolism and leptin production in vitro. *J Clin Endocrinol Metab* 2004; 89(11):5577–82.
12. Parish R, Petersen KF. Mitochondrial dysfunction and type 2 diabetes. *Curr Diab Rep* 2005; 5 (3):177–83.
13. Klaassen CD, ed. *Cassert & Doull's Toxicology: The Basic Science of Poison,* 6th edition. New York: McGraw-Hill, 2004.
14. Beutler E. Nutritional and metabolic aspects of glutathione. *Annual Review of Nutrition* 1989; 9:287–302.
15. Bland JS, Benum S. *The 20-Day Rejuvenation Diet Program.* New Canaan, CT: Keats Publishing, 1997.
16. Nichols TW. *Optimal Digestive Health,* 2nd ed. Rochester, VT: Healing Arts Press, 2005;598.
17. Chaparro M et al. Angiogenesis in chronic inflammatory liver disease. *Hepatology* 2004; 39(5):1185–95.
18. Vidali M et al. Interplay between oxidative stress and hepatic steatosis in the progression of chronic hepatitis C. *J Hepatol* 2008; 48(3):399–406.
19. Diehl AM, Poordad,F. Nonalcoholic Fatty Liver Disease, in *Sleisenger & Fordtran's Gastrointestinal and Liver Disease,* 7th ed., ed. M. Feldman, L.S. Friedman, and M.H. Sleisinger, Vol. II. Philadelphia: Saunders, 2002; 1393–1401.
20. McLaughlin T et al. Use of metabolic markers to identify overweight individuals who are insulin resistant. *Ann Int Med* 2003; 139(10):802–9.
21. Sumner A et al., Fasting triglyceride and the trigylceride-HDL cholesterol ratio are not markers of insulin resistance in African Americans. *Arch Intern Med* 2005; 165(12):1395–400.
22. Bonora E et al. Homeostasis model assessment closely mirrors the glucose clamp technique in the assessment of insulin sensitivity. *Diab Care* 2000; 23(1):57–63.
23. *Hepatic Detox Profile*: www.doctorsdata.com/test_info.asp?id = 153.
24. Yang C et al. Lymphocytic microparticles inhibit angiogenesis by stimulating oxidative stress and negatively regulating VEGF-induced pathways. *Am J Physiol Regul Integr Comp Physiol,* 2007; 294(2):R467–76.

25. Fan Y et al. Oxidative stress in patients with chronic hepatitis B before and after interferon alpha-2b treatment. *Zhonghua Shi Yan He Lin Chuang Bing Du Xue Za Zhi* 2007; 21(10):23–5.

26. Mayer RP et al. Silymarin treatment of viral hepatitis: A systematic review. *J Viral Hepatitis* 2005; 12:559–67.

27. Levent G et al. Oxidative stress and antioxidant defense in patients with chronic hepatitis C patients before and after pegylated interferon alfa-2b plus ribavirin therapy. *J Transl Med* 2006; 4:25.

28. Gabbay E et al. Antioxidant therapy for chronic hepatitis C after failure of interferon: Results of phase II randomized, double-blind placebo controlled clinical trial. *World J Gastroenterol* 2007; 13(40): 5317–23.

29. Berkson B. A conservative triple antioxidant approach to the treatment of hepatitis C. Combination of alpha lipoic acid (thioctic acid), silymarin, and selenium: Three case histories. *Med Klin* (Munich) 1999; 94(Suppl 3):84–9.

30. Berkson B. Thiotic acid in treatment of hepatotoxic mushroom (Phalloides) poisoning. *N Engl J Med* 1979; 300(7):371.

31. Nichols TW. Alpha lipoic acid: biological effect and clinical implications. *Alternative Medicine Review* 1997; 2(3):177–83.

32. Nugent C, Younossi ZM. Evaluation and Management of Obesity-Related Nonalcoholic Fatty Liver Disease *Nat Clin Pract Gastroenterol Hepatol* 2007; 4(8):432–41.

33. Bosworth T. Targetting the Trigger of Metabolic Syndrome, in *Gatroenterology & Endoscopy News*. New York: McMahon Publishing, 2007; 1–24

34. Solga S et al. Dietary composition and nonalcoholic fatty liver disease. *Dig Dis Sci* 2004; 49(10):1578–83.

35. Luyckx F et al. Nonalcoholic steatohepatitis: Association with obesity and insulin resistance, and influence of weight loss. *Diabetes Metab* 2000; 26(2):98–106.

36. Sabuncu T et al. The effects of sibutramine and orlistat on the ultrasonographic findings, insulin resistance and liver enzyme levels in obese patients with nonalcoholic steatohepatitis. *Rom J Gastroenterol* 2003; 12(3):189–92.

37. Clements RH. Gastric bypass surgery significantly improves NASH, in *Medscape Gastroenterology*. 2005, Medscape: 22nd Annual Meeting of American Society of Bariatric Surgery.

38. El-Zayadi A. Heavy smoking and liver. *World J Gastroenterol* 2006; 12(38):6098–101.

39. Life Extension Web Site. *Liver degenerative disease: Toxic damage to the liver.* http://www.lef.org/protocols/prtcl-125a.shtml.

40. Marmugi A et al. Low doses of bisphenol A induce gene expression related to lipid synthesis and trigger triglyceride accumulation in adult mouse liver. *Hepatology* 2012; Feb:55(2):395–407.

41. Iwashita K, Nagashima H. Rubratoxin B reduces signs of fatty acid oxidation disorders (FAODs) in mice. *Toxicol Lett* 2011 Oct 10; 206(2):238–43. Epub 2011.

42. Peraica M et al. Toxic effects of mycotoxins in humans. *Bull World Health Org* 1999; 77(9):754–66.

43. Poullis A et al. Alcohol, obesity and TNF-a. *Gut*, 2001; 49:313–14.

44. Storlien LH et al. Fish oil prevents insulin resistance induced by high-fat feeding in rats. *Science* 1987; 237:885–8.

45. Vega GL et al. Effects of N-3 fatty acids on hepatic triglyceride content in humans. *J Investig Med* 2008; 56(5):780–5.

46. Capanni M et al. Prolonged n-3 polyunsaturated fatty acid supplementation ameliorates hepatic steatosis in patients with nonalcoholic fatty liver disease: A pilot study. *Aliment Pharmacol Ther* 2006; 23:1143–51.

47. Abdelmalek MF et al. Betaine, a promising new agent for patients with nonalcoholic steatohepatitis: results of a pilot study. *Am J Gastroemterol* 2001; 96(9):27111–7.

48. Ueland PM et al. Betaine a key modulator of one-carbon metabolism and homocysteine status. *Clin Chem Lab Med* 2005; 43(10):1069–75.

49. Song Z et al. Involvement of AMP-activated protein kinase in beneficial effects of betaine on high-sucrose diet-induced hepatic steatosis. *Am J Physiol Gastrointestinal Liver Physiol* 2007; 2924(4):G894–902.

50. Dufour JF et al. Randomized placebo-controlled trial of ursodeoxycholic acid with vitamin e in nonalcoholic steatohepatitis. *Clin Gastroenterol Hepatol* 2006; 12:1537–43.

51. Thong-Ngam D et al. N-acetylcysteine attenuates oxidative stress and liver pathology in rats with nonalcoholic steatohepatitis. *World J Gastroenterol* 2007; 13(38):5127–32.

52. Oz H. et al. Glutathione-enhancing agents protect against steatohepatitis in a dietary model. *J Biochem Mol Toxicol* 2006; 20:2714–24.

53. Spenser MD et al. Association between composition of the human gastrointestinal microbiome and development of fatty liver with choline deficiency. *Gastroenterology* 2011; 140(3):976–86.

54. Buang Y et al. Dietary phosphatidylcholine alleviates fatty liver induced by orotic acid. *Nutrition* 2005; 21(7–8):867–73.

55. Agrawal S et al. Management of nonalcoholic steatohepatitis: An analytic review. *J Clin Gastroenterol* 2002; 35(3):253–61.

56. Munter K et al. Characterization of a transporting system in rat hepatocytes. Studies with competitive and non competitive inhibitors of phalloidin transport. *Biochem Biophys Acta* 1986; 860:91–8.

57. Rolo AP et al. Protection against post-ischemic mitochondrial injury in rat liver by silymarin or TUDC. *Hepato Res* 2003; 26:217–24.

58. Boigk G et al. Silymarin retards collagen accumulation in early and advanced biliary fibrosis secondary to complete bile duct obliteration in rats. *Hepatology* 1997; 26:643–9.

59. Loguercio C. The effect of a silybin-vitamin e-phospholipid complex on nonalcoholic fatty liver disease: A pilot study. *Dig Dis Sci* 2007; 52(9):2387–95.

60. Morazzoni P et al. Comparative bioavailability of silipide, a new flavolignan complex, in rats. *Eur J Drug Metab Pharmacokinet* 1992; 17:39–44. 615.

61. Phase II Trial of Silymarin for Non-Cirrhotic Patients With Non-Alcoholic Steatohepatitis (SyNCH). http://clinical trials.gocv/ct2/show/NCT00680407: 2011.

62. Tappenden K et al. The physiological relevance of the intestinal microbiota—contributions to human health. *J Am Coll Nutr* 2007; 26(6):679S–83S.

63. Nardone G et al. Probiotics: A potential target for the prevention and treatment of steatohepatitis. *J Clin Gastroenterol* 2004; 38(6 Suppl):S121–2.

64. Sachan D et al. Ameliorating effects of carnitine and its precursors on alcohol-induced fatty liver. *Am J Clin Nutr* 1984; 39(5):738–44.

65. Leuschner UO et al. *Steatohepatitis (NASH and ASH)*. Falk Symposium No 121. Dordrecht, Netherlands: Kluwer Academic Publishers, 2001.

66. Farrell G et al. *Fatty Liver Disease: NASH and Related Disorders*. Blackwell Publishing, 2005; Massachusetts: Blackwell Publishing Ltd., 337.

67. Rajasekar P et al. Effect of L-carnitine on skeletal muscle lipids and oxidative stress in rats fed high-fructose diet. *Exp Diabetes Res* 2007; 2007(72741).

68. Liska D et al. Detoxification and Biotranformational Imbalances, in *Text Book of Functional Medicine*, ed. Jones, DS. Gig Harbor, WA: Institute of Functional Medicine, 2005.

69. Sazci A et al. Methlyenetetrahydrofolate gene polymorphisms in patients with nonalcoholic steatohepatitis (NASH). *Cell Biochem Funct* 2007.

70. Miller A. The methionine-homocysteine cycle and its effects on cognitive disease. *Altern Med Rev* 2003; 1:7–19.

71. Shim JY et al. Protective effects of chlorella vulgaris on the liver toxicity in cadmium-administered rats. *J Emd Foo* 2008; 11(3):479–85.

72. Rossi F et al. Use of branched chain amino acids for treating hepatic encephalopathy: Clinical experience. *Gut* 1986; (3)27 (Suppl 1):111–5.

73. Als-Nielsen B et al. Branched-chain amino acids for hepatic encephalopathy. *Cochrane Database of Systematic Reviews* 2003; Issue 2. Art. No.: CD001939. DOI: 10.1002/14651858.CD001939.

14 Irritable Bowel Syndrome

Linda A. Lee, M.D., and Octavia Pickett-Blakely, M.D.

INTRODUCTION

Irritable bowel syndrome (IBS) is a complex, chronic disorder characterized by abdominal pain or discomfort and altered bowel habits. IBS is symptom defined, not associated with gross [1] anatomic abnormality, and is thought to arise from a perturbance in the brain-gut axis. The diagnosis of IBS rests on fulfillment of the Rome III clinical criteria established by a multinational consensus group. The diagnosis requires the following: recurrent abdominal pain or discomfort of at least six months' duration relieved by defecation and associated with changes in stool consistency or frequency (Table 14.1). Patients are subgrouped into different categories based on their primary symptoms: constipation predominant (IBS-C), diarrhea predominant (IBS-D), or mixed (IBS-M). The diagnosis of IBS is further supported by the age of symptom onset, which typically is prior to the fifth decade of life, the lack of nocturnal symptoms, and the absence of weight loss, anemia, or rectal bleeding. The diagnosis of IBS is characterized by the absence of clinically measurable diagnostic tests.

Therapy for IBS is thus directed toward addressing individual dietary patterns, food and nutrient intake, psychological factors, and comorbidities. Patients with IBS are more likely to have other functional gastrointestinal (GI) disorders, such as dyspepsia, which has some overlapping symptoms [2,3]. Patients with IBS are likely to have other comorbid disorders that affect a variety of organ systems, such as cystitis, chronic pelvic pain, fibromyalgia, migraine headaches, and chronic fatigue syndrome [4,5]. There is a high prevalence of IBS among patients with psychiatric illness [6], and up to 94% of IBS patients who present for medical care have evidence of psychiatric illness [5]. A history of sexual or physical abuse can be elicited in many patients with functional gastrointestinal disorders [7]. Despite an association with psychiatric comorbidity, it should be emphasized that IBS is not a psychiatric disorder but a disorder of the brain-gut axis, as will be described here.

EPIDEMIOLOGY

IBS is a frequently diagnosed gastrointestinal condition with an estimated US prevalence of 10–15% [8]. Symptoms of IBS are among the most common reasons for office visits with primary care physicians and specialists. In 2002, more than two million clinic visits were made for IBS [9]. Symptoms can be mild or severe and can fluctuate in frequency and intensity. Studies have repeatedly demonstrated that functional GI disorders perturb quality of life more significantly than organic GI disorders and other chronic diseases such as rheumatoid arthritis [10,11].

IBS occurs worldwide but is less prevalent in Asia compared to the United States [12]. Women are affected three times more often than men. In the United States, Caucasians are 2.5 times more likely than African Americans to have IBS [13]. However, IBS has the same impact on health-related quality of life across ethnic groups [14,13]. The impact of socioeconomic status on IBS

TABLE 14.1

Rome III Criteria for Irritable Bowel Syndrome

At least three months, with onset at least six months previously of recurrent abdominal pain or discomfort** associated with two or more of the following:

- Improvement with defecation and/or
- Onset associated with a change in frequency of stool and/or
- Onset associated with a change in form (appearance) of stool

**Discomfort means an uncomfortable sensation not described as pain.

---

prevalence is less clearly defined. Some studies associate IBS with affluence and others implicate poverty as a risk factor [15,16,17,18].

The economic impact of IBS is astonishing. IBS-related costs rose to $1.35 billion in the United States in 2003 [19,20,21]. The predicted costs are likely an underestimation because expenditures for prescription or over-the-counter medications were not included. Quality of life and work productivity are also adversely impacted by IBS symptoms. Consequently, IBS continues to be the second most common reason for work absenteeism [22]. For example, a survey of over 5000 persons from US households found that IBS patients missed an average of 13.4 days per year from work or school due to illness, whereas the average subject without a GI disorder missed only 4.9 days [23].

Risk factors for IBS may include environmental as well as genetic ones. A family aggregation study, which surveyed relatives of individuals with IBS, demonstrated a prevalence of 17% in patients' relatives versus 7% in spouses' relatives [24]. Other studies have also shown a familial aggregation of IBS, but this could be complicated by environmental factors, such as sharing acquired responses to abdominal symptoms or, as some investigators believe, nutrition in fetal life [25]. Twin studies are conflicting, with some demonstrating concordance of IBS is twice as great in monozygotic compared to dizygotic twins [26,27].

PATHOPHYSIOLOGY

The pathophysiology of IBS is complex and still poorly understood. However, visceral hypersensitivity, disordered cortical pain processing, small bowel bacterial overgrowth, and increased intestinal permeability recently have been implicated and will be discussed here.

VISCERAL HYPERSENSITIVITY

Visceral hypersensitivity is defined as having a low threshold to painful stimuli arising from the gastrointestinal tract. In research settings, this has traditionally been assessed by measuring the pain response to inflation of a balloon within the digestive tract; IBS patients tend to experience more pain compared to controls for a given volume inflated. This was first documented in 1973 when inflation of a sigmoid balloon to 60 ml caused pain in 6% of controls but in 55% of patients with IBS [28]. Thus, luminal distention, triggered post prandially and exacerbated by gas-producing foods, may trigger symptoms as a result of enhanced perception of bloating and abdominal pain in those with IBS.

Increased pain perception could be mediated at the level of extrinsic gut afferent nerves responsible for sensory perception as well as by cortical processing that affects pain inhibition. Visceral hypersensitivity is thought to arise from a disruption in normal serotonin (also known as 5-hydroxytriptamine or 5-HT) signaling. Ninety-five percent of the serotonin in the human body is found in the gastrointestinal tract, mostly produced by enterochromaffin cells in the gastrointestinal epithelium [29]. Enterochromaffin cells act as sensory transducers that release 5-HT after meals.

5-HT binds 5-HT4 receptors present on visceral motor afferent nerves, which control gastrointestinal reflexes that govern intestinal motility and secretion. By binding 5-HT3 receptors present on extrinsic gut afferent neurons, 5-HT also regulates visceral sensation, which is responsible for transmitting sensory signals from gut to cortical regions [29]. The amount of 5-HT that is functionally active at any one time is determined by the rate of production by enterochromaffin cells and the rate of reuptake into mucosal enterocytes via serotonin reuptake transporters (SERT), where it is then catabolized. It has been postulated that defects in 5-HT production, SERT reuptake, or metabolism can affect the pool of 5-HT available and lead to alterations in visceral motility, secretion, and sensation. Thus, increased 5-HT bioavailability has been implicated in IBS-D, whereas reduced 5-HT bioavailability has been implicated for IBS-C [30,31].

Data supporting a critical role of intestinal serotonin signaling in the pathogenesis of IBS have emerged from both animal and human studies. Postprandial plasma 5-HT levels are lower in individuals with IBS-C and higher in IBS-D patients compared to controls [30,31]. A transgenic mouse with SERT gene knockout demonstrates increased rectal transit time resulting in wetter stools [32]. A recent study of IBS-D and IBS-C patients revealed no differences in expression of SERT in colonic mucosa. Instead, expression of p11, a molecule that increases serotonergic receptor function (5-HT1B), was increased in IBS [33]. Further identification of additional factors regulating 5-HT signaling may lead to the development of novel therapeutic agents.

Studies on postinfectious IBS (PI-IBS) also support the role of serotonin in IBS. Up to 17% of individuals with IBS report the first onset of IBS symptoms following a bout of infectious colitis [34]. Predictors of developing PI-IBS include gender (female), prolonged diarrhea (greater than 15 days), psychological factors, and severity of initial illness [35]. PI-IBS has been reported following outbreaks of giardiasis [36], salmonellosis [35], shigellosis [37,38,39], and *Campylobacter jejuni* infection [40]. In a rodent model of 2,4,6-trinitrobenzene sulfonic acid (TNBS)–induced colitis, 5-HT gut mucosal content, number of 5-HT-immunoreactive cells, and the proportion of epithelial cells that were 5-HT-immunoreactive was twofold higher than in control animals [41]. Increased levels of enterochromaffin cells and 5-HT levels have been identified in the rectal mucosa of individuals suffering from PI-IBS [40,34].

In addition to abnormalities in serotonin processing and function, alterations in central processing of pain signaling have now been demonstrated using positron emission tomography (PET) and cortical functional magnetic resonance imaging (fMRI). Cortical fMRI indirectly measures cognitive activity and neuronal activation by assessing changes in oxyhemoglobin that occur as a result of fluctuations in cerebral blood flow [42]; fMRI has demonstrated that a painful rectal stimulus activates the anterior cingulate cortex (ACC), the central nervous system pain center, to a greater degree in IBS patients than controls [43]. A concern raised about interpretation of IBS fMRI studies is that anticipation of pain and somatization may contribute to the patterns of neuronal activation seen, so that alterations in cognitive response rather than visceral hypersensitivity may contribute to the fMRI results [44,45].

For many individuals with IBS, there is a clear association between emotional stress and severity of symptoms. CRH, released by the hypothalamus, is a mediator of the stress response. CRH not only triggers cortisol release, but it also activates the autonomic nervous system to slow small bowel transit and accelerate colonic motility. In addition, CRH appears to have a direct effect in increasing visceral hypersensitivity in normal volunteers when administered intravenously [46]. Persistent elevation of cerebrospinal fluid (CSF) corticotropin-releasing factor (CRF) concentrations following early-life adversity [47] may provide an explanation for the link between severe types of abuse in many with IBS [48].

Peripheral administration of αhCRH, a nonselective CRH receptor antagonist, reduced abdominal pain and anxiety induced by rectal electrical stimulation in a small group of IBS patients [1], but most subjects experienced drowsiness. However, a recent randomized, double-blind, placebo-controlled, two-week study to evaluate an oral selective CRF(1) receptor antagonist in patients with IBS-D did not significantly alter colonic or other regional transit or bowel function [49].

INCREASED INTESTINAL PERMEABILITY

Postinfectious IBS (PI-IBS) may result from an increase in intestinal permeability as a result of inflammation triggered by infection. Intestinal permeability is detected noninvasively by measuring the urinary excretion of orally consumed probe molecules, such as mannitol and lactulose [50,51]. Increased intestinal permeability is more frequently encountered among patients with diarrhea-predominant (IBS-D) and PI-IBS, particularly in those with a history of atopy [52]. Although IBS has been classified as a functional disorder not typically associated with anatomic defects, some investigators have now identified an inflammatory component among those with PI-IBS or IBS-D. An increased number of activated T lymphocytes and mast cells have been noted in the colonic [53] and jejunal mucosa [54] of patients with IBS-D, and the presence of these mast cells near enteric nerves may account for visceral pain or sensitivity. Increased intestinal permeability may also be related to elevated proinflammatory cytokine production as has been noted in peripheral blood monocytes of IBS-D patients [55].

SMALL INTESTINAL BACTERIAL OVERGROWTH

Increased intestinal permeability has been attributed by some to small intestinal bacterial over-growth (SIBO), which may occur in about 10% of IBS patients. The percentage of those with IBS with SIBO has been disputed in part because the diagnosis is difficult to establish; the most commonly used tests, the glucose or lactulose hydrogen breath tests, have a relatively low specificity. Interpretation of the breath tests is based on an assumption that small bowel transit is more than one hour; however, studies have demonstrated that in more than 50% of individuals, small bowel transit is less than one hour. This means that abnormal findings on the breath tests could be due to fermentation of the substrate by colonic bacteria rather than small intestinal organisms. Regardless, some investigators have demonstrated antibiotics significantly improve IBS symptoms in those with IBS-diarrhea or IBS-mixed [56,57].

Although the mechanism of SIBO development in IBS is not entirely clear, SIBO can aggravate symptoms of bloating, cramping, and diarrhea, which in the setting of visceral hyperalgesia can lead to significant distress. These symptoms arise from malabsorption of ingested fat, protein carbohydrates, and vitamins as a result of bacterial utilization of these macro- and micronutrients. Impaired intestinal motility or diminished gastric-acid secretion are risk factors for the development of SIBO. Pimentel et al. demonstrated that patients with IBS and SIBO have reduced phase III of the migrating motor complex, the component of fasting-gut motility responsible for clearing the small intestinal lumen of contents from the last meal [58]. These data implicate impaired motility as a possible etiology of SIBO and, thus, IBS symptoms in some patients. Furthermore, treatment of IBS symptoms with antibiotics and/or probiotics in an effort to restore the equilibrium of enteric flora has yielded promising results [56,59,60]. A widely publicized, randomized, placebo-controlled study compared rifaximin, a poorly absorbed antibiotic to placebo for the treatment of symptoms in individuals with IBS-D or IBS-M [61]. Outcome was measured by symptomatic improvement in at least two of the four weeks the study drug was consumed. Although there was a statistically significant improvement in the group that received the antibiotic, it should be noted that only 41% of the study subjects responded (compared to 31% improvement in the placebo group). Moreover, no assessment for SIBO was performed in this study, so it is entirely probable that symptomatic improvement was the result of altering colonic flora rather than treating SIBO.

ALTERATIONS IN THE INTESTINAL MICROBIOTA

Recent investigation of the human gut microbiome has revealed that the microbiota composition of IBS patients differs from normal controls, as shown by several investigators. Global and deep molecular analysis of fecal samples from 62 patients with IBS and 46 healthy individuals showed that those with IBS had a twofold increased ratio of the firmicutes to bacteroidetes, two of the dominant phyla in the gut microbiome [62], Alterations in the numbers of specific bacterial species was assessed, raising intriguing hypotheses about the role of the microbiome in the pathogenesis of IBS. Although it still remains to be determined whether the documented changes are the cause or a consequence of IBS, it is interesting to speculate as to how differences in the intestinal flora might contribute to bacterial fermentation of poorly digested carbohydrates and how the production of fermentation by products might affect visceral sensitivity or gut motility.

PHARMACOLOGY

Few therapies exist with documented efficacy in the treatment of IBS. Interpretation of efficacy in clinical trials is hampered by the large placebo effect among IBS patients [63]. Some commonly used therapies are directed toward symptom management of abdominal cramping, constipation, diarrhea, and/or bloating. Others specifically target serotonin metabolism, which is now thought to be in part responsible for visceral hyperalgesia. Given the broad range in symptom severity and frequency, treatment of IBS must be individualized.

CONSTIPATION

Often a first-line therapy is to prescribe a high-fiber diet; increasing fiber intake to 25–30 gms per day is thought to increase gastrointestinal transit, although data in this area are conflicting. A typical serving of a given fruit or vegetable may contain anywhere from 2–5 grams of fiber. Fiber is also available as a dietary supplement, in both soluble and insoluble forms. Soluble fiber such as psyllium and partially hydrolyzed guar gum derived from plants is extensively fermented by colonic bacteria leading to the production of substantial amounts of gas and volatile fatty acids. As a consequence, stool content is heavy in bacterial mass and low in fiber residue. Conversely, insoluble fiber such as wheat or oat bran is minimally metabolized by colonic flora and thus produces less gas. However, in a patient with visceral hypersensitivity, even minimal amounts of gas in the setting of altered visceral hypersensitivity and motility, may be perceived as significant abdominal cramping and bloating. Despite being widely prescribed, a recent meta-analysis found that bulking agents were no better than placebo in improving IBS [64]. Few data exist as to the efficacy of other laxatives in the treatment of IBS-C. Lubiprostone, a locally acting chloride channel activator currently FDA-approved for the treatment of constipation, is now being investigated for use in IBS-C [65].

Anecdotal use of 5-hydroxytryptophan (5-HTP), the precursor to serotonin, is widely described on the Internet; 5-HTP is often used with vitamin B6, which is a cofactor needed for conversion of 5-HTP to 5-HT. Although it is debatable that 5-HTP may have a future role in the treatment of depression [66], there are no published clinical trials in the medical literature regarding its efficacy in IBS. However, a tryptophan 5-hydroxylase (TPH) inhibitor that reduces serotonin (5-HT) synthesis peripherally, is currently under development and investigation for the treatment of IBS-D [67,68].

Lubiprostone, a chloride channel activator, is a laxative that has been FDA approved for the treatment of IBS-constipation. It increases small intestinal fluid secretion, thus potentially enhancing the movement of stool. The dose used for IBS-constipation is lower than that approved for the treatment of functional constipation.

Tegaserod is a 5-HT4 receptor agonist that was shown in clinical trials to be more effective than placebo in improving IBS symptoms in women with predominant constipation [69]. Tegaserod stimulated intestinal and colonic transit and reduced abdominal discomfort while improving constipation. Its manufacturer withdrew Tegaserod from the US market in 2007 because of safety concerns. Renzapride is a 5-HT(4) receptor full agonist/5-HT(3) receptor antagonist currently being investigated for efficacy in the treatment of constipation predominant IBS. Despite being shown to accelerate colonic transit in an early trial [70], in a more recent phase II clinical trial, however, no significant difference in relief from abdominal pain occurred between renzapride and placebo [71].

ABDOMINAL CRAMPING

Anticholinergic agents, such as dicyclomine or hyoscyamine, are often prescribed to reduce smooth muscle spasm, although well-designed clinical trials are lacking that have proven their efficacy in reducing global IBS symptoms [72]. Nevertheless, some patients report symptomatic improvement if taken before triggering events or before ingestion of meals. In addition to its use in foods and fragrances, peppermint oil extract derived from the peppermint leaf has long been thought to have medicinal properties. Particular to the gastrointestinal tract, it has been shown to result in smooth muscle relaxation possibly via a calcium channel antagonist mechanism [73]. The effect of peppermint oil on gastrointestinal motility has not been completely elucidated. There are data showing decreased small intestinal transit time as well as increased gastric emptying time [73]. Colonic spasm relief has also been demonstrated with peppermint oil [74]. The literature is sparse, however, on clinical trials examining the effect of peppermint oil on IBS symptoms. A small study in the pediatric literature showed dramatic symptom improvement after a 14-day trial of peppermint oil [75]. However, moderate symptom improvement was observed in the placebo group to a greater extent than the treatment group. A large placebo effect hampers many IBS clinical trials. In the adult population, peppermint oil was effective in improving overall IBS scores in another trial [76]. Side effects reported in clinical trials with peppermint oil are heartburn and anal/perianal burning [77]. Heartburn may be reduced if an enteric-coated preparation is used [75].

DIARRHEA

Antidiarrheal agents are used to manage diarrhea in patients with diarrhea-predominant IBS, but they do not necessarily address the global symptoms of IBS. Alosetron, a 5-HT3 receptor antagonist, has been shown to improve global symptoms of IBS-D [78,79]. Alosetron increases stool frequency, stool consistency, and abdominal discomfort. Reports of ischemic colitis and severe constipation requiring bowel resection have led to its availability only on a restricted basis. Among IBS patients, specific polymorphisms have been identified more frequently in the serotonin transporter gene SLC6A4, whose gene product is responsible for reuptake of serotonin from the synaptic cleft. Some polymorphisms are associated with increased colonic transit time in response to alosetron [80]. The SERT-deletion/deletion-promoter polymorphism is more common among those with diarrhea-predominant IBS in Koreans [81] and Caucasians [82], suggesting the possibility of identifying individuals who might respond more readily to pharmacologic agents that modify serotonin signaling.

ABDOMINAL PAIN, BLOATING

Because visceral hypersensitivity is central to IBS pathophysiology, there is increased interest in the use of antidepressants, which may be effective in dampening visceral pain perception. Typically, anti depressant doses used for IBS are lower than those used for the treatment of depression. Tricyclic antidepressants may help to improve abdominal pain but may not improve IBS [72,83]. A disadvantage is that some patients cannot tolerate side effects associated with some of these agents. In a study of IBS patients without depression, the selective serotonin receptor inhibitor, citalopram, improved abdominal pain, bloating, impact of symptoms on daily life, and overall well-being [84].

As a role for mucosal inflammation has emerged in IBS, and with increased recognition that intestinal microflora can modulate the host immune response, probiotics have been pursued as a possible treatment strategy for managing IBS symptoms. Probiotics consist of live microorganisms, which are used to confer health benefits. Support for the use of probiotics comes from several randomized, placebo-controlled trials using highly specific bacterial strains in which some individual symptoms of IBS, such as abdominal pain or bloating, improved after four or eight weeks of therapy [60,85,86,87]. In a randomized placebo-controlled study using B infantis 35624 in 77 IBS patients, symptomatic improvement was associated with normalization of the ratio of an anti-inflammatory to proinflammatory cytokines [88], suggesting that certain bacterial strains may indeed modulate cytokine production. Highly specific bacterial strains are used in clinical trials, and a response to one strain does not mean that the same response will be achieved with any commercially available probiotic. Probiotic preparations abound, and manufacturing of these compounds is not subject to regulation by the Food and Drug Administration, making difficult the selection of an appropriate preparation by consumers and healthcare providers.

For symptomatic relief of their symptoms, 51.9% of IBS patients use complementary therapies [89]. Among the most popular therapies are digestive enzymes—commercially available preparations of enzymes normally produced by the stomach, pancreas, or intestine. In a study of 314 IBS-D patients, 6.1% were found to have pancreatic insufficiency as demonstrated by depressed fecal elastase levels [90]. Pancreatic enzyme supplementation has been shown to reduce postprandial bloating, gas, and fullness in 18 healthy volunteers when administered with a high-calorie, high-fat meal [90]. The mechanism underlying this symptomatic improvement was not elucidated, but the authors noted there was no discernable change in hydrogen breath testing in response to lactulose. No studies of pancreatic enzyme supplementation have been published in IBS patients.

COMORBID CONDITIONS

Self-described food intolerance by IBS patients is complicated because there are several potential causes of food intolerance including food allergy and carbohydrate malabsorption. Even normal physiologic responses of the GI tract to the ingestion of food may trigger the gastrocolonic reflex, which is sufficient to provoke symptoms in some individuals with visceral hypersensitivity [92]. Food composition itself may also precipitate symptoms; for example, ingestion of caffeine or foods with high-fat content may provoke colonic motility and GI symptoms in an IBS patient.

Some patients mistakenly believe the symptoms of food intolerance indicate true food allergy. Food allergy is less common than IBS and has an estimated prevalence up to 4% in adults and up to 8% of children [93] and is discussed in detail in chapter 16 of this text. The most common food allergens in US adults are tree nuts, peanuts, shellfish, and fish, and in children are egg, wheat, and soybean. Food allergies can be mediated by immunoglobulin E, which leads to an immediate reaction or can be triggered by cell-mediated mechanisms that account for delayed responses. Negative skin-prick testing in adults has a negative predictive value > 95%, but a positive response unfortunately has a positive predictive value of only 30–40% [94], leaving food withdrawal and challenge still the most common way of diagnosing food allergy. Nevertheless, some studies have attempted to use the increased presence of IgG antibodies over baseline to food allergens to guide food withdrawal with some improvement in a subset of IBS patients [95–97]. However, tests that measure IgE or IgG antibodies to specific foods are of questionable utility, especially when IgG antibodies against various food substances are prevalent even among the non-IBS population [98,99]. Food elimination diets still remain the primary tool for evaluating food allergy. Interpretation of a clinical response to food elimination in IBS patients, however, can be challenging when one considers that most elimination diets involve the withdrawal of wheat, eggs, soy, fish, and milk [95–97,100,101]. The elimination of milk and wheat may improve IBS symptoms if the individual also suffers from lactose intolerance or experiences gassiness with fiber (which contains fructans) ingestion. Practitioners and patients should recognize that an elimination diet that is devoid of wheat by-products, milk, soy, and eggs, often means shifting from a diet rich in processed foods to one comprised of whole foods. The elimination of processed foods does indeed get rid of potential food allergens but also decreases the intake of poorly absorbed carbohydrates, such as fructose, fructans, and sorbitol, that ultimately are fermented by colonic bacteria to produce gas. Thus, symptomatic improvement achieved by food elimination may really reflect a response to reduced dietary intake of poorly absorbed carbohydrates rather than exclusion of a food allergen.

Food allergy may be responsible for symptoms in 13–25% of adult patients who have the rare inflammatory condition, eosinophilic gastroenteritis [102]. The primary symptoms of eosinophilic gastroenteritis depend on which organs it affects, but can consist of dysphagia, diarrhea, and/or abdominal pain. A relationship between IBS and eosinophilic gastroenteritis has not yet been established despite some overlap in symptoms. Eosinophilic gastroenteritis is characterized by the histologic presence of increased eosinophils within the gastrointestinal mucosa; this finding is absent in those with IBS. Eosinophilic infiltration can be patchy, occur at different tissue depths, and any portion of the entire GI tract is vulnerable such that some individuals will present only with esophageal involvement and others with primarily gastric involvement. Given the role of eosinophils in this disease, one would assume that the pathogenesis is solely an IgE dependent process. However, one rationale for why allergens are not always identified on routine allergen testing is that eosinophilic gastroenteritis is in fact a delayed hypersensitivity reaction (cell mediated) [103]. Therefore, eosinophilic gastroenteritis is thought to be a polygenic allergic disorder. Half of affected individuals will have a history of atopy and peripheral eosinophilia may be present. The diagnosis can only be established by endoscopic biopsy of the involved segment of the GI tract [104].

A discussion about food allergy and IBS always includes the topic of celiac disease. There is symptomatic overlap of IBS and celiac disease (CD). Bloating, abdominal pain, and diarrhea are observed in patients who suffer with either, or both, of these disorders. This overlap has been reported in the literature with one study finding up to 5% of newly diagnosed IBS patients having CD, while another report found 20% of patients with CD meeting Rome I criteria for IBS [105,106]. Furthermore, CD serologies and HLA DQ2 positivity in IBS-D patients are predictors of gluten-free diet responsiveness [107] even in the absence of overt celiac disease. Given the symptom overlap, it is quite reasonable and cost effective to screen patients with IBS for CD in populations where the prevalence is above 1% [108]. Current guidelines recommend screening by serologic testing for tissue transglutaminase IgA, which has a specificity greater than 95% and a sensitivity in the range of 90%–96% [109].

PATIENT EVALUATION

The patient history is the most important component in making the diagnosis of IBS as there are no physical exam findings that are diagnostic of IBS. Rather, it is the absence of significant physical exam findings that is most consistent with IBS. A clinical presentation that fulfills the Rome III criteria may alone be diagnostic in the absence of alarm symptoms. The criteria for IBS are distinct from that of functional constipation, namely that the latter is not associated with abdominal pain or discomfort. A history of weight loss, nocturnal awakening for diarrhea or abdominal pain, anemia, or rectal bleeding should prompt a search for an alternative diagnosis. Similarly, if the onset of symptoms occurs after age 50, the diagnosis of IBS should be questioned. Screening questionnaires for IBS primarily exist to measure symptom severity and impact on quality of life once the diagnosis of IBS is made. Such questionnaires, such as the IBSQOL, are used primarily for research purposes. The IBS Severity Scale is the tool recommended to assess responsiveness to an intervention in clinical trials [110].

Serum laboratory tests in IBS typically are normal. Laboratory testing is done to exclude the possibility of other underlying disorders, such as thyroid or celiac disease. Stool tests should be considered to rule out active intestinal infection in those with diarrhea. Testing for visceral hypersensitivity with balloon manometry and functional MRI or PET scanning are only done primarily for research purposes; no role for these tests as yet have been established in clinical practice. In a 2002 position statement, the American College of Gastroenterology Functional Gastrointestinal Disorders Task Force stated because IBS patients do not have an increased incidence of organic disease, "available data do not support the performance of diagnostic tests amongst patients with IBS" in the absence of alarm symptoms such as rectal bleeding or weight loss [111].

TREATMENT RECOMMENDATIONS

Once the diagnosis of IBS is made, treatment begins by obtaining a thorough dietary history, in part to identify symptom aggravators, especially because most patients with IBS will describe intolerance to specific foods [112]. Particular attention should be paid to medications and supplements, as many agents are known to precipitate or aggravate constipation or diarrhea even in those without IBS. Common medications and supplements that cause altered bowel habits are listed in Table 14.2. It is important to obtain a food diary to understand what components in the diet could be responsible for symptom aggravation in IBS [100]. The diet should be reviewed for dietary sources of fructose and sorbitol, which could easily aggravate symptoms in an individual with visceral hypersensitivity. Caffeine intake or a high-fat diet should be monitored as both are known to stimulate colonic motility. Carbohydrate malabsorption is another cause of symptom exacerbation in IBS.

Gibson and Shepherd coined the term FODMAPS to refer to the highly fermentable but poorly absorbed short-chain carbohydrates and polyols (fermentable oligo-, di-, and monosaccharides and polyols) found in the diets of highly industrialized areas [113]. They originally hypothesized that ingestion of FODMAPS could increase susceptibility to Crohn's disease, an inflammatory bowel disease that is distinct from IBS. They later observed that dietary restriction of FODMAPs in patients with inflammatory bowel disease improved functional GI symptoms, such as abdominal pain, bloating, flatulence, and diarrhea [114]. FODMAPs presumably trigger gastrointestinal symptoms in people with visceral hypersensitivity by inducing luminal distension via a combination of osmotic effects and gas production related to their rapid fermentation by bacteria in the small and proximal large intestine. Rodent studies have suggested that butyrate, a fermentation by product, might contribute to the development to visceral hypersensitivity, at least when administered as an enema [115]. In some studies, a low-FODMAP diet is defined as one that contains < 9 gms of FODMAPs [116]. FODMAPS food sources are provided in detail by Gibson and Shepherd in their excellent review [117].

TABLE 14.2
Common Causative Agents of Constipation and Diarrhea

Agent	Constipation	Diarrhea
Supplements	Calcium	Magnesium
	Iron	Vitamin C
		Niacin
Herbals	St. John's Wort (*Hypercum perforatum*)	Goldenseal (*Hydrastasis canadenis*)
		Aloe Vera
Prescription Drugs	Anticholinergics (oxybutynin)	Cholinesterase Inhibitors (pyridostigmine)
	Opiods Analgesics (morphine)	Biguanides (metformin)
	Calcium Channel Blockers (diltiazem)	Calcinuerin Inhibitors (tacrolimus)
	Nonopioid Analgesics (tramadol)	Immunosuppressants (mycophenolate mofetil)
	Psychotropics (lithium)	Colchicine
	Antidepressants (sertraline)	Stimulants (amphetamine)
	Beta Blockers (atenolol)	Proton Pump Inhibitors (pantoprazole)
	Stimulants (dextroamphetamine)	Antibiotics (flouroquinolones)
		Laxative Agents (lactulose)
		HAART Therapy
		Chemotherapy Agents (fluorouracil)
		Anti-Parkinson's (Tolcapone)

Lactose intolerance is a common cause of milk-related symptoms. Lactose is hydrolyzed in the small intestine by the enzyme, lactase, expressed by the enterocytes found in intestinal villi. Lactase activity is highest during infancy. Downregulation of lactase enzyme activity within the small intestine is a normal occurrence in the vast majority of adults, but the rate of loss is dependent on race and ethnicity [118]. Because milk is pervasive in the Western diet, many individuals are unaware that undigested lactose can trigger their gastrointestinal symptoms. Undigested lactose delivered to the colon increases the osmotic load producing a more watery stool. In addition, undigested lactose undergoes fermentation by luminal bacteria to produce diarrhea and gas. Systemic symptoms of lactose intolerance may also include headache, fatigue, and myalgias.

Lactose intolerance is measurable by lactose hydrogen breath testing, which has a specificity between 89% and 100% and sensitivity 69%–100% [119]. Although many IBS patients self-report lactose intolerance, lactose hydrogen breath testing has demonstrated no increased prevalence of lactose malabsorption in IBS patients compared to controls in various geographic populations [120,121] though other studies suggest otherwise. Whether adherence to a lactose-free diet improves IBS symptoms in those who are lactose intolerant has been debated. Differences in response to a lactose-free diet reflects regional prevalence of lactose malabsorption and dietary compliance; regions with high prevalence of lactose malabsorption report clinical improvement in response to a low-lactose diet [122–124]. Foods fermented with lactic acid–producing organisms, such as yogurt or kefir, may be better tolerated in individuals with lactose intolerance because these bacteria hydrolyze lactose. This may explain why food fermentation, an ancient practice to preserve food that occurs in every culture, produces foods that are widely held to be more easily digestible [125].

Fructose malabsorption may also aggravate IBS symptoms, particularly in combination with ingested sorbitol [126,127]. Fructose is a monosaccharide absorbed by carrier-mediated facilitated diffusion. Fructans are polymers of fructose. Both are found in many types of fruits, vegetables, legumes, wheat, and rye. Most humans have an intestinal absorption capacity of less than 50 g per day [128] even though it has been estimated the average American ingests about 100 g of fructose daily. Intestinal fructose absorption is enhanced when ingested with glucose [128], and therefore ingestion of fruits and foods in which glucose is present in equal or greater concentrations than fructose are less likely to trigger. When not absorbed in the small intestine, fructose exerts an osmotic effect and is fermented by colonic bacteria to produce hydrogen, carbon dioxide, and short-chain fatty acids [129]. In a small study of normal volunteers, 50% of individuals were found to malabsorb fructose after ingesting only 25 g, and two-thirds malabsorbed fructose after ingesting 50 gms as measured by fructose hydrogen breath testing [130]. Gastrointestinal symptoms from fructose malabsorption may be more prevalent among both the normal and IBS populations when one considers fructose ingestion has increased more than 1000% in the United States over the past 20 years with the addition of high-fructose corn syrup used to sweeten soft drinks and fruit juices, candy, cereals, and many processed foods [131]; 25–50 g of fructose are equivalent to > 500 mL of a high-fructose, corn syrup–sweetened soft drink [132]. Fructose malabsorption may not be more common among the IBS population [133] and does not have an etiologic role in IBS, but fructose malabsorption may indeed aggravate IBS symptoms. In two small studies of IBS patients with documented fructose intolerance, improvement in pain, belching, bloating, fullness, indigestion, and diarrhea were reported in response to dietary avoidance of fructose [134,135]. Dietary guidelines to reduce symptoms of fructose malabsorption have been proposed and may be effective in managing patients with IBS [117,129].

In an effort to reduce caloric intake, patients may resort to consuming sugar-free products, which contain polyols, such as sorbitol, maltitol, or xylitol. Such artificial sweeteners may add to bloating and diarrhea symptoms in patients with IBS simply because they are poorly absorbed in the small intestine but fermented by colonic bacteria. Thus, patients are well advised to avoid these artificial sweeteners; they are pervasive in chewing gum and soft drinks in particular.

Sucralose is a nonnutritive sweetener found in a variety of foods. Although some GI complaints have been attributed to sucralose ingestion, it is unclear as to how it causes these symptoms. Most ingested sucralose is excreted intact in the feces [136], so that colonic bacterial fermentation should not be a significant issue [137].

DIETARY RESTRICTION OF GLUTEN

Most individuals with IBS do not meet the clinical criteria for the diagnosis of celiac disease. However, many with IBS will report symptom improvement in response to a gluten-free diet. Gluten sensitivity is defined as symptoms developing after the ingestion of gluten in the absence of definitive evidence of celiac disease or food allergy. Ingestion of gluten has been shown to aggravate IBS symptoms compared to when it was eliminated from the diet in individuals that did not have celiac disease [137]. While some individuals with gluten sensitivity may indeed have latent celiac disease [107], it is highly probable that some symptomatic improvement occurs because wheat is a major source of poorly absorbed and highly fermentable fructans [114].

OTHER THERAPIES

Recognition that IBS represents a disorder of the brain-gut axis has raised a possible role for psychological therapies in the management of IBS. Cognitive behavior therapy (CBT), a form of psychotherapy used to modify maladaptive thinking, has been successfully used for the treatment of several psychiatric disorders, such as anxiety and depression. CBT has been studied in multiple clinical trials, and is now recommended as an IBS treatment option by the United Kingdom Department of Health [138]. Hutton states in his review, "CBT is most appropriate for patients who are significantly distressed by their symptoms, are open to the idea that psychological factors play some role in their difficulties, are willing to take part in an intervention that requires their active participation and have already had reasonable medical investigations and interventions" [139].

Although a Cochrane review to evaluate the efficacy of hypnotherapy in the treatment of IBS identified few studies of sufficient quality or size for meta-analysis [140], there are some studies demonstrating that hypnotherapy may also help to improve abdominal pain and global IBS symptoms in those who have failed medical therapy [141–144]. Relaxation therapies have also been studied in clinical trials as adjunctive therapy to medical therapy with promising results [145]. Thus, psychological therapies could play a more significant role in the management of IBS as the understanding of brain-gut interaction increases.

SUMMARY

The treatment of IBS begins with the recognition that there is tremendous variability in symptom severity, frequency, and triggering events. Thus, successful management of IBS requires an effective physician-patient relationship and an individualized biopsychosocial approach [146]. Dietary counseling is essential as is attention to the role of psychological therapy in management of symptoms. Among the standard pharmacologic therapies currently used in the management of IBS, only alosetron and tegaserod have been shown to improve global IBS symptoms; but some therapies listed here have been shown to be helpful in improving a specific symptom for which they are listed. Some listed therapies still lack proven efficacy in clinical trials, but are often used in clinical practice given their low side-effect profiles.

APPROACH TO IBS

History and Physical Exam
- History: Note absence of alarm symptoms (rectal bleeding, anemia, weight loss)
- Note presence of comorbid illnesses (e.g., fibromyalgia, chronic pelvic pain, cystitis, chronic fatigue)

- Note history of sexual or physical abuse
- Physical exam—normal
- Laboratory tests—usually normal, including thyroid function tests; serum tissue transglutaminase IgA (celiac disease screen) negative, normal stool studies

Management

IBS-C

- Dietary and medication history
- Increase dietary fiber to 25–30 g per day (improves stool bulk but may worsen bloating)
- Add bulk laxative, such as insoluble or soluble fiber (improves stool bulk but may worsen bloating)
- Increase daily water intake, physical exercise
- Consider osmotic laxative (PEG 3350, but may worsen bloating)
- Consider Lubiprostone—currently under investigation
- Consider stimulant laxative (may worsen cramping)

IBS-D

- Dietary history
- Consider lactose intolerance
- Consider fructose malabsorption
- Reduce caffeine
- Reduce dietary fat intake
- No meal skipping
- Antidiarrheal agents (e.g., loperamide) to decrease stool frequency and improve consistency
- Antispasmodics taken prior to triggering events (e.g., work, social events) or foods
- Alosetron—improves abdominal discomfort and diarrhea
- Bloating, abdominal cramping/pain

Dietary recommendations: Consider FODMAPs diet and/or restrict the following:

- Carbonated beverages
- Chewing gum
- Artificial sweeteners
- High fructose consumption
- High-fat diet
- Consider testing for lactose intolerance (lactose hydrogen breath test)
- Consider testing for small intestine bacterial overgrowth (lactulose hydrogen breath test) if positive, trial of antibiotic therapy (e.g., rifaximin, norfloxacin, amoxicillin-clavulinic acid)
- Antispasmodics (hyoscyamine, dicyclomine, or peppermint oil) preferably taken prior to triggering events or foods
- Tricyclic antidepressants, SSRIs, SNRIs
- Cognitive behavior therapy, gut-directed hypnotherapy, relaxation therapy

REFERENCES

1. Sagami, Y., Y. Shimada, J. Tayama, T. Nomura, M. Satake, Y. Endo, T. Shoji, K. Karahashi, M. Hongo, and S. Fukudo. 2004. Effect of a corticotropin releasing hormone receptor antagonist on colonic sensory and motor function in patients with irritable bowel syndrome. *Gut* 53 (7):958–64.
2. Talley, N. J., E. H. Dennis, V. A. Schettler-Duncan, B. E. Lacy, K. W. Olden, and M. D. Crowell. 2003. Overlapping upper and lower gastrointestinal symptoms in irritable bowel syndrome patients with constipation or diarrhea. *Am J Gastroenterol* 98 (11):2454–59.

3. Whitehead, W. E., N. A. Gibbs, Z. Li, and D. A. Drossman. 1998. Is functional dyspepsia just a subset of the irritable bowel syndrome? *Baillieres Clin Gastroenterol* 12 (3):443–61.
4. Whitehead, W. E., O. S. Palsson, R. R. Levy, A. D. Feld, M. Turner, and M. Von Korff. 2007. Comorbidity in irritable bowel syndrome. *Am J Gastroenterol* 102 (12):2767–76.
5. Whitehead, W. E., O. Palsson, and K. R. Jones. 2002. Systematic review of the comorbidity of irritable bowel syndrome with other disorders: What are the causes and implications? *Gastroenterology* 122 (4):1140–56.
6. Garakani, A., T. Win, S. Virk, S. Gupta, D. Kaplan, and P. S. Masand. 2003. Comorbidity of irritable bowel syndrome in psychiatric patients: A review. *Am J Ther* 10 (1):61–67.
7. Drossman, D. A., J. Leserman, G. Nachman, Z. M. Li, H. Gluck, T. C. Toomey, and C. M. Mitchell. 1990. Sexual and physical abuse in women with functional or organic gastrointestinal disorders. *Ann Intern Med* 113 (11):828–33.
8. Thompson, W. G. 1986. A strategy for management of the irritable bowel. *Am J Gastroenterol* 81 (2):95–100.
9. Shaheen, N. J., R. A. Hansen, D. R. Morgan, L. M. Gangarosa, Y. Ringel, M. T. Thiny, M. W. Russo, and R. S. Sandler. 2006. The burden of gastrointestinal and liver diseases. *Am J Gastroenterol* 101 (9):2128–38.
10. Simren, M., J. Svedlund, I. Posserud, E. S. Bjornsson, and H. Abrahamsson. 2006. Health-related quality of life in patients attending a gastroenterology outpatient clinic: Functional disorders versus organic diseases. *Clin Gastroenterol Hepatol* 4 (2):187–95.
11. Frank, L., L. Kleinman, A. Rentz, G. Ciesla, J. J. Kim, and C. Zacker. 2002. Health-related quality of life associated with irritable bowel syndrome: Comparison with other chronic diseases. *Clin Ther* 24 (4):675–89; discussion 674.
12. Cremonini, F., and N. J. Talley. 2005. Irritable bowel syndrome: Epidemiology, natural history, health care seeking and emerging risk factors. *Gastroenterol Clin North Am* 34 (2):189–204.
13. Wigington, W. C., W. D. Johnson, and A. Minocha. 2005. Epidemiology of irritable bowel syndrome among African Americans as compared with whites: A population-based study. *Clin Gastroenterol Hepatol* 3 (7):647–53.
14. Gralnek, I. M., R. D. Hays, A. M. Kilbourne, L. Chang, and E. A. Mayer. 2004. Racial differences in the impact of irritable bowel syndrome on health-related quality of life. *J Clin Gastroenterol* 38 (9):782–89.
15. Minocha, A., W. D. Johnson, T. L. Abell, and W. C. Wigington. 2006. Prevalence, sociodemography, and quality of life of older versus younger patients with irritable bowel syndrome: A population-based study. *Dig Dis Sci* 51 (3):446–53.
16. Icks, A., B. Haastert, P. Enck, W. Rathmann, and G. Giani. 2002. Prevalence of functional bowel disorders and related health care seeking: A population-based study. *Z Gastroenterol* 40 (3):177–83.
17. Howell, S., N. J. Talley, S. Quine, and R. Poulton. 2004. The irritable bowel syndrome has origins in the childhood socioeconomic environment. *Am J Gastroenterol* 99 (8):1572–78.
18. Olafsdottir, L. B., H. Gudjonsson, and B. Thjodleifsson. 2005. Epidemiological study of functional bowel disorders in Iceland. *Laeknabladid* 91 (4):329–33.
19. Leong, S. A., V. Barghout, H. G. Birnbaum, C. E. Thibeault, R. Ben-Hamadi, F. Frech, and J. J. Ofman. 2003. The economic consequences of irritable bowel syndrome: A US employer perspective. *Arch Intern Med* 163 (8):929–35.
20. Inadomi, J. M., M. B. Fennerty, and D. Bjorkman. 2003. Systematic review: The economic impact of irritable bowel syndrome. *Aliment Pharmacol Ther* 18 (7):671–82.
21. Hulisz, D. 2004. The burden of illness of irritable bowel syndrome: Current challenges and hope for the future. *J Manag Care Pharm* 10 (4):299–309.
22. Quigley, E. M. 2006. Changing face of irritable bowel syndrome. *World J Gastroenterol* 12 (1):1–5.
23. Drossman, D. A., Z. Li, E. Andruzzi, R. D. Temple, et al. 1993. U.S. householder survey of functional gastrointestinal disorders. Prevalence, sociodemography, and health impact. *Dig Dis Sci* 38 (9):1569–80.
24. Kalantar, J. S., G. R. Locke III, A. R. Zinsmeister, C. M. Beighley, and N. J. Talley. 2003. Familial aggregation of irritable bowel syndrome: A prospective study. *Gut* 52 (12):1703–7.
25. Bengtson, M. B., T. Ronning, M. H. Vatn, and J. R. Harris. 2006. Irritable bowel syndrome in twins: Genes and environment. *Gut* 55 (12):1754–59.
26. Park, M. I., and M. Camilleri. 2005. Genetics and genotypes in irritable bowel syndrome: Implications for diagnosis and treatment. *Gastroenterol Clin North Am* 34 (2):305–17.
27. Wojczynski, M. K., K. E. North, N. L. Pedersen, and P. F. Sullivan. 2007. Irritable bowel syndrome: A co-twin control analysis. *Am J Gastroenterol* 102 (10):2220–29.
28. Ritchie, J. 1973. Pain from distension of the pelvic colon by inflating a balloon in the irritable colon syndrome. *Gut* 14 (2):125–32.

29. Gershon, M. D. 2004. Review article: Serotonin receptors and transporters—roles in normal and abnormal gastrointestinal motility. *Aliment Pharmacol Ther* 20 Suppl 7:3–14.

30. Atkinson, W., S. Lockhart, P. J. Whorwell, B. Keevil, and L. A. Houghton. 2006. Altered 5-hydroxytryptamine signaling in patients with constipation- and diarrhea-predominant irritable bowel syndrome. *Gastroenterology* 130 (1):34–43.

31. Dunlop, S. P., N. S. Coleman, E. Blackshaw, A. C. Perkins, G. Singh, C. A. Marsden, and R. C. Spiller. 2005. Abnormalities of 5-hydroxytryptamine metabolism in irritable bowel syndrome. *Clin Gastroenterol Hepatol* 3 (4):349–57.

32. Chen, J. J., Z. Li, H. Pan, D. L. Murphy, H. Tamir, H. Koepsell, and M. D. Gershon. 2001. Maintenance of serotonin in the intestinal mucosa and ganglia of mice that lack the high-affinity serotonin transporter: Abnormal intestinal motility and the expression of cation transporters. *J Neurosci* 21 (16):6348–61.

33. Camilleri, M., C. N. Andrews, A. E. Bharucha, P. J. Carlson, et al. 2007. Alterations in expression of p11 and SERT in mucosal biopsy specimens of patients with irritable bowel syndrome. *Gastroenterology* 132 (1):17–25.

34. Spiller, R. C. 2007. Role of infection in irritable bowel syndrome. *J Gastroenterol* 42 Suppl 17:41–47.

35. Mearin, F., M. Perez-Oliveras, A. Perello, J. Vinyet, A. Ibanez, J. Coderch, and M. Perona. 2005. Dyspepsia and irritable bowel syndrome after a salmonella gastroenteritis outbreak: One-year follow-up cohort study. *Gastroenterology* 129 (1):98–104.

36. Dizdar, V., O. H. Gilja, and T. Hausken. 2007. Increased visceral sensitivity in giardia-induced postinfectious irritable bowel syndrome and functional dyspepsia. Effect of the 5-HT3-antagonist ondansetron. *Neurogastroenterol Motil* 19 (12):977–82.

37. Ji, S., H. Park, D. Lee, Y. K. Song, J. P. Choi, and S. I. Lee. 2005. Post-infectious irritable bowel syndrome in patients with Shigella infection. *J Gastroenterol Hepatol* 20 (3):381–86.

38. Kim, H. S., M. S. Kim, S. W. Ji, and H. Park. 2006. The development of irritable bowel syndrome after Shigella infection: 3 year follow-up study. *Korean J Gastroenterol* 47 (4):300–305.

39. Wang, L. H., X. C. Fang, and G. Z. Pan. 2004. Bacillary dysentery as a causative factor of irritable bowel syndrome and its pathogenesis. *Gut* 53 (8):1096–101.

40. Dunlop, S. P., D. Jenkins, K. R. Neal, and R. C. Spiller. 2003. Relative importance of enterochromaffin cell hyperplasia, anxiety, and depression in postinfectious IBS. *Gastroenterology* 125 (6):1651–59.

41. Linden, D. R., J. X. Chen, M. D. Gershon, K. A. Sharkey, and G. M. Mawe. 2003. Serotonin availability is increased in mucosa of guinea pigs with TNBS-induced colitis. *Am J Physiol Gastrointest Liver Physiol* 285 (1):G207–16.

42. Amaro, E., Jr., and G. J. Barker. 2006. Study design in fMRI: Basic principles. *Brain Cogn* 60 (3):220–32.

43. Mertz, H., V. Morgan, G. Tanner, D. Pickens, R. Price, Y. Shyr, and R. Kessler. 2000. Regional cerebral activation in irritable bowel syndrome and control subjects with painful and nonpainful rectal distention. *Gastroenterology* 118 (5):842–48.

44. Lawal, A., M. Kern, H. Sidhu, C. Hofmann, and R. Shaker. 2006. Novel evidence for hypersensitivity of visceral sensory neural circuitry in irritable bowel syndrome patients. *Gastroenterology* 130 (1):26–33.

45. Naliboff, B. D., and E. A. Mayer. 2006. Brain imaging in IBS: Drawing the line between cognitive and non-cognitive processes. *Gastroenterology* 130 (1):267–70.

46. Lembo, T., V. Plourde, Z. Shui, S. Fullerton, H. Mertz, Y. Tache, B. Sytnik, J. Munakata, and E. Mayer. 1996. Effects of the corticotropin-releasing factor (CRF) on rectal afferent nerves in humans. *Neurogastroenterol Motil* 8 (1):9–18.

47. Carpenter, L. L., A. R. Tyrka, C. J. McDougle, R. T. Malison, M. J. Owens, C. B. Nemeroff, and L. H. Price. 2004. Cerebrospinal fluid corticotropin-releasing factor and perceived early-life stress in depressed patients and healthy control subjects. *Neuropsychopharmacology* 29 (4):777–84.

48. Drossman, D. A., Z. Li, J. Leserman, T. C. Toomey, and Y. J. Hu. 1996. Health status by gastrointestinal diagnosis and abuse history. *Gastroenterology* 110 (4):999–1007.

49. Sweetser, S., M. Camilleri, S. J. Linker Nord, D. D. Burton, L. Castenada, R. Croop, G. Tong, R. Dockens, and A. R. Zinsmeister. 2009. Do corticotropin releasing factor-1 receptors influence colonic transit and bowel function in women with irritable bowel syndrome? *Am J Physiol Gastrointest Liver Physiol* 296 (6):G1299–306.

50. Camilleri, M., and H. Gorman. 2007. Intestinal permeability and irritable bowel syndrome. *Neurogastroenterol Motil* 19 (7):545–52.

51. Bjarnason, I., A. MacPherson, and D. Hollander. 1995. Intestinal permeability: An overview. *Gastroenterology* 108 (5):1566–81.

52. Dunlop, S. P., J. Hebden, E. Campbell, J. Naesdal, L. Olbe, A. C. Perkins, and R. C. Spiller. 2006. Abnormal intestinal permeability in subgroups of diarrhea-predominant irritable bowel syndromes. *Am J Gastroenterol* 101 (6):1288–94.

53. Barbara, G., V. Stanghellini, R. De Giorgio, C. Cremon, et al. 2004. Activated mast cells in proximity to colonic nerves correlate with abdominal pain in irritable bowel syndrome. *Gastroenterology* 126 (3):693–702.

54. Guilarte, M., J. Santos, I. de Torres, C. Alonso, M. Vicario, L. Ramos, C. Martinez, F. Casellas, E. Saperas, and J. R. Malagelada. 2007. Diarrhoea-predominant IBS patients show mast cell activation and hyperplasia in the jejunum. *Gut* 56 (2):203–9.

55. Liebregts, T., B. Adam, C. Bredack, A. Roth, et al. 2007. Immune activation in patients with irritable bowel syndrome. *Gastroenterology* 132 (3):913–20.

56. Pimentel, M., S. Park, J. Mirocha, S. V. Kane, and Y. Kong. 2006. The effect of a nonabsorbed oral antibiotic (rifaximin) on the symptoms of the irritable bowel syndrome: A randomized trial. *Ann Intern Med* 145 (8):557–63.

57. Yang, J., H. R. Lee, K. Low, S. Chatterjee, and M. Pimentel. 2008. Rifaximin versus other antibiotics in the primary treatment and retreatment of bacterial overgrowth in IBS. *Dig Dis Sci* 53 (1):169–74.

58. Pimentel, M., E. E. Soffer, E. J. Chow, Y. Kong, and H. C. Lin. 2002. Lower frequency of MMC is found in IBS subjects with abnormal lactulose breath test, suggesting bacterial overgrowth. *Dig Dis Sci* 47 (12):2639–43.

59. Sharara, A. I., E. Aoun, H. Abdul-Baki, R. Mounzer, S. Sidani, and I. Elhajj. 2006. A randomized double- blind placebo-controlled trial of rifaximin in patients with abdominal bloating and flatulence. *Am J Gastroenterol* 101 (2):326–33.

60. Whorwell, P. J., L. Altringer, J. Morel, Y. Bond, D. Charbonneau, L. O'Mahony, B. Kiely, F. Shanahan, and E. M. Quigley. 2006. Efficacy of an encapsulated probiotic Bifidobacterium infantis 35624 in women with irritable bowel syndrome. *Am J Gastroenterol* 101 (7):1581–90.

61. Pimentel, M., A. Lembo, W. D. Chey, S. Zakko, Y. Ringel, J. Yu, S. M. Mareya, A. L. Shaw, E. Bortey, and W. P. Forbes. 2011. Rifaximin therapy for patients with irritable bowel syndrome without constipation. *N Engl J Med* 364 (1):22–32.

62. Rajilic-Stojanovic, M., E. Biagi, H. G. Heilig, K. Kajander, R. A. Kekkonen, S. Tims, and W. M. de Vos. 2011. Global and deep molecular analysis of microbiota signatures in fecal samples from patients with irritable bowel syndrome. *Gastroenterology* 141 (5):1792–801.

63. Patel, S. M., W. B. Stason, A. Legedza, S. M. Ock, et al. 2005. The placebo effect in irritable bowel syndrome trials: A meta-analysis. *Neurogastroenterol Motil* 17 (3):332–40.

64. Schoenfeld, P. 2005. Efficacy of current drug therapies in irritable bowel syndrome: What works and does not work. *Gastroenterol Clin North Am* 34 (2):319–35, viii.

65. Johanson, J. F., D. A. Drossman, R. Panas, A. Wahle, and R. Ueno. 2008. Clinical trial: Phase 2 trial of lubiprostone for irritable bowel syndrome with constipation. *Aliment Pharmacol Ther*.

66. Shaw, K., J. Turner, and C. Del Mar. 2002. Tryptophan and 5-hydroxytryptophan for depression. *Cochrane Database Syst Rev* (1):CD003198.

67. Camilleri, M. 2011. LX-1031, a tryptophan 5-hydroxylase inhibitor, and its potential in chronic diarrhea associated with increased serotonin. *Neurogastroenterol Motil* 23 (3):193–200.

68. Camilleri, M. 2010. LX-1031, a tryptophan 5-hydroxylase inhibitor that reduces 5-HT levels for the potential treatment of irritable bowel syndrome. *IDrugs* 13 (12):921–28.

69. Evans, B. W., W. K. Clark, D. J. Moore, and P. J. Whorwell. 2007. Tegaserod for the treatment of irritable bowel syndrome and chronic constipation. *Cochrane Database Syst Rev* (4):CD003960.

70. Camilleri, M., S. McKinzie, J. Fox, A. Foxx-Orenstein, D. Burton, G. Thomforde, K. Baxter, and A. R. Zinsmeister. 2004. Effect of renzapride on transit in constipation-predominant irritable bowel syndrome. *Clin Gastroenterol Hepatol* 2 (10):895–904.

71. George, A. M., N. L. Meyers, and R. I. Hickling. 2008. Clinical trial: Renzapride therapy for constipation-predominant irritable bowel syndrome—a multicentre, randomised, placebo-controlled, double-blind study in the primary healthcare setting. *Aliment Pharmacol Ther*

72. {, 2002 #310}

73. McKay, D. L., and J. B. Blumberg. 2006. A review of the bioactivity and potential health benefits of peppermint tea (Mentha piperita L.). *Phytother Res* 20 (8):619–33.

74. Leicester, R. J., and R. H. Hunt. 1982. Peppermint oil to reduce colonic spasm during endoscopy. *Lancet* 2 (8305):989.

75. Kline, R. M., J. J. Kline, J. Di Palma, and G. J. Barbero. 2001. Enteric-coated, pH-dependent peppermint oil capsules for the treatment of irritable bowel syndrome in children. *J Pediatr* 138 (1):125–28.

76. Cappello, G., M. Spezzaferro, L. Grossi, L. Manzoli, and L. Marzio. 2007. Peppermint oil (Mintoil) in the treatment of irritable bowel syndrome: A prospective double blind placebo-controlled randomized trial. *Dig Liver Dis* 39 (6):530–36.

77. Grigoleit, H. G., and P. Grigoleit. 2005. Peppermint oil in irritable bowel syndrome. *Phytomedicine* 12 (8):601–6.

78. Andresen, V., V. M. Montori, J. Keller, C. P. West, P. Layer, and M. Camilleri. 2008. Effects of 5-ydroxy-tryptamine (serotonin) type 3 antagonists on symptom relief and constipation in nonconstipated irritable bowel syndrome: A systematic review and meta-analysis of randomized controlled trials. *Clin Gastroenterol Hepatol.*

79. Krause, R., V. Ameen, S. H. Gordon, M. West, A. T. Heath, T. Perschy, and E. G. Carter. 2007. A randomized, double-blind, placebo-controlled study to assess efficacy and safety of 0.5 mg and 1 mg alosetron in women with severe diarrhea-predominant IBS. *Am J Gastroenterol* 102 (8):1709–19.

80. Camilleri, M., E. Atanasova, P. J. Carlson, U. Ahmad, H. J. Kim, B. E. Viramontes, S. McKinzie, and R. Urrutia. 2002. Serotonin-transporter polymorphism pharmacogenetics in diarrhea-predominant irritable bowel syndrome. *Gastroenterology* 123 (2):425–32.

81. Park, J. M., M. G. Choi, J. A. Park, J. H. Oh, Y. K. Cho, I. S. Lee, S. W. Kim, K. Y. Choi, and I. S. Chung. 2006. Serotonin transporter gene polymorphism and irritable bowel syndrome. *Neurogastroenterol Motil* 18 (11):995–1000.

82. Yeo, A., P. Boyd, S. Lumsden, T. Saunders, et al. 2004. Association between a functional polymorphism in the serotonin transporter gene and diarrhoea predominant irritable bowel syndrome in women. *Gut* 53 (10):1452–58.

83. Drossman, D. A., D. L. Patrick, W. E. Whitehead, B. B. Toner, N. E. Diamant, Y. Hu, H. Jia, and S. I. Bangdiwala. 2000. Further validation of the IBS-QOL: A disease-specific quality-of-life questionnaire. *Am J Gastroenterol* 95 (4):999–1007.

84. Tack, J., D. Broekaert, B. Fischler, L. Van Oudenhove, A. M. Gevers, and J. Janssens. 2006. A controlled crossover study of the selective serotonin reuptake inhibitor citalopram in irritable bowel syndrome. *Gut* 55 (8):1095–103.

85. Kim, H. J., M. I. Vazquez Roque, M. Camilleri, D. Stephens, D. D. Burton, K. Baxter, G. Thomforde, and A. R. Zinsmeister. 2005. A randomized controlled trial of a probiotic combination VSL# 3 and placebo in irritable bowel syndrome with bloating. *Neurogastroenterol Motil* 17 (5):687–96.

86. Niedzielin, K., H. Kordecki, and B. Birkenfeld. 2001. A controlled, double-blind, randomized study on the efficacy of lactobacillus plantarum 299V in patients with irritable bowel syndrome. *Eur J Gastroenterol Hepatol* 13 (10):1143–47.

87. O'Mahony, L., J. McCarthy, P. Kelly, G. Hurley, et al. 2005. Lactobacillus and bifidobacterium in irritable bowel syndrome: Symptom responses and relationship to cytokine profiles. *Gastroenterology* 128 (3):541–51.

88. Nobaek, S., M. L. Johansson, G. Molin, S. Ahrne, and B. Jeppsson. 2000. Alteration of intestinal microflora is associated with reduction in abdominal bloating and pain in patients with irritable bowel syndrome. *Am J Gastroenterol* 95 (5):1231–38.

89. Kong, S. C., D. P. Hurlstone, C. Y. Pocock, L. A. Walkington, N. R. Farquharson, M. G. Bramble, M. E. McAlindon, and D. S. Sanders. 2005. The incidence of self-prescribed oral complementary and alternative medicine use by patients with gastrointestinal diseases. *J Clin Gastroenterol* 39 (2):138–41.

90. Leeds, J. S., A. D. Hopper, R. Sidhu, A. Simmonette, N. Azadbakht, N. Hoggard, S. Morley, and D. S. Sanders. 2010. Some patients with irritable bowel syndrome may have exocrine pancreatic insufficiency. *Clin Gastroenterol Hepatol* 8 (5):433–38.

91. Suarez, F., M. D. Levitt, J. Adshead, and J. S. Barkin. 1999. Pancreatic supplements reduce symptomatic response of healthy subjects to a high fat meal. *Dig Dis Sci* 44 (7):1317–21.

92. Whorwell, P., and R. Lea. 2004. Dietary treatment of the irritable bowel syndrome. *Curr Treat Options Gastroenterol* 7 (4):307–16.

93. Sampson, H. A. 2004. Update on food allergy. *J Allergy Clin Immunol* 113 (5):805–19; quiz 820.

94. Nowak-Wegrzyn, A., and H. A. Sampson. 2006. Adverse reactions to foods. *Med Clin North Am* 90 (1):97–127.

95. Zar, S., M. J. Benson, and D. Kumar. 2005. Food-specific serum IgG4 and IgE titers to common food antigens in irritable bowel syndrome. *Am J Gastroenterol* 100 (7):1550–57.

96. Zar, S., L. Mincher, M. J. Benson, and D. Kumar. 2005. Food-specific IgG4 antibody-guided exclusion diet improves symptoms and rectal compliance in irritable bowel syndrome. *Scand J Gastroenterol* 40 (7):800–807.

97. Atkinson, W., T. A. Sheldon, N. Shaath, and P. J. Whorwell. 2004. Food elimination based on IgG antibodies in irritable bowel syndrome: A randomised controlled trial. *Gut* 53 (10):1459–64.

98. Zar, S., D. Kumar, and M. J. Benson. 2001. Food hypersensitivity and irritable bowel syndrome. *Aliment Pharmacol Ther* 15 (4):439–49.

99. Shanahan, F., and P. J. Whorwell. 2005. IgG-mediated food intolerance in irritable bowel syndrome: A real phenomenon or an epiphenomenom? *Am J Gastroenterol* 100 (7):1558–59.

100. Drisko, J., B. Bischoff, M. Hall, and R. McCallum. 2006. Treating irritable bowel syndrome with a food elimination diet followed by food challenge and probiotics. *J Am Coll Nutr* 25 (6):514–22.

101. Zuo, X. L., Y. Q. Li, W. J. Li, Y. T. Guo, X. F. Lu, J. M. Li, and P. V. Desmond. 2007. Alterations of food antigen-specific serum immunoglobulins G and E antibodies in patients with irritable bowel syndrome and functional dyspepsia. *Clin Exp Allergy* 37 (6):823–30.

102. Arora, A. S., and K. Yamazaki. 2004. Eosinophilic esophagitis: Asthma of the esophagus? *Clin Gastroenterol Hepatol* 2 (7):523–30.

103. Swoger, J. M., C. R. Weiler, and A. S. Arora. 2007. Eosinophilic esophagitis: Is it all allergies? *Mayo Clin Proc* 82 (12):1541–49.

104. Heine, R. G. 2004. Pathophysiology, diagnosis and treatment of food protein-induced gastrointestinal diseases. *Curr Opin Allergy Clin Immunol* 4 (3):221–29.

105. O'Leary, C., P. Wieneke, S. Buckley, P. O'Regan, C. C. Cronin, E. M. Quigley, and F. Shanahan. 2002. Celiac disease and irritable bowel-type symptoms. *Am J Gastroenterol* 97 (6):1463–67.

106. Sanders, D. S. 2003. Celiac disease and IBS-type symptoms: The relationship exists in both directions. *Am J Gastroenterol* 98 (3):707–8.

107. Wahnschaffe, U., J. D. Schulzke, M. Zeitz, and R. Ullrich. 2007. Predictors of clinical response to gluten-free diet in patients diagnosed with diarrhea-predominant irritable bowel syndrome. *Clin Gastroenterol Hepatol* 5 (7):844–50; quiz 769.

108. Spiegel, B. M., V. P. DeRosa, I. M. Gralnek, V. Wang, and G. S. Dulai. 2004. Testing for celiac sprue in irritable bowel syndrome with predominant diarrhea: A cost-effectiveness analysis. *Gastroenterology* 126 (7):1721–32.

109. AGA Institute Medical Position Statement on the Diagnosis and Management of Celiac Disease. 2006. *Gastroenterology* 131 (6):1977–80.

110. Camilleri, M., A. W. Mangel, S. E. Fehnel, D. A. Drossman, E. A. Mayer, and N. J. Talley. 2007. Primary endpoints for irritable bowel syndrome trials: A review of performance of endpoints. *Clin Gastroenterol Hepatol* 5 (5):534–40.

111. Evidence-based position statement on the management of irritable bowel syndrome in North America. 2002. *Am J Gastroenterol* 97 (11 Suppl):S1–5.

112. Monsbakken, K. W., P. O. Vandvik, and P. G. Farup. 2006. Perceived food intolerance in subjects with irritable bowel syndrome—etiology, prevalence and consequences. *Eur J Clin Nutr* 60 (5):667–72.

113. Gibson, P. R., and S. J. Shepherd. 2005. Personal view: Food for thought—western lifestyle and susceptibility to Crohn's disease. The FODMAP hypothesis. *Aliment Pharmacol Ther* 21 (12):1399–409.

114. Gearry, R. B., P. M. Irving, J. S. Barrett, D. M. Nathan, S. J. Shepherd, and P. R. Gibson. 2009. Reduction of dietary poorly absorbed short-chain carbohydrates (FODMAPs) improves abdominal symptoms in patients with inflammatory bowel disease—A pilot study. *J Crohns Colitis* 3 (1):8–14.

115. Bourdu, S., M. Dapoigny, E. Chapuy, F. Artigue, M. P. Vasson, P. Dechelotte, G. Bommelaer, A. Eschalier, and D. Ardid. 2005. Rectal instillation of butyrate provides a novel clinically relevant model of noninflammatory colonic hypersensitivity in rats. *Gastroenterology* 128 (7):1996–2008.

116. Ong, D. K., S. B. Mitchell, J. S. Barrett, S. J. Shepherd, P. M. Irving, J. R. Biesiekierski, S. Smith, P. R. Gibson, and J. G. Muir. 2010. Manipulation of dietary short chain carbohydrates alters the pattern of gas production and genesis of symptoms in irritable bowel syndrome. *J Gastroenterol Hepatol* 25 (8):1366–73.

117. Gibson, P. R., and S. J. Shepherd. 2010. Evidence-based dietary management of functional gastrointestinal symptoms: The FODMAP approach. *J Gastroenterol Hepatol* 25 (2):252–58.

118. Jarvela, I. E. 2005. Molecular genetics of adult-type hypolactasia. *Ann Med* 37 (3):179–85.

119. Arola, H., and A. Tamm. 1994. Metabolism of lactose in the human body. *Scand J Gastroenterol Suppl* 202:21–25.

120. Farup, P. G., K. W. Monsbakken, and P. O. Vandvik. 2004. Lactose malabsorption in a population with irritable bowel syndrome: Prevalence and symptoms. A case-control study. *Scand J Gastroenterol* 39 (7):645–49.

121. Vernia, P., V. Marinaro, F. Argnani, M. Di Camillo, and R. Caprilli. 2004. Self-reported milk intolerance in irritable bowel syndrome: What should we believe? *Clin Nutr* 23 (5):996–1000.

122. Parker, T. J., J. T. Woolner, A. T. Prevost, Q. Tuffnell, M. Shorthouse, and J. O. Hunter. 2001. Irritable bowel syndrome: Is the search for lactose intolerance justified? *Eur J Gastroenterol Hepatol* 13 (3):219–25.

123. Vernia, P., M. R. Ricciardi, C. Frandina, T. Bilotta, and G. Frieri. 1995. Lactose malabsorption and irritable bowel syndrome. Effect of a long-term lactose-free diet. *Ital J Gastroenterol* 27 (3):117–21.

124. Bohmer, C. J., and H. A. Tuynman. 2001. The effect of a lactose-restricted diet in patients with a positive lactose tolerance test, earlier diagnosed as irritable bowel syndrome: A 5-year follow-up study. *Eur J Gastroenterol Hepatol* 13 (8):941–44.

125. Caplice, E., and G. F. Fitzgerald. 1999. Food fermentations: Role of microorganisms in food production and preservation. *Int J Food Microbiol* 50 (1–2):131–49.

126. Rumessen, J. J., and E. Gudmand-Hoyer. 1988. Functional bowel disease: Malabsorption and abdominal distress after ingestion of fructose, sorbitol, and fructose-sorbitol mixtures. *Gastroenterology* 95 (3):694–700.

127. Rumessen, J. J., and E. Gudmand-Hoyer. 1991. Functional bowel disease: The role of fructose and sorbitol. *Gastroenterology* 101 (5):1452–53.

128. Rumessen, J. J., and E. Gudmand-Hoyer. 1986. Absorption capacity of fructose in healthy adults. Comparison with sucrose and its constituent monosaccharides. *Gut* 27 (10):1161–68.

129. Shepherd, S. J., and P. R. Gibson. 2006. Fructose malabsorption and symptoms of irritable bowel syndrome: Guidelines for effective dietary management. *J Am Diet Assoc* 106 (10):1631–39.

130. Beyer, P. L., E. M. Caviar, and R. W. McCallum. 2005. Fructose intake at current levels in the United States may cause gastrointestinal distress in normal adults. *J Am Diet Assoc* 105 (10):1559–66.

131. Bray, G. A., S. J. Nielsen, and B. M. Popkin. 2004. Consumption of high-fructose corn syrup in beverages may play a role in the epidemic of obesity. *Am J Clin Nutr* 79 (4):537–43.

132. Gibson, P. R., E. Newnham, J. S. Barrett, S. J. Shepherd, and J. G. Muir. 2007. Review article: Fructose malabsorption and the bigger picture. *Aliment Pharmacol Ther* 25 (4):349–63.

133. Nelis, G. F., M. A. Vermeeren, and W. Jansen. 1990. Role of fructose-sorbitol malabsorption in the irritable bowel syndrome. *Gastroenterology* 99 (4):1016–20.

134. Choi, Y. K., N. Kraft, B. Zimmerman, M. Jackson, and S. S. Rao. 2008. Fructose intolerance in IBS and utility of fructose-restricted diet. *J Clin Gastroenterol.*

135. Shepherd, S. J., F. C. Parker, J. G. Muir, and P. R. Gibson. 2008. Dietary triggers of abdominal symptoms in patients with irritable bowel syndrome: Randomized placebo-controlled evidence. *Clin Gastroenterol Hepatol* 6 (7):765–71.

136. Roberts, A., A. G. Renwick, J. Sims, and D. J. Snodin. 2000. Sucralose metabolism and pharmacokinetics in man. *Food Chem Toxicol* 38 Suppl 2:S31–41.

137. Biesiekierski, J. R., E. D. Newnham, P. M. Irving, J. S. Barrett, M. Haines, J. D. Doecke, S. J. Shepherd, J. G. Muir, and P. R. Gibson. 2011. Gluten causes gastrointestinal symptoms in subjects without celiac disease: A double-blind randomized placebo-controlled trial. *Am J Gastroenterol* 106 (3):508–14; quiz 515.

138. Department of Health. 2001. Treatment choice in psychological therapies and counselling: Evidence based clinical practice guidelines. In *NHS Executive*. London.

139. Hutton, J. 2005. Cognitive behaviour therapy for irritable bowel syndrome. *Eur J Gastroenterol Hepatol* 17 (1):11–14.

140. Webb, A. N., R. H. Kukuruzovic, A. G. Catto-Smith, and S. M. Sawyer. 2007. Hypnotherapy for treatment of irritable bowel syndrome. *Cochrane Database Syst Rev* (4):CD005110.

141. Palsson, O. S., M. J. Turner, D. A. Johnson, C. K. Burnelt, and W. E. Whitehead. 2002. Hypnosis treatment for severe irritable bowel syndrome: Investigation of mechanism and effects on symptoms. *Dig Dis Sci* 47 (11):2605–14.

142. Whorwell, P. J., A. Prior, and E. B. Faragher. 1984. Controlled trial of hypnotherapy in the treatment of severe refractory irritable-bowel syndrome. *Lancet* 2 (8414):1232–34.

143. Galovski, T. E., and E. B. Blanchard. 1998. The treatment of irritable bowel syndrome with hypnotherapy. *Appl Psychophysiol Biofeedback* 23 (4):219–32.

144. Roberts, L., S. Wilson, S. Singh, A. Roalfe, and S. Greenfield. 2006. Gut-directed hypnotherapy for irritable bowel syndrome: piloting a primary care-based randomised controlled trial. *Br J Gen Pract* 56 (523):115–21.

145. van der Veek, P. P., Y. R. van Rood, and A. A. Masclee. 2007. Clinical trial: Short- and long-term benefit of relaxation training for irritable bowel syndrome. *Aliment Pharmacol Ther* 26 (6):943–52.

146. Drossman, D. A. 2006. The functional gastrointestinal disorders and the Rome III process. *Gastroenterology* 130 (5):1377–90.

15 Inflammatory Bowel Disease

Integrating Food and Nutrients into Disease Management

*Gerard E. Mullin, M.D., Colleen Fogarty Draper,
M.S., R.D., and Melissa A. Munsell, M.D.*

INTRODUCTION

Inflammatory bowel disease (IBD) is a chronic illness that is characterized by unremitting intestinal inflammation with tissue injury caused by increased oxidative and metabolic stress. Increased energy, macronutrient, micronutrient, and electrolyte requirements result from thermodynamic demands of inflammation and tissue losses from intestinal injury. Consequent protein-calorie malnutrition and micronutrient deficiencies are common among these patients and require close supervision and corrective supplementation (Table 15.1) [1]. Along these lines, food harbors nutrients that are vital for optimal cellular function (i.e., antioxidants, polyphenols, omega-3-fatty acids, etc.) and that regulate key components of the inflammatory cascade. Diet plays an important role in downregulating the unresolved inflammation of IBD while optimizing healing and immunity. Thus, dietary and nutrient strategies have been studied as primary treatment in IBD. We review the nutritional consequences and therapy of inflammatory bowel disease.

EPIDEMIOLOGY

Incidence of IBD increased after 1940 when Westernized diets were broadly adopted in the United States and Europe. Since that time, rates have plateaued with the prevalence of ulcerative colitis estimated at 214 cases per 100,000 and Crohn's disease at 174 per 100,000 [2]. However the incidence of IBD has recently increased in Asian countries concurrent with increasing Westernized diets [3]. High–animal fat, high-sugar, and low-fiber diets are proinflammatory and have been implicated in the development of IBD [4–6]. Though IBD has remained an idiopathic disease, it has been proposed that genetically susceptible individuals develop disease in response to an exaggerated immune response to an environmental trigger (i.e., infectious, dietary) in the gut microbiota. Since IBD is believed to be the result of a complex interaction between genetic, immune, microbial, and environmental factors as noted here, it is highly plausible that diet, as an environmental factor, may contribute to the pathogenesis of these diseases. For example, *Mycobacterium paratuberculosis* has reemerged as a possible infectious etiology for Crohn's disease. This infectious pathogen is found in unpasteurized cow's milk in Europe [7]. Furthermore, elemental diets will produce

279

TABLE 15.1
Malnutrition in Inflammatory Bowel Disease

Deficiency	Crohn's Disease	Ulcerative Colitis	Treatment
Negative nitrogen balance	69%	Unknown	Adequate energy and protein
Vitamin B12	48%	5%	1000 mcg/day × seven days, then monthly
Folate	67%	30–40%	1 mg/day
Vitamin A	11%	Unknown	5000–25,000 IU/day
Vitamin D	75%	35%	5000–25,000 IU/day
Calcium	13%	Unknown	1000–1200 mg/day
Potassium	5–20%	Unknown	Variable
Iron	39%	81%	Iron Gluconate 300 mg TID
Zinc	50%	Unknown	Zn Sulfate 220 mg qd or BID

symptomatic relief and objective remission in up to 90% of patients, and may be considered as a first line in therapy for pediatric patients [8]. Elemental diets contain no intact protein and dietary nitrogen is supplied as amino acids, while polymeric diets contain intact protein. In animal models of IBD, dietary protein increased intestinal permeability, which resolved with the institution of an elemental diet [9]. Since dietary constituents influence the composition and function of the intestinal microflora and the clinical course of IBD, nutrition appears to be an integral role in the pathogenesis and treatment.

Gene polymorphisms confer susceptibility to IBD, Crohn's, and ulcerative colitis (UC). These genes can be categorized into those responsible for bacterial recognition, immunity response, and epithelial barrier integrity [10]. Other gene polymorphisms are associated with suboptimal nutrient metabolism that may exacerbate nutrition insufficiencies or deficiencies, which already exist in the setting of IBD. Of note, IBD susceptibility and risk of nutrient deficiencies is both polygenic and polyenvironmental. Thus, interactions between multiple genes and various environmental exposures, including nutrition, need to be contemplated in order to understand the origins of disease.

PATHOPHYSIOLOGY

OVERVIEW OF INFLAMMATORY BOWEL DISEASE PRESENTATION

Ulcerative colitis (UC) affects the colonic mucosa diffusely and is characterized by diarrhea, abdominal pain, and hematochezia. UC is categorized as distal disease (affecting rectum and/or sigmoid), left-sided colitis (up to splenic flexure), extensive colitis (up to hepatic flexure), or pancolitis (entire colon). Crohn's disease (CD) is characterized by transmural inflammation, which is discontinuous and may affect any part of the gastrointestinal tract. The most common location of disease involvement is the small bowel, whereby most nutrients are assimilated and absorbed. Endoscopically, the mucosa is described as cobblestoned with evidence of apthous ulcerations. Radiographically, evidence of fistulae or stricturing disease may be present. Crohn's disease is classified by location of disease and the pattern of disease (inflammatory, fibrostenotic, or fistulizing) [11]. Patients with CD often have symptoms of abdominal pain that limit nutrient intake, diarrhea from severe mucosal injury causing malabsorption of fat and lipid-soluble vitamins, loss of fluids electrolytes minerals, and consequent weight loss. Despite aggressive evaluation with clinical, endoscopic, radiological, and pathological criteria, about 5% of patients with IBD affecting the colon are termed indeterminate colitis, whereby the disease is indistinguishable from either UC or CD.

CHRONIC INFLAMMATION

Chronic inflammation in IBD is characterized by infiltration of mononuclear cells and polymorpho-nuclear neutrophils into the wall of the intestine [13]. The inflammatory response is amplified as these cells are proinflammatory mediators and activate and recruit more inflammatory cells to the bowel. It is believed that mononuclear cells mediate this immune response via secretion of tumor necrosis factor (TNF), interferon-γ, interleukins, and eicosanoids (prostaglandin class 2, throm-boxanes, leukotrienes class 4) [14]. Activation of NFκB stimulates expression of these molecules, which are increased in active IBD, yet also stimulates expression of protective molecules that inhibit inflammatory responses [15].

Genetics and dietary nutrient intake influence NFκB activation. Studies have shown that poly-phenols, n-3 fatty acids, and short-chain fatty acids (SCFAs) such as butyrate can reduce NFκB activity and become possible nutraceutical therapeutic modalities for IBD [16–18].

Tumor necrosis factor (TNF)-α, interleukin (IL)-6, and interleukin (IL)-10 are inflammatory cyto-kines associated with inflammatory disease. Individuals with certain TNF-α and IL-6 gene polymor-phisms are at higher risk of disease activity, particularly with a high dietary intake of saturated and monounsaturated fats, or a high dietary n-6/n-3 polyunsaturated fatty acid (PUFA) ratio [19]. TNF-α gene polymorphisms are, also, associated with ulcerative colitis progression [20] Certain interleukin (IL)-10 gene polymorphisms are associated with the risk of CD development, early age at diagnosis, structuring CD behavior, bowel resection requirement, and elevation of serum IL-10 levels [5].

Linoleic acid is an essential PUFA and is a substrate for eicosanoids. PUFAs are categorized into two main families: n-6 and n-3. Linoleic acid is the parent compound to the proinflammatory n-6 fatty acids and is found in fairly high concentrations in corn, soybean, and safflower oils [14]. The other class of essential fatty acids are n-3 PUFAs of which the parent compound is α-linoleic acid that is synthesized into fatty acids important in immunomodulatory and anti-inflammatory effects via the production of prostaglandin class 3 and leukotriene B_5, and by inhibiting production of ara-chidonic acid [21] (Figure 15.1). The n-3 fatty acids are believed to compete with n-6 fatty acids as precursors for eicosanoid synthesis [22]. N-3 fatty acids also reduce TNF-α production by inhibiting protein kinase C activity [23]. N-3 PUFAs are found in flaxseed, canola, and walnuts, but oils from deep-sea fish are a more advantageous source of n-3 PUFAs since humans do not readily transform

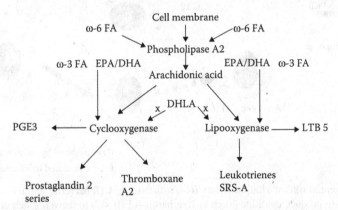

FIGURE 15.1 Modulation of the arachidonic acid cascade: ω-6 Fatty acids appear to promote the produc-tion of phospholipase A2 (PLP A2), arachidonic acid (AA), and production of noxious proinflammatory eico-sanoids such as prostaglandin-2 series (PGE2), leukotrienes (LTB) such as slow reactive releasing substance (SRS-A), and thromboxane A2 (TXA2). ω-3 Fatty acids, in contrast, downregulate production of proinflam-matory eicosanoids by competitive inhibition of the enzymes cyclooxygenase-2 (COX-2) and 5-Lipoxygenase (5-LPO) for AA, thus leading to preferential production of the prostaglandin-3 series (PGE3) and leukot-riene-5 series (LTB5). Adapted from Clarke JO, Mullin GE. A review of complementary and alternative approaches to immunomodulation. *Nutr Clin Pract*. 2008;23(1):49–62.

α-linoleic acid to eicosapentanoic acid and docosahexaenoic acid, which are the main precursors for desirable eicosanoids [14]. Fish oil affects the gut immune system by suppressing T-cell signaling, inhibiting proinflammatory cytokine synthesis, reducing inflammatory cell recruitment, and enhancing epithelial barrier function [24,25]. (See Figure 15.2.)

Along with PUFAs, short-chain fatty acids (SCFAs) are thought to play a role in IBD pathogenesis. SCFAs are monocarboxylic hydrocarbons produced by the endogenous bacterial flora digestion of nonabsorbable carbohydrates reaching the colon, and include acetate, proprionate, and butyrate [26]. Nonabsorbable carbohydrates such as dietary fibers include, but are not limited to, nonstarch polysaccharides, resistant starch, cellulose, and pectins [27]. Butyrate is a major source of energy for colonocytes and early studies demonstrated that rectal epithelial cells in patients with UC have impaired oxidation of butyrate that may be caused by elevated levels of TNF [28–30]. Other studies have shown that SCFAs such as butyrate may have an anti-inflammatory effect by downregulating cytokines [31]. Furthermore, SCFAs may promote colonic sodium absorption [32]. SCFAs therapeutic potential has been shown in both animal and human studies in IBD [33]. Butyrate and other SCFAs may be mediated by epigenetic modification of some IBD susceptibility genes. Butyrate increases gene expression through histone deactylase inhibition [33–35].

Various fields of research inform the complex interplay between genetic, immune, and environmental factors. While diets high in animal fats and sugar and low in fiber have been implicated in IBD, studies on the dietary role in IBD are challenging to interpret as other lifestyle or environmental factors may play a role. [34] Dietary microparticles have also been theorized to be involved in the etiology of IBD. Microparticles are bacterial-sized inorganic particles such as titanium, aluminum,

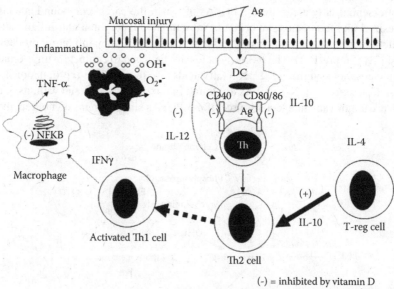

(-) = inhibited by vitamin D

(+) = stimulated by vitamin D

FIGURE 15.2 Potential role of vitamin D in Crohn's disease: In CD, bacterial antigens drive antigen-presenting cells (DCs) to produce cytokines such as interleukin-12 (IL-12) to drive a T-helper (Th1) proinflammatory response to induce macrophages that produce TNF-α and neutrophil chemoattractive agents, which ultimately result in the production of noxious agents and tissue injury. The damaged intestinal tissue is more permeable to antigens, which drive the vicious cycle of antigen-presentation, local immune activation and tissue injury. Anti-inflammatory cytokines such as interleukin-10 (IL-10), made by regulatory T cells (T regs), antagonize Th1 proinflammatory processes by stimulating T-helper 2 function. Vitamin D antagonizes Th1 proinflammatory responses by interfering with antigen presentation and Th1 activation, upregulating Th2 cytokines and downregulating NFκB in macrophages. Adapted from Mullin GE, Dobs A. Vitamin D and its role in cancer and immunity: A prescription for sunlight. *Nutr Clin Pract.* 2007;22(3):305–322.

and silicone that are found in Western diets, often in food additives. They have been proposed to exacerbate inflammation via antigen-mediated immune responses and by increasing intestinal permeability leading to increased immune exposure to antigens [36,37]. Specific foods can aggravate gastrointestinal symptoms in IBD but do not indicate a causative role. Currently, there is no definitive evidence linking specific foods as a direct cause in IBD; therefore, a diet rich in polyphenols, omega-3 fatty acids, along with prebiotic-rich foods coupled with a healthful lifestyle is recommended to patients with UC and CD to minimize the risk of malnutrition.

MALNUTRITION

Hospitalized patients with IBD have a higher prevalence of malnutrition than patients hospitalized with other benign conditions [38] (see Table 15.1). CD patients, in particular, are susceptible to protein-calorie malnutrition, which contributes to both increased length of stay and hospital costs [39,40]. Protein-calorie malnutrition in IBD is often manifested clinically by weight loss [41]. Up to 70% of adult patients with CD are underweight while fewer patients with UC experience weight loss, and weight loss is more commonly seen in hospitalized UC patients [42–44].

Not only do hospitalized CD patients experience weight loss, but it is common in outpatients as well, and up to 75% of patients with CD experience weight loss [1, 45–47]. CD patients have significantly lower lean body mass [48]. Even when CD patients are in remission, 20% of patients were more than 10% below their ideal body weight [49]. Patients with IBD lose fat stores, and male patients with CD have been shown to have significantly lower percentage of body fat and hamstring muscle strength compared to healthy controls [44,50]. The reasons for protein-calorie malnutrition in IBD stem from ongoing inflammation and catabolic cytokine production, hypothalamic pituitary adrenal (HPA), HPA-axis dysregulation, and malabsorption of nutrients along with diminished intake from abdominal discomfort.

While malnutrition is common, obesity can be seen that can lead to protein-calorie malnutrition. Often fat occurs in a distribution of mesenteric fat, although this is often independent of body mass index. "Creeping fat" is seen in CD and is described as fat hypertrophy and visceral fat wrapping around the small and large bowel [1]. It was originally thought that creeping fat simply results from transmural inflammation, but emerging data shows that mesenteric fat itself is proinflammatory with increased synthesis of TNF-α and proinflammatory adipocytokines [51]. Hyperinsulinism, cortisol and catecholamine imbalance, along with enhanced proinflammatory cytokines make obesity a special consideration in the setting of concurrent IBD. Prednisone therapy can contribute to weight gain by decreasing lipid oxidation and increasing protein oxidation while increasing fatty mass and depleting muscle protein [52,53]. Together, hypercortisolism, corticosteroids, and obesity are a dangerous combination for the IBD patient from both a nutritional and disease-outcome point of view.

MECHANISMS OF GROWTH RETARDATION AND MALNUTRITION

Growth impairment in IBD is multifactorial with poor nutrition, mediators of chronic inflammation, and complications of therapy all contributing [54,55]. Decreased oral intake is frequently seen in those with high disease activity, which may be due to anorexia or sitophobia [56]. Even while in remission, patients may have lower daily intake of nutrients such as fiber and phosphorus [50]. In addition to reduced dietary intake, maldigestion, malabsorption, enteric loss of nutrients, and rapid GI transit contribute to malnutrition, particularly in CD, as do increased basal caloric requirements from active inflammation with inherent catabolic proinflammatory cytokine production or sepsis. Disease activity and extent can markedly influence the prevalence and degree of malnutrition in CD [46]. Patients with diffuse small bowel involvement typically are at more risk for malnutrition due to impaired absorption of nutrients that can be similarly seen in small bowel resection and small bowel bacterial overgrowth [49,57,58]. Genetic susceptibility may also play a role as children with NOD2/CARD15 variants in CD had lower height and weight percentiles [59]. The growth hormone, insulin-like growth factor (IGF)-1, has been found to be involved in metabolic derangements in both children and adults with IBD. Total and free IGF-1 levels are reduced in patients with both Crohn's disease (CD) and ulcerative colitis (UC) when compared to healthy controls and may be partially, but not completely, reversed by steroid therapy and TNF inhibitors [60–62]. Once inflammation and disease activity is controlled, a patient's nutritional status usually improves. Biologic therapies improve weight and BMI in children with active CD who respond to treatment [63]. Four to six years after patients with UC undergo total proctocolectomy with ileal pouch-anal anastomosis, muscular strength is increased by 11%, total tissue mass by 4.5%, and bone mineral density by almost 2% suggesting the role of inflammation in metabolic disturbance [58].

IMPLICATIONS OF MALNUTRITION

Malnutrition has many detrimental effects. It is associated with deterioration in muscle, respiratory, and immune function, as well as delayed wound healing and recovery from illness [64]. In children, malnutrition leads to stunted growth, and in all ages leads to weight loss [65,66]. CD patients have a greater loss of muscle than fat, particularly in ileal and ileocolic disease [46]. Patients often develop hypoalbuminemia, which results from increased catabolism and decreased synthesis due to ongoing inflammation, intestinal protein loss, reduced hepatic protein synthesis, malabsorption, and anorexia [67]. In the hospitalized setting, hypoalbuminemia portends an adverse prognosis for the IBD patient. Villous atrophy may occur as a result of malnutrition leading to poor nutrient absorption [68]. Malnourished patients may experience a low quality of life, depression, and anxiety [69,70]. Malnutrition on admission to a hospital has been correlated with longer length of stays, higher costs, and increased mortality [71–73]. IBD patients admitted with hypoalbuminemia and evidence of malnutrition require a prompt nutritional evaluation and early intervention. Individuals who undergo an aggressive correction of their underlying malnutrition in the hospital setting have improved outcomes, lower morbidity, lower mortality rates, and shorter hospital stays [74,75].

NUTRITION AND BONE HEALTH

Bone loss is an early systemic process and occurs even before clinical disease manifests. Bone disease is attributed to vitamin D deficiency, steroid use, and/or systemic inflammation. Malnutrition and systemic inflammation contribute to the decreased bone mineral density that occurs in patients with IBD though other factors such as corticosteroid use likely contribute [76–80]. In IBD, the prevalence of osteopenia is 50% while the prevalence is 15% for osteoporosis [81]. Though both patients with CD and UC are at risk for decreased bone density, those with CD carry greater risk [82]. Studies have shown that osteopenia may be seen in newly diagnosed patients with IBD, prior to any steroid therapy [83]. This is contrasted, however, with a study demonstrating that women who developed IBD prior to age 20 were likely to have normal bone mineral density as adults [84]. Though steroid use has often been blamed for reduced bone mineral density in IBD, it has been shown to be a weak predictor of osteopenia in Crohn's disease patients. Age, body mass index, serum magnesium, and history of bowel resections appear to be more important predictors for low bone mineral density [85,86]. The overall relative risk of fractures is 40% greater in IBD than in the general population—the prevalence of osteopenia and osteoporosis are 50% and 15%, respectively. The risk of fracture is similar for Crohn's disease and ulcerative colitis and for both males and females with IBD. In relation to bone health, calcium, vitamin D, vitamin K, and magnesium deficiency occur. Calcium and vitamin D supplementation have been shown to maintain and increase bone mineral density in patients with CD [87,88].

Vitamin D is not only important in bone health, but appears to have a role in immunomodulation as well. Vitamin D can help regulate cytokine responses and dampen inflammatory responses

[89]. The ability of vitamin D to influence the immunopathogenesis of IBD is reviewed elsewhere and show in Figure 15.1 [90,91]. Vitamin D exerts its effects via vitamin D receptors on T cells and antigen-presenting cells. Vitamin D can antagonize T-helper 1 proinflammatory responses by interfering with antigen presentation and Th1 activation, upregulating Th2 cytokines, and downregulating NFκB in macrophages [35,92,93].

Vitamin D receptor (VDR) gene polymorphisms have a variety of effects on the immune system and have, also, been linked to IBD [94–97]. VDR functions as an intracellular hormone receptor, which binds to vitamin D or calcitrol to facilitate calcium absorption. The vitamin D3 receptor gene, VDR, is one of the first genes found to be associated with osteoporosis susceptibility [98]. The VDR-gene variations inhibit transcription activity of the VDR gene, which limit calcium absorption and thereby impair bone turnover, decrease bone mineral density [99,100], reduce bone mineral content [101], and lower serum vitamin D [102].

Biologic therapy with infliximab is associated with increased markers of bone formation without increasing bone resorption [103]. Weight-bearing exercise should be encouraged, while smoking should be avoided. All women with IBD should be supplemented with calcium and vitamin D according to the Dietary Reference Intakes. However, most experts agree that, given the prevalence of vitamin D insufficiency (25[OH]D levels < 32 mcg/mL) in Crohn's disease, supplementation should be individualized to meet individual needs. Finally, a recent study showed a trend for vitamin D3 (daily dose of 1200 IU) maintaining remission of quiescent Crohn's disease (p = 0.06) [104].

NUTRIENT DEFICIENCIES

Vitamin and mineral deficiencies are commonly seen in IBD. Overall, low calcium and phosphorus levels occur in IBD as well as deficiencies in niacin, zinc, copper, and vitamins A and C [105]. In IBD, increased oxidative stress, oxidative damage to proteins and DNA, along with impaired antioxidant defenses in the form of mucosal zinc, copper, and super oxide dismutase have been shown in both serum and in the involved intestinal mucosa [106].

Gene polymorphisms associated with vitamin and mineral metabolism, as well as oxidative defense and xenobiotic metabolism, can exacerbate these nutritional deficiencies; for example, glutathione-S-transferase involved in phase I detoxification. Genetic expression is upregulated by cruciferous vegetables. Polymorphisms of this gene are associated with lower serum vitamin C and susceptibility to IBD [107,108]. Additionally, there is an epigenetic association with XRCC1, involved in DNA repair, and glutathione s transferase polymorphisms and CPG island hypermethylation of the colonic mucosa [109]. Thus, every patient with IBD should be screened at least annually for vitamin and mineral deficiencies and closely monitored for response to nutrition therapies to individualize and titrate the therapies necessary to overcome deficiencies since response to therapy may vary according to genotype.

ANEMIA

Anemia is frequently seen in inflammatory bowel disease and may be related to iron, B12, and folic acid deficiency. Measurement of serum B12 should be performed annually in patients with ileal disease [110]. Methylmalonic acid can be used as a more sensitive test for the diagnosis of cobalamin deficiency [111]. Hyperhomocysteinemia is seen in IBD and is associated with decreased levels of vitamin B12 and folate [112].

Methylenetetrahydrofolate reductase (MTHFR) is an enzyme that metabolizes folate to facilitate homocysteine remethylation to methionine, is related to certain key epigenetic mechanisms, and its gene is highly polymorphic [113]. MTHFR-gene polymorphisms lead to decreased enzyme activity and are associated with low serum folate, vitamin B12 and riboflavin deficiencies and hyperhomocysteinemia, and are responsive to increased dietary intake and supplementation [114–117]. Certain MTHFR genotypes with hyperhomocysteinemia respond to riboflavin supplementation with a reduction in homocsteine levels, as well as folate [118]. While MTHFR genotypes are not specifically related to IBD susceptibility, individuals with certain MTHFR genotypes are at greater risk of developing hyperhomocsteinemia and should be monitored closely for B vitamin deficiencies.

ROLE OF PARENTERAL NUTRITION

Previously, total parenteral nutrition (TPN)—now called central parenteral nutrition (CPN)—was used as an adjunct to bowel rest and has been used as primary therapy for Crohn's disease. However, a key study in 1988 demonstrated that complete bowel rest was not a major factor in achieving clinical remission; thus CPN is no longer used as primary therapy of IBD [119]. However, CPN is used in IBD to manage enterocutaneous fistulas (ECF), short bowel syndrome, and preoperative nutrition support in the setting of malnutrition [120]. When feeding the gastrointestinal tract is not feasible, then CPN is used to provide nutritional support. CPN carries risks of sepsis and cholestatic liver disease (see Table 15.2). Complications are increased by overfeeding [121]. In animal models, long-term CPN use is associated with small intestinal atrophy and increased intestinal permeability, while villous atrophy is not seen with enteral feeds, though this has not been uniformly seen in human studies [122–125]. A recent study of nationwide patterns of inpatient CPN utilization showed that usage was associated with higher in-hospital mortality, length of stay, and hospital costs ($51,729 vs. $19,563) [126]. Total enteral nutrition can prevent malnutrition as well as CPN in patients with adequate bowel length and thus should be favored over CPN due to preservation of mucosal integrity and favorable adverse effect profile relative to parenteral infusion [127,128].

ROLE OF ENTERAL NUTRITION

The role of enteral nutrition as primary therapy is uncertain, particularly in adults. While enteral nutrition as primary therapy for active CD is less successful in inducing remission than steroid therapy, it has a better response than placebo [129–131]. Meta-analyses have shown that remission rates with enteral feeds in Crohn's disease are approximately 60% [130,132]. Oral diet supplementation with low-residue nutrition has also been shown to improve nutritional status and decrease disease activity in CD [133,134]. One randomized control study showed that having patients obtain half of calories from an elemental diet and the remaining half from a polymeric diet was an effective strategy for reducing relapse compared to patients receiving all calories from a normal diet [135]. Often these studies are challenging to perform due to a large dropout rate from poor palatability or intolerance of the diet [22]. In terms of type of enteral feeds, elemental (amino acid–based) diets have not been shown to be more successful in inducing remission than nonelemental diets [132,136]. This is

---

TABLE 15.2

Complications of TPN

Catheter-related infections
Venous thrombosis
Occlusion of catheter lumen
Gallbladder stasis
Hyperoxaluria
Hepatic dysfunction

Adapted from Montalvo-Jave EE, Zarraga JL, Sarr MG.
Specific topics and complications of parenteral nutrition.
Langenbecks Arch Surg. 2007;392(2):119–126.

an important clinical pearl since elemental formulations are not palatable and noncompliance is an issue. In children, enteral nutritional support has a positive effect on growth and development and may help children avoid steroid use [137,138]. In the maintenance of remission in CD, controlled data demonstrate that defined enteral nutrition reduces the risk of relapse requiring steroid treatment. Elemental formulations do not provide an advantage over polymeric regimens in maintaining remission in Crohn's disease. Finally, there are no data in support of primary nutrition therapy in UC either in management of the acute flare or in maintenance.

MODE OF ACTION OF ENTERAL NUTRITION

It is unclear by what mechanism enteral nutrition acts to affect the inflammatory process in Crohn's disease. Proposed mechanisms include provision of essential nutrients, reduction of antigenic load, alteration of bowel flora, and improved immune function [139]. The enteral diet may have an anti-inflammatory effect on the gastrointestinal mucosa that may be related to the fatty acids in the feed or alteration of gut flora [1,140,141]. The feeds studied (AL110, Modulen IBD, and ACD004 [Nestle, Vevey, Switzerland]) all have casein as the protein source, are lactose free, and are rich in transforming growth factor beta (TGF-beta). They have all been shown to induce clinical remission associated with mucosal healing [142]. In the case of Modulen IBD, in addition to mucosal macroscopic and histological healing, there was a fall in mucosal proinflammatory cytokines: interleukin-1 mRNA in colon and ileum, interleukin-8 mRNA in colon, and interferon gamma mRNA in ileum, but a rise in the regulatory cytokine TGF-beta mRNA in the ileum. Taken together, these results indicate that these formulas are influencing the disease process itself and thus suggest that the clinical remission achieved is a result of a reduction in inflammation, rather than a consequence of some other nutrition effect.

Clinical response to enteral nutrition is associated with mucosal healing and downregulation of proinflammatory cytokines [140]. Modulen supplementation provided statistically significant protection against weight loss, hypoalbuminemia, acidosis, and GI damage in a rat model of IBD [143]. Though illustrative, future animal research of the mechanism of action of Modulen's protective effects is needed before further human trials are considered.

Glutamine

The nonessential amino acid glutamine is a source of energy for intestinal epithelial cells, and it stimulates proliferation of intestinal epithelial cells [144]. Glutamine sufficiency is crucial for the colonic epithelium to mount a cell-protective, antiapoptotic, and anti-inflammatory response against inflammatory injury. In animal models of IBD, glutamine-enriched parenteral nutrition decreased bacterial translocation and stimulated IgA mucosal secretion [145,146]. New animal data has suggested that parenteral glutamine may have anti-inflammatory effects via the NFκB pathway with anti-TNF-α properties [147]. These findings led to the hypothesis that glutamine-enriched parenteral nutrition may improve outcomes in patients with CD. Glutamine-enriched parenteral nutrition has failed to show a clinical benefit in patients with inflammatory bowel disease compared to standard parenteral nutrition [148]. However, intestinal utilization of glutamine is impaired, thus mitigating attempts for restorative therapy [149]. A recent trial of glutamine for patients with Crohn's disease showed improvement in intestinal morphology and permeability [37]. Finally, glutamine has been shown to be a "pharmacologically acting nutrient" in the setting of experimental IBD in animal models [150]. Thus, the jury is still out whether glutamine may be beneficial for the treatment of IBD.

OTHER DIETARY THERAPY IN INFLAMMATORY BOWEL DISEASE

As stated previously, though diet has been implicated in the pathogenesis of IBD, there is no definitive evidence linking a specific food or additive as a cause of IBD. Therefore, most patients are recommended to follow a healthful, well-balanced diet. Following are dietary strategies and management that have been studied further.

POLYUNSATURATED FATTY ACIDS

Dietary fat has been proposed to have a role in disease activity. One proposed mechanism for the efficacy of low-fat elemental diets is insufficient n-6 fatty acids to synthesize proinflammatory eicosanoids [151]. The family of n-3 fatty acids have the parent compound α-linoleic acid, which is synthesized into fatty acids important in immunomodulatory and anti-inflammatory effects via the production of prostaglandin class 3 and leukotriene B5, and by inhibiting production of arachidonic acid and TNF-α production [21–23]. These findings would suggest that a diet rich in n-3 PUFAs may be protective against IBD while those rich in n-6 PUFAs would promote inflammation. PUFAs may reduce the risk of recurrence in CD and may also have a role in UC [152,153] (see Figure 15.3). A controlled trial evaluated a polymeric enteral diet high in oleate acid (monounsaturated fat) versus an identical diet high in linoleate acid and demonstrated that remission rates were better with the linoleate diet [141]. Elemental diets with increasing amounts of long-chain triglycerides (LCTs) had lower remission rates in active Crohn's disease than the same diet with lower LCTs [154]. Soybean oil was used as the LCT with the principal fatty acids being oleic acid and linoleic acid. Based on the *Cochrane* review, omega-3 fatty acids might be effective for maintenance therapy in CD, though this was not supported in UC (Figure 15.3) [155,156]. Most recently, though, two randomized, placebo-controlled trials showed omega-3 fatty acids were not effective in the prevention of relapse in CD [157]. However, two subsequent meta-analyses demonstrated a statistical benefit for consuming omega-3 fatty acids in the maintenance of remission of Crohn's disease [158,159]. A formulation using fish oils, antioxidants, and gum arabic (prebiotic) showed significant weaning in

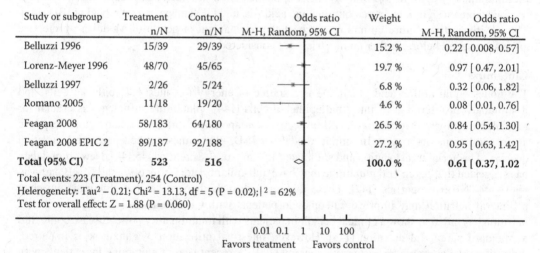

Study or subgroup	Treatment n/N	Control n/N	Odds ratio M-H, Random, 95% CI	Weight	Odds ratio M-H, Random, 95% CI
Belluzzi 1996	15/39	29/39		15.2 %	0.22 [0.008, 0.57]
Lorenz-Meyer 1996	48/70	45/65		19.7 %	0.97 [0.47, 2.01]
Belluzzi 1997	2/26	5/24		6.8 %	0.32 [0.06, 1.82]
Romano 2005	11/18	19/20		4.6 %	0.08 [0.01, 0.76]
Feagan 2008	58/183	64/180		26.5 %	0.84 [0.54, 1.30]
Feagan 2008 EPIC 2	89/187	92/188		27.2 %	0.95 [0.63, 1.42]
Total (95% CI)	**523**	**516**		**100.0 %**	**0.61 [0.37, 1.02**

Total events: 223 (Treatment), 254 (Control)
Heterogeneity: Tau^2 – 0.21; Chi^2 = 13.13, df = 5 (P = 0.02);|^2 = 62%
Test for overall effect: Z = 1.88 (P = 0.060)

0.01 0.1   1   10   100
Favors treatment   Favors control

FIGURE 15.3 Omega-3 fatty acids for maintenance of remission in Crohn's disease: six studies were eligible for inclusion. There was a marginal significant benefit of n-3 therapy for maintaining remission (RR 0.77 0; 95% CI 0.61 to 0.98; P = 0.03). However, the studies were both clinically and statistically heterogeneous (P = 0.03, I^2 = 58%). Two large studies showed negative results. When considering the estimated rather than the observed one-year relapse rate of these two studies, the benefit was no longer statistically significant (RR 0.59; 95% CI 0.34 to 1.03; P = 0.06). No serious adverse events were recorded in any of the studies but in a pooled analyses there was a significantly higher rate of diarrhea (RR 1.36 95% CI 1.01 to 1.84) and symptoms of the upper gastrointestinal tract (RR 1.98 95% CI 1.38 to 2.85) in the n-3 treatment group. Adapted from Turner, D., et al., Omega 3 fatty acids (fish oil) for maintenance of remission in Crohn's disease. *Cochrane Database Syst Rev*, 2009(1): CD006320.

steroid-dependent ulcerative colitis and lowering of the Crohn's disease activity index along with improving the quality of life [160,161].

SHORT-CHAIN FATTY ACIDS, LOW-PARTICLE DIETS, AND POLYPHENOLS

In addition to PUFAs, other dietary strategies in IBD include SCFAs, low-particle diets, and polyphenols [17,31,152,153,162]. The majority of studies on SCFAs have been performed in animals, but human studies have been performed. Though the studies were small, many prospective studies demonstrated clinical response or improvement with SCFA enemas (Table 15.3) [163–167]. One small, randomized, controlled trial demonstrated a decrease in clinical index activity scores in patients with ulcerative colitis treated with 30 grams of germinated barley that increased luminal butyrate production [168].

Microparticles have been proposed to exacerbate inflammation via antigen-mediated immune responses [36]. An initial pilot study of 20 patients showed that those on a diet low in microparticles had a significant improvement in Crohn's disease activity index, though a follow-up multi-center, randomized, controlled trial showed no improvement in Crohn's disease activity with reduced microparticle intake in the diet [169,170].

Polyphenols are phytochemicals found in food substances produced from plants and have been found to be potentially immunomodulating [171]. Examples of polyphenols include resveratrol, epigallocatechin, and curcumin. Resveratrol is found most abundantly in the skin of red grapes [172]. Resveratrol appears to have anti-inflammatory and immunomodulatory effects though the mechanism has not been clearly established [17]. In rodent models of inflammatory colitis, resveratrol has been shown to reverse weight loss, increase stool consistency, improve mucosal appearance, improve histology, decrease inflammatory infiltrate, and decrease mucosal levels of

TABLE 15.3
Prospective Studies of Short-Chain Fatty Acids for Left-Sided Ulcerative Colitis

Study	Design	No. Patients (Treatment)	Study Duration (wk)	Butyrate Dose	Results
Scheppach	Single blind	10 (Butyrate enema)	2	100 mM	↓ Stool frequency, hematochezia, ↓Endoscopic histologic score
Breuer	Crossover Open label	10 (Placebo) 10 (SCFA enema)	6	100 mL bid 40 mM 100 mL bid	No change with placebo ↓ Disease activity index ↓Mucosal histology score
Steinhart	Open label	10 (Butyrate enema)	6	80 mM 60 mL qd	↓ Disease activity index 60% Response 40% Complete remission
Patz	Open label	10 (SCFA enema)	6	40 mM 100 mL bid	5/10 Endoscopic and clinical improvement
Vernia	Open label	10 (Butyrate + 5-ASA enema)	6	80 mM 100 mL bid	7/9 Endoscopic, clinical, and histologic improvement

Adapted from Scheppach W, Sommer H, Kirchner T, et al. Effect of butyrate enemas on the colonic mucosa in distal ulcerative colitis. *Gastroenterology*. 1992;103(1):51–56; Breuer RI, Buto SK, Christ ML, et al. Rectal irrigation with short-chain fatty acids for distal ulcerative colitis: Preliminary report. *Dig Dis Sci*. 1991;36(2):185–187; Steinhart AH, Brzezinski A, Baker J. Treatment of refractory ulcerative proctosigmoiditis with butyrate enemas. *Am J Gastroenterol*. 1994;89(2):179–183; Patz J, Jacobsohn WZ, Gottschalk-Sabag S, Zeides S, Braverman DZ. Treatment of refractory distal ulcerative colitis with short-chain fatty acid enemas. *Am J Gastroenterol*. 1996;91(4):731–734; Vernia P, Cittadini M, Caprilli R, Torsoli A. Topical treatment of refractory distal ulcerative colitis with 5-ASA and sodium butyrate. *Dig Dis Sci*. 1995;40(2):305–307.

interleukin-1β, COX-2, and prostaglandin D2 [173]. To date, resveratrol has not been studied in human subjects with IBD.

Catechins such as gallocatechin gallate (EGCG) are abundant in green (nonfermented) tea [174]. Green tea has been linked to beneficial effects in prevention or treatment of cancer such as breast, lung, ovarian, prostate, and stomach, as well as in diseases such as hypertension and cardiovascular health [17]. EGCG can modulate and inhibit NFκB activity, which may affect inflammation [175]. Similar to resveratrol, green tea has been shown to improve disease activity in murine models of colitis [176–178]. An in vitro study involving human colonic tissues showed that EGCG administration resulted in decreased proinflammatory cytokine production, but to date, there are no in vivo human studies to evaluate the role of green tea extract in IBD [179].

Another phytonutrient studied for its anti-inflammatory role is curcumin. Turmeric, from the herb *Curcuma longa*, is the major spice found in curry. Curcumin is the major chemical constituent of turmeric. Curcumin has been used as an oral and topical agent to treat a variety of ailments and has had an excellent safety profile [180,181]. Curcumin appears to have multiple mechanisms of action including NFκB inhibition, thereby, likely downregulating proinflammatory genes and cytokines [182]. Overall, in animal models of colitis, curcumin has demonstrated positive effects [183–188]. A randomized controlled trial of 89 patients with quiescent ulcerative colitis were administered 1 gram of curcumin twice daily and had clinical improvement and a significant decrease in the rate of relapse [189].

SUPPORTING COLONIC MICROBES

PREBIOTICS AND PROBIOTICS

The relevance of diet in both the pathogenesis and the therapy of inflammatory bowel disease is an evolving science. Disturbance of intestinal microflora (dysbiosis) is putatively a key element in the environmental component causing inflammatory bowel disease. Disturbances in bacterial intestinal flora have been purported as a triggering factor for IBD [190]. Therapy with prebiotics and probiotics may present a treatment option with few side effects. Animal models suggest probiotics may be useful in the treatment of UC and CD [191,192]. Probiotics are living microbes that can benefit the host once introduced. Examples include lactobacilli, bifidobacteria, and yeast species such as *Saccharomyces boulardii* [193]. Based on animal models, probiotics can alter gastrointestinal flora and ameliorate disease [194]. Prebiotics also produce SCFAs [195]. Pouchitis is a complication of surgery for UC and is typically treated effectively with antibiotics, suggesting a role of bacteria [196]. In patients with chronic pouchitis induced to remission with antibiotic therapy, VSL#3 (a well-studied probiotic) was successful in maintaining remission [197]. VSL#3 may also have a role as primary prophylaxis of pouchitis in patients with ileal pouch-anal anastomosis [198].

Probiotics have been shown to be efficacious in maintenance therapy but not in the treatment of active ulcerative colitis as supported by meta-analyses [199,200]. The benefit appeared to be equal for single-strain and multistrain species.

Prebiotics are among the dietary components used in an attempt to counteract dysbiosis. Such predominantly carbohydrate dietary components exert effects on the luminal environment by physicochemical changes through pH alteration, by production of short-chain fatty acids, and by selectively promoting putatively "health-beneficial" bacteria. Prebiotics are compounds that promote intestinal proliferation of probiotic bacteria (also metabolized into SCFAs). Most prebiotics are from the group of dietary fibers found in foods such as legumes, artichokes, onions, garlic, banana, soya, and other beans [201]. Examples of prebiotics are inulin and oligofructose. When these prebiotics are given in sufficient amounts they selectively promote the growth of *bifidobacteria* [202]. Animal models of IBD have shown inulin to reduce inflammatory mediators and reduce histological damage scores [203]. Along with inulin, other prebiotics such as oligofructose and lactulose have shown anti-inflammatory effects in animal models of IBD [204,205]. Prebiotics may also have a role in antibiotic-refractory or antibiotic-dependent pouchitis. In clinical studies, inulin as compared to placebo was associated with improvement in inflammation in chronic pouchitis [206]. Combining probiotics and prebiotics as synbiotics may play a role in the treatment of IBD. In mild ulcerative colitis, a synbiotic preparation (oligofructose-enriched inulin and *Bifidobacterium lon-gum*) compared to placebo showed a trend in reduction of mucosal expression of proinflammatory cytokines (TNF-α), improvement in inflammation on a histological level, and by clinical activity indices [207].

Probiotics have been studied in CD as well. One studied showed patients using *S. boulardii* plus mesalazine had fewer relapses than using mesalazine alone [208]. There have been other studies, however, that did not demonstrate probiotics to be effective in a maintenance strategy in Crohn's disease [209,210]. A recent meta-analysis showed that probiotics are not effective for preventing postoperative recurrence of Crohn's disease [211]. Prebiotics and synbiotics have not been extensively studied in the maintenance of Crohn's disease. In treating active Crohn's disease, probiotics have not been shown to significantly have a role in treatment, though one study showed that prebiotics may reduce disease activity in active CD [212]. Research on probiotics and prebiotics in this area is limited for a number of reasons, including enrollment of small number of patients, variability in choice of probiotic or prebiotic used, and variability in patients' diets. Larger randomized controlled trials are needed to determine the role of probiotics and prebiotics in the treatment of IBD.

FOOD INTOLERANCE AND INFLAMMATORY BOWEL DISEASE

Irritable bowel syndrome (IBS) occurs with increased frequency and severity given the underlying chronic inflammation in IBD, and physicians need to recognize this in order to avoid use of IBD therapy to treat symptoms resulting from IBS [213]. Patients may have intolerance to many foods, including but not limited to dairy products, caffeine, fried foods, and foods with high fiber content [214]. It is important to note that food intolerance is not a true allergic reaction. If foods cause a true allergic reaction they need to be completely avoided. Patients who have intolerance to certain foods should try to avoid specific triggers in order to minimize their symptoms.

GLUTEN

Celiac disease has been noted with increased frequency among patients with CD [215]. Rather than recommending a gluten-free diet for all, if patients continue to have ongoing symptoms despite treatment for CD, testing for celiac disease should ensue. In general, only those with celiac disease should be given a gluten-free diet. Given that there is not enough data to support or refute a recommendation concerning gluten-sensitivity testing for IBD, it is reasonable as experts for us to suggest that clinicians query patients as to their possible intolerance to gluten and if suspicious-IgG$_1$/IgG$_4$ antibody testing should be considered.

CELIAC SUSCEPTIBILITY GENETIC TESTING

Human leukocyte antigens (HLAs) help discriminate between host and foreign cells. HLAs are highly polymorphic with the HLA DQ2 and 8 genotypes associated with celiac disease susceptibility. In fact, 95% of individuals with celiac disease are positive for HLA DQ2 and/or 8 gene markers [216]. Also, non-celiac related HLA DR/DQ alleles are associated with ulcerative colitis and Crohn's disease susceptibility and various clinical presentation phenotypes [217,218]. However, 40% of the population possesses a celiac disease susceptibility HLA genotype, and only 1% of the population has been diagnosed with the disease [219]. Gluten intolerance in the absence of celiac disease is becoming increasingly common; however, it is unknown whether or not this is related to celiac disease susceptibility and the high proportion of gluten-containing foods in Western diets. However, genetic testing for HLA DQ2 and 8 may be helpful for individuals with

IBD who may suspect gluten intolerance in the absence of traditional confirmatory evidence of celiac disease.

IBD, particularly CD, can result in complications of intestinal strictures, fistulas, high-output ostomy, as well as short bowel syndrome. Though patients with nonstricturing CD do not benefit universally from a low-residue diet, most experts in IBD would recommend a low-residue diet in patients who have ongoing intestinal strictures [220]. While continued intake of adequate soluble and insoluble fiber is helpful for patients with both forms of IBD, tolerance can limit intake based upon disease manifestations. For example, Crohn's disease patients with luminal narrowing from strictures can become obstructed from fiber plugging. Patients with intestinal fistula, high-output ostomy, and short bowel syndrome often are difficult to manage from a nutrition standpoint. Careful management of fluid and electrolyte disturbances is essential, and parenteral nutrition may be necessary in some cases [221].

PATIENT EVALUATION

INFLAMMATION AND DISEASE ACTIVITY

In the evaluation of the patient with IBD, disease activity needs to be assessed. Inflammation plays a role in malnutrition as well as in potential complications of IBD such as osteoporosis and colorectal cancer. Medications need to be adjusted to maintain patients in remission. Often, if disease flare is suspected, markers of inflammation may be ordered, including erythrocyte sedimentation rate (ESR) and C-reactive protein (CRP).

MALNUTRITION

At each visit, the patient's weight and body mass index should be recorded to assess for weight loss as a marker of protein-calorie malnutrition.

VOLUME DEPLETION/DEHYDRATION

Patients with intestinal fistula, high-output ostomy, and short bowel syndrome often are difficult to manage from a nutrition standpoint. Careful management of fluid and electrolyte disturbances is essential, and parenteral nutrition may be necessary in some cases [221]. If patients with CD have these complications, orthostatic vital signs should be performed to assess for adequate fluid hydration.

NUTRIENT DEFICIENCIES

Laboratory studies that should be followed periodically include vitamin B12 levels, particularly in patients with ileal Crohn's disease. If there is evidence of anemia, iron studies and folic acid levels may need to be assessed. Since patients with IBD are at risk for osteoporosis, vitamin D levels should be ordered, and dual-energy X-ray absorptiometry (DEXA) should be assessed soon after diagnosis and repeated in about one year. Other fat-soluble vitamins may be deficient such as vitamin A, E, and K. Minerals other than iron may be deficient in IBD, and these include magnesium, selenium, zinc, and copper. Zinc is commonly deficient in Crohn's disease and copper status is unknown. In ulcerative colitis, these trace minerals are unlikely to be deficient unless patients have profuse diarrhea [222]. Selenium deficiency may be seen in patients on long-term parenteral nutrition or in patients who have undergone significant small bowel resections [223]. Serum levels should be checked because selenium is an essential cofactor for glutathione peroxidase, which helps detoxify hydroxyl free radicals that are overabundant in inflamed tissues.

TREATMENT APPROACHES

AVOID UNNECESSARY FOOD RESTRICTION

Most patients and some providers believe that diet influences their disease; this can lead to excessive food restriction [224]. It is important to establish food intolerance as a separate entity, not part of IBD itself. As such, one patient's food intolerance should not be generalized to a recommendation appropriate for IBD at large. For example, there is no evidence that a gluten-free diet is efficacious in CD if celiac disease is absent; however, if gluten sensitivity is suspected and confirmed via IgG testing or an elimination trial, removal is warranted [225]. Patients with IBD need to eat healthful diets with as few restrictions as possible. Unnecessary food restrictions can result in elimination of health-promoting foods beneficial to gastrointestinal and immunological functioning:

- Removing spicy foods from the diet would lessen the phytonutrient curcumin and other less studied nutrients known to temper inflammation.
- Removing gluten-containing foods as a general rule has been shown to result in unhealthful food selection that the patient may mistakenly consider healthful solely because it is gluten free. Confirmation of gluten sensitivity, if suspected, should be done prior to removal from the diet.
- Avoiding foods containing lactose is important when lactose intolerance is established. If patients tolerate lactose, following a lactose-free diet may unnecessarily reduce their intake of highly absorbable minerals, and fermented dairy products are a source of probiotics. Breath hydrogen testing should be performed if lactose intolerance is suspected.
- Avoiding nuts and seeds as a potential IBD trigger in patients who have not demonstrated they have allergies or sensitivities to these foods results in unnecessary restriction of mono-unsaturated fats, minerals, and protein. For example, walnuts are a rich source of omega-3 fatty acids, which are anti-inflammatory in nature and can benefit patients with IBD. Nuts and seeds are often substituted for processed snack foods known to be proinflammatory. Nuts and seeds may need to be avoided in patients with stricturing disease or ostomies.

USE CAUTION WITH RED MEAT, DUE TO COLORECTAL CANCER RISK

Topical nutrients are preferentially used by the gut mucosa to maintain structure and function. With the colon, topical nutrients are generated by the colonic microbiota to maintain mucosal health. As previously mentioned, short-chain fatty acids control proliferation and differentiation, thereby reducing colon cancer risk. Unfortunately, the microbiota may also elaborate toxic products from food residues such as genotoxic hydrogen sulfide by sulfur-reducing bacteria in response to a high-meat diet. Most nutritionists suggest abundant red meat in the diet of IBD patients due to microscopic blood loss from the chronic inflammation. Iron, although important to maintain sufficiency, can be a pro-oxidant by catalyzing superoxide anion formation. Thus, caution needs to be exercised with regard to iron intake in IBD patients [106]. Patients with both forms of IBD have an increased risk of acquiring colorectal cancer. Given the connection of red meat and processed meats to colorectal cancer, advising patients to consume an ad-lib diet of red meat and or processed meats as is done in most hospital centers is concerning and should be scrutinized [226–228].

BONE HEALTH

To minimize bone loss, calcium supplements should be given at doses of 1200 mg/day with vitamin D supplementation at 800 IU/day. If vitamin D deficiency is found, repletion and maintenance will be needed. Finally, patients may need bisphosphonates to treat osteoporosis.

REPLETION OF NUTRIENT DEFICIENCIES

Hypovitaminosis D

IBD, particularly small bowel CD, patients are susceptible to vitamin D deficiency. This often is manifested by low 25(OH) D levels. A target serum level of 32 ng/ml or greater is considered the optimal serum 25(OH) D level. For vitamin D deficiency, (25[OH]D < 20 ng/ml), initial treatment should be 50,000 IU of vitamin D2 or D3 orally once per week for six to eight weeks, then 800 to 1000 IU of vitamin D3 daily, thereafter [229]. For vitamin D insufficiency, 25(OH) D 20–30 ng/ml, 800 to 1000 IU of vitamin D3 should be given daily and this should bring levels within the target range in approximately three months. Vitamin D (25[OH]D) should be measured three months after beginning therapy. In patients with malabsorption, repletion will vary. These patients may need higher doses of vitamin D of 10,000 to 50,000 IU daily. Calcium supplementation of 1000 to 1200 mg should be given with vitamin D. Vitamin D toxicity can occur at levels of 88 ng/ml or greater, and the first signs of toxicity include hypercalciuria and hypercalcemia [230,231].

Iron Deficiency

Anemia is frequently seen in IBD, and iron status should be assessed. Iron deficiency in IBD is typically caused by chronic blood loss. Though oral iron supplementation has not been shown to worsen disease activity, patients may develop gastrointestinal side effects [232]. With oral supplementation, usually ferrous sulfate 325 mg three times daily is given, though if patients develop gastrointestinal upset, ferrous gluconate may be substituted. Other tips for patients suffering from side effects of iron therapy include gradually increasing the dose from one time per day to three times per day or taking it with food, though absorption will be decreased. Parenteral iron is usually given to patients who do not tolerate oral iron or where blood loss exceeds the ability of the GI tract to absorb iron.

Vitamin B12 Deficiency

Patients with B12 deficiency do not always have evidence of anemia, or it may be mild. Therefore, serum cobalamin should be assessed periodically, particularly in patients with ileal CD or following ileal resection. If the serum cobalamin level is greater than 300 pg/ml, this is normal and cobalamin deficiency is unlikely. Levels less than 200 pg/ml are consistent with cobalamin deficiency. If the level ranges between 200 to 300 pg/ml, cobalamin deficiency is possible and further testing may be needed with measurement of methylmalonic acid (MMA) and homocysteine levels. If both tests are normal with MMA levels of 70–270 nmol/L and homocysteine of 5–14 μmol/L, then cobalamin deficiency is unlikely. If MMA and homocysteine levels are increased, then cobalamin deficiency is likely, though folate deficiency may be present as well. If MMA is normal, but homocysteine is elevated, then folate deficiency is likely [111]. Patients with cobalamin deficiency are treated with a dose of cobalamin 1000 μg or 1 mg daily for one week followed by 1 mg per week for four weeks, then 1 mg per month. Serum cobalamin levels should be monitored after therapy.

Folate Deficiency

Folate deficiency is frequently seen in both UC and CD and is multifactorial with insufficiency dietary amounts of folic acid and side effects of medicine contributing. Serum folate levels reflect short-term folate balance while red blood cell (RBC) folate is a more accurate measure of tissue folate [233]. However, if the serum folate is > 4 ng/ml folate deficiency is unlikely. If serum folate is between 2 to 4 ng/ml then RBC folate can be measured along with the metabolites described earlier (MMA and homocysteine). Serum folate < 2 ng/ml is essentially diagnostic of deficiency in the absence of recent fasting or anorexia, which may be frequent, particularly in hospitalized patients. Typically, folate is repleted with 1 mg of folic acid daily for one to four months or longer if needed. It is important to rule out cobalamin deficiency before treating a patient with folic acid. Recent literature suggests that repletion with folate in doses greater than 1 mg per day can actually be harmful [234].

Patients Receiving Specialized Nutrition Support

In patients receiving TPN, serum electrolytes, glucose, calcium, magnesium, phosphate, amino-transferases, bilirubin, and triglycerides should be measured regularly. The catheter site needs to be monitored to assess for signs of infection. (See Table 15.2 for complications related to TPN use.) Avoid overfeeding to "catch up" as many patients with IBD are malnourished in the hospitalized setting. Overzealous feeding, termed refeeding syndrome, is a particularly deadly complication of TPN that is under recognized by physicians worldwide.

RECOMMENDATIONS

Across the digestive disease and nutrition societies, no clear guidelines exist for the dietary management of inflammatory bowel disease, however evidence-based recommendations can be offered [235,236]:

- In order to prevent excessive food restriction, patients should be encouraged to follow a healthful diet as tolerated but be mindful to follow an anti-inflammatory Mediterranean type diet whenever possible and pursue appropriate testing and clinical analysis to rule out food sensitivities.
- When supplemental nutrition is necessary, enteral therapy should be used over parenteral therapy if the gut can be used.
- Medical therapy needs to be initiated to achieve remission to minimize inflammation and improve gastrointestinal function. Medications vary from 5-ASA medications to infliximab.
- Supplementation with polyphenols, probiotics, and fish oils should be considered as adjuncts to care.
- Patients should be counseled on the risk of osteopenia and osteoporosis and be encouraged to take calcium and vitamin D, if deficient.
- Other nutrients may be deficient as well and should be evaluated and repleted when deficient.

FINANCIAL DISCLOSURES

Gerard E. Mullin is an advisor to Abbott Laboratories and Prometheus Laboratories. Colleen Fogarty Draper is the owner of Nugenso Nutrition & Company. Dr. Munsell does not have any relevant financial disclosures or conflicts of interest to state.

REFERENCES

1. O'Sullivan M, O'Morain C. Nutrition in inflammatory bowel disease. *Best Practice & Research Clinical Gastroenterology.* 2006;20(3):561–573.
2. Loftus CG, Loftus EV, Jr., Harmsen WS, et al. Update on the incidence and prevalence of Crohn's disease and ulcerative colitis in Olmsted county, Minnesota, 1940–2000. *Inflamm Bowel Dis.* 2007;13(3):254–261.
3. Shoda R, Matsueda K, Yamato S, Umeda N. Epidemiologic analysis of Crohn's disease in Japan: Increased dietary intake of n-6 polyunsaturated fatty acids and animal protein relates to the increased incidence of Crohn disease in Japan. *Am J Clin Nutr.* 1996;63(5):741–745.
4. Jarnerot G, Jarnmark I, Nilsson K. Consumption of refined sugar by patients with Crohn's disease, ulcerative colitis, or irritable bowel syndrome. *Scand J Gastroenterol.* 1983;18(8):999–1002.
5. Sakamoto N, Kono S, Wakai K, et al. Dietary risk factors for inflammatory bowel disease: A multicenter case-control study in Japan. *Inflamm Bowel Dis.* 2005;11(2):154–163.
6. Kelly DG, Fleming CR. Nutritional considerations in inflammatory bowel diseases. *Gastroenterol Clin North Am.* 1995;24(3):597–611.
7. Behr MA, Kapur V. The evidence for mycobacterium paratuberculosis in Crohn's disease. *Curr Opin Gastroenterol.* 2008;24(1):17–21.

8. Akobeng AK, Thomas AG. Enteral nutrition for maintenance of remission in Crohn's disease. *Cochrane Database Syst Rev*. 2007;(3)(3):CD005984.

9. Suzuki H, Hanyou N, Sonaka I, Minami H. An elemental diet controls inflammation in indomethacinin-duced small bowel disease in rats: The role of low dietary fat and the elimination of dietary proteins. *Dig Dis Sci*. 2005;50(10):1951–1958.

10. Ferguson LR, et al. Genetic factors in chronic inflammation: single nucleotide polymorphisms in the STAT-JAK pathway, susceptibility to DNA damage and Crohn's disease in a New Zealand population. *Mutation research*, 2010;690(1–2):108–115.

11. Hagymasi K, Tulassay Z. Genotype-phenotype associations in inflammatory bowel disease. *Orv Hetil*, 2005;146(34):1767–1773.

12. Chutkan RK. Inflammatory bowel disease. *Prim Care*. 2001;28(3):539–556, vi.

13. Podolsky DK. Inflammatory bowel disease. *N Engl J Med*. 2002;347(6):417–429.

14. Razack R, Seidner DL. Nutrition in inflammatory bowel disease. *Curr Opin Gastroenterol*. 2007;23(4):400–405.

15. Sartor RB. Mechanisms of disease: Pathogenesis of Crohn's disease and ulcerative colitis. *Nat Clin Pract Gastroenterol Hepatol*. 2006;3(7):390–407.

16. Hodin R. Maintaining gut homeostasis: The butyrate-NF-kappaB connection. *Gastroenterology*. 2000;118(4):798–801.

17. Clarke JO, Mullin GE. A review of complementary and alternative approaches to immunomodulation. *Nutr Clin Pract*. 2008;23(1):49–62.

18. Hudert CA, Weylandt KH, Lu Y, et al. Transgenic mice rich in endogenous omega-3 fatty acids are pro-tected from colitis. *Proc Natl Acad Sci USA*. 2006;103(30):11276–11281.

19. Guerreiro CS, et al. Fatty acids, IL6, and TNFalpha polymorphisms: An example of nutrigenetics in Crohn's disease. *The American Journal of Gastroenterology*. 2009;104(9):2241–2249.

20. Petronis A, Petroniene R. Epigenetics of inflammatory bowel disease. *Gut*. 2000;47(2):302–306.

21. Miura S, Tsuzuki Y, Hokari R, Ishii H. Modulation of intestinal immune system by dietary fat intake: Relevance to Crohn's disease. *J Gastroenterol Hepatol*. 1998;13(12):1183–1190.

22. Wild GE, Drozdowski L, Tartaglia C, Clandinin MT, Thomson AB. Nutritional modulation of the inflam-atory response in inflammatory bowel disease— from the molecular to the integrative to the clinical. *World J Gastroenterol*. 2007;13(1):1–7.

23. Caughey GE, Mantzioris E, Gibson RA, Cleland LG, James MJ. The effect on human tumor necrosis factor alpha and interleukin 1 beta production of diets enriched in n-3 fatty acids from vegetable oil or fish oil. *Am J Clin Nutr*. 1996;63(1):116–122.

24. Zhang P, Kim W, Zhou L, et al. Dietary fish oil inhibits antigen-specific murine Th1 cell development by suppression of clonal expansion. *J Nutr*. 2006;136(9):2391–2398.

25. Whiting CV, Bland PW, Tarlton JF. Dietary n-3 polyunsaturated fatty acids reduce disease and colonic proinflammatory cytokines in a mouse model of colitis. *Inflamm Bowel Dis*. 2005;11(4):340–349.

26. Kles KA, Chang EB. Short-chain fatty acids impact on intestinal adaptation, inflammation, carcinoma, and failure. *Gastroenterology*. 2006;130(2 Suppl 1):S100–105.

27. James SL, Muir JG, Curtis SL, Gibson PR. Dietary fibre: A roughage guide. *Intern Med J*. 2003; 33(7):291–296.

28. Dray X, Marteau The use of enteral nutrition in the management of Crohn's disease in adults. *JPEN J Parenter Enteral Nutr*. 2005;29(4 Suppl):S166–169; discussion S169–172, S184–188.

29. Roediger WE. The colonic epithelium in ulcerative colitis: An energy-deficiency disease? *Lancet*. 1980;2(8197):712–715.

30. Yamamoto T, Nakahigashi M, Umegae S, Kitagawa T, Matsumoto K. Impact of elemental diet on muco-sal inflammation in patients with active Crohn's disease: Cytokine production and endoscopic and histo-logical findings. *Inflamm Bowel Dis*. 2005;11(6):580–588.

31. Segain JP, Raingeard de la Bletiere D., Bourreille A, et al. Butyrate inhibits inflammatory responses through NFkappaB inhibition: Implications for Crohn's disease. *Gut*. 2000;47(3):397–403.

32. Binder HJ, Mehta Short-chain fatty acids stimulate active sodium and chloride absorption in vitro in the rat distal colon. *Gastroenterology*. 1989;96(4):989–996.

33. Sealy L, Chalkley R. The effect of sodium butyrate on histone modification. *Cell*. 1978;14(1): 115–121.

34. Andersen V, et al. Diet and risk of inflammatory bowel disease. *Dig Liver Dis*, , 2012;44(3):185–194.

35. Mullin GE, Turnbull LK, Kines K. Vitamin D: A D-lightful health supplement: Part II. *Nutr Clin Pract*. 2009;24(6):738–740.

36. Lomer MC, Thompson RP, Powell JJ. Fine and ultrafine particles of the diet: Influence on the mucosal immune response and association with Crohn's disease. *Proc Nutr Soc*. 2002;61(1):123–130.

37. Korzenik JR. Past and current theories of etiology of IBD: Toothpaste, worms, and refrigerators. *J Clin Gastroenterol*. 2005;39(4 Suppl 2):S59–65.

38. Pirlich M, Schutz T, Kemps M, et al. Prevalence of malnutrition in hospitalized medical patients: Impact of underlying disease. *Dig Dis*. 2003;21(3):245–251.

39. O'Sullivan M, O'Morain C. Nutritional therapy in inflammatory bowel disease. *Curr Treat Options Gastroenterol*. 2004;7(3):191–198.

40. Harries AD, Jones L, Heatley RV, Rhodes J, Fitzsimons E. Mid-arm circumference as simple means of identifying malnutrition in Crohn's disease. *Br Med J (Clin Res Ed)*. 1982;285(6351):1317–1318.

41. Silk DB, Payne-James J. Inflammatory bowel disease: Nutritional implications and treatment. *Proc Nutr Soc*. 1989;48(3):355–361.

42. O'Keefe SJ. Nutrition and gastrointestinal disease. *Scand J Gastroenterol Suppl*. 1996;220:52–59.

43. Burke A, Lichtenstein G, Rombeau J. Nutrition and ulcerative colitis. *Bailliére's Clinical Gastroenterology*. 1997;11(1):153–174.

44. Powell-Tuck J. Protein metabolism in inflammatory bowel disease. *Gut*. 1986;27 Suppl 1:67-71.

45. Dyer NH, Dawson AM. Malnutrition and malabsorption in Crohn's disease with reference to the effect of surgery. *Br J Surg*. 1973;60(2):134–140.

46. Lanfranchi GA, Brignola C, Campieri M, et al. Assessment of nutritional status in Crohn's disease in remission or low activity. *Hepatogastroenterology*. 1984;31(3):129–132.

47. Heatley RV. Assessing nutritional state in inflammatory bowel disease. *Gut*. 1986;27 Suppl 1:61–66.

48. Jahnsen J, Falch JA, Mowinckel P, Aadland E. Body composition in patients with inflammatory bowel disease: A population-based study. *Am J Gastroenterol*. 2003;98(7):1556–1562.

49. Harries AD, Jones LA, Heatley RV, Rhodes J. Malnutrition in inflammatory bowel disease: An anthropometric study. *Hum Nutr Clin Nutr*. 1982;36(4):307–313.

50. Geerling BJ, Badart-Smook A, Stockbrugger RW, Brummer RJ. Comprehensive nutritional status in patients with long-standing Crohn's disease currently in remission. *Am J Clin Nutr*. 1998;67(5):919–926.

51. Schaffler A, Scholmerich J, Buchler C. Mechanisms of disease: Adipocytokines and visceral adipose tissue—emerging role in intestinal and mesenteric diseases. *Nat Clin Pract Gastroenterol Hepatol*. 2005;2(2):103–111.

52. Al-Jaouni R, Schneider SM, Piche T, Rampal P, Hebuterne X. Effect of steroids on energy expenditure and substrate oxidation in women with Crohn's disease. *Am J Gastroenterol*. 2002;97(11):2843–2849.

53. Cabre E, Gassull MA. Nutritional and metabolic issues in inflammatory bowel disease. *Curr Opin Clin Nutr Metab Care*. 2003;6(5):569–576.

54. Baldassano RN, Piccoli DA. Inflammatory bowel disease in pediatric and adolescent patients. *Gastroenterol Clin North Am*. 1999;28(2):445–458.

55. Reilly J, Ryan J, Strole W, Fischer J. Hyperalimentation in inflammatory bowel disease. *American Journal of Surgery*. 1976;131(2):192–200.

56. Rigaud D, Angel LA, Cerf M, et al. Mechanisms of decreased food intake during weight loss in adult Crohn's disease patients without obvious malabsorption. *Am J Clin Nutr*. 1994;60(5):775–781.

57. Sandstrom B, Davidsson L, Bosaeus I, Eriksson R, Alpsten M. Selenium status and absorption of zinc (65Zn), selenium (75Se) and manganese (54Mn) in patients with short bowel syndrome. *Eur J Clin Nutr*. 1990;44(10):697–703.

58. Jensen MB, Houborg KB, Vestergaard P, Kissmeyer-Nielsen P, Mosekilde L, Laurberg S. Improved physical performance and increased lean tissue and fat mass in patients with ulcerative colitis four to six years after ileoanal anastomosis with a J-pouch. *Dis Colon Rectum*. 2002;45(12):1601–1607.

59. Tomer G, Ceballos C, Concepcion E, Benkov KJ. NOD2/CARD15 variants are associated with lower weight at diagnosis in children with Crohn's disease. *Am J Gastroenterol*. 2003;98(11):2479–2484.

60. Gronb.k H, Thogersen T, Frystyk J, Vilstrup H, Flyvbjerg A, Dahlerup JF. Low free and total insulinlike growth factor I (IGF-I) and IGF binding protein-3 levels in chronic inflammatory bowel disease: Partial normalization during prednisolone treatment. *American Journal of Gastroenterology*. 2002;97(3):673–678.

61. Eivindson M, Gronb.k H, Flyvbjerg A, Frystyk J, Zimmermann-Nielsen E, Dahlerup JF. The insulinlike growth factor (IGF)-system in active ulcerative colitis and Crohn's disease: Relations to disease activity and corticosteroid treatment. *Growth Hormone & IGF Research*. 2007;17(1):33–40.

62. Eivindson M, Gronbaek H, Skogstrand K, et al. The insulin-like growth factor (IGF) system and its relation to infliximab treatment in adult patients with Crohn's disease. *Scand J Gastroenterol*. 2007;42(4):464–470.

63. Walters TD, Gilman AR, Griffiths AM. Linear growth improves during infliximab therapy in children with chronically active severe Crohn's disease. *Inflamm Bowel Dis*. 2007;13(4):424–430.

64. O'Sullivan MA, O'Morain CA. Nutritional therapy in Crohn's disease. *Inflamm Bowel Dis*. 1998;4(1):45–53.

65. Burbige EJ, Shi-Shung Huang, Bayless TM. Clinical manifestations of Crohn's disease in children and adolescents. *Pediatrics*. 1975;55(6):866.

66. McCaffery TD, Nasr K, Lawrence AM, Kirsner JB. Severe growth retardation in children with inflamatory bowel disease. *Pediatrics*. 1970;45(3):386.

67. Stokes MA. Crohn's disease and nutrition. *Br J Surg*. 1992;79(5):391–394.

68. Winter TA, Lemmer ER, O'Keefe SJ, Ogden JM. The effect of severe undernutrition, and subsequent refeeding on digestive function in human patients. *Eur J Gastroenterol Hepatol*. 2000;12(2):191–196.

69. Norman K, Kirchner H, Lochs H, Pirlich M. Malnutrition affects quality of life in gastroenterology patients. *World J Gastroenterol*. 2006;12(21):3380–3385.

70. Addolorato G, Capristo E, Stefanini GF, Gasbarrini G. Inflammatory bowel disease: A study of the association between anxiety and depression, physical morbidity, and nutritional status. *Scand J Gastroenterol*. 1997;32(10):1013–1021.

71. Weinsier RL, Hunker EM, Krumdieck CL, Butterworth CE, Jr. Hospital malnutrition. A prospective evaluation of general medical patients during the course of hospitalization. *Am J Clin Nutr*. 1979;32(2):418–426.

72. Chima C, Barco K, Dewitt MA, Maeda M, Teran JC, Mullen K. Relationship of nutritional status to length of stay, hospital costs, and discharge status of patients hospitalized in the medicine service. *Journal of the American Dietetic Association*. 1997;97(9):975–978.

73. Nguyen GC, Munsell M, Harris ML. Nationwide prevalence and prognostic significance of clinically diagnosable protein-calorie malnutrition in hospitalized inflammatory bowel disease patients. *Inflamm Bowel Dis*. 2008.

74. Executive summary: Management of the critically ill patient with severe acute pancreatitis. *Proc Am Thorac Soc*. 2004;1(4):289–290.

75. Brugler L, DiPrinzio MJ, Bernstein L. The five-year evolution of a malnutrition treatment program in a community hospital. *Jt Comm J Qual Improv*. 1999;25(4):191–206.

76. Silvennoinen JA, Karttunen TJ, Niemela SE, Manelius JJ, Lehtola JK. A controlled study of bone mineral density in patients with inflammatory bowel disease. *Gut*. 1995;37(1):71–76.

77. Abitbol V, Roux C, Chaussade S, et al. Metabolic bone assessment in patients with inflammatory bowel disease. *Gastroenterology*. 1995;108(2):417–422.

78. Bjarnason I, Macpherson A, Mackintosh C, Buxton-Thomas M, Forgacs I, Moniz C. Reduced bone density in patients with inflammatory bowel disease. *Gut*. 1997;40(2):228–233.

79. Semeao EJ, Jawad AF, Stouffer NO, Zemel BS, Piccoli DA, Stallings VA. Risk factors for low bone mineral density in children and young adults with Crohn's disease. *J Pediatr*. 1999;135(5):593–600.

80. Ardizzone S, Bollani S, Bettica P, Bevilacqua M, Molteni P, Bianchi Porro G. Altered bone metabolism in inflammatory bowel disease: There is a difference between Crohn's disease and ulcerative colitis. *J Intern Med*. 2000;247(1):63–70.

81. Bernstein CN, Blanchard JF, Metge C, Yogendran M. The association between corticosteroid use and development of fractures among IBD patients in a population-based database. *Am J Gastroenterol*. 2003;98(8):1797–1801.

82. Jahnsen J, Falch JA, Aadland E, Mowinckel Bone mineral density is reduced in patients with Crohn's disease but not in patients with ulcerative colitis: A population based study. *Gut*. 1997;40(3):313–319.

83. Lamb EJ, Wong T, Smith DJ, et al. Metabolic bone disease is present at diagnosis in patients with inflammatory bowel disease. *Aliment Pharmacol Ther*. 2002;16(11):1895–1902.

84. Bernstein CN, Leslie WD, Taback S. Bone density in a population-based cohort of premenopausal adult women with early onset inflammatory bowel disease. *Am J Gastroenterol*. 2003;98(5):1094–1100.

85. Habtezion A, Silverberg MS, Parkes R, Mikolainis S, Steinhart AH. Risk factors for low bone density in Crohn's disease. *Inflamm Bowel Dis*. 2002;8(2):87–92.

86. Jong DJ, Corstens FHM, Mannaerts L, Rossum LGM, Naber AHJ. Corticosteroid-induced osteoporosis: Does it occur in patients with Crohn's disease? *Am J Gastroenterol*. 2002;97(8):2011–2015.

87. Vogelsang H, Ferenci P, Resch H, Kiss A, Gangl A. Prevention of bone mineral loss in patients with Crohn's disease by long-term oral vitamin D supplementation. *Eur J Gastroenterol Hepatol*. 1995;7(7):609–614.

88. Siffledeen JS, Fedorak RN, Siminoski K, et al. Randomized trial of etidronate plus calcium and vitamin D for treatment of low bone mineral density in Crohn's disease. *Clin Gastroenterol Hepatol*. 2005;3(2):122–132.

89. Leal JY, Romero T, Ortega P, Amaya D. Serum values of interleukin-10, gamma-interferon and vitamin A in female adolescents. *Invest Clin*. 2007;48(3):317–326.

90. Ginanjar E, Sumariyono, Setiati S, Setiyohadi B. Vitamin D and autoimmune disease. *Acta Med Indones.* 2007;39(3):133–141.

91. Mullin GE, Dobs A. Vitamin D and its role in cancer and immunity: A prescription for sunlight. *Nutr Clin Pract.* 2007;22(3):305–322.

92. Mullin GE, Turnbull L, Kines K. Vitamin D: A D-lightful health supplement. *Nutr Clin Pract.* 2009;24(5):642–644.

93. Mullin GE, Dobs A. Vitamin D and its role in cancer and immunity: A prescription for sunlight. *Nutr Clin Pract.* 2007;22(3):305–322.

94. Pei FH, et al. Vitamin D receptor gene polymorphism and ulcerative colitis susceptibility in Han Chinese. *Journal of Digestive Diseases.* 2011;12(2):90–98.

95. Naderi N, et al. Association of vitamin D receptor gene polymorphisms in Iranian patients with inflamatory bowel disease. *Journal of Gastroenterology and Hepatology.* 2008;23(12):1816–1822.

96. Dresner-Pollak R, et al. The BsmI vitamin D receptor gene polymorphism is associated with ulcerative colitis in Jewish Ashkenazi patients. *Genetic Testing.* 2004;8(4): 17–20.

97. Simmons JD, et al. Vitamin D receptor gene polymorphism: Association with Crohn's disease susceptibility. *Gut.* 2000;47(2):211–214.

98. Eisman JA. Genetics of osteoporosis. *Endocr Rev.* 1999;20(6):788–804.

99. Dennison EM, et al. Birthweight, vitamin D receptor genotype and the programming of osteoporosis. *Paediatr Perinat Epidemiol.* 2001;15(3):211–219.

100. Ferrari S, et al. Bone mineral mass and calcium and phosphate metabolism in young men: Relationships with vitamin D receptor allelic polymorphisms. *J Clin Endocrinol Metab.* 1999;84(6):2043–2048.

101. Abrams SA, et al. Vitamin D receptor Fok1 polymorphisms affect calcium absorption, kinetics, and bone mineralization rates during puberty. *J Bone Miner Res.* 2005;20(6):945–953.

102. Theodoratou E, et al. Modification of the inverse association between dietary vitamin D intake and colorectal cancer risk by a FokI variant supports a chemoprotective action of vitamin D intake mediated through VDR binding. *International Journal of Cancer. Journal International du Cancer.* 2008;123(9):2170–2179.

103. Abreu MT, Geller JL, Vasiliauskas EA, et al. Treatment with infliximab is associated with increased markers of bone formation in patients with Crohn's disease. *J Clin Gastroenterol.* 2006;40(1): 55–63.

104. Jorgensen SP, et al.,Clinical trial: Vitamin D3 treatment in Crohn's disease—a randomized double-blind placebo-controlled study. *Aliment Pharmacol Ther.* 2010;32(3):377–383.

105. Dudrick SJ, LatifiR, Schrager R. Nutritional management of inflammatory bowel disease. *Surg Clin North Am.* 1991;71(3):609–623.

106. Lih-Brody L, Powell SR, Collier KP, et al. Increased oxidative stress and decreased antioxidant defenses in mucosa of inflammatory bowel disease. *Dig Dis Sci.* 1996;41(10):2078–2086.

107. Horska A, et al. Vitamin C levels in blood are influenced by polymorphisms in glutathione S-transferases. *European journal of nutrition.* 2011;50(6):437–446.

108. Cahill LE, Fontaine-Bisson B, El-Sohemy A. Functional genetic variants of glutathione S-transferase protect against serum ascorbic acid deficiency. *American Journal of Clinical Nutrition.* 2009;90(5): 1411–1417.

109. Tahara T. et al. Association between polymorphisms in the XRCC1 and GST genes, and CpG island methylation status in colonic mucosa in ulcerative colitis. *Virchows Archiv: An International Journal of Pathology.* 2011;458(2):205–211.

110. Carter MJ, Lobo AJ, Travis SPL. Guidelines for the management of inflammatory bowel disease in adults. *Gut.* 2004;53(S5):v1–16.

111. Savage DG, Lindenbaum J, Stabler SP, Allen RH. Sensitivity of serum methylmalonic acid and total homocysteine determinations for diagnosing cobalamin and folate deficiencies. *Am J Med.* 1994;96(3):239–246.

112. Romagnuolo J, Fedorak RN, Dias VC, Bamforth F, Teltscher M. Hyperhomocysteinemia and inflamatory bowel disease: Prevalence and predictors in a cross-sectional study. *Am J Gastroenterol.* 2001;96(7):2143–2149.

113. Curtin K, et al. Genetic polymorphisms in one-carbon metabolism: Associations with CpG island methylator phenotype (CIMP) in colon cancer and the modifying effects of diet. *Carcinogenesis.* 2007;28(8):672–679.

114. Zittan E, et al. High frequency of vitamin B12 deficiency in asymptomatic individuals homozygous to MTHFR C677T mutation is associated with endothelial dysfunction and homocysteinemia. *American Journal of Physiology. Heart and Circulatory Physiology.* 2007;293(1):H860–5.

115. Powers HJ, et al. Responses of biomarkers of folate and riboflavin status to folate and riboflavin supplementation in healthy and colorectal polyp patients (the FAB2 Study). *Cancer Epidemiology, Biomarkers & Prevention: A Publication of the American Association for Cancer Research,Ccosponsored by the American Society of Preventive Oncology.* 2007;16(10):2128–2135.

116. Hung J, et al. Additional food folate derived exclusively from natural sources improves folate status in young women with the MTHFR 677 CC or TT genotype. *Journal of Nutritional Biochemistry.* 2006;17(11):728–734.

117. Guinotte CL, et al. Methylenetetrahydrofolate reductase 677C→T variant modulates folate status response to controlled folate intakes in young women. *Journal of Nutrition.* 2003;133(5): 272–280.

118. McNulty H, et al. Riboflavin lowers homocysteine in individuals homozygous for the MTHFR 677C→T polymorphism. *Circulation.* 2006;113(1):74–80.

119. Greenberg GR, Fleming CR, Jeejeebhoy KN, Rosenberg IH, Sales D, Tremaine WJ. Controlled trial of bowel rest and nutritional support in the management of Crohn's disease. *Gut.* 1988;29(10): 1309–1315.

120. Sepehripour S,. Papagrigoriadis S. A systematic review of the benefit of total parenteral nutrition in the management of enterocutaneous fistulas. *Minerva Chir.* 2010;65(5):577–585.

121. Jeejeebhoy KN. Enteral and parenteral nutrition: Evidence-based approach. *Proc Nutr Soc.* 2001;60(3):399–402.

122. Hughes CA, Bates T, Dowling RH. Cholecystokinin and secretin prevent the intestinal mucosal hypoplasia of total parenteral nutrition in the dog. *Gastroenterology.* 1978;75(1):34–41.

123. Guedon C, Schmitz J, Lerebours E, et al. Decreased brush border hydrolase activities without gross morphologic changes in human intestinal mucosa after prolonged total parenteral nutrition of adults. *Gastroenterology.* 1986;90(2):373–378.

124. Rossi TM, Lee PC, Young C, Tjota A. Small intestinal mucosa changes, including epithelial cell proliferative activity, of children receiving total parenteral nutrition (TPN). *Dig Dis Sci.* 1993;38(9): 1608–1613.

125. Sedman PC, MacFie J, Palmer MD, Mitchell CJ, Sagar PM. Preoperative total parenteral nutrition is not associated with mucosal atrophy or bacterial translocation in humans. *Br J Surg.* 1995;82(12):1663–1667.

126. Nguyen GC, LaVeist TA, Brant SR. The utilization of parenteral nutrition during the in-patient management of inflammatory bowel disease in the United States: A national survey. *Aliment Pharmacol Ther.* 2007;26(11–12):1499–1507.

127. Dickinson RJ, Ashton MG, Axon AT, Smith RC, Yeung CK, Hill GL. Controlled trial of intravenous hyperalimentation and total bowel rest as an adjunct to the routine therapy of acute colitis. *Gastroenterology.* 1980;79(6):1199–1204.

128. Gonzalez-Huix F, Fernandez-Banares F, Esteve-Comas M, et al. Enteral versus parenteral nutrition as adjunct therapy in acute ulcerative colitis. *Am J Gastroenterol.* 1993;88(2):227–232.

129. King T. Meta-analysis of enteral nutrition as a primary treatment of active Crohn's disease. *Clinical Nutrition..* 1995;14(6):388–389.

130. Griffiths AM, Ohlsson A, Sherman PM, Sutherland LR. Meta-analysis of enteral nutrition as a primary treatment of active Crohn's disease. *Gastroenterology..* 1995;108(4):1056–1067.

131. Messori A, Trallori G, D'Albasio G, Milla M, Vannozzi G, Pacini F. Defined-formula diets versus steroids in the treatment of active Crohn's disease: A meta-analysis. *Scand J Gastroenterol.* 1996;31(3):267–272.

132. Fernandez-Banares F, Cabre E, Esteve-Comas M, Gassull M. How effective is enteral nutrition in inducing clinical remission in active Crohn's disease? A meta-analysis of the randomized clinical trials. *JPEN J Parenter Enteral Nutr.* 1995;19(5):356–364.

133. Harries AD, Danis V, Heatley RV, et al. Controlled trial of supplemented oral nutrition in Crohn's disease. *Lancet.* 1983;321(8330):887–890.

134. Koga H, Iida M, Aoyagi K, Matsui T, Fujishima M. Long-term efficacy of low residue diet for the maintenance of remission in patients with Crohn's disease. *Nippon Shokakibyo Gakkai Zasshi.* 1993;90(11):2882–2888.

135. Takagi S, Utsunomiya K, Kuriyama S, et al. Effectiveness of an "half elemental diet" as maintenance therapy for Crohn's disease: A randomized-controlled trial. *Aliment Pharmacol Ther.* 2006;24(9):1333–1340.

136. Verma S, Kirkwood B, Brown S, Giaffer MH. Oral nutritional supplementation is effective in the maintenance of remission in Crohn's disease. *Dig Liver Dis.* 2000;32(9):769–774.

137. Wilschanski M, Sherman P, Pencharz P, Davis L, Corey M, Griffiths A. Supplementary enteral nutrition maintains remission in paediatric Crohn's disease. *Gut.* 1996;38(4):543–548.

138. Newby EA, Sawczenko A, Thomas AG, Wilson D. Interventions for growth failure in childhood Crohn's disease. *Cochrane Database Syst Rev.* 2005;(3):CD003873.

139. Lewis JD, Fisher RL. Nutrition support in inflammatory bowel disease. *Med Clin North Am.* 1994;78(6):1443–1456.

140. Fell JM, Paintin M, Arnaud-Battandier F, et al. Mucosal healing and a fall in mucosal pro-inflammatory cytokine mRNA induced by a specific oral polymeric diet in paediatric Crohn's disease. *Aliment Pharmacol Ther.* 2000;14(3):281–289.

141. Gassull MA, Fernandez-Banares F, Cabre E, et al. Fat composition may be a clue to explain the primary therapeutic effect of enteral nutrition in Crohn's disease: Results of a double blind randomised multicentre European trial. *Gut.* 2002;51(2):164–168.

142. Fell JM. Control of systemic and local inflammation with transforming growth factor beta containing formulas. *JPEN J Parenter Enteral Nutr.* 2005;29(4 Suppl):S126–128; discussion S129–133, S184–188.

143. Harsha WT, Kalandarova E, McNutt P, Irwin R, Noel J. Nutritional supplementation with transforming growth factor-beta, glutamine, and short chain fatty acids minimizes methotrexate-induced injury. *J Pediatr Gastroenterol Nutr.* 2006;42(1):53–58.

144. Bamba T, Kanauchi O, Andoh A, Fujiyama Y. A new prebiotic from germinated barley for nutraceutical treatment of ulcerative colitis. *J Gastroenterol Hepatol.* 2002;17(8):818–824.

145. Kudsk KA, Wu Y, Fukatsu K, et al. Glutamine-enriched total parenteral nutrition maintains intestinal interleukin-4 and mucosal immunoglobulin A levels. *JPEN J Parenter Enteral Nutr.* 2000;24(5):270–274.

146. Chen K, Okuma T, Okamura K, Torigoe Y, Miyauchi Y. Glutamine-supplemented parenteral nutrition improves gut mucosa integrity and function in endotoxemic rats. *JPEN J Parenter Enteral Nutr.* 1994;18(2):167–171.

147. Singleton KD, Beckey VE, Wischmeyer PE. Glutamine prevents activation of NF-kappaB and stress kinase pathways, attenuate inflammatory cytokine release, and prevents acute respiratory distress syndrome (ARDS) following sepsis. *Shock.* 2005;24(6):583–589.

148. Ockenga J, Borchert K, Stuber E, Lochs H, Manns MP, Bischoff SC. Glutamine-enriched total parenteral nutrition in patients with inflammatory bowel disease. *Eur J Clin Nutr.* 2005;59(11):1302–1309.

149. Sido B, Seel C, Hochlehnert A, Breitkreutz R, Droge W. Low intestinal glutamine level and low glutaminase activity in Crohn's disease: A rational for glutamine supplementation? *Dig Dis Sci.* 2006;51(12):2170–2179.

150. Xue H, Sufit AJ, Wischmeyer, PE. Glutamine therapy improves outcome of in vitro and in vivo experimental colitis models. *JPEN J Parenter Enteral Nutr.* 2011;35(2):188–197.

151. Fernandez-Banares F, Cabre E, Gonzalez-Huix F, Gassull MA. Enteral nutrition as primary therapy in Crohn's disease. *Gut.* 1994;35(1_Suppl):S55–59.

152. Belluzzi A, Brignola C, Campieri M, Pera A, Boschi S, Miglioli M. Effect of an enteric-coated fish-oil preparation on relapses in Crohn's disease. *N Engl J Med.* 1996;334(24):1557–1560.

153. Shimizu T, Fujii T, Suzuki R, et al. Effects of highly purified eicosapentaenoic acid on erythrocyte fatty acid composition and leukocyte and colonic mucosa leukotriene B4 production in children with ulcerative colitis. *J Pediatr Gastroenterol Nutr.* 2003;37(5):581–585.

154. Bamba T, Shimoyama T, Sasaki M, et al. Dietary fat attenuates the benefits of an elemental diet in active Crohn's disease: A randomized, controlled trial. *Eur J Gastroenterol Hepatol.* 2003;15(2):151–157.

155. Turner D, Zlotkin SH, Shah PS, Griffiths AM. Omega 3 fatty acids (fish oil) for maintenance of remission in Crohn's disease. *Cochrane Database Syst Rev.* 2007;(2):CD006320.

156. Turner D, Steinhart AH, Griffiths AM. Omega 3 fatty acids (fish oil) for maintenance of remission in ulcerative colitis. *Cochrane Database Syst Rev.* 2007;(3):CD006443.

157. Feagan BG, Sandborn WJ, Mittmann U, et al. Omega-3 free fatty acids for the maintenance of remission in Crohn disease: The EPIC randomized controlled trials. *JAMA.* 2008;299(14):1690–1697.

158. Turner D, et al., Maintenance of remission in inflammatory bowel disease using omega-3 fatty acids (fish oil); A systematic review and meta-analyses. *Inflamm Bowel Dis.* 2011;17(1):336–345.

159. Turner D, et al. Omega 3 fatty acids (fish oil) for maintenance of remission in Crohn's disease. *Cochrane Database Syst Rev.* 2009(1):CD006320.

160. Wiese DM, et al. The effects of an oral supplement enriched with fish oil, prebiotics, and antioxidants on nutrition status in Crohn's disease patients. *Nutr Clin Pract.* 2011;26(4):463–473.

161. Seidner DL, et al. An oral supplement enriched with fish oil, soluble fiber, and antioxidants for corticosteroid sparing in ulcerative colitis: a randomized, controlled trial. *Clin Gastroenterol Hepatol.* 2005;3(4):358–369.

162. Lomer MC, Harvey RS, Evans SM, Thompson RP, Powell JJ. Efficacy and tolerability of a low microparticle diet in a double blind, randomized, pilot study in Crohn's disease. *Eur J Gastroenterol Hepatol.* 2001;13(2):101–106.

163. Scheppach W, Sommer H, Kirchner T, et al. Effect of butyrate enemas on the colonic mucosa in distal ulcerative colitis. *Gastroenterology*. 1992;103(1):51–56.

164. Breuer RI, Buto SK, Christ ML, et al. Rectal irrigation with short-chain fatty acids for distal ulcerative colitis: Preliminary report. *Dig Dis Sci*. 1991;36(2):185–187.

165. Steinhart AH, Brzezinski A, Baker JTreatment of refractory ulcerative proctosigmoiditis with butyrate enemas. *Am J Gastroenterol*. 1994;89(2):179–183.

166. Patz J, Jacobsohn WZ, Gottschalk-Sabag S, Zeides S, Braverman DZ. Treatment of refractory distal ulcerative colitis with short chain fatty acid enemas. *Am J Gastroenterol*. 1996;91(4):731–734.

167. Vernia P, Cittadini M, Caprilli R, Torsoli A. Topical treatment of refractory distal ulcerative colitis with 5-ASA and sodium butyrate. *Dig Dis Sci*. 1995;40(2):305–307.

168. Kanauchi O, Suga T, Tochihara M, et al. Treatment of ulcerative colitis by feeding with germinated barley foodstuff: First report of a multicenter open control trial. *J Gastroenterol*. 2002;37 Suppl 14:67–72.

169. Lomer MC, Harvey RS, Evans SM, Thompson RP, Powell JJ. Efficacy and tolerability of a low microparticle diet in a double blind, randomized, pilot study in Crohn's disease. *Eur J Gastroenterol Hepatol*. 2001;13(2):101–106.

170. Lomer MC, Grainger SL, Ede R, et al. Lack of efficacy of a reduced microparticle diet in a multi-centered trial of patients with active Crohn's disease. *Eur J Gastroenterol Hepatol*. 2005;17(3):377–384.

171. Mullin GE. Comment on: Black and green tea consumption and the risk of coronary artery disease: A meta-analysis. *Nutr Clin Pract,* 2011;26:356.

172. Athar M, Back JH, Tang X, et al. Resveratrol: A review of preclinical studies for human cancer prevention. *Toxicol Appl Pharmacol*. 2007;224(3):274–283.

173. Martin AR, Villegas I, La Casa C, de la Lastra CA. Resveratrol, a polyphenol found in grapes, suppresses oxidative damage and stimulates apoptosis during early colonic inflammation in rats. *Biochem Pharmacol*. 2004;67(7):1399–1410.

174. Cabrera C, Artacho R, Gimenez R. Beneficial effects of green tea—a review. *J Am Coll Nutr.* 2006;25(2):79–99.

175. Nomura M, Ma W, Chen N, Bode AM, Dong Z. Inhibition of 12-O-tetradecanoylphorbol-13-acetate-induced NF-kappaB activation by tea polyphenols-epigallocatechin gallate and theaflavins. *Carcinogenesis*. 2000;21(10):1885–1890.

176. Mazzon E, Muia C, Paola RD, et al. Green tea polyphenol extract attenuates colon injury induced by experimental colitis. *Free Radic Res*. 2005;39(9):1017–1025.

177. Oz HS, Chen TS, McClain CJ, de Villiers WJ. Antioxidants as novel therapy in a murine model of colitis. *J Nutr Biochem*. 2005;16(5):297–304.

178. Varilek GW, Yang F, Lee EY, et al. Green tea polyphenol extract attenuates inflammation in interleukin-2-deficient mice, a model of autoimmunity. *J Nutr*. 2001;131(7):2034–2039.

179. Porath D, Riegger C, Drewe J, Schwager J. Epigallocatechin-3-gallate impairs chemokine production in human colon epithelial cell lines. *J Pharmacol Exp Ther*. 2005;315(3):1172–1180.

180. Bengmark S. Curcumin, an atoxic antioxidant and natural NFkappaB, cyclooxygenase-2, lipooxygenase, and inducible nitric oxide synthase inhibitor: A shield against acute and chronic diseases. *JPEN J Parenter Enteral Nutr*. 2006;30(1):45–51.

181. Cheng AL, Hsu CH, Lin JK, et al. Phase I clinical trial of curcumin, a chemopreventive agent, in patients with high-risk or pre-malignant lesions. *Anticancer Res*. 2001;21(4):2895–2900.

182. Jobin C, Bradham CA, Russo MP, et al. Curcumin blocks cytokine-mediated NF-kappa B activation and proinflammatory gene expression by inhibiting inhibitory factor I-kappa B kinase activity. *J Immunol*. 1999;163(6):3474–3483.

183. Jian YT, Mai GF, Wang JD, Zhang YL, Luo RC, Fang YX. Preventive and therapeutic effects of NF-kappaB inhibitor curcumin in rats' colitis induced by trinitrobenzene sulfonic acid. *World J Gastroenterol*. 2005;11(12):1747–1752.

184. Ukil A, Maity S, Karmakar S, Datta N, Vedasiromoni JR, Das PK. Curcumin, the major component of food flavour turmeric, reduces mucosal injury in trinitrobenzene sulphonic acid-induced colitis. *Br J Pharmacol*. 2003;139(2):209–218.

185. Sugimoto K, Hanai H, Tozawa K, et al. Curcumin prevents and ameliorates trinitrobenzene sulfonic acidinduced colitis in mice. *Gastroenterology*. 2002;123(6):1912–1922.

186. Zhang M, Deng C, Zheng J, Xia J, Sheng D. Curcumin inhibits trinitrobenzene sulphonic acid-induced colitis in rats by activation of peroxisome proliferator-activated receptor gamma. *Int Immunopharmacol*. 2006;6(8):1233–1242.

187. Salh B, Assi K, Templeman V, et al. Curcumin attenuates DNB-induced murine colitis. *Am J Physiol Gastrointest Liver Physiol*. 2003;285(1):G235–243.

188. Deguchi Y, Andoh A, Inatomi O, et al. Curcumin prevents the development of dextran sulfate sodium (DSS)-induced experimental colitis. *Dig Dis Sci*. 2007;52(11):2993–2998.

189. Hanai H, Iida T, Takeuchi K, et al. Curcumin maintenance therapy for ulcerative colitis: Randomized, multicenter, double-blind, placebo-controlled trial. *Clin Gastroenterol Hepatol*. 2006;4(12):1502–1506.

190. Campieri M, Gionchetti P. Probiotics in inflammatory bowel disease: New insight to pathogenesis or a possible therapeutic alternative? *Gastroenterology*. 1999;116(5):1246–1249.

191. Schultz M, Sartor RB. Probiotics and inflammatory bowel diseases. *American Journal of Gastroenterology*. 2000;95(1):S19–S21.

192. Shanahan F. Probiotics in inflamatory bowel disease. *Gut*. 2001;48(5):609.

193. Fuller R. Probiotics in man and animals. *J Appl Bacteriol*. 1989;66(5):365–378.

194. Sartor RB. Therapeutic manipulation of the enteric microflora in inflammatory bowel diseases: Antibiotics, probiotics, and prebiotics. *Gastroenterology*. 2004;126(6):1620–1633.

195. Probert HM, Apajalahti JH, Rautonen N, Stowell J, Gibson GR. Polydextrose, lactitol, and fructooligo-saccharide fermentation by colonic bacteria in a three-stage continuous culture system. *Appl Environ Microbiol*. 2004;70(8):4505–4511.

196. Sandborn W, Waters G, Gregory S, Pemberton J. Ileal pouch anal anastomosis and the problem of pouchitis. *Curr Opin Gastroenterol*. 1997;13(1):34–40.

197. Gionchetti P, Rizzello F, Venturi A, et al. Oral bacteriotherapy as maintenance treatment in patients with chronic pouchitis: A double-blind, placebo-controlled trial. *Gastroenterology*. 2000;119(2):305–309.

198. Gionchetti P, Rizzello F, Helwig U, et al. Prophylaxis of pouchitis onset with probiotic therapy: A double-blind, placebo-controlled trial. *Gastroenterology*. 2003;124(5):1202–1209.

199. Mallon P, et al. Probiotics for induction of remission in ulcerative colitis. *Cochrane Database Syst Rev*. 2007(4):CD005573.

200. Sang LX, et al. Remission induction and maintenance effect of probiotics on ulcerative colitis: A meta-analysis. *World J Gastroenterol*. 2010;16(15):1908–1915.

201. Bengmark S. Pre-, pro- and synbiotics. *Curr Opin Clin Nutr Metab Care*. 2001;4(6):571–579.

202. Roberfroid MB. Introducing inulin-type fructans. *Br J Nutr*. 2005;93 (S1):S13–25.

203. Videla S, Vilaseca J, Antolin M, et al. Dietary inulin improves distal colitis induced by dextran sodium sulfate in the rat. *Am J Gastroenterol*. 2001;96(5):1486–1493.

204. Hoentjen F, Welling GW, Harmsen HJ, et al. Reduction of colitis by prebiotics in HLA-B27 transgenic rats is associated with microflora changes and immunomodulation. *Inflamm Bowel Dis*. 2005;11(11):977–985.

205. Madsen KL, Doyle JS, Jewell LD, Tavernini MM, Fedorak RN. Lactobacillus species prevents colitis in interleukin 10 gene-deficient mice. *Gastroenterology*. 1999;116(5):1107–1114.

206. Welters CF, Heineman E, Thunnissen FB, van den Bogaard AE, Soeters PB, Baeten CG. Effect of dietary inulin supplementation on inflammation of pouch mucosa in patients with an ileal pouch-anal anastomosis. *Dis Colon Rectum*. 2002;45(5):621–627.

207. Furrie E, Macfarlane S, Kennedy A, et al. Synbiotic therapy (Bifidobacterium longum/Synergy 1) initiates resolution of inflammation in patients with active ulcerative colitis: A randomised controlled pilot trial. *Gut*. 2005;54(2):242–249.

208. Guslandi M, Mezzi G, Sorghi M, Testoni PA. Saccharomyces boulardii in maintenance treatment of Crohn's disease. *Dig Dis Sci*. 2000;45(7):1462–1464.

209. Prantera C, Scribano ML, Falasco G, Andreoli A, Luzi C. Ineffectiveness of probiotics in preventing recurrence after curative resection for Crohn's disease: A randomised controlled trial with lactobacillus GG. *Gut*. 2002;51(3):405–409.

210. Schultz M, Timmer A, Herfarth HH, Sartor RB, Vanderhoof JA, Rath HC. Lactobacillus GG in inducing and maintaining remission of Crohn's disease. *BMC Gastroenterol*. 2004;4:5.

211. Doherty GA, et al. Meta-analysis: Targeting the intestinal microbiota in prophylaxis for post-operative Crohn's disease. *Aliment Pharmacol Ther*. 2010;31(8):802–809.

212. Lindsay JO, Whelan K, Stagg AJ, et al. Clinical, microbiological, and immunological effects of fructooligosaccharide in patients with Crohn's disease. *Gut*. 2006;55(3):348–355.

213. Bayless TM, Harris ML. Inflammatory bowel disease and irritable bowel syndrome. *Med Clin North Am*. 1990;74(1):21–28.

214. MacDermott RTreatment of irritable bowel syndrome in outpatients with inflammatory bowel disease using a food and beverage intolerance, food and beverage avoidance diet. *Inflamm Bowel Dis*. 2007;13(1):91–96.

215. Tursi A, Giorgetti GM, Brandimarte G, Elisei W. High prevalence of celiac disease among patients affected by Crohn's disease. *Inflamm Bowel Dis*. 2005;11(7):662–666.

216. Kagnoff MF. Celiac disease: Pathogenesis of a model immunogenetic disease. *Journal of Clinical Investigation.* 2007;117(1):41–49.
217. Bouzid D, et al. Inflammatory bowel disease: Susceptibility and disease heterogeneity revealed by human leukocyte antigen genotyping. *Genet Test Mol Biomarkers,* 2012;16(6):482–487.
218. Waterman M, et al. Distinct and overlapping genetic loci in Crohn's disease and ulcerative colitis: Correlations with pathogenesis. *Inflammatory Bowel Diseases.* 2011;17(9):1936–1942.
219. Fasano A, et al. Prevalence of celiac disease in at-risk and not-at-risk groups in the United States: A large multicenter study. *Archives of Internal Medicine.* 2003;163(3):286–292.
220. Levenstein S, Prantera C, Luzi C, D'Ubaldi A. Low residue or normal diet in Crohn's disease: A prospective controlled study in Italian patients. *Gut.* 1985;26(10):989–993.
221. Misiakos EP, Macheras A, Kapetanakis T, Liakakos T. Short bowel syndrome: Current medical and surgical trends. *J Clin Gastroenterol.* 2007;41(1):5–18.
222. Goldschmid S, Graham M. Trace element deficiencies in inflammatory bowel disease. *Gastroenterol Clin North Am.* 1989;18(3):579–587.
223. Rannem T, Ladefoged K, Hylander E, Hegnhoj J, Jarnum S. Selenium status in patients with Crohn's disease. *Am J Clin Nutr.* 1992;56(5):933–937.
224. Jowett SL, Seal CJ, Phillips E, Gregory W, Barton JR, Welfare MR. Dietary beliefs of people with ulcerative colitis and their effect on relapse and nutrient intake. *Clin Nutr.* 2004;23(2):161–170.
225. Schedel J, Rockmann F, Bongartz T, Woenckhaus M, Scholmerich J, Kullmann F. Association of Crohn's disease and latent celiac disease: A case report and review of the literature. *Int J Colorectal Dis.* 2005;20(4):376–380.
226. Kuhnle GG, Bingham SA. Dietary meat, endogenous nitrosation and colorectal cancer. *Biochem Soc Trans.* 2007;35(Pt 5):1355–1357.
227. Ryan-Harshman M, Aldoori W. Diet and colorectal cancer: Review of the evidence. *Can Fam Physician.* 2007;53(11):1913–1920.
228. Santarelli RL, Pierre F, Corpet DE. Processed meat and colorectal cancer: A review of epidemiologic and experimental evidence. *Nutr Cancer.* 2008;60(2):131–144.
229. Dawson-Hughes B, Heaney RP, Holick MF, Lips P, Meunier PJ, Vieth R. Estimates of optimal vitamin D status. *Osteoporos Int.* 2005;16(7):713–716.
230. Gertner JM, Domenech M. 25-hydroxyvitamin D levels in patients treated with high-dosage ergo- and cholecalciferol. *J Clin Pathol.* 1977;30(2):144–150.
231. Vieth R. Vitamin D supplementation, 25-hydroxyvitamin D concentrations, and safety. *Am J Clin Nutr.* 1999;69(5):842–856.
232. de Silva AD, Mylonaki M, Rampton DS. Oral iron therapy in inflammatory bowel disease: Usage, tolerance, and efficacy. *Inflamm Bowel Dis.* 2003;9(5):316–320.
233. Galloway M, Rushworth L. Red cell or serum folate? Results from the national pathology alliance benchmarking review. *J Clin Pathol.* 2003;56(12):924–926.
234. Kim YI. Does a high folate intake increase the risk of breast cancer? *Nutr Rev.* 2006;64(10 Pt 1):468–475.
235. Brown AC, Rampertab SD, Mullin GE. Existing dietary guidelines for Crohn's disease and ulcerative colitis. *Expert Rev Gastroenterol Hepatol.* 2011;5(3):411–425.
236. Brown AC, Roy M. Does evidence exist to include dietary therapy in the treatment of Crohn's disease? *Expert Rev Gastroenterol Hepatol.* 2010;4(2):191–215.

16 Celiac Disease and Non-Celiac Gluten Sensitivity

The Evolving Spectrum

Thomas O'Bryan, D.C., Rodney Ford, M.D., M.B.B.S., and Cynthia Kupper, R.D.

INTRODUCTION

Underneath the umbrella of gluten-related disorders, celiac disease and non-celiac gluten sensitivity have an immune reaction to gluten in common and often present with overlapping clinical symptoms. Differentiating among gluten-related disorders allows clinicians to give patients specific nutritional and other medical recommendations; however, clinical and laboratory diagnosis is complex and evolving as presented in this chapter. Nutrition holds the potential to advance medical care for patients with gluten-related disorders in several ways: A dietary history can prompt diagnosis in a clinical setting. A gluten-free diet is a medical therapy. Nutritional interventions can restore nutrients depleted by disease-associated malabsorption. Lastly, nutritional therapies have been shown to improve gastrointestinal health.

BACKGROUND

Adverse reactions to the toxic family of gluten proteins found in wheat, barley, rye, and their derivatives may trigger a heterogeneous set of conditions, including wheat allergy, gluten sensitivity (GS), and celiac disease (CD), that, combined, affect between 10–15% of the general population [1–5]. Once believed to fall exclusively into the domain of allergic conditions (e.g., wheat allergy), it is now clear that the intestinal and extraintestinal manifestations of CD are different entities other than allergy, mediated by innate and adaptive immune pathways [6,7]. Gluten sensitivity is a state of heightened immunological responsiveness to ingested gluten in genetically susceptible people. It represents a spectrum of diverse manifestations, of which gluten-sensitive enteropathy also known as CD is one of many [8].

In both wheat allergy and CD, the immune reaction to gluten is mediated via the adaptive immune system by T-cell activation in the gastrointestinal mucosa. However, in wheat allergy, it is the crosslinking of immunoglobulin E (IgE) by repeat sequences in gluten peptides that triggers the release of chemical mediators, such as histamine, from basophils and mast cells [9]. In contrast, CD, which affects approximately 1% of the general population, is an autoimmune disorder evidenced by recognition of antibodies to self (tissue transglutaminase 2 and/or endomysium), the autoimmune enteropathy identified commonly by the Marsh classification system (Table 16.1), and numerous associated autoimmune comorbidities [10].

TABLE 16.1

Stages of Small Intestine Histopathology in Crohn's Disease

Histopathology	Normal Mucosa (Intact Villous)	Normal Villous Crypt Morphology with IEL	Crypt Hyperplasia Infiltrative	Partial Villous Atrophy Enterocyte Loss Crypt Hyperplasia	Subtotal/Total Villous Atrophy Crypt Hyperplasia	Mucosal Atrophy
Marsh Classification	Preinfiltrative	Infiltrative	Infiltrative Hyperplastic	Infiltrative Hyperplastic Partial Destructive	Flat Destructive	Atrophic Hyperplastic
Characteristic	Type O	Type I	Type II	Type IIIa	Type IIIb	Type IIIc
Villous Atrophy	–	–	–	+	++	+++
IEL#	–	+	+	+	+	+
Crypt Hyperplasia	–	–	+	+	++	++
Enterocyte Degradation	–	–	–	+	++	+++

Source: Adapted from [128]

Understanding of immune reactions to the toxic family of glutens found in wheat, rye, and barley has been rapidly growing because of significant advances in knowledge about pathogenic, epidemiological, clinical, and diagnostic aspects [11]. Over the past 20 years, the diagnostic accuracy of serology for GS and CD has progressively increased with the development of highly reliable tests such as the detection of IgA tissue transglutaminase and antiendomysial and IgG antideamidated gliadin peptide antibodies [12]. As a result, what was once considered a rare disease of childhood (CD) has ballooned in the last two decades to be classified as "one of the most common life-long disorders in both Europe and the U.S. [13]."

Gluten is a generic term for storage proteins naturally found in grains. The toxic proteins of gluten have been recognized as a common environmental trigger in the initiation, development, and propagation of autoimmune pathology [14–16]. Extraintestinal manifestations of GS can occur (Table 16.2) with or without gut involvement and physicians are recommended to become familiar with the common presentations (Table 16.3) and means of diagnosis of these conditions [17–20,113]. Epidemiological studies, performed by accurate serological screening in the general population, have radically changed our knowledge about GS and CD prevalence, showing that the conditions occur much more frequently than previously thought (Table 16.4) [21–28].

Autoimmune disease, the third leading cause of morbidity and mortality in the industrialized world [29], is 10 times more common in those with the gluten-sensitive enteropathy (CD) than in the general population [30]. Thus, the burden on society from GS cannot be overestimated. Earlier identification might result in earlier treatment, better quality of life, and an improved prognosis for these patients [31].

EPIDEMIOLOGY

Once considered a rare food-intolerance condition, CD is now generally considered "one of the most common lifelong disorders in both the U.S. and Europe" [8,32]. The prevalence of celiac disease has increased fivefold overall since 1974. This increase was not due to increased sensitivity

TABLE 16.2

Presenting Symptoms of Celiac Disease

General	**Weakness***, lassitude, malaise, weight loss, short stature, failure to thrive
Gastrointestinal	**Diarrhea/constipation**, anorexia, nausea and vomiting, **flatulence and abdominal distension, abdominal pain, motility disturbance**, glossitis/apthous ulcers
Metabolic	Anemia features, bleeding tendency, edema, **cramps/tetany**, dental enamel hypoplasia, fat malabsorption, nutrient insufficiencies/deficiencies
Musculoskeletal	**Bone pain** and fractures, **myopathy, osteopenia/osteoporosis**
Neuropsychiatric	**Depression, anxiety, schizophrenia, paresthesia, peripheral neuropathy, cerebrospinal degeneration**
Reproductive	Menstrual irregularities, recurrent miscarriages, abnormalities of sperm morphology and motility, infertility, intrauterine growth retardation
Skin	Variety of rashes, petechiae

*Bold font indicates symptoms also associated with non-celiac gluten sensitivity.
Source: Adapted from [25,26,32]

TABLE 16.3

Disorders Associated with Celiac Disease

Autoimmune	**Idiopathic**	**Chromosomal**	**Miscellaneous**
IDDM	Dilated cardiomyopathy	Down syndrome	Female and male infertility,
Antiphospoholipid syndrome	**Epilepsy with or without**	Turner syndrome	IUGR
IgA nephropathy*	**occipital calcifications**	Williams syndrome	Miscarriages
Sjögren's syndrome	Sarcoidosis		
Hashimoto thyroiditis	**Myalgia/myositis**		Depression
Graves' disease	Hypertransaminasemia		Anxiety
Addison's disease	Atopy		Social phobia
Autoimmune hemolytic disease	Recurrent pancreatitis		**Psychiatric disease**
Myasthenia gravis	**Cerebellar ataxia**		**(Schizophrenia)**
Autoimmune hepatitis	**Peripheral neuropathy**		Fat malabsorption
Primary biliary cirrhosis	Multiple myoclonus		Nutrient insufficiencies
Primary sclerosing cholangitis	Multiple sclerosis		Nutrient deficiencies
Alopecia	**Brain atrophy**		
Vitiligo	Inflammatory bowel disease		
Psoriases	**Irritable bowel syndrome**		
Dermatitis herpetiformis			
IgA deficiency			
Autoimmune atrophic gastritis			

*Bold font indicates symptoms also associated with non-celiac gluten sensitivity.
Abbreviations: IDDM: Insulin Dependent Diabetes Mellitus. Adapted from (29, 35)
IUGR: Intrauterine Growth Retardation
Source: Adapted from [26,32]

TABLE 16.4

Groups at Risk for Celiac Disease

Condition	Estimated Prevalence of Celiac Disease
Elderly	2.5%
Anemia in celiac disease	46–50%
Celiac disease in anemia	5.2%
Osteopenia/Osteoporosis in celiac disease	47–80%
Celiac disease in osteoporosis	3.4–5.5%
Insulin-dependent diabetes mellitus	8–12%
Multiple sclerosis	11%
Thyroiditis	3–5%
Autoimmune thyroid disease	3.3–7.7%
Sjogren's syndrome (and other connective tissue disease)	3–4%
Down syndrome	10–12%
Williams syndrome	5%
Turner syndrome	5%
Psoriasis	4.34%
Chronic unexplained hypertransaminasemia	9%
Primary biliary cirrhosis	0–11%
Autoimmune hepatitis (type 1 and 2)	4–6.4%
Liver transplantation	4.3%
Diet-resistant non-alcoholic fatty liver disease	3.4%
Recurrent pancreatitis	7%

Group	Estimated Prevalence of Celiac Disease
Siblings	
First-degree relatives	5–20%
Family members with positive tTG	11%
Monozygotic twins	75%
HLA-identical siblings	40%
Relatives	21.3%
Relatives of Two Siblings with Celiac Disease	
Offspring	14.7%
First-degree relatives	17.2%
Second-degree relatives	19%

There is a male preponderance among families of new cases, and many have "silent CD" despite severe histological injury.
Source: Adapted from [23,51,53,54,55,64]

of testing, but rather due to an increasing number of subjects that lost the immunological tolerance to gluten in their adulthood [33].

The prevalence of celiac disease in elderly people was higher than what has been reported in the population in general but the symptoms were subtle (intestinal and extraintestinal). The total frequency of biopsy-proven CD and seropositive cases without histological confirmation in the elderly was more than double (2.45%) that in the general population [34]. The prevalence of CD in first-degree relatives is increasing worldwide and recognized to be as high as 1 in 22 [35–40] (Table 16.5). The presence of the gene HLA-DQ2 and being a sibling are the greatest risk factors for CD in first-degree relatives. Active case finding of suspected cases by serologic screening is encouraged, since undetected cases may be prone to increased morbidity and mortality. Increased

TABLE 16.5

Clinical Manifestations of Celiac Disease (CD) in Pediatrics

Manifestations Secondary to Untreated CD	Associated Diseases	Genetic-Associated Diseases
CD with classic symptoms	Autoimmune diseases	Down syndrome
Abdominal distension/gas	Type-1 diabetes	Turner syndrome
Anorexia	Thyrioditis	Williams syndrome
Chronic or recurrent diarrhea	Sjogren's syndrome	IgA deficiency
Failure to thrive or weight loss	Neurologic and	
Constipation	psychological disturbances	
Irritability	Ataxia	
Lethargy	Autism	
Muscle wasting	Depression	
Short stature	Epilepsy with intracranial	
Celiac crises (rare)	calcifications	
Hepatitis	IgA nephropathy	
Iron-deficient anemia	Osteopenia/osteoporosis	
CD with nonclassic symptoms		
Arthritis		
Aphthous stomatitis		
Dental enamel defects		
Dermatitis herpetiformis		
Pubertal delay		
Recurrent abdominal pain		
Vomiting		

Source: Adapted from [46,47].

alertness and repeat screening is recommended in at-risk individuals as the disorder may develop at any age [41].

PATHOPHYSIOLOGY

CD is a chronic immune-mediated disease caused by a genetically determined, permanent intolerance to ingested gluten proteins of wheat, barley, and rye (and their derivatives) resulting in inflammatory damage of the small-intestinal mucosa [42]. CD is the only autoimmune trait with a known environmental trigger (gluten). Also known as celiac sprue or gluten-sensitive enteropathy, the most recognized expression of the disorder is characteristic, though not specific, small intestine lesions that impair nutrient absorption and improve upon withdrawal of the responsible grain [43].

Because of the heterogeneity among clinical signs and the lack of specificity of many presenting symptoms, the clinical diagnosis of CD is a challenge even for experts. The presentation can be misleading because the symptoms vary tremendously from patient to patient and appear to depend largely on the length and the severity of small intestine damage [26]. Many cases remain undiagnosed and thus carry a risk of long-term complications, including osteoporosis [44], a multitude of autoimmune diseases [45], psychiatric syndromes [46], infertility and reproductive disorders [47], various neurologic conditions including peripheral neuropathy, ataxia, seizures [25,48], and cancer [8]. The classic presentation of diarrhea and malabsorption is now less common, and atypical and silent presentations are increasing [49].

The routine use of antibody markers has allowed researchers to discover a very high number of borderline cases, characterized by positive serology and mild intestinal lesions or normal small intestine architecture, which can be classified as potential CD. It is evident that the old celiac disease with flat mucosa is only a part of the spectrum of CD [26]. In North America, comparing the time periods 1990–96 and 2000–6, antibody testing of children for celiac disease tripled the incidence and quadrupled the median age at diagnosis. One in four children were diagnosed as having celiac disease as a result of case finding of associated conditions, including gastrointestinal symptoms, chronic fatigue, short stature, delayed puberty, dental enamel defects, elevated liver transaminase levels, dermatitis herpetiformis, and nutritional anemias [50]. Occult celiac disease seems to start in childhood, even in those who are subsequently diagnosed as adults [51].

Every time the disease is clinically diagnosed in an adult, that person has for decades had disease in a latent or silent stage [52]. Multiple studies suggest that patients with CD should be treated, whether or not they have symptoms or associated conditions [33].

CLINICAL PRESENTATION

Celiac disease was originally described as a pediatric syndrome of diarrhea, steatorrhea, and weight loss. This symptomatic presentation in which gastrointestinal manifestations predominate is known as the classic presentation [53]. Although defined by the small intestine injury and resulting malabsorption, more recently it has been recognized to be a multisystem disorder that may affect other organs, such as the nervous system, bones, skin, heart, and, the liver [27,54,55,56]. Before 2000, the primary clinical presentation recognized was diarrhea. After 2000, recognition of multiple clinical presentations became evident. These are:

- Typical, characterized mostly by gastrointestinal signs and symptoms;
- Atypical or extraintestinal, noted by minimal or absent gastrointestinal signs/symptoms;
- Various extraintestinal, characterized by present manifestations, ranging from short stature to iron-deficient anemia, and from dermatitis herpetiformis to female infertility;
- Silent, where the small intestinal mucosa is damaged and CD autoimmunity can be detected by serology, but there are minimal or no symptoms; silent CD is commonly found in patients that come to be diagnosed by screening, often belonging to high-risk groups [22].

Half of pregnancies of mothers with celiac disease are complicated by unfavorable fetal outcomes or miscarriages [32]. In a case-control study, comparison of 94 untreated and 31 treated celiac women indicated that the relative risk of spontaneous abortion was 8.9 times higher, the relative risk of low birth weight baby was 5.84 times higher and duration of breast feeding was 2.54 times shorter in untreated mothers. The high incidence of spontaneous abortion, low birth weight babies, and shortened duration of breastfeeding was effectively corrected with a gluten-free diet [57,58]. CD diagnosed prior to pregnancy does not constitute as great a risk as undiagnosed CD [44]. Fetal growth restriction is a major pregnancy complication responsible for a 5–20-fold increase in perinatal mortality and perinatal morbidity [45]. There is a growing body of evidence supporting the association between undiagnosed CD and fetal growth restriction, odds ratios varying between 1.3 and 6 [59,60]. Treatment of maternal CD reduces the risk of fetal growth restriction to that of the general population [44].

Pediatric presentations are varied from classic symptoms to short stature, pubertal delay, dental enamel defects, epilepsy with intracranial calcifications, Turners syndrome, Down syndrome, and others (see Table 16.5) [61,62].

PATIENT EVALUATION

Historically, the diagnosis of celiac disease was made by a gastroenterologist in 52.7% of cases [63]. Given the multitude of presentations of CD, clinicians across specialties are evaluating patients [64].

For every classic symptomatic patient with CD, there are eight patients with CD and no gastrointestinal symptoms [65,66]. A recent meta-analysis indicated that the ratio of known to undiagnosed cases of celiac disease was 1:7 [62]. This suggests a failure in case finding for this extremely common disease [67,68,69]. Although celiac disease was traditionally considered a childhood disease, most patients are diagnosed in adulthood [59,70]. The median delay in diagnosis after presenting symptoms are recognized ranges from 4.9 to 11 years [64,65]. Investigating the metabolic function of intestinal microflora, fecal short-chain fatty acid (SCFA) patterns in children with untreated classic CD (diarrhea, steatorrhea, and weight loss), screening-detected CD, and asymptomatic CD were discovered to all differ significantly from healthy reference children. This common pathogenic mechanism of aberrant gut-floral patterns in children with various presentations of CD emphasizes the necessity of a wider criterion of inclusion for CD-differential diagnosis than just the classic presentation [71,72].

The National Institutes of Health consensus statement on celiac disease states that "the single most important step in diagnosing celiac disease is to first consider the disorder by recognizing its myriad clinical features" [73].

Understanding about CD has progressed, and currently there is a general consensus that it is a heterogeneous autoimmune disorder, the diagnosis of which relies not only on histological findings but also on increasingly important serological and genetic tests. Serology has become increasingly relevant to CD diagnosis [74]. The availability of immunologic tests that confirm symptoms to be related to food sensitivity has definitively changed the diagnostic algorithm for CD. CD-related antibodies have allowed researchers to confirm a great number of borderline cases in patients with mild intestinal lesions and positive serology, diagnosing the so-called potential and "silent" CD before the appearance of severe intestinal damage [26].

GENETICS

Over 97% of CD patients will carry one or both of two genes, HLA-DQ2 and/or HLA-DQ8. Each of these genes will carry two subunits—an alpha subunit typically designated A1 and a beta subunit typically designated B1. The beta subunit is the most prognostic component of the DQ molecule, but the alpha subunit has also been shown to carry an increased risk for celiac disease. Some think that since the beta subunit carries most of the risk and the alpha unit only minor risk, testing for only the beta subunit is adequate. Thus, some laboratories offer genetic testing of the entire HLA-DQ2/8 profile and some only offer HLA-DQ2/8 beta subunit. Comprehensive testing will diminish false-negatives. The genetic risk of developing CD varies with the combination of HLA-DQ genes and the subunits (Table 16.6) [75].

SEROLOGY

There is general agreement that the best strategy for CD serological screening is the detection of IgA tissue transglutaminase antibodies (tTGA). These antibodies are the most sensitive test for CD (up to 97%), whereas IgA EmA are employed as a confirmatory test in tTGA positive cases due to their higher specificity (about 100%)(see Table 16.7) [71]. IgG tTGA may be used for detecting CD in patients with IgA deficiency, a condition ten times more common in CD than in the general population [76]. IgA anti-gliadin (AGA) is an obsolete test for identifying CD, due to its associated low sensitivity and specificity; the search for these antibodies is relevant for non-celiac gluten sensitivity (NCGS) [77,78] but not for CD. The exception to this is in very young children (under two years of age) when EMA, anti-tTG, and IgA-class AGA may fluctuate, whereas IgG-class AGA usually remains positive [79].

A new antibody test has been introduced into the serological workup of CD [80]. This test consists of antibodies binding to deamidated gliadin peptides (DGP-AGA). Both IgG and IgA DGP-AGA show a lower sensitivity for CD with total villous atrophy than IgA tTGA, and IgG DGP-AGA

TABLE 16.6
Estimated Celiac Risk from Associated HLA-DQB Genotypes

Genotype	Risk
DQ2+DQ8	1:7 (14.3%)
DQ2+DQ2 or DQ2 Homozygous DQB1*02	1:10 (10%)
DQ8+DQ8	1:12 (8.42%)
DQ8+DQB1*02	1:24 (4.2%)
Homozygous DQB1*02	1:26 (3.8%)
DQ2 alone	1:35 (2.9%)
DQ8 alone	1:89 (1.1%)
General population risk (genotype unknown)	1:100 (1%) [1/3]
½ DQ2:DQB1*02	1:210 (0.5%)
½ DQ2:DQA1*05	1:1842 (0.05%)
No HLA-DQA/DQB susceptibility alleles	1:2518 (< 0.04%)

Note: Actual risk for celiac disease may be greater than shown here when there are symptoms of celiac disease, positive results for celiac antibody tests or small bowel biopsy, or if there is a family history of celiac disease.

Source: Adapted from [74].

displays a very high specificity for CD (higher than tTGA and similar to EmA); moreover, these antibodies have a higher sensitivity with lesser degrees of villous atrophy [81] and allow for the identification of all CD cases in IgA-deficient patients with a very high sensitivity in young children less than two years of age [82].

Negative serology should not reassure the clinician of negative immune activity nor pathology [83]. Several reports show that in the majority of CD patients, antibodies to gliadin, endomysium, and transglutaminase may be negative [84–88]. In particular, seronegative CD seems to be frequent in patients with milder intestinal damage (Marsh I-IIIa lesions) [89]. Some reports identify the sensitivity with lesser degrees of villous atrophy as low as 27–31% [90]. Patients with nonvillous atrophy GS (Marsh I, Marsh II) are more likely than others to test negative for tissue transglutaminase and endomysial antibodies [91].

TABLE 16.7
Performance of Serological Markers for Celiac Disease Diagnosis (Cohorts Identified with Marsh III Villous Atrophy)

	Sensitivity (%)	Specificity (%)	PPV (%)	NPV (%)	Diagnostic accuracy (%)
IgA tTGA	97	91	91	97	98
IgA EmA	94	100	100	94	97
IgA AGA	73	87	84	77	80
IgA AGA	73	77	75	75	75
IgA DGP-AGA	84	90	89	85	87
IgG DGP-AGA	84	99	98	87	92

Abbreviations: AGA, antigliadin antibodies; DGP-AGA, antibodies to deamidated gliadin peptides; EmA, antiendomysial antibodies; tTGA, antibodies to tissue transglutaminase.
Source: Modified from [26].

Within the endoscopy unit, a prebiopsy algorithm accomplished a rare milestone. The algorithm is simple—a positive serological test for IgA antibody to tTGA combined with being at high risk (defined as having weight loss, diarrhea, or anemia) achieved 100% sensitivity in CD detection. The rule identified every patient with the disease in a cohort of 2000 patients, all of whom underwent intestinal biopsy as the gold standard and the final diagnostic step [92,93]. Thus, in the subset of patients presenting with weight loss, diarrhea, or anemia, this algorithm is of value.

Multiple peptides of the incompletely digested proteins of wheat have the potential to be antigenic and stimulate an immune response in an individual. The protease-resistant 33-mer peptide (α-gliadin) is the immunodominant antigen identified in half of CD patients [94]. Only approximately half of CD patients demonstrate elevated antigliadin antibodies [95]. Antigenic peptides of wheat consist of alpha-gliadin, omega-gliadin, glutenin, gluteomorphin, prodynorphin, and agglutinins, any of which has a capacity to challenge the immune system [96]. Because of this heterogeneity of gluten proteins and peptides, multiple variations in T-cell responses may occur against them.

Exorphins are peptides that may have activity similar to that of morphine and other opioids [97]. Exorphins in wheat and dairy include gluteomorphins, prodynorphins, and casomorphins. In order for exorphins to function as opioid peptides in the central nervous system in vivo, they must: (a) be produced in the gastrointestinal tract, (b) survive degradation by intestinal proteases, (c) be absorbed—without degradation—into the bloodstream, (d) cross the blood-brain barrier and thereby reach central opiate receptors, and (e) interact as opiates with these receptors [98]. Five distinct exorphins of gluten and eight distinct exorphins in dairy have been identified and referred to as food hormones [99,100]. After passing through an abnormally permeable intestinal membrane, these food-derived exorphins reach both binding sites in the intestinal submucosa and endogenous tissue interacting with a wide variety of proteins [101]. If they penetrate through the blood–brain barrier and enter the central nervous system, they may exert an effect on neurotransmission, as well as producing other physiologically based symptoms [102]. The inhibitory action of the exorphins in wheat have a specific opiate effect [103,104]. The morphine-like psychoactive nature of the peptides results from the incomplete digestion of these dietary ligand–proteins binding to the opiate receptors in the brain and offers a possible explanation for some of the reported psychiatric reactions to these gluten proteins, including the opioid theory of autism, schizophrenia, and the sense of "brain fog" that often accompanies immune reactions to these foods [105].

A review of the history of research examining the effectiveness of gluten- and casein-free diets to ameliorate the symptoms of autism demonstrates an overall beneficial effect in a subgroup of children [106]. Although to date there have been no double-blind, cross-over trials of the use of this type of intervention in autism, there have been several open trials of various combinations of the diets. All studies that have excluded gluten and/or casein from the diet have demonstrated significant improvements in the behavior of subgroups of people with autism and related spectrum disorders. The types of behavioral changes reported include improvements in language, emotional responses, and cognitive functioning with subsequent regression in skills when the diet is challenged. Although no formal explanation has been provided for these phenomena, several studies have found an association between gluten withdrawal and affective disorders in CD, notably depression and anxiety [107].

A large number of gluten epitopes may be implicated in the development of gluten sensitivity and CD. Although the majority of immune reactions to gluten peptides are due to binding to HLA-DQ2 (90%) and/or HLA-DQ8 (10%), some gluten peptides have a different antigenic specificity from that of CD and are independent of the action of tTG enzyme and HLA-DQ2/DQ8; therefore, they are directly presented by antigen presenting cells to T cells [108].

The repertoire and hierarchy of gluten peptides stimulate the intestinal T cells and result in a significant elevation of IgG and IgA production. Up to 86% of CD patients recognize a different array of gluten peptides [109]. And yet, until recently, the only commercially available peptide for testing has been alpha-gliadin 33 MER. With the advent of testing for a panel of gluten peptides, which includes a number of the more common immunodominant antigens, new tools have appeared to screen, prevent disease development in individuals at risk [110], and increase the sensitivity of the test to identify GS with or without CD. Early detection of immune activation, IgA and IgG against multiple gluten epitopes, is anticipated to facilitate clinical diagnosis [95].

RECOGNIZING GLUTEN-RELATED DISORDERS

Russell Jaffe, M.D., Ph.D., presents an emerging, integrative view based on his experience in regenerative medicine. While more studies are needed, this comprehensive approach shows promise in distinguishing those who need to avoid gluten absolutely from those who need to avoid mostly and from those who lose and then restore digestive competence with regard to glutens.

Overlapping Pathophysiologies with Distinct Treatments

With "true" celiac disease careful avoidance of gluten may allow the inflammatory, repair-deficit process to be corrected as part of a digestive healing and rehabilitation program. Rehabilitation goes beyond implementation of a gluten-free diet (GFD). Dietary and nutritional insufficiencies need be addressed. Even with restoration of healthy digestion, current best practice guidelines suggest lifelong substitution for the provocative substances.

By contrast, for people with non-celiac gluten sensitivity, incompletely digested molecular remnants irritate the delicate lining of the digestive track. Restoring digestive competence may require identification of all sources of digestive irritants. Digestive intolerances are mostly acquired maldigestions that resolve when digestive health is fully restored. Theoretically, reintroduction of a modest amount of wheat or gluten products in non-celiac gluten sensitivity may sometimes be tolerated after avoidance has led to both repair of the small intestine, improvement in digestion, and is reflected in restoration of immune tolerance.

The high amplification within the immune system to true gluten hypersensitivities requires vigilant, meticulous avoidance to quench immune reactions. This means that foods labeled "gluten free" and that are permitted to include 20 ppm gluten may still be provocative for such people whose immune systems are hypervigilant around gluten exposures. For type I, IgE immediate reactions, immunotherapy's goal is to raise IgG4 levels to balance the IgE and reduce histaminic cascades. For type II–V delayed reactions, identification of other reactive foods and chemicals is important for sustained remission and restoration of immune defenses.

While wheat components such as gluten and gliadin are linked to many chronic illnesses, a primary focus on gluten is often clinically incomplete. The importance of complete rather than relative gluten avoidance depends on which of the different mechanisms is responsible. Symptoms can be difficult to differentiate among these conditions in part because the symptoms themselves are varied, overlapping, and broad. Additionally, some immune responses may be specific for wheat, rye, rice, or oats, or cross reactive to all glutens.

On Antibody Testing

Antibodies and T cells are how the immune system "remembers" and is able to respond to foreign invaders. A useful analogy is to antibodies that occur from childhood infectious illnesses. These are almost always protective and helpful rather than harmful; as long as healthy immune systems produce those IgG antibodies, the body is protected.

The presence or absence of an antibody that may be helpful or harmful is a piece of information to be interpreted in light of clinical experience and the individual case. In the less than typical cases where discrimination among possibilities is most difficult is exactly where conventional serology or standard ELISA assays become less helpful. Quantitative antibody tests, such as IgG ELISA or EIA IgG, do not assess function and therefore do not distinguish between helpful and harmful antibodies. Querying the laboratory as to methods of determination in established reference ranges may bring a level of confidence to the clinician as to interpretation.

Another limitation to interpreting antibody tests for celiac disease is establishing normal values. Lab ranges generally represent two standard deviations around the mean of the population tested. Most lab tests do not have ranges for healthy and asymptomatic people. This leaves room for much interpretation through the lens of clinical experience and the individual patient. Querying the laboratory as to methods of determination in established reference ranges may bring a level of confidence to interpretation.

Diagnostic Approaches

A brief review of each of the three conditions follows, including comments about the reliability of available tests and evidence-based integrative clinical management once the diagnosis has been confirmed.

Celiac Disease

Celiac disease is an autoimmune attack particularly on the first portion of the small intestine, the duodenum. Screening tests include tTG IgA and the more recently introduced DGP-AGA IgG antibody quantification tests. These tests were initially reported to have high sensitivity, specificity, and predictive index based on small numbers of people tested. Reports using larger groups report appreciable decline in sensitivity and specificity as well as predictive significance [6]. Both tests have predictive significance between 72–84% depending on how the lab sets their reference range. Predictive significance in the 72–84% range qualifies tTG and DGP-AGA as screening assessments and not as diagnostic tests where higher predictive significance is needed. Sensitivity has been identified to be correlated with the degree of villous atrophy. Milder degrees of villous atrophy correlate with sensitivity from 27–84%. Higher degrees of villous atrophy correlate with 92–100%.

To confirm the diagnosis of celiac disease, a small bowel biopsy is required, preferably with ultra structure analysis, according to most celiac specialists [111].

In carefully biopsied, proven celiac disease cases, 80+% react to gluten or gliadin while 10–20% of cases are atypical and due to delayed reactions to other foods or chemicals.

Once the cause of a particular case of celiac disease has been confirmed, current best practice guidelines suggest lifelong substitution for the provocative substances.

"A variety of hematologic and biochemical abnormalities may be found in individuals with untreated celiac disease including iron deficiency, folic acid deficiency, and vitamin D deficiency. These abnormalities reflect nutritional deficiency states secondary to enteropathy-induced malabsorption. Although relevant to patient evaluation and management, none is sufficiently sensitive or specific to serve as useful screening or diagnostic tools. An oral xylose and/or lactulose absorption test, fecal fat evaluation, small bowel radiographic study, or capsule endoscopy may also be abnormal in untreated celiac disease, but will not provide a specific diagnosis" [112]. Transport-enhanced tabsules and sublingual forms of nutrients are recommended because of the higher risk of intestinal uptake block in this population from enteropathic repair deficit inflammation.

Non-celiac Gluten Sensitivity

Non-celiac gluten sensitivity may be due to acquired maldigestion, particularly of hard-to-digest proteins like gluten with focal repair deficit inflammation found along the GI tract and without evidence of immune reactivity. Fifty percent of non-celiac gluten sensitive patients have elevated antibodies to gluten [113]; tTG and DGP-AGA tests are sometimes positive.

Reactivity of these antibody tests across different clinical categories is part of what makes these tests less predictive and thus less discriminating in light of the different management.

Non-celiac gluten sensitivity is often accompanied by dysbiosis. Clinical best outcomes include repletion of balanced microflora, 40+ grams per day of prebiotic dietary fiber, and attention to stimulating intestinal repair through supplemental use of recycled glutamine that avoids glutamate buildup, calibrated vitamin C (100% l-ascorbate fully buffered and reduced), polyphenolics such as quercetin dehydrate and LMW orthoproanthocyanidins (OPCs), enhanced-uptake magnesium, and sublingual vitamin D. Starting each meal with something warm such as a broth or fresh vegetable juice helps improve digestion. In addition, abdominal breathing, rhythmic stretching, and relaxation response-enhancing activities are associated with improved digestive transit and competence.

Sustained restoration of digestive competence and transit is associated with ability to restore digestive competence and subsequently to safely include grains.

Gluten hypersensitivity may be either immediate or delayed. Immediate reactions are known as type I, histaminic, and mediated by a high IgE to IgG4 ratio. The goal of successful immunotherapy for immediate reactions is to raise IgG4 levels to balance the elevated IgE and thus quench symptomatic histamine amplified degranulation reactions of dendritic cells such as mast cells, basophils, and eosinophils. Immediate reactions are measurable either by radioallergosorbent serum tests (RAST) or standardized skin-prick tests.

Delayed reactions are known [7] as type II (reactive antibody), type III (immune complex), and type IV (T-cell mediated), and are mediated by reactive antibodies (IgM, IgA, sIgA, or IgG), immune complexes (IgM anti-IgG-antigen), and T-cell activation in the absence of circulating antibody.

Other food or chemical hypersensitivities can provoke symptoms and are important to identify in order to achieve sustained remissions and clinical improvement. Immune function tests (such as lymphocyte response assay), are available for determination of which foods or chemicals create immune system burdens and to which items the individual is tolerant. This allows development of personalized plans for what to eat, what to substitute, and how to do so, as well as which physical and mental activities and which targeted supplements are most likely to restore that individual to good health.

Clinically, all gluten-related disorders are complex and chronic—often with diffuse presentations. Each of the conditions needs different therapeutic emphases to achieve better outcomes. For now, distinguishing various types of digestive issues related to gluten takes considerable clinical skill, with more informative tests on the horizon.

DIAGNOSING NON-CELIAC GLUTEN SENSITIVITY

A number of morphological, functional, and immunological disorders that are lacking one or more of the key CD criteria (enteropathy, associated HLA haplotypes, presence of anti-TG2 antibodies) but respond to gluten exclusion are included under the umbrella of gluten sensitivity [114]. Non-celiac gluten sensitivity (GS) is indeed associated with multisystemic symptoms and disease [12,88,113,115,116].

Reports of GS without CD date to 1978, with the report of a woman who had normal small bowel biopsies and whose chronic diarrhea improved within days of beginning a GFD [76]. It is now accepted that GS is a systemic illness that can manifest in a range of organ systems. Such manifestations can occur independently of the presence of the classic small-bowel lesion [105] or positive celiac serology that defines CD. GS is now recognized as a systemic autoimmune condition with diverse manifestations and reports of at least sixfold more frequency than CD [117–119]. That GS is regarded as principally a disease of the small bowel is a historical misconception [105].

To date, identifying GS has been a challenge. Gluten sensitivity is a common disease that can manifest in diverse ways. As screening for gluten sensitivity has become a reality in clinical practice, and as more details of the individual genetic background that leads to aberrant immune responses are being revealed [120], emphasis is likely to shift toward the early identification of patients who are specifically at risk of severe, and sometimes permanent, complications (e.g., T-cell lymphoma, liver failure, neurological deficits). New diagnostic tools are becoming available (e.g., detection of antibodies against multiple peptides of gluten, antibodies against multiple isoenzymes of tissue transglutaminase, such as TG3, TG6) [121], which will enable identification of, for example, patients with neurological manifestations without enteropathy.

There is confusion about the role of antigliadin antibodies as a screening tool. With the recognition of deamidated gliadin antibodies as a more sensitive and specific marker of CD than gliadin antibodies, the role of antigliadin antibodies in identifying CD is no longer supported. However, given that GS can exist without an identifiable enteropathy, it is inappropriate to ignore antigliadin antibodies due to their lack of sensitivity and specificity against the presence of enteropathy [122]. Although the mechanisms of gluten sensitivity's extraintestinal manifestations are yet to be clearly identified, the associations between an immune reaction to multiple peptides of gluten and various neurological/cognitive presentations is undeniable. To assert that antigliadin antibodies lack specificity based on the fact that 10% of the healthy population may have them is a misconception. It is entirely plausible that 10% of the healthy population with circulating antigliadin antibodies have gluten sensitivity without recognized enteropathy [123]. For example, in a tertiary neurology center, when the cause of a neurological disease was known, the percentage of those patients with elevated antibodies to gliadin was 5%. When the cause of a neurological disease was unknown, the percentage of those patients with elevated antibodies to gliadin was 57% [124]. Only a third of patients presenting with neurological dysfunction due to gluten sensitivity will have evidence of an enteropathy on duodenal biopsy [117]. When comparing serology of multiple sclerosis patients against controls, a fourfold (IgA) to sixfold (IgG) increase in antigliadin antibodies was noted [125]. Antigliadin antibodies are especially noxious as shown for cerebellar atrophy and ataxia [126], CD, and gluten/gliadin related epilepsy [127,128], and these antibodies have a high affinity for the blood–brain barrier vasculature [129]. Recognition of this immune response to gliadin may be of therapeutic value to the patient.

Morbidity and mortality are increased with celiac disease and gluten sensitivity. In one of the largest (10,000 CD patients) and longest (29-year) observational studies of standard mortality ratios (SMR) with CD, mortality risks were elevated for a wide array of diseases including non-Hodgkin's lymphoma (SMR, 11.4), cancer of the small intestine (SMR, 17.3), autoimmune diseases (including rheumatoid arthritis (SMR, 7.3) and diffuse diseases of connective tissue (SMR 17.0), allergic disorders (such as asthma, SMR, 2.8), inflammatory bowel diseases (including Crohn's disease and ulcerative colitis (SMR, 70.9), diabetes mellitus (SMR, 3.0), disorders of immune deficiency (SMR, 20.9), tuberculosis (SMR, 5.9), pneumonia (SMR, 2.9), and nephritis (SMR, 5.4) [130]. Higher risks were observed for a wide array of conditions characterized by disturbances of immune function.

And in the largest study to date (351,403 biopsy reports in 287,586 unique individuals), mortality was compared between CD (biopsy-diagnosed Marsh III villous atrophy), latent CD (positive serology, negative histology), and inflammation (increased intraepithelial lymphocytes (Marsh stage I or II). An increased hazard ratio (HR) for death was observed in celiac disease (HR, 1.39; 95% confidence interval [CI], 1.33–1.45; median follow-up, 8.8 years), latent celiac disease (HR, 1.35; 95% CI, 1.14–1.58; median follow-up, 6.7 years), and inflammation (HR, 1.72; 95%; CI, 1.64–1.79; median follow-up, 7.2 years) [131]. The similarity of HR mortality between CD and latent CD suggests an equal recognition and call for treatment to either stage of the disease. And the twofold increased mortality in patients with inflammation without villous atrophy emphasizes the necessity for clinical aggressiveness with every stage of the disease.

It has been hypothesized that the immune-mediated disease mechanisms that may predispose to autoimmune diseases in patients with celiac disease may result from gluten-stimulated production of certain antibodies, such as tTG and fibroblast-derived extracellular matrix protein (actin, myosin) [132]. Increased mortality in patients with celiac disease may also be related to reduced absorption of important nutrients, including vitamin A (linked with cancer of the upper gastrointestinal tract) and vitamin E (linked with neurologic disorders) [133,134]. These complications may be worse among patients with a delayed diagnosis or those not following a strict gluten-free diet.

GS is a state of heightened immunological responsiveness to ingested gluten in genetically susceptible people. It represents a spectrum of diverse manifestations, of which the gluten sensitive enteropathy CD is one of many [1].

DIETARY TREATMENT

At this time, there are no pharmacological therapies for gluten-reactive conditions. Avoiding gluten is a necessary component of the treatment plan for anyone with a gluten-reactive condition. The NIH consensus statement on CD underscored with an acronym the six patient elements essential to treating CD once it is diagnosed:

C Consultation with a skilled dietician (nutritionist)
E Education about the disease
L Lifelong adherence to a gluten-free diet
I Identification and treatment of nutritional deficiencies
A Access to an advocacy group
C Continuous long-term follow-up [71]

REASONS TO EMPHASIZE WHOLE FOODS OVER GLUTEN-FREE REPLACEMENT PRODUCTS

A common approach to the GFD is to introduce commercially prepared gluten free (GF)-replacement products. Patients commonly replace gluten-containing excess carbohydrate, high-glycemic index foods, with gluten-free versions of the same breads, cookies, and salted, fried snacks. There are several limitations to such an approach and, instead, a healthful GFD is encouraged.

1. GF is an opportunity. Changing to a GFD creates the opportunity for patients to revisit their association with foods. Implementing a GF lifestyle can be an opportunity for the patient to embrace the association of food choices and a healthy functioning body. Focusing on colorful fresh fruits and vegetables, herbs and spices, lean protein sources, plentiful healthy fats and limited sugars, salt and processed foods, lifestyle habits can transition from one of disease to health [135].

   There are many gluten-free grains with nutritional profiles better than wheat. Listed alphabetically, they include: amaranth, arrowroot, buckwheat, corn, hemp, Indian rice grass, legumes (also called dry beans), mesquite, millet, nut flours, potato and sweet potato, quinoa, rice (brown or wild), sorghum, soy, tapioca, and teff. Alternating gluten-free whole grains increases protein, calcium, iron, and fiber [136].

2. Replacement products may have a lower nutrient density than their non-GF equivalents. Commercially prepared GF products are predominantly not fortified or enriched, whereas their gluten containing counterparts may have been, thus possibly creating a nutrient intake loss with the implementation of the GFD. GF products often contain higher amounts of salt, sugar, and additives to increase palatability; thus, these foods pose the risk of further nutrient insufficiency.

3. Patients gain weight on a GFD emphasizing replacement products. Processed gluten-free foods often are much higher in calories, high glycemic-index refined carbohydrates, sugar, and salt; they lack substantial fiber sources and may be higher in trans and other processed fats. Longitudinal studies have shown that one year after implementation of the GFD,

percentage of body fat was higher in celiac disease patients than in control subjects and lipid intakes tended to be higher than before treatment. Untreated patients preferentially utilized carbohydrates as a fuel substrate, probably as a consequence of both lipid malabsorption and a high carbohydrate intake, and lipid utilization increased with the restoration of the intestinal mucosa [137].

4. Some gluten-free replacement products are not required to be 100% gluten-free. Labeling differs among regulatory agencies, which can lead to confusion costly to a patient's health.

SPECIFICS ON GLUTEN-FREE LABELING

Threshold studies on gluten intake are based on celiac disease, not gluten sensitivity. One study, reviewed by the World Health Organization (WHO), was instrumental in establishing a safety threshold for gluten-free foods, indicating that up to 100 mg gluten/1 kg may be safe; however, histological changes have been shown with 50 mg gluten intake [138]. Thus, the WHO established an upper limit threshold for foods labeled gluten-free at 20 ppm gluten and low-gluten foods at less than 100 ppm gluten. The world, with a couple of exceptions, has accepted an upper limit of 20 ppm gluten in foods labeled gluten free. This low level of gluten is difficult to see and even more difficult for consumers to understand. Gluten is difficult to avoid completely. An important message for consumers is that it is so small you cannot see it. It is less than crumbs (1/90th of a slice of bread). So being diligent about avoiding cross contamination is critical. Even minute traces of immunogenic peptides of gluten are capable of triggering a state of heightened immunological activity in gluten sensitive people [9].

There are some important differences between the various regulatory agencies related to labeling. All regulating agencies are being encouraged to adopt common regulations related to allergens and gluten, but this is not in place at this time. The category of goods—such as food, cosmetics, or alcohol—will determine if federal guidelines ensure accurate labeling.

The Food and Drug Administration (FDA) enacted the Food Allergy Labeling and Consumer Protection Act (FALCPA) in 2006, which requires that the top eight allergens (wheat, soy, eggs, milk, peanuts, tree nuts, fish, and shellfish) be clearly marked in common language on food and nutritional supplements. The FDA will also define gluten free for labeling purposes and have promised final rulings in late 2012. FALCPA does not apply to pharmaceutical products where potential sources of gluten contamination come primarily from the addition of the excipient (filler) ingredients to the active drug in order to make a particular dosage [139]. A recommendation for patients to check with their pharmacist when filling prescriptions is warranted.

The U.S. Department of Agriculture (USDA), which regulates meats, eggs, and poultry, does not currently enforce allergen labeling. USDA products may have potential gluten sources and only be listed as dextrin or starch (i.e., a turkey may be injected with hydrating juices containing gluten—thus in reality, a hidden, potentially toxic source of gluten). This is not true of FDA-regulated products, where dextrin and starch are required to be labeled as containing wheat if they do so. Allergen labeling on products with a USDA seal may voluntarily comply with the FDA allergen regulations.

Alcohol is marked with an ingredient list. The Bureau of Alcohol, Tobacco, Firearms and Explosives (ATF), which regulates alcoholic products, does not allow gluten-free claims on labels. The exception is beer labeled gluten free, which is regulated by the FDA. The issue with alcohol is whether it has been fermented or distilled. Fermented beverages, such as beer, some hard ciders, and ales, are not processed to remove protein from them. Distillation does not allow protein into the finished product, no matter what the starting materials are, leaving hard spirits safe in the GF diet.

In sum, with FDA-regulated products, wheat will always be labeled on a product. This eliminates the need to be concerned about such things as modified food starch, vinegar, and flavorings containing gluten. This is not true of pharmaceuticals, and USDA- and ATF-regulated products. At this time, there is no universal definition for gluten-free labeling in the United States, and the FDA-proposed ruling is applicable to foods and nutritional products regulated by the FDA itself.

CROSS CONTAMINATION

Review tips to avoid cross contamination when dining. Soap, water, and good cleaning will remove gluten from equipment and surfaces. Sanitation with chemicals will simply sanitize gluten on surfaces not necessarily remove it. Creating contact barriers with a piece of parchment paper, napkin, or plate can avoid contamination from surfaces. Avoid double dipping in condiments. Wash hands. Handle GF foods first. These are all simple yet effective ways to avoid cross contamination.

PERSPECTIVE/COUNSELING

Patients often react with grief and many have a hard time understanding or accepting that something so fundamental to their diet could be injuring them [140]. The GFD diet can be overwhelming and difficult initially. Resources are available [141–146]. CD is treatable: a positive attitude from health care providers along with sound dietary information are the tools necessary for the patient to take control. Close follow-up to assess for correction of nutrient deficiencies are generally scheduled within one to three months [147].

OPTIMIZING FOOD AND NUTRIENTS

Through any clinical lens, recovery from celiac disease takes time, but watchful waiting on a gluten-free diet is not the most comprehensive treatment. Furthermore, a gluten-free diet alone may not be adequate in resolving villous blunting, inflammation, and increased intestinal permeability, which may take many months to years to resolve. Other conditions also factor into celiac disease in higher proportion than the general population. For example, children diagnosed with celiac disease have a threefold increase in long-term (> 5 years) mortality from causes such as accidents, suicide, violence, cancer, and cerebrovascular disease. Underlying and associated medical conditions should be identified [148]. (See Tables 16.2 and 16.3.)

NUTRITIONAL DEFICIENCIES PERSIST ON GLUTEN-FREE DIET

Inflammation and damage to the small intestine can lead to a number of nutritional issues in gluten-related conditions. The Academy of Nutrition and Dietetics Practice Guidelines for Celiac Disease indicates that many vitamins, minerals, and macronutrients may be deficient in the gluten-free diet [149]. These nutrient deficiencies may be due to dietary choices, malabsorption, or inadequate digestion. The Academy Evidence Analysis Library for Celiac Disease recommends that the patient's dietary intake be carefully analyzed for calcium, iron, vitamin B complex, and vitamin D and encourages the following biochemical data be reviewed: anemia (folate, ferritin, and vitamin B12), vitamin profile (thiamin, vitamin B6, and 25-hydroxy vitamin D), and a mineral profile (copper and zinc).

Because the proximal small intestine is the predominant site of inflammation and also the site of iron absorption, malabsorption of iron is markedly impaired and the association of celiac disease to refractory iron deficiency anemia is well established [150]. Nutrients such as fat-soluble vitamins; fat-soluble phytonutrients such as lycopene, lutein, resveratrol, and zeaxanthin; B-complex vitamins; and minerals should be closely evaluated. Nutritional deficiencies may or may not be corrected by strict compliance with a gluten-free lifestyle [151]. Fifty percent of the adult celiac patients carefully treated with a GFD for 8–12 years showed signs of poor vitamin status [152]. The Academy of Nutrition and Dietetics recommends periodic review of these nutrients and appropriate supplementation, if needed. There are not generally accepted practice guidelines for dosage of nutrients in persons with celiac disease and gluten sensitivity beyond dietary reference intakes (DRI). Monitoring patient progress with periodic laboratory testing insures safety (Table 16.8).

TABLE 16.8

Laboratory Tests for Celiac-Associated Genetics, Food-Related Disorders, and Nutrient Insufficiencies/Deficiencies

Assessment/Diagnosis	Specimen	Laboratory Resources	Comment/Notes
Genetics HLADQ2 (DQA1*0501) (DQA1*0505) (DQB1*0201) (DQB1*0202) HLADQ8	Buccal swab or Lavender top tube Lavender top tube	Kimball Genetics www.kimballgenetics.com Lab Corp www.labcorp.com Prometheus Labs www.prometheuslabs.com	Buccal swab (Kimball) convenient for patient
Transglutaminase Endomysium Deamidated gliadin	Serum	Lab Corp www.labcorp.com Kimball www.kimballgenetics.com Most Hospital Labs	
Multiple peptides of gluten	Serum	Genova Labs www.gdx.net Cyrex Labs www.cyrexlabs.com	
Native gliadin	Serum	Lab Corp www.labcorp.com Genova Labs www.gdx.net Cyrex Labs www.cyrexlabs.com Metametrix www.metametrix.com	
Lymphocyte response assays (LRAs)	Whole blood	ELISA/ACT Biotechnologies Lab; www.elisaact.com	
Vitamin D (25- Hydroxy Vit D) 25 (OH) D	Serum	Lab Corp www.labcorp.com Most specialty labs	Ref. Range 32-100 NG/ML Optimal 50-80 NG/ML
Comprehensive nutrient evaluations, including niacin, folate, vitamin B12, calcium, vitamin D, phosphorus, iron, zinc, and magnesium	Serum, urine	Genova Labs www.gdx.net	NutriEval provides a framework of core nutrients in five key areas: antioxidants, B vitamins, digestive support, essential fatty acids, and minerals
		Metametrix Laboratory www.metametrix.com	I.O.N. (Individual Optimal Nutrition) measures levels of organic acids, fatty acids, amino acids, vitamins, minerals, and antioxidants.
		Spectacell Laboratory www.spectracell.com	Comprehensive nutritional panel measures levels of vitamins, minerals, amino acids, antioxidants, carbohydrate metabolism, fatty acids, and metabolites

Some authors have suggested that, despite a GFD, treated CD patients continue to show mild malnutrition in terms of low body weight and reduced body mass index, which may be due to incomplete intestinal mucosal recovery, poor digestive efficiency, or to the gluten-free diet itself [153]. AND recommends a review of the nutritional status of gluten-free consumers on an ongoing basis.

A common finding in CD is decreased bone mineral content with adults [154], youth [155], and children untreated or newly diagnosed [156]. The gluten-free diet has a remineralization effectiveness of over 50% [157], usually within one to two years. However, monitoring of bone mineral density may demonstrate the need for additional therapy (calcium, vitamin D, or hormone replacement therapy) in some situations.

Treated Celiac Disease is a Risk Factor for Weight Gain

Some forms of malnutrition during infancy impose epigenetic effects observed to predispose the child to obesity as nutritional resources are improved. This observation may apply to celiac disease. Two reports have been published of adolescents with known CD who became obese despite being malnourished as babies. This obesity had developed despite the persistence of villous atrophy on jejunal biopsy. It is postulated that as the surface area of the small bowel increases with age, children develop the ability to ingest adequate compensatory energy [158,159].

Cross Reactivity with Other Foods is Common

The current consensus is that proteins with > 35% identity over 80 amino acids or with identity of six consecutive amino acids have the possibility of inducing cross reactivity [160]. Commonly associated cross reactivities and food sensitivities may include dairy, egg, soy, coffee, fructose, or other carbohydrates. These intolerances may be transient and resolve with time on the gluten-free diet or linger for years. These further restrictions compound the need to monitor closely long-term nutritional deficiencies.

Digestive Inefficiency

Thirty to 40% of CD patients suffer from dyspepsia [161]. CD should be included in the differential diagnosis of patients with non–*Helicobacter pylori* peptic disease (PD) [162].

Investigators have reported abnormal intraesophageal pH in 30% of subjects with celiac disease; thus, gastroesophageal acid reflux is suspected as the cause of symptoms [163]. In population studies, body mass index correlates closely with risk for gastroesophageal reflux disease (GERD) symptoms [164]. Conversely, in this study, the subjects with newly diagnosed celiac disease had low initial body mass index (median, 20.2 kg/cm2) despite the high frequency of GERD. Furthermore, GERD symptoms resolved upon treatment with the gluten-free diet, whereas the mean body mass index in the celiac group increased (median, 24.0 after 12 months of gluten avoidance). Although not conclusive, these observations suggest that the pathophysiology of GERD symptoms in untreated celiac disease may be different from those of GERD in the general population.

In a clinical long-term follow-up of nonerosive GERD in CD patients on a gluten-free diet and controls, GERD symptoms were resolved in 86.2% of CD patients and in 66.7% controls after eight weeks of proton pump inhibitors (PPI) treatment. In the CD group, recurrence of GERD symptoms was found in 20% at 6 months but in none at 12, 18, and 24 months, while in the control group recurrence was found in 30%, 60%, 75%, and 85% at 6, 12, 18, and 24 months, respectively, suggesting that GFD could be a useful approach in reducing GERD symptoms and in the prevention of recurrence [165].

HYPOCHLORHYDRIA

Four percent of CD patients are identified with antigastric parietal cell antibodies [166]. Inadequate stomach acid secretion predisposes to food allergies such as gluten sensitivity, presumably because peptides are not fully disassembled into amino acids in the stomach when acidity is low.

CD is associated with:

- A deficiency in the duodenal output of pancreatic enzymes [167],
- Increased fasting gallbladder volume,
- Reduced gallbladder emptying (50%) in response to meals [168].

This is likely due to impaired meal-induced release of gut hormones such as cholecystokinin secondary to villous atrophy and increased somatostatin levels. Insufficient digestive function (from inadequate secretion of hydrochloric acid or bile acids or pancreatic enzymes) may predispose to food allergies and sensitivities.

NUTRIENT SUPPORT

Nutritional supplements are medically indicated in celiac disease [147,169,170]. Not only is there a significant dietary restriction that can, in many settings, pose a barrier to achieving a healthful diet, but nutrients have been poorly absorbed for years and the body has had extra metabolic demands from the associated inflammatory response.

A multivitamin and mineral supplement containing no gluten is a starting point, not a solution. Refer to the chapter on inflammatory bowel disease for specific nutrient requirements that are similar to those in celiac disease. Table 16.8 lists nutritional evaluation and diagnostic testing that can inform decisions surrounding osteoporosis prevention, anemia treatment, cardiovascular health, and healthful weight maintenance.

CLINICAL SUMMARY

Gluten and related proteins found in grains contribute to a cluster of diseases, not limited to CD and not always substantiated by clinical symptoms. Diagnostic tools extend beyond the small bowel biopsies for villous atrophy characteristic of classic CD. They include patient-reported improvement in symptoms on a gluten-free-diet, comorbid conditions extending beyond the small bowel, testing for genetic haplotypes associated with CD, and an expanded number of serologic autoimmune markers.

An area of forthcoming research is the ability of gluten products to exert opioid-like effects in the central nervous system. Patients with autism, attention-deficit hyperactivity disorder, and cognitive decline may be particularly vulnerable to these exorphins, apart from CD or GS.

A GFD is more effectively achieved with a diet rich in fruits and vegetables including non-gluten containing whole grains. Among the reasons to minimize gluten-free prepackaged foods are: gluten-free labeling does not mean 100% gluten-free, these foods are not as likely to be fortified with nutrients as are their gluten-containing counterparts, and the opportunity to choose an overall more healthful diet may be lost.

For CD, a GFD is often insufficient to meet nutrient needs given the nutrient deficit following malabsorption and less-understood epigenetic effects. Screening for and correcting nutrient deficiencies may improve immune tolerance.

The increased prevalence of diseases is not attributable to increased case detection alone but rather to a more pervasive loss of immune tolerance in Western countries. There are many possible reasons for the changes in immune tolerance, some of which are discussed in the toxicology section of this book.

REFERENCES

1. Catassi, C., and Fasano, A. 2008. Celiac disease. *Curr Opin Gastroenterol* 24: 687–91.
2. Anderson, L.A., McMillan, S.A., Watson, R.G., et al. 2007. Malignancy and mortality in a population based cohort of patients with coeliac disease or "gluten sensitivity." *World J Gastroenterol* 13: 146–51.
3. Ferguson, A., Gillett, H., Humphreys, K., and Kingstone, K. 1998. Heterogeneity of celiac disease: Clinical, pathological, immunological, and genetic. *Intestinal Plasticity in Health and Disease* 859: 112–20.
4. Hadjivassiliou, M., Grunewald, R.A., and Davies-Jones, G.A.B. 2002. Gluten sensitivity as a neurological illness. *J Neurol Neurosurg Psychiatry* 72: 560–63.
5. Constantin, C., Huber, W.D., Granditsch, G., Weghofer, M., and Valenta, R. 2005. Different profiles of wheat antigens are recognised by patients suffering from coeliac disease and IgE-mediated food allergy. *Int Arch Allergy Immunol* 138: 257–66.
6. Vermeersch, P., Geboes, K., Mariën, G., Hoffman, I., Hiele, M., and Bossuyt, X. 2010. Diagnostic performance of IgG anti-deamidated gliadin peptide antibody assays is comparable to IgA anti-tTG in celiac disease. *Clin Chim Acta* Jul 4;411(13–14): 931–35.
7. According to the Gel and Coombs suggested nomenclature, 1967.
8. Marsh, M.N. 1995. The natural history of gluten sensitivity: Defining, refining and redefining. *Q J Med* 85: 9–13.
9. Tanabe, S. 2008. Analysis of food allergen structures and development of foods for allergic patients. *Biosci Biotechnol Biochem* 72: 649–59.
10. Sapone, A., Lammers, K.M., Mazzarella, G., et al. Differential mucosal IL-17 expression in two gliadin-induced disorders: Gluten sensitivity and the autoimmune enteropathy celiac disease. *Int Arch Allergy Immunol* 152 (1): 75–80.
11. Di Sabatino, A., and Corazza, G.R. 2009. Coeliac disease. *Lancet* 373: 1480–93.
12. Volta, U. 1999. Coeliac disease: Recent advances in pathogenesis, diagnosis and clinical signs. *Rec Prog Med* 1: 37–44.
13. Fasano, A. 2003. Celiac disease—how to handle a clinical chameleon. *N Engl J Med* 348: 2568–70.
14. Hadjivassiliou, M., Chattopadhyay, A., Davies-Jones, A., et al. 1997. Neuromuscular disorder as a presenting feature of coeliac disease. *Journal of Neurology, Neurosurgery, and Psychiatry* 63: 770–75.
15. Brannagan, T., III, Hays, A., Chin, S., et al. 2005. Small-fiber neuropathy/neuronopathy associated with celiac disease. *Arch Neurol* 62: 1574–78.
16. Tye-Din, J., Stewart, J., Dromey, J., et al. 2010. Comprehensive, quantitative mapping of T-cell epitopes in gluten in celiac disease. *Sci Transl Med* 2 (41): 41–51.
17. Biesiekierski, J., Newnham, E., Irving, P., et. al. 2011. Gluten causes gastrointestinal symptoms in subjects without celiac disease: A double-blind randomized placebo-controlled trial. *Am J Gastroenterol* 106 (3): 508–14.
18. Barton, S., and Murray, J. 2008. Celiac disease and autoimmunity in the gut and elsewhere. *Gastroenterol Clin N Am* 37: 411–28.
19. Hadjivassiliou, M., Aeschlimann, D., Grünewald, R.A., Sanders, D. S., Sharrack, B. and Woodroofe, N. 2011. GAD antibody-associated neurological illness and its relationship to gluten sensitivity. *Acta Neurol Scand* 123(3): 175–80.
20. Pittschieler, K., and Ladinser, B. 1996. Coeliac disease screened by a new strategy. *Acta Paediatr Suppl* 412: 42–45.
21. Corazza, G.R., Andreani, M.L., Biagi, F., et al. 1997. The smaller size of the "coeliac iceberg" in adults. *Scand J Gastroenterol* 32: 917–19.
22. Johnston, S.D., Watson, R.G., McMillan, S.A., Sloan, J., and Love, A.H. 1997. Prevalence of celiac disease in Northern Ireland. *Lancet* 350: 1370.
23. Kolho, K.L., Farkkila, M.A., and Savilahti, E. 1998. Undiagnosed coeliac disease is common in Finnish adults. *Scand J Gastroenterol* 33: 1280–83.
24. Ivarsson, A., Persson, L.A., Juto, P., Peltonen, M., Suhr, O., and Hernell, O. 1999. High prevalence of undiagnosed coeliac disease in adults: A Swedish population-based study. *J Intern Med* 245: 63–68.
25. Riestra, S., Fernandez, E., Rodrigo, L., Garcia, S., and Ocio, G. 2000. Prevalence of coeliac disease in the general population of Northern Spain. *Scand J Gastroenterol* 35: 398–402.
26. Volta, U., Bellentani, S., Bianchi, F.B., et al. 2001. High prevalence of celiac disease in Italian general population. *Dig Dis Sci* 46: 1500–1505.
27. Maki, M., Mustalahti, K., Kokkonen, J., et al. 2003. Prevalence of celiac disease among children in Finland. *N Engl J Med* 348: 2517–24.

28. Guandalini, S., and Newland, C. 2011. Differentiating food allergies from food intolerances. *Curr Gastroenterol Rep* 13 (5): 426–34.

29. Arnson, Y., Amital, H., and Shoenfeld, Y. 2005. Vitamin D and autoimmunity: New aetiological and therapeutic considerations. *J of Immunology* 175: 4119–26.

30. Green, P., Alaedini, A., Sander, H.W., Brannagan, T.H., III, Latov, N., and Chin, R. 2005. Mechanisms underlying Celiac disease and its neurologic manifestations. *Cell Mol Life Sci.* 62: 791–99.

31. Volta, U., and Villanacci, V. 2011. Celiac disease: Diagnostic criteria in progress. *Cellular & Molecular Immunology* 8: 96–102.

32. Cascella, N., and Kryszak, D. 2011. Prevalence of celiac disease and gluten sensitivity in the United States clinical antipsychotic trials of intervention effectiveness study population. *Schizophr Bull* 37 (1): 94–100.

33. Catassi, C., Kryszak, D., Bhatti, B., et al. 2010. Natural history of celiac disease autoimmunity in a USA cohort followed since 1974. *Ann Med* 42 (7): 530–38.

34. Vilppula, A., Collin, H., Maki, M., et al. 2008. Undetected coeliac disease in the elderly. A biopsy-proven population-based study. *Digestive and Liver Disease* 40: 809–13.

35. Vilppula, A., Kaukinen, K., Luostarinen, L., et al. 2009. Increasing prevalence and high incidence of celiac disease in elderly people: A population-based study. *BMC Gastroenterology* 9: 49.

36. Barton, S.H., and Murray, J.A. 2008. Celiac disease and autoimmunity in the gut and elsewhere. *Gastroenterol Clin North Am* 37:411–28.

37. Rubio-Tapia, A., Kyle, R., Kaplan, E., et al. 2009. Increased prevalence and mortality in undiagnosed celiac disease, *Gastroenterology* 137:88–93.

38. Almeida, P.L., Gandolfi, L., Modelli, I.C., Martins, R.D.C., Almeida, R.C., and Pratesi, R. 2008. Prevalence of celiac disease among first degree relatives of Brazilian celiac patients. *Arq Gastroenterol* 45 (1): 69–72.

39. Dube, C., Rostom, A., Sy, R., et al. 2005. The prevalence of celiac disease in average-risk and at-risk Western European populations: A systematic review. *Gastroenterology* 128 (4 Suppl 1): S57–67.

40. Vilppula, A., Kaukinen, K., Luostarinen, L., et.al. 2011. Clinical benefit of gluten-free diet in screen-detected older celiac disease patients. *BMC Gastroenterol* 11 (1): 136.

41. Rubio-Tapia, A., Van Dyke, C., Lahr, B., et al. 2008. Predictors of family risk for celiac disease: A population-based study. *Clin Gastroenterol Hepatol* 6 (9): 983–87.

42. Rubio-Tapia, A., and Murray, J., The liver in celiac disease, *Hepatology* 46: 1650–58.

43. Choi, J.M., Lebwohl, B., Wang, J., et al. 2011. Increased prevalence of celiac disease in patients with unexplained infertility in the U.S. *J Reprod Medicine* 56: 199–203.

44. Stenson, W., Newberry, R., Lorenz, R., et al. 2005. Increased prevalence of celiac disease and need for routine screening among patients with osteoporosis. *Arch Intern Med* 165: 393–99.

45. Alaedini, A., and Green, P. 2008. Autoantibodies in celiac disease. *Autoimmunity* 41(1): 19–26.

46. De Santis, A., Addolorato, G., Romito, A., et al. 1997. Schizophrenic symptoms and SPECT abnormalities in a coeliac patient: Regression after a gluten-free diet. *J Intern Med* 242: 421–23.

47. Bast, A., O'Bryan, T., and Bast, E. 2009. Celiac disease and reproductive disorders. *Practical Gastroenterology* XXXIII (10).

48. Hadjivassiliou, M., Gibson, A., Davies-Jones, G.A., et al. 1996. Does cryptic gluten sensitivity play a part in neurological illness? *Lancet* 347: 369–71.

49. Ellis, A., and Linaker, B.D. 1978. Non-coeliac gluten sensitivity? *Lancet* 1: 1358–59.

50. McGowan, K.E., Castiglione, D.A., and Butzner, J.D. 2009. The changing face of childhood celiac disease in North America: Impact of serological testing. *Pediatrics* 124: 1572–78.

51. Bingley, P.J., Williams, A.J., Norcross, A.J., et al. 2004. Undiagnosed coeliac disease at age seven: Population based prospective birth cohort study. *BMJ* 328: 322–23.

52. Mäki, M., Mustalahti, K., Kokkonen, J., et al. 2003. Screening for celiac disease. *N Engl J Med* 349: 1673–74.

53. Schuppan, D. 2000. Current concepts of celiac disease pathogenesis. *Gastroenterology* 119: 234–42.

54. Frustaci, C., Cuoco, L., Chimenti, C., et al. 2002. Celiac disease associated with autoimmune myocarditis. *Circulation* 105: 2611–18.

55. Hu, W.T., Murray, J.A., Greenaway, M.C., Parisi, J.E., and Josephs, K.A. 2006. Cognitive impairment and celiac disease. *Arch Neurol* 63: 1440–46.

56. Zone, J.J. 2005. Skin manifestations of celiac disease. *Gastroenterology* 128 (Suppl 1): S87–S89.

57. Ludvigsson, J.F., Montgomery, S.M., and Ekbom, A. 2005. Celiac disease and risk of adverse fetal outcome: A population-based cohort study. *Gastroenterology* 129: 454–63.

58. Ciacci, C., Cirillo, M., Auriemma, G., Di Dato, G., Sabbatini, F., and Mazzacca, G. 1996. Celiac disease and pregnancy outcome. *Am J Gastroenterol* 91(4): 718–22.

59. Salvatore, S., Finazzi, S., Radaelli, G., Lotzniker, M., and Zuccotti, GV. 2007. Prevalence of undiagnosed celiac disease in the parents of preterm and/or small for gestational age infants. *Am J Gastroenterol* 102: 168–73.

60. McCarthy, F., Khasan, A., Kenny, L., Quigley, E., and Shanahan, F. 2009. Don't forget increased risk of fetal growth restriction. *BMJ* 338: b1069.

61. Fasano, A. 2005. Clinical presentation of celiac disease in the pediatric population. *Gastroenterology* 128: S68–S73.

62. Hoffenberg, E.J., Emery, L.M., Barriga, K.J., and Bao, F. 2004. Clinical features of children with screening-identified evidence of celiac disease. *Pediatrics* 113: 1254–59.

63. Sanders, D.S., Hurlstone, D.P., Stokes, R.O., et al. 2002. Changing face of adult coeliac disease: Experience of a single university hospital in South Yorkshire. *Postgrad Med J* 78: 31–33.

64. McGowan, K.E., Castiglione, D.A., and Butzner, J.D. 2009. The changing face of childhood celiac disease in North America: Impact of serological testing. *Pediatrics* 124: 1572–78.

65. van Heel, D., and West, J. 2006. Recent advances in coeliac disease. *Gut* 55: 1037–46.

66. Fasano, A., and Catassi, C. 2001. Current approaches to diagnosis and treatment of celiac disease: An evolving spectrum. *Gastroenterology* 120: 636–51.

67. Mitka, M. 2004. Higher profile needed for celiac disease: Underdiagnosis fosters treatment delays, says panel. *JAMA* 292 (8): 913–14.

68. Green, P.H.R., Stavropolous, S.N., Panagi, S.G., et al. 2001. Characteristics of adult celiac disease in the USA: Results of a national survey. *Am J Gastro* 96: 126–31.

69. Graber, M.L., and Kumar, A. 2007. Commentary: Reaching a milestone in diagnosing coeliac disease. *BMJ* 334 (7596): 732.

70. Rubio-Tapia, A., and Murray, J. 2010. Celiac disease. *Current Opinion in Gastroenterology* 26: 116–22.

71. Tjellström, B., Stenhammar, L., Högberg, L., et al. 2010. Screening-detected and symptomatic untreated celiac children show similar gut microflora-associated characteristics. *Scandinavian Journal of Gastroenterology* 45: 1059–62.

72. Tjellström, B., Stenhammar, L., Högberg, L., et al. 2005. Gut microflora associated characteristics in children with celiac disease. *Am J Gastroenterol* 100: 2784–88.

73. Mitka, M. 2004. Higher profile needed for celiac disease: Underdiagnosis fosters treatment delays, says panel. *JAMA* 292 (8): 913–14.

74. Dieterich, W., Laag, E., Schopper, H., et al. 1998. Autoantibodies to tissue transglutaminase as predictors of celiac disease. *Gastroenterology* 115: 1317–21.

75. Downloaded from Labcorp.com 2-1-12. https://www.labcorp.com/wps/portal/!ut/p/c1/04_SB8K8xLLM9MSSzPy8xBz9CP0os_hACzO_QCM_IwMLXyM3AyNjMycDU2dXQwN3M6B8JG55AwMCuv088nNT9SP1o8zjQ11Ngg09LY0N_N2DjQw8g439TfyM_MzMLAz0Q_QjnYCKIvEqKsiNKDfUDVQEAOrk-dE!/dl2/d1/L0lJWXBwZyEhL3dIRUJGUUFoTWFBRUJyQ0svWUk1eWx3ISEvN19VRTRTMUk5MzBPR1MyMElTM080TjJONjY4MC92aWV3V3VGVzdA!!/?testId=407634#\7_UE4S1I930OGS20IS3O4N2N6680.

76. Cataldo, F., Marino, V., Ventura, A., Bottaro, G., and Corazza, G.R. 1998. Prevalence and clinical features of selective immunoglobulin A deficiency in coeliac disease: An Italian multicentre study. *Gut* 42: 362–65.

77. Wahnschaffe, U., Schulzke, J.D., Zeitz, M., and Ullrich, R. 2007. Predictors of clinical response to gluten-free diet in patients diagnosed with diarrhea-predominant irritable bowel syndrome. *Clin Gastroenterol Hepatol* 5 (7): 844–50.

78. Biesiekierski, J.R., Newnham, E.D., Irving, P.M., and Barrett, J.S. 2011. Gluten causes gastrointestinal symptoms in subjects without celiac disease: A double-blind randomized placebo-controlled trial. *Am J Gastroenterol* 106 (3): 508–14.

79. Bizzaro, N., Tozzoli, R., Villalta, D., et al. 2012. Cutting-edge issues in celiac disease and in gluten intolerance. *Clin Rev Allergy Immunol* 42(3):279–87.

80. Niveloni, S., Sugai, E., Cabanne, A., and Vazquez, H. 2007. Antibodies against synthetic deamidated gliadin peptides as predictors of celiac disease: Prospective assessment in an adult population with a high pretest probability of disease. *Clinical Chemistry* 53 (12): 2186–92.

81. Kurppa, K., Lindfors, K., Collin, P., et al. 2011. Antibodies against deamidated gliadin peptides in early-stage celiac disease. *J Clin Gastroenterol* 45: 673–78.

82. Lagerqvist, C., Dahlbom, I., Hansson, T., et al. 2008. Antigliadin immunoglobulin A best in finding celiac disease in children younger than 18 months of age. *J Pediatr Gastroenterol Nutr* 47: 428–35.

83. Sanders, D.S., Hurlstone, D.P., McAlindon, M.E., et al. 2005. Antibody negative Coeliac disease presenting in elderly people—an easily missed diagnosis. *BMJ* 330 (7494): 775–76.

84. Rostami, K., Kerckhaert, J., Tiemessen, R., von Blomberg, M.E., Meijer, J.W.R., and Mulder, C.J.J. 1999. Sensitivity of antiendomysium and antigliadin antibodies in untreated celiac disease: Disappointing in clinical practice. *Am J Gastroenterol* 94: 888–94.

85. Dickey, W., Hughes, D.F., and McMillan, S.A. 2000. Reliance on serum endomysial antibody testing underestimates the true prevalence of coeliac disease by one fifth. *Scand J Gastroenterol* 35: 181–83.

86. Tursi, A., Brandimarte, G., Giorgetti, G., Gigliobianco, A., Lombardi, D., and Gasbarrini, G. 2001. Low prevalence of antigliadin and anti-endomysium antibodies in subclinical/silent coeliac disease. *Am J Gastroenterol* 96: 1507–10.

87. Tursi, A., Brandimarte, G., and Giorgetti, G. 2003. Prevalence of anti-tissue transglutaminase antibodies in different degrees of intestinal damage in celiac disease. *J Clin Gastroenterol* 36: 219–21.

88. Abrams, J.A., Diamone, B., Rotterdam, H., and Green, P.H.R. 2004. Seronegative celiac disease: Increased prevalence with lesser degrees of villous atrophy. *Dig Dis Sci* 49: 546–50.

89. Tursi, A. 2005. Seronegative coeliac disease—a clinical challenge. *BMJ* 330:775.

90. Lebwohl, B., and Green, P. 2003. Screening for celiac disease. *N Engl J Med* 349: 1673–74.

91. Dickey, W. 2009. Symposium 1: Joint BAPEN and British Society of Gastroenterology symposium on coeliac disease: Basics and controversies. *Proceedings of the Nutrition Society* 68 (3): 234–41.

92. Dickey, W., and Hughes, D. 1999. Prevalence of celiac disease and its endoscopic markers among patients having routine upper gastrointestinal endoscopy. *Am J Gastroenterol* 94: 2182–86.

93. Hopper, A., Cross, S., Hurlstone, D., and McAlindon, M. 2007. Pre-endoscopy serological testing for coeliac disease: Evaluation of a clinical decision tool. *BMJ* 334 (7596): 729.

94. Tye-Din, J.A., Stewart, J.A., Dromey, J.A., et.al. 2010. Comprehensive, quantitative mapping of T-cell epitopes in gluten in celiac disease. *Sci Transl Med* 2(41): 41ra51.

95. Vader, W., Kooy, Y., Van Veelen, P., et al. 2002. The gluten response in children with celiac disease is directed toward multiple gliadin and glutenin peptides. *Gastroenterology* 122: 1729–37.

96. Vojdani, A., O'Bryan, T., and Kellerman, G. 2008. The immunology of immediate and delayed hypersensitivity reaction to gluten. *European Journal of Inflammation* 6(1).

97. Vader, W., Kooy, Y., Van Veelen, P., et. al. 2002. The gluten response in children with celiac disease is directed toward multiple gliadin and glutenin peptides. *Gastroenterology* 122 (7): 1729–37.

98. Zioudrou, C., Streaty, R., and Klee, W. 1979. Opioid peptides derived from food proteins. *Journal of Biological Chemistry* 254 (7) 2446–49.

99. Teschemacher, T. 2003. Opioid receptor ligands derived from food proteins. *Current Pharmaceutical Design* 9: 1331–44.

100. Fukudome, S., and Yoshikawa, M. 1992. Opioid derived from wheat gluten: Their isolation and characterization. *Febs* 296: 107–11.

101. Artemova, N., Bumagina, N., Kasakov, A., et al. 2010. Opioid peptides derived from food proteins suppress aggregation and promote reactivation of partly unfolded stressed proteins. *Peptides* 31: 332–38.

102. Shattock, P., and Whiteley, P. 2002. Biochemical aspects in autism spectrum disorders: Updating the opioid-excess theory and presenting new opportunities for biomedical intervention. *Expert Opin Ther Targets* 6(2).

103. Fukudome, S., Shimatsu, A., Suganuma, H., and Yoshikawa, M. 1995. Effect of gluten exorphins A5 and B5 on the postprandial plasma insulin level in conscious rats. *Life Sci* 57 (7): 729–34.

104. Mycroft, F.J., Wei, E.T., Bernardin, J.E., and Kasarda, D.D. 1982. MIF-like sequences in milk and wheat proteins. *N Engl J Med* 307 (14): 895.

105. Dohan, F.C. 1988. Genetic hypothesis of idiopathic schizophrenia: Its exorphin connection. *Schizophr Bull* 14 (4): 489–94.

106. Knivsberg, A., Reichelt, K.L., and Nodland, M. 2001. Reports on dietary intervention in autistic disorders. *Nut Neurosci* 4: 25–37.

107. Addolorato, G., Leggio, L., D'Angelo, C., et al. 2008. Affective and psychiatric disorders in celiac disease. *Dig Dis* 26: 140–48.

108. Samaroo, D., Dickerson, F., Kasarda, D.D., et.al. 2010. Novel immune response to gluten in individuals with schizophrenia. *Schizophr Res* 118(1–3): 248–55.

109. Camarca, A., Anderson, R.P., Mamone, G., et al. 2009. Intestinal T-cell responses to gluten peptides are largely heterogeneous: Implications for a peptide-based therapy in celiac disease. *J Immunol* 182 (7): 4158–66.

110. Vader, W., Kooy, Y., Van Veelen, P., et al. 2002. The gluten response in children with celiac disease is directed toward multiple gliadin and glutenin peptides. *Gastroenterology* 122 (7): 1729–37.

111. Presutti, R.J., Cangemi, J.R., Cassidy, H.D., and Hill, D.A. 2007. Celiac disease. *Am Fam Physician* 76(12):1795–1802 and UpToDate Diagnosis of Celiac Syndrome, 2011 update.

112. UpToDate Diagnosis of Celiac Disease, 2011 update.
113. Samaroo, D., et al., 2010. Novel immune response to gluten in individuals with schizophrenia, *Schizophr Res* May;118(1–3): 248–55.
114. Troncone, R., and Jabri, B. 2011. Coeliac disease and gluten sensitivity. *J Intern Med* 269 (6):582–90.
115. Hadjavassilios, M. 2010. GS: From gut to brain. *Lancet Neurol* 9: 318–30.
116. Verdu, E. 2011. Can gluten contribute to irritable bowel syndrome? *Am J Gastroenterol* 106: 516–18.
117. Ford, R.P. 2009. The gluten syndrome: A neurological disease. *Med Hypotheses* 73 (3): 438–40.
118. El-Chammas, K., and Danner, E. 2011. Gluten-free diet in nonceliac disease. *Nutrition in Clinical Practice* 26 (3): 294–99.
119. Cascella, N., and Kryszak, D. 2011. Prevalence of celiac disease and gluten sensitivity in the United States clinical antipsychotic trials of intervention effectiveness study population. *Schizophr Bull* 37 (1): 94–100.
120. Hadjavassilios, M., 2010. GS: From gut to brain. *Lancet Neurol* 9: 318–30.
121. Thomas, H., Beck, K., Adamczyk, M., et.al. 2011. Transglutaminase 6: A protein associated with central nervous system development and motor function. *Amino Acids*.
122. Hadjivassiliou, M., Grünewald, R.A., Sharrack, B., et al. 2003. Gluten ataxia in perspective: Epidemiology, genetic susceptibility and clinical characteristics. *Brain* 126: 685–91.
123. Hadjivassiliou, M., and Grünewald, R.A 2004. The neurology of gluten sensitivity: Science vs. conviction. *Practical Neurology* 4: 124–27.
124. Hadjivassiliou, M., Grünewald, R.A., and Davies-Jones, G.A. 2002. GS as a neurological illness. *J Neurol Neurosurg Psychiatry* 72 (5): 560–63.
125. Reichelt, K.L., and Jensen, D. 2004. IgA antibodies against gliadin and gluten in multiple sclerosis, *Acta Neurol Scand.* 110 (4): 239–41.
126. Hadjivassiliou, M., Boscolo, S., Davies-Jones, G.A.B., et al. 2002. The humoral response in the pathogenesis of gluten ataxia. *Neurology* 58: 1221–26.
127. Chapman, R.W.G., Laidlow, J.M., Colin-Jones, D., et al. 1978. Increased prevalence of epilepsy in celiac disease. *BMJ* 22: 250–51.
128. Gobbi, G., Bouquet, F., Gicco, L., et al. 1992. Coeliac disease, epilepsy, and cerebral calcifications. *Lancet* 340: 439–43.
129. Pratesi, R., Gandolfi, L., Friedman, H., et al. 1998. Serum IgA antibodies from patients with celiac disease react strongly with human brain blood-vessel structures. *Scand J Gastroenterol* 33: 817–21.
130. Peters, U., Askling, J., Gridley, G., et al. 2003. Causes of death in patients with celiac disease in a population-based Swedish cohort. *Arch Intern Med* 163 (13): 1566–72.
131. Ludvigsson, J., Montgomery, S., Ekbom, A., et al. 2009. Small-intestinal histopathology and mortality risk in celiac disease. *JAMA* 302 (11): 1171–78.
132. Maki, M. 1996. Coeliac disease and autoimmunity due to unmasking of cryptic epitopes? *Lancet* 348: 1046–47.
133. Wright, D.H. 1995. The major complications of coeliac disease. *Baillieres Clin Gastroenterol* 9: 351–69.
134. Hermaszewski, R.A., Rigby, S., and Dalgleish, A.G. 1991. Coeliac disease presenting with cerebellar degeneration. *Postgrad Med J* 67: 1023–24.
135. Fera, T., Cascio, B., Angelini, G., and Martini, S. 2003. Affective disorders and quality of life in adult coeliac disease patients on a gluten-free diet. *Eur J Gastroenterol Hepatol* 15 (12): 1287–92.
136. Lee, A.R., Ng, D.L., Dave, E., Ciaccio, E.J., and Green, P.H. 2009. The effect of substituting alternative grains in the diet on the nutritional profile of the gluten-free diet. *J Hum Nutr Diet* 22(4): 359–63.
137. Capristo, E., Addolorato, G., Mingrone, G., et al. 2000. Changes in body composition, substrate oxidation, and resting metabolic rate in adult celiac disease patients after a 1-y gluten-free diet treatment. *Am J Clin Nutr* 72: 76–81.
138. Catassi, C., Fabiani, E., Iacono, G., et al. 2007. A prospective, double-blind, placebo-controlled trial to establish a safe gluten threshold for patients with celiac disease. *Am J Clin Nutr* 85 (1): 160–66.
139. Parish, C. 2007. Medications and celiac disease—tips from a pharmacist. *Practical Gastroenterology*.
140. Murray, J. 1999. The widening spectrum of celiac disease. *Am J Clin Nutr* 69: 354–65.
141. Celiac Disease Foundation–Los Angeles, 13251 Ventura Boulevard, Suite 1, Studio City, CA 91604–1838, 818–990–2354. www.celiac.org.
142. Gluten Intolerance Group of North America (GIG), 15110 10th Avenue SW, Suite A, Seattle, WA 98166, 206–246–6652. www.gluten.net.
143. Celiac Sprue Association–USA, Inc., P. O. Box 31700, Omaha, NE 68131–0700, 402–558–0600. www.csaceliacs.org.

144. National Foundation for Celiac Awareness (NFCA), 224 South Maple Street, Ambler, PA 19002, 215–325–1306. www.celiaccentral.org

145. Raising Our Celiac Kids (R. O. C. K.), 3527 Fortuna Rand Road, Encinitas, CA 92024. 858-395-5421. www.celiackids.com (for kids); www.glutenfreedom.net (for adults).

146. Canadian Celiac Association, 5170 Dixie Road, Suite 204, Mississauga, ON L4W1E3, Canada 905–507–6208; 800–363–7296 (Canada only). www.celiac.ca.

147. See, J., and Murray, J. A. 2006. Gluten-free diet: The medical and nutrition management of celiac disease. *Nutr Clin Pract* 21 (1): 1–15.

148. Solaymani-Dodaran, M., West, J., and Logan, R.F.A. 2007. Long-term mortality in people with celiac disease diagnosed in childhood compared with adulthood: A population-based cohort study. *Am J Gastroenterol* 102: 864–70.

149. Academy of Nutrition and Dietetics (formerly the American Dietetic Association). Evidence Analysis Library, 2010. Guidelines for Celiac Disease. http://www.adaevidencelibrary.com/topic.cfm?cat=4519.

150. Barton, S., Kelly, D., and Murray, J. 2007. Nutritional deficiencies in celiac disease. *Gastroenterol Clin N Am* 36: 93–108.

151. Botero-López, J.E., Araya, M., Parada, A., et. al. 2011. Micronutrient deficiencies in patients with typical and atypical celiac disease. *Pediatr Gastroenterol Nutr* 53 (3): 265–70.

152. Hallert, C., Grant, C., Grehn, S., and Grännö C. 2002. Evidence of poor vitamin status in coeliac patients on a gluten-free diet for 10 years. *Aliment Pharmacol Ther* 16 (7): 1333–39.

153. Bardella, M., Fredella, C., Prampolini, L., Molteni, N. 2000. Body composition and dietary intakes in adult celiac disease patients consuming a strict gluten-free diet. *Am J Clin Nutr* 72: 937–39.

154. McFarlane, X., Bhalla, A., Reeves, D., et al. 1995. Osteoporosis in treated adult coeliac disease. *Gut* 36: 710–14.

155. Jatla, M., Zemel, B.S., Bierly, P., and Verma, R. 2009. Bone mineral content deficits of the spine and whole body in children at time of diagnosis with celiac disease. *J Pediatr Gastroenterol Nutr* 48 (2): 175–80.

156. Olmos, M., Antelo, M., Vazquez, H., Smecuol, E., and Mauriño, E. 2008. Systematic review and meta-analysis of observational studies on the prevalence of fractures in coeliac disease. *Dig Liver Dis* 40 (1): 46–53.

157. Hopman, E.G., von Blomberg, M.E., Batstra, M.R., and Morreau, H. 2008. Gluten tolerance in adult patients with celiac disease 20 years after diagnosis? *Eur J Gastroenterol Hepatol* 20 (5):423–29.

158. Conti Nibali, S., Magazzu, G., and De Luca, F. 1987. Obesity in a child with untreated coeliac disease. *Helv Paediat Acta* 42: 45–48.

159. Czaja-Bulsa, G., Garanty-Bogacka, B, Syrenicz, M., and Gebala, A. 2001. Obesity in an 18-year-old boy with untreated celiac disease [letter]. *J Pediatr Gastroenterol Nutr* 32: 226.

160. Bondsa, R., Midoro-Horiutib, T., and Goldblum, R. 2008. A structural basis for food allergy: The role of cross-reactivity. *Current Opinion in Allergy and Clinical Immunology* 8: 82–86.

161. Fasano, A., and Catassi C. 2001. Current approaches to diagnosis and treatment of celiac disease: An evolving spectrum. *Gastroenterology* 120 (3): 636–51.

162. Levine, A., Domanov, S., Sukhotnik, I., et al. 2009. Celiac-associated peptic disease at upper endoscopy: How common is it? *Scandinavian Journal of Gastroenterology* 44: 1424–28.

163. Usai, P., Usai-Satta, P., Lai, M., et al. 1997. Autonomic dysfunction and upper digestive functional disorders in untreated adult celiac disease. *Eur J Clin Invest* 27: 1009–15.

164. Jacobson, B.C., Somers, S.C., Fuchs, C.S., et al. 2006. Body-mass index and symptoms of gastroesophageal reflux in women. *N Engl J Med* 354: 2340–48.

165. Usai, P., Manca, R., Cuomo, R., et al. 2008. Effect of gluten-free diet on preventing recurrence of gastroesophageal reflux disease-related symptoms in adult celiac patients with nonerosive reflux disease. *J Gastroenterol Hepatol* 23 (9): 1368–72.

166. da Rosa Utiyama, S.R., da Silva Kotze, L.M., Nisihara, M., and Carvalho, R.F. 2001. Spectrum of auto-antibodies in celiac patients and relatives. *Dig Dis Sci* 46 (12): 2624–30.

167. Freeman, H. 2007. Pancreatic endocrine and exocrine changes in celiac disease. *World J Gastroenterol* 13 (47): 6344–46.

168. Brown, A., Bradshaw, M., Richardson, R., et al. 1987. Pathogenesis of the impaired gall bladder contraction of coeliac disease. *Gut* 28: 1426–32.

169. Barton, S., Kelly, D., and Murray, J. 2007. Nutritional deficiencies in celiac disease. *Gastroenterol Clin N Am* 36: 93–108.

170. Hallert, C., Grant, C., Grehn, S., et al. 2002. Evidence of poor vitamin status in coeliac patients on a gluten-free diet for 10 years. *Aliment Pharmacol Ther* 16: 1333–39.

17 Bariatric Surgery and Post–Bariatric Surgery Nutrition Needs

Mark DeLegge, M.D., Debbie Petitpain, M.S., R.D., and Nina Crowley, M.S., R.D.

INTRODUCTION

Primary care physicians have a unique and important role in the continuum of a patient's consideration of bariatric surgery and subsequent postsurgical course. The decision to have a bariatric surgical procedure is a complex one for the patient and the physician. In addition to weight loss, the effects of bariatric surgery on a patient's mortality and medical comorbidities need to be evaluated. This chapter will help the primary care physician understand the surgical options available for morbidly obese patients, how to help patients select the appropriate type of surgery, how surgery alters appetite signaling, and what dietary and lifestyle changes are expected after surgery. In addition, this chapter identifies lifelong changes in nutrient needs due to the physiologic changes in absorption. Evaluation of nutrient status of a patient who has undergone bariatric surgery even decades earlier may reveal treatable deficiencies exacerbating seemingly unrelated medical conditions.

INDICATIONS FOR BARIATRIC SURGERY

Bariatric surgical procedures have been performed in increasing numbers over the past two decades both in the United States and internationally. While surgery is not the solution to the obesity epidemic, weight-loss surgery is currently the only effective way for morbidly obese individuals to achieve substantial weight loss and keep it off long term [1]. Although these procedures can have a tremendous impact on appropriate patients, they are not without risk. Therefore, attempts have been made to identify which patients are appropriate for surgical intervention. Published criteria for the appropriate bariatric surgery patient vary somewhat depending on the recommending body and/or requirements of third-party payers. In 1991, the National Institutes of Health (NIH) recommended bariatric surgery for patients with a body mass index (BMI) above 40 kg/m^2 or for patients with a BMI above 35 kg/m^2 with two or more medical comorbidities [2]. Recently, the Food and Drug Administration approved the use of a bariatric surgical medical device, the laparoscopic adjustable gastric band (LAGB), for patients with a BMI of 30 kg/m^2 or greater with one or more medical comorbidities. The use of the LAGB in the adolescent population has become a topic of discussion although no definitive consensus has been obtained [3]. Additional recommendations outline the need for evaluation by a multidisciplinary team of psychologists, dietitians, and a surgeon.

Although bariatric surgical procedures primarily focus on weight-loss outcomes, one of the other major goals is to improve or eliminate medical comorbidities that are related to obesity and reduce obesity-related mortality. In a Swedish prospective matched controlled study, obese patients who received bariatric surgery had a 23.7% reduction in mortality compared to obese controls [4]. In a retrospective study from the United States, patients were followed for seven years after gastric bypass surgery and compared to control, those receiving bariatric surgery had a 33% reduction in mortality [5]. Bariatric surgery has been shown to be a cost-effective treatment of medical comorbidities, particularly type 2 diabetes [6]. The most impressive effect of bariatric surgical procedures is on the improvement or elimination of type 2 diabetes. Improvement in diabetes is seen before weight loss occurs and is believed to be secondary to the "bypassing" of the normal food stream from the duodenum (e.g., in Roux-en-Y gastric bypass). Ten-year follow-up studies have also shown an improvement in hypertriglyceridemia, hypertension, and hyperuricemia in obese patients receiving bariatric surgery as compared to similar control patients [7]. A meta-analysis in 2004 of 137 published trials on the effects of bariatric surgical procedures on medical comorbidities confirmed major improvements in hypertension, diabetes, and hypertriglyceridemia following bariatric surgical procedures; it also noted a major improvement in obstructive sleep apnea [2].

While researchers continue to search for ways to help define who might be an appropriate surgical candidate, studies are beginning to examine alterations in genetic material, commonly referred to as single-nucleotide polymorphisms (SNPs), which can alter absorption, metabolism, elimination, or biochemical effects of nutrients. There is an effect of gene composition on nutrient use and an effect of nutrients on gene expression [8]. Obesity, because of its complex changes in the expression of thousands of genes, is both an ideal·candidate and a puzzle for the development of genetic screening tests that are able to identify those at risk for obesity as well as specific nutrient effects on the expression of "obesity" genes in an individual. Although still in its infancy, nutrigenomics is an intriguing science that would allow those at risk of obesity to choose foods and other nutrients that would have the least impact of causing obesity, or in the ideal world, preventing obesity entirely.

One of the most important functions of the relationship a primary care physician has with an obese patient is to continually have a conversation about weight and BMI. Many patients are waiting for their doctor to suggest surgery as a medical treatment for their obesity. Patients with a BMI ≥ 35 with an obesity-related comorbidity are appropriate for consideration of bariatric surgery [1]. Understanding treatment options for obese patients who have spent years trying and failing at non-surgical efforts at weight loss is critical for primary care physicians today.

BARIATRIC SURGICAL PROCEDURES

Bariatric surgical procedures are generally divided into three groups: restrictive, malabsorptive, and a combination of restrictive/malabsorptive. The decision of which procedure to use can be influenced by the patient's degree of obesity and medical comorbidities, the surgeon's preference and skill set, and other factors such as the age of the patient, the desire to have a reversible procedure, the cost of the procedure, and insurance coverage.

It is important to make the distinction between weight loss that can be achieved with purely restrictive procedures like the LAGB and the vertical banded gastroplasty, and hybrid procedures that combine restriction and malabsorption like the biliopancreatic diversion, duodenal switch, and the Roux-en-Y gastric bypass (RYGB) [9]. While most bariatric surgery procedures are generally accepted as effective treatments for morbid obesity, the RYGB is considered to be most efficacious in producing long-term weight loss, which may be due in part to the neural and hormonal mechanisms that are unique to the rerouting of the small intestine and the loss of appetite that RYGB patients experience [10].

Restrictive procedures today are best exemplified by the LAGB (LAP-BAND® or Realize® band) and the sleeve gastrectomy. (See Figures 17.1a and 17.1b.) The band is a silicone ring placed around the proximal portion of the stomach and inflated to create a small proximal gastric pouch

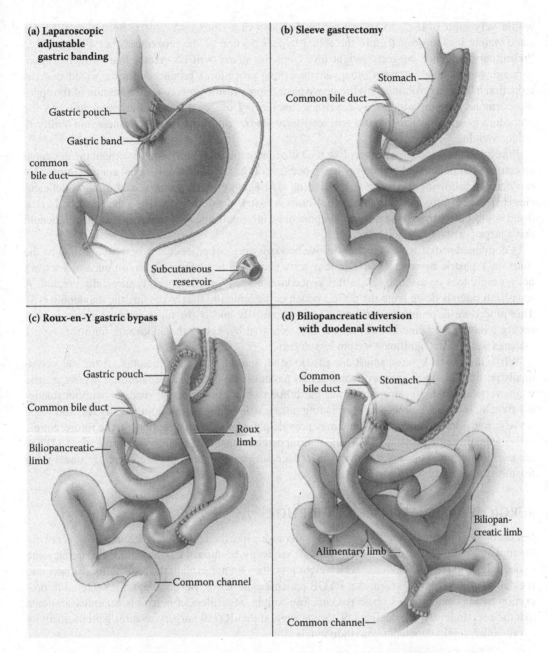

FIGURE 17.1 Common bariatric surgeries. (From DeMaria EJ 2007. Reproduced with permission.)

and a narrowed opening between the proximal and distal stomach [11]. This procedure is reversible because the band can be removed. However, weight regain is likely; therefore it is recommended only if there is a complication. This procedure has been advocated for obese adolescents or those with a lower BMI. It also involves much less complicated surgery, thus creating an option for those who desire a less risky procedure. Weight loss occurs more slowly than with other procedures, and most patients can expect to lose 30–50% of excess body weight over three to five years, with an average of 47% [2,12].

Sleeve gastrectomy involves removing a large portion of the stomach leaving only a sleeve (tunnel) between the esophagus and the pylorus. This procedure is sometimes advocated for patients with a very high BMI (> 55 kg/m^2) as the first step in a Roux-en-Y gastric bypass to allow for some weight loss to occur before the actual bypass portion of the procedure. (See Figure 17.1c.) Preliminary evidence suggests weight loss from the sleeve will be greater than with the band, although not as much as what other malabsorptive procedures produce. It is theorized that the reduction in stomach volume with the sleeve gastrectomy results in greater suppression of the appetite hormone ghrelin, which may explain its increasing use as a stand-alone procedure. As the procedure gains popularity, so too will long-term studies outlining its effectiveness and ability to reduce weight.

Purely malabsorptive procedures like the biliopancreatic diversion (with or without the duodenal switch) are not performed commonly today because of the significant nutritional complications that can develop following the procedure including significant protein, vitamin, and mineral deficiencies [13]. (See Figure 17.1d.) In these procedures, a gastric pouch is created and then attached to the distal small bowel bypassing a large component of the small intestine that includes the duodenum and a large portion of the jejunum [14].

A combined restrictive and malabsorptive bariatric surgical procedure is best exemplified by the Roux-en-Y gastric bypass (RYGB). In long-term studies, it has been noted to produce 61% excess body weight loss on average [2]. In this procedure, a small gastric pouch is surgically created. A roux-limb extends down from the gastric pouch to the jejunum, thus bypassing the duodenum [15]. This procedure is primarily performed laparoscopically and is the most common bariatric procedure today in the United States [16]. It is of note that bypassing the duodenum improves type 2 diabetes well before significant weight loss occurs.

While the gastric bypass, adjustable gastric band, and the sleeve gastrectomy are the most commonly performed, physicians will come across patients who have had the intestinal bypass, gastric wrap, vertical banded gastroplasty, and the biliopancreatictic diversion (with or without duodenal switch). Innovative procedures, including intragastric balloons, intraluminal sleeves, and vagal nerve stimulators are under study and may provide patients with more options in the future. Single incision laparoscopic surgery (SILS) and natural orifice transluminal endoscopic surgery (NOTES) are exciting surgical approaches that will reduce surgical trauma, and are currently undergoing feasibility and safety studies in animals [17].

SURGICAL ALTERATION OF GUT PEPTIDES

Gut hormones are not affected by restrictive operations like the LAGB and therefore do not contribute to weight loss [18]. (See Table 17.1.) While adiposity hormones leptin and insulin are elevated in obese individuals and decrease with weight loss, they do not explain the reduction in hunger and regulation of lower body weight that RYGB patients experience. Because leptin is secreted in proportion to adipose tissue, as obese patients lose weight, regardless of how, it is generally assumed that their leptin levels will decline [19]. Some suggest that RYGB surgery restores leptin sensitivity to previously leptin deficient obese individuals [18].

TABLE 17.1

Gastrointestinal Hormones and Their Effects

Gastrointestinal Hormones	Principal Site of Release	Hunger/Appetite	Gastric Emptying	Insulin Release	Satiety
Glucagon-like peptide-1 (GLP-1)	Distal gut	↓	↓	↑	↑
Peptide YY (PYY)	Distal gut	↓	↓	-	↑
Leptin	Adipocytes	↓	-	-	-
Ghrelin	Gastric mucosa	↑	↑	↓	↓

Ghrelin, an enteric peptide hormone, is a known appetite stimulant produced by the stomach and duodenum; in the unaltered stomach, endogenous levels increase before eating and decrease afterwards [20]. (See Figure 17.2.) Ghrelin is thought to stimulate mealtime hunger and is associated with initiating a meal. In people who experience nonsurgical weight loss, ghrelin levels increase; the increase of ghrelin is thought to be an adaptive response to weight loss, which allows an individual to maintain long-term energy homeostasis and weight regain after weight loss [21]. Paradoxically, those who have had RYGB surgery do not have the increase in ghrelin levels associated with the weight loss that they experience [22]. After RYGB surgery, most of the ghrelin producing tissue from the stomach and duodenum is permanently separated from contact with ingested nutrients, which disrupts production of ghrelin and may result in suppressed ghrelin levels [10]. Subtle differences in surgical technique have been implicated in contradictory findings in postoperative levels of ghrelin. These differences are related to the location of the staple line and how effectively the surgery excludes the fundus from food and severs the vagus nerve [10,21]. Whether or not the surgeon can sever the vagus nerve and disrupt autonomic nerve fibers that innervate the foregut is thought to be associated with variable ghrelin secretion and weight loss [18]. While research on ghrelin is ongoing, changes in ghrelin levels are currently not correlated with bariatric surgery weight-loss success [23].

The glucagon-like peptide-1 (GLP-1) hormone is an incretin produced by intestinal L cells in the hindgut after ingestion of food that stimulates insulin secretion, improves pancreatic beta cell function, inhibits gastric acid secretion and motility, and decreases food intake [24]. After gastric bypass, ingested nutrients bypass most of the foregut without the barrier of the pylorus and reach the hindgut more readily, increasing GLP-1 levels [10]. Peptide tyrosine tyrosine (PYY) is another satiety hormone that is secreted postprandially from L cells in the distal ileum inhibiting neuropeptide Y (NPY) and decreasing food intake [25]. After gastric bypass, patients experience an exaggerated PYY and GLP-1 response and decreased ghrelin levels after a carbohydrate meal, which contributes to their early satiety, reduced gastric emptying, reduced food intake, and subsequent weight loss [26]. Similar elevations of PYY are seen after other procedures that allow rapid delivery of nutrients to the distal small bowel, but such elevations are not seen following purely restrictive bariatric operations like the LAGB [23].

It seems that exclusion of the hormonally active foregut from the digestive process after surgery explains why RYGB and biliopancreatic diversion result in the quickest and most effective weight loss and diabetes resolution. Compared to restrictive operations like the LAGB, patients who

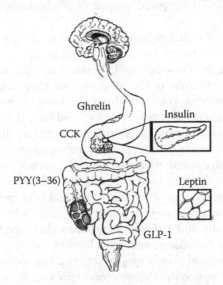

FIGURE 17.2   Gastrointestinal hormones and their primary sites of release. (From Crowell MD, Decker GA, Levy R, Jeffrey R, Talley NJ 2006. Reproduced with permission.)

undergo RYGB have elevated levels of postprandial GLP-1 and PYY, and lower levels of postprandial ghrelin [19]. Bariatric surgeries that do not bypass the stomach may not lower ghrelin levels or increase GLP-1 and PYY levels enough to promote reduced hunger, early satiety, and reduced intake and, therefore, may explain why RYGB surgery continues to have the strongest data supporting long-term weight maintenance [19].

PERIOPERATIVE NUTRITION RECOMMENDATIONS AND EXPECTATIONS FOR WEIGHT LOSS

Since the 1991 NIH consensus conference, guidelines have existed to help define who would be an appropriate candidate for surgery. These guidelines suggest that patients who cannot comprehend the nature of the surgical intervention and the lifelong measures required to maintain an acceptable level of health should be excluded from surgery [27]. In practice, multidisciplinary bariatric surgery teams discuss patients on an individual basis to decide who would be an appropriate surgical candidate. Often, while someone may be deemed appropriate for surgery, the patient may be limited by insurance policy benefits. A growing trend is the requirement that a patient show documentation of a "six-month physician supervised weight loss program" [28]. Primary care providers can assist patients in obtaining insurance coverage for surgery by documenting weight, BMI, and dietary counseling at monthly visits.

Preoperative weight loss has been evaluated for its association with postoperative weight loss and improved outcomes, but definitive answers are not available. While heavier patients are less likely to lose as much of their excess weight as patients with lower body mass indices, there are very few reliable predictors of success after all bariatric surgery procedures [29]. Surgeons may believe that by requiring patients to lose weight preoperatively, they will lower their BMI, therefore increasing their chances of achieving a nonobese BMI postoperatively [30]. Based on the assertion that those who can prove their ability to lose weight preoperatively are more motivated, better adapted, and have a better understanding of postoperative guidelines, many insurance companies and bariatric programs require 5–10% of total body weight loss prior to surgery [31]. A recent meta-analysis found no significant benefit of preoperative weight loss one year after bariatric surgery but did find that weight loss prior to surgery was associated with shorter operative times, less blood loss, and slightly fewer complications [32]. Another found that while weight loss did not differ postsurgery in a very low-calorie diet (VLCD) compared to controls, 30-day complication rates were fewer in the VLCD group [33].

Because obesity is associated with nonalcoholic fatty liver disease, instead of focusing on weight loss prior to surgery, some programs focus on low carbohydrate diets to reduce liver fat content and liver size, making the surgery itself less difficult [34]. Based on equivocal evidence, it is suggested to rely on the judgment and expertise of the bariatric team regarding preoperative weight loss. Comprehensive bariatric surgery programs involve a registered dietitian who works closely with patients to assess their nutritional status before, during, and after bariatric surgery. The nutrition evaluation encompasses multidisciplinary factors affecting a patient's diet such as their readiness to change their eating behaviors, setting realistic goals for eating and weight loss, assessment of their self-care, and other behavioral, cultural, psychosocial, and economic issues [35].

Optimizing micronutrition before surgery is emphasized, especially given the nutritional demands, reduced intake, and reduced absorption associated with bariatric surgery. Occurrence of iron deficiency of up to 44% and vitamin B12 deficiency of up to 29% has been described in the preoperative patient. In one study, 100% of presenting patients had suboptimal (< 32ng/mL) vitamin D levels [36]. This can be done by ordering nutritional labwork preoperatively, treating any deficiencies, starting the patient on a multivitamin prophylactically, and individualizing supplementation based on the patient and the procedure. Patients considering bariatric surgery may also want to know what they will be able to eat for the weeks following surgery. While there is no standardized "post-RYGB surgery diet," most patients follow a similar staged approach. Approximately 24 hours after surgery, patients are initiated on a clear liquid diet to start the staged meal progression from clear liquids, to full liquids, to pureed foods, to regular textured foods about a month after surgery. See Table 17.2 for the standard diet progression.

During the first six months, also known as the rapid weight-loss phase, patients typically consume fewer than 800 calories and by one year approximately 900–1000 calories per day [37]. General guidelines encourage all bariatric surgery patients to take small bites and thoroughly chew their food, avoid drinking beverages about 30–60 minutes after eating, sip consistently on about 64 ounces of noncaloric, noncarbonated fluids, and avoid concentrated sweets or anything made with added sugars.

Weight-loss outcomes can be quantified in a number of ways but are typically reported as percent excess weight lost (% EWL = pounds of weight lost divided by the pounds of excess weight one was carrying preoperatively, which is the difference between baseline weight and ideal body weight). Percent change in BMI and weight loss as a percent of initial body weight are also used. A successful outcome is generally considered the loss of 50% EWL [38]. A meta-analysis of 22,000 patients demonstrating long-term outcomes reported a weight loss of -61.6% EWL for RYGB and -47.5% EWL for LAGB [2]. Some degree of weight regain after bariatric surgery is considered normal, as

TABLE 17.2
Suggested Diet Progression after Gastric Bypass Surgery

Postoperative Stage	Timeline	Diet Recommendation	Specific Types of Foods Included	Recommended Amounts
I	Postop days 1–2	Clear liquids Noncarbonated, non-caloric, no added sugar	Sugar-free popsicles, low-sodium broth, powdered add ins (like Crystal Light) to water, diet Jello, clear protein supplements	Aim for 48–64 oz/day (total fluid)
II	Postop days 2–3	Full liquids Protein-rich, non-carbonated, noncaloric, no added sugar	Skim milk, lactaid milk, unsweetened soy milk, nonfat milk powder mixed in, whey or soy protein powder-based supplements, fat free	Aim for 48–64 oz/day (both clear and full liquids)
III	Postop days 3–30	Pureed foods Soft, moist, blended, or pureed foods that are the consistency of pudding or applesauce, emphasis on protein sources	No added-sugar yogurt or plain nonfat Greek yogurt, eggs/egg substitute, blended meats, poultry, fish, beans, soups, peanut butter, low-fat cheese, cottage cheese	Aim for 4–6 mini-meals per day (meal may be a couple tablespoons) Start with protein choices first (meats/milks), then add vegetables and fruits, limiting starches and added fats
IV	4 weeks postop and beyond	Transition to regular textured foods Same foods as tolerated on pureed diet, just not pureed anymore (encourage moist methods of cooking)	Begin with chopped/mashed/flaked foods, then add well-cooked, soft protein choices, soft fruits and vegetables, and once tolerated, all textures of foods are appropriate	Continue to strive for 4–6 mini-meals but include a source of protein (1–2 oz) at each eating occasion, along with fruit, vegetable, or whole grain starches (¼–½ cup) Avoid added sugars, carbonation, added trans fats, and alcohol for life.

it occurs in approximately 30–50% of patients, but significant weight regain (> 15% of total weight lost) is only seen in about 15–20% of patients [39,40]. Few patients have surgical factors like a dilated gastric pouch or stoma, which explain weight regain. More commonly, factors contributing to regain include less frequent dumping syndrome, resolution of food intolerances, and a return to the preoperative eating and lifestyle behaviors that contributed to obesity prior to surgery.

DUMPING SYNDROME

Patients who have had the RYGB or other gastric surgeries that bypass the pylorus and/or interfere with gastric innervation are at risk for dumping syndrome. The term itself describes the rapid emptying of gastric contents into the small bowel, which leads to a variety of symptoms, both gastrointestinal and vasomotor [41]. While up to 70% of RYGB patients report dumping in the early postoperative period, a minority experience debilitating symptoms and the sensitivity to dumping decreases over time. Dumping syndrome can occur anywhere from a few minutes to several hours after eating and is categorized as "early dumping" versus "late dumping" [9,41].

While the pathophysiology of dumping syndrome is not completely understood, the crucial component of "early dumping" is accelerated gastric emptying of hyperosmolar contents into the upper small intestines, which forces a shift in fluid from the intravascular compartment into the intestinal lumen that leads to bowel distention and intestinal hypermotility [41,42]. The primary symptoms include weakness, dizziness, palpitations, diaphoresis, and the urgent need to lie down. Although not a necessary part of this syndrome, gastrointestinal distress may occur including epigastric fullness, bloating, nausea, abdominal cramps, and explosive diarrhea. Most patients are affected by early dumping, which occurs within 10–30 minutes after a meal. By contrast, late dumping occurs one to three hours after a meal as a consequence of reactive hypoglycemia from an exaggerated release of insulin. Only approximately 25% of patients experience late dumping syndrome, although it may be harder to diagnose. The symptoms are more systemic and include the symptoms of early dumping syndrome as well as extreme fatigue, difficulty with concentration, tremor, hunger, syncope, and decreased consciousness. Orthostatic changes such as a drop in blood pressure or increased heart rate as well as low blood sugar levels may be measurable by a physical exam. A better understanding of the enteric nervous system and mediating GI hormones, which regulate gastric emptying, will help describe why some patients experience dumping syndrome and others do not, why some experience debilitating symptoms while others experience only mild symptoms, and why some patients develop complete immunity to dumping over time while others remain sensitive [41,42].

Due to the breadth of symptoms experienced and length of time postprandial, diagnosing dumping syndrome has its challenges. A food journal with detailed information on foods consumed and when corresponding symptoms occur is critical. A trained professional such as a registered dietitian can evaluate the data and look for trends. A simple elimination test of potentially offending foods is an easy place to start. An oral glucose challenge (using 50 g glucose), following a 10-hour fast, may be used to diagnose early dumping. An increase in heart rate of 10 beats per minute after ingestion or a positive hydrogen breath test indicate early dumping. Late dumping can be diagnosed by sampling blood glucose levels after the oral glucose challenge. Within the first hour, plasma levels should rise, followed by decreased levels one to two hours later. Evaluation of the GI tract by upper endoscopy, barium study, or gastric emptying scintigraphy may be warranted to rule out other postgastrectomy syndromes [42].

Dietary modification is the first line of treatment for dumping syndrome. Simple sugars and concentrated sweets, high-fat foods, and alcohol should be eliminated. Some patients may also be sensitive to lactose and will need to avoid certain dairy foods. A meal plan with low-volume, high-protein, carbohydrate-controlled mini-meals, spaced equally throughout the day, as well as separating the intake of food and fluid by an hour or more, may be necessary [35]. The addition of soluble fiber from guar gum, glucomannan, or pectins (starting at 500 mg per meal) can delay gastric emptying and increase transit time in the bowel, therefore slowing glucose absorption. Drug therapy may provide relief for patients who do not respond completely to dietary modification. Some medications that have been studied include tolbutamide, propranolol, cyproheptadine, methysergide maleate, verapamil, and acarbose; acarbose has been more studied than the others but with inconsistent results. By slowing the conversion of polysaccharides and disaccharides into monosaccharides, acarbose ameliorates symptoms of late dumping. However, short-term side effects of acarbose include flatulence and diarrhea. Octreotide, a somatostatin analog, is a well-established treatment option. It works through several mechanisms including delay of gastric emptying and transit time through the bowel and inhibition of the release of insulin and gut-derived hormones. Octreotide that is administered in subcutaneous doses at 25 to 50 mcg approximately 15–30 minutes before a meal relieves the vasomotor and gastrointestinal symptoms of dumping, although doses as high as 100–200 mcg may be required [42]. Surgical options are limited for the treatment of dumping syndrome and often are not curative [41].

PREGNANCY IN THE POST–BARIATRIC SURGERY PATIENT

Approximately 80% of weight-loss surgery patients are women of childbearing age (ages 18–45 years) [43,4]. Literature shows no significant differences in maternal or neonatal outcomes for patients who underwent bariatric surgery versus the general obstetric population [44]. Children born to mothers who had surgery have a lower weight at birth and later in life compared to siblings born prior to the mother's weight-loss surgery [9,35]. This evidence should reassure the patient that bariatric surgery is not a contraindication to pregnancy.

Rapid weight loss occurs in the first one to two years following the RYGB and sleeve gastrectomy and at a more moderate pace following placement of the LAGB. During the rapid weight-loss phase, pregnancy is discouraged because it is difficult to meet the demands of mother and fetus. However, rapid weight loss also increases fertility and may improve polycystic ovary syndrome (PCOS), increasing the possibility of pregnancy after bariatric surgery [43]. Oral contraceptives may be poorly absorbed and therefore less effective following a malabsorptive weight-loss procedure. Intrauterine device (IUD) and barrier methods may offer the best protection if used correctly and may be used in combination with oral contraceptives. Transdermal methods (i.e., Depo-Provera and Implanon) may be less effective in patients heavier than 195 lbs [45].

While the bariatric patient may have lost a significant amount of weight, her BMI may still put her in the obese (BMI > 30 kg/m^2) or overweight (BMI 25–30 kg/m^2) category. Above and beyond the risk associated with being overweight or obese during pregnancy, there are some risks unique to the pregnant bariatric surgery patient.

One risk underscored here is hyperemesis gravidarum (HG) because it mimics the presentation of problems unique to the surgery patient [46]. In the LAGB patient, HG may mask problems with the band such as gastric prolapse or gastric slip or even contribute to such a complication. Additionally, the pregnant gastric band patient may experience pain at the port site due to the growing abdomen. The pregnant patient should be monitored for adequate oral intake, routine labs, and fetal growth, deflating the band as needed to improve nutritional status or for patient preference. HG may cause ulceration of the gastric pouch in patients who have had the RYGB or sleeve that may be perceived as heartburn. Additionally, there is a risk of small bowel obstruction or internal herniation as a result of anatomical changes that occur with surgery, weight loss, and uterine changes. These may present as peri-umbilical or epigastric pain radiating to the back, acute weight loss, poor oral intake, and nausea—common pregnancy concerns. Such symptoms should not be dismissed as normal pregnancy symptoms until other surgical etiologies can be ruled out [43,45].

LIFELONG CONSIDERATIONS FOR NUTRIENT NEEDS

Restrictive procedures, such as vertical banded gastroplasty and LAGB, by definition, decrease the amount of nutrition consumed making it difficult to ingest optimal amounts of nutrients. However, needs are usually met with supplementation of a multivitamin-mineral supplement. In comparison, restrictive-malabsorptive procedures including RYGB reduce dietary intake as well as absorption pathways, thus requiring adherence to strict vitamin-mineral supplementation to reduce the risk of nutritional deficiencies [35]. Currently, there is a paucity of data on the micronutrition of patients who have had the sleeve gastrectomy but current literature demonstrates rates of deficiencies similar to the RYGB versus the LAGB; therefore, sleeve patients are advised to follow the more prudent supplement routine of RYGB patients [47]. Patients with older procedures, including the biliopancreatic diversion with or without the duodenal switch, may be at even greater risk for deficiencies. The remainder of this section focuses on deficiencies among patients who undergo restrictive-malabsorptive procedures because micronutrition deficiencies are more common among this group.

Bariatric surgery patients are advised to have nutritional labs (Table 17.3) drawn at least twice per year postoperatively until weight stabilizes and then at least annually [9]. These labs can be ordered by physicians other than those at the surgical center, preferably in a primary care setting.

Patients are also instructed to adhere to taking micronutrient supplements as individualized for them. Minimal nutritional supplementation should include: one to two adult multivitamin-mineral supplements containing iron, zinc, folic acid, and thiamin; 1500–2000 mg of elemental calcium citrate plus vitamin D in divided doses; and at least 350 mcg crystalline vitamin B12 or, as an alternative, intramuscular supplementation with 1000 mcg vitamin B12 monthly (Table 17.4) [9,35].

Iron deficiency anemia has been reported in up to 50% of postoperative patients [48]. In addition to a multivitamin-mineral supplement containing iron, additional iron from ferrous sulfate, ferrous fumarate, or ferrous gluconate to achieve a total intake of 50–100 mg of elemental iron may be required to prevent anemia in the post-bariatric patient, particularly among menstruating women. Iron supplements should be taken with a source of vitamin C to enhance absorption and taken separately from calcium supplements, which inhibit absorption [35]. Intravenous iron infusions may be warranted in patients who do not tolerate or do not respond to oral iron [49].

Serum vitamin B12 deficiency has been reported in one-third of RYGB patients two years out from surgery, defined as levels < 150 pg/ml [50]; however, vitamin B12 deficiency may take years to develop because body stores are generally greater than daily needs [35]. Although serum vitamin B12 is the routine screening method, clinical signs and symptoms of deficiency such as megaloblastic anemia and paresthesias may present at levels above 200 pg/mL; elevated levels of methylmalonic acid and homocysteine would confirm vitamin B12 deficiency [49].

Vitamin D deficiency, measured as serum 25-hydroxyvitamin D, in the post-RYGB patient has been reported in 50–63% of cases [51,52]. This is despite the fact that vitamin D is fat soluble and the relationship between serum vitamin D and vitamin D stored in adipose tissue is currently unclear [53,54]. Optimal intake of calcium and vitamin D is important in the development of peak bone mass and prevention of metabolic bone disease; routine bone density scans are appropriate. Adherence to supplementation of calcium citrate with vitamin D is difficult due to the amount required (generally six tablets per day). Taking calcium citrate supplements with food may bind oxalate and decrease risk of forming kidney stones in susceptible patients. Patients with severe vitamin D malabsorption may need additional vitamin D2 (ergocalciferol) or vitamin D3 (cholecalciferol) as high as 15,000

TABLE 17.3

Routine Laboratory Analysis for Common Micronutrient Deficiencies

Complete blood count (CBC), basic metabolic panel (BMP)

Iron (hemoglobin, hematocrit, serum iron, percent iron saturation, unsaturated iron-binding capacity [UIBC], total iron-binding capacity [TIBC], ferritin, transferrin)

25-hydroxy vitamin D, PTH

B vitamins (folate, vitamin B12, thiamin)

TABLE 17.4

Micronutrient Supplementation for Post Malabsorptive Surgery Patient (Gastric Bypass and Sleeve Gastrectomy)

Supplement	Dosage
Multivitamin-mineral with iron, zinc, folic acid and thiamin	Two daily for first six months or until cessation of rapid weight-loss phase; one daily for life
Calcium	1200–1500 mg of elemental calcium, from calcium citrate, in divided doses plus 400–800 IU vitamin D, daily
Vitamin D	400–800 IU daily, in calcium citrate supplement
Folic acid	400 mcg daily, in multivitamin
Vitamin B12	At least 350 mcg daily taken orally in crystalline form, or 1000 mcg intramuscularly once per month
Iron	Ferrous sulfate, ferrous fumarate, or ferrous gluconate in amounts needed for total daily supplementation of 50–100 mg elemental iron for patients at risk of anemia (i.e., menstruating females)

IU to 50,000 IU daily. Vitamin D can also be made by the body after skin exposure to ultraviolet-B radiation, which triggers a cascade of reactions to yield a biologically active form of vitamin D [55]. For early identification and treatment of secondary hyperthyroidism, periodically measure parathyroid hormone (PTH) levels [49].

Thiamin deficiency can occur quickly in patients with persistent vomiting after any bariatric procedure. Symptoms of Wernicke's syndrome, dry beriberi, and wet beriberi have been reported in bariatric surgery patients [49]. These patients should be screened for thiamin deficiency, aggressively treated with thiamin supplementation, and should avoid intravenous fluid containing dextrose without thiamin as this can aggravate the deficiency [35].

Deficiencies of zinc, copper, selenium, folate, and vitamins A, C, E, and K have been described [56]. Treatment of micronutrient deficiencies should be referred to a bariatric surgery center of excellence or a physician who specializes in this area as many factors play a role including patient compliance, food intolerances or aversions, nausea, vomiting, diarrhea, and other medical complications. In extreme cases, repletion through parenteral nutrition may be required. Supplementation, in addition to annual review of laboratory values, is required for life [35]. However, recommendation updates are expected as advances are made in the field of bariatrics and nutrition; one should be familiar with the signs and symptoms of micronutrient deficiencies since these can occur at any point after bariatric surgery (Table 17.5).

Prior practice was a prophylactic cholecystectomy during bariatric surgery to prevent the occurrence of symptomatic gallstone disease following weight loss. However, over time this practice has changed because the risk of receiving a prophylactic cholecystectomy was determined to be greater than any benefit received by the patient in the prevention of symptomatic gallstones [57]. Another supplement of interest is omega-3 fatty acids; however, routine use of fatty acid chromatography to detect essential fatty acid deficiency is not cost effective and is not recommended because this deficiency has not been reported in the literature [35].

All patients should aim to eat lean protein sources, low-fat dairy, whole fruits and vegetables, high-fiber foods, and omega-3 fatty acids. Protein intake is generally recommended at 60–80 grams per day, or 1.0–1.5 grams protein per kg of ideal body weight [35], which represents approximately 30–40% of total calories consumed. This is in comparison to the recommended dietary allowance (RDA) for normal adults of 50 grams per day [61]. Over time, total caloric intake tends to increase and percent of calories from protein decreases. Protein intake is important to promote healing, protect lean body mass during the weight-loss phase, and to promote satiety. Since approximately 17%

TABLE 17.5

Signs and Symptoms of Micronutrient Deficiencies

Signs and Symptoms	Suspect Deficiency	Laboratory Test
Skin and mucosal changes	All B vitamins, vitamins A, C, E, zinc	Serum thiamin, serum pyrixodoxal-5'-phosphate, serum vitamin B12, serum folate and/or homocysteine, retinol, ascorbic acid, plasma vitamin C, plasma alpha-tocopherol, serum zinc
Cardiac failure and cardiomyopathy	Selenium, vitamin D	Serum selenium, serum 25-hydroxyvitamin D
Anemia	Iron, vitamin B12, folate, copper	Serum iron, ferritin, serum vitamin B12, complete blood count, serum folate, serum copper
Muscle pain and cramps	Vitamin D, selenium	Serum 25-hydroxyvitamin D, serum selenium
Bone pain	Vitamin D	Serum 25-hydroxyvitamin D
Neurological manifestations	Thiamine, niacin, copper, vitamin B12, folate, vitamin E	Serum thiamin, serum copper, serum vitamin B12, serum folate
Visual symptoms	Vitamin A, vitamin E	Retinol, plasma alpha-tocopherol

Source: Adapted from [56].

of patients report intolerance to protein-rich foods—such as intolerances to dry, tough meats—many patients explore nonmeat alternative protein sources from soy or vegetable proteins or experiment with fish, shellfish, beans, eggs, and low-fat dairy products. Caution should be used when recommending protein supplements; if the protein source does not supply all nine of the indispensable amino acids (IAA) and/or adequate substrate for the eleven dispensable amino acids that compose body protein, an IAA deficiency may occur [35]. However, protein malnutrition is still considered rare. In fact, protein malnutrition is usually associated with other factors, unrelated to the malabsorptive component of the surgery, such as anorexia, prolonged vomiting, diarrhea, fear of weight regain, substance abuse, or other factors related to decreased intake [35].

The recommended daily allowance (RDA) for carbohydrates is 130 grams per day for adults [61]. Preference should be given to high-fiber foods such as whole grains, vegetables, and fruits, and low-nutrient, calorie-dense foods should be avoided. However, getting in the recommended average of 25 grams of fiber per day [61] can be challenging and constipation may occur. While an adequate intake level of total fat has not been established for adults, preference should be given to foods rich in polyunsaturated fats and specifically foods rich in the essential omega-3 fatty acids EPA, DHA, and ALA such as fish, flax seed, walnuts, and canola oil. During pregnancy and lactation, a supplement may be required to reach the recommended dose of at least 300 mg of EPA+DHA per day of which at least 200 mg are from DHA [60].

SUMMARY

Familiarity with the various bariatric surgical procedures, their expected outcomes, and their potential complications can inform clinical decisions on suitability of bariatric surgery and nutritional approaches preoperatively.

Since bariatric surgery is becoming an increasingly more common therapy for the obese patient, clinicians may also want to be aware of the associated changes in nutritional needs long term. Evaluation of nutrient status of a patient who has undergone bariatric surgery even decades earlier may reveal treatable deficiencies exacerbating seemingly unrelated medical conditions.

SUMMARY LIST OF CLINICAL RECOMMENDATIONS

- Bariatric surgery procedures can have a tremendous impact on appropriate patients, although they are not without risk.
- Consider bariatric surgery for patients with a BMI > 40 kg/m2 or for patients with a BMI > 35 kg/m2 with two or more medical comorbidities.
- Currently, the most commonly performed procedures are the Roux-en-Y gastric bypass (RYGB), the adjustable gastric band, and the sleeve gastrectomy; RYGB produces the greatest percent excess body weight lost.
- There are no definitive answers on the benefits of preoperative weight loss; however, it may be most beneficial for patients with nonalcoholic fatty liver disease.
- Patients who have had a RYGB or a similar procedure may experience dumping syndrome, characterized by gastrointestinal and vasomotor symptoms; thus patients should avoid simple sugars and concentrated sweets, high-fat foods, and alcohol.
- A large percentage of bariatric surgery patients are women of childbearing age and special consideration is needed for the postsurgery pregnant patient.
- Strict adherence to vitamin-mineral supplementation to reduce the risk of nutritional deficiencies is required for life. The most common micronutrient deficiencies are iron, vitamin B12, vitamin D, and vitamin B1, although other deficiencies have been described. Nutritional lab work should be evaluated at least annually.
- All patients should aim to eat lean protein sources, low-fat dairy, whole fruits and vegetables, high-fiber foods, and omega-3 fatty acids. Patients should eat 60–80 grams of high-quality protein, at least 130 grams of high fiber carbohydrates, and some unsaturated fats.

REFERENCES

1. Deveney CW, Martindale RG. Factors in selecting the optimal bariatric procedure for a specific patient and parameters by which to measure appropriate response to surgery. *Curr Gastroenterol Rep.* 2010;12:296–303.
2. Buchwald H, Avidor Y, Braunwald E, Jensen MD, Pories W, Fahrbach K, Schoelles K. Bariatric surgery. A systemic review and meta-analysis. *J Am Med Assoc.* 2004;292:1724–1734.
3. O'Brien PE, Sawyer SM, Laurie C, et al. Laparoscopic adjustable gastric banding in severely obese adolescents. A randomized trial. *J Am Med Assoc.* 2010;303:519–526.
4. Sjostrom L, Narbro K, Sjorstrom CD, et al. Effects of bariatric surgery on mortality in Swedish obese patients. *N Engl J Med.* 2007;357:741–752.
5. Adams TD, Gress RE, Smith SC, et al. Long-term mortality after gastric bypass surgery. *N Engl J Med.* 2007;357:741–752.
6. Keating CL, Dixon JB, O'Brien PE. Bariatric surgery was dominant over conventional therapy for lifetime management of type 2 diabetes in obese patients. *Ann Intern Med.* 2009;151:JC2–JC15.
7. Sjorstrom L, Lindroos A-K, Peltonen M, et al. Lifestyle, diabetes and cardiovascular risk factors 10 years after bariatric surgery. *N Engl J Med.* 2004;351:2683–2693.
8. Key TJ, Schatzkin A, Willett WC, Allen NE, Spencer EA, Travis RC. Diet, nutrition and the prevention of cancer. *Publ Health Nutr.* 2004;7:187–200.
9. Mechanick JI, Kushner RF, Sugerman HJ, et al. American Association of Clinical Endocrinologists, The Obesity Society, and American Society for Metabolic and Bariatric Surgery medical guidelines for clinical practice for the perioperative nutritional, metabolic, and nonsurgical support of the bariatric surgery patient. *Surg Obes Rel Dis.* 2008;4:S109–S184.
10. Cummings DE, Overduin J, Foster-Schubert KE. Gastric bypass for obesity: Mechanisms of weight loss and diabetes resolution. *J Clin Endocrinol Metab.* 2004;89:2608–2615.
11. Shikora SA, Kim J, Tanoff ME. Nutritional and gastrointestinal complications of bariatric surgery. *Nutr Clin Prac.* 2007;22:29–40.
12. Chapman AE, Kiroff G, Game P, Foster B, O'Brien P, Ham J, Maddern GJ. Laparoscopic adjustable gastric banding in the treatment of obesity: A systematic literature review. *Surgery.* 2004;135:326–51.
13. Scopinaro N, Marinari G, Camerini G, Papadia F; 2004 ABS Consensus Conference. Biliopancreatic diversion for obesity: State of the art. *Surg Obes Relat Dis.* 2005;317–328.

14. Doolen JL, Miller SK. Primary care management of patients following bariatric surgery. *J Am Acad Nurse Pract.* 2005;17(11)446–450.

15. Higa K, Ho T, Tercero F, Yunus T, Boone KB. Laparoscopic roux-en-y gastric bypass: 10 year follow-up. *Surg Obes Rel Dis.* 2011;7:516–525.

16. Shinogle JA, Owings MF, Kozak LJ. Gastric bypass as treatment for obesity: Trends, characteristics, and complications. *Obes Res.* 2005. 13;2202–2209.

17. Abeles D, Shikora SA. Bariatric surgery: Current concepts and future directions. *Aesthetic Surgery Journal.* 2008; 28(1):79–84.

18. Korner J, Inabnet W, Conwell IM, et al. Differential effects of gastric bypass and banding on circulating gut hormones and leptin levels. *Obesity.* 2006;14(9):1553–1561.

19. Beckman LM, Beckman TR, Earthman CP. Review: Changes in gastrointestinal hormones and leptin after roux-en-y gastric bypass procedure: A review. *J Am Diet Assoc.* Apr 2010;110(4):571–584.

20. Kojima M, Hosoda H, Date Y, Nakazato M, Matsuo H, Kangawa K. Ghrelin is a growth-hormone-releasing acylated peptide from stomach. *Nature.* Dec 1999;402(6762):656–660.

21. Cummings DE, Shannon MH. Ghrelin and gastric bypass: Is there a hormonal contribution to surgical weight loss? *J Clin Endocrinol Metab.* 2003;88:2999–3002.

22. Cummings DE, Weigle DS, Frayo RS, Breen PA, Ma MK, Dellinger EP, Purnell JQ. Human plasma ghrelin levels after diet-induced weight loss and gastric bypass surgery. *N Engl J Med.* 2002;346: 1623–1630.

23. Aylwin S. Gastrointestinal surgery and gut hormones. *Curr Opin Endocrinol Diabetes.* 2005;12:89–98.

24. Drucker DJ. Enhancing incretin action for the treatment of type 2 diabetes. *Diabetes Care.* 2003;26:2929–2940.

25. Tadross JA, Le Roux CW. Review: The mechanisms of weight loss after bariatric surgery. *Int J Obesity.* 2009;33:S28–S32.

26. le Roux CW, Aylwin SJB, Batterham RL, Borg CM, Coyle F, Prasad V, Shurey S, Ghatei MA, Patel AG, Bloom SR. Gut hormone profiles following bariatric surgery favor an anorectic state, facilitate weight loss, and improve metabolic parameters. *Ann Surg.* 2006;243:108–114.

27. Consensus Development Conference Panel. NIH conference: Gastrointestinal surgery for severe obesity. *Ann Intern Med.* 1991;115:956–961.

28. Brethauer S. ASMBS position statement on preoperative supervised weight loss requirements. *Surg Obes Rel Dis.* 2011;7:257–260.

29. Van der Weijgert EJHM, Russler CH, Elte JWF. Long term follow up after gastric bypass surgery for morbid obesity: Preoperative weight loss improves the long term control of morbid obesity after vertical banded gastroplasty. *Obes Surg.* 1999;9:426 –432.

30. Alami RS, Morton JM, Schuster R, Lie J, Sanchez BR, Peters A, Curet MJ. Is there a benefit to pre-operative weight loss in gastric bypass patients? A prospective randomized trial. *Surg Obes Rel Dis.* 2007;3:141–145.

31. Sadhasivam S, Larson CJ, Lambert PJ, Mathiason MA, Kothari SN. Refusals, denials, and patient choice: Reasons prospective patients do not undergo bariatric surgery. *Surg Obes Relat Dis.* 2007;3:531– 536.

32. Edholm D, Kullberg J, Haenni A, Karlsson FA, Ahlstrom A, Hedberg J, Ahlstrom H, Sundbom, M. Preoperative 4-week low-calorie diet reduces liver volume and intrahepatic fat, and facilitates laparo-scopic gastric bypass in morbidly obese. *Obes Surg.* 2011;21:345–350.

33. Van Nieuwenhove Y, Dambrauskas Z, Campillo-Soto A, van Dielen F, Wiezer R, Janssen I, Kramer M, Thorell. Preoperative very low-calorie diet and operative outcome after laparoscopic gastric bypass. *Arch Surg.* 2011;146(11):1300–1305.

34. Benjaminov O, Beglaibter N, Gindy L, Spivak H, Singer P, Wienberg M, Stark A, Rubin M. The effect of a low-carbohydrate diet on the nonalcoholic fatty liver in morbidly obese patients before bariatric surgery. *Surg Endosc.* 2007;21:1423–1427.

35. Aills, L., Blankenship, J., Buffington, C., Furtado, M., Parrott, J. ASMBS allied health nutritional guide-lines for the surgical weight loss patient. *Surg Obes Rel Dis.* 2008;4, S73–S108.

36. Petitpain D, Budak A, DesMarteau J, Durkalski V, Byrne TK. Preoperative vitamin D status in potential bariatric surgery patients. *Bariatric Nursing and Surgical Patient Care.* 2010:5(3):255–260.

37. Kim J, Tarnoff M, Shikora S. Surgical treatment for extreme obesity: Evolution of a rapidly growing field. *Nutrition in Clinical Practice.* 2003;18:109–123.

38. Coleman KJ, Toussi R, Fujioka K. Do gastric bypass patient characteristics, behavior, and health differ depending upon how successful weight loss is defined? *Obes Surg.* 2010;20:1385–1392.

39. Magro DO, Geloneze B, Delfini R, Pareja BC, Callejas F, Pareja JC. Long-term weight regain after gas-tric bypass: A 5-year prospective study. *Obes Surg.* 2008;18:648–651.

40. Hsu LK, Benotti PN, Dwyer J, Roberts SB, Saltzman E, Shikora S, Rolls BJ, Rand W. Nonsurgical factors that influence the outcome of bariatric surgery: A review. *Psychosom Med.* 1998;60: 338–346.

41. Vogel SB. Remedial operations for postgastrectomy and postvagotomy syndromes. In: *Current Surgical Therapy* (6th ed.), ed J.L. Cameron. St. Louis: Mosby, Inc., 1998.

42. Ukleja, A. Dumping syndrome. *Pract Gastroenterol.* 2006; 35:32–46.

43. Maggard MA, Yermilov I, Li Z, et al. Pregnancy and fertility following gastric bypass surgery: A systematic review. *J Am Med Assoc.* 2008;300(19):2286–2296.

44. Wax JR, Cartin A, Wolff R, Lepich S, Pinette MG. Pregnancy following gastric bypass surgery for morbid obesity: Maternal and neonatal outcomes. *Obes Surg.* 2008;18:540–544.

45. Harris AA, Barger MK. Specialized care for women pregnant after bariatric surgery. *J Midwifery Womens Health.* 2010;55:529–539.

46. American College of Obstetritians and Gynecologists. ACOG practice bulletin no. 105: Bariatric surgery and pregnancy. *Obstet Gynecol.* 2009;113:1405–1413.

47. Aarts EO, Janssen IMG, Berends FJ. The gastric sleeve: Losing weight as fast as micronutrients? *Obes Surg.* 2011; 21:207–211.

48. Brolin RE, Gorman JH, Gorman RC, et al. Prophylactic iron supplementation after roux-en-y gastric bypass: A prospective, double-blind, randomized study. *Arch Surg.* 1998;133:740–744.

49. Kushner R. Managing micronutrient deficiencies in the bariatric surgical patient. *Obesity Management.* 2005; 203–206.

50. Vargus-Ruiz AG, Hernandez-Rivera G, Herrera MF. Prevalence of iron, folate and vitamin B12 deficiency anemia after laparoscopic roux-en-y gastric bypass. *Obes Surg.* 2008;18:288–293.

51. Slater GH, Ren CJ, Seigel N, et al. Serum fat-soluble vitamin deficiency and abnormal calcium metabolism after malabsorptive bariatric surgery. *J Gasrointest Surg.* 2004;8:48–55.

52. Sanchez-Hernandez J, Ybarra J, Gich I, De Leiva A, Rius X, Rodriguez-Espinosa J, Perez A. Effects of bariatric surgery on vitamin D status and secondary hyperparathyroidism: A prospective study. *Obesity Surgery.* 2005; 15:1389–1395.

53. Lin E, Armstrong-Moore D, Liang Z, Sweeney JF, Torres WE, Ziegler TR, Tangpricha V, Gletsu-Miller N. Contribution of adipose tissue to plasma 25-hydroxyvitamin D concentrations during weight loss following gastric bypass surgery. *Obesity.* 2011;19(3):588–594.

54. Pramyothin P, Biancuzzo RM, Lu Z, Hess DT, Apovian CM, Holick MF. Vitamin D in adipose tissue and serum 25-hydroxyvitamin D after roux-en-y gastric bypass. *Obesity.* 2011;19(11):2228–2234.

55. Holick MF. Vitamin D deficiency. *N Engl J Med.* 2007;357:266–281.

56. Valentino D, Sriram K, Shankar P. Update on micronutrients in bariatric surgery. *Curr Opin Clinic Nutr Metab Care.* 2011; 14:635–641.

57. Taylor J, Leitman IM, Horowitz M. Is routine cholecystectomy necessary at the time of roux-en-Y gastric bypass? *Obes Surg.* 2006;16:759–761.

58. DeMaria EJ. Bariatric surgery for morbid obesity. *N Engl J Med.* 2007;356(21):2176–2183.

59. Crowell MD, Decker GA, Levy R, Jeffrey R, Talley NJ. Gut-brain neuropeptides in the regulation of ingestive behaviors and obesity. *Am J Gastroenterol.* 2006;101:2848–2856.

60. Brenna JT, Lipillonne A. Background paper on fat and fatty acid requirements during pregnancy and lactation. *Ann Nutr Metab.* 2009;55:97–122.

61. Institute of Medicine. *Dietary Reference Intakes for Energy, Carbohydrate, Fiber, Fat, Fatty Acids, Cholesterol, Protein and Amino Acids.* Washington, DC: National Academy Press, 2005.

Section IV

Endocrine and Dermatologic Disorders

18 Obesity

Primary Care Approaches to Weight Reduction

Ingrid Kohlstadt, M.D., M.P.H.

INTRODUCTION

Experts agree on two critical aspects of obesity. A 5–10% reduction in weight improves overall health among obese and overweight individuals. Combining proven strategies for weight reduction increases success.

These points of agreement amidst a controversial epidemic raise discussion about the physician's role in helping patients lose weight. Since advice from healthcare professionals can significantly increase patient motivation and a medical doctor is perceived as the best source of health information [1], it is sometimes recommended that physicians add dietary counseling to already full office visits. The U.S. Preventive Services Task Force found fair to good evidence for intensive behavioral dietary counseling where obesity increases disease risk [2]. However, nutritionists, dieticians, and specifically trained nurses also provide dietary counseling, often more cost effectively than physicians [2]. This chapter refocuses the physician's role in weight management, underscoring the evidence base for diagnosing and treating underlying metabolic disturbances with food and nutrient therapies.

EPIDEMIOLOGY

Epidemiologic tools have reshaped the understanding of obesity and underscore the importance of early intervention including food and nutrient therapies.

Women of childbearing age with type 2 diabetes have offspring who are at greater risk of childhood obesity and insulin resistance [3]. While risk was previously viewed as genetic [4], it is now appreciated that the risk is also conferred by potentially modifiable environmental factors beginning in utero. Twin studies do not fully distinguish between genetic and in utero environmental factors [5]. Barker's epidemiologic study of a food embargo during World War II was the first of several to show that maternal starvation during the first half of pregnancy confers a greater risk of obesity and diabetes among the adult offspring [6]. Subsequently demonstrated in population studies, Jirtle and Dolinoy's research in animal models demonstrated that bisphenol-A can cause an obesity gene to be expressed, while genisten found in soy and folate found in vegetables can counteract the toxin and switch the obesity gene off [7,8]. Lactation, often considered an extension of the in utero environment, is protective against obesity.

Epidemiologic research tools have also demonstrated that weight recidivism is common, and prevention commensurately more critical. Because of the redundant biologic systems in place to defend body weight, treatment plans are multifaceted, combining lifestyle strategies [9] with medical and surgical approaches.

The population at risk for obesity has broadened. All racial and ethnic groups appear vulnerable despite unique dietary and genetic factors. Women and men are now almost equally affected. Onset is occurring at younger ages, giving rise to sub-epidemics of previously rare medical conditions such as slipped capital femoral epiphysis, polycystic ovary syndrome, precocious puberty, and childhood onset of type 2 diabetes.

PATHOGENESIS

CALORIC INTAKE VERSUS DIETARY QUALITY

Potentially the most scientifically contentious aspect of the pathophysiology of obesity is the calorie intake and expenditure equation. To what extent is weight a function of calories? Animal studies and clinical trials in free-living humans have shown a tight correlation with caloric balance and weight reduction. Consequently, calorie counting became the center of dietary strategies and the term "overnutrition" was previously used to describe obesity. Current evidence demonstrates that not only caloric balance but dietary quality is important, especially in preventing diabetes, insulin resistance, and nonalcoholic fatty liver disease. The emerging refocus on dietary quality is merited on several lines of reasoning:

- Diets that are proinflammatory increase insulin resistance and predispose to unfavorable body composition, essentially lowering an individual's metabolic rate over time.
- Diets influence the microbiome, which has recently been shown to be a measurable, quantifiable risk factor of obesity [10].
- Dietary quality influences appetite both short term through glycemic index and fiber content, and long term through insulin resistance and dyslipidemia. From a practical clinical vantage point, food cravings, hunger, and delayed satiety limit a patient's ability to maintain a reduced-calorie diet. The most successful diets are those to which patients can adhere [11].
- Processed foods can introduce noncaloric food components such as sweeteners, allergens, preservatives, xenobiotics, and metal toxicants. Such components, even though they do not contribute to calorie intake directly, are neuroactive (Chapter 28: Migraine Headaches and Chapter 29: Attention Deficit Hyperactivity Disorder) and promote weight gain across different mechanisms.
- Obesity increases the pretest probability of micronutrient deficiencies [12,13] attributed in part to overconsumption of nutrient-sparse foods.
- Diet quality influences concurrent medical conditions that can directly promote weight gain or indirectly promote weight gain through medications, immobility, or metabolic dysfunction [14].
- Poor diets can lead to fatigue and reduced energy expenditure (Chapter 34: Fibromyalgia).

In sum, various lines of research converge suggesting that an emphasis on diet quality is merited in weight management.

SARCOPENIA

Muscle loss contributes to obesity. Because skeletal muscle at rest burns six calories per pound per day compared to the two calories per pound per day of adipose tissue, mathematically muscle loss without reduced calorie intake would lead to weight gain.

Muscle loss often heralds obesity clinically. The biologic bases for this observation are many.

- Obesity is associated with inflammation, nutrient deficiencies, inefficient use of dietary protein, and impaired insulin-like growth factor 1 (IGF-1), all of which damage muscle tissue.
- Obesity may limit the physical activity needed for maintenance of lean tissue.
- Losing weight and regaining it, sometimes called "yo-yo dieting" or weight recidivism, nets muscle loss because adipose is regained more quickly than is muscle.
- Obesity can mask muscle atrophy and delay diagnosis of sarcopenic obesity.
- Obesity may have resulted from medications that simultaneously increase adipose and decrease lean tissue.
- Obesity alters protein usage, leaving inadequate protein for anabolic functions.
- In striking contrast to dieting humans, hibernating mammals and aestivating frogs do not lose skeletal muscle. The esoteric observation suggests there is much more for science to learn about the molecular controls of muscle and fat accumulation [15].

BIOPHYSICAL PARAMETERS

Obesity poses biophysical challenges directly related to the increase in adipose tissue relative to lean tissue. The biophysical changes may help explain why obesity is a diabetes risk factor apart from insulin resistance and fatty liver disease [16]. Biophysical changes associated with obesity include:

Paucity of body water: Fat is relatively anhydrous. While a healthy weight adult has 60–65% body water, someone who is extremely obese tends to have a total body water of 35–45%. Disproportionate (allometric) growth of adipose may increase vulnerability to dehydration [17], which is strikingly common [18].

Suppressed metabolic rate: Body water is involved in removing heat and chemical byproducts from metabolic reactions. In order to satisfy the physiologic priorities of temperature and pH, exothermic, acid-producing pathways such as fat oxidation are suppressed, a mechanism that could help explain lower-than-predicted metabolic rates observed with extreme obesity [19].

Impaired transport of fat-soluble nutrients and toxins: Vitamin D travels from the epidermis where it is synthesized to the liver where it becomes partially activated. Obesity is associated with low levels of vitamin D in the serum and adequate levels in adipose tissue. Other fat-soluble vitamins such as lutein, xeoxanthin, and lycopene may be similarly stored in adipose, rendering the nutrients unavailable elsewhere. Also inadequately studied are the adverse effects of fat-soluble toxins [20], which become released into circulation during weight reduction.

In sum, biophysical effects influence metabolic parameters. Biophysical effects of obesity underscore the need for hydration, adequate electrolytes, incorporation of alkalinizing foods such as most minimally processed fruits and vegetables, and monitoring and possible supplementation of fat-soluble vitamins and phytonutrients.

DISRUPTED CHRONOBIOLOGY

Successful weight reduction must overcome the body's internal workings and create "unhomeostasis" until a new benchmark can be obtained and maintained. Subtle cues of circadian patterns, neurotransmitter sufficiency, meal timing, rate of eating, and the aroma of foods influence food intake—often bypassing the neocortex and the corresponding awareness associated with neocortical stimulation.

During unhomeostasis patients are thought to be more vulnerable to external and internal cues. Shift work and jet lag are associated with obesity [21]. Melatonin may mediate some of these effects [22]. Sunlight and full-spectrum lighting favorably influence melatonin release. Cell phone use has been shown to alter brain protein configurations [23] and glucose metabolism [24], sufficient to disrupt appetite-related chronobiology. The findings merit further research.

PATIENT EVALUATION

OFFICE ENVIRONMENT

The office environment helps communicate to patients that it is indeed safe and appropriate to discuss their weight problem during the physician encounter. A screening checklist is as follows: chairs accommodate patients with weight issues, office scales are discretely placed, large exam gowns are provided, large-size blood pressure cuffs are used when needed, and staff uses neutral words such as "weight issue" or "excess weight."

PATIENT HISTORY

Questions to establish baseline parameters and guide discussions about diet and weight loss include the following.

What do you eat for breakfast? Eating breakfast improves metabolic rate. Patients who skip breakfast miss out on boosting their metabolic rate and may have underlying insulin resistance and elevated triglycerides. Food selection at breakfast can prevent or promote food cravings throughout the day.

How is your digestion? Irregular bowel patterns, heartburn, and constipation influence food selection. Impaired digestion can point to gallbladder disease, use of artificial sweeteners, food allergies or intolerances, and an opportunity to increase fiber, magnesium, vitamin C, and hydration.

What has helped you lose weight in the past (if they have tried)? Diet patterns, nutritional programs, supplements, prescription medications, surgeries, and fitness programs that have been helpful in the past are likely to be helpful again as the patient's metabolism is optimized. Nonmedically advised weight loss, eating disorders, depressed mood, and risks for muscle atrophy might also be identified.

Practitioners may want to address specific risk factors for weight gain, especially those with an iatrogenic component. Examples that arise with some frequency include:

- Recently quitting smoking
- Orthopedic injury
- Discontinuation of a stimulant medication such as methylphenidate (Ritalin)
- Initiation of any centrally acting medication
- Fertility treatments in women
- Treatment of celiac disease

PHYSICAL EXAM

Monitoring Fat and Muscle Mass

Reduction in adipose tissue can be estimated by monitoring waist circumference, waist to hip ratio, bioimpedence (BIA) [25], and resting metabolic rate. Clinical assessment can be supported by imaging studies such as dual energy X-ray absorptiometry (DEXA). DEXA technically assesses bone densitometry and body composition, although not all facilities utilize this feature. Obesity and muscle atrophy coexist in a condition known as sarcopenic obesity, which predicts mortality [26] and often responds to treatment (Chapter 33: Surgery).

Neck Circumference

Neck circumference is a predictor of sleep apnea and its severity [27]. Since obstructive sleep apnea is obesogenic [28] [29], treatment with positive airway pressure should not be delayed due to intended weight reduction but used in conjunction [30].

First Cranial Nerve Assessment

First cranial nerve (CNI) impairment can be diagnosed by holding an alcohol swab a measured distance from the patient's nose as described in Chapter 2: Chemosensory Disorders. Making patients aware of their deficit in olfaction and taste helps them avoid inadvertent over sweetening or over salting of food.

Oral Cavity

Xerostomia, periodontal disease, tooth decay, amalgam fillings, and odor may indicate barriers to weight reduction, including dehydration, unfavorable microbiota, inadequate mastication, under-methylation, and insulin resistance.

Hydration Status

Dry mucus membranes, pedal edema, poor skin turgor, and a dry mouth generally indicate intra-cellular dehydration, and can be corroborated with urine specific gravity. Since muscle is more hydrous than fat and therefore conducts a current more quickly, poor hydration is associated with less favorable BIA.

Moderate Pressure to Shin Bones

Applying moderate pressure to an adult patient's shin bones or ribs is associated with discomfort when osteomalacia is present. Osteomalacia is a late but not rare manifestation of vitamin D deficiency and obesity elevates risk [31,12]. Clinical findings should be corroborated with laboratory testing and treated. Even moderately low vitamin D levels forestall weight loss by perpetuating insulin resistance, possibly lowering mood, and limiting physical activity [12,32,33].

TREATMENT: OVERVIEW

Diagnostic tests that inform the treatment of obesity are presented in Table 18.1.

Primary care is viewed as central to the nexus of choices for weight reduction. Asking patients about their perceived weight and willingness to lose weight when indicated is well aligned with current treatment options. Figure 18.1 presents a conventional algorithm for approaching weight reduction.

One in three patients sustained clinically meaningful weight loss following behavioral counseling from their primary care physician [34]. Counseling included quarterly physician visits with education on weight management, monthly sessions with a lifestyle coach on behavioral weight control, and either a meal replacement or a weight-loss medication.

Pharmacotherapy can augment the treatment results. New agents are anticipated to receive a Food and Drug Administration (FDA)–approved treatment indication for obesity. Currently available drug treatment results show but modest benefit [35] and opportunity costs can be significant. For example, expense precludes some patients from using both nutrients and medications, medications may unfavorably alter food selection, and medications impair absorption in patients with preexisting nutrient depletion.

Physician referral to community programs can be viewed as an effective early intervention [36,37]. Internet-delivered interventions are being studied [38].

Referral to obesity treatment centers may be region specific. Considerations for surgical treatment are presented in Chapter 17: Bariatric Surgery.

TREATMENT—MINIMIZING OBESOGENIC EFFECTS OF MEDICATIONS

Food-drug interactions are covered only modestly in the medical literature, suggesting that they may be under recognized [39,40]. Informing patients of the possibility of appetite deregulation may prompt a joint decision to choose another medication, use a lower dose, or modify environmental

TABLE 18.1
Nutritional Diagnostic Tests to Guide Weight Reduction

Test	Interpretation	Mechanism(s)	Treatment	Relevance to Weight Loss
Albumin (serum)	Low suggests protein malnutrition	Inadequate intake; malabsorption potentially from prior bariatric surgery	Dietary protein; supplemental amino acids; digestive enzymes	Maintain lean body mass
C-Reactive Protein (CRP)	High sensitivity CRP should be below 10 mg/L	Inflammation from various sources including food allergies and weight reduction	Supplemental fiber; alkaline diet; avoidance of food allergens; supplemental curcumin 2–4 g/d	Inflammation exacerbates preexisting sarcopenic obesity
Carnitine	Deficiency if low plasma carnitine or elevated urinary excretion of adipic, suberic, and ethylmalonic acids	Impaired absorption; decreased synthesis; high demand during fat metabolism	Supplemental L-carnitine 2 grams/ day	Fat metabolism increases demand for carnitine
Carotenes (fractionated serum or plasma)	a-Carotene: 9–101 µg/L b-Carotene: 42–373 µg/L Lutein: 50–250 µg/L Zeaxanthin: 8–80 µg/L	Impaired absorption; reduced intake; increased oxidative stress; sequestration in excess adipose tissue	Green leafy vegetables; cooking with spices and phytonutrient-rich cooking oils; phytonutrient supplements	Obesity is a risk factor for reduced fat-soluble nutrients
Coenzyme Q10	Low serum CoQ10 signifies depletion of tissue CoQ10; high levels of pyruvate, succinate, fumarate, and malate in the urine suggest insufficient CoQ10 to meet energy pathway demands	Nutrient deficiencies and medications can interfere with synthesis	Supplemental CoQ10 up to 300 mg/day	Fat metabolism increases demand for coenzyme Q10
DEXA	Evaluate for sarcopenic obesity and adequate bone mineral density	Sarcopenic obesity and osteopenia from various causes	Dietary protein during weight reduction; supplemental amino acids; digestive enzymes to increase protein absorption; alkaline diet for bone and muscle health during weight reduction; coordinate with medically supervised physical activity	Used to diagnose and monitor sarcopenic obesity
Fatty Acid Profile (various)	Erythrocyte fatty acid profiles can identify omega-3, omega-6, trans, very long chain and saturated fatty acids	Skewed dietary intake; inappropriate supplement use; reduced delta-6 desaturase enzyme activity; fat malabsorption	Balance mono- and polyunsaturated fatty acids with diet and supplements	Guides strategic use of dietary and supplemental fatty acids for weight reduction; fatty acid imbalances may stem from prior medical or surgical treatment of obesity

TABLE 18.1 (*continued*)
Nutritional Diagnostic Tests to Guide Weight Reduction

Test	Interpretation	Mechanism(s)	Treatment	Relevance to Weight Loss
Homocysteine	Elevation signifies deficiency in vitamin B12, folate or vitamin B6.	Impaired absorption and inadequate intake of vitamin B12, folate or vitamin B6	Supplementation of folate and vitamin B12 to improve methylation	Maintain energy metabolism
Iron Studies	Low ferritin and % saturation < =15 suggest iron deficient erythropoesis even when HCT is normal; elevation suggests hemochromatosis.	Deficiency from impaired absorption; inadequate intake; excess from primary hemochromatosis, a nutrient-gene interaction	Treat deficiency with supplemental minerals, dietary iron, and cooking with an iron skillet; hemochromatosis is managed medically and by minimizing dietary iron intake	Deficiency tends to coexist with other mineral deficiencies, exacerbated by some diets; iron, zinc, and chromium alter food preferences; hemochromatosis contributes to the inflammatory component of obesity
Magnesium	Erythrocyte (RBC) magnesium below laboratory-specified range	Impaired absorption, inadequate dietary intake, competitive absorption with calcium	Increase fruit and vegetable intake; supplement calcium and magnesium in a ratio of 2:1	Optimizing magnesium supports hydration and fat metabolism
Resting Metabolic Rate (RMR)	RMR lower than predicted may suggest thyroid dysfunction or loss of lean tissue. Various medications may influence RMR	Low RMR may suggest sarcopenia.	Establish plan for preventing further muscle atrophy with exercise and adequate protein.	Allows diagnosis and treatment of a low metabolic rate
Thyroid Stimulating Hormone	Above 2 mIU/L, further evaluation	Lowered metabolic rate and marked decrease in exercise tolerance	If Hashimoto's, treat as per Chapter 20: Hashimoto's Thyroiditis	Maintain optimal metabolic rate; reduce myalgias, fatigue and gastrointestinal symptoms
Triglycerides	Fasting values above 100 mg/dl or even 75 mg/dl suggest impaired fat metabolism	Steatosis, increased oxidative stress, consumption of synthetic fats, and refined carbohydrates	Diet low in refined carbohydrates and no trans or highly processed fats; liver support; supplemental l-carnitine 2 g/d	Elevated triglycerides represent a treatable impairment in fat metabolism.
Urinalysis	A specific gravity above 1.025 suggests inadequate hydration; the presence of protein may require further evaluation	Medical barriers to adequate hydration may be present; urinary protein losses can suggest chronic kidney disease	Address medical barriers to hydration; diet may need to be modified if chronic kidney disease is present.	Hydration facilitates weight reduction. Urine protein loss may require modifying a patient's diet.
Vitamin B12	Serum concentration under 540 pg/ml and elevated urine methylmalonate, homocysteine, and mean cell volume suggest deficiency	Impaired absorption partly from drug interactions; reduced intake from some diets	Oral, sublingual, or IM supplementation	Maintain energy metabolism

continued

TABLE 18.1 (*continued*)
Nutritional Diagnostic Tests to Guide Weight Reduction

Test	Interpretation	Mechanism(s)	Treatment	Relevance to Weight Loss
Vitamin D	25(OH)D in the range of 30–40 ng/ml throughout the year	Malabsorption; inadequate sun exposure; obesity increase demand for preactivated vitamin D	50,000 IU of vitamin D2 weekly for eight weeks to achieve 30 ng/ml 25(OH)D; sunlight and dietary sources of fish, dairy, and mushrooms	Obesity is a risk factor for reduced fat-soluble nutrients. Optimizing vitamin D may facilitate weight reduction.

Note that only some tests are applicable for most patients, and their use depends on concurrent medical conditions or clinical suspicion.

factors. Collective decision making can improve adherence to pharmacotherapy. In contrast, patients not informed may skip their needed medication in order to lose weight, or they may gain weight, which could have been averted.

Medications that act in the central nervous system tend to influence appetite and satiety as detailed in Table 18.2. However, given the extensive input into the loci of appetite control, patients vary in their sensitivity to potentially obesogenic drugs. Table 18.3 highlights the effects of top-selling and commonly prescribed medications on appetite and weight. The following section presents obesogenic medications, mechanisms of action, and potential methods to reduce risk of weight gain.

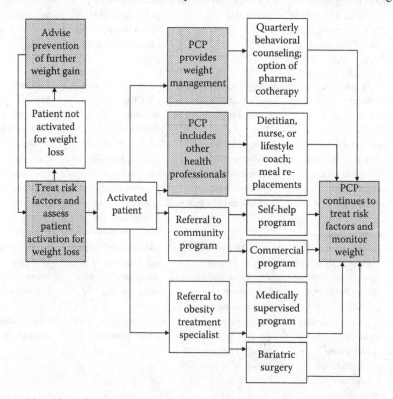

FIGURE 18.1. Algorithm of conventional treatment options in the primary care setting [34,117]. Shaded boxes symbolize the points in the algorithm where adjunctive food and nutrient therapies may be effectively included.

TABLE 18.2

Neuroendocrine Messengers of Appetite Regulation

Neuroendocrine Messenger	Increase Appetite Promote Weight Gain	Decrease Appetite Promote Weight Loss
Neuropeptides	• Neuropeptide Y (NPY) • Galanin	• Bombesin • Enterostatin (central action) • Corticotrophin releasing hormone (CRH) • Melanocyte stimulating hormone • Peptide analogues and antagonists (under development)
Neurotransmitters	• Serotonin antagonists • Dopamine antagonists • Mu and kappa opioids • Gamma amino butyric acid (GABA) • Histamine H1 antagonists • Norepinephrine α receptor agonists	• Serotonin agonists and reuptake inhibitors • Dopamine agonists and reuptake inhibitors • Mu and kappa opioid antagonists (under development) • Histamine H1 receptor agonists • Norepinephrine β receptor agonists
Central Action of Peripheral Hormones	• Insulin • Ghrelin (potentiating role) • Glucocorticoids • Adipocytokines (other than adiponectin) • Androgens • Progestins	• Glucagon-like peptide-1 • Leptin • Cholecystokinin (CCK) • Adiponection • Estrogen • Gut hormone peptide YY (PYY)

Source: Adapted from [114]. With permission.

MEDICATIONS FOR TYPE 2 DIABETES MELLITUS

Insulin increases appetite, whether it is exogenously administered or endogenously synthesized. An endogenous effect can occur when a diet high in refined carbohydrates or high-glycemic index foods is ingested. These foods rapidly raise blood glucose, which, in turn, induces insulin production. When the blood glucose drops as rapidly as it rose, the lingering insulin stimulates appetite, leading to weight gain.

Exogenous insulin similarly stimulates appetite, and the tighter the glucose control, the greater the effect of insulin on appetite and weight gain [41]. Patients receiving hypoglycemic medications for tight glucose control have gained statistically more weight than those whose diabetes was managed by diet alone.

Three classes of medications stimulate endogenous insulin release, with varied effects on weight: sulfonylureas, incretin mimetics, and gliptins. Sulfonylureas increase appetite by stimulating endogenous insulin secretion from the beta cells of the pancreas. Sulfonylureas have been associated with weight gain.

Incretin mimetics are long-acting analogs of the gastric hormones called incretins such as glucagons-like peptide-1 (GLP-1) that stimulate insulin release. However, in addition to stimulating insulin release, which would promote appetite and weight gain, they delay gastric emptying, which results in a net reduction of food intake. Their use in treatment of type 2 diabetes mellitus (DM), has not been associated with weight gain when combined with either metformin or a sulfonylurea [42].

A newer class of drugs that stimulates insulin release is the dipeptidyl peptidase-4 (DPP-4) inhibitors or gliptins. They inhibit the enzyme DDP-4, which inactivates GLP-1, thereby potentiating

TABLE 18.3

Most Commonly Prescribed Medicines and Top-Selling Medications in the United States in 2010 and Potential Effects on Body Weight

Medication	Prescriptions	Potential Effects on Weight
Hydrocodone (combined with acetaminophen)	131.2 million	None for short-term use
Generic Zocor (simvastatin)	94.1 million	May reduce exercise tolerance, promote insulin resistance, and deplete coenzyme Q10
Lisinopril (brand names include Prinivil and Zestril)	87.4 million	Weight neutral antihypertensive
Generic Synthroid (levothyroxine sodium)	70.5 million	Appropriate use optimizes metabolic rate
Generic Norvasc (amlodipine besylate)	57.2 million	Calcium channel blockers increase appetite centrally in some patients
Generic Prilosec (omeprazole)	53.4 million	May contribute to vitamin B12 deficiency and diet indiscretion
Azithromycin (brand names include Z-Pak and Zithromax)	52.6 million	None for short-term use
Amoxicillin (various brand names)	52.3 million	None for short-term use
Generic Glucophage (metformin)	48.3 million	Weight neutral but may lower vitamin B12
Hydrochlorothiazide (various brand names)	47.8 million	Promotes weight gain by several mechanisms [116]

Medication	Sales	Potential Effects on Weight
Lipitor—a cholesterol-lowering statin drug	$7.2 billion	May reduce exercise tolerance, promote insulin resistance, and deplete coenzyme Q10
Nexium—an antacid medication	$6.3 billion	May contribute to vitamin B12 deficiency (fatigue and impaired methylation) and diet indiscretion
Plavix—a blood thinner	$6.1 billion	Likely to be weight neutral
Advair Diskus—an asthma inhaler	$4.7 billion	Potentially protects against weight gain by reducing need for corticosteroids, however a boxed warning appears on the drug label
Abilify—an antipsychotic drug	$4.6 billion	Increases appetite centrally
Seroquel—an antipsychotic drug	$4.4 billion	Increases appetite centrally
Singulair—an oral asthma drug	$4.1 billion	Potentially protects against weight gain by reducing need for corticosteroids
Crestor—a cholesterol-lowering statin drug	$3.8 billion	May reduce exercise tolerance, promote insulin resistance, and deplete coenzyme Q10
Actos—a thiazolidinedione diabetes drug	$3.5 billion	Associated with weight gain
Epogen—an injectable anemia drug	$3.3 billion	Likely to be weight neutral

Source: Adapted from [115].

endogenous incretin and GLP-1. The advantage of gliptins over incretins is oral rather than subcutaneous administration. As with incretin mimetics, the delay in gastric emptying and resulting satiety may offer the net benefit of appetite reduction. Muscle pain that limits physical activity is cited among the common adverse effects and may emerge as a significant barrier to achieving lifestyle modification.

Thiazolidinediones contribute to adiposity and cardiovascular disease by encouraging the division and differentiation of fat cells [41]. The weight gain observed with thiazolidinediones has been more pronounced than with insulin [43]. In addition to promoting adipocyte cell differentiation, thiazolidinediones cause fluid retention and edema by reducing sodium excretion and increased capillary permeability [44]. More weight gain occurs with thiazolidinediones when they are combined with insulin therapy [45].

Metformin is a biguanide, a class of medications that acts by decreasing glucose production and improving liver sensitivity to insulin. One correctable effect is that metformin depletes vitamin B12 [46]. Metformin is a plant extract, as is the dietary supplement berberine, that is gaining scientific merit in both diabetes and weight management [47,48].

In summary, potential weight gain associated with hypoglycemic agents can be lessened by:

- Counseling patients on the potential effects of appetite, so they can anticipate and prevent weight gain with lifestyle modifications for both obesity and diabetes.
- Initiating metformin earlier in the course of diabetes and including incretins and DPP-4 inhibitors, where indicated.
- Diagnosing drug-nutrient interactions such as suboptimal vitamin B12.
- Treating comorbidities shown to exacerbate obesity such as sleep apnea, liver disease, and peripheral vascular disease.

MEDICATIONS FOR DYSLIPIDEMIA

Statins are the group of lipid-lowering medications that work by inhibiting the enzyme HMG-CoA reductase, the rate-limiting enzyme in the biosynthesis of cholesterol. A reduction in cholesterol synthesis leads to decrease in blood LDL levels. Despite the fact that statins are generally well tolerated drugs, their use is associated with myalgias and muscle atrophy [49], depletion of coenzyme Q10 (CoQ10) [50], and heightened risk of diabetes [51]. Nutritional approaches to treating dyslipidemia are detailed in Chapter 4: Dyslipidemia.

MEDICATIONS FOR HYPERTENSION

Thiazide diuretics [52], loop diuretics, calcium channel blockers, beta blockers, and alpha-adrenergic blockers can promote weight gain, generally by increasing appetite. Beta blockers reduce the cardiac response to exercise and can cause electrolyte abnormalities and predispose to nutritional deficiencies, including calcium and vitamin D depletion [53]. Generally the less centrally acting medications in a class tend to be less obesogenic. The angiotensin-converting enzyme (ACE) inhibitors and angiotensin receptor blockers used to treat hypertension appear to be weight neutral. In addition to lifestyle management, several foods, spices, nutrients, and dietary supplements act as diuretics, calcium channel blockers, and ACE inhibitors as elaborated in Chapter 6: Hypertension.

MEDICATIONS FOR GASTROESOPHAGEAL REFLUX

H2 blockers and proton-pump inhibitors alter appetite indirectly. When gastroesophageal reflux (GERD) stems from unhealthful dietary choices, medication is permissive. It removes the discomfort associated with having made a poor choice. Reducing stomach acid reduces absorption of nutrients vital to energy balance including vitamin B12, minerals such as magnesium and chromium [54], and amino acids.

ANTIHISTAMINES

Histamine potentiates leptin and its anorexigenic effect. Medications that block H1 or activate H3 receptors increase appetite by reducing leptin's central activity [55]. Patients may benefit from this information as they selection over-the-counter medications for rhinosinusitis and as sleep aides. Optimal hydration and select phytonutrients have been shown to reduce allergic rhinitis [56] and can be used alone or in conjunction with pharmacotherapy when needed.

STEROID HORMONES

Corticosteroids promote fat gain [39] and reduce muscle mass, thereby exerting two unfavorable influences on body composition. The orally inhaled steroids used in the treatment of asthma exert antiobesogenic effects. High-dose steroids used to prevent nausea from chemotherapy adversely influence body composition among cancer survivors who are a group at high risk for insulin resistance and weight gain. Nutrients modify inflammatory response and are used in adjunct to corticosteroid medications (Chapter 10: Asthma, and Chapter 15: Inflammatory Bowel Disease).

Sex steroids influence appetite, as demonstrated by the monthly fluctuation in hormone levels among women of childbearing age (Figure 18.2). During the luteal premenstrual phase, women take in 270 kcal more per day than during the preceding periovulatory phase [57]. Sex hormone imbalances arising from disease or medication exacerbate the normal variation in caloric intake. Through similar mechanisms xenoestrogenic toxins are obesogenic [58,59]. Therefore, hormonal contraceptives, agents that promote fertility, and medications to prevent prostate or breast cancer recurrence are appropriately anticipated to influence appetite.

Obesity in turn exacerbates sex hormone imbalances. Adipose tissue is an endocrine organ that converts androgens to estrogen. Steatohepatitis, if present, compromises the liver's ability to neutralize foreign estrogens and interconvert endogenous hormones. Polycystic ovary syndrome is associated with dietary obstacles such as sweet cravings, obesogenic fertility medications, bulimia nervosa, central adiposity, low cholecystokinin (a satiety peptide), and insulin resistance [60]. Once diagnosed, nutritional and pharmacologic strategies can improve insulin sensitivity and facilitate weight reduction.

ANTICONVULSANTS

Historically medications used to treat epilepsy increased appetite and weight [61]. For example, carbamazepine increases appetite and contributes to weight gain by causing fluid retention and fat deposition [62]. Several newer anticonvulsants can have the opposite effect; they are appetite stabilizing or even appetite suppressing and are being considered for the treatment of obesity. The ketogenic diet, used to treat epilepsy since the 1920s, is appetite suppressing, but safety and difficulty of use limited the suitability in many patients. The modified ketogenic diet is effective, better tolerated, and provides a more balanced nutrient intake [63] making diet a viable treatment option.

PSYCHOACTIVE MEDICATIONS

Psychotherapeutic agents that act on neurotransmitters cannot be assumed to be appetite neutral, and some can induce profound increases in appetite and subsequent increases in adiposity. For many

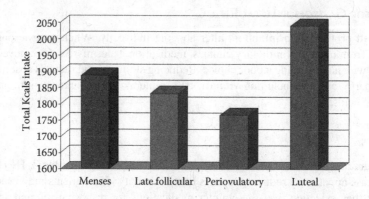

FIGURE 18.2. Calorie intake fluctuates with the phases of the menstrual cycle. (Adapted from [57]. With permission.)

patients, each viable pharmacotherapy is likely to increase appetite, compounding already serious clinical consequences. Patients with mental illness are at increased risk for metabolic syndrome [64] and a 10- to 15-year shorter life expectancy attributable to chronic medical illness [65].

The neuroactive metal lithium, a mood stabilizer, exerts its therapeutic effects centrally, where it also promotes accumulation of adipose through a yet to be elucidated mechanism. First generation antipsychotics such as haloperidol have long been implicated in creating oxidative stress and inducing apoptosis in the liver. Atypical antipsychotics such as risperidone can cause steatohepatitis and marked weight gain; among the mechanisms is upregulation of neuropeptide Y, an inducer for food intake [66].

Clinicians are not without options. Discussing the anticipated effects on weight may help prevent weight gain in some patients. Appetite stimulation does not necessarily translate into weight gain, although it is extremely difficult to prevent. An illustration of this point stems from the early clinical trials of atypical antipsychotics. The appetite stimulation and obesogenic potential of these medications were not fully appreciated in the first trials because participants were institutionalized patients who were served fixed-portion meals. An increase in intake is required for the obesogenic effects to manifest as weight gain. Weight gain is a common reason why patients discontinue their antipsychotic therapy, resulting in disease relapse [67]. Routinely monitoring body weight, liver function, fasting blood glucose, and lipid profiles in patients, as described in the drug labeling of atypical antipsychotic medications, can allow for prompt detection of nutritionally responsive adverse drug effects [68].

Some medications have fewer metabolic effects and may be used preferentially. The Clinical Antipsychotic Trials for Intervention Effectiveness study, a comparative effectiveness trial for the treatment of schizophrenia in adults, demonstrated that medications differ in their adverse metabolic profiles [67]. This research has been combined with other data to extrapolate the findings to pediatrics [68,69]. Pharmacological modalities are being considered to counteract weight gain. Among these are amantidine [70], fluoxetine [71], metformin [72], and topiramate. Additional approaches relevant to some patients are the modified ketogenic diet and the nutritional and environmental approach to bipolar illness described in Chapter 32: Bipolar Disorder.

TREATMENT—SPECIAL CIRCUMSTANCES

LACTATION

Breastfeeding helps mothers shed weight gained during pregnancy. At the same time breastfeeding protects the infant from obesity later in life. However, mothers with a BMI over 30 are more likely to decline lactation, have delayed onset of lactation, experience less prolactin response to suckling, and are prone to early cessation of breastfeeding. Methods to address these potential barriers to lactation include optimizing prenatal weight gain, limiting maternal-newborn separation, and massage or pumping of the breasts [73].

CHILDHOOD OBESITY

Treating obesity in childhood is a vital investment in a child's future: 80% of obese children become obese adults, comorbidities appear earlier in adults who were obese as children, and obesity in childhood reduces overall life expectancy [3]. Although special attention to the social and behavioral components of eating is necessary, food and nutrient interventions should be as early and intensive as possible.

When young children are unable to innately regulate calorie intake, it usually signals a metabolic disturbance. Causes of a metabolic disturbance and energy imbalance reach beyond dietary indiscretion. Common and often amenable disturbances include delayed healing time from injuries [74], depression, asthma, sleep disorders, and vitamin D deficiency.

Medications should be viewed through the lens of these findings: Children are receiving more medications to treat chronic diseases [75]. Some drug effects are unique to children [76]. Children are more vulnerable to central drug effects such as the effects on appetite and satiety [77]. Preexisting childhood obesity increases the vulnerability to adverse metabolic drug effects [77]. While only a few medications treat childhood obesity, many medications with pediatric indications [78] are relevant to weight management. For example, medications may increase appetite centrally, promote weight gain peripherally, represent a less obesogenic alternative, be prescribed alongside diet and exercise, or be contraindicated if obesity is present.

PRIOR BARIATRIC SURGERY

Surgical treatment of obesity extends life [79,80]. A 10-year follow-up study identified surgical weight reduction as tenfold more effective than lifestyle intervention and medication [35]. Bariatric surgery is no longer limited to permanent procedures. Reversible banding has achieved successful results as part of a comprehensive treatment of lifestyle modification, nutritional medicine, and surgery. Addressing nutrient deficiencies following bariatric surgery can help prevent weight recidivism [81,82]. Future bariatric surgery does not exclude nutritional interventions. On the contrary, surgical outcomes are enhanced by nutrient optimization and presurgical weight loss [82].

TREATMENT—DIETARY RESOURCES

SELECTING A DIET

Patients tend to know what diet plan or program they would like to try, only some of their selections are healthful and new diets emerge frequently, preventing a practitioner from becoming familiar with all diet options. Criteria by which to assess a diet's underlying metabolic effects are presented to help practitioners navigate the array of dietary options.

Criteria 1. Alkalinizing

Alkalinizing is a biochemical term for a diet that is bicarbonate generating instead of hydrogen ion donating [83]. As a generality, fruits and vegetables are alkalinizing and lean meats, grains, salt, and sugar—including fruit sugar—are acidifying. In practice, an alkaline diet includes more alkaline foods and accompanies healthful acidifying foods with alkalinizing ones. The Mediterranean, DASH, and Prudent (Chapter 37: Cancer and Insulin) are generally alkaline, and an alkalinizing diet can be assembled from most ethnic foods.

Criteria 2. Fatty Acid Strategic

Processed fats [84] and reduced-calorie fat substitutes [85] are associated with obesity in humans. Furthermore, processing removes the naturally occurring fat-soluble vitamins and fat-soluble phytonutrients recognized as insulin sensitizing, and supplemented or fortified nutrients do not confer equivalent antioxidant protection. Healthful fats promote weight reduction: Unprocessed fats add flavor to food potentially reducing the need for sweeteners and salt. Coconut and other tropical oils contain medium chain triglycerides shown to improve weight reduction [86]. A diet with a balanced omega-3 and omega-6 ratio [87] will reduce inflammation, improve cell signaling to convey appropriate satiety messages, and minimize the need for fatty acid supplements that are an overlooked source of calories.

Criteria 3. Compatible

Some diets may contain food allergens, are unlikely to meet nutritional needs, or can exacerbate an existing medical condition. For example, a patient with chronic kidney disease should exclude diets high in protein, while a dieting athlete is unlikely to achieve adequate protein or mineral intake on a nonsupplemented vegan diet.

USING SUBSTITUTIONS

An effective method for shifting a patient's dietary pattern is by implementing a series of substitutions. Substitutions can break down a complex shift in diet into small manageable steps and are among the least difficult forms of change. Ideally these changes will be implemented by all those who share meals with the patient.

- Replace trans and other processed fats with unrefined oils.
- Replace starches with whole grains, vegetables, berry fruits, and other fiber sources [88].
- Replace sugar with flavor.
- Replace calories with volume [89,90].
- Replace caloric beverages with water, herbal tea, and highly diluted juices [91] .
- Replace routine with variety by rotating diets, meal plans, and dining venues to help eating remain an enjoyable, portion-appropriate, and multisensory experience.

APPROACHES TO SWEETENERS

Eliminate sugar-sweetened beverages. Even though a meta-analysis demonstrated that fructose does not promote weight gain in short-term isocaloric diet studies [92], it increases appetite and people gain weight from using it [93]. Sports drinks emphasize the benefits of repleting electrolytes, however these beverages average 6% glucose. Only 2% glucose is needed for maximum uptake of water by enterocytes.

One commonly used substitution that is unlikely to be beneficial long term is replacing sugar with a low-calorie, high-intensity (artificial) sweetener. Several medically related problems can arise:

- The first ingredient in the sweetener packets is usually dextrose. Consuming several packets a day can impede glucose control in patients with diabetes.
- Artificial sweeteners are orders of magnitude sweeter than sugar. They tend to accustom the palette to a very sweet taste and may thereby increase total calorie intake long term.
- People may not be aware that certain diet foods contain artificial sweeteners, making potential side effects such as flatus and diarrhea difficult to diagnose.
- Nonabsorbed chemicals in the intestinal lumen create an osmotic effect that commonly contributes to dehydration. Sweeteners do not facilitate water uptake by enterocytes in contrast to glucose.
- Weight control during pregnancy is important, but the safety and potential side effects of sweeteners on fetal development is poorly established.
- Artificial sweeteners and other poorly understood additives may underlie or trigger migraine headaches, attention deficit hyperactivity disorder, food intolerances, and irritable bowel syndrome.

Natural sweeteners such as honey, pure agave, and maple syrup contain a variety of sugars, impart complex flavors, and satisfy taste more effectively than sugar alone. Stevia is a natural sweetener that has the added benefit of reduced calories [94], although population use and therefore safety data is limited. Polyols are sugar alcohols, such as sorbitol and xylitol, that may have a direct favorable effect on metabolic syndrome and the microbiome [95], although their use is limited to unheated beverages and by gastrointestinal symptoms. Ribose (see Chapter 34: Fibromyalgia) is an effective sweetener with added health benefits. Spices such as vanilla and cinnamon can also infuse sweet flavors, requiring less sugar.

SUPPORTING HYDRATION

Drinking water assists weight reduction [96,97]. In this context, addressing medically related barriers to hydration such as edema, prolonged urination with prostate hypertrophy, bladder incontinence, and urinary frequency are one aspect of treating obesity. Additional strategies are avoiding dry indoor air and drinking more water when at higher elevation and hydrating with noncaloric beverages.

Perspiration may be an overlooked advantage of exercise because it promotes hydration to adipose tissue. For patients unable to work up a sweat, steam rooms and saunas may have some, albeit unstudied, benefit to hydrating tissue and facilitating removal of toxicants.

REDUCING CALORIC INTAKE

- Eating breakfast reduces total calorie intake and late-night eating increases it. Meal timing may extend beyond calorie intake, with breakfast favoring fat metabolism and late-night eating reducing fat metabolism [98].
- Eating mindfully reduces total calorie intake, mostly by giving the body sufficient time to experience satiety before overeating.
- Increasing dietary fiber to 40 grams a day increases the volume of food, which increases satiety and reduces overall food intake.
- Choosing meals low in both their glycemic index and glycemic load facilitates adherence to a diet plan by stabilizing blood sugar.
- Eating calories rather than drinking calories also reduces total calorie intake.
- Women of childbearing age can monitor calorie intake more closely as menses approaches (see Figure 18.2) [57].

Additional strategies for reducing caloric intake and balancing energy expenditure are presented in Chapter 19: Diabetes and Chapter 37: Cancer and Insulin.

TREATMENT—MEDICAL FOODS AND SUPPLEMENTAL NUTRIENTS

Dietary supplements are not evaluated for safety and efficacy by the FDA before marketing. Physicians can correct patient misperceptions about dietary supplements [99] and recommend patients discontinue dietary supplements, which increase metabolic rate at the expense of lean tissue, may be of compromised quality, or are taken at inappropriately high doses. Supplemental nutrients used appropriately can help patients achieve weight maintenance. Appropriate supplemental nutrients are not intended to "rev up" metabolism. Instead they are used by skilled clinicians to restore optimal metabolic functioning. Supplemental nutrients can be used short term to correct underlying deficiencies and transition patients to nutrient-rich foods.

FIBER

Supplemental fiber can help transition patients to a fiber-rich diet. Low fiber intake is a key mediator of the obesity epidemic. In the United States, the population averages 10–15 grams of fiber a day, less than half of the recommended 25 grams for women and 38 grams for men. Reversing the low-fiber trend can be an effective component of weight loss [100]:

- Low glycemic index foods are generally high in fiber [101].
- Fiber adds volume to food. Mechanically stretching the stomach releases gut-synthesized satiety peptides [89,90].
- Fiber improves lipid profiles and insulin sensitivity, which enables patients to improve comorbidities and avoid obesogenic nutrient-drug interactions [102].

- Fiber reduces inflammation directly and indirectly by modulating the gut microbiata [103,104].
- There are other hypothesized benefits that are not easy to quantify. Fiber may reduce intake of endocrine-disrupting fat-soluble toxicants by the same mechanism by which fiber reduces colon cancer risk.
- Fiber acts as a prebiotic, favorably influencing gastrointestinal microflora, which exert satiety signals, modify host nutrients, and preserve the gastrointestinal barrier [105].

Gastrointestinal symptoms frequently limit fiber's therapeutic use. Like a fitness program, one can work up to higher fiber intake—often called improving bowel tolerance. Supplemental fiber can be gradually introduced to improve bowel tolerance and make use of fiber's appetite-reducing benefits. Consumption of fermented foods and supplemental probiotics may be additionally beneficial.

LIPID SUPPLEMENTS

Supplementing polyunsaturated fats as a weight-reduction strategy may be reasonable since obesity is associated with inflammation and the reduced ability to convert the essential fatty acids into eicosapentaenoic acid (EPA) and docosahexaenoic acid (DHA). A reasonable starting dose is EPA 240 mg, DHA 160 mg, and gamma linolenic acid (GLA) 160 mg. Fish oil and evening primrose oil can be used in combination. Recommend fish and evening primrose oils over flax oil, which contains alpha-linolenic acid and linoleic acid. GLA is an omega-6 fatty acid, which is supplemented along with EPA and DHA, because it, too, depends on the delta-6-desaturase enzyme. Chlorella has added advantages as a source of EPA and DHA: as an alga it is a nonanimal source, it is a food rather than an isolated nutrient, and it facilitates removal of metals, xenoestrogen, and biotoxins as detailed in Chapter 44: Biotoxins.

Coconut oil is encouraged as a cooking oil and as a supplement as a medium-chain triglyceride; however, the gastrointestinal side effects can limit use, usually to 1–2 grams a day. Coconut oil improves weight reduction through several mechanisms [86,106], including that microbiota metabolized it into short-chain fatty acids such as butyrate. Reduced intake of fermentable carbohydrates among dieters can lead to inadequate butyrate [107], with potential changes in the microbiome and satiety signaling. Supplementation with magnesium or calcium butyrate at 3 grams a day may be merited. The related prodrug, sodium phenylbutyrate (Buphenyl) is a prescription medication used to treat urea cycle disorders. Sodium phenylbutyrate and sodium butyrate represent potentially significant sources of sodium for some patients with obesity.

Optimizing phosphatidylcholine (PC) through supplementation merits consideration. Most patients have suboptimal PC [108] for important metabolic functions such as balancing cholesterol, improving membrane pliability for neuronal signaling, and enhancing the uptake of magnesium. Risk factors for PC deficiency include: reduced dietary intake of nuts, seeds, and egg yolks, prior cholecystectomy, and inadequate digestive enzymes. Patients tend to prefer supplementing with glycerophosphocholine and citicoline over soy-lecithin-derived PC and report reduced food cravings and improved mental focus.

PROTEIN AND AMINO ACID SUPPLEMENTS

Obesity makes achieving adequate dietary protein more difficult: greater total protein requirement due to larger size, calorie restriction for weight loss, decreased absorption from impaired enzyme function, increased demand due to inflammation and exercise, and reallocation for energy production rather than anabolic functions. However, protein is metabolically expensive. Protein sources are usually acidifying, high in saturated fat, and energy dense.

Some amino acid combinations are utilized more readily for anabolic function than others, a concept sometimes referred to as net nitrogen utilization (NNU). Eggs, eaten as the white and yolk together, are the food source with the highest NNU, where the protein is most likely to be used for anabolic functions during weight reduction. Lean meats in turn have a higher NNU than whey and soy protein powders. Supplemental essential amino acids are well absorbed, low calorie, and more readily utilized for anabolic functions. Five grams can be taken twice daily on an empty stomach. Amino acids are neurotransmitter precursors. Insufficient amino acid precursors for dopamine, serotonin, and possibly GABA may be a significant component of food cravings. Medications that promote the action of neurotransmitters are sometimes used in weight reduction [109].

MINERALS

General mineral depletion is common and compounded by reduced intake. Inclusion of kelps, seafood, and lean meats improve mineral status as can mineral supplements. Magnesium and chromium merit specific consideration during weight reduction.

Magnesium plays a critical role in fat oxidation. Suboptimal dietary intake, competitive absorption with supplemental calcium, and impaired absorption with various gastrointestinal conditions make magnesium deficiency common. Pedal edema and constipation are often responsive to supplemental magnesium [74]. Magnesium supplementation can be initiated at 250 mg a day, generally as chelated minerals, especially magnesium citrate, which is highly alkalinizing.

Chromium facilitates glucose uptake by the muscles. Body stores of chromium are two orders of magnitude less than iron and too small to measure clinically. Chromium is found in diverse foods, making a diet history minimally useful in establishing chromium deficiency. Chromium uptake is competitively inhibited by iron, posing hypotheses that supplemental iron and hemochromatosis may lower body stores of chromium. Stress and steroid medications appear to increase urinary loss of chromium, another mechanism by which a deficiency state may occur. Deficiency is likely in diabetes where urinary losses of chromium may be significant. A randomized clinical trial found that chromium reduces body fat in those with diabetes, when added to conventional therapy [110]. There was no demonstrated benefit in women with a healthy weight on a balanced diet [111]. The average chromium dose in clinical trials is 400 mcg/day and duration of treatment 79 days [112]. Patients with insulin resistance and polycystic ovary syndrome may find chromium helpful in managing food cravings. Rather than on a scheduled dosing, 200 mcg can be taken twice daily as needed for food cravings.

CARNITINE

L-carnitine is an organic acid that transports fatty acids to the inner mitochondria for fat oxidation. The body's ability to synthesize adequate L-carnitine may not be sufficient during the phase of active weight reduction. While found primarily in meats, it can also be supplemented during weight reduction where it has been shown beneficial [82]. L-carnitine can be dosed at 1 gram twice daily and avoid the gastrointestinal symptoms common at higher doses. Purified L-carnitine should be chosen, not a racemic mixture. L-carnitine should be combined with avoidance of trans fats and refined carbohydrates.

L-carnitine is most likely to benefit patients with impaired fat oxidation, identified early as triglycerides in excess of 100 mg/dl. Vegetarians may benefit from L-carnitine due to low dietary intake. A clinical assay for L-carnitine is available (see Table 18.1).

CURCUMIN

Curcumin is a phytonutrient that reduces the inflammation associated with weight reduction, is protective of joints strained from the mechanical stress of excess weight, and may protect against obesity-associated cognitive decline [113]. Curcumin can be initiated at a dose of 400 mg per day and taken with food.

SUMMARY

Tools are available to clinical practitioners to buttress their patients' weight-loss initiatives.

Some medical conditions can be diagnosed and treated to help patients achieve their diet and exercise goals. These are:

- Chemosensory disorders
- Periodontal disease
- Sleep apnea
- Osteomalacia
- Dehydration and pedal edema
- Muscle atrophy
- Elevated triglycerides
- Sex hormone imbalances
- Difficulty with lactation
- Nutrient deficiencies from prior bariatric surgery

The obesogenic effects of medications can be identified and sometimes minimized. Medications that are centrally acting are especially likely to cause resistance to weight reduction, mostly by unfavorably altering hunger and satiety signaling. Medications are increasingly being implicated as a risk factor in childhood obesity.

While addressing a patient's specific questions on diet and weight reduction, general principles emerge:

- Choose diets that are alkalinizing, strategically use dietary fats, and are medically compatible.
- Substitutions can be useful but artificial (high-intensity) sweeteners are not a beneficial substitute for sugar. Natural sweeteners, polyols, and ribose may confer some metabolic benefits when used sparingly.
- Practitioners can help patients hydrate, especially by addressing medical conditions that can sometimes unknowingly reduce hydration.
- Diet strategies on meal timing, mindfulness, fiber intake, carbohydrate selection, and beverage calories assist in maintaining a reduced calorie diet.

Dietary supplements sometimes appropriate as adjuncts to weight reduction include: fiber, chlorella, or fish oil alongside gamma-linolenic acid, coconut oil or butyrate, glycerophosphocholine or citicoline, amino acids, minerals with specific attention to magnesium and chromium, carnitine, and curcumin.

ACKNOWLEDGMENTS

Thank you for your insights Eileen Wright, M.D.; Jonathan Salo, M.D.; Yuliya Klopouh, Pharm.D.; and Mark Houston, M.D., M.S.

REFERENCES

1. Hiddink, G.J., et al., *Consumers' expectations about nutrition guidance: The importance of primary care physicians.* Am J Clin Nutr, 1997. 65(6 Suppl): p. 1974S–1979S.
2. *Screening for obesity in adults: Recommendations and rationale.* Ann Intern Med, 2003. 139(11): p. 930–932.
3. Salbe, A., M.B. Schwartz, and I. Kohlstadt, Childhood obesity, in *Scientific evidence for musculoskeletal, bariatric, and sports nutrition*, I. Kohlstadt, Editor 2006, Boca Raton, FL.: CRC Press, Taylor & Francis Group, p. 253–269.

4. Stunkard, A.J., *Genetic contributions to human obesity.* Res Publ Assoc Res Nerv Ment Dis, 1991. 69: p. 205–218.

5. Poulsen, P. and A. Vaag, *Glucose and insulin metabolism in twins: Influence of zygosity and birth weight.* Twin Res, 2001. 4(5): p. 350–355.

6. Gluckman, P.D. and M.A. Hanson, *The fetal matrix: Evolution, development, and disease.* 2005, Cambridge, UK ; New York: Cambridge University Press. xiv, 257 p.

7. Dolinoy, D.C. and R.L. Jirtle, *Environmental epigenomics in human health and disease.* Environ Mol Mutagen, 2008.

8. Dolinoy, D.C., et al., *Maternal genistein alters coat color and protects Avy mouse offspring from obesity by modifying the fetal epigenome.* Environ Health Perspect, 2006. 114(4): p. 567–572.

9. Kushi, L.H., et al., *American Cancer Society Guidelines on nutrition and physical activity for cancer prevention: Reducing the risk of cancer with healthy food choices and physical activity.* CA Cancer J Clin, 2012. 62(1): p. 30–67.

10. Fava, F., et al., *The type and quantity of dietary fat and carbohydrate alter faecal microbiome and short-chain fatty acid excretion in a metabolic syndrome "at-risk" population.* Int J Obes (Lond), 2012.

11. Badman, M.K. and J.S. Flier, *The gut and energy balance: Visceral allies in the obesity wars.* Science, 2005. 307(5717): p. 1909–1914.

12. Kimmons, J.E., et al., *Associations between body mass index and the prevalence of low micronutrient levels among US adults.* MedGenMed, 2006. 8(4): p. 59.

13. Ruottinen, S., et al., *High sucrose intake is associated with poor quality of diet and growth between 13 months and 9 years of age: The special Turku Coronary Risk Factor Intervention Project.* Pediatrics, 2008. 121(6): p. e1676–1685.

14. Kohlstadt, I., *Safeguarding muscle during weight reduction.* Medscape J Med, 2008. 10(8): p. 199.

15. Shavlakadze, T. and M. Grounds, *Of bears, frogs, meat, mice and men: complexity of factors affecting skeletal muscle mass and fat.* Bioessays, 2006. 28(10): p. 994–1009.

16. Sung, K.C., et al., *Combined influence of insulin resistance, overweight/obesity, and Fatty liver as risk factors for type 2 diabetes.* Diabetes Care, 2012. 35(4): p. 717–722.

17. Batmanghelidj, F., and I. Kohlstadt, Water: A driving force in the musculoskeletal system, in *Scientific Evidence for Musculoskeletal, Bariatric, and Sports Nutrition*, I. Kohlstadt, Editor 2006, Boca Raton, FL.: CRC Press, Taylor & Francis, p. 127–136.

18. Stookey, J.D., et al., *What is the cell hydration status of healthy children in the USA? Preliminary data on urine osmolality and water intake.* Public Health Nutr, 2012: p. 1–9.

19. Livingston, E.H. and I. Kohlstadt, *Simplified resting metabolic rate-predicting formulas for normal-sized and obese individuals.* Obes Res, 2005. 13(7): p. 1255–1262.

20. World Health Organization, *Persistent Organic Pollutants: Impact on Child Health.* 2010. www.who.int/ceh.

21. Stempfer, M.O., et al., *Sleep alterations of obese night shiftworkers.* C R Seances Soc Biol Fil, 1989. 183(5): p. 449–456.

22. Nduhirabandi, F., E.F. du Toit, and A. Lochner, *Melatonin and the metabolic syndrome: A tool for effective therapy in obesity-associated abnormalities?* Acta Physiol (Oxf), 2012.

23. Fragopoulou, A.F., et al., *Brain proteome response following whole body exposure of mice to mobile phone or wireless DECT base radiation.* Electromagn Biol Med, 2012. [Epub ahead of print.]

24. Volkow, N.D., et al., *Effects of cell phone radiofrequency signal exposure on brain glucose metabolism.* Jama, 2011. 305(8): p. 808–813.

25. Heber, D., et al., *Clinical detection of sarcopenic obesity by bioelectrical impedance analysis.* Am J Clin Nutr, 1996. 64(3 Suppl): p. 472S–477S.

26. Sui, X., et al., *Cardiorespiratory fitness and adiposity as mortality predictors in older adults.* Jama, 2007. 298(21): p. 2507–2516.

27. Pinto, J.A., et al., *Anthropometric data as predictors of obstructive sleep apnea severity.* Braz J Otorhinolaryngol, 2011. 77(4): p. 516–521.

28. Punjabi, N.M. and V.Y. Polotsky, *Disorders of glucose metabolism in sleep apnea.* J Appl Physiol, 2005. 99(5): p. 1998–2007.

29. Al Mamun A, L., et al. *Do childhood sleeping problems predict obesity in young adulthood? Evidence from a prospective birth cohort study.* Am J Epidemiol, 2007. 12(166): p. 1368–1373.

30. Trenell, M.I., et al., *Influence of constant positive airway pressure therapy on lipid storage, muscle metabolism and insulin action in obese patients with severe obstructive sleep apnoea syndrome.* Diabetes Obes Metab, 2007. 9(5): p. 679–687.

31. Olson, M.L., et al., *Vitamin D deficiency in obese children and its relationship to glucose homeostasis.* J Clin Endocrinol Metab, 2012. 97(1): p. 279–285.

32. Holick, M., Vitamin D: Importance for musculoskeletalfunction and health, in *Scientific Evidence for Musculoskeletal, Bariatric and Sports Nutrition*, I. Kohlstadt, Editor. 2006, New York: Taylor and Francis.

33. Wicherts, I.S., et al., *Vitamin D status predicts physical performance and its decline in older persons.* J Clin Endocrinol Metab, 2007. 92(6): p. 2058–2065.

34. Wadden, T.A., et al., *A two-year randomized trial of obesity treatment in primary care practice.* N Engl J Med, 2011. 365(21): p. 1969–1979.

35. Sjostrom, L., et al., *Lifestyle, diabetes, and cardiovascular risk factors 10 years after bariatric surgery.* N Engl J Med, 2004. 351(26): p. 2683–2693.

36. Jolly, K., et al., *Comparison of range of commercial or primary care led weight reduction programmes with minimal intervention control for weight loss in obesity: Lighten Up randomised controlled trial.* BMJ, 2011. 343: p. d6500.

37. Jebb, S.A., et al., *Primary care referral to a commercial provider for weight loss treatment versus standard care: A randomised controlled trial.* Lancet, 2011. 378(9801): p. 1485–1492.

38. Arem, H. and M. Irwin, *A review of web-based weight loss interventions in adults.* Obes Rev, 2011. 12(5): p. e236–243.

39. Cheskin, L.J., et al., *Prescription medications: A modifiable contributor to obesity.* South Med J, 1999. 92(9): p. 898–904.

40. Kohlstadt, I., M. Murphy, and L. Osmond. Continuing education programs can assess practitioner knowledge of drug labeling. in *The 11th International Congress on Obesity*. 2010. Stockholm, Sweden: Wiley-Blackwell.

41. *Intensive blood-glucose control with sulphonylureas or insulin compared with conventional treatment and risk of complications in patients with type 2 diabetes (UKPDS 33). UK Prospective Diabetes Study (UKPDS) Group.* Lancet, 1998. 352(9131): p. 837–853.

42. Kendall, D.M., et al., *Effects of exenatide (exendin-4) on glycemic control over 30 weeks in patients with type 2 diabetes treated with metformin and a sulfonylurea.* Diabetes Care, 2005. 28(5): p. 1083–1091.

43. Zangeneh, F., Y.C. Kudva, and A. Basu, *Insulin sensitizers.* Mayo Clin Proc, 2003. 78(4): p. 471–479.

44. Nesto, R.W., et al., *Thiazolidinedione use, fluid retention, and congestive heart failure: A consensus statement from the American Heart Association and American Diabetes Association.* Diabetes Care, 2004. 27(1): p. 256–263.

45. Isley, W.L., *Glitazones, glycemia, and global health status.* Diabetes Care, 2001. 24(12): p. 2158–2159.

46. de Jager, J., et al., *Long term treatment with metformin in patients with type 2 diabetes and risk of vitamin B-12 deficiency: Randomised placebo controlled trial.* BMJ, 2010. 340: p. c2181.

47. Kim, W.S., et al., *Berberine improves lipid dysregulation in obesity by controlling central and peripheral AMPK activity.* Am J Physiol Endocrinol Metab, 2009. 296(4): p. E812–819.

48. Yin, J., H. Xing, and J. Ye, *Efficacy of berberine in patients with type 2 diabetes mellitus.* Metabolism, 2008. 57(5): p. 712–717.

49. Alberton, M., et al., *Adverse events associated with individual statin treatments for cardiovascular disease: An indirect comparison meta-analysis.* QJM, 2012. 105(2): p. 145–157.

50. Bliznakov, E.G. and W. D.J., *Biochemical and clinical consequences of inhibiting coenzyme Q10 biosynthesis by lipid lowering HMG-CoA reductase inhibitors (statins): A critical overview.* . Adv Therapy, 1998. 15: p. 218–228.

51. FDA. *FDA Drug Safety Communication: Important safety labeling changes to cholesterol-lowering statin drugs.* 2012.

52. Cooper-DeHoff, R.M., et al., *Impact of abdominal obesity on incidence of adverse metabolic effects associated with antihypertensive medications.* Hypertension, 2010. 55(1): p. 61–68.

53. Dunn, S.P., et al., *Nutrition and heart failure: Impact of drug therapies and management strategies.* Nutrition in clinical practice: Official publication of the American Society for Parenteral and Enteral Nutrition, 2009. 24(1): p. 60–75.

54. Anderson, R., Chromium: Roles in the regulation of lean body mass and body weight, in *Scientific evidence for musculoskeletal, bariatric and sports nutrition*, I. Kohlstadt, Editor. 2006, Boca Raton, FL.: CRC Press, p. 175–192.

55. Jorgensen, E.A., et al., *Histamine and the regulation of body weight.* Neuroendocrinology, 2007. 86(3): p. 210–214.

56. Hardy, M. and E. Volkmann, Rhinosinusitis, in *Food and Nutrients in Disease Management*, I. Kohlstadt, Editor. 2009, Boca Raton, FL.: CRC Press, p. 29–42.

57. Gong, E.J., D. Garrel, and D.H. Calloway, *Menstrual cycle and voluntary food intake.* Am J Clin Nutr, 1989. 49(2): p. 252–258.

58. Lind, P.M., et al., *Serum concentrations of phthalate metabolites related to abdominal fat distribution two years later in elderly women.* Environ Health, 2012. 11(1): p. 21.

59. Garcia-Mayor, R.V., et al., *Endocrine disruptors and obesity: obesogens.* Endocrinol Nutr, 2012. 59(4): p. 261–267.

60. Hirschberg, A.L., et al., *Impaired cholecystokinin secretion and disturbed appetite regulation in women with polycystic ovary syndrome.* Gynecol Endocrinol, 2004. 19(2): p. 79–87.

61. Jallon, P. and F. Picard, *Bodyweight gain and anticonvulsants: a comparative review.* Drug Saf, 2001. 24(13): p. 969–978.

62. Lampl, Y., et al., *Weight gain, increased appetite, and excessive food intake induced by carbamazepine.* Clin Neuropharmacol, 1991. 14(3): p. 251–255.

63. Kossoff, E.H. and A.L. Hartman, *Ketogenic diets: New advances for metabolism-based therapies.* Curr Opin Neurol, 2012. 25(2): p. 173–178.

64. McEvoy, J.P., et al., *Prevalence of the metabolic syndrome in patients with schizophrenia: Baseline results from the Clinical Antipsychotic Trials of Intervention Effectiveness (CATIE) schizophrenia trial and comparison with national estimates from NHANES III.* Schizophr Res, 2005. 80(1): p. 19–32.

65. Colton, C.W. and R.W. Manderscheid, *Congruencies in increased mortality rates, years of potential life lost, and causes of death among public mental health clients in eight states.* Prev Chronic Dis, 2006. 3(2): p. A42.

66. Holtmann, M., et al., *Risperidone-associated steatohepatitis and excessive weight-gain.* Pharmacopsychiatry, 2003. 36(5): p. 206–207.

67. Lieberman, J.A., et al., *Effectiveness of antipsychotic drugs in patients with chronic schizophrenia.* N Engl J Med, 2005. 353(12): p. 1209–1223.

68. Kohlstadt, I. and B. Vitiello, *Use of atypical antipsychotics in children: Balancing safety and effectiveness.* Am Fam Physician, 2010. 81(5): p. 585.

69. Correll, C.U., *Antipsychotic use in children and adolescents: Minimizing adverse effects to maximize outcomes.* J Am Acad Child Adolesc Psychiatry, 2008. 47(1): p. 9–20.

70. Floris, M., J. Lejeune, and W. Deberdt, *Effect of amantadine on weight gain during olanzapine treatment.* Eur Neuropsychopharmacol, 2001. 11(2): p. 181–182.

71. Poyurovsky, M., et al., *Olanzapine-induced weight gain in patients with first-episode schizophrenia: A double-blind, placebo-controlled study of fluoxetine addition.* Am J Psychiatry, 2002. 159(6): p. 1058–1060.

72. Klein, D.J., et al., *A randomized, double-blind, placebo-controlled trial of metformin treatment of weight gain associated with initiation of atypical antipsychotic therapy in children and adolescents.* Am J Psychiatry, 2006. 163(12): p. 2072–2079.

73. Jevitt, C., I. Hernandez, and M. Groer, *Lactation complicated by overweight and obesity: Supporting the mother and newborn.* J Midwifery Womens Health, 2007. 52(6): p. 606–613.

74. Kohlstadt, I., *Scientific evidence for musculoskeletal, bariatric, and sports nutrition.* 2006, Boca Raton: CRC Taylor & Francis, 621 p.

75. Medco's, *Drug Trend Report.* Drugtrend.com, 2010. 12.

76. Smith, P.B., et al., *Safety monitoring of drugs receiving pediatric marketing exclusivity.* Pediatrics, 2008. 122(3): p. 628–633.

77. Correll, C.U., et al., *Cardiometabolic risk of second-generation antipsychotic medications during first-time use in children and adolescents.* Jama, 2009. 302(16): p. 1765–1773.

78. Kohlstadt, I. and M. Murphy, *Pediatric drug research informs prevention of childhood obesity.* 2012 in review.

79. Sjostrom, L., et al., *Effects of bariatric surgery on mortality in Swedish obese subjects.* N Engl J Med, 2007. 357(8): p. 741–752.

80. Adams, T.D., et al., *Long-term mortality after gastric bypass surgery.* N Engl J Med, 2007. 357(8): p. 753–761.

81. Bralley JA, L.R., *Laboratory evaluations in molecular medicine.* 2001, <add city> Institute for Advances in Molecular Medicine. p. 365.

82. Kohlstadt, I., Bariatric surgery: More effective with nutrition, in *Scientific Evidence for Musculoskeletal, Bariatric, and Sports Nutrition,* I. Kohlstadt, Editor. 2006, Boca Raton, FL.: CRC Taylor&Francis Group: p. 271–282.

83. Frassetto, L. and S. Berkemeyer, Osteoporosis: The scientific basis of the alkaline diet, in *Food and Nutrients in Disease Management,* I. Kohlstadt, Editor. 2009, Boca Raton, FL.: CRC Press, p. 503–520.

84. Dahm, C.C., et al., *Adipose tissue fatty acid patterns and changes in anthropometry: A cohort study.* PLoS One, 2011. 6(7): p. e22587.

85. Swithers, S.E., S.B. Ogden, and T.L. Davidson, *Fat substitutes promote weight gain in rats consuming high-fat diets.* Behav Neurosci, 2011. 125(4): p. 512–518.

86. Clegg, M.E., *Medium-chain triglycerides are advantageous in promoting weight loss although not beneficial to exercise performance.* Int J Food Sci Nutr, 2010. 61(7): p. 653–679.

87. Yehuda, S., *Omega-6/omega-3 ratio and brain-related functions.* World Rev Nutr Diet, 2003. 92: p. 37–56.

88. Ledikwe, J.H., et al., *Dietary energy density is associated with energy intake and weight status in US adults.* Am J Clin Nutr, 2006. 83(6): p. 1362–1368.

89. Rolls, B.J., E.A. Bell, and M.L. Thorwart, *Water incorporated into a food but not served with a food decreases energy intake in lean women.* Am J Clin Nutr, 1999. 70(4): p. 448–455.

90. Rolls, B.J., L.S. Roe, and J.S. Meengs, *Reductions in portion size and energy density of foods are additive and lead to sustained decreases in energy intake.* Am J Clin Nutr, 2006. 83(1): p. 11–17.

91. Rolls, B.J. and L.S. Roe, *Effect of the volume of liquid food infused intragastrically on satiety in women.* Physiol Behav, 2002. 76(4–5): p. 623–631.

92. Sievenpiper, J.L., et al., *Effect of fructose on body weight in controlled feeding trials: A systematic review and meta-analysis.* Ann Intern Med, 2012. 156(4): p. 291–304.

93. Malik, V.S. and F.B. Hu, *Sweeteners and risk of obesity and type 2 diabetes: The role of sugar-sweetened beverages.* Curr Diab Rep, 2012.

94. Anton, S.D., et al., *Effects of stevia, aspartame, and sucrose on food intake, satiety, and postprandial glucose and insulin levels.* Appetite, 2010. 55(1): p. 37–43.

95. Amo, K., et al., *Effects of xylitol on metabolic parameters and visceral fat accumulation.* J Clin Biochem Nutr, 2011. 49(1): p. 1–7.

96. Stookey, J.D., et al., *Drinking water is associated with weight loss in overweight dieting women independent of diet and activity.* Obesity (Silver Spring), 2008. 16(11): p. 2481–2488.

97. Daniels, M.C. and B.M. Popkin, *Impact of water intake on energy intake and weight status: A systematic review.* Nutr Rev, 2010. 68(9): p. 505–521.

98. de Castro, J.M., *The time of day of food intake influences overall intake in humans.* J Nutr, 2004. 134(1): p. 104–111.

99. Pillitteri, J.L., et al., *Use of dietary supplements for weight loss in the United States: Results of a national survey.* Obesity (Silver Spring), 2008. 16(4): p. 790–796.

100. Rigaud, D., et al., *Effect of psyllium on gastric emptying, hunger feeling and food intake in normal volunteers: A double blind study.* Eur J Clin Nutr, 1998. 52(4): p. 239–245.

101. Thomas, D.E., E.J. Elliott, and L. Baur, *Low glycaemic index or low glycaemic load diets for overweight and obesity.* Cochrane Database Syst Rev, 2007(3): p. CD005105.

102. Jenkins, D.J., et al., *Dietary fibres, fibre analogues, and glucose tolerance: Importance of viscosity.* Br Med J, 1978. 1(6124): p. 1392–1394.

103. King, D.E., et al., *Effect of psyllium fiber supplementation on C-reactive protein: The trial to reduce inflammatory markers (TRIM).* Ann Fam Med, 2008. 6(2): p. 100–106.

104. King, D.E., et al., *Effect of a high-fiber diet vs a fiber-supplemented diet on C-reactive protein level.* Arch Intern Med, 2007. 167(5): p. 502–506.

105. Nicholson, J.K., et al. Science, 2012. 336(6086):1262–1267.

106. Hargrave, K.M., M.J. Azain, and J.L. Miner, *Dietary coconut oil increases conjugated linoleic acid-induced body fat loss in mice independent of essential fatty acid deficiency.* Biochim Biophys Acta, 2005. 1737(1): p. 52–60.

107. Duncan, S.H., et al., *Reduced dietary intake of carbohydrates by obese subjects results in decreased concentrations of butyrate and butyrate-producing bacteria in feces.* Appl Environ Microbiol, 2007. 73(4): p. 1073–1078.

108. Zeisel, S.H. and K.A. da Costa, *Choline: An essential nutrient for public health.* Nutr Rev, 2009. 67(11): p. 615–623.

109. Miller, S., *Pharmacotherapy for weight loss.* US Pharmacist, 2006. 12: p. 75–85.

110. Martin, J., et al., *Chromium picolinate supplementation attenuates body weight gain and increases insulin sensitivity in subjects with type 2 diabetes.* Diabetes Care, 2006. 29(8): p. 1826–1832.

111. Lukaski, H.C., W.A. Siders, and J.G. Penland, *Chromium picolinate supplementation in women: Effects on body weight, composition, and iron status.* Nutrition, 2007. 23(3): p. 187–195.

112. Pittler, M.H., C. Stevinson, and E. Ernst, *Chromium picolinate for reducing body weight: Meta-analysis of randomized trials.* Int J Obes Relat Metab Disord, 2003. 27(4): p. 522–529.

113. Scapagnini, G., et al., *Modulation of Nrf2/ARE pathway by food polyphenols: A nutritional neuroprotective strategy for cognitive and neurodegenerative disorders.* Mol Neurobiol, 2011. 44(2): p. 192–201.

114. Contoreggi, C., and I Kohlstadt, Neuroendocrine regulation of appetite, in *Scientific Evidence for Musculoskeletal, Bariatric, and Sports Nutrition*, I. Kohlstadt, Editor. 2006, Boca Raton, FL.: CRC Press, p. 211–229.

115. The use of medicines in the United States: Review of 2010, in *IMS Institute for Healthcare Informatics.* 2011, Parsipanny, NJ: IMS Health Incorporated: p. 37.

116. Manrique, C., M. Johnson, and J.R. Sowers, *Thiazide diuretics alone or with beta-blockers impair glucose metabolism in hypertensive patients with abdominal obesity.* Hypertension, 2010. 55(1): p. 15–17.

117. Tsai, A.G. and T.A. Wadden, *Treatment of obesity in primary care practice in the United States: A systematic review.* J Gen Intern Med, 2009. 24(9): p. 1073–1079.

19 Diabetes and Insulin Resistance

Food and Nutrients in Primary Care

Mark Hyman, M.D., Jayashree Mani, M.S., and Russell Jaffe, M.D., Ph.D.

INTRODUCTION

This chapter focuses on solutions to obesity and diabetes that are cost and outcome effective, evidence based, and encouraging in their potential to improve health while lowering health care costs. These two disorders now exceed malnutrition in global public health costs and life lost. Recent National Health and Nutrition Examination Survey (NHANES) data of Americans 2003–8 show that nearly 75% of the US population is now overweight [1]. Childhood obesity has increased three- to fourfold since the 1960s [2]. In 1980, no states had obesity rates over 15%; by 2010, every state had an obesity rate greater than 20% [3].

EPIDEMIOLOGY AND PATHOGENESIS

Diabetes prevalence has risen sevenfold since 1983. In 2010, diabetes was diagnosed in approximately 25 million adults in the United States, including a prevalence rate of 26.9% in seniors > 65 years [4]. Diabetes and obesity together also place an enormous economic burden on our society. The direct and indirect annual costs of obesity in the United States are $113 billion and $174 billion for diabetes, cumulatively $3 trillion over the past decade [5]. The problem is also expanding globally. In China, 92 million individuals have diabetes, 60% of whom are undiagnosed. Another 148 million have metabolic syndrome, 100% of whom are undiagnosed [6].

Overweight and obesity are, for the majority, markers of a single unifying metabolic dysfunction. Population wide, risk stratification is based on profiles of body weight associated with increased risk. Overweight is expressed as a body mass index (BMI) > 25; obesity is defined by a BMI > 30. Health risks increase progressively with higher BMI. Clinically, this profile is less useful than considering metabolic dysfunctions as a continuum from optimal insulin sensitivity to end-stage diabetes.

In childhood, both low weight and accelerated weight gain affect glucose tolerance and the risk of type 2 diabetes [7]. In adulthood, weight gain is the primary precursor to diabetes. This spectrum

373

has been referred to as "diabesity" and is a more useful clinical concept, focusing on mechanism rather than phenotype for obesity.

MORTALITY AND MORBIDITY

Obesity shortens lifespan by nine years of life for the average person [8]. In adolescence, obesity creates the same risk of premature death as heavy smoking [9]. Diabesity along the entire continuum of metabolic dysfunction is the primary driver of diabetes, cardiovascular disease [10], stroke, dementia [11], cancer [12], and most chronic disease mortality [13]. A recent 40-year prospective study of 4857 Pima Indian children found that the major predictor of premature death was insulin resistance, not hypertension or hyperlipidemia. Pima Indians in the highest quartile of glucose intolerance had a 73% increase in early death rate compared to those in the lowest quartile [14]. In the past, when these same Native Americans lived an active nomadic life they showed little evidence of insulin resistance. This suggests that insulin resistance is a classic epigenetic or lifestyle-acquired condition, based largely on how we eat, drink, think, and live.

MAJOR STUDIES ON LIFESTYLE FACTORS

We know from the evidence that lifestyle is an important factor in the development of insulin resistance. In one diabetes prevention trial, evidence for the importance of exercise and nutrition became so compelling that it was deemed unethical to deny exercise and good nutrition to the control group and the study was halted [15]. As a result of this type of data, we no longer take lifestyle for granted [16]. In the 27-center study cited here, researchers found that when patients at risk for diabetes lost just eight pounds through regular exercise, the incidence of type 2 diabetes was reduced by 58%.

RISK FACTORS OR CAUSES: CHANGING THE FOCUS OF CLINICAL INTERVENTION

Medical focus has primarily emphasized medications or bariatric surgical approaches to correct downstream risk factors in addressing this epidemic and its primary disease sequela (diabetes, heart disease, and stroke) at great cost and yet little or no benefit.

The recent ACCORD [17] and NAVIGATOR trials provided evidence that aggressive pharmacologic intervention for lipids [18], glucose [19], and blood pressure [20] did *not* decrease cardiac or overall mortality and in some cases increased adverse cardiac events and mortality.

The problem may be that our model or paradigm is obsolete. Despite a rich evidence base from major clinical trials [21], few resources are currently devoted to the lifestyle, biological, social, and policy drivers of obesity and overweight presented in Figure 19.1. Metabolic disease and social networks predict disease and outcomes more effectively than risk factors alone [22].

DIETARY FACTORS

Nutrigenomics is the study of the effects of macronutrients, micronutrients, phytonutrients, and glycemic load on gene expression, which provides an important lens for viewing the impact of nutrition on obesity and insulin resistance [23,24].

GLYCEMIC INDEX AND GLYCEMIC LOAD

The continued intake of high-glycemic load meals is associated with an increased risk of adaptive insulin resistance [25]. Glycemic index (GI) is a measure of the effects of carbohydrates on blood sugar levels. Carbohydrates that break down quickly during digestion and release glucose rapidly

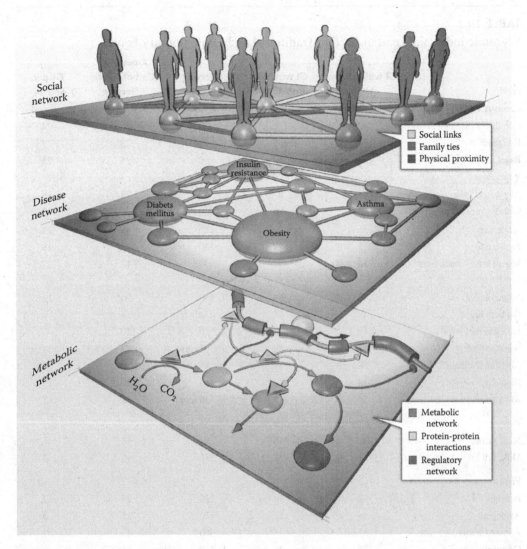

FIGURE 19.1 Complex networks of direct relevance to network medicine. (Reproduced with permission from the Massachusetts Medical Society.)

into the bloodstream have a high rating on the glycemic index. Examples of high GI foods include sugar, white flour products, and instant rice, as well as corn and potatoes (Table 19.1). Glycemic load (GL) is another way to assess the impact of carbohydrate consumption that provides a fuller picture than the glycemic index alone. While the GI value depicts how rapidly a particular carbohydrate breaks down into pure glucose, the GL indicates how much of that kind of carbohydrate is contained in a prepared food (for example, the refined flour content of white bread). GL calculations also reflect glycemic impact based on serving size.

Carbohydrates with a high glycemic index and high glycemic load produce substantial increases in blood glucose and insulin levels after ingestion. Within a few hours after their consumption, blood sugar levels begin to decline rapidly from peak concentration, due largely to an increase in insulin secretion. A profound state of hunger (experienced as food cravings) is created as the brain senses this precipitous drop in glucose energy supply. The continued intake of high glycemic load meals is associated with an increased risk of adaptive insulin resistance.

TABLE 19.1

Glycemic Index and Load of Certain Traditional and Contemporary Foods

Food	GI with Glucose as 100	GI with White Bread as 100	Serving Size (g)	Amount of Carbohydrate g/Serving	GL per Serving
Grains/Cereals					
Cornflakes (Kellogg's)	92	130	30	26	24
Doughnut	76	108	47	23	17
Bagel, white	72	103	70	35	25
White flour	70	100			
Angel food cake	67	95	50	29	19
Coca Cola, soft drink	63	90	250 mL	26	16
White rice	56	80	150	41	23
Brown rice	55	79	150	33	18
Muesli bread, made from packet mix	54	77	30	12	7
Bulgur wheat	48	68	150	26	12
Oat bran bread	47	68	30	18	9
Barley kernel bread	43	62	30	20	9
Whole wheat	41	59	50 (dry)	34	14
All-Bran (Kellogg's)	38	54	45	30	23
High amylose rice	38	54	150	39	15
Rye kernels	34	48	50 (dry)	38	13
Dairy					
Milk, skim	32	46	250	13	4
Milk, full fat	27	38	250	12	3
Fruits					
Banana	52	74	120	24	12
Apple, raw	38	52	120	15	6
Apricot (dried)	31	44	60	28	9
Grapefruit, raw	25	36	120	11	3
Pulses/Peas/Beans					
Chick peas	28	39	150	30	8
Kidney beans	28	39	150	25	7
Red lentils	26	36	150	18	5
Soya beans	18	25	150	6	1
Sweeteners					
Sucrose (table sugar)	68	97	10	10	7
Honey	55	78	25	18	10
Fructose	19	27	10	10	2
Organic agave cactus nectar	10	14	10	8	1
Xylitol	8	11	10	10	1
Lactitol	2	3	10	10	0

TABLE 19.1 (*continued*)

Glycemic Index and Load of Certain Traditional and Contemporary Foods

Food	GI with Glucose as 100	GI with White Bread as 100	Serving Size (g)	Amount of Carbohydrate g/Serving	GL per Serving
Vegetables					
Russet potato	85	121	150	30	26
Instant mashed potato	85	122	150	20	17
Peas	48	68	80	7	3
Carrots	47	68	80	6	3

Glycemic index is based on whole foods. Food components should be evaluated in the context of the foods in which they are eaten. Variation in food preparations also alter glycemic index.

DIETARY SUGARS, REFINED FLOURS

Dietary sugars and refined flours are significant triggers of immune dysfunction that clinically present as inflammation and result in compromised repair functions in the body. Our Paleolithic ancestors ate 22 teaspoons of sugars in the form of natural sweeteners such as honey, totaling approximately one-quarter pound of sugar a year [26]. By 1800, the average person was consuming 10 pounds of sugar annually (less than a pound a month). Current consumption rates average 150–180 pounds per person per year (almost one-half pound a day).

Liquid calories are another major factor, increasing obesity even more than calories from solid foods [27]. These risks are compounded by lack of exercise: hours of television watched are second only to consumption of liquid sugar calories as a risk factor for obesity [28]. This lifestyle is reflected in the latest NHANES data on American teenagers, which show that from 2003 to 2008, fewer than 20% of teen respondents consumed a healthful diet (Figure 19.2) [29].

Hyperinsulinemia leads to a biochemical cascade that alters genetic expression, reflected in repair deficit [30]. Too often, an avoidable downward spiral into further inflammation and insulin resistance is reinforced by food cravings, counterproductive daily choices, compromised microflora, impaired energy levels, sedentary habits of daily living, and poor quality of life.

FIBER CONTENT OF FOOD

Glycemic load and nutrient density are also controlled by fiber content of food. Paleolithic fiber consumption averaged 100 grams a day. Today it is less than 8 grams per day [31]. Lack of fiber has been associated with obesity, diabetes, heart disease, cancer, and numerous other chronic diseases [32]. Consumption of 50 grams of fiber per day has been found to lower hemoglobin A1c as effectively as diabetic medication [33].

PROTEIN CONSUMPTION

Diabetes is associated with impaired protein synthesis and wound healing, resulting in compromised repair functions. Higher protein intake can improve glycemic control. However, when protein is ingested at levels above 50–60 grams per day (approximately 15% of caloric intake), that has an increasing metabolic cost, as protein-containing foods tend to increase net acid load. Protein is therefore necessary but metabolically costly. Protein choices should be wise. Whey protein, for example, has been found effective in reducing body fat. A reduction of just 5% in body fat mass can lower the risk of obesity-related diseases significantly. Whey protein also appears to have a

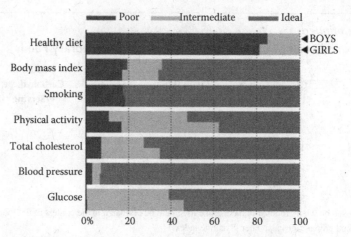

FIGURE 19.2 NHANES survey of health habits in American teenagers. (Courtesy: National Center for Health Statistics).

beneficial effect on glucose control and insulin responses [34]. A novel, whey-based whole meal has been found in outcome research to have a glycemic load below 10 [35].

ARTIFICIAL SWEETENERS

Artificial sweeteners promote obesity by increasing hunger, motivating food consumption beyond satiety. In a recent study, rats were fed yogurt sweetened either with sugar or artificial sweetener for 14 days. The rats that consumed artificially sweetened yogurt increased their total food consumption, but not total calories, yet body fat and weight increased, elevating their risk of diabesity, while body temperature and thermogenesis decreased [36].

RESULTING MALNUTRITION AND NUTRITIONAL INTERVENTIONS

Today obesity is often associated with malnutrition in industrial societies. Obese children in North America are increasingly diagnosed with nutritional deficits such as scurvy, kwashiorkor, pellagra, and rickets. Nutrient-poor, calorie-dense diets are resulting in a society of overfed and undernourished people.

Comprehensive care using patient-specific functional therapies is more cost and outcome effective than current conventional diabetes care alone.

DIGESTIVE FUNCTION AND DYSFUNCTION

Metabolic dysfunction and insulin resistance have recently been linked to disturbances in intestinal ecology or microbiome [37]. The evolutionary shift from a Paleolithic diet to a highly processed, low-fiber, high-sugar, and high-fat diet has commensurately altered gut microflora.

COMPROMISED FLORA

The modern-day microbiome is no longer a symbiotic one that is mutually beneficial to the microflora and human host. There have been homeodynamic shifts to dysbiosis, a harmful interaction between microflora and host. These altered flora, when present in high concentration, create metabolic endotoxemia through an increase in levels of bacterial endotoxins. Higher levels of lipopolysaccharides (LPS) binding to lymphocytes trigger the release of tumor necrosis factor alpha (TNF-α), which blocks peroxisome proliferator activated receptors (PPARs) that control inflammation, insulin sensitivity, and mitochondrial function. This can trigger a cascade of inflammation, insulin resistance, and weight gain [38].

SLOW TRANSIT TIME

Assessment of transit time and hydration are important as systemic indicators of digestive health. Healthy transit time is typically 12–18 hours. Hydration improves transit time. A digestive system without sufficient fluid results in constipation. With adequate hydration, sufficient fluid is present in the digestive track to support healthy transit time and the effective distribution of nutrients.

FOOD SENSITIVITIES AND ALLERGIES

Delayed food sensitivities have been confirmed to play a role in the development of insulin resistance and diabesity due to the effects of chronic low-grade systemic inflammation. Immune reactivities to food and environmental antigens in diabetics are patient specific and clinically important.

Response to dairy products is a case in point. Diabetes is less common in nonmilk drinkers and insulin resistance is more common in milk drinkers. Since food reactivities to dairy are statistically common, a clinical trial was conducted to evaluate this potential correlation. In a study comparing obese children to normal weight children, the obese children had a two-and-a-half-fold higher level of IgG antibodies (in response to 277 different foods tested) and threefold higher levels of C-reactive protein [39]. In addition, the obese children had increased carotid intimal thickness, indicating systemic inflammation. Individuals with low antigen reactivity typically have low levels of inflammation, with lab values of hsCRP below 0.5 mg/L.

A community-based randomized clinical trial to identify reactivities employed lymphocyte-based delayed testing in cohorts of patients with type 1 ($n = 27$) and type 2 diabetes ($n = 26$) [40]. Patients undertook conventional best practices diabetes management alone or additionally carried out a patient-specific comprehensive care protocol (test arm, 14 type 1 and 13 type 2 diabetes). Test patients substituted nonreactive foods for their reactive antigens and were advised to follow a repair-stimulating diet including nutrient supplementation. Glycemic control, assessed by changes in hemoglobin A1c (HbA1c) levels, showed clear improvement following the six-month comprehensive care protocol.

The reduction in average HbA1c levels was significant among type 2 diabetics: 13.3% reduction in test subjects and 2.6% in control subjects ($P < 0.05$). Decreases in HbA1c levels in the type 1 groups were greater in the test group: 8.7% reduction compared with reductions in control subjects of 5.2%.

MITOCHONDRIAL AND REDUCTION-OXIDATION DYSFUNCTION

Obesity and diabetes have been linked to defects in mitochondrial function [41]. An evaluation of first-degree relatives of diabetics found that relatives who were healthy and maintained normal weight had mitochondria that were 50% less active than those of individuals without a family history of diabetes [42]. Additional research has linked obesity and diabetes with oxidative stress [43] that holds implications for antioxidant supplementation to meet oxidative stress load plus what is needed for healthy metabolic function. Mitochondria can be conserved by the use of fully reduced and buffered, 100% l-ascorbates. Ascorbates prevent or repair from oxidative stress in the cell due to free-radical oxidation of one or another kind [44,45]. They increase production of nitric oxide [46] and decrease lipid peroxide generation thereby retaining functionality and resilience; consequently, adequate native ascorbates' intake is essential for sustainable health. For individualized care, we suggest the ascorbate calibration protocol to determine individual ascorbate need and thus assess the global cell antioxidant need using ascorbate as a surrogate marker for antioxidant network status. The ascorbate calibration protocol allows needs for vitamins C to be measured regularly since antioxidant requirement is so dynamic [47].

HORMONAL DYSREGULATION: INSULIN, THYROID, ADRENAL, AND SEX HORMONES

Obesity both results from and drives neurohormonal immune dysregulation [48]. Common features of diabesity include impairment in insulin sensitivity, thyroid metabolism, adrenal hormone levels, sex hormones, and neuroendocrine appetite regulation. Undiagnosed thyroid disease worsens insulin resistance [49], and insulin resistance worsens thyroid function [50].

CORTISOL

Chronic stress drives chronically elevated cortisol, which promotes insulin resistance, central adiposity, dyslipidemia, depression, and even dementia [51]. Elevated cortisol also lowers testosterone levels, promoting muscle loss. High cortisol interferes with thyroid and growth hormones and negatively impacts sleep, all of which lead to problems with weight gain.

Measurement of salivary cortisol and dehydroepiandrosterone can identify underlying adrenal stress and aid in diabetes management [52]. Saliva is an ultrafiltrate and therefore may more closely reflect tissue levels, although certain conditions common among those with diabetes may limit its accuracy in some circumstances.

SLEEP AND APPETITE

Sleep deprivation or impaired sleep, in turn, can cause hormonal imbalances that underlie obesity and diabetes. Sleep debt increases appetite, as well as cravings for sugars and refined carbohydrates. A study of healthy young men found that when they were deprived of just two hours of sleep, their blood levels of ghrelin (a hunger hormone) increased and Peptide YY (PYY—the brake on appetite) decreased [53]. Obestatin, a ghrelin antagonist, appears to act as an anorectic hormone, decreasing food intake and reducing body weight gain. The ghrelin/obestatin ratio is modified in anorexia nervosa and obesity and continues to be studied as a potential drug target [54].

ESTROGEN AND ANDROGEN IMBALANCES

Diabesity also drives sex hormone dysregulation. Insulin resistance has been identified as a factor in both infertility [55] and polycystic ovarian syndrome [56]. In men, insulin resistance can result in androgen deficiency and impaired sexual function [57]. Successful outcomes research on both type 2 and type 1 diabetes has confirmed these hypotheses as valid in community-based, real world studies.

IMMUNE DEFENSE AND REPAIR DEFICITS IN INFLAMMATION

Silent inflammation is a final common pathway in most chronic diseases from diabesity to heart disease [58], cancer [59], and Alzheimer's senility [60]. Elevated levels of inflammatory markers such as high sensitivity C-reactive protein (hsCRP) and interleukin 6 (IL-6) confer an increased risk of developing diabetes [61]. Inflammation is a cumulative repair deficit. Elevated hsCRP occurs when enhanced repair is required and remains elevated until the repair deficit has been corrected. These underlying causes of inflammation need to be understood and addressed if diabesity risk is to be effectively treated. Anti-inflammatory medications do not address the more important question, "What is causing the inflammation and how do we treat it most effectively?"

Obesogens is a term for inflammatory agents associated with weight gain and results from environmental exposures such as diet and allergens. Obesogens are implicated in the 73% increase in obesity in six-month-old infants since 1980 [62]. The increasing load of persistent organic pollutants or POPs (including polychlorinated biphenyls and other biocides) and heavy metals (such as arsenic, mercury, cadmium, nickel, and lead) act as obesogens and have been linked to obesity [63], diabetes [64], and insulin resistance [65], in part through increased cytokine production. Chronic infections can also trigger inflammation and cause persistent weight gain. New studies show that chronic viral infections such as adenovirus may be linked to obesity and insulin resistance [66].

PERIPHERAL NEUROPATHY AS A DIABETIC SEQUELA

Peripheral neuropathy is characterized by pain, numbness, and tingling in the extremities and slow nerve conduction, with debilitating effects. Diabetes remains the most common etiological factor. In the United States alone, it has been estimated that there are more than five million patients suffering from diabetic peripheral neuropathy (DPN), with the total annual cost of treating the disease and its complications topping $10 billion.

The pathophysiology of diabetic neuropathy includes increased oxidative stress yielding advanced glycosylated end products, polyol accumulation, and homocysteinemia [67]. Functionally, neuropathy results in decreased protective nitric oxide activity, impaired endothelial function, and compromised sodium-potassium intercellular transport reflecting impaired Na+/K+ -ATPase activity. Diabetes alters the myelin's phospholipid content, deranging fatty acids and healthy cholesterol components in a pattern that can modify membrane fluidity. Diabetes can induce sciatic nerve myelin abnormalities [68]. High blood pressure and reduced beneficial high-density lipoprotein (HDL) cholesterol coexist in DPN [69].

Nutritionally, vitamins C and E as antioxidants have proven to be very helpful in DPN. Acetyl-L-carnitine, carnitine fumarate, benfotiamine, and the combination of active B vitamins such as natural folates, hydroxocobalamin, and methylcobalamin, as well as pyridoxal-6-phosphate show promise [70]. Universally, treatment with 600 mg alpha lipoic acid (ALA) administered via IV or orally daily for 5–12 weeks presents an effective solution for DPN [71,72]. Recent success in animal-based, gene-related therapies such as electro-gene therapy demonstrated significant amelioration of sensory deficits in peripheral nerves suggesting potential for remediation in human subjects [73].

INTERVENTIONS FOR RISK REDUCTION

The causes of diabesity are not the same for every person. For some, diabesity may be simply a result of poor diet. For others, it may be due to environmental toxins, chronic inflammation, digestive imbalances, chronic stress, or even food sensitivities. Recent population-based cohort studies show a significant combined effect of lifestyle changes on diabetes risk reduction.

EVALUATION OF LIFESTYLE MARKERS

The effect of lifestyle factors on the development of diabetes has been studied in large clinical trials, with an emphasis on:

- BMI of ≤ 25
- An alkaline forming diet high in cereal fiber, probiotics, and nutrient-dense whole foods
- Low glycemic load nutrition and targeted supplementation as needed to reach healthy goal values (see Table 19.3 later in this chapter)
- Increasing intake of detoxifying, sulfur rich foods: garlic, onions, ginger, broccoli sprouts, and eggs

- Shifting intake toward polyunsaturated, unoxidized fats and away from omega-6 rich and/
  or trans fats
- Exercising regularly to include low-impact weight bearing and cardio training
- Abstaining from smoking
- Consuming alcohol moderately, if at all.

This profile of health habits is associated with a 90% lower incidence of type 2 diabetes risks compared with women who did not observe a healthy lifestyle [74]. Type 2 diabetes can thus be prevented by the adoption of this healthful lifestyle [75]. Chemical control of blood sugar alone does not achieve the same benefits [17–20].

LAB TESTING

Aggregate risk reduction is associated with more favorable values for:

- Serum high sensitivity C-reactive protein (serum hsCRP): healthful value is < 0.5 mg/L. Usual lab ranges are statistical and not predictive.
- Plasma homocysteine: healthy goal value is < 6 µmol/L.
- Serum oxidized LDL/HDL and urine 8-hydroxy-2'-deoxyguanosine (8OHdG): healthful goal values are undetectable indicating adequate antioxidants to prevent free-radical oxidation.
- Saliva free cortisol/dehydroepiandrosterone (DHEA) ratio: healthful stress hormone rhythm means a peak in the early morning and a trough in the afternoon within the upper half of the lab reference range.
- First morning urine pH to assess cellular metabolic acidosis. This can be accomplished easily at home with high-sensitivity pH test strips with a range from 5–8 with a healthful goal value of 6.5–7.5 after six hours of rest to allow the urine to equilibrate with the cells in the bladder and kidney.

We suggest measuring and interpreting these tests annually for people over the age of 30 who want to maintain, enhance, or restore their functional vitality, immune tolerance, and neurohormone resilience (see Table 19.3 later in this chapter). We reinforce the points made earlier regarding nutritional sufficiency, including hydration.

DIETARY INTERVENTIONS

Shifting from a nutrient-poor diet to a nutrient-dense diet that is abundant in plant foods such as fresh, whole fruits, vegetables, nuts, seeds, beans, and whole grains improves the function of hundreds of genes that control insulin function and obesity. This approach is characteristic of the Alkaline Way [76] and Mediterranean diets [47,77], particularly the Greek Mediterranean diet [78].

Improved glycemic control is the goal of modern diabetes management and translates to better long-term outcomes. We have found that reducing immunologic load for the individual while providing nutrient sufficiency and neurohormonal distress reduction improves glycemic control.

Calorie restriction helps to improve mitochondrial function [79]. However, simply modifying lifestyle, engaging in interval training and exercise, eating a nutrient-dense diet, and appropriate use of dietary supplements can enhance mitochondrial function and reduce oxidative stress [80].

In the clinical setting, it is important to be aware of interactions between medications and nutritional supplements that can either support or limit successful therapies. Oral antidiabetic agents and nutrient interactions are reviewed in Table 19.2.

TABLE 19.2
Food and Nutrient Consideration with Diabetes Pharmacotherapy

Pharmacological Agent	Mechanism of Action	Clinical Considerations	Nutrient Considerations	Food/Diet Interactions
Sulfonylureas First generation (chlorpropamide, tolbutamide) and second generation (glyburide, glipizide, and glimepiride)	Stimulate insulin secretion by binding to receptors on pancreatic beta cells Metabolized in the liver via the cytochrome P450 system	Secondary benefit: decrease LDL, increase HDL to normal levels Risks include weight gain, hypoglycemic episodes.	Minor acetohexamide, glyburide and tolazamide may inhibit CoQ10 synthesis	To be avoided with alcohol; for glipizide: recommended taking 30 minutes before a meal for optimum results
Meglitinides repaglinide and nateglinide (glinides)	Similar to sulfonylureas Metabolized in the liver via the cytochrome P450 system	More favorable safety profile than sulfonylureas, especially in patients with renal failure Specific caution with the following medications: rifampicin, ciclosporin, gemfibrozil, and repaglinide: also with statins such as simvastatin and lovastatin	Minor	Have a rapid elimination rate, so recommended to be taken at the beginning of a meal Not to be taken with grapefruit juice as the juice can enhance its effect precipitating hypoglycemia
Biguanides (metformin)	Reduces hepatic glucose production	Reduction in TG, LDL, total cholesterol, HbA1C, and insulin, reducing oxidative stress GI discomfort, rare lactic acidosis	Folate and vitamin B12; intrinsic factor is calcium dependent so calcium supplementation may be indicated. Increase in homocysteine levels	To minimize GI disturbances, recommended to be taken with food,
Thiazolidinediones (rosglitazone, pioglitazone)	Improve insulin action Metabolized in the liver via the cytochrome P450 system	Decrease in homocysteine Rosglitazone: reduction in TG, LDL, total cholesterol, HbA1C, and insulin, reducing oxidative stress 1. Increased risk of myocardial infarction and heart failure 2. Fracture risk in women, and, for rosiglitazone, more rapid bone loss 3. To be used with caution in people with hepatic dysfunction Specific caution when combined with statins	Due to risk of bone loss, bone-nutrient supplementation is recommended, particularly for women postmenopause	No effect of food on action
Incretin analogues exenatide and rimonabant (injectable)	Stimulate insulin secretion from pancreatic beta cells Slower absorption of carbohydrates from the gut	Accelerated weight loss; possible nausea, diarrhea, vomiting	No specific interactions yet identified	Not to be taken after meals

NUTRITIONAL SUPPLEMENTATION

A number of nutrients are particularly important in the prevention and treatment of diabesity, including such repair promoting:

- Antioxidants: 100% reduced and buffered l-ascorbates (vitamins C) [81], polyphenolics (especially quercetin dihydrate, low molecular weight orthoproanthocyanidins, and resveratrols) [82], and alpha-lipoic acids [83,84]
- Vitamins: vitamin D [85], and B complex including biotin and para amino benzoic acid (PABA)
- Minerals: chromium [86,87], magnesium [88], zinc [89], and vanadium [90]
- Beneficial fats: omega-3 fats—eicosapentaenoic acid (EPA) and docosahexaenoic acid (DHA) being more helpful; conversion from alpha-linoleic acid is often blocked or impaired) [91]
- Amino acids: 100% L-carnitine fumarate [92], gamma-amino butyric acid (GABA) [93]

These nutrients regulate glucose metabolism and insulin sensitivity [94,95]. In patients with diabetes, supplementing with nutrients is prudent because modern agricultural and processing practices have greatly diminished the nutrient content and density of our diet, while lifestyle in urban society has increased the demand [96]. Probiotics are important to restore gut flora and reduce the burden of systemic inflammation. Table 19.3 presents an overview of nutrients important in the regulation of diabetes and the association between adequate supplementation and favorable primary marker lab values.

Low-level nutrient and antioxidant deficiencies promote inflammation. Some studies suggest that taking a multivitamin and mineral supplement can be as effective in enhancing repair and lowering inflammation as a statin, though at lesser expense with fewer side effects [97,98].

Hydration is important and continues to be underappreciated in the clinical setting, despite its being essential to reduce food cravings and reverse diabesity. Hydration can be assessed and quantified in different ways. One is the "back of palm skin pinch" test for skin turgor. With adequate hydration, the skin should go flat within one second after releasing the pinch. For those whose skin relaxation time is longer, we suggest having the patient drink a glass of water, possibly with electrolytes if available, and doing a retest in 30–45 minutes.

PSYCHOSOCIAL/SPIRITUAL BALANCE

Stress has been shown to promote central obesity, insulin resistance, and diabetes due to the elevation of cortisol, insulin, and cytokines. Mice bred to be obese and diabetic show improved metabolic function and lost weight through adrenalectomy, though admittedly not an optimum strategy for weight loss [99]. Depression and diabetes are linked [100] and may be interactive.

Chronic stress is yet another cause of chronic inflammation [101]. Lack of regular exercise promotes low-grade inflammation while regular exercise reduces inflammation [102]. Management of stress, including relaxation therapies, meditation, deep breathing, biofeedback, massage, saunas, exercise, yoga, dancing, and laughter, as well as social and group support can reduce the frequency of the stress response, normalizing adrenal function and neuroendocrine signaling [103].

CONCLUSION

Risk evaluation and intervention are most effectively addressed in the context of the upstream drivers of disease. Distinguishing between risk factors and causes is essential for effective primary prevention and treatment of chronic disease.

Treatment must focus on the system, not the symptom. Obesity and its chronic disease consequences commonly referred to as risk factors, dyslipidemia, hyperglycemia, and hypertension are

TABLE 19.3

Supplemental Nutrients in Diabetes with Associated Primary Health Markers

Nutrients	Dosage/Function	Primary Markers with Favorable Range
Marine lipids as EPA/DHA distilled under nitrogen	1–4 grams daily total omega-3 fats as mix of EPA and DHA	Antioxidant status: favorable omega-3/omega-6 ratio and no oxidized HDL/LDL cholesterol
Magnesium in fully ionized forms	400–1000 mg of elemental magnesium daily as glycinate, citrate, malate, succinate, fumarate, aspartate, and/or ascorbate, or other fully ionized forms; avoid chelates and pulverized rocks Uptake is uniquely enhanced with concurrent choline citrate to form neutral charge droplets easily taken up by small intestine. No other choline form is helpful (e.g., choline bitartrate is not effective in enhancing magnesium uptake)	Metabolic status after six or more hours of rest, 1st a.m. urine pH: 6.5–7.5
Potassium	3–4 g total daily intake	Maintain healthy plasma potassium (serum can be misleading)
Chromium: uptake enhanced with concurrent biotin, taurine, and/or vanadium	500–1000 mcg/day as picolinate or citrate; improves lean body mass and insulin sensitivity; works synergistically with vanadium	Included in d-penicillamine provocation tests for essential and toxic minerals
Vitamin B12 (hydroxocobalamin preferred) and folates (all eight natural forms)	Help maintain healthy homocysteine levels Improve endothelial dysfunction in diabetes	Sufficient to bring homocysteine < 6 μmol/L; methionine and sulfur rich foods may also be needed.
Carotenoids: alpha and beta carotene, zeaxanthin, cryptoxanthin, pseudoxanthin, lutein, astaxanthin, lycopene Only natural mixed forms such as from D.Salina recommended. Free lycopene is active while lycopene complex is barely active if at all.	Improve cognitive health and memory-induced learning; serum carotenoid levels are inversely proportional to insulin resistance.	
Iodine and iodide	Thyroid disorders associated with adrenal dysfunction more likely with diabetes Need for adequate iodine levels	Free thyroid hormone tests depend upon functionally available iodine Adrenal health; saliva free DHEA/ free cortisol balance
Ascorbate (Vitamin C)	Adequate to quench free radicals; ascorbate calibration recommended to determine individual need	Repair deficit and inflammation: sufficient to bring high sensitivity C- reactive protein (hsCRP) < 0.5 mg/L
Vitamin E	400–3200 IU/day only as mixed natural tocopherols and tocotrienols; d-alpha tocopherol acetate or succinate not recommended	Include 250–1,000 mcg per day of selenomethionine to activate vitamin E

continued

TABLE 19.3 (*continued*)

Supplemental Nutrients in Diabetes with Associated Primary Health Markers

Nutrients	Dosage/Function	Primary Markers with Favorable Range
Alpha-lipoic acid	600 mg alpha lipoic acid twice daily can be neuroprotective in diabetes	Adequate ascorbate protects and regenerates alpha lipoic acid; all eight forms recommended
100% L-Carnitine fumarate and acetyl L-carnitine	500–1000 mg/day can support improvement in nerve conduction and pain reduction while improving fat metabolism	
Rice bran oil and gamma oryzanol; pure rice bran oil will include gamma oryzanol content, a beneficial ergogenic compound; recommended for most softgels to enhance uptake and benefit	Improve hyperglycemia, insulin resistance, and overall lipid metabolism	
Essential minerals	With other antioxidants; useful for diabetic retinopathy	D-penicillamine provocation to assess essential and toxic mineral status on 24° urine; metabolic acidosis increases beneficial mineral loss and increases retention of toxic minerals
Vitamin D3	2000 IU cholecalciferol per day or enough to bring 25-hydroxyvitamin D3 into beneficial range	25-hydroxyvitamin D3 levels: goal value is 50–80 ng/ml

only downstream symptoms of upstream biological causes. They are the smoke, not the fire. A comprehensive solution involves a systems approach to risk factors rather than symptoms alone, addressing diet, exercise, stress management, and detoxification to reduce the effects of toxic environmental exposures.

The research reflects consensus that comprehensive lifestyle medicine has the potential to stem the impending tsunami of obesity and chronic disease. A systems approach that includes lifestyle interventions also has the potential to reduce the incidence of cardiovascular disease and diabetes by more than 90%. Diabetes, more a lifestyle than a disease, can be avoided or managed more successfully with comprehensive, evidence-based integrative approaches.

REFERENCES

1. Flegal, K. M., Carroll M. D., Ogden, C. L., and L. R. Curtin. 2010. Prevalence and trends in obesity among US adults, 1999–2008. *JAMA* Jan 20;303(3):235–41.
2. Hedley, A. A., Ogden C. L., Johnson, C. L., Carroll, M. D., Curtin, L. R., and K. M. Flegal. 2004. Prevalence of overweight and obesity among US children, adolescents, and adults, 1999–2002. *JAMA* Jun 16;291(23):2847–50.
3. http://www.cdc.gov/obesity/index.html.
4. Centers for Disease Control and Prevention. 2011. National diabetes fact sheet: National estimates and general information on diabetes and prediabetes in the United States. U.S. Department of Health and Human Services, CDC, Atlanta.
5. Fradkin, J., and G. P. Rodgers. 2008. The economic imperative to conquer diabetes. *Diabetes Care* March 2008 31:624–25.
6. Yang, W., Lu, J., Weng, J., et al. 2010. China National Diabetes and Metabolic Disorders Study Group. Prevalence of diabetes among men and women in China. *N Engl J Med* Mar 25;362(12):1090–1101.

7. Power, C., and C. Thomas. 2011. Changes in BMI, duration of overweight and obesity, and glucose metabolism: 45 years of follow-up of a birth cohort. *Diabetes Care* 34:1986–91.

8. Olshansky, S. J., Passaro, D. J., Hershow, R.C., et al. 2005. A potential decline in life expectancy in the United States in the 21st century. *N Engl J Med* Mar 17;352(11):1138–45.

9. Bibbins-Domingo, K., Coxson, P., Pletcher, M. J., et al. 2007. Adolescent overweight and future adult coronary heart disease. *N Engl J Med* Dec 6;357(23):2371–79.

10. Lakka, H. M., Laaksonen, D. E., Lakka, T. A., et al. 2002. The metabolic syndrome and total and cardiovascular disease mortality in middle-aged men. *JAMA* Dec 4;288(21):2709–16.

11. Ott, A., Stolk, R. P., van Harskamp, F., Pols, H. A., Hofman, A., and M. M. Breteler. 1999. Diabetes mellitus and the risk of dementia: The Rotterdam Study. *Neurology* Dec 10;53(9):1937–42.

12. Key, T. J., Spencer, E. A., and G. K. Reeves. 2009. Symposium 1: Overnutrition: Consequences and solutions for obesity and cancer risk. *Proc Nutr Soc* Dec 3:1–5.

13. National Center for Chronic Disease. Centers for Disease Control. 2007. National diabetes fact sheet. U.S. Department of Health and Human Services, CDC, Atlanta. Available at http://apps.nccd.cdc.gov/DDTSTRS/FactSheet.aspx.

14. Franks, P. W., Hanson, R. L., Knowler, W. C., Sievers, M. L., Bennett, P. H., and H. C. Looker. 2010. Childhood obesity, other cardiovascular risk factors, and premature death. *N Engl J Med.* Feb 11;362(6):485–93.

15. Tuomilehto, J., Lindstrom, J., Eriksson, J. G., et al., and the Finnish Diabetes Prevention Study Group. 2001. Prevention of type 2 diabetes mellitus by changes in lifestyle among subjects with impaired glucose tolerance. *N Engl J Med* 344(18):1343–50.

16. Rakel, D. P. 2006. Perspectives on integrative practice. In *Complementary Medicine in Clinical Practice,* ed. D. P. Rakel and N. J. Faass, 3–8. Burlington, MA: Jones & Bartlett Learning.

17. Gerstein, H. C., Miller, M. E., Byington, R. P., et al., and the Action to Control Cardiovascular Risk in Diabetes Study Group. 2008. Effects of intensive glucose lowering in type 2 diabetes. *N Engl J Med* Jun 12;358(24):2545–59.

18. The ACCORD Study Group. 2010. Effects of combination lipid therapy in type 2 diabetes mellitus. *N Engl J Med* 2010 May 6;362(18):1748.

19. The NAVIGATOR Study Group. 2010. Effect of nateglinide on the incidence of diabetes and cardiovascular events. *N Engl J Med* 2010 Apr 22;362(16):1463–76. Epub Mar 14, 2010.

20. The ACCORD Study Group. 2010. Effects of intensive blood-pressure control in type 2 diabetes mellitus. *N Engl J Med* 2010 Apr 9;362(17):1575–85. Epub Mar 14, 2010.

21. American College of Preventive Medicine. *Lifestyle Medicine: Evidence Review.* June 30, 2009. Available at: http://www.acpm.org/LifestyleMedicine.htm. Accessed September 18, 2009.

22. Barabasi, A.L. 2007. Network medicine: From obesity to the "diseasome." *N Engl J Med* Jul 26;357(4):404–7.

23. Kligler, B., and D. Lynch. 2003. An integrative approach to the management of type 2 diabetes mellitus. *Altern Ther Health Med* Nov–Dec;9(6):24–32; quiz 33. Review.

24. Kelly, G. S. 2000. Insulin resistance: Lifestyle and nutritional interventions. *Altern Med Rev* Apr;5(2):109–32. Review.

25. Barclay, A. W., Petocz, P., McMillan-Price, J., et al. 2008. Glycemic index, glycemic load, and chronic disease risk: A meta-analysis of observational studies. *Am J Clin Nutr* Mar;87(3):627–37.

26. Cordain L, et al. 2005. Origin and evolution of the Western diet: Health implications for the 21st century. *Am J Clin Nutr* 8 (2):341–54. Review.

27. Ludwig, D. S., Peterson, K. E., and S. L. Gortmaker. 2001. Relation between consumption of sugar-sweetened drinks and childhood obesity: A prospective, observational analysis. *Lancet* Feb 17;357(9255):505–8.

28. Hu, F. B., Li, T. Y., Colditz, G. A., Willett, W. C., and J. E. Manson. 2003. Television watching and other sedentary behaviors in relation to risk of obesity and type 2 diabetes mellitus in women. *JAMA* Apr 9;289(14):1785–91; Hyman, M. 2007. Systems biology, toxins, obesity, and functional medicine. *Altern Ther Health Med.* Mar–Apr;13(2):S134–39. Review.

29. Centers for Disease Control. National Health and Nutrition Examination Surveys 2003–8. U.S. Department of Health and Human Services, CDC, Atlanta.

30. Tzanavari, T., Giannogonas, P., and K. P. Karalis. 2010. TNF-alpha and obesity. *Curr Dir Autoimmun* 11:145–56.

31. Eaton, S.B., and M. Konner. 1985. Paleolithic nutrition. A consideration of its nature and current implications. *N Engl J Med* Jan 31;312(5):283–89. Review.

32. Robson, A. A. 2009. Preventing diet induced disease: Bioavailable nutrient-rich, low-energy-dense diets. *Nutr Health* 20(2):135–66. Review.

33. Chandalia, M., Garg, A., Lutjohann, D., von Bergmann, K., Grundy, S. M., and L. J. Brinkley. 2000. Beneficial effects of high dietary fiber intake in patients with type 2 diabetes mellitus. *N Engl J Med* May 11;342(19):1392–98.

34. Frid, A. H., Nilsoon, M., Holst, J. J., and I. M. Bjorck. 2005. Effect of whey on blood glucose and insulin responses to composite breakfast and lunch meals in type 2 diabetic subjects. *Am J Clin Nutr* Jul;82(1):69–75.

35. Jaffe, R., and J. Mani. 2012. Effect of novel whey based low glycemic load meal replacement. Washington, DC, Weight of the Nation Conference, April 2012. Poster submission.

36. Swithers, S. E., and T. L. Davidson. 2008. A role for sweet taste: Calorie predictive relations in energy regulation by rats. *Behav Neurosci* Feb;122(1):161–73.

37. Tsai, F., and W. J. Coyle. 2009. The microbiome and obesity: Is obesity linked to our gut flora? *Curr Gastroenterol Rep* Aug;11(4):307–13. Review.

38. Cani, P. D., Amar, J., Iglesias, M. A., et al. 2007. Metabolic endotoxemia initiates obesity and insulin resistance. *Diabetes* Jul;56(7):1761–72.

39. Jaffe, R., Mani, J., DeVane, J., and H. Mani. 2006. Tolerance loss in diabetics: Association with foreign antigen exposure. *Diabet Med* Aug;23(8):924–25.

40. Deuster P. A., and R. Jaffe. 2000. Autoimmunity: Clinical relevance of biological response modifiers in diagnosis, treatment, and testing, part I and part II. *Intl J Integrative Med* 2 (2):16–22 & 58–65.

41. Hampton, T. 2004. Mitochondrial defects may play role in the metabolic syndrome. *JAMA* Dec 15;292(23):2823–24.

42. Petersen, K. F., Dufour, S., Befroy, D., Garcia, R., and G. I. Shulman. 2004 Impaired mitochondrial activity in the insulin-resistant offspring of patients with type 2 diabetes. *N Engl J Med* Feb 12;350(7):664–71.

43. Chuang, K. J., Chan, C. C., Su, T. C., Lee, C. T., and C. S. Tang. 2007. The effect of urban air pollution on inflammation, oxidative stress, coagulation, and autonomic dysfunction in young adults. *Am J Respir Crit Care Med* Aug 15;176(4):370–76.

44. Valko, M., Morris, H., and M. T. Cronin. 2005. Metals, toxicity and oxidative stress. *Curr Med Chem* 12(10):1161–208.

45. Li, X., Cobb, C. E., Hill, K. E., Burk, R. F., and J. M. May. 2001. Mitochondrial uptake and recycling of ascorbic acid. *Arch Biochem Biophys* Mar 1;387(1):143–53.

46. Barone, M. C., Darley-Usmar, V. M., and P. S. Brookes. 2003. Reversible inhibition of cytochrome c oxidase by peroxynitrite proceeds through ascorbate-dependent generation of nitric oxide. *J Biol Chem* Jul 25;278(30): 27520–24.

47. Giugliano, D., and K. Esposito. 2008. Mediterranean diet and metabolic diseases. *Curr Opin Lipidol* Feb;19(1):63–68. Review.

48. Hyman, M. A. 2006. Systems biology: The gut-brain-fat cell connection and obesity. *Altern Ther Health Med* Jan–Feb;12(1):10–16. Review.

49. Maratou, E., Hadjidakis, D. J., Kollias, A., et al. 2009. Studies of insulin resistance in patients with clinical and subclinical hypothyroidism. *Eur J Endocrinol* May;160(5):785–90.

50. Ayturk, S., Gursoy, A., Kut, A., Anil, C., Nar, A., and N. B. Tutuncu. 2009. Metabolic syndrome and its components are associated with increased thyroid volume and nodule prevalence in a mild-to-moderate iodine-deficient area. *Eur J Endocrinol* Oct;161(4):599–605.

51. Golden, S. H. 2007. A review of the evidence for a neuroendocrine link between stress, depression and diabetes mellitus. *Curr Diabetes Rev* Nov;3(4):252–9. Review.

52. Gallagher, P., Leitch, M. M., Massey, A. E., Hamish McAllister-Williams, R., and A. H. Young. 2000. Assessing cortisol and dehydroepiandrosterone (DHEA) in saliva: Effects of collection method. *J Psychopharma* 20(5): 643–49.

53. Van Cauter, E., Holmback, U., Knutson, K., et al. 2007. Impact of sleep and sleep loss on neuroendocrine and metabolic function. *Horm Res* 67 Suppl 1:2–9.

54. Hassouna R, Zizzari P, Tolle V. 2010. The ghrelin/obestatin balance in the physiological and pathological control of growth hormone secretion, body composition and food intake. *J Neuroendocrinol* Jul;22(7):793–804.

55. Chavarro, J. E., Rich-Edwards, J. W., Rosner, B. A., and W. C. Willett. 2007. Diet and lifestyle in the prevention of ovulatory disorder infertility. *Obstet Gynecol* Nov;110(5):1050–58.

56. Garruti, G., Depalo, R., Vita, M. G., et al. 2009. Adipose tissue, metabolic syndrome and polycystic ovary syndrome: From pathophysiology to treatment. *Reprod Biomed Online* Oct;19(4):552–63.

57. Zitzmann, M. 2009. Testosterone deficiency, insulin resistance and the metabolic syndrome. *Nat Rev Endocrinol* Dec;5(12):673–81.

58. Lopez-Pedrera, C., Perez-Sanchez, C., Ramos-Casals, M., Santos-Gonzalez, M., Rodriguez-Ariza, A., and M. J. Cuadrado. 2012. Cardiovascular risk in systemic autoimmune diseases: Epigenetic mechanisms of immune regulatory functions. *Clin Dev Immunol* Epub Sep 14, 2011.

59. Harvey, A. E., Lashinger, L.M., and S. D. Hursting. 2011. The growing challenge of obesity and cancer: An inflammatory issue. *Ann N Y Acad Sci* Jul;1229:45–52.

60. Johnston, H., Boutin, H., and S. M. Allan. 2011. Assessing the contribution of inflammation in models of Alzheimer's disease. *Biochem Soc Trans* Aug;39(4):886–90.

61. Pradhan, A. D., Manson, J. E., Rifai, N., Buring, J. E., and P. M. Ridker. 2001. C-reactive protein, interleukin 6, and risk of developing type 2 diabetes mellitus. *JAMA* Jul 18;286(3):327–34.

62. Chuang, K.J., Chan, C. C., Su, T. C., Lee, C. T., and C. S. Tang. 2007. The effect of urban air pollution on inflammation, oxidative stress, coagulation, and autonomic dysfunction in young adults. *Am J Respir Crit Care Med* Aug 15;176(4):370–76.

63. Ronn, M., Lind, L., van Bavel, B., Salihovic, S., Michaelsson, K., and P. M. Lind. 2011. Circulating levels of persistent organic pollutants associate in divergent ways to fat mass measured by DXA in humans. *Chemosphere* 85: 335–43.

64. Jones, O. A., Maguire, M. L., and J. L. Griffin. 2008. Environmental pollution and diabetes: A neglected association. *Lancet* Jan 26;371(9609):287–88.

65. Navas-Acien, A., Silbergeld, E. K., Pastor-Barriuso, R., and E. Guallar. 2008. Arsenic exposure and prevalence of type 2 diabetes in US adults. *JAMA* Aug 20;300(7):814–22.

66. Atkinson, R. L. 2007. Viruses as an etiology of obesity. *Mayo Clin Proc* Oct;82(10):1192–98. Review.

67. Head, K. A. 2006. Peripheral neuropathy: Pathogenic mechanisms and alternative therapies. *Altern Med Rev* Dec;11(4):294–329.

68. Cermenati, G., Abbiati, F., Cermenati, S., et al. 2012. Diabetes induced myelin abnormalities are associated with an altered lipid pattern: Protective effects of LXR activation. *J Lipid Res* 53(2):300–310.

69. Al-Ani, F. S., Al-Nimer, M. S., and F. S. Ali. 2011. Dyslipidemia as a contributory factor in etiopathogenesis of diabetic neuropathy. *Indian J Endocrinol Metab* Apr;15(2):110–14.

70. Miranda-Massari, J. R., Gonzalez, M. J., Jimenez, F. J., Allende-Vigo, M. A., and J. Duconge. 2011. Metabolic correction in the management of diabetic peripheral neuropathy: Improving clinical results beyond symptom control. *Curr Clin Pharmacol* Nov 1;6(4):260–73.

71. McIlduff, C. E., Rutkove, S. B., and Zhonghua Yi Xue Za Zhi. 2011. Critical appraisal of the use of alpha lipoic acid (thioctic acid) in the treatment of symptomatic diabetic polyneuropathy. *Ther Clin Risk Manag* 7:377–85.

72. Gu, X. M., Zhang, S. S., Wu, J. C., et al. 2010. Efficacy and safety of high-dose α-lipoic acid in the treatment of diabetic polyneuropathy [article in Chinese]. *Zhonghua Yi Xue Za Zhi* Sep 21;90(35):2473–76.

73. Murakami, T., Imada, Y., Kawamura, M. et al. 2011. Placental growth factor-2 gene transfer by electroporation restores diabetic sensory neuropathy in mice. *Exp Neurol* Jan;227(1):195–202. Epub Nov 5, 2010.

74. Hu, F. B., Manson, J. E., Stampfer, M. J. et al. 2001. Diet, lifestyle, and the risk of type 2 diabetes mellitus in women. *N Engl J Med* 345(11):790–97.

75. Nilsen, V., Bakke, P. S., and F. Gallefoss. 2011. Effects of lifestyle intervention in persons at risk for type 2 diabetes mellitus: Results from a randomized, controlled trial. *BMC Public Health* 11:893.

76. Health Studies Collegium Foundation. 2010. *Joy of Eating the Alkaline Way,* 14th Edition. Ashburn: VA, 1–56.

77. Rumawas, M. E., Meigs, J. B., Dwyer, J. T., McKeown, N. M., and P. F. Jacques. 2009. Mediterraneanstyle dietary pattern, reduced risk of metabolic syndrome traits, and incidence in the Framingham Offspring Cohort. *Am J Clin Nutr* Dec;90(6):1608–14.

78. Simopoulos, A.P. 2001. Mediterranean diets: What is so special about the diet of Greece? The scientific evidence. *J Nutr* 131;3065S–73S.

79. Fontana, L. 2009. The scientific basis of caloric restriction leading to longer life. *Curr Opin Gastroenterol* Mar;25(2):144–50. Review.

80. Ames, B. N. 2003. The metabolic tune-up: metabolic harmony and disease prevention. *J Nutr* May;133(5 Suppl 1):1544S–48S.

81. Badr, G., Bashandy, S., Ebaid H., Mohany, M. and D. Sayed. 2012. Vitamin C supplementation reconstitutes polyfunctional T cells in streptozotocin-induced diabetic rats. *Eur J Nutr* Aug;51(5):623–33.

82. Kim, J. H., Kang, M. J., Choi, H. N., Jeong, S. M., Lee, Y. M., and J. I. Kim. 2011. Quercetin attenuates fasting and postprandial hyperglycemia in animal models of diabetes mellitus. *Nutr Res Pract* Apr;5(2):107–11.

83. Shay, K. P., Moreau, R. F., Smith, E. J., Smith, A. R., and T. M. Hagen. 2009. Alpha-lipoic acid as a dietary supplement: Molecular mechanisms and therapeutic potential. *Biochim Biophys Acta* Oct;1790(10):1149–60. Epub Aug 4, 2009.

84. Poh, Z., and K. P. Goh. 2009. A current update on the use of alpha lipoic acid in the management of type 2 diabetes mellitus. *Endocr Metab Immune Disord Drug Targets* Dec;9(4):392–98.

85. Reis, J. P., von Mühlen, D., Miller, E. R. III, Michos, E. D., and L. J. Appel. 2009. Vitamin D status and cardiometabolic risk factors in the United States adolescent population. *Pediatrics* Sep;124(3):e371–79. Epub Aug 3, 2009.

86. A scientific review: the role of chromium in insulin resistance.[No authors listed.] 2004. *Diabetes Educ* Suppl:2–14. Review.

87. Lau, F. C., Bagchi, M., Sen, C. K., and D. Bagchi. 2008. Nutrigenomic basis of beneficial effects of chromium(III) on obesity and diabetes. *Mol Cell Biochem* Oct;317(1–2):1–10. Epub Jul 18, 2008. Review.

88. Chaudhary, D. P., Sharma, R., and D. D. Bansal. 2010. Implications of magnesium deficiency in type 2 diabetes: A review. *Biol Trace Elem Res* May;134(2):119–29.

89. Masood, N., Baloch, G. H., Ghori, R. A., Memon, I. A., Memon, M. A., and M. S. Memon. 2009. Serum zinc and magnesium in type-2 diabetic patients. *J Coll Physicians Surg Pak* Aug;19(8):483–86.

90. Thompson, K. H., Lichter, J., LeBel, C., Scaife, M. C., McNeill, J. H., and C. Orvig. 2009. Vanadium treatment of type 2 diabetes: A view to the future. *J Inorg Biochem* Apr;103(4):554–58.

91. Flachs, P., Rossmeisl, M., Bryhn, M., and J. Kopecky. 2009. Cellular and molecular effects of n-3 poly-unsaturated fatty acids on adipose tissue biology and metabolism. *Clin Sci* (Lond) Jan;116(1):1–16. Review.

92. Ringseis, R., Keller, J., and K. Eder. 2012. Role of carnitine in the regulation of glucose homeostasis and insulin sensitivity: Evidence from in vivo and in vitro studies with carnitine supplementation and carnitine deficiency. *Eur J Nutr* Feb;51(1):1–18.

93. Tian, J. et al. 2004. Gamma-aminobutyric acid inhibits T cell autoimmunity and the development of inflammatory responses in a mouse type 1 diabetes model. *J Immunol* 173(8):5298–304.

94. Kligler, B., and D. Lynch. 2003. An integrative approach to the management of type 2 diabetes mellitus. *Altern Ther Health Med* Nov–Dec;9(6):24–32; quiz 33. Review.

95. Kelly, G.S. 2000. Insulin resistance: Lifestyle and nutritional interventions. *Altern Med Rev* Apr;5(2):109–32. Review.

96. Benbrook, C., Zhao, X., Yanez, J., Davies, and P. Andrews. 2008. New evidence confirms the nutritional superiority of plant-based organic foods. *State of Science Review* March, available at: http://www.organic-center.org/science.nutri.php?action=view&report_id=126.

97. Church, T. S., Earnest, C. P., Wood, K. A., and J. B. Kampert. 2003. Reduction of C-reactive protein levels through use of a multivitamin. *Am J Med* Dec 15;115(9):702–7.

98. Jaffe, R. 2012. Diabetes as an immune dysfunction syndrome. In *Bioactive Foods as Dietary Interventions for Diabetes*. Eds. R. R. Watson and Victor R. Preedy. Academic Press: *in press*.

99. Makimura, H., Mizuno, T. M., Bergen, H., and C. V. Mobbs. 2002. Adiponectin is stimulated by adrenalectomy in ob/ob mice and is highly correlated with resistin mRNA. *Am J Physiol Endocrinol Metab* Dec;283(6):E1266–71.

100. Holt, R. I., Phillips, D. I., Jameson, K. A., Cooper, C., Dennison, E. M., and R. C. Peveler; Hertfordshire Cohort Study Group. 2009. The relationship between depression and diabetes mellitus: Findings from the Hertfordshire Cohort Study. *Diabet Med* Jun;26(6):641–48.

101. Munhoz, C. D., García-Bueno, B., Madrigal, J. L., Lepsch, L. B., Scavone, C., and J. C. Leza. 2008. Stress-induced neuroinflammation: Mechanisms and new pharmacological targets. *Braz J Med Biol Res* Dec;41(12):1037–46. Review.

102. Smith, J. K., Dykes, R., Douglas, J. E., Krishnaswamy, G., and S. Berk. 1999. Long-term exercise and atherogenic activity of blood mononuclear cells in persons at risk of developing ischemic heart disease. *JAMA* May 12;281(18):1722–27.

103. Bijlani R. L., Vempati, R. P., Yadav, R. K., Ray, R. B., Gupta, V., Sharma, R., Mehta, N., and S. C. Mahapatra. 2005. A brief but comprehensive lifestyle education program based on yoga reduces risk factors for cardiovascular disease and diabetes mellitus. *J Altern Complement Med.* Apr;11(2):267–74.

20 Hashimoto's Thyroiditis

Optimizing Thyroid Function with Nutrition

Sheila George, M.D.

INTRODUCTION

Hashimoto's thyroiditis, an autoimmune disease, is the most common cause of primary hypothyroidism in the United States [1]. Despite supplementation with thyroid hormone, whether thyroxine or thyroxine and triioothyronine, some patients continue to have symptoms of hypothyroidism.

Many factors can impact on the proper functioning of the thyroid gland and thyroid hormone metabolism, including nutrient deficiencies, toxins, infections, food intolerances and food allergies, poor liver function, and chronic stress.

This chapter discusses foods and nutrients that address these challenges, thereby helping to optimize thyroid hormone metabolism and improve symptoms in the patient with hypothyroidism.

EPIDEMIOLOGY

Hashimoto's thyroiditis affects up to 3.7% of the general population [2]. According to the National Health and Nutrition Examination Survey (NHANES III) study, the prevalence of subclinical and clinical hypothyroidism in the US population is 4.3% and 0.3%, respectively [3]. The study demonstrated that the average serum thyroid-stimulating hormone (TSH) concentrations and the prevalence of antithyroid antibodies are greater in women and increase with age. These values are higher in whites and Mexican Americans than in blacks. In addition, the study revealed that the serum TSH levels were slightly higher in children aged 12–19 years than in young adults aged 20–29 years.

The National Health and Nutrition Examination Survey (NHANES 1999–2002) revealed that hypothyroid prevalence in women of reproductive age (12–49 years) is 3.1%. And individuals aged 80 years and older had five times greater odds for hypothyroidism compared to 12 to 49 year olds.

THYROID HORMONE METABOLISM

Thyroid hormone production is controlled by feedback mechanisms within the hypothalamic-pituitary-thyroid axis. In response to low thyroid hormone, the hypothalamus stimulates the pituitary gland via thyrotropin-releasing hormone (TRH) to release thyroid-stimulating hormone (TSH). TSH signals the thyroid gland to upregulate thyroid hormone production.

The synthesis of thyroid hormone requires tyrosine and iodine. Iodide enters the thyroid via the sodium-iodide symporter and becomes iodine through the process of organification. This is catalyzed by thyroid peroxidase enzyme (TPO), accompanied by hydrogen peroxide. The iodine is incorporated into the tyrosine residue of the thyroglobulin molecule at the third and fifth positions forming 3, 5–diiodotyrosine (DIT). This is again catalyzed by TPO. The coupling of two DIT molecules creates thyroxine/T4 (3, 5, 3' 5' –tetraiodothyronine). The coupling of a DIT molecule with a MIT (3-monoiodotyrosine) molecule forms T3 (3, 5, 3' –triiodothyronine) and reverse T3 (3, 3', 5' –triiodothyronine). Proteases cleave the thyroid hormone from the thyroglobulin molecule releasing it into the blood.

T4 is quantitatively the major hormone produced and secreted by the thyroid gland. Both T4 and T3 are primarily in the bound form with thyroid-binding globulin (TBG), with lesser amounts bound to albumin and transthyretin. Approximately 80% of T4 is converted to T3 or reverse T3 (rT3) in the peripheral tissues, primarily the liver and kidneys, and catalyzed by selenium-dependent deiodinase enzyme. The brain and nervous system convert T4 to T3 for their own local use.

The cellular activity of thyroid hormone is mediated by the interaction of T3 with nuclear T3 receptors. T3 binds to the nuclear T3 receptor and influences intracellular gene expression and basal metabolic rate.

PATHOGENESIS OF HASHIMOTO'S THYROIDITIS

Hashimoto's thyroiditis is a chronic autoimmune disorder in which the immune system attacks and destroys the thyroid gland. Susceptibility to the disease is due to a combination of genetics and environmental factors [4]. Among the major susceptibility genes that have been identified are the HLA-DR and HLA-DQ (human leukocyte antigen) gene loci, non-MHC (major histocompatibility) genes, including cytotoxic T-lymphocyte-associated factor 4 (CTLA-4), and thyroid specific genes [5,6]. Some of the major environmental triggers include iodine (subsequently discussed), infections, and pollutants.

Some of the infectious agents that have been implicated include *Yersinia enterocolitica* [6], hepatitis C virus [7], and *Helicobacter pylori* [8]. There are two main theories that have been proposed for the induction of autoimmunity by infectious agents:

1. The molecular mimicry theory suggests that there are sequence similarities between infectious proteins and self-proteins. And this can induce a cross-over immune response to the self-proteins/antigens [9].
2. The bystander activation theory suggests that infections of certain tissues can induce local inflammation through cytokine release, resulting in activation of auto-reactive T cells that were suppressed by peripheral regulatory mechanisms [10].

Genetic susceptibility coupled with environmental triggers lead to a breakdown of immune system tolerance. The environmental triggers induce antigen-presenting cells (APC). Self-antigenic peptides within the gland combine with the APCs [5]. This complex travels to lymph nodes and stimulates T cells and B cells. This produces an infiltration into the thyroid gland of T cells and B cells reactive to the thyroid auto-antigens and the production of thyroid antibodies [5]. Consequently, T cells, B cells, and macrophages accumulate in the thyroid gland. Eventually, clinical hypothyroidism develops due to the antibody-dependent, cytokine-mediated, and apoptotic mechanisms of cytotoxicity [5].

CLINICAL PRESENTATION

Hypothyroidism is not always so apparent and can mimic other diseases and conditions, especially subclinical hypothyroidism. It is a master of disguises and the condition can go for years without detection.

Hypothyroidism may present as chronic fatigue with symptoms of malaise and signs of low iron or low vitamin B12 and can be accompanied by depression. Carpal tunnel syndrome, joint pains, and arthralgias may also be due to low thyroid hormone. It may present as hypercholesterolemia only modestly responsive to dietary interventions. Chronic constipation is a common symptom due to diminished motility in the colon and tends to be less responsive to the dietary recommendations to increase fiber and water intake.

In young women, it can present as infertility, menorrhagia, or frequent miscarriages. In older women, symptoms of hypothyroidism may be similar to perimenopausal or menopausal symptoms such as fatigue, poor memory, insomnia, depression, and difficulty losing weight. If hypothyroidism is underlying the symptoms, hormone replacement therapy (HRT) can make symptoms worse because elevations in estrogen block thyroid hormone metabolism.

Gastroesophageal reflux (GERD) can be an early symptom of hypothyroidism due to the associated lower esophageal sphincter tone and slow gastric emptying. When hypothyroidism is the underlying perturbation, pharmacotherapy for GERD can compound poor digestion and reduce absorption of the trace minerals such as iodine and selenium important for thyroid function.

Hashimoto's thyroiditis may also manifest in different ways biochemically. In overt hypothyroidism, individuals have high TSH, low fT4, and low fT3 levels on laboratory tests. With subclinical hypothyroidism, individuals have a high TSH level with normal fT4 and fT3 [1]. However, individuals who present with normal TSH and fT4 levels but low fT3 may also have hypothyroidism. T3 has a higher affinity for the thyroid nuclear receptor. And it is the binding of T3 to the nuclear receptor that initiates gene transcription and regulates metabolism and energy production [11].

In addition, Hashimoto's thyroiditis is an autoimmune condition. It commonly is associated with anti-thyroid peroxidase antibodies, anti-thyroglobulin antibodies, or both. Therefore, in addition to replacing thyroid hormone, addressing the basis for the heightened and aberrant immune response is merited. In some patients, nutritional needs, potentially stemming from thyroid metabolism itself, can be identified and treated. Also triggering the autoimmune disease, can be ongoing environmental exposures.

NUTRIENTS FOR THYROID METABOLISM

Minerals such as iodine, iron, selenium, and zinc, and vitamins such as D and A are essential for optimal thyroid hormone metabolism. Often with thyroid disease, gastrointestinal absorption can be impaired and metabolic pathways can be altered placing additional importance on adequate dietary intake.

Iodine

Iodine deficiency results in impaired thyroid hormone synthesis and eventual hypothyroidism. Iodine deficiency is a global problem that temporarily improved with the initiation of the universal salt iodization program. By the 1970s, the United States was a country with iodine sufficiency, with a median urinary iodine level of 320 mcg/L. However, the NHANES survey III of 1988–94 revealed a median urinary iodine value of 145 mcg/L. In less than two decades, iodine intake appears to have been reduced by half.

The NHANES survey for 2003–4 showed a median urinary iodine (UI) level of 160 mcg/L. Women of reproductive age had a median UI level of 139 mcg/L and non-Hispanic blacks in this group had a lower UI level than other racial/ethnic groups [12]. The NHANES surveys for 2005–6 and 2007–8 revealed that the mean UI level had stabilized at 164 mg/L. However, pregnant women had a mean UI level of 125 mcg/L with over 55% less than 150 mcg/L [13]. Adequate UI levels for pregnant women are 150 mcg/L–249 mcg/L.

TABLE 20.1

Factors That Reduce Body Iodine Stores

Cause for Iodine Deficiency	Reason
Decreased table salt consumption	Reducing sodium chloride for positive health considerations
Decreased egg consumption	Concerns over cholesterol
Decreased fish consumption	Food preference and concerns over mercury
Decreased iodine in milk	Changes in dairy industry and milk processing
Removal of iodine from bread products	Commercial bread production replacement of iodine with potassium bromate
Minimal access to sea vegetables	Unaware or no access to the food; dislike of food
Soil iodine depletion	Accelerated deforestation and soil erosion
Heavy daily sweating through athletic training	May be part of a physician-prescribed fitness program
Frequent use of saunas and steam rooms	Sweat loss can range from 11.6 mcg to 99.8 mcg for one hour of heavy sweating during activity.
Chronic inflammatory bowel disease and gluten-related disorders and pharmacotherapy for gastroesophageal reflux	Decreased absorption of iodine and other minerals

Adapted from Tenpenny, S., *Hypothyroidism: Optimizing function with nutrition* in Food and Nutrients in Disease Management, 2009.

There are likely to be several reasons that iodine intake and body stores are lower now than they were in the 1970s, shortly after iodization of salt was initiated (Table 20.1).

Food Sources

The best sources for iodine are found in seaweed, such as kelp, nori, kombu, hijiki, wakame, and ocean fish (Table 20.2). Two grams of iodized salt (about one-half teaspoon) provides approximately 150 mcg of iodine. Salt found in commercially prepared food should only be considered fortified with iodine if so stated on the food labeling.

The Dietary Reference Intakes (DRIs) are the most recent set of dietary recommendations established by the Food and Nutrition Board of the Institute of Medicine, 1997–2001. They include the recommended dietary allowances (RDAs), adequate intake (AI), estimated average requirement (EAR), and tolerable upper-intake level (UL). The RDA for iodine is as follows:

- Adults and adolescents—150 mcg/day
- Pregnant women—220 mcg/day
- Lactating women—290 mcg/day
- Children aged 1–8 years—90 mcg/day
- Children aged 9–13—120 mcg/day

The tolerable upper-intake level (UL) is 1,100 mcg/day (1.1 mg/day) for adults [14]. However, individuals with autoimmune thyroid disease (AITD) are susceptible to high intakes of iodine and may not be protected by the UL for iodine intake for the general population [14].

Goitrogens

The consumption of goitrogen foods may interfere with the way the body utilizes iodine. They competitively inhibit iodine uptake by the thyroid gland and block its incorporation into the thyroglobulin molecule [15].

TABLE 20.2

Sea Vegetables and Iodine Content

Sea Vegetable	How Provided	How Used	Amount of Iodine in a Serving	Amount Needed to Provide 150 mcg/day
Sea salt	Formed from evaporation of ocean water; contains trace minerals; unlike salt mined from land sources, sea salt does not contain added sugar.	Beyond food, sea salt is also used in cosmetics, deodorants, antiperspirants, and other skin care products.	0.065 mg per 1 gram	About 1/2 teaspoon
Dulce	Can be powdered in a condiment, used in chunks for cooking	Plain food source; used in soups and stews; chewy texture when cooked; often included in packaged foods as a thickener or stretcher	0.135mg per 1 gram	About 1/5 teaspoon
Whole leaf kelp	There are many different kinds of kelp, constituting around 30 genera.	Used as a flavoring, a garnish, a vegetable, or a snack food; dried sheets used to wrap sushi and in other foods such as broth	0.450 mg per 1 gram	About 1/10 teaspoon
Nori	Type of edible red algae; dried into thin sheets.	Wrap for sushi, edible garnish, flavoring in noodles and soups	40 mcg per sheet	4 sheets
Kombu	Edible kelp from China, Korea, and Japan; comes as green, thick strips	Soup stock, eaten fresh as sashimi	1,450 mcg per 1-inch piece	1/10 inch
Wakame	Edible kelp from China, Korea, and Japan; green leaves, sweet flavor, slippery texture	Miso soup, salads, served alone like a cucumber; high in calcium, thiamine, niacin, vitamin B12, and omega-3 essential fatty acids	82 mcg per tablespoon	2 tablespoon
Arame	Edible kelp from China, Korea, and Japan; brown strands, mild flavor, firm texture	Soups, muffins, rice dishes; high in iron and calcium.	732 mcg per tablespoon	1/2 teaspoon

Adapted from Tenpenny, S., *Hypothyroidism: Optimizing function with nutrition* in Food and Nutrients in Disease Management, 2009.

Cruciferous vegetables contain thiocyanate and isothiocyanates that have goitrogenic properties. Thiocyanates are also present in cassava root. Thiocyanate compounds primarily inhibit the iodine concentrating mechanism of the thyroid and their goitrogenic activity can be overcome by iodine administration [16]. However, isothiocyanates also interfere with the organification of iodine and the formation of active thyroid hormone [16]. And their action usually cannot be antagonized by iodine. Cooking inactivates goitrogen activity in cruciferous vegetables and cassava root when properly prepared [15].

Soy has isoflavones, which inhibit TPO activity. Therefore, if ingested at high levels, it may cause hypothyroidism—particularly in iodine-deficient individuals. The fermentation of soy deactivates its goitrogen activity. There are other foods that have small amounts of goitrogenic compounds. However, unless they are consumed in large amounts, they do not impact on thyroid synthesis. In addition, adequate selenium in the diet also decreases the impact of goitrogenic foods on the thyroid.

Iodine Excess

Too much dietary iodine intake can trigger thyroid autoimmunity, but the exact mechanism of action is not clear.

1. Iodine may stimulate B-lymphocytes to increase the production of immunoglobulin and thus induce autoimmune thyroid disease (AITD) by enhancing the activity of lymphocytes that have been primed by thyroid-specific antigens [17,18].
2. Iodine may enhance the antigen presenting capabilities of macrophages, resulting in increased macrophage activity and enhanced lymphocyte stimulation.
3. A high iodine intake increases the iodine content of the thyroglobulin molecule, which may increase its immunogenicity [19].
4. Iodine may provoke thyroid follicular cells to become antigen-presenting cells and potentiate AITDs by turning genetically predisposed normal thyrocytes into antigen-presenting thyrocytes [18].

Selenium may protect the thyroid from damage from excess iodine exposure. And, if both iodine and selenium are deficient, they should be replenished simultaneously.

Iodine in Other Tissues

Peroxidase and iodide symporter activity also incorporate iodide into salivary glands, gastric mucosa, ovaries, thymus, joints, the choroid plexus, and the ciliary body of the eye. In addition, both lactating and nonlactating mammary tissue accumulates iodine. And studies have shown that iodine supplementation exerts a suppressive effect on neoplasms in the breast [20]. So, the previously listed RDAs may be optimal for thyroid hormone synthesis, but the total body needs for iodine remains unknown.

Testing for Iodine Deficiency

Most (> 90%) of iodine excretion is through the kidneys, which is why the 24-hour urine iodine collection has conventionally been used as the diagnostic tool for iodine stores and for establishing the recommended dietary allowances. Also, the diurnal variation of both iodine and creatinine urinary excretion makes the 24-hour urine iodine collection more ideal than the random urine iodine-to-creatinine ratio to assess iodine stores [21].

Iron

Thyroid peroxidase, the enzyme required for organification of iodide and incorporation of iodine into the thyroglobulin molecule, is a heme protein and requires iron for its synthesis and activity. Iron deficiency reduces the activity of heme-dependent thyroid peroxidase [22]. Menorrhagia, which can deplete iron stores, is a common symptom of hypothyroidism.

Food Sources

Food sources of heme iron include chicken liver, oysters, beef liver, beef, turkey, and chicken. The absorption of heme iron from meat proteins is very efficient, ranging from 15% to 35% [23]. Nonheme iron compounds are found in plants and animal food and include meat, fish, poultry, lentils, beans, peas, spinach, beetroot, and broccoli. Absorption of nonheme iron in plant foods is 2% to 20% [23]. Meat protein will improve nonheme iron absorption because heme enhances the bioavailability of nonheme iron. In addition, using a cast iron skillet will increase iron stores [24].

SELENIUM

Selenoenzymes such as glutathione peroxidase (GXP) and thioredoxin reductase (TR), within the thyroid gland, act as antioxidants and detoxify peroxides. Iodination of thyroglobulin is catalyzed by TPO and requires the generation of high hydrogen peroxide concentrations, which are potentially harmful to the thyrocyte. Generation of H_2O_2 is regulated through the action of TSH. The iodination of thyroglobulin and generation of H_2O_2 takes place on the luminal surface of the apical membrane of the thyrocyte. Intracellular GXP, TR, and catalase systems degrade any harmful hydrogen peroxide that diffuses into the thyrocyte [25]. Thus, when selenium intake is adequate, the intracellular GPX and TR systems protect the thyrocyte from peroxides.

The thyroid hormone deiodinases are also selenium dependent. Type I iodothyronine deiodinase, found mainly in the liver and kidney, is responsible for the peripheral conversion of T4 to the active T3 thyroid hormone. It is also involved in the degradation of rT3. Type II iodothyronine deiodinase, found mainly in the brain, is responsible for local conversion of T4 to T3. Type III iodothyronine deiodinase, found mainly in fetal tissue, can also be found in pathological condition. It is responsible for catalyzing T4 to rT3, the inactive hormone. If selenium is deficient, T4 is more likely to be converted to rT3. This increase in rT3 can block T3 receptors and decrease thyroid hormone activity. Therefore, adequate selenium intake is required for optimal T4 metabolism.

Food Sources

Foods typically rich in selenium include Brazil nuts, meat, and seafood, but the selenium content in food depends on the selenium content in the soil where the plants grow and animals graze (grass-fed animals). Most human research studies dose selenium at 200 mcg/day of selenium. The tolerable upper intake level (UL) is 400 mcg/day [26].

ZINC

Often zinc deficiency occurs when some type of stress is placed on the body. This includes stress due to increased gut permeability, dysbiosis, infection, and the release of stress hormones.

Normally, mechanisms are in place to prevent zinc deficiency, including increased absorption and decreased excretion through the modification of zinc transporters. In addition, there is the induction of metallothionein, which modulates zinc absorption and transport. However, inflammation and the release of stress hormones may cause a decrease in serum zinc level mediated in part by changes in the zinc transporters [27].

Zinc deficiency can decrease the activity of type I deiodinase and the conversion of T4 to T3. In addition, zinc is a component of the thyroid hormone nuclear receptor and thus necessary to activate intracellular gene expression and regulate cellular metabolism.

Resolving increased permeability, dysbiosis, and infection in the gut will decrease the release of stress hormones. A stool analysis to measure digestive capability and microbial imbalance will assist in identifying the necessary steps needed to restore the gut to health. It may also be necessary to make lifestyle changes to reduce overall stress.

Food Sources

Excellent food sources for zinc include seafood, especially oysters, red meats, and organ meats. Whole grains, nuts, and legumes are relatively good plant sources for zinc, but phytates may inhibit its absorption.

VITAMIN D

Vitamin D insufficiency is due primarily to reduced ability to synthesize this prohormone from ultraviolet rays. Only in high-latitude environments has dietary intake and absorption historically been important. However, in modern indoor dwelling inadequate vitamin D is prevalent. Vitamin D influences the activity of T-regulatory cells and the balance of Th1 and Th2 cells [28]. It is immunosuppressant, but does not interfere with the ability to act defensively against infections [29]. It can markedly suppress autoimmune diseases in the presence of sufficient calcium [30]. Vitamin D insufficiency is a common finding in Hashimoto's thyroiditis, both overt and subclinical [31]. Moreover, many individuals with Hashimoto's have a genetic defect in the vitamin D receptor (VDR) making it difficult for vitamin D to get into the cells and modulate gene transcription [32]. Therefore, it is best to keep vitamin D levels in the upper range of normal.

Vitamin A

Vitamin A insufficiency can stem from inadequate dietary intake or poor digestion and absorption of fat-soluble nutrients. Severe vitamin A deficiency (VAD) has multiple effects on thyroid metabolism [33]. It decreases iodide uptake, impairs thyroglobulin synthesis and coupling of iodotyrosine residues to form thyroid hormone, and increases thyroid size.

Peripherally, VAD increases free- and total-circulating thyroid hormone and binding of transthyretin (TTR). TTR is a carrier of thyroid hormone and a carrier of retinol-binding protein bound to retinol. Centrally, the retinoic acid-activated retinoid X receptor coupled with the thyroid hormone activated receptor suppress transcription of the pituitary TSH β gene. With severe VAD, the pituitary gland with elevated TSH becomes insensitive to feedback control by thyroid hormone. Combined deficiencies of VA and iodine have greater adverse effects on the pituitary-thyroid axis than single deficiencies of VA or iodine. Moderate VAD alone does not adversely affect the pituitary-thyroid axis. What is not established is the extent to which vitamin A would need to be deficient in order to have an unfavorable impact on thyroid function.

ENVIRONMENTAL TOXINS

Toxicants can block thyroid hormone synthesis and metabolism. Therefore, it is important to obtain an environmental, occupational, and dietary exposure history to determine the potential impact of toxicants on the body.

Chemical toxins such as polyhalogenated compounds can bind to thyroid hormone receptors, thus inducing or exacerbating Hashimoto's thyroiditis [34]. Polychlorinated biphenols (PCBs) toxins, which are no longer commercially produced in the United States, can still be found in our environment and food supply. They are commonly found in fish at the top of the food chain because they bioaccumulate. Bisphenol A (BPA), a chemical found in some food containers and in the epoxy resin liner of most canned products, has been shown to leech out into food.

PCBs, BPA, and other compounds such as polybrominated diphenylethers (PBDEs) and triclosan bind to thyroid hormone receptors. Organochlorine pesticides such as hexachlorobenzene (HCB) and dioxin may decrease the serum T4 half-life by activating hepatic enzymes (diphosphate glucuronyltransferases/UDPGTs), which glucuronidates T4 [35]. This may result in hypothyroidism in individuals unable to maintain an increased production of T4.

Dietary choices can reduce exposure to these "organic" toxicants. For example, concentrations of PCBs, dioxins, polybrominated diphenylethers, and pesticides are significantly lower in wild Pacific salmon than in farm-raised salmon [36]. It is the feed of farmed salmon that is the source of the increased organic contaminants [36]. And this may reduce the net health benefits derived from its consumption.

Toxic metals may also trigger or exacerbate Hashimoto's thyroiditis. For example, mercury binds strongly to sulfhydryl (SH) groups that are found on thiol-containing amino acids and enzymes/proteins, blocking their normal physiological function. Methyl mercury cation exhibits a high affinity for sulfhydryl group radicals in cell membranes and can alter permeability [37]. This bond does not induce metallothionein, which is protective to the individual [38]. Intestinal permeability is increased and leads to inflammation and dysbiosis, which triggers an immune response and may trigger Hashimoto's thyroiditis. Also, there may be direct interaction of mercury and thyroid antigenic self-proteins that trigger Hashimoto's thyroiditis [38].

Mercury can also inhibit iodide uptake, TPO activity, and T4 conversion to T3. In addition, it has a high affinity for the brain. And, it can accumulate in the hypothalamus and pituitary gland and affect TSH levels and the feedback mechanism.

The majority of mercury exposure comes from the burning of coal for electricity. Dental amalgams account for the largest percent of nonoccupational mercury exposure. Among seafood, mackerel, swordfish, and tilefish have the highest levels of mercury. A 24-hour provoked urine excretion test may be helpful to detect toxic metals.

THE LIVER

The liver has an important role in thyroid hormone metabolism and thyroid hormone is important for normal hepatic function.

Thyroid hormone increases the expression of LDL receptors on the hepatocytes [39] and increases the activity of lipid-lowering liver enzymes, resulting in a reduction in low-density lipoprotein levels [40]. Thyroid hormone also increases the expression of apolipoprotein A1, a major component of high-density lipoprotein [41]. Hypothyroid patients usually have an increase in low-density lipoprotein cholesterol that is reduced with thyroid hormone treatment.

Hypothyroidism is associated with cholestatic jaundice due to reduced bilirubin and bile excretion. The reduction in part may be due to an increase in membrane cholesterol-phospholipid ratio and diminished membrane fluidity [42]. The reduced bilirubin excretion, hypercholesterolemia, along with hypotonia of the gall bladder increases the incidence of gallstones [43]. These abnormalities can be reversed with thyroid hormone replacement [44].

Autoimmune thyroiditis occurs in 10%–25% of patients with primary biliary cirrhosis (PBC) [45] and 18% [46] with autoimmune hepatitis. Primary sclerosing cholangitis is also associated with autoimmune thyroiditis [47]. In addition, hepatitis C virus and nonalcoholic fatty liver disease [48] have been associated with thyroid abnormalities. Thus, clinical consideration of hypothyroidism may be merited with liver test abnormalities.

GASTROINTESTINAL TRACT AND HASHIMOTO'S THYROIDITIS

Hashimoto's thyroiditis affects the gastrointestinal tract at multiple levels. With Hashimoto's thyroiditis, dysmotility in the esophagus may develop along with decreased lower esophageal sphincter pressure causing dysphagia and GERD. Symptoms improve with thyroid hormone replacement [49]. Reduced gastric acid secretion seen in Hashimoto's may be due to gastric mucosal changes, reduction in gastrin levels [50], or an association with parietal cell antibodies [51]. The decreased gastric acid may cause protein, vitamin B12, and mineral deficiencies. Gastric emptying is delayed in some individuals due to smooth muscle dysfunction or pylorospasm [52]. Small intestinal overgrowth is found in more than 50% of individuals with hypothyroidism [53]. The symptoms improve with antibiotics.

Diminished motility of the esophagus, stomach, small intestines, and large intestine typically reverses with thyroid hormone replacement. And the ascites in myxedema, which can also be associated with pleural and pericardial effusions, disappears with thyroid hormone replacement [54].

An intact gastrointestinal barrier is critical to arresting environmental triggers in AITD [55]. The intestinal defense system and intestinal permeability govern the interplay between environmental triggers and the host. The gut-associated lymphoid tissue (GALT) regulates intestinal defense, and intercellular tight junctions regulate intestinal epithelial permeability.

The balance between immunity and tolerance is necessary for a healthy gut. Abnormal immune responses to environmental triggers/antigens such as certain microbes and possibly gluten in genetically susceptible individuals can result in an influx of inflammatory/immune cells [55]. This can alter epithelial tight junctions and increase permeability triggering autoimmune thyroiditis.

The dysfunctional barrier allows for a continued influx of antigens and a continued immune response that targets the thyroid gland. Therefore, it is important to not only identify and remove the environmental triggers but also restore the intestinal barrier.

ESTROGEN, CORTISOL, AND HASHIMOTO'S THYROIDITIS

It is estimated that approximately 5% of all postmenopausal women receive treatment with both hormone replacement therapy (HRT) (estrogen-progesterone) and thyroid hormone replacement [56]. Oral estrogen therapy raises the circulating levels of thyroid-binding globulin, thus increasing bound thyroid hormone and decreasing free thyroid hormone. Consequently, individuals receiving oral HRT may require a dose adjustment in their thyroid medication.

Estrogen dominance (progesterone deficiency) inhibits thyroid action. And hypothyroidism lowers the clearance rate of estrogen in women [57]. Therefore, in addition to thyroid hormone support, estrogen dominance should be addressed. According to a 2002 study by the National Cancer Institute, exercising five days a week, including just walking two of the five days, lowered blood estrogen levels in postmenopausal women described as sedentary, overweight, and not taking HRT. Avoiding xenoestrogens and eating organic fresh vegetables, including cooked cruciferous vegetables, grass-fed meats, and PCB-free and mercury-free fish will all contribute to lowering excess estrogen. Supplements to improve estrogen metabolism include DIM (diindolylmethane) and calcium D-glucarate.

Cortisol acts in synergy with thyroid hormone at the receptor-gene level. At physiological levels, cortisol makes thyroid hormone work more efficiently in turning on gene expression and increasing metabolic activity and energy [58]. When cortisol levels are low, as with adrenal fatigue, thyroid hormone activity is less efficient in increasing metabolic activity and energy. When cortisol levels are high, as with chronic stress, it can inhibit the conversion of T4 to T3 (active hormone) [59]. Thus, thyroxine hormone levels can be normal, but the individual has symptoms of hypothyroidism.

Nutrition and lifestyle changes can be used to support both conditions. To improve adrenal fatigue, the patient should eat within one hour of arising in the morning and then every three hours while awake. Main meals should consist of high-quality protein, fresh vegetables, nonallergic whole grain, and healthful fats. Snacks can include nuts and seeds. There should be a minimum of processed and concentrated sugar and no coffee or alcohol. Supplements to support the adrenals include pantothenic acid and vitamin B-complex. Siberian ginseng (*Eleutherococcus senticosus*) is characterized as an adaptogen and improves the body's ability to adapt to stress. Licorice root (*Radix glycyrrhizae*) will extend the half-life of cortisol. Adequate sleep is also important in restoring the adrenals. Phosphatidylserine, a phosphorylated lipid component of cellular membranes, has been shown to reduce high cortisol levels [60].

In sum, hypothyroidism may be coupled with estrogen and cortisol imbalances, but dietary and lifestyle approaches can make a difference.

CLINICAL SUMMARY

Diagnosing hypothyroidism and restoring thyroid hormone levels can be an important intervention from a nutrition standpoint. For some patients, it may provide the energy they needed to exercise, the improvement in cholesterol to accompany their heart-healthful diet, the restored gastrointestinal functioning, or an improved mood to adopt a can-do approach to dieting.

However, normalizing thyroid levels alone may not be sufficient to restore patients' well-being, especially with autoimmune thyroiditis. A dietary history and the metabolic laboratory tests detailed in Table 20.3 can identify nutritional and hormonal imbalances, food allergies, dysbiosis, and infectious agents.

TABLE 20.3
Laboratory Diagnostic Tests for Hashimoto's Thyroiditis Based on Clinical Practice

Laboratory Test	Rationale for Hashimoto's	Preferred Lab and Other Notes
Amino acid (20) profile—serum	Amino acid deficiencies can impact on availability of enzymes and proteins important to thyroid hormone synthesis and metabolism.	Metametrix Clinical Lab Genova Diagnostics
Red blood cell (RBC) elemental analysis	Detect intracellular nutrient status including selenium and zinc; selenium is a component of the deiodinases. Zinc is a component of the thyroid hormone (TH) nuclear receptor.	Genova Diagnostics
Iron, Ferritin, Total iron binding capacity	Thyroid peroxidase enzyme function is heme dependent.	Lab Corp; Quest
24-hr urine iodine collection	Iodine insufficiency can impact on thyroid hormone synthesis.	Hakala Labs
Fat-soluble vitamin serum analysis	Vitamin D impacts on Th1 and Th2 balance and autoimmunity; vitamin A impacts on thyroid hormone synthesis and TH nuclear receptor.	Increased incidence of vitamin D receptor defect with Hashimoto's; Metametrix Clinical Lab
IgG food antibody assessment	Detects delayed food reactions, which impact on the gastrointestinal tract and the immune system	Genova Diagnostics; Metametrix Clinical Lab
Gastrointestinal stool profile	Identifies pathogenic bacteria, parasites, overgrowth of yeast; identifies need for digestive support and detects antigliadin sIGA	Metametrix Clinical Lab has increased sensitivity over microscopy for parasite detection and traditional cultures for microbes (DNA analysis).
Adrenal stress profile using saliva specimen	Assess the need for cortisol support for optimal thyroid function; detect cortisol excess that inhibits thyroid metabolism	Metametrix Clinical Lab; Genova Diagnostics; four timed salivary collections in one day
Estrogen profile using urine specimen	Detects imbalance in estrogen metabolism, which can impede thyroid hormone metabolism	Metametrix Clinical Lab; first morning urine

REFERENCES

1. Thyroid Guidelines Committee. 2002. AACE clinical practice for the evaluation and treatment of hyperthyroidism and hypothyroidism. Endocr Pract. 8(6): 451–67.
2. Yutaka, A., Belin, R. M., Clickner, R. et al. 2007. Serum TSH and total T4 in the United States population and their association with participant characteristics: National Health and Nutrition Examination Survey (NHANES 1999–2002).
3. Hollowell, J. G., Staehling, N. W., Flanders, W. D. et al. Feb 1, 2002. Serum TSH, T4, and thyroid antibodies in the United States population (1988 to 1994): National Health and Nutrition Examination Survey (NHANES III). J Clin Endocrinol Metab. 87(2): 489–99.
4. Tomer, Y., Huber, A. 2009. The etiology of autoimmune thyroid disease: A story of genes and environment. J of Autoimmunity 32: 231–239.
5. Chistiakov, D. 2005. Immunogenetics of Hashimoto's thyroiditis. J of Autoimmune Diseases. 2:1.
6. Corapcioglu, D., Tonyukuk, V., Kiyan, M., et al. 2002. Relationship between thyroid autoimmunity and Yersinia enterocolitica antibodies. Thyroid. 12(7): 613–17.

7. Antonelli, A., Ferri, C., Pampana, A. et al. 2004. Thyroid disorders in chronic hepatitis C. Am J Med. 117 (1): 10–13.

8. de Luis, D. A., Varela, C., de La Calle, H. et al. 1998. Heliobacter pylori infection is markedly increased in patients with autoimmune atrophic thyroiditis. J Clin Gastroenterol. 26(4): 259–63.

9. Oldstone, M. B. A. 1987. Molecular mimicry and autoimmune disease. Cell. 50:819–20.

10. Fournie, G. J., Mas, M., Cautain, B. et al. 2001. Induction of autoimmunity through bystander effects. Lessons from immunological disorders induced by heavy metals. J Autoimmun. 16(3): 319–26.

11. Baynes, J. and M. Dominiczak. 1999. *Medical Biochemistry*: Chapter 35. Mosby, 451–67.

12. Caldwell, K. L., Miller, G. A., Wang, R. Y., Jain, R. B., Jones, R. L. 2008 Nov. Iodine status of the U.S. population, National Health and Nutrition Examination Survey 2003–2004. Thyroid. 18(11): 1207–14.

13. Caldwell, K. L., Makhmudov, A., Ely, E., Jones, R. L., Wang, R. Y. 2011 Apr. Iodine status in the U.S. population, National Health and Nutrition Examination Survey, 2005–2006 and 2007–2008. Thyroid. 21(4): 419–27.

14. Food and Nutrition Board, Institute of Medicine. 2001. Iodine. In *Dietary Reference Intake for Vitamin A, Vitamin K, Boron, Chromium, Copper, Iodine, Iron, Manganese, Molybdenum, Nickel, Silicon, Vanadium, and Zinc*. Washington, DC: National Academy Press; 258–59.

15. Greer, M. A. 1957. Goitrogenic Substances in Food. Amer J Clin Nutri. 5(4): 440–40.

16. Gaitan, E., 1990. Goitrogens in food and water. Annu Rev Nutri. 10:21–39.

17. Weetman, A. P., McGregor, A. M. 1984. Autoimmune thyroid disease: Developments in our understanding. Endocr Rev. 5: 309–55.

18. Saranac, S., Zivanovic, B., Bjelakovic, B. et al. 2011. Why is the thyroid so prone to autoimmune disease? Horm Res Paediatr. 75: 157–65.

19. Carayanniotis, G. Rao, V. P. 1997. Searching for pathogenic epitopes in thyroglobulin: Parameters and caveats. Immunol Today. 18: 83–88.

20. Aceves, C., Anguiano, B. Delgado, G. 2005 Apr. Is iodine the gatekeeper of the integrity of the mammary gland? J Mammary Gland Biol Neoplasia. 10(2): 189–96.

21. Amdur, R. J. and Mazzaferri, E. L. 2005, Part 5B, Measuring urinary iodine. In *Essentials of Thyroid Cancer Management*, ed. R. J. Amdur, and E. L. New York: Mazzaferri, Springer Science + Business Media, Inc., 215–19.

22. Baynes, R., Stipanuk, M. 2000. Iron. In *Biochemical and Physiological Aspects of Human Nutrition*. Ed. M. H. Stipanuk, W. B. Saunders Co., 711–40.

23. Food and Nutrition Board, Institute of Medicine. 2001. Iron. In *Dietary Reference Intake for Vitamin A, Vitamin K, Boron, Chromium, Copper, Iodine, Iron, Manganese, Molybdenum, Nickel, Silicon, Vanadium, and Zinc*. Washington, DC: National Academy Press; 290–393.

24. Kroger-Ohlsen, M. V., Trugvason, T., Sklbsted, L. H., Michaelsen, K. F. Nov. 2002. Release of iron into foods cooked in an iron pot: Effect of pH, salt, and organic acids. Journal of Food Science 67(9): 3301–03.

25. Beckett, G. J., Arthur, J. R. 2005. Selenium and endocrine systems. J of Endocr. 184: 455–65.

26. Food and Nutrition Board, Institute of Medicine. 2000. Selenium. In *Dietary Reference Intakes for Vitamin C, Vitamin E, Selenium, and Carotenoid*. Washington, DC: National Academy Press. 284–324.

27. Mohommad, M.K., Zhou, Z., Cave, M., Barve, A., McClain, C. J. 2012 Feb. Zinc and liver disease. Nutr Clin Pract. 27(1): 8–20.

28. Drugarin, D. 2000. The pattern of Th1 cytokine in autoimmune thyroiditis. Immunol Letts. 71: 73–77.

29. DeLuca, H. F., Cantorna, M. T. 2001. Vitamin D: Its role and uses in immunology. FASEB Journal. 15: 2579–85.

30. Cantorna, M. T., Zhu, Y., Froicu, M., Wittke, A. 2004. Vitamin D status, 1, 25–dihydroxyvitamin D3, and the immune system. Am J Clin Nutr. 80 (suppl): 1717S–20S.

31. Tamer, G., Arik, S., Tamer, I., Coksert, D. 2011. Relative vitamin D insufficiency in Hashimoto's thyroiditis. Thyroid. 21(8): 891–96.

32. Lin, W., Wan, L., Tsai, C., Chen, R., Lee, C., Tsai, F. 2006. Vitamin D receptor gene polymorphisms are associated with risk of Hashimoto's thyroiditis in Chinese patients in Taiwan. J Clin Lab Analysis. 20: 109–12.

33. Biebinger, R., Arnold, M., Koss, M. et al. 2006. Effects of concurrent vitamin A and iodine deficiencies on the thyroid-pituitary axis in rats. Thyroid. 16(10): 961–65.

34. Pearce, E. N., Braverman, L. E. 2009. Environmental pollutants and the thyroid. Best Practice and Research Clinical Endocrinology and Metabolism. 23: 801–13.

35. Howdeshell K. L. 2002. A model of the development of the brain as a construct of the thyroid system. Environmental health Perspectives. 110 (suppl. 3): 337–48.

36. Foran, J. A., Carpenter, D. O., Hamilton, M. C., Knuth, B. A., Schwager, S. J. May 2005. Risk-based consumption advice for farmed Atlantic and wild Pacific salmon contaminated with dioxins and dioxin-like compounds. Environmental Health Perspectives. 113(5): 552–56.

37. Ochiai, E. 2011. Environmental issues: Heavy metal pollutants and others. In *Chemicals for Life and Living*, ed Eiichiro Ochiai. Springer, 177–86.

38. Powell, J. J., Van de Water, J., Gershwin, M. E. 1999. Evidence for the role of environmental agents in the initiation or progression of autoimmune conditions. Environmental health perspectives. 107 (suppl. 5): 667–72.

39. Ness, G. C., Loez, D., Chambers, C. M. et al. 1998. Effects of L-triiodothyronine and the thyromimetic L-94901 on serum lipoprotein levels and hepatic low-density lipoprotein receptor, 3-hydroxy-3-methylglutaryl coenzyme A reductase, and apo A-1 gene expression. Biochem Pharmocol 56:121–29.

40. Ness, G. C., Lopez, D. 1995. Transcriptional regulation of rat hepatic low-density lipoprotein receptor and cholesterol 7 alpha hydroxylase by thyroid hormone. Arch Biochem Biophys. 323: 404–8.

41. Taylor, A. H., Stephan, Z. F., Steele, R. E., Wong, N. C. 1997. Beneficial effects of a novel thyromimetic on lipoprotein metabolism. Mol Pharmacol. 52: 542–47.

42. Van Steenbergen, W., Fevery, J., De Vos, R., Heirwegh, K. P., De Groote, J. 1989. Thyroid hormones and the hepatic handling of bilirubin. I. Effects of hypothyroidism and hyperthyroidism on the hepatic transport of bilirubin mono- and diconjugates in the Wistar rat. Hepatology. 9: 314–21.

43. Inkinen, J., Sand, J., Nordback, I. 2000. Association between common bile duct stones and treated hypothyroidism. Hepatogastroenterology. 47: 919–21.

44. Gaitan, E. Cooper, D. S. 1997. Primary hypothyroidism. Curr Ther Endocrinol Metab. 6: 94–98.

45. Sherlock, S., Scheuer, P. J., 1973. The presentation and diagnosis of 100 patients with primary biliary cirrhosis. N Engl J Med. 289: 674–78.

46. Krawitt, E. L. 1996. Autoimmune hepatitis. N Engl J Med. 334: 897–903.

47. Saarinen, S., Olerup, O., Broome, U. 2000. Increased frequency of autoimmune diseases in patients with primary sclerosing cholangitis. Am J Gastroenterol. 95:3195–99.

48. Pagadala, M. R., Zein, C. O., Dasrathy, S., Yerian, L. M., Lopez, R., McCullough, A. J. 2012 Feb. Prevalence of hypothyroidism in nonalcoholic fatty liver disease. Dig Dis Sci. 57(2): 528–34.

49. Eastwood, G. I., Braverman, L. E., White, E. M. et al. 1982. Reversal of lower espophageal hypotension and esophageal aperistalsis after treatment for hypothyroidism. J Clin Gastroenterol. 4: 307–10.

50. Seino, Y. Matsukura, S., Inoue, Y. et al. 1978. Hypogastronemia in hypothyroidism. Am J Dig Dis. 23: 189–91.

51. Markson, J. L., Moore, J. M. 1962. Thyroid auto-antibodies in pernicious anemia. Brit Med J. 2: 1352.

52. Gunsar, F., Yilmaz, S., Bor, S. et al. 2003. Effect of hypo- and hyperthyroidism on gastric myoelectric activity. Dig Dis Sci. 48: 706–12.

53. Lauritano, B. C., Bilotta, A. L., Gabrielli, M., et al. 2007. Association between hypothyroidism and small intestinal bacterial overgrowth. J Clin Endocrinol Metab. 92: 4180–84.

54. Haley, H. B., Leigh, C., Bronsky, D., et al. 1962. Ascites and intestinal obstruction in myxedema. Arch Surg. 85: 328–32.

55. Fasano, A., Shea-Donohue, T. Sept 2005, Mechanism of disease: The role of intestinal barrier function in the pathogenesis of gastrointestinal autoimmune diseases. Nat Clin Pract Gastroenterol Hepatol. 2(9): 416–22.

56. Mazer, N. A. 2004. Interaction of estrogen therapy and thyroid hormone replacement in postmenopausal women. Thyroid. 14 Supp.: S27–34.

57. Arafah, B. M. 2001. Increased need for thyroxine in women with hypothyroidism during estrogen therapy. N Engl J Med. 344(23): 1743–49.

58. Shigemasa, C., Kouchi, T., Ueta, Y., Mitani, Y., Yoshida, A., Mashiba, H. 1992 Nov. Evaluation of thyroid function in patients with isolated adrenocorticotropin deficiency. Am J Med Sci. 304(5): 279–84.

59. Hida, J. T., Kaplan, M. M. 1988 Jul. Inhibition of thyroxine 5'-deiodination type II in cultured human placental cells by cortisol, insulin, 3', 5'-cyclic adenosine monophosphate, and butyrate. Metabolism. 37(7): 664–68.

60. Jager, R., Purpura, M., Kingsley, M. 2007 Jul. Phospholipids and sports performance. J Int Soc Sports Nutri. 4:5.

21 The Hyperparathyroidisms

Michael F. Holick, M.D., Ph.D.

INTRODUCTION

Parathyroid hormone (PTH) is essential for maintaining calcium homeostasis [1–8]. It accomplishes this by regulating calcium mobilization from the skeleton, controlling calcium excretion in the kidney, and stimulating the kidneys to activate vitamin D. Hyperparathyroidism is a consequence of the excess production of PTH by the parathyroid glands. This can be caused by a benign or malignant tumor in the parathyroid gland(s), or stimulation of the parathyroid glands by vitamin D deficiency, hypocalcemia, or hyperphosphatemia. The consequences of hyperparathyroidism include hypercalciuria, hypercalcemia, hypophosphatemia, osteopenia/osteoporosis, osteomalacia, and kidney stones [1–7]. The major causes of hyperparathyroidism are a benign adenoma in a parathyroid gland causing primary hyperparathyroidism, and vitamin D deficiency and chronic kidney disease (CKD) causing secondary hyperparathyroidism [1–5].

PARATHYROID PHYSIOLOGY

The chief cells in the parathyroid glands produce PTH. The calcium sensor (calcium receptor, CaR) in the plasma membrane of the chief cells is constantly monitoring blood ionized calcium levels [4–6]. In response to a decrease in serum ionized calcium, there is an immediate increase in the receptor activity leading to signal transduction resulting in the stimulation of nuclear expression of the PTH mRNA that increases the transcription and translation for PTH [2,6]. PTH is transcribed into a 115 amino acid peptide often called the prepro form [2,6]. It undergoes posttranslational modification to the 84 amino acid PTH and is then incorporated into secretionary granules that release PTH into the circulation. The first 34 amino acids in the N-terminal region of PTH are responsible for most if not all of the calcium regulating properties of PTH [2,6]. PTH interacts with its receptor PTH receptor 1 (PTHR-1) in the kidneys, which stimulates proximal and distal tubular reabsorption of calcium from the ultrafiltrate and decreases tubular reabsorption of phosphorus (Figure 21.1). PTH interacts with its receptor on the osteoblasts to increase the expression of RANKL (receptor activator of NFκB ligand) [8]. RANKL, which is on the plasma membrane of the osteoblast, interacts with its receptor RANK present on the monocytic precursor of the osteoclast and stimulates it to become a mature osteoclast to mobilize calcium from the skeleton (Figure 21.2).

PTH enhances the renal adenylate cyclase to increase cAMP for inducing signal transduction in the renal tubular cell. This results in an increase in urinary levels of cAMP. PTH also stimulates the kidneys to convert 25-hydroxyvitamin D (25[OH]D) to its active form 1,25-dihydroxyvitamin D (1,25[OH]$_2$D) [3,10]. 1,25(OH)$_2$D interacts with its nuclear receptor (VDR) in the small intestine to increase the efficiency of intestinal calcium absorption. Thus, PTH indirectly is responsible for enhancing intestinal calcium absorption to help maintain serum calcium levels within the normal physiologic range of 8.6–10.2 mg% [3,10].

This work was supported in part by NIH grant M01RR00533.

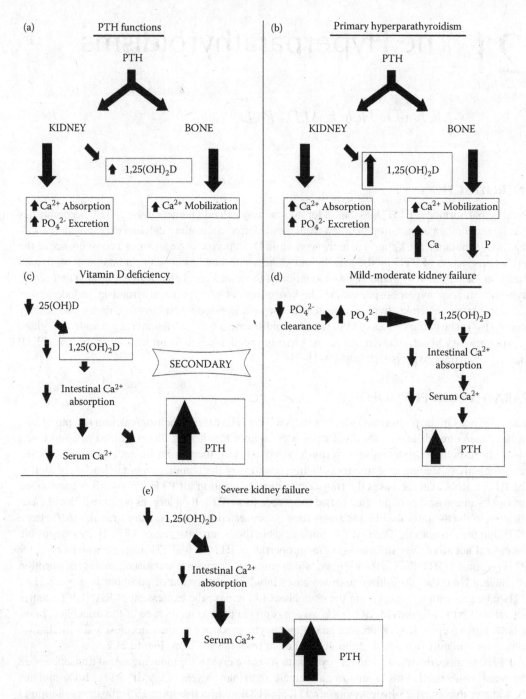

FIGURE 21.1 The physiologic functions of parathyroid hormone (PTH) on calcium, phosphorus, and vitamin D metabolism. The schematic presents the consequences of vitamin D deficiency and chronic kidney disease (CKD) on PTH levels and PTH effects on calcium and phosphorus metabolism. Used with permission from Holick, M.F., Biancuzzo, R.M., Chen, T.C., et al. 2008.

The CaR that is present in the parathyroid glands is a seven transmembrane receptor [4,6]. Unlike most receptors, where binding its ligand stimulates receptor activity and signal transduction, the CaR works in an opposite manner: The less calcium binding to the CaR the more active

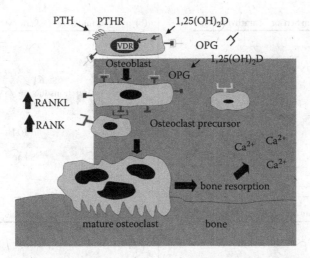

FIGURE 21.2 Parathyroid hormone (PTH) and 1,25-dihydroxyvitamin D [1,25(OH)₂D] interact with their respective receptors in osteoblasts resulting in the expression of RANKL. The receptor RANK on the pre-osteoclast interacts with RANKL inducing the cell to become a mature osteoclast. The mature osteoclasts release collagenases and hydrochloric acid to destroy the matrix and release calcium into the extra cellular space. Osteoprotegerin (OPG) is an endogenously produced decoy RANKL that can bind to the RANK of the preosteoclast preventing it from becoming a mature osteoclast. Used with permission from Holick, M.F., Biancuzzo, R.M., Chen, T.C., et al. 2008.

CaR is in enhancing signal transduction for stimulating the parathyroid cell to produce PTH (Figure 21.3).

MAGNESIUM AND PARATHYROID FUNCTION AND ACTIVITY

Magnesium plays a major role in parathyroid function [11]. The CaR recognizes magnesium. If the magnesium is elevated, it will shut down the production of PTH similar to high serum calcium (as shown in Figure 21.3). However, more important is that hypomagnesemia leads to a marked decrease in the production and secretion of PTH and also prevents PTH from acting on the skeleton (see Figure 21.3) [11]. As a result, hypomagnesemia causes functional hypoparathyroidism; that is, the parathyroid glands cannot increase the production of PTH and the PTH that is made is unable to carry out its physiologic functions on both the skeleton and in the kidneys [11]. Alcohol causes magnesium loss into the urine. Alcoholics who present to an emergency room with seizure, carpal pedal spasms, and severe hypocalcemia are also severely magnesium deficient. Thus, repleting the calcium as well as the magnesium deficits is important in restoring calcium metabolism. Most magnesium is intracellular, and, thus, a serum magnesium level does not provide any insight into the magnesium status of an individual. The only method to determine whether a patient is magnesium deficient or sufficient is to give them a loading dose of 1 gram of magnesium oxide and then to collect the 24-hour urine magnesium. If magnesium is spilled into the urine, then the magnesium tank is likely to be full and the magnesium status normal. However, if there is very little magnesium excreted into the urine, then there is a magnesium deficit even if the serum magnesium is normal.

It is often advertised that it is necessary to take magnesium with calcium in order to maximize calcium absorption. Magnesium does not directly influence calcium absorption in the small intestine. However, it indirectly affects intestinal calcium absorption by maintaining the production of PTH, which stimulates the kidneys to produce 1,25(OH)₂D, in turn enhancing intestinal calcium absorption. Magnesium also is important for PTH and 1,25(OH)₂D to stimulate bone calcium mobilization when dietary sources of calcium are inadequate to satisfy the body's calcium needs [12].

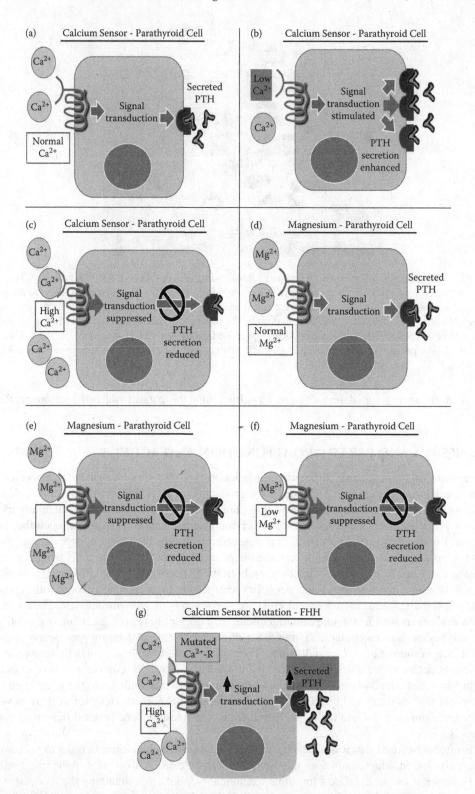

FIGURE 21.3 These schematics portray how calcium and magnesium interact with the calcium sensor (calcium receptor; CaR) on the parathyroid cell resulting in either an increase, decrease, or normal expression and secretion of PTH. Reproduced with permission, copyright 2008.

PRIMARY HYPERPARATHYROIDISM AND ITS HEALTH CONSEQUENCES

Primary hyperparathyroidism is the third most common endocrine disorder with the highest incidence in postmenopausal women [13]. Approximately one in 1000 adults will develop a benign tumor in one or more of their parathyroid glands resulting in the autonomous production of PTH [1,13,14]. The chronic elevation in PTH results in an increase in osteoclastic activity that causes loss of matrix and mineral from the skeleton. Cortical bone is more sensitive to PTH than trabecular bone and, thus, cortical bone wasting is greater than trabecular bone wasting. The consequence for patients with primary hyperparathyroidism is that they are at higher risk of fracturing their wrist or hip than their spine (Figure 21.4) [1, 7, 13]. Thus, primary hyperparathyroidism will precipitate and exacerbate osteopenia and osteoporosis. The elevated serum calcium and increased calcium in the urine can increase risk of nephrocalcinosis and kidney stones [13,14].

Patients with hyperparathyroidism have elevated PTH, which is associated with fasting hypercalcemia, hypophosphatemia, and high normal or elevated levels of $1,25(OH)_2D$. Since the PTH increases the metabolism of $25(OH)D$ to $1,25(OH)_2D$, often the patients with hyperparathyroidism have vitamin D deficiency, low serum levels of $25(OH)D$ (see Figures 21.2 and 21.5) [3,10]. The presumed mechanism is that $1,25(OH)_2D$ enhances 25-hydroxyvitamin D-24-hydroxylase (cyp24A1), which metabolizes $25(OH)D$ to 24,25-dihydroxyvitamin D [$24,25(OH)_2D$], which is then catabolized to a water-soluble inactive calcitroic-like metabolite.

Approximately 75–85% of patients with primary hyperparathyroidism have a benign tumor (i.e., a single adenoma). Two to 12% of these patients can have a second adenoma in a different parathyroid gland [13]. Most people have four parathyroid glands; however, as many as six can be present. Thus 4–16% of cases have an ectopic adenoma in the mediastinum near or associated with the thymus, esophagus, or angle of the jaw as well as being embedded in the thyroid gland. Less than 1% is due to carcinoma. Often the parathyroid adenoma can be visualized by using a sestamibi scan that helps the surgeon locate and easily remove the adenoma [1,13,14]. Once the adenoma is removed, these patients often have remarkable improvement in their bone mineral density and restoration of the calcium metabolism to normal.

INHERITED CAUSES OF HYPERPARATHYROIDISM

Approximately 15% of patients who present with hyperparathyroidism have hyperplasia of all four parathyroid glands. The two major inherited causes for parathyroid gland hyperplasia are the multiple endocrine neoplasia (MEN) syndromes type 1 and type 2 [15] and familial hypocalcuric hypercalcemia (FHH) [4, 16]. The MEN syndromes are due to a mutation in the genes that regulate the proliferation and differentiation not only of parathyroid cells but other cells of endocrine origin [15].

When evaluating patients with mild to moderate elevation in serum calcium with elevated PTH, it is important to rule out FHH. Although this autosomal dominant disease is relatively rare

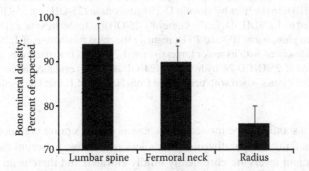

FIGURE 21.4 Bone mineral density in postmenopausal women with primary hyperparathyroidism. Adapted from Silverberg, S.J., Shane, E., de la Cruz, L., et al. 1989 with permission.

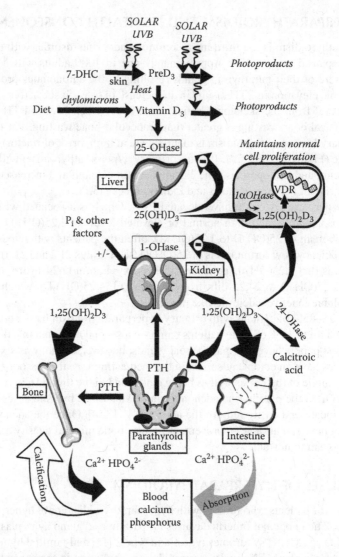

FIGURE 21.5. Schematic diagram of cutaneous production of vitamin D and its metabolism and regulation for calcium homeostasis and cellular growth. During exposure to sunlight 7-dehydrocholesterol (7-DHC) in the skin absorbs solar UVB radiation and is converted to previtamin D_3 (preD_3). PreD_3 undergoes thermally induced transformation to vitamin D3. Additional exposure to sunlight converts preD_3 and vitamin D3 to biologically inert photoproducts. Vitamin D originating from the diet or from the skin enters the circulation and is metabolized to 25(OH)D_3 in the liver by vitamin D 25-hydroxylase (25-OHase), 25(OH)D_3 reenters the circulation and is converted to 1,25(OH)$_2D_3$ in the kidney by 25(OH)D_3 1α-hydroxylase (1-OHase). A variety of factors, including serum phosphorus (P$_i$) and PTH, regulate the renal production of 1,25(OH)$_2$D and calcium metabolism through interactions with its major target tissues; 1,25(OH)$_2D_3$ also induces its own destruction by enhancing the expression of 25(OH)D 24-hydroxylase (24-OHase). For regulation of cellular growth, 25(OH) D is metabolized in other tissues. Used with permission from Holick, M.F. and Garabedian, M. 2006.

(~1/15,000–30,000), it should not be missed. The cause is due to a point mutation of the CaR in the parathyroid glands making the parathyroid glands less responsive to serum calcium levels. As a result, the serum calcium levels are chronically mildly elevated and there is an elevation in serum PTH levels. Since the calcium sensor in the kidney is also defective, this results in a marked increase in tubular resorption of calcium in the kidney. Thus, distinguishing primary hyperparathyroidism from FHH can be accomplished by obtaining a 24-hour urine for calcium and creatinine and a blood for calcium and creatinine at the same time. A calcium clearance should be determined. A calcium clearance of < 1% is considered consistent with FHH and not primary hyperparathyroidism. The reason for this is that patients with FHH have hyperplasia of all their hyperparathyroid glands. If the surgeon removes three-and-a-half glands, remnant parathyroid tissue will once again become hyperplastic and cause the same problem. Most patients with FHH do not have any deleterious effects on either their skeleton or calcium metabolism and, thus, do not need any intervention. The only intervention is to make the diagnosis and prevent the patient from seeing a surgeon to have a parathyroidectomy.

SECONDARY HYPERPARATHYROIDISM ASSOCIATED WITH VITAMIN D DEFICIENCY AND ITS HEALTH CONSEQUENCES

The major cause of hyperparathyroidism is due to vitamin D deficiency. Vitamin D deficiency is defined as a low circulating level of 25(OH)D of < 20 ng/ml [3,17–19]. This results in a decrease of efficiency of intestinal calcium absorption leading to a decrease of ionized calcium, which is recognized by the CaR in the parathyroid glands resulting in an increase in the synthesis and secretion of PTH (see Figure 21.1).

Like primary hyperparathyroidism, the elevated PTH levels result in increased osteoclastic activity. This causes osteopenia and osteoporosis and increases risk of fracture. The secondary hyperparathyroidism also causes a loss of phosphorus into the urine resulting in low normal or low serum phosphorus. The consequence is an inadequate calcium-phosphate product in the circulation preventing the normal mineralization of the collagen matrix laid down by osteoblasts. The defect is known as osteomalacia [3,10]. Patients with osteomalacia often present with isolated or generalized aches and pains in their bones and muscles. These patients have a normal sedimentation rate and, thus, no rheumatologic disorder and often are misdiagnosed as having fibromyalgia, chronic fatigue syndrome, or depressive symptoms [20–22]. The unmineralized collagen matrix is hydrated and, thus, is pushing upward on the periosteal covering of the bones, which is heavily innervated with sensory fibers. These patients complain of throbbing, aching bone pain, and when their periosteum is depressed, they complain of bone pain. This can happen when patients are sitting or lying in bed and complain of painful bones. The diagnosis can be made by pressing with a thumb or forefinger with moderate pressure on the sternum or anterior tibia. If the patient winches with pain, it is likely that their periosteal bone discomfort is caused by osteomalacia [3,22].

To make the diagnosis of secondary hyperparathyroidism associated with vitamin D deficiency, a fasting blood chemistry reveals a normal serum calcium, low normal or low serum phosphorus, elevated PTH, and a low 25(OH)D of < 20 ng/ml (see Figure 21.1). The $1,25(OH)_2D$ levels are often normal or elevated for several reasons [3]; $1,25(OH)_2D$ levels are 1000 times less in concentration compared to 25(OH)D. The elevated PTH levels stimulate the kidneys to produce $1,25(OH)_2D$. The reason that patients are vitamin D deficient is that there is an inadequate amount of $1,25(OH)_2D$ that is being made to satisfy the small intestine's requirement. Thus, even though the blood level of $1,25(OH)_2D$ can be normal or elevated, it is not a reflection of the intestinal levels of $1,25(OH)_2D$. This is the reason why measurement of $1,25(OH)_2D$ should never be used in evaluating patients for vitamin D deficiency [3].

SECONDARY HYPERPARATHYROIDISM ASSOCIATED WITH CHRONIC KIDNEY DISEASE

It is outside the scope of this chapter to review in any detail the causes and treatment for secondary hyperparathyroidism associated with chronic kidney disease. See Kidney Disease Outcomes

Quality Initiative (K/DOQI) Guidelines and Kidney Disease Improving Global Outcomes (KDIGO) and recent reviews for more details [3,23–28]. It was obvious once it was realized that the kidneys were responsible for producing $1,25(OH)_2D$ why patients with severe chronic kidney disease had severe abnormalities in their calcium metabolism and had associated metabolic bone disease [3,26,28]. However, patients with mild to moderate CKD also have abnormalities in their calcium and bone metabolism and often suffer from secondary hyperparathyroidism. There are several reasons for this. In mild to moderate CKD, the patients are unable to efficiently excrete phosphorus (see Figure 21.1). The increase in serum phosphorus levels results in a marked inhibition in renal production of $1,25(OH)_2D$ [3,21,22]. This is thought to be due to an increase in fiberblast growth factor 23 that is produced by the osteoblasts and osteocytes and causes a suppression of the production of $1,25(OH)_2D$ in the kidneys. In addition, the high serum phosphorus suppresses the expression of the CaR in the parathyroid cell, and enhances tumor growth factor α/epidermal growth factor receptor (TGFα/EGFR) activation to enhance proliferation and stimulate the parathyroid glands to produce PTH [26]. Thus, most patients with mild to moderate CKD use a phosphate binder such as calcium carbonate or a resin to prevent excess dietary phosphorus from being absorbed to help keep the serum phosphorus level within the normal range [3,23–27].

In CKD where more than ~60% of the kidney function is lost, the kidneys no longer have the capacity to produce an adequate amount of $1,25(OH)_2D$ to satisfy the body's requirement. As a result, intestinal calcium absorption is decreased, resulting in a decrease in ionized calcium stimulating the parathyroid glands to produce PTH. These patients benefit by receiving either $1,25(OH)_2D_3$ or one of its active analogues (see Figure 21.1) [3,23–28].

Patients with CKD disease benefit from maintaining a serum 25(OH)D of > 30 ng/ml, which is what is recommended by the K/DOQI and KDIGO guidelines [3, 23–25]. There are at least two reasons for this. The first is that the parathyroid glands have the enzymatic machinery, 25-hydroxyvitamin D-1-hydroxylase (1-OHase), to produce $1,25(OH)_2D$ in the parathyroid cells, which locally suppress PTH expression and production (see Figure 21.5) [3,26]. Increasing serum 25(OH)D > 30 ng/ml suppresses PTH synthesis [26–30]. In addition, 25(OH)D may be converted to $1,25(OH)_2D$ in many other tissues in the body including the colon, breast, and prostate for the purpose of regulating cell growth and a wide variety of other cellular functions [3,10,28,29]. Thus, maintaining serum 25(OH)D > 30 ng/ml helps reduce risk of cancers, infectious diseases, heart disease, and autoimmune diseases [3,10,31–34].

TERTIARY HYPERPARATHYROIDISM AND HEALTH CONSEQUENCES

Chronic secondary hyperparathyroidism leads to marked hyperplasia, increased cellular growth of the parathyroid glands, which can markedly boost their size [35]. Often these glands become hypercellular and develop islands of nodules [36]. The cells within these nodules have less CaR expression and also lack a vitamin D receptor (VDR), making the cells less responsive to the regulatory activities that calcium and $1,25(OH)_2D$ have on suppressing PTH production [3,10,21,23,24,26]. Thus, patients with chronic severe secondary hyperparathyroidism due to vitamin D deficiency or CKD can have autonomous activity within the parathyroid glands. As a result, the serum calcium becomes elevated, and with an elevated PTH level, this is now no longer considered to be secondary hyperparathyroidism, but tertiary hyperparathyroidism [3,10,26,34,35]. By definition, tertiary hyperparathyroidism is associated with an elevated serum calcium, elevated PTH, low normal or low phosphorus with a low or normal serum 25(OH)D level. For patients with CKD, their serum calcium can be controlled by dialysis three times a week with a low calcium dialysis bath [23–25]. When these patients receive a renal transplant, their transplanted kidney makes $1,25(OH)_2D$. Some of these patients who have marked parathyroid gland hyperplasia will have autonomous parathyroid cell activity resulting in hypercalcemia, and, thus, tertiary hyperparathyroidism [3,23–25,34,35].

TREATMENT STRATEGIES

Most patients with primary hyperparathyroidism who have a single or multiple adenomas often schedule surgery to have the adenoma(s) removed with good outcomes [1,2,13,14]. The availability of intraoperative PTH measurements before and immediately after surgery has been a tremendous help to surgeons. If they observe a dramatic intraoperative drop in the PTH level (~50% 10–15 minutes) after excising the adenoma(s) then the surgeon has a high degree of confidence that the problem has been cured [13]. However, if the patient has hyperplasia, three-and-a-half glands are removed. This usually preserves parathyroid function, but markedly diminishes the parathyroid tissue burden resulting in reduced or normal levels of PTH with normal calcium homeostasis [13]. Less than 1% of patients with primary hyperparathyroidism have a malignant carcinoma that needs to be aggressively treated [13]. Sometimes these patients with metastatic disease and who have elevated PTH levels benefit by using a CaR mimetic cinacalcet [13,14].

There is no need to treat FHH unless the hypercalcemia causes nonspecific constitutional symptoms including fatigue, depression, constipation, and so on. From my clinical experience, a trial of cinacalcet may be helpful. Patients with MEN 1 and 2 require parathyroid surgery and need to be evaluated for other endocrine tumors [15].

Patients with mild to moderate CKD should control their serum phosphorus levels with a calcium binder [3,23–25]. In addition, they need to be vitamin D sufficient with 25(OH)D of > 30 ng/ml. Patients with more severe kidney disease and who are unable to produce adequate $1,25(OH)_2D$ need to be treated with either $1,25(OH)_2D_3$ therapy or one of its active analogues including paricalcitol and doxercalciferol [3,23–25]. There is no advantage to using an active analog over $1,25(OH)_2D$. They suppress PTH to the same degree and have the same incidence of hypercalcemia [23–25,37].

The most common cause of hyperparathyroidism is due to vitamin D deficiency. Vitamin D deficiency is defined as a 25(OH)D of < 20 ng/ml [17–19]. However, many studies have reported that PTH levels will continue to decrease until 25(OH)D levels are > 30 ng/ml [38–40]. Thus, vitamin D sufficiency is now considered to be a 25(OH)D of > 30 ng/ml. This level is believed to maximize children and adult bone health and prevent secondary hyperparathyroidism [3,40–42]. To achieve this level, at least 1500–2000 IU of vitamin D a day is needed for adults when inadequate sun exposure cannot provide the body with its vitamin D requirement [3,10,19]. The rule of thumb is that for every 100 IU of vitamin D ingested, there is an increase in 25(OH)D of ~1 ng/ml [3,43,44]. Although it has been reported that vitamin D_2 is less effective than vitamin D_3 in maintaining serum 25(OH)D levels [45] and that vitamin D_2 enhanced the destruction of vitamin D_3 [46], several reports suggest that vitamin D_2 is equally as effective as vitamin D_3 in maintaining serum 25(OH)D levels [18,19,44].

Patients who are vitamin D deficient need to be aggressively repleted. This can be accomplished by giving 50,000 IU of vitamin D_2 once a week for eight weeks to fill the empty vitamin D tank [3,17,16,47] If the blood level of 25(OH)D does not reach above 30 ng/ml, the tank may be so empty that it requires an additional eight-week course of 50,000 IU of vitamin D_2. Since treatment for vitamin D deficiency does not correct the cause of the vitamin D deficiency, I give all of my patients—once I have corrected their vitamin D deficiency and raised their blood level of 25(OH)D > 30 ng/ml—50,000 IU of vitamin D_2 once every two weeks forever. A recent analysis of more than 100 of my patients who received this therapy for up to six years, maintained blood levels of 25(OH)D of between 30–60 ng/ml with no untoward consequences [47]. An alternative is to give 5000–6000 IU of vitamin D_2 or vitamin D_3 a day for at least two to three months, followed by 1500–2000 IU of vitamin D_2 or vitamin D_3 daily thereafter [19,47]. It has also been reported that taking 100,000 IU of vitamin D_3 every three months can help reduce risk of fracture and maintain 25(OH)D above 20 ng/ml [48].

Patients with chronic kidney disease with a renal transplant who develop tertiary hyperparathyroidism and patients with chronic vitamin D deficiency and tertiary hyperparathyroidism often benefit by treating their vitamin D deficiency and raising blood levels of 25(OH)D > 30 ng/ml [3]. There has been concern that patients with primary or tertiary hyperparathyroidism who have elevated levels of serum calcium would increase their serum calcium to a greater extent if vitamin D were given to the patient. Patients with primary hyperparathyroidism who received vitamin D to treat their vitamin D deficiency did not experience a significant increase in their serum calcium levels [3,19,49]. From my own experience, patients with both primary and tertiary hyperparathyroidism often benefit by correcting their vitamin D deficiency. Correcting vitamin D deficiency can significantly reduce PTH levels, especially in patients with early onset tertiary hyperparathyroidism and can sometimes prevent the need for surgical debulking of the parathyroid glands.

CONCLUSION

Patients are routinely screened with their blood chemistries for a serum calcium level. Most patients with a primary hyperparathyroidism are picked up by the primary care physician finding an elevated serum calcium that is corrected to their albumin levels [13]. If further workup reveals an elevated PTH level, this is diagnostic of primary hyperparathyroidism. The only time this is not true is when a patient has tertiary hyperparathyroidism or FHH.

The major cause of secondary hyperparathyroidism is vitamin D deficiency. Besides causing osteopenia and osteoporosis with increased risk of fracture, most patients with vitamin D deficiency and secondary hyperparathyroidism have nonspecific aches and pains in their bones and muscles due to osteomalacia [3,20–22]. These patients often have dramatic improvement of their nonspecific complaints with correction of their vitamin D deficiency. Since the serum calcium is normal in patients with secondary hyperparathyroidism, primary care physicians will not easily pick up this diagnosis unless they screen for 25(OH)D levels. From a cost-benefit perspective, it would be much better to obtain a 25(OH)D on patients suspected of vitamin D deficiency and to forego the PTH analysis unless there is an extenuating circumstance that requires it. Only when the calcium is elevated, should a PTH level be determined to rule out primary or tertiary hyperparathyroidism.

REFERENCES

1. Silverberg, S.H., Bilezikian, J.P. 1997. Primary hyperparathyroidism: Still evolving? *J Bone Miner Res* 12(5):856-862.
2. Kronenberg, H.M., Bringhurst, F.R., Segre, G.V., Potts, J.T., Jr., 1994. Parathyroid hormone biosynthesis and metabolism. In *The Parathyroids Basic and Clinical Concepts*, ed. J.P. Bilezikian, R. Marcus, M.A. Levine, 125–137. New York: Raven Press.
3. Holick, M.F. 2007. Vitamin D deficiency. *N Eng J Med* 357:266–281.
4. Tfelt-Hansen, J., Yano, S., Brown, E.M., Chattapadyay, N. 2002. The role of the calcium-sensing receptor in human pathophysiology. *Current Medicinal Chemistry–Immunology, Endocrine & Metabolic Agents* 2(3):175–193.
5. Slatopolsky, E., Brown, A., Dusso, A. 2001. Role of phosphorus in the pathogenesis of secondary hyperparathyroidism. *Am J Kidney Dis* 37(1 suppl 2):S54–57.
6. Brown, E.M., Juppner, H. 2006. Parathyroid horone: Synthesis, secretion, and action. In *Primer on the Metabolic Bone Diseases and Disorders of Mineral Metabolism*, ed. M.J. Favus, MD, 6th edition, 90–99. Washington, DC: American Society for Bone and Mineral Research.
7. Silverberg, S.J., Shane, E., de la Cruz, L., et al. 1989. Skeletal disease in primary hyperparathyroidism. *J Bone Miner Res* 4(3)283–291.
8. Bell, N.H. 2003. RANK ligand and the regulation of skeletal remodeling. *J Clin Invest* 111(3)1120–1122.
9. Holick, M.F. 2004. Sunlight and vitamin D for bone health and prevention of autoimmune diseases, cancers, and cardiovascular disease. *Am J Clin Nutr* 80:1678S–1688S.
10. Holick, M.F., and Garabedian, M. 2006. Vitamin D: Photobiology, metabolism, mechanism of action, and clinical applications. In *Primer on the Metabolic Bone Diseases and Disorders of Mineral Metabolism*, ed. M.J. Favus, MD, 6th edition, 129–137. Washington, DC: American Society for Bone and Mineral Research.
11. Rude, R.K. 2006. Magnesium depletion and hypermagnesemia. In *Primer on the Metabolic Bone Diseases and Disorders of Mineral Metabolism*, ed. M.J. Favus, MD, 6th edition, 230–233. Washington, DC: American Society for Bone and Mineral Research.

12. Holick, M.F. 1996. Evaluation and treatment of disorders in calcium, phosphorus, and magnesium metabolism. In *Primary Care and General Medicine*, ed. J. Noble, 2nd edition, Chapter 37, 545–557. St. Louis: Mosby.

13. Fraser, W.D. 2009. Hyperparathyroidism. *Lancet* 374:145–158.

14. Bilezikins, J.P., Silverberg, S.J. 2006. Primary hyperparathyroidism. In *Primer on the Metabolic Bone Diseases and Disorders of Mineral Metabolism*, ed. M.J. Favus, MD, 6th edition, 181–185. Washington, DC: American Society for Bone and Mineral Research.

15. Arnold, A. 2006. Familial hyperparathyroid syndromes. In *Primer on the Metabolic Bone Diseases and Disorders of Mineral Metabolism*, ed. M.J. Favus, MD, 6th edition, 185–188. Washington, DC: American Society for Bone and Mineral Research.

16. Marx, S. 2006. Familial hypocalciuric hypercalcemia. In *Primer on the Metabolic Bone Diseases and Disorders of Mineral Metabolism*, ed. M.J. Favus, MD, 6th edition, 188–190. Washington, DC: American Society for Bone and Mineral Research.

17. Malabanan, A., Veronikis, I.E., Holick, M.F. 1998. Redefining vitamin D insufficiency. *Lancet* 351: 805–806.

18. IOM (Institute of Medicine). 2011. Dietary reference intakes for calcium and vitamin D. *Committee to Review Dietary Reference Intakes for Calcium and Vitamin D*. Washington DC: National Academies Press.

19. Holick, M.F., Binkley, N.C., Bischoff-Ferrari, H.A., Gordon, C.M., Hanley, D.A., Heaney, R.P., Murad, M.H., and Weaver, C.M. 2011. Evaluation, treatment & prevention of vitamin D deficiency: An endocrine society clinical practice guideline. *J Clin Endocrinol Metab* 96(7):1911–1930.

20. Glerup, H., Middelsen, K., Poulsen, L., et al. 2000. Hypovitaminosis D myopathy without biochemical signs of osteomalacia bone involvement. *Calcif Tissue Int* 66:419–424.

21. Plotnikoff, G.A., and Quigley, J.M. 2003. Prevalence of severe hypovitaminosis D in patients with persistent, nonspecific musculoskeletal pain. *Mayo Clin Proc* 78:1463–1470.

22. Holick, M.F. 2003. Vitamin D deficiency: What a pain it is. *Mayo Clin Proc* 78(12):1457–1459.

23. K/DOQI. 2003. Clinical practice guidelines for bone metabolism and disease in chronic kidney disease. *Am J Kidney Dis* 42:(suppl 3)S1–S201.

24. KDIGO Clinical Practice Guideline for the Diagnosis, Evaluation, Prevention, and Treatment of Chronic Kidney Disease-Mineral and Bone Disorder (CKD-MBD). 2009. Suppl. to *Kidney International* 76:S113.

25. KDOQI US Commentary on the 2009 KDIGO Clinical Practice Guidelines for the Diagnosis, Evaluation, and Treatment of CKD-Mineral and Bone Disorder (CKD-MBD). 2010. *Am J Kidney Disease* 55:773–799.

26. Dusso, A.S., Sato, T., Arcidiacono, M.V., et al. 2006. Pathogenic mechanisms for parathyroid hyperplasia. *Kidney Int Suppl* 70:S8–S11.

27. Martin, K.J. Al-Aly, Z., Gonzalez, E. 2006. Renal osteodystrophy. In *Primer on the Metabolic Bone Diseases and Disorders of Mineral Metabolism*, ed. M.J. Favus, MD, 6th edition, 359–368. Washington, DC: American Society for Bone and Mineral Research.

28. Dusso, A.S., Brown, A.J., Slatopolsky, E. 2005. Vitamin D. *Am J Physiol Renal Physiol.* 289(1):F8–F28.

29. Jones, G. 2007. Expanding role for vitamin D in chronic kidney disease: Importance of blood 25-OH-D levels and extra-renal 1α-hydroxylase in the classical and nonclassical actions of 1α,25-dihydroxyvitamin D_3. *Seminars in Dialysis* 20(4):316–324.

30. Correa, P., Segersten, U., Hellman, P., Akerstrom, G., Westin, G. 2002. Increased 25-hydroxyvitamin D_3, 1α-hydroxylase and reduced 25-hydroxyvitamin D_3, 24-hydroxylase expression in parathyroid tumors—new prospects for treatment of hyperparathyroidism with vitamin D. *J Clin Endorcrinol Metab* 87:5826–5829.

31. Holick, M.F. Vitamin D: Extraskeletal health. *Endo Metab Clin North America* 2010. 39(2):381–400.

32. Holick, M.F. The vitamin D deficiency pandemic: A forgotten hormone important for health. *Public Health Reviews* 2010. 32(1):267–283.

33. Adams, J.S., and Hewison, M. Update in vitamin D. *J Clin Endocrinol Metab* 2010. 95(2):471–478.

34. Holick, M.F. 2005. Vitamin D for health and in chronic kidney disease. *Seminars in Dialysis* 18:266–75.

35. Prince, R.L. 2006. Secondary and tertiary hyperparathyroidism. In *Primer on the Metabolic Bone Diseases and Disorders of Mineral Metabolism*, ed. M.J. Favus, MD, 6th edition, 190–195. Washington, DC: American Society for Bone and Mineral Research.

36. Fukuda, N., Tanaka, Y., Tominaga, Y., Fukagawa, M., Kurokawa, K., and Seino, Y. Decreased 1,25-dihydroxyvitamin D_3 receptor density is associated with a more severe form of parathyroid hyperplasia in chronic uremic patients. 1993. *J. Clin. Invest* 92:1436–1443.

37. Wesseling-Perry, et al. Calcitriol and doxecalciferol are equivalent in controlling bone turnover, suppressing parathyroid hormone, and increasing fibroblast growth factor-23 in secondary hyperparathyroidism. 2010. *Kidney International* 79:1–8.

38. Chapuy, M.C., Preziosi, P., Maaner, M., et al. 1997. Prevalence of vitamin D insufficiency in an adult normal population. *Osteopor Int* 7: 439–443.

39. Thomas, K.K., Lloyd-Jones, D.M., Thadhani, R.I., et al. 1998. Hypovitaminosis D in medicine in patients. *N Engl J Med* 3 38:777–783.

40. Holick, M.F., Siris, E.S., Binkley, N., et al. 2005. Prevalence of vitamin D inadequacy among postmenopausal North American women receiving osteoporosis therapy. *J Clin Endocrinol Metab* 90:3215–3224.

41. Vieth, R., Bischoff-Ferrari, H., Boucher, B.J., et al. 2007. The urgent need to recommend an intake of vitamin D that is effective. *Am J Clin Nutr* 85(3):649–650.

42. Bischoff-Ferrari, H.A., Giovannucci, E., Willett, W.C., Dietrich, T., and Dawson-Hughes, B. 2006. Estimation of optimal serum concentrations of 25-hydroxyvitamin D for multiple health outcomes. *Am J Clin Nutr* 84:18–28.

43. Heaney, R.P., Davies, K.M., Chen, T.C., Holick, M.F., Barger-Lux, M.J. 2003. Human serum 25-hydroxycholecalciferol response to extended oral dosing with cholecalciferol. *Am J Clin Nutr* 77:204–210.

44. Holick, M.F., Biancuzzo, R.M., Chen, T.C., et al. 2008. Vitamin D2 is as effective as vitamin D3 in maintaining circulating concentrations of 25-hydroxyvitamin D. *J Clin Endocrinol Metab* 93(3):677–681.

45. Tang, H.M., Cole, D.E.C., Rubin, L.A., Pierratos, A., Siu, S., and Vieth, R. 1998. Evidence that vitamin D_3 increases serum 25-hydroxyvitamin D more efficiently than does vitamin D2. *Am J. Clin. Nutr* 68:854–858.

46. Armas, L.A.G., Hollis, B., and Heaney, R.P. 2004. Vitamin D2 is much less effective than vitamin D3 in humans. *J Clin Endocrino Metab* 89:5387–5391.

47. Pietras, S.M., Obayan, B.K., Cai, M.H., and Holick M.F. Research letter: Vitamin D2 treatment for vitamin D deficiency and insufficiency for up to 6 years. 2009. *Arch Intern Med* 169(19):1806–1808.

48. Trivedi, D.P., Doll, R., Khaw, K.T. 2003. Effect of four monthly oral vitamin D_3 (cholecalciferol) supplementation on fractures and mortality in men and women living in the community: Randomized double blind controlled trial. *BMJ* 326:469–475.

49. Grey, A.G., Lucas, J., Horne, A., Gamble, G., Davidson, J.S., Reid, I.R. 2005. Vitamin D repletion in patients with primary hyperparathyroidism and coexistent vitamin D insufficiency. *J Clin Endocrinol Metab* 90:2122–2126.

22 Acne and Diet

Valori Treloar, M.D.

INTRODUCTION

In the early twentieth century, dermatologists believed that diet could have a profound influence on acne [1]. However, in 1969 and 1971, two studies authored by prominent dermatologists proclaimed the opposite [2,3], and since that time the major textbooks of dermatology [4,5] have denied that diet affects acne by citing those two papers. In 2012, the website of the American Academy of Dermatology links to a patient information site that declares: "There's no need to worry about food affecting the acne" [6]. The pendulum has remained suspended in that position, defying the gravity of scrutiny for nearly 40 years. However, the drumbeat of studies challenging the acne-diet dogma has grown louder and corroborated by increasingly more sophisticated science. This chapter reviews the scientific evidence, much of it outside the dermatology literature, for the acne-diet link and concludes with a dietary treatment program for acne patients.

EPIDEMIOLOGY

Observational and epidemiologic studies support a diet-acne connection. Schaeffer, who worked among the Inuit for 30 years, observed that acne, which had been absent in that population became prevalent as the people acculturated from a fish-based diet to one rich in bread, sweets, pastries, and soft drinks [7]. The low rate of acne among Japanese teens, half that of American teens in 1964 [8], could be attributed to genetics except that a 2001 study shows that with the displacement of part of the traditional Japanese diet by Western fast foods, the rates equalized [9]. Acne is nearly unknown in the Kitavan and Ache tribes still living in their hunter-gatherer tradition with a diet rich in wild game, fish, and plants [10]. Ghanaian school children in urban areas have a strikingly higher prevalence of acne (12.9%) compared to those in rural areas (0.2%). The authors attributed this to the Westernization of urban areas. The concomitant increase in obesity seen in this study suggests that "dietary Westernization" plays a critical role [11]. A study comparing more than 800 Korean acne patients to approximately 500 controls correlated a high glycemic load diet, processed cheese, a high-fat diet, and iodine with the exacerbation of acne. In addition, those with acne were more likely to skip breakfast [12]. Low raw vegetable intake correlated with increased acne in females in a Norwegian study [13]. A Chinese study found no dietary difference between subjects with acne and those without until they divided them into a Yin-predominant group and a Yang-predominant group. In the latter, those who ate desserts and fresh fruit juices were more likely to have acne, whereas those who ate dairy and soy had a lower incidence of acne. In the former group, intake of food from street stalls correlated with a lower incidence of acne [14]. A cross-sectional study of 2300 Turkish youths found fat, sugar, and fast food consumption to be positively correlated with acne prevalence [15].

In Western cultures, acne appears to be increasing in incidence, occurring in older age groups and sometimes lasting longer. Goulden et al. noted that the mean age of their acne patients increased from 20.5 to 26.5 from 1989 to 1999 [16]. A British retrospective cohort study in 1998–99 found the prevalence of acne to be more than twice that previously reported for 1991–92, 3.1% compared to 1.3% respectively [17]. A study of male students at the University of Glasgow found an increase in the incidence of acne over the period 1948 to 1968. The authors state, "We suggest that environmental exposure may underlie this, as changes in the prevalence of germ-line genetic variants are very unlikely to occur in such a short time period [18]." If human genes have not changed, some change in the environment must account for the striking increase in acne. The uniform worldwide response does not correlate with any known industrial pollutant.

On the other hand, diet, one of the most powerful influences on physiology, has changed dramatically over the past few decades around the world. This "nutrition transition," characterized by "the introduction of fast-food chains and Westernized dietary habits . . . seems to be a marker of the increasing prevalence of obesity" and its related complications [19]. Acne as a complication or comorbidity of obesity is supported by a number of studies [20–22].

The dietary lifestyle therapy for acne seems to compete with conventional teaching; however, the concepts actually weave nicely into the matrix the pathophysiology of acne provides.

OVERVIEW OF ACNE PATHOPHYSIOLOGY

The pathophysiology of acne encompasses four problems:

1. Abnormal hyperkeratinization in the hair follicle lumen;
2. Increased sebum production by the sebaceous glands;
3. Overgrowth of *Propionobacterium acnes* (*P. acnes*) within the follicle; and
4. Inflammation [23].

Conventional dermatology seeks pharmaceutical agents that quell the symptoms. For example, retinoids slow hyperkeratosis and decrease sebum production while the tetracycline antibiotics suppress both *P. acnes* and inflammation (see Figure 22.1) A systems biology approach, analyzing the relationships among the elements in a system in response to genetic or environmental perturbations in order to understand the system [24], might instead pose the question: Why do hyperkeratinization, excessive sebum, bacterial overgrowth, and inflammation occur in the first place? Understanding the antecedents and triggers of the disease process may give us insight into the mechanisms of the dietary effects on acne.

Increased proliferation of the basal keratinocytes and decreased apoptosis and separation of the corneocytes contribute to the abnormal follicular hyperkeratinization that plugs the follicle. Rather than being shed, the cells remain in place and thicken the follicular lining. This crowding of the follicular lumen may contribute to tearing and rupture of the wall with attendant inflammation. Plugging also seals the lumen contributing to the anaerobic environment ideal for *P. acnes*. As with all biological processes, the cause of the hyperkeratosis is multifactorial and still incompletely understood. Possible contributors to the process have included, but are not limited to: localized insufficient action of vitamin A [25], localized deficiency of linoleic acid (LA) [26], increased insulin-like growth factor (IGF-1) action [27], decreased peroxisome-proliferator activated receptor-gamma (PPAR gamma) [28], disturbance of desmosomes and tonofilaments [29], increased dihydroepiandrostendione sulfate (DHEA-S) [30], oxidized squalene [31], and increased inflammation [32,33], particularly IL-1alpha [34]. Already the dance of interaction and complexity begins with one of the four factors, inflammation, cited as a cause of one of the others, hyperkeratosis.

The increased sebaceous gland activity seen in acne leads to not only an increase in the amount of sebum but also alters the composition of the secretion. The amount of LA decreases as the quantity of lipid increases (contributing to follicular hyperkeratinization). As a nutrient source for the bacteria, sebum feeds an increasing population of *P. acnes*. Breakdown of the oils by the bacteria produces inflammatory free fatty acids. Oxidation of squalene, the lipid found nowhere in the human body except in the sebum, produces by-products that induce comedones and increase inflammatory mediators [31]. The increased and altered sebum that produces the oiliness of the skin so characteristic of acne has been ascribed to increased testosterone and dihydrotestosterone

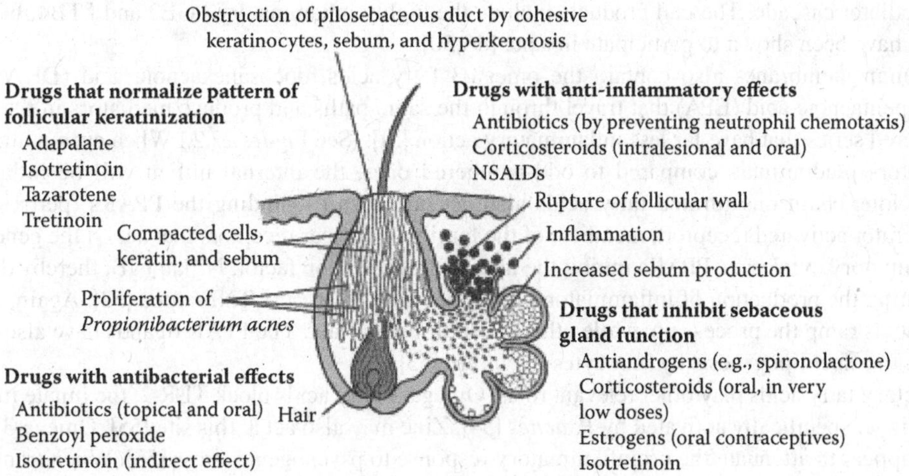

Obstruction of pilosebaceous duct by cohesive
keratinocytes, sebum, and hyperkerotosis

**Drugs that normalize pattern of
follicular keratinization**
Adapalane
Isotretinoin
Tazarotene
Tretinoin

Compacted cells,
keratin, and sebum

Proliferation of
Propionibacterium acnes

Drugs with antibacterial effects
Antibiotics (topical and oral)   Hair
Benzoyl peroxide
Isotretinoin (indirect effect)

Drugs with anti-inflammatory effects
Antibiotics (by preventing neutrophil chemotaxis)
Corticosteroids (intralesional and oral)
NSAIDs

Rupture of follicular wall
Inflammation
Increased sebum production

**Drugs that inhibit sebaceous
gland function**
Antiandrogens (e.g., spironolactone)
Corticosteroids (oral, in very
low doses)
Estrogens (oral contraceptives)
Isotretinoin

FIGURE 22.1 The four elements of acne pathophysiology: hyperkeratosis, increased sebum production, proliferation of *P. acnes*, and inflammation are targets for pharmacologic and nutrient-based treatment. (From www.merck.com, accessed Mar ch 31, 2008, used with permission.)

(DHT) [35], increased insulin [36], increased IGF-1 [37], increased PPAR alpha and decreased PPAR gamma [38], increased corticotropin releasing hormone (CRH) [39], increased substance P [29], and localized, insufficient action of vitamin A [25].

P. acnes, the "bug" thought to contribute to acne, is a normal inhabitant of our skin and its role in acne is not well understood. However, the numbers of this organism increase in acne and tend to decrease as treatment produces clinical improvement. Recent research shows that *P. acnes* activates Toll-like receptor 2 (TLR2) in the innate immune system, triggering an inflammatory cascade [40]. *P. acnes* can also induce hyperkeratinization by activating the IGF-1/IGF-1 receptor system [41]. Overgrowth of *P. acnes* appears to be triggered by: decreased LA, increased sebum (which is its nutrient supply), and abnormally desquamated follicular keratinocytes, which increases anaerobic conditions [42].

Inflammation accounts for the characteristic redness, swelling, and pustule and nodule formation in acne. Originally thought to be a late player in the process, recent evidence suggests that inflammation may be a primary initiator of the acne lesion [43]. The following factors, among others, may account for the inflammation seen in acne: TLR-2 activation by *P. acnes* [40], omega-6 fatty acids and eicosanoids [44], oxidative stress [45,46], insulin [47], adiposity [48], and testosterone [49].

Note that these lists tend to overlap; that is, the same proximate causes contribute to more than one of the four pathophysiologic factors of acne. Not only do the same elements repeat, the causes and factors interact. Inflammation increases the hyperproliferation of keratinocytes; the excess cellular debris makes a more anaerobic environment optimal for *P. acnes*; *P. acnes* binds TLR-2, triggering further inflammation. The recurring themes that deserve particular attention include disturbances of: fatty acids and fatty acid signaling, insulin/IGF-1, and oxidative and psychogenetic stress. These triggers of the pathophysiology of acne are responsive to environmental input, namely diet and lifestyle.

PATHOPHYSIOLOGY TRIGGERS AND DIET

FATTY ACIDS AND FATTY ACID SIGNALING

Fatty acids serve as precursors for inflammatory mediators, the prostaglandins (PG) and leukotrienes (LT). Classically, the omega-6 fatty acid arachidonic acid (AA) is the most prevalent fatty acid in cellular membranes and is most likely to be plucked out by phospholipase A and shunted down the mediator cascade. The end products include the highly inflammatory PGE2 and LTB4, both of which have been shown to participate in acne [46,50].

Human membranes also contain the omega-3 fatty acids, docosahexaenoic acid (DHA) and eicosapentaenoic acid (EPA) that travel through the same paths and produce mediators in the odd-numbered series that have far less inflammatory action [51]. (See Figure 22.2.) When even-numbered mediators predominate compared to odd-numbered ones, the internal milieu will be inflamed. These long-chain unsaturated fatty acids also act on genes by binding the PPARs (peroxisone-proliferator activated receptor), members of the family of nuclear receptors that act on the genes for inflammatory cytokines. PPARs inhibit the nuclear transcription factor, NFkappaB, thereby down-regulating the production of inflammatory cytokines IL-1, IL-6, and TNF-alpha [52]. Again, some fatty acids ramp the process up, while others keep things calmer. The PPAR ligands have also been shown to affect lipogenesis by sebocytes in culture [53].

Dietary fatty acids play other relevant roles. Omega-3 fatty acids block TLR-2, the innate immunity trigger specifically activated by *P. acnes* [54]. Zinc may also act at this site [55]. Omega-3 fatty acids appear to attenuate the proinflammatory response to psychogenic stress [56]. When trans fats exacerbate essential fatty acid deficiency, they both increase hyperkeratosis, as demonstrated in a rat model, and contribute to inflammation [57].

The role played by linoleic acid (LA) is complex and incompletely understood. LA suppresses *P. acnes* growth. *P. acnes* protects itself by biohydrogenating LA, rendering it incapable of its suppressive action [58]. LA also controls keratinocyte proliferation and, in its absence, hyperkeratosis occurs. The proportion of LA decreases as sebum production increases. The follicular plugging of

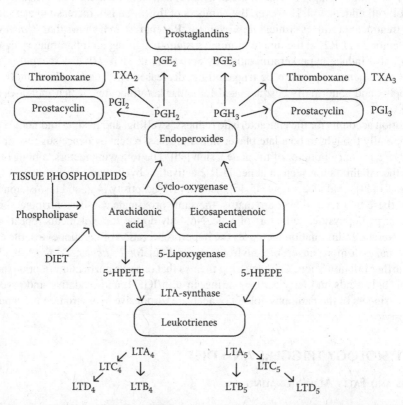

FIGURE 22.2 Arachidonic acid (AA) and eicosapentaenoic acid follow parallel pathways in the production of inflammatory mediators, but mediators derived from AA have greater inflammatory activity. (From [65]. With permission.)

acne has been attributed to "localized LA deficiency" [59]. On the other hand, LA increases sebum production in cell culture [60].

In summary, fatty acids and fatty acid signaling via PPARs play important roles in all four of the components of acne pathogenesis: hyperkeratinization, sebum overproduction, *P. acnes* overgrowth, and inflammation.

Diet and Fatty Acids

Fats in the diet end up in the skin. The lipid bilayer cell membranes can be envisioned as sacks made from fatty acid fabric composed of the fats in the diet. Arachidonic acid, dominant in the US diet, is the dominant fatty acid in the bodies of most Americans. LA from vegetable oils converts readily to AA. Enriching the diet with foods containing omega-3 fatty acids will incorporate more EPA and DHA in cell membranes while decreasing AA [61]. A diet rich in hydrogenated vegetable oils will weave a stiff fabric containing straight trans fatty acids.

Since cell membranes serve as the reservoir for the building blocks of inflammatory mediators, a stockpile of AA will produce a wealth of inflammatory even-numbered eicosanoids. Omega-3 fatty acids compete for the same enzyme pathways and produce odd-numbered eicosanoids with lower activity. The PPAR and TLR-2 actions of fatty acids may also help explain why higher serum levels of omega-3 fatty acids correlate with lower serum levels of proinflammatory markers and higher levels of anti-inflammatory markers [51,62]. Eating fish and seaweed and taking omega-3 supplements will create a less inflammatory internal milieu.

Man-made hydrogenated vegetable oils brought trans fatty acids into our food supply in the early twentieth century and have achieved a dominant position over the past few decades. Intake of hydrogenated vegetable oil, the major source of dietary trans fats, has increased from 10 g/day in 1960 to 30 g/day in 1993 [63]. In women, trans fatty acid intake correlates directly with serum levels of inflammatory markers [64]. The same eicosanoid and PPAR mechanisms previously discussed probably explain why eating less hydrogenated vegetable oil will help decrease inflammation.

Concurrent with increased intake of trans fat, the dietary ratio of omega-6 to omega-3 fatty acids changed. When human metabolism evolved, diets were rich in hunted wild animal and bird meat, fish, and gathered root vegetables, greens, fruits, nuts, seeds, and eggs. The whole vegetable, nut, or seed accompanied by fiber and antioxidant vitamins and plant polyphenols served as the dietary source of omega-6 fats. The ratio of omega-6 to omega-3 was about 1:1. Today much of the fat in the American diet comes from sophisticated, powerful presses squeezing omega-6-rich oils from plant seeds: canola, safflower, sunflower, peanut, soy, and cottonseed. LA, one of the dominant plant seed fatty acids, is an omega-6 fatty acid that is readily converted to AA in our bodies. The heat from the pressing produces oxidized moieties, many not found in nature.

Further processing includes degumming, refining, bleaching, deodorizing, additives, and winterization in order to produce the clear oil with a prolonged shelf life that we find in the grocery stores. It is devoid of the polyphenolic compounds that provide color, flavor, and antioxidant protection. The modern dietary omega-6 to omega-3 ratio is about 16:1 [65]. In genetic terms the dietary shift is extremely recent, because a 1% change in the human genome occurs approximately every 10,000 years. Given the acneigenic effects of an increased omega-6 to omega-3 ratio and increased dietary trans fats, knowledgeable observers might have predicted the "acne epidemic" [66] that has accompanied this change in the Western diet over the past several decades.

INSULIN/INSULIN-LIKE GROWTH FACTOR-1

A little-recognized, but well-documented phenomenon of adolescence is the rise and fall of insulin resistance that mirrors acne activity. Insulin resistance peaks at about Tanner stage 3 and returns to normal at the end of the teen years [67]. Insulin is one of our major anabolic hormones and tends to rise with elevation of growth hormone (GH); an increase in insulin levels during a period of rapid growth and development should come as no surprise. Insulin, GH, and insulin-like growth factor-1

(IGF-1) interweave in their physiologic activity. Insulin and IGF-1 can bind each other's receptors and may stimulate similar processes, albeit in different concentrations [36].

IGF-1 levels reflect GH levels and are used as the surrogate marker for the elusive GH. Elevation during adolescence is normal and expected. Less expected is the elevation of IGF-1 in adult women with acne that was noted by Cappel and colleagues [68]. While men's IGF-1 levels do not correlate with acne severity, they do match DHEA-S and androstendione levels. Cappel and colleagues go on to suggest that the effects of androgens were "dependent on the influence of IGF-1" [67]. Patients with longstanding acne have increases in IGF-1 and decreased levels of the protein that binds IGF-1 and takes it out of the action, IGF binding protein-3 (IGFBP-3) [69].

What roles do these factors play in acne? Insulin appears to decrease hepatic production of SHBG, which leads to higher circulating levels of unbound, active androgen triggering all the well-established androgen effects of proliferation and differentiation of the sebocytes as well as upregulation of lipid production [70]. The activity of 5 alpha-reductase, the follicular enzyme that converts testosterone to its more active form, dihydrotestosterone, correlates with fasting insulin levels [71]. Although the correlation has not been shown in acne, insulin can increase systemic inflammatory markers [47]. Insulin and IGF-1 directly increase sebum production, insulin largely through differentiation, and IGF-1 through proliferation of the sebocytes [36]. Free IGF-1 directly stimulates basal keratinocyte proliferation, thereby contributing to the follicular hyperkeratosis, whereas IGFBP-3 inhibits it [27,72]. Also, IGFBP-3 and tretinoin, a mainstay of acne therapy, bind the same retinoid X nuclear receptor (RXR alpha) [73].

An interesting side note illustrates the web-like interaction of the elements of acne pathophysiology. In vitro, *P. acnes* membrane fraction increases IGF-1 secretion and activates the IGF-1 receptor inducing keratinocyte proliferation. This process is blocked by preincubation of cell cultures with zinc gluconate [74]. Insulin/IGF-1 affects three of the four pathophysiologic steps in acne: hyperkeratinization, inflammation, and sebum overproduction.

Diet and Insulin/Insulin-Like Growth Factor-1

Insulin levels are driven by diet. Sugars digested and absorbed into the bloodstream must be directed into cells to be used as energy or stored. The health ravages of diabetes show why our bodies strive to keep blood glucose levels within a tight range, and this is insulin's primary job. Insulin levels chase blood sugar levels, rising fast and high in response to rapidly absorbed refined carbohydrates and more slowly and lower when foods contain more fiber, fat, and protein, all of which slow the absorption of sugar into the blood.

The glycemic index (GI) measures how fast and high blood sugar is pushed by different foods. The glycemic load (GL) takes the usual size of a portion into consideration. The insulinemic response tends to track the glycemic response, so low GI foods eaten at regular intervals will help keep insulin levels moderated throughout the day. A typical American diet tends to result in spiking insulin levels and the area under the curve tends to be high [75]. A diet with decreased fat and refined carbohydrates, an increased ratio of omega-3 to omega-6, fewer saturated fatty acids, and an increase in foods rich in "phytoestrogens" and fiber not only lowered insulin levels but also lowered serum testosterone and raised SHBG [76]. While insulin has a prominent effect on SHBG, dietary monosaccharides, especially fructose, may also slow SHBG production allowing higher testosterone levels [77]. In the only randomized clinical trial of diet and acne, young men with acne were randomized to either a low GI diet or a standard Western diet. Statistically significant clinical improvement in acne paralleled improved insulin sensitivity, BMI, decreased free androgen index, and increased IGFBP-1 [78,79].

Dairy products are a special case; the insulinemic response is higher than predicted from the GI [80]. In prepubertal boys, casein supplementation increased IGF-1 by 15% with no effect on insulin. Whey supplementation increased insulin by 20% with no effect on IGF-1 [81]. The effect of these milk proteins on insulin and IGF-1 may help explain the association between dairy intake and acne found in a series of studies from the Harvard School of Public Health [82–84].

Diet clearly affects IGF-1 and IGFBP-3. Insulin raises IGF-1 levels. IGFBP-3, on the other hand, falls after ingestion of high GI foods and rises after eating low GI foods [85]. Lower levels of IGF-1 and higher levels of IGFBP-3 are associated with greater intake of omega-3 fatty acids, tomatoes, vegetables, and dietary fiber. In contrast, higher levels of IGF-1 are associated with dietary saturated fat, vegetable oils, milk, and dairy products [86,87].

STRESS, OXIDATIVE, AND PSYCHOGENIC

The link between oxidative and psychogenic stress is not readily apparent, but the following discussion identifies inflammation with its attendant generation of reactive oxygen species as the connection between the two. Using McEwen's concept of allostatic load, stress becomes problematic when the forces impinging on an individual overwhelm the capacity to compensate for the disturbance or when the compensatory mechanisms begin to cause problems themselves [88]. For example, UV light causes oxidative damage to squalene in cell membranes in the dermis. Vitamin E can reduce the oxidized lipid, but unless the vitamin E is replaced or reduced back to its normal state by vitamin C, the capacity to compensate for the oxidative damage becomes overwhelmed and injury/ acne ensues. The compensatory mechanism of cortisol levels rising in response to sleep deprivation keeps the metabolism running fairly smoothly in the short term, but over time, excessive cortisol causes central obesity, peripheral muscle wasting, hyperglycemia, and acne. One night of sleep deprivation causes insulin resistance [89]. This is another example of the web-like patterns of acne pathophysiology.

Several lines of evidence suggest that psychogenic stress plays a role in acne. Examination stress appears to increase acne severity [90,91]. Stress has been shown to elicit the release of the neuropeptide, substance P, which appears to increase lipogenesis in sebocytes and also increases inflammation via mast cell release of IL-6 and TNF-alpha [92]. CRH generated in the sebaceous gland increases sebocyte lipogenesis. This is thought to be a localized stress response analogous to that of the central hypothalamic-pituitary adrenal axis [39]. CRH released centrally may have a similar effect. Higher levels of urinary cortisol, a marker of stress, correlate with higher 8-hydroxy-guanosine levels, a marker of DNA oxidation illustrating the connection between psychogenic stress and oxidative stress [93]. Those who practiced a relaxation response–eliciting exercise (RR), such as meditation, progressive relaxation, or Qi gong, had different gene expression profiles compared to those without RR. The specific functional group expression suggested a greater capacity to respond to oxidative stress. The genes COX7B, UQCRB, and CASP2 responded in the opposite direction from that seen in the stress response [94].

More than 20 years ago, Swedish researchers noted that in men with severe acne, red blood cells carried far less of one of our most powerful antioxidants, glutathione [95]. More recently, the stratum corneum in acne patients bore significantly less glutathione than that of subjects without acne [96]. Measurement of markers of oxidative injury and activity of antioxidant enzymes showed significant oxidative damage in acne patients compared to controls [45,97]. Reactive oxygen species (ROS) generated by neutrophils contribute to follicular wall injury and inflammation. ROS can serve as regulators of NFkappaB, a transcription factor that upregulates expression of genes for inflammatory cytokines including TNF-alpha, IL-1, IL-8, and IL-6. AP-1 is another redox-sensitive transcription factor that generates inflammatory cytokines [98]. Among the genes reported to be upregulated in acne, the most strongly induced included IL-1, IL-8, and MMP1— all known to be generated through ROS activated pathways. IL-1 may actually "trigger the keratinocyte activation cycle" perhaps serving as one of the very first steps in the formation of an acne lesion [66]. Matrix metalloproteinases (MMPs) degrade IGFBP-3, preventing its protective effect against hyperkeratinization and its action at the retinoid X receptor [99]. Inflammation is triggered by and generates ROS; oxidation and inflammation intimately interconnect. And psychogenic stress, via substance P, spirals into the mix as well.

Stress impacts three of four components of acne pathophysiology: hyperkeratinization, sebum overproduction, and inflammation.

Diet and Stress (Oxidative and Psychogenic)

Psychological stress induces the production of proinflammatory cytokines, IFN-gamma, TNF-alpha, and IL-6. University students with lower serum omega-3 levels or with a higher omega-6/omega-3 ratio had significantly greater examination-induced TNF-alpha and IFN-gamma responses [56]. Given that the gene for TNF-alpha is one of those found to be activated in acne, that the fact that examination stress increases acne is not surprising. Dietary intake of different fatty acids can alter the immunologic response to stress, broadening the scope of treatment options.

Oxidative stress is a condition of life in our earthly atmosphere. Food serves as an important source of antioxidants to contend with the ROS generated by metabolism. The richest dietary sources of antioxidants are vegetables and fruits. Not only do they contain high levels of antioxidant vitamins, but the polyphenolic compounds that give produce its colors, fragrances, and tastes appear to have even more powerful antioxidant activity than vitamins do [100].

While some foods offer antioxidant benefit, other foods are pro-oxidants, compounding the problem. Dietary trans fats increase markers of oxidative damage [101]. High fructose intake enhances ROS generation and the protein and lipid damage it causes [102]. In fact, a high fructose diet is used in experimental models to create insulin resistance in rats. Zinc alone and in combination with selenium and vitamin E decreased both the degree of insulin resistance and the oxidative damage sustained [103]. To round out the discussion, oxidative stress appears to be instrumental in triggering insulin resistance, the biochemical finding in teens that most closely parallels acne [104]. Following the syllogism, high fructose intake from food and especially beverages increases ROS generation and exacerbates the normal insulin resistance of adolescence, perhaps contributing to acne. Based on their findings of increased oxidation markers and decreased antioxidant enzyme activity in acne patients, the researchers stated: "Drugs with antioxidative effects might be valuable in treatment" [105]. More prudent perhaps would be the suggestion to increase intake of foods rich in antioxidants and decrease intake of pro-oxidative foods.

DRUG-NUTRIENT INTERACTIONS

While some effects of diet and nutrients on medications are well recognized, less known is the converse, the effect drugs can have on nutrient status. The systemic medications used in the treatment of acne include: antibiotics (particularly tetracycline, doxycycline, minocycline), oral contraceptives (for women), and isotretinoin. All are often given for months, even years, at a time. Isotretinoin is usually prescribed for 20 weeks. All have been reported to interact with nutrients.

Antibiotics in general alter the colonic flora and can interfere with production by these organisms of vitamin K, vitamins B1, B2, and B3, biotin, and folic acid [106], although this has not resulted in clinical reports of vitamin deficiency. A number of antibiotics cause decrease in serum vitamin C levels; the tetracylines were not evaluated in the study [107]. Interaction between the tetracyclines and high-dose vitamin A can cause pseudotumor cerebri [108].

Oral contraceptives can deplete vitamin B6, at least temporarily [109], as well as vitamins B12, B2, C, zinc, and folic acid [110]. Iron, copper, and vitamins A and K can be elevated [111]. Clinical consequences are not well documented and supplementation is controversial.

Isotretinoin is a vitamin A analog used in a 20-week course of therapy to treat severe nodulocystic acne. It significantly lowers serum retinol levels in women but not in men [112]. While isotretinoin causes symptoms of hypervitaminosis A, such as dry, peeling skin and angular cheilitis, it can also cause nightblindness, a condition of retinol deficiency. Isotretinoin slows rhodopsin regeneration in the retina; one likely mechanism is competition with 11-cis-retinal for binding proteins in the rhodopsin system [113]. This suggests that patients on isotretinoin may suffer deficiency of some forms of vitamin A while showing signs of excess of other isoforms, making supplementation problematic. Supplementation with vitamin A during isotretinoin therapy is specifically proscribed, but ensuring a vitamin A-rich diet especially from plant-sourced beta-carotene may be beneficial. Some researchers recommend assuring that patients are replete with vitamin A prior to instituting a course of isotretinoin treatment [114]. The activity of biotinidase, the enzyme that recycles biotin, appears to be impaired by isotretinoin [115]. Although biotin levels do not seem to decline, the hair loss suffered by some patients suggests that this may be clinically relevant for them. Two studies assessing the effect of isotretinoin on vitamin D metabolism produced contradictory results, but both demonstrate significant alterations in serum levels of different forms of vitamin D [116,117]. Elevation of serum triglycerides and cholesterol is fairly common with isotretinoin and responds to fish oil supplementation [118]. L-carnitine levels tend to fall during a course of isotretinoin and the decline correlates with myalgia. Supplementation with L-carnitine 100 mg/kg/day (compared to placebo) caused resolution of myalgias within five to six days and by day 45 of the study normalized both L-carnitine levels and LFTs that had risen during isotretinoin therapy [119]. Isotretinoin raises homocysteine levels perhaps due to suppression of cystathione-beta-synthase [120]. Elevated homocysteine levels are found in a subgroup of subjects with depression [121] and may play a role in the connection seen between isotretinoin and depression. Supplementation with vitamin B12 and folic acid can improve homocysteine levels but may not have clinical effect.

LABORATORY/DIAGNOSTIC TESTS

If the patient shows signs of hyperinsulinemia, insulin resistance, or polycystic ovarian syndrome, insurance may cover fasting and Two-hour Postprandial Insulin Testing. Given the acneigenic role insulin plays, a positive test result supports an action plan of diet and lifestyle to improve insulin metabolism.

The Zinc Taste Test correlates well with serum zinc levels and can be performed easily and inexpensively in the office. Several nutrient supplement companies offer zinc solution products. The one study that evaluated this phenomenon used 2 ml of a 1% solution of zinc sulfate (approximately 4 mg test dose) held in the mouth for 10 seconds. Taste test scores of one (no particular taste sensation within 10 seconds) and two (perception of a peculiar taste within a few seconds) correlated with zinc deficiency with a serum level < 90 mcg/dl. Zinc taste test scores of three (distinctive taste is perceived immediately but is not a nasty one) and four (perception of a very nasty, distinctive taste straightaway) correlated with normal serum zinc levels, 90-110 mcg/dl. Zinc supplementation increased serum levels and zinc taste test scores significantly and in parallel [122].

Given that the ratio of omega-3 to omega-6 fatty acids in cell membranes influences inflammation, measurement of this parameter, and trans fatty acid levels, can help guide decisions on dietary changes and fish oil supplementation. Several fatty acid profile tests are available including a recently introduced fingerstick blood draw.

NUTRIGENOMICS

Taking the definition from the University of California, Davis Nutrigenomics Center, "nutritional genomics, or nutrigenomics, is the study of how foods affect our genes and how individual genetic differences can affect the way we respond to nutrients and other naturally occurring compounds in the foods we eat" [123]. Individual genetic differences can unveil how foods affect our genes. Single nucleotide polymorphisms in genes can result in protein products with altered function.

In human subjects with substitution of codon 1013 G to A in the IGF-1 receptor gene, free blood levels of IGF-1 are lower than normal. While this polymorphism has not been studied in acne, those with the variant gene showed prolonged lifespan, a physiologic response that does, like acne, correlate with IGF-1 levels [124]. A study of subjects with Laron Syndrome, congenital IGF-1 deficiency, found only 1 of 22 had acne, a mild case. "Among the 6 treated female patients, 3 had signs of hyperandrogenism (oligo-amenorrhea) and acne during IGF-1 over-dosage. On reduction of the IGF-1 dose (to 50 mg/kg/day) or cessation of treatment, the acne disappeared in all 3 patients" [125]. Individual genetic differences in IGF-1 clearly affect the risk of acne in response to foods.

Using diet to lower insulin/IGF-1 may mimic the effects seen in those with genetically low levels and improve acne (and longevity, too).

Melnik [126] elucidates the genomic effects of increased insulin/IGF-1 by tracing its activation of the phosphoinositide-3-kinse/Akt pathway and the subsequent reduction of nuclear transcription factor Fox 01. Nuclear Fox 01 suppresses nuclear androgen receptors and PPAR gamma as well as "key genes and transcription factors of cell proliferation (cyclin D2), lipid biosynthesis (sterol response element binding protein-1) and inflammatory signaling (NF kappa-B)" [126]. Loss of nuclear Fox 01 de-represses these genes and receptors increasing androgen signaling, cell proliferation, sebum production, and inflammation—expressions of the pathophysiology of acne. Following this line of reasoning, the insulingenic effects of milk provide a genetic mechanism that accounts for the epidemiologic correlation between milk intake and acne.

PPARs are gene transcription factors activated by ligands that include EPA and DHA. Their actions are complex and sometimes contradictory. Activation of PPARs increases sebum production [127]. On the other hand, PPAR alpha activation represses NFkappaB transcription decreasing production of inflammatory cytokines [128]. Activation of PPAR gamma also promotes epidermal differentiation, restoring epidermal homeostasis in hyperproliferative mouse skin [129]. Most studies of PPAR agonists have used pharmaceuticals; evidence suggests that fatty acids, among the endogenous ligands, may have similar activities [130].

A twin study of acne genetics found only one striking difference between twins with and without acne—decreased ApoA1 in those with acne [131]. This lipoprotein fraction is associated with decreased cardiovascular risk and can be raised by exercise, diet, and weight control [132]. The dietary advice offered in the study was as follows: avoid excessive consumption of high-fat foods, reduce portion sizes, and increase daily intake of complex carbohydrates, lean meats, dairy products, fruits, and vegetables. Of note, the program also improved insulin sensitivity and decreased serum markers of lipid oxidation.

A Medline search for "nutrigenomics" produced 619 references in January 2012; the number dropped to zero when the term was crossed with "acne." This field of study is in its infancy. Our food speaks to our genes; gene expression is dictated by the environment washing over our cells and our diet is the major ruler of that environment. Other elements of lifestyle, such as stress and exercise, also modify the environment that dictates gene expression. Recognition of the critical roles these elements play in our health and disease is dawning in medicine. Soon the need to control for these variables, a rare occurrence in the gold standard, double-blind, placebo-controlled studies we revere, will alter research dramatically. Until then, lower level evidence and common sense guide our use of diet and nutrients in disease management.

CONCLUSION AND CLINICAL SUMMARY

Diet can influence the antecedents and triggers of acne—the proximate causes behind the four pathophysiologic elements of acne. Why did two widely accepted clinical trials conclude otherwise? We return to these two landmark studies that turned the tide away from the acne-diet connection. Through the lens of modern nutritional science, the two studies that form the foundation of the current diet-acne dogma demonstrate significant weaknesses, the most glaring being that neither took the underlying diet into consideration. Anderson's open study included only 27 subjects and no controls; it would not be accepted for publication under today's more stringent peer review [3]. Fulton and colleagues [2] concluded that chocolate had no influence on acne by comparing a chocolate bar to a pseudochocolate bar composed of 28% hydrogenated vegetable oil, a food known to increase inflammatory markers, and 14% nonfat milk solids, the acneigenic potential of which is demonstrated by three studies from the Harvard School of Public Health. The sugar content of the bars was 44.3% and 53% respectively; both likely to induce a rapid and high insulin response. The evidence for a dietary effect on acne is a young and growing body of knowledge, but it is far more robust than the evidence against such an effect. In spite of the dearth of the controlled, blinded, human trials that clinicians rely on most heavily, the risk-benefit ratio of dietary strategies for acne remains far more favorable than any pharmaceutical agent. The implementation of a dietary treatment for acne does not preclude conventional treatment and is likely to complement it. Even when advised that these suggestions are based on biochemistry and physiology, cell culture and animal studies, but very few human clinical trials, many patients will take the opportunity to incorporate lifestyle modification. A summary clinical approach is presented in Table 22.1.

One final note: evidence that increased IGF-1 and decreased IGFBP-3 levels are associated with increased prostate cancer [133] dovetails with the increased risk of prostate cancer seen in those

---

TABLE 22.1
Food, Nutrient, and Lifestyle Approaches to Managing Acne

Diet

1. Try a dairy-free diet for three to six months. No milk, cream, yogurt, ice cream, cheese of any kind (including cream and cottage). Decrease your use of butter or switch to ghee (clarified butter).
2. Eat three nutrient-dense meals and two "mini-meal" snacks daily.
3. Eat five to eight servings of vegetables and two servings of fruit per day, all colors of the rainbow.
4. Eat 2.5 to 3 palm-sized servings of protein-rich foods (meat, poultry, eggs, fish) daily; include fish one to two times weekly.
5. Minimize refined carbohydrates, such as candy, sweets, baked goods, crackers, white bread, white rice, white potatoes, pasta. (Unless you are performing very high intensity exercise more than an hour a day on a regular basis.)
6. Eat vegetable carbohydrates, such as squash, sweet potatoes, root vegetables and, if you tolerate them, legumes and grains.
7. Eliminate hydrogenated vegetable oil; decrease liquid oil rich in omega-6 fatty acids (safflower, sunflower, peanut, soy, cottonseed).
8. Eliminate high fructose corn syrup (HFCS).
9. Do not drink liquid calories, such as soda, sports drinks, undiluted juice, chocolate.
10. Drink filtered water, sparkling water, green tea, diluted juice, herbal teas, juiced vegetables.
11. Limit alcohol intake. (If you are under legal drinking age, do not drink.)

Supplements

Consider nutritional supplements on a patient-by-patient basis:

High-quality fish oil capsules, 2 to 4 gm (600 to 4000 mg EPA/DHA) daily
Zinc gluconate (or other readily absorbed form), 15 to 30 mg daily
Vitamin E with natural mixed tocopherols, 100 to 200 IU daily
Pyridoxal-5-phosphate (B6), 25 to 50 mg daily
Vitamin C 500 mg daily
N-acetyl cysteine 500 mg daily
Selenium 100 micrograms daily
Vitamin A 5000 IU daily

Lifestyle

Complement nutritional intervention with a lifestyle that helps reduce adrenal stress and improve insulin action.

1. Aim to sleep seven to eight uninterrupted hours nightly. If you awaken wishing you could sleep more, you may have a sleep deficit and may need more than eight hours nightly for a while to make it up.
2. Practice an exercise that induces the relaxation response every day, such as meditation, yoga, tai chi, self-hypnosis, biofeedback, or progressive muscle relaxation.
3. Participate in strength, aerobic, and flexibility exercise at least three times weekly. Aim to do at least one of the three every day.

For clinical recommendations specifically written for patients refer to *The Clear Skin Diet* [137].

with more severe acne treated with tetracycline [134]. While the connection to breast cancer is less clear, hyperinsulinaemia, subsequent insulin resistance, and stimulation of the insulin-like growth factor-1 axis all promote tumor progression [135] and type 2 diabetes has been described as an independent negative prognostic factor for breast cancer [136]. Addressing dysregulated IGF-1/IGFBP-3/insulin to treat the underlying mechanisms of acne improves our patients' long-term health by decreasing cancer risk as well.

REFERENCES

1. Stokes, J. H. Fundamentals of Medical Dermatology. 7th rev. ed. 1942, Philadelphia: University of Pennsylvania Department of Dermatology Book Fund.
2. Fulton, J. E., Jr., Plewig, G., Kligman, A. M. Effect of chocolate on acne vulgaris. JAMA, 1969. 210(11): 2071–74.
3. Anderson, P.C. Foods as the cause of acne. Am Fam Physician, 1971. 3(3): 102–3.
4. Freedberg, I. et al. Fitzpatrick's Dermatology in General Medicine. 6th ed. 2003, New York: McGraw-Hill.
5. Burns, T., Breathnach, S., Cox, N., Griffiths, C. Rook's Textbook of Dermatology, 7th ed. 2004, Hoboken, NJ: John Wiley & Sons, Inc.
6. Acne Myths [website]. Available from: http://www.skincarephysicians.com/acnenet/myths.html.
7. Schaefer, O. When the Eskimo comes to town. Nutr Today, 1971. 6: 8–16.
8. Hamilton, J. B., Terada, H., Mestler, S. E. Greater tending to acne in white Americans than in Japanese populations. J Clin Endocrinol Metab, 1964. 24: 267–72.
9. Hayashi, N., Kawashima, M., Watanabe, S., Nakata, T. An epidemiological study of Acne vulgaris in Japan by questionnaire. Jpn J Dermatol, 2001. 111: 1347–55.
10. Cordain, L., et al. Acne vulgaris: A disease of Western civilization. Arch Dermatol, 2002. 138(12): 1584–90.
11. Hogewoning, A. A., Koelemij, I., Amoah, A. S., Bouwes Bavinck, J. N., Aryeetey, Y., Hartgers, F., Yazdanbakhsh, M., Willemze, R., Boakye, D. A., Lavrijsen, A. P. Prevalence and risk factors of inflammatory acne vulgaris in rural and urban Ghanaian schoolchildren. Br J Dermatol, 2009. 161(2): 475–77.
12. Jung, J. Y., Yoon, M. Y., Min, S. U., Hong, J. S., Choi, Y. S., Suh, D. H. The influence of dietary patterns on acne vulgaris in Koreans. Eur J Dermatol, 2010. Nov-Dec;20(6): 768–72.
13. Halvorsen, J. A. , Dalgard F., Thoresen, M., Bjertness, E., Lien, L. Is the association between acne and mental distress influenced by diet? Results from a cross-sectional population study among 3775 late adolescents in Oslo, Norway. BMC Public Health, 2009. Sep 16;9: 340.
14. Law, M. P., Chuh, A. A., Molinari, N., Lee, A. An investigation of the association between diet and occurrence of acne: A rational approach from a traditional Chinese medicine perspective. ClinExpDermatol. 2010. Jan;35(1): 31–35.
15. Koku Aksu, A. E., Metintas, S., Saracoglu, Z. N., Gurel, G., Sabuncu, I., Ankan, I., Kalyoncu, C. Acne prevalence and relationship with dietary habits in Eskisehir, Turkey. J Eur Acad Dermatol Venereol. 2011. Nov 10. First published online, 10 November, 2011.
16. Goulden, V., Stables, G. I., Cunliffe, W. J. Prevalence of facial acne in adults. J Am Acad Dermatol, 1999. 41(4): 577–80.
17. Purdy, S., Langston, J., Tait, L. Presentation and management of acne in primary care: A retrospective cohort study. Br J Gen Pract. 2003. Jul;53(492): 525–29.
18. Galobardes, B., et al. Has acne increased? Prevalence of acne history among university students between 1948 and 1968. Glasgow Alumni Cohort Study. Br J Dermatol, 2005. 152(4): 824–25.
19. Astrup, A., et al. Nutrition transition and its relationship to the development of obesity and related chronic diseases. Obes Rev, 2008. 9 Suppl 1: 48–52.
20. Al-Mutairi, N. Associated cutaneous diseases in obese adult patients: A prospective study from a skin referral care center. Med Princ Pract. 2011. 20(3): 248–52.
21. Tsai, M. C., Chen, W., Cheng, Y. W., Wang, C. Y., Chen, G. Y., Hsu, T. J. Higher body mass index is a significant risk factor for acne formation in schoolchildren. Eur J Dermatol. 2006. May-Jun;16(3): 251–53.
22. Hogewoning, A. A., Koelemij, I., Amoah, A. S., BouwesBavinck, J. N., Aryeetey, Y., Hartgers, F., Yazdanbakhsh, M., Willemze, R., Boakye, D. A., Lavrijsen, A. P. Prevalence and risk factors of inflammatory acne vulgaris in rural and urban Ghanaian schoolchildren. BrJDermatol. 2009. Aug;161(2):475–77.
23. Degitz, K., Placzek, M., Borelli, C., Plewig G. Pathophysiologyofacne.J Dtsch Dermatol Ges. 2007. Apr;5(4): 316–23.

24. Weston, A. D., Hood, L. Systems biology, proteomics, and the future of health care: Toward predictive, preventative, and personalized medicine. Journal of Proteome Research 2004. 3:179–96.

25. Orfanos, C.E., et al. Current use and future potential role of retinoids in dermatology. Drugs, 1997. 53(3): 358–88.

26. Cunliffe, W. J., et al. Comedogenesis: Some aetiological, clinical and therapeutic strategies. Dermatology, 2003. 206(1): 11–16.

27. Bol, D. K., et al. Overexpression of insulin-like growth factor-1 induces hyperplasia, dermal abnormalities, and spontaneous tumor formation in transgenic mice. Oncogene, 1997. 14(14): 1725–34.

28. Demerjian, M., et al. Topical treatment with thiazolidinediones, activators of peroxisome proliferatoractivated receptor-gamma, normalizes epidermal homeostasis in a murine hyperproliferative disease model. Exp Dermatol, 2006. 15(3): 154–60.

29. Toyoda, M., Morohashi, M. Pathogenesis of acne. Med Electron Microsc, 2001. 34(1): 29–40.

30. Harper, J.C., Thiboutot, D. M. Pathogenesis of acne: Recent research advances. Adv Dermatol, 2003. 19: 1–10.

31. Chiba, K., Yoshizawa, K., Makino, I., Kawakami, K., Onoue, M. Comedogenicity of squalene monohydroperoxide in the skin after topial application. J Toixol Sci. 2000. 25: 77–83.

32. Plewig, G. Follicular keratinization. J Invest Dermatol, 1974. 62(3): 308–20.

33. Jeremy, A.H., et al. Inflammatory events are involved in acne lesion initiation. J Invest Dermatol, 2003. 121(1): 20–27.

34. Guy, R., Green, M. R., Kealey, T. Modeling acne in vitro. J Invest Dermatol. 1996. Jan; 106(1):176–82.

35. Deplewski, D., Rosenfield, R. L. Role of hormones in pilosebaceous unit development. Endocr Rev, 2000. 21(4): 363–92.

36. Deplewski, D., Rosenfield, R. L. Growth hormone and insulin-like growth factors have different effects on sebaceous cell growth and differentiation. Endocrinology, 1999. 140(9): 4089–94.

37. Smith, T. M., et al. Insulin-like growth factor-1 induces lipid production in human SEB-1 sebocytes via sterol response element-binding protein-1. J Invest Dermatol, 2006. 126(6): 1226–32.

38. Trivedi, N.R., et al. Peroxisome proliferator-activated receptors increase human sebum production. J Invest Dermatol, 2006. 126(9): 2002–9.

39. Zouboulis, C.C., et al. Corticotropin-releasing hormone: An autocrine hormone that promotes lipogenesis in human sebocytes. Proc Natl Acad Sci U S A, 2002. 99(10): 7148–53.

40. Jugeau, S., et al. Induction of toll-like receptors by Propionibacterium acnes. Br J Dermatol, 2005. 153(6): 1105–13.

41. Isard, O., Knol, A. C., Aries, M. F., Nquyen, J. M., Khammari, A., Castex-Rizzi, N., Dreno, B. Propionibacterium acnes activates the IGF-1/IGF-1R system in the epidermis and induces kertinocyte proliferation. J Invest Dermatol, 2011. 131: 59–66.

42. Leyden, J.J., K.J. McGinley, Vowels, B. Propionibacterium acnes colonization in acne and nonacne. Dermatology, 1998. 196(1): 55–58.

43. Jeremy, A. H., Holland, D. B., Roberts, S. G., Thomson, K. F., Cunliffe, W. J. Inflammatory events are involved in acne lesion initiation. J Invest Dermatol. 2003. Jul;121(1): 20–27.

44. Alestas, T., et al. Enzymes involved in the biosynthesis of leukotriene B4 and prostaglandin E2 are active in sebaceous glands. J Mol Med, 2006. 84(1): 75–87.

45. Arican, O., Kurutas, E.B., Sasmaz, S. Oxidative stress in patients with acne vulgaris. Mediators Inflamm, 2005. (6): 380–84.

46. Ottaviani, M., et al. Peroxidated squalene induces the production of inflammatory mediators in HaCaT keratinocytes: A possible role in acne vulgaris. J Invest Dermatol, 2006. 126(11): 2430–37.

47. Fishel, M. A., et al. Hyperinsulinemia provokes synchronous increases in central infl ammation and betaamyloid in normal adults. Arch Neurol, 2005. 62(10): 1539–44.

48. Pou, K. M., et al. Visceral and subcutaneous adipose tissue volumes are cross-sectionally related to markers of inflammation and oxidative stress: The Framingham Heart Study. Circulation, 2007. 116(11): 1234–41.

49. Gilliver, S. C., et al. Androgens modulate the infl ammatory response during acute wound healing. J Cell Sci, 2006. 119(Pt 4): 722–32.

50. Tehrani, R., Dharmalingam, M. Management of premenstrual acne with Cox-2 inhibitors: A placebo controlled study. Indian J Dermatol Venereol Leprol, 2004. 70(6): 345–48.

51. Bagga, D., et al. Differential effects of prostaglandin derived from omega-6 and omega-3 polyunsaturated fatty acids on COX-2 expression and IL-6 secretion. Proc Natl Acad Sci USA, 2003. 100(4): 1751–56.

52. Jump, D. B. The biochemistry of n-3 polyunsaturated fatty acids. J Biol Chem, 2002. 277(11): 8755–58.

53. Downie, M. M., et al. Peroxisome proliferator-activated receptor and farnesoid X receptor ligands differentially regulate sebaceous differentiation in human sebaceous gland organ cultures in vitro. Br J Dermatol, 2004. 151(4): 766–75.

54. Lee, J. Y., et al. Differential modulation of Toll-like receptors by fatty acids; Preferential inhibition by n-3 polyunsaturated fatty acids. J Lipid Res, 2003. 44(3): 479–86.

55. Jarrousse, V., et al. Zinc salts inhibit in vitro Toll-like receptor 2 surface expression by keratinocytes. Eur J Dermatol, 2007. 17(6): 492–96.

56. Maes, M., et al. In humans, serum polyunsaturated fatty acid levels predict the response of proinflammatory cytokines to psychologic stress. Biol Psychiatry, 2000. 47(10): 910–20.

57. Hill, E.G., Johnson, S. B., Holman, R. T. Intensification of essential fatty acid deficiency in the rat by dietary trans fatty acids. J Nutr, 1979. 109(10): 1759–65.

58. Verhulst, A., Janessen, G. Parmentier, G., Eyssen, H. Isomerization of polyunsaturated long chain fatty acids by propionobacteria. System Appl Microbiol, 1987. 9: 12–15.

59. Downing, D.T., et al. Essential fatty acids and acne. J Am Acad Dermatol, 1986. 14(2 Pt 1): 221–25.

60. Makrantonaki, E., Zouboulis, C. C. Testosterone metabolism to 5alpha-dihydrotestosterone and synthesis of sebaceous lipids is regulated by the peroxisome proliferator-activated receptor ligand linolenic acid in human sebocytes. Br J Dermatol, 2007. 156(3): 428–32.

61. Calder, P.C. Dietary modification of inflammation with lipids. Proc Nutr Soc, 2002. 61(3): 345–58.

62. Ferrucci, L., et al. Relationship of plasma polyunsaturated fatty acids to circulating inflammatory markers. J Clin Endocrinol Metab, 2006. 91(2): 439–46.

63. Enig, M. Trans fatty acids in the food supply: A comprehensive report covering 60 years of research. 2nd ed. 1995, Silver Spring, MD: Enig Associates, Inc.

64. Mozaffarian, D., et al. Dietary intake of trans fatty acids and systemic inflammation in women. Am J Clin Nutr, 2004. 79(4): 606–12.

65. Simopoulos, A. P. Essential fatty acids in health and chronic disease. Am J Clin Nutr, 1999. 70(3 Suppl): 560S–69S.

66. Silverberg, N. B., Weinberg, J. M. Rosacea and adult acne: A worldwide epidemic. Cutis, 2001. 68(2): 85.

67. Moran, A., et al. Insulin resistance during puberty: Results from clamp studies in 357 children. Diabetes, 1999. 48(10): 2039–44.

68. Cappel, M., D. Mauger, and D. Thiboutot. Correlation between serum levels of insulin-like growth factor 1, dehydroepiandrosterone sulfate, and dihydrotestosterone and acne lesion counts in adult women. Arch Dermatol, 2005. 141(3): 333–38.

69. Kaymak, Y., et al. Dietary glycemic index and glucose, insulin, insulin-like growth factor-I, insulin-like growth factor binding protein 3, and leptin levels in patients with acne. J Am Acad Dermatol, 2007. 57(5): 819–23.

70. Rosignoli, C., et al. Involvement of the SREBP pathway in the mode of action of androgens in sebaceous glands in vivo. Exp Dermatol, 2003. 12(4): 480–89.

71. Tomlinson, J. W., Finney, J., Gay, C., Hughes, B. A., Hughes, S. V., Stewart, P.M. Impaired glucose tolerance and insulin resistance are associated with increased adipose 11beta-hydroxysteroid dehydrogenase type 1 expression and elevated hepatic 5alpha-reductase activity. Diabetes, 2008. Oct;57(10): 2652–56.

72. Edmondson, S. R., et al. Epidermal homeostasis: The role of the growth hormone and insulin-like growth factor systems. Endocr Rev, 2003. 24(6): 737–64.

73. Cordain, L. Implications for the role of diet in acne. Semin Cutan Med Surg, 2005. 24(2): 84–91.

74. Isard, O., Knol, A. C., Aries, M. F., Nguyen, J. M., Khammari, A., Castex-Rizzi, N., Dreno, B. Propionibacterium acnes activates the IGF-1/IGF-1R system in the epidermis and induces keratinocyte proliferation. Journal of Investigative Dermatology, 2011. 131: 59–66.

75. Brand-Miller, J. C., et al. Physiological validation of the concept of glycemic load in lean young adults. J Nutr, 2003. 133(9): 2728–32.

76. Kaaks, R., et al. Effects of dietary intervention on IGF-I and IGF-binding proteins, and related alterations in sex steroid metabolism: The Diet and Androgens (DIANA) Randomised Trial. Eur J Clin Nutr, 2003. 57(9): 1079–88.

77. Selva, D. M., et al. Monosaccharide-induced lipogenesis regulates the human hepatic sex hormonebinding globulin gene. J Clin Invest, 2007. 117(12): 3979–87.

78. Smith, R. N., et al. The effect of a high-protein, low glycemic-load diet versus a conventional, high glycemic-load diet on biochemical parameters associated with acne vulgaris: A randomized, investigator masked, controlled trial. J Am Acad Dermatol, 2007. 57(2): 247–56.

79. Smith, R. N. et al. A low-glycemic-load diet improves symptoms in acne vulgaris patients: A randomized controlled trial. Am J Clin Nutr, 2007. 86(1): 107–15.

80. Hoyt, G., Hickey, M. S., Cordain, L. Dissociation of the glycaemic and insulinaemic responses to whole and skimmed milk. Br J Nutr, 2005. 93(2): 175–77.

81. Hoppe, C., Mølgaard, C., Dalum, C., Vaag, A.. Michaelsen, K. F. Differential effects of casein versus whey on fasting plasma levels of insulin, IGF-1 and IGF-1/IGFBP-3: Results from a randomized 7-day supplementation study in prepubertal boys. European Journal of Clinical Nutrition, 2009. 63: 1076–83.

82. Adebamowo, C. A., et al. Milk consumption and acne in teenaged boys. J Am Acad Dermatol, 2008. 58(5): 787-93.

83. Adebamowo, C. A., et al. Milk consumption and acne in adolescent girls. Dermatol Online J, 2006. 12(4): 1.

84. Adebamowo, C. A., et al. High school dietary dairy intake and teenage acne. J Am Acad Dermatol, 2005. 52(2): 207–14.

85. Brand-Miller, J. C., et al. The glycemic index of foods infl uences postprandial insulin-like growth factor binding protein responses in lean young subjects. Am J Clin Nutr, 2005. 82(2): 350–54.

86. Gunnell, D., et al. Are diet-prostate cancer associations mediated by the IGF axis? A cross-sectional analysis of diet, IGF-I and IGFBP-3 in healthy middle-aged men. Br J Cancer, 2003. 88(11): 1682–86.

87. Probst-Hensch, N. M., et al. Determinants of circulating insulin-like growth factor I and insulin-like growth factor binding protein 3 concentrations in a cohort of Singapore men and women. Cancer Epidemiol Biomarkers Prev, 2003. 12(8): 739–46.

88. McEwen, B. Protective and damaging effects of stress mediators. New England J Med, 1998. 338: 171–79.

89. Donga, E., van Dijk, M., van Dijk, J. G., Biermasz, N. R., Lammers, G. J., van Kralingen, K. W., Corssmit, E. P., Romijn, J. A. A single night of partial sleep deprivation induces insulin resistance in multiple metabolic pathways in healthy subjects. J Clin Endocrinol Metab, 2010. 95: 2963–68.

90. Chiu, A., Chon, S. Y., Kimball, A. B. The response of skin disease to stress: Changes in the severity of acne vulgaris as affected by examination stress. Arch Dermatol, 2003. 139(7): 897–900.

91. Yosipovitch, G., et al. Study of psychological stress, sebum production and acne vulgaris in adolescents. Acta Derm Venereol, 2007. 87: 135–39.

92. Toyoda, M., Morohashi, M. New aspects in acne infl ammation. Dermatology, 2003. 206(1): 17–23.

93. Joergensen, A., Broedbaek, K., Weimann, A., Semba, R. D., Ferrucci, L., Joergensen, M. B., Poulsen, H. E. Association between urinary excretion of cortisol and markers of oxidatively damaged DNA and RNA in humans. P LoS One, 2011. 6(6): e20795.

94. Dusek, J. A., et al. Genomic counter-stress changes induced by the relaxation response. PLoSONE, 2008. 3(7): e2576.

95. Michaelsson, G., Edqvist, L. E. Erythrocyte glutathione peroxidase activity in acne vulgaris and the effect of selenium and vitamin E treatment. Acta Derm Venereol, 1984. 64(1): 9–14.

96. Ikeno, H., Tochio, T., Tanaka, H., Nakata, S. Decrease in glutathione may be involved in pathogenesis of acne vulgaris. JCosmetDermatol, 2011. Sep;10(3): 240–44.

97. Kurutas, E.B., Arican, O., Sasmaz, S. Superoxide dismutase and myeloperoxidase activities in polymorphonuclear leukocytes in acne vulgaris. Acta Dermatovenerol Alp Panonica Adriat, 2005. 14(2): 39–42.

98. Briganti, S., Picardo, M. Antioxidant activity, lipid peroxidation and skin diseases. What's new. JEADV, 2003. 17: 663–69.

99. Fowlkes, J.L., et al. Matrix metalloproteinases degrade insulin-like growth factor-binding protein-3 indermal fibroblast cultures. J Biol Chem, 1994. 269(41): 25742–46.

100. Arts, I.C., Hollman, P. C. Polyphenols and disease risk in epidemiologic studies. Am J Clin Nutr, 2005. 81(1 Suppl): 317S–25S.

101. Tomey, K. M., et al. Dietary fat subgroups, zinc, and vegetable components are related to urine F2a isoprostane concentration, a measure of oxidative stress, in midlife women. J Nutr, 2007. 137(11): 2412–19.

102. Sakai, M., Oimomi, M., Kasuga, M. Experimental studies on the role of fructose in the development of diabetic complications. Kobe J Med Sci, 2002. 48(5–6): 125–36.

103. Faure, P., et al. Comparison of the effects of zinc alone and zinc associated with selenium and vitamin E on insulin sensitivity and oxidative stress in high-fructose-fed rats. J Trace Elem Med Biol, 2007. 21(2): 113–19.

104. Evans, J. L., et al. Are oxidative stress-activated signaling pathways mediators of insulin resistance and beta-cell dysfunction? Diabetes, 2003. 52(1): 1–8.

105. Basak, P.Y., Gultekin, F., Kilinc, I. The role of the antioxidative defense system in papulopustular acne. J Dermatol, 2001. 28(3): 123–27.

106. Klipstein, F. A., Samloff, I. M. Folate synthesis by intestinal bacteria. Am J Clin Nutr, 1966. Oct;19(4):237–46.

107. Alabi, Z. O., Thomas, K. D., Ogunbona, O., Elegbe, I. A. The effect of antibacterial agents on plasma vitamin C levels. AfrJMedMedSci, 1994. Jun;23(2): 143–46.

108. Walters, B. N., Gubbay, S. S. Tetracycline and benign intracranial hypertension: Report of five cases. Br Med J (Clin Res Ed), 1981. 282 (6257): 12–20.

109. van der Vange, N., van der Berg, H., Kloosterboer, H. J., Haspels, A. A. Effects of seven low-dose combined contraceptives on vitamin B6 status. Contraception, 1989. Sep;40(3): 377–84.

110. Lussana, F., Zighett, M. L., Bucciarelli, P., Cugno, M., Cattaneo, M. Blood levels of honocysteine, folate, vitamin B6 and B12 in women using oral contraceptives compared to non-users. Throm Res, 2003. 112: 37–41.

111. Webb, J. L. Nutritional effects of oral contraceptive use: A review. J Reprod Med, 1980. 25: 150–56.

112. Lippman, S. M., Benner, S. E., Fritsche, H. A. Jr., Lee, J. S., Hong, W. K. The effect of 13-cis-retinoic acid chemoprevention on human serum retinol levels, Cancer Detect Prev, 1998. 22(1): 51–56.

113. Sieving, P. A., Chaudhry, P., Kondo, M., Provenzano, M., Wu, D., Carlson, T. J., Bush, R. A., Thompson, D. A. Inhibition of the visual cycle in vivo by 13-cis retinoic acid protects from light damage and provides a mechanism for night blindness in isotretinoin therapy. Proc Natl Acad Sci USA, 2001. Feb 13;98(4): 1835–40.

114. Welsh, B. M., Smith, A. L., Elder, J. E., Varigos, G. A. Night blindness precipitated by isotretinoin in the setting of hypovitaminosis A. Australas J Dermatol, 1999. Nov;40(4): 208–10.

115. Schulpis, K. H., Georgala, S., Papakonstantinou, E. D., Michas, T., Karikas, G. A. The effect of isotretinoin on biotinidase activity, Skin Pharmacol Appl Skin Physiol, 1999. Jan-Apr;12(1-2): 28–33.

116. Rødland, O., Aksnes, L., Nilsen, A., Morken, T. Serum levels of vitamin D metabolites in isotretinoin-treated acne patients. Acta Derm Venereol, 1992. 72(3): 217–19.

117. Ertugrul, D. T., Karadag, A. S., Tutal, E., Akin, K. O. Therapeutic hotline. Does isotretinoin have effect on vitamin D physiology and bone metabolism in acne patients? Dermatol Ther, 2011. Mar–Apr;24(2): 291–95.

118. Marsden, J. R. Effect of dietary fish oil on hyperlipidaemia due to isotretinoin and etretinate. Hum Toxicol, 1987. May;6(3): 219–22.

119. Georgala, S., Schulpis, K. H., Georgala, C., Michas, T. L-carnitine supplementation in patients with cystic acne on isotretinoin therapy. J Eur Acad Dermatol Venereol, 1999. Nov;13(3): 205–9.

120. Roodsari, M. R., Akbari, M. R., Sarrafi-rad, N., Saeedi, M., Gheisari, M., Kavand, S. The effect of isotretinoin treatment on plasmahomocysteine levels in acne vulgaris. Clin Exp Dermatol, 2010. Aug;35(6): 624–26.

121. Bottiglieri, T., Laundy, M., Crellin, R., Toone, B. K., Carney, M. W., Reynolds, E. H. Homocysteine, folate, methylation and monoamine metabolism in depression. J Neurol Neurosurg Psychiatry, 2000. 69: 228–32.

122. Garg, H. K., Singal, K. C., Arshad, Z. Zinc taste test in pregnant women and its correlation with serum zinc level. Indian J Physol Pharmacol, 1993. 37: 318–22.

123. http://nutrigenomics.ucdavis.edu/?page=Information. Accessed January 10, 2012.

124. Bonafe, M., Barbieri, M., Marchegiani, F. O., Ragno, E., Giampieri, C., Mugianesi, E., Centruelli, M., Franceschi, C., Paolisso, G. Polymorphic variants of IGF-1 receptor and phosphoinositide 3-kinase genes affect IGF-1 plasma levels and human longevity: Cues for an evolutionarily conserved mechanism of life span control. J Clin Endocrinol Metabol, 2003. 88: 3299–304.

125. Ben-Amitai, D., Laron, Z. Effect of insulin-like growth factor-1 deficiency or administration on the occurrence of acne. JEADV, 2011. 25: 950–54.

126. Melnik, B. C. Evidence for acne-promoting effects of milk and other insulinotropic dairy products. Nestle Nutr Workshop Ser Pediatr Program, 2011. 67: 131–45.

127. Trivedi, N. R., Cong, Z., Nelson, A. M., Albert, A. J., Rosamilia, L. L., Sivarajah, S., Gilliland, K. L., Liu, W., Mauger, D. T., Gabbay, R. A., Thiboutot, D. M. Peroxisome proliferator-activated receptors increase human sebum production. Journal of Investigative Dermatology, 2006. 126: 2002–9.

128. Cernuda-Morollón, E., Rodríguez-Pascual, F., Klatt P., Lamas, S., Pérez-Sala, D. PPAR agonists amplify iNOS expression while inhibiting NF-kappaB: Implications for mesangial cell activation by cytokines. JAmSocNephrol, 2002. Sep;13(9): 2223–31.

129. Demerjian, M., Man, M. Q., Choi, E. H., Brown, B. E., Crumrine, D., Chang, S., Mauro, T., Elias, P. M., Feingold, K. R. Topical treatment with thiazolidinediones, activators of peroxisome proliferator-activated receptor-gamma, normalizes epidermal homeostasis in amurine hyperproliferative disease model. Exp Dermatol, 2006. Mar;15(3): 154–60.

130. Gani, O. A. et al. Are fish oil omega-3 long-chain fatty acids and their derivatives peroxisome proliferator-activated receptoragonists? Cardiovascular Diabetology, 2008. 7: 6.

131. Bataille, V., Snieder, H., MacGregor, A. J., Sasieni, P. Spector, T. D.The influence of genetics and environmental factors in the pathogenesis of acne: A twin study of acne in women. J Invest Dermatol, 2002. Dec;119(6): 1317–22.

132. Williams, P. T., Krauss, R. M., Vranizan, K. M., Albers, J. J., Wood, P. D. Effects of weight-loss by exercise and by diet on apolipoproteins A-I and A-II and the particle-size distribution of high-density lipoproteins in men. Metabolism, 1992. Apr;41(4): 441–49.

133. Chan, J. M., Stampfer, M. J., Giovannucci, E., Gann, P. H., Ma, J., Wilinson, P., Hennekens, C. H., Pollak, M. Plasma insulin-like growth factor-1 and prostate cancer risk: A prospective study. Science, 1998. Jan 23;279(5350): 563–66.

134. Sutcliffe, S., et al. Acne and risk of prostate cancer. Int J Cancer, 2007. December 15;121(12): 2688–92.

135. Doyle, S. L., Donohoe, C. L., Lysaght, J., Reynolds, J. V. Visceral obesity, metabolic syndrome, insulin resistance and cancer. Proc Nutr Soc, 2011. Nov 3: 1–9.

136. Kaplan, M. A., Pekkolay, Z., Kucukoner, M., Inal, A., Urakci, Z., Ertugrul, H., Akdogan, R., Firat, U., Yildiz, I., Isikdogan, A. Type 2 diabetes mellitus and prognosis in early stage breast cancer in women. MedOncol, 2011. Nov 15. First published online, 15 November, 2011.

137. Logan, A.C., Treloar, V. The Clear Skin Diet: A Nutritional Plan for Getting Rid of and Avoiding Acne. 2007, Nashville, TN: Cumberland House Publishing Company.

23 Atopic Dermatitis and Diet

Jose M. Saavedra, M.D.

INTRODUCTION

Atopic dermatitis (AD) is the most common chronic disease of the skin, as well as the most common chronic illness of infants. Today it affects about 20% of all infants in developed countries, and is increasing dramatically. Together with allergic rhinitis and asthma, AD is part of the global epidemic of chronic noncommunicable diseases.

AD is strongly linked to food allergies. And while its exact pathophysiologic mechanisms remain to be elucidated, AD is associated with food in its etiology, in its management, and in its potential preventive measures. This chapter reviews the relationship between diet and AD, with focus on pathophysiologic links to food allergies, and the role of diet in treatment and prevention of AD.

DEFINITION AND DIAGNOSIS

Atopic dermatitis is a chronic inflammatory and intensely pruritic skin disease, with characteristic patterns of distribution. It is generally considered a type of eczema, a group of chronic skin conditions, often with genetically determined skin barrier defects. Seborrheic dermatitis, contact dermatitis, nummular eczema, dyshidrotic eczema, and lichen simplex chronicus are all in the eczema family [1]. The terms atopic dermatitis and atopic eczema are often used interchangeably.

The etiology, as well as the nomenclature, of AD has been a source of confusion and ongoing debate. In the early 1900s it was referred to as neurodermatitis, terminology that subsequently lead to its conceptualization as a condition associated with psychologic instability [2]. While the dermatitis (skin inflammation) component has been consistent, the term atopic may incompletely characterize the condition as allergy related, and not fully encompass the pathophysiologic events in the skin of these patients, characterized by loss of barrier function, as will be described here.

There is no universal consensus for the meaning of the term atopy, although it is often used to refer to an inherited tendency to develop allergic conditions, such as asthma, hay fever, and AD (the atopic triad). In some, but not all of these conditions, there is elevated IgE reactivity, as part of the atopic response, pointing to a role for allergens as triggers in this disease [1–3].

DIAGNOSIS

There is no laboratory test that is diagnostic of AD. However, there is some consensus around the recommendation that only the eczema occurring in patients with elevated total serum IgE (> 150 kU/l) and with specific IgE responses to aero- and food-derived allergens should be called atopic dermatitis, whereas the previously called intrinsic eczema should be called nonatopic eczema or nonatopic dermatitis [4]. The great majority of AD patients demonstrate elevated total serum IgE, although up to 30% of these patients have normal total serum IgE and show no allergic sensitization to food or aeroallergens [5].

The diagnosis of AD is based on clinical criteria. Generally speaking, AD is a disease of infancy and early childhood, with more than 95% of cases occurring before five years of age [6], and pruritus is a defining symptom. Infantile AD is characterized by generalized xerosis and erythematous scaly exudative plaques affecting the cheeks, forehead, scalp, and extensor surfaces of the extremities. The diaper area is usually spared. As the disease progresses into childhood, lesions tend to migrate to the flexure areas, particularly the antecubital and popliteal fossae, and the creases of the buttocks and thighs. The clinical criteria for diagnosis, recommended by the American Academy of Dermatology consensus conference on pediatric AD [7] are indicated in Table 23.1. In general pediatric practice, a simplified approach is helpful [8]. An infant with AD can be recognized as having three or more of the following criteria:

- Visible rashes on the flexural areas (elbows, back of knees, front of neck, or eyelids); in infants, the rash may be present on the cheeks or extensor areas of the knees or elbows
- History of rashes on the flexural areas;
- Personal or family history of respiratory allergies (asthma or allergic rhinitis);
- History of dry skin in the past year;
- Onset before two years of age.

AD, particularly when severe, can have significant, and sometimes profound, effects on quality of life. It will disrupt the establishment of normal sleep patterns, behavior, and family relationships. The physiologic and psychological effects of AD not only change the life of the affected child but

---

TABLE 23.1
Universal Criteria for the Diagnosis of Atopic Dermatitis

A. Essential features; must be present and, if complete, are sufficient for diagnosis
1. Pruritus
2. Eczematous changes that are acute, subacute, or chronic:
    a. Typical and age-specific patterns
       (i)   Facial, neck, and extensor involvement in infants and children
       (ii)   Current or prior flexural lesions in adults/any age
       (iii)   Sparing of groin and axillary regions
    b. Chronic or relapsing course

B. Important features that are seen in most cases, adding support to the diagnosis
1. Early age at onset
2. Atopy (IgE reactivity)
3. Xerosis

C. Associated features
Clinical associations; help in suggesting the diagnosis of AD but are too nonspecific to be used for defining or detecting AD for research and epidemiologic studies
1. Keratosis pilaris/Ichthyosis/Palmar hyperlinearity
2. Atypical vascular responses
3. Perifollicular accentuation/Lichenification/Prurigo
4. Ocular/periorbital changes
5. Perioral/periauricular lesions

D. Exclusions
Firm diagnosis of AD depends on excluding conditions such as scabies, allergic contact dermatitis, seborrheic dermatitis, cutaneous lymphoma, ichthyoses, psoriasis, and other primary disease entities.

Source: Adapted from [7].

also affect the physical, social, and emotional functioning of parents [9,10]. Infants who develop AD are at increased risk for mental health, emotional, and behavioral problems up to at least 10 years of age, even if the AD resolves by two years of age. The strength of this association increases with the length of persistence of signs and symptoms of AD [11].

INCIDENCE

AD is not only the most common skin disorder, but also the most common chronic disease of early life, affecting up to 1:5 of all infants. AD affects 10% to 20% of children and approximately 1% to 3% of adults [12]. It is primarily a disease of infancy, with more than 60% to 80% of AD cases presenting before the first year of life, and in 95% of cases occurs before age five years [6]. Patients with severe AD, particularly those with early sensitization to allergens typically have persistent illness, which may last through adulthood. AD occurs in all ethnicities [13]. A recent prospective study showed a cumulative incidence of 17% by six months of age, with an increased risk in African American and Asian infants, and males vs. females [14].

Another lens by which to view AD is the financial burden it places on patients, their families, and society as a whole. Healthcare costs of AD to the health system in the United States has been estimated to be between $1 billion [15], up to $3.8 billion [16], with few studies measuring the indirect cost of disease.

The global prevalence of AD is higher in developed countries, and is increasing dramatically, similar to that of other atopic disorders, particularly asthma [7,17]. Globally, in developed countries, approximately 25% to 30% of the population suffers from AD, food allergy, or allergic rhinitis. Data from the Centers for Disease Control and Prevention National Health Information survey confirm a rise in all atopic diseases in North America. AD prevalence increased from 7% in 1998 to 10% in 2006, and the reported prevalence of asthma has gone from 3% in 1990 to 7.7% in 2007 [18]. More recently, we have witnessed an even more dramatic rise in GI allergic disorders. These eosinophilic gastrointestinal disorders share common pathophysiologic mechanisms and linkages to the atopic triad of AD, allergic rhinitis, and asthma [19], and to IgE mediated food allergies [20]. Eosinophilic esophagitis has increased in some series from 18-fold to 35-fold rise over the last 10 years [21,22].

The reason for the higher prevalence of AD, allergic rhinitis, asthma, and food allergies in developed countries is unclear. The hygiene hypothesis was first proposed by Strachan in 1989 [23]. It suggested that early childhood infections "protected" children from development of allergic diseases. This explained the higher prevalence of allergies in urban areas compared to rural. In addition, its frequency is increased in patients who immigrate to developed countries from underdeveloped countries [24]. Reinforcing the hypothesis were subsequent observations that showed a higher incidence in Western countries, in urban rather than rural areas, and also linking antibiotic use in the first years of life with significant increases of allergic disease, including AD [25]. The concept, which has increasingly gathered momentum, suggests that increasingly hygienic measures, including food cleanliness and pasteurization lead to a decreased "microbial experience" in early life, which may prevent maturation of the child's developing immune system, thereby skewing immune response toward exaggerated Th2 immune responses and allergy development [26,27].

PATHOGENESIS

The pathogenesis of AD is still poorly understood, and undoubtedly complex, involving genetic factors, inherited and acquired skin barrier defects, and immune dysfunction [28]. A family history of allergic disorders strongly correlates with risk of AD [29] and high concordance has been documented in monozygotic twin pairs [30]. The lesions observed in AD result in significant part from an imbalance between Th2 and Th1 lymphocytes. Acute AD lesions exhibit reduced expression of IL-12 and increased production of IL-10, which increases Th2 activity and suppresses Th1 activity.

This mechanism results in cytokine production of IL-4, -5, -12, and -13, which causes an increase in IgE and a decrease in interferon (IFN)-g levels [31]. Thus, patients with acute AD have a cutaneous immunodeficiency that makes them more susceptible to infection, such as herpes simplex virus and molluscum. In addition, epidermal Langerhans cells in atopic skin have several high-affinity IgE receptors that, when triggered, further promote the IgE-mediated hypersensitivity and inflammatory responses seen in AD. Genetic polymorphisms in AD patients have been associated with chromosome 5q22-23, which contains a cluster of T helper type 2 (Th2) cytokine genes (IL-4 and IL-13). Those genes play a significant role in IgE production and allergic sensitization. Th1/Th2 cell dysregulation, IgE production, mast cell hyperactivity, and dendritic cell signaling abnormalities have been described in the pathogenesis of atopic dermatitis [32,33].

More recently, gene mutations were associated with deficiencies in filaggrin, a protein essential to the normal barrier function of the skin, suggesting a role of skin barrier defects in the pathogenesis of AD [34]. Filaggrin is essential to the formation of the cornified envelope, which is the basis of normal barrier function in the skin. Filaggrin deficiency contributes to physical barrier defects in AD, predisposes patients to increased trans-epidermal water loss, infections, and inflammation, as well as exposure of cutaneous immune cells to allergens [35,36]. A defective epidermal barrier in AD could potentially lead to epicutaneous delivery of both food and aeroallergens that induces asthma and allergic rhinitis, explaining the predisposition of patients with AD to the later development of rhinitis and asthma, what is known as the "atopic march" discussed in this chapter.

Most food-related allergic sensitization in infants occurs via the oral route, and this leads to a host of allergic conditions associated with food proteins, including skin, gastrointestinal, and respiratory manifestations. However, epicutaneous sensitization is also possible. For example, children who have never been exposed to peanut during the prenatal period and with negative tests for peanut-specific IgE in the cord blood were documented to have been sensitized to peanut allergens as a result of application of skin preparations containing peanut oil on inflamed skin [37]. The observations regarding skin barrier disruption have led many investigators to conclude that this epidermal disruption is the primary cause of AD; and that in fact, the breakdown of the skin barrier is what drives food allergic sensitization and allergic response in AD, rather than the other way around. Clearly, the relationship to antigen in early life in the sequence of events in AD is yet to be fully understood.

In summary, deficiencies in innate and adaptive immunity based on a genetic predisposition result in skin barrier dysfunction with hyper-reactivity to environmental stimuli and susceptibility to skin infections, which in turn influence the course and severity of AD [38]. Regardless, whether primarily or secondarily, allergens—and particularly food allergens—contribute to the development of the perpetuation of the allergic component of the disease in the majority of patients.

FOOD ALLERGY AND ATOPIC DERMATITIS

Since AD and food allergy are highly associated, patients with AD exhibit a much higher rate of food allergy than the general population. Elevated titers of IgE to specific allergens can be found in up to 85% of patients with AD [39]. The incidence of food allergy documented in patients with AD, using double-blind, placebo-controlled food challenges (DBPCFC), ranges from 33 to 63% [3]. Thus, roughly one-third to one-half of patients with moderate to severe AD have food allergies. Younger children with more severe cases of AD show higher rates.

FOOD ALLERGENS IN ATOPIC DERMATITIS

Food allergens are defined as those specific components of food or ingredients within food (typically proteins, but sometimes also chemical haptens) that are recognized by allergen-specific immune cells and elicit specific immunologic reactions resulting in allergic manifestations, including AD, rhinitis, asthma, gastrointestinal allergy (eosiniphilic esophagitis), urticaria (hives), and anaphylaxis. In some cases, food allergens may share structural or sequence similarity with other allergens, including aeroallergens; thus, the adverse reaction may be caused by cross-reaction to the other allergen [40].

The number of foods implicated in food allergy is rather limited, and the frequency as an allergen also varies somewhat with age. In fact, milk, soy, egg, wheat, peanut, tree nuts, and fish account for more than 90% of all documented food allergies. Cow's milk proteins are universally found to be the most common food allergen in infants who develop symptoms in the first year of life. Table 23.2 lists the most commonly implicated allergenic foods [41].

The documentation of specific food allergens as a causative factor in AD has gradually and significantly increased. Studies showing avoidance of allergenic foods leading to AD improvement [42–45], or development of symptoms with allergen intake [46–49], have increasingly reinforced this relationship. Recent large prospective studies are better defining the risk of AD in relation to early sensitization to food allergens [50]. At one year of age, almost 9.8% of infants are sensitized to at least one food allergen, while only 2.3% are sensitized to aeroallergens. And this early sensitization (at 12 months) was associated with a higher prevalence of atopic disease at six years, with AD present in 10.6% of the children, allergic rhinitis in 8.1%, and asthma in 3.4%. Even though two-thirds of the children with early sensitizations in this study did not develop an atopic disease, they had a twofold to fourfold increased risk of doing so in comparison to children without sensitization. As opposed to infants and young children, in adults, food hypersensitivity plays a very minor role in AD [51,52]. Of note, in older children and adults, birch pollen sensitization with cross-reacting foods, such as apple (with its peel), can lead to exacerbation of AD or trigger responses in food challenges [53].

Milk, soy, and egg, by far the most common food sensitizing proteins in infants, are strongly associated with development of AD up to six years of age. Twenty-two percent of children with early egg allergen sensitization and 23% of those with early milk allergen sensitization develop AD at the age of six. Early aeroallergen sensitization occurs with significant lower frequency. When it

---

TABLE 23.2

Most Common Allergenic Foods by Age

Infants

Cow's milk

Egg

Wheat

Soy

Children (2–10 Years)

Cow's milk

Egg

Peanut

Tree nuts

Fish

Shellfish

Sesame

Kiwi fruit

Adolescents and Young Adults

Peanut

Tree nuts

Fish

Shellfish

Sesame

Source: Adapted from [41].

---

does, it correlates even more strongly than food allergen sensitization with AD, allergic rhinitis, and asthma by age six [50].

Allergies to multiple foods are not uncommon in infants with AD. In a study of infants between three and 18 months of age, 60% were allergic to a single food, 28% were allergic to two foods, 8% were allergic to three foods, and 4% were allergic to four foods. Milk, peanut, and egg were the most likely to produce positive food challenges in this study [54].

Adding to the causative relation of food allergens to AD are studies in breast-fed infants with maternal dietary avoidance of allergens, which suggest a varying level of protection from AD [55–57]. More recently, a number of studies have shown that the risk of development of AD can be significantly reduced in infants with a family history of allergy by utilizing specific hydrolyzed cow's milk protein formulas instead of intact cow's milk protein infant formulas [58,59]. These studies are the strongest evidence for the potential for dietary intervention for the prevention of AD in infants who do not exclusively breast-feed, discussed here.

PATTERNS OF CLINICAL REACTIONS TO FOOD IN ATOPIC DERMATITIS

AD associated to IgE mediated food allergy is most common in infants. Nonatopic dermatitis (non-IgE mediated), including irritant or contact dermatitis, with all the clinical features of AD, is more common in preschool children and adults. Studies have shown a prevalence of 45% to 64% in older children [60,61]. Nonatopic children with eczema have been reported to have a lower risk of developing asthma than atopic children with eczema.

The best data regarding allergic responses to food in patients diagnosed with AD comes from oral food challenge studies. About 70% of patients with AD in challenge studies will demonstrate skin reactions. These include pruritic, morbilliform, or macular eruptions, in areas typically common in AD (head, neck, and creases). Gastrointestinal and respiratory symptoms occur less frequently, 50% and 45%, respectively [51]. While less common, eczematous-delayed reactions can occur on food challenges six to 48 hours later, suggesting a non-IgE–mediated skin reaction [62,63].

In formal food challenge testing, acute IgE-mediated reactions can occur. However, these cases are significantly less common with normal dietary exposure to allergens, potentially from down-regulation from repeated exposures, in a more dilute and less acute post-fasting state that is used in food challenge tests [51].

NATURAL HISTORY OF FOOD ALLERGY IN ATOPIC DERMATITIS

Most children with IgE mediated food allergies (including those with AD), particularly to cow's milk and egg, will develop tolerance by late childhood and "outgrow" their allergy symptoms; allergies to peanut, sesame, and tree nuts are more persistent, with less than 20% developing tolerance [64]. Thus, in adults, cow's milk and egg allergies are uncommon, and allergies to peanuts, tree nuts, fish, and shellfish predominate. A high initial level of allergen-specific IgE (sIgE) against a food is associated with a lower rate of resolution of clinical allergy over time [40].

In children, a drop in IgE levels is often a marker for the onset of tolerance to the food allergens. However, in adult onset of allergy, food allergies may persist despite a drop in sIgE levels. AD resolution is considered a useful marker for the onset of tolerance to food allergens [40]. Cow's milk protein allergy (CMPA) is of particular interest, in that virtually all infants who develop CMPA will do so in the first year of life, and clinical tolerance will develop in about 80% by age five years. More recent studies suggest these rates of clinical tolerance may be decreasing [40,65].

DIAGNOSIS OF FOOD ALLERGIES IN ATOPIC DERMATITIS

While the immediate connection between food ingestion and AD may not be readily apparent, food allergy should be suspected in infants and young children diagnosed with moderate to severe AD.

Children less than five years of age with moderate to severe AD should be considered for allergy to milk, egg, peanut, wheat, and soy, particularly if the child has persistent AD in spite of optimized management and topical therapy, or a reliable history of an immediate reaction after ingestion of a specific food [40].

The criteria and tools for diagnosis of food allergy have been recently set out by an Expert Panel from National Institute of Allergy and Infectious Disease (NIAID) and the National Institutes of Health (NIH)[40]. Aside from adequate medical history and physical examination, the panel concluded that skin prick tests, serum IgE, and atopy patch tests are useful adjuvants, but not individually diagnostic of food allergy. It suggested that elimination of one, or a few, specific foods from the diet may be useful in the diagnosis of food allergy, especially in identifying foods responsible for some non-IgE–mediated food allergic disorders, particularly GI allergic conditions, but cautioned against prolonged and complicated elimination diets which can lead to nutrient deficiencies. Finally, it recommends using oral food challenges for diagnosis—with the double-blind, placebo-controlled food challenge considered as the "gold standard." The single-blind and open food challenge may be considered diagnostic in the clinical setting when the food challenge elicits no symptoms (i.e., negative challenge), or when there are objective symptoms (i.e., positive challenge) that correlate with medical history and are supported by laboratory tests.

DIET IN THE TREATMENT OF ATOPIC DERMATITIS

Standard management of AD is directed principally to diminishing pruritus and improving the skin barrier, with emollients, topical anti-inflammatory medications, antibiotics, and avoidance of environmental triggers. For new patients, or flares of disease, the objectives usually include an induction phase—often relying on topical steroids, a maintenance phase, including emollients, topical steroids, and occasionally topical calcineurin inhibitors, and ultraviolet (UV) light [2].

The only currently available treatment for patients with AD and food allergy, whether IgE or non-IgE mediated, is a strict dietary avoidance of the causative food. As mentioned earlier, prolonged dietary avoidance should only be prescribed to patients with a well-documented diagnosis of food hypersensitivity.

For infants who have developed AD and are exclusively breast-fed, there is limited evidence that maternal avoidance diets reduce severity or eliminate AD signs and symptoms, compared to those of mothers following nonexclusionary diets [57]. For infants who receive infant formulas during their first six months, and have documented food allergy, cow's milk proteins being the most common offender, exclusion of allergens can be most easily accomplished with the use of hypoallergenic infant formulas. Currently, casein based, extensively hydrolyzed formulas (with approximate median molecular weight of casein peptides of 450 Daltons) are the most common approach. A subset of infants may not fully respond to these formulas, and this has led to an increased use of amino acid–based infant formulas.

After weaning foods have been introduced, the management of food allergic manifestations, including AD, becomes more complicated, since infant formula (exclusively, or in combination with breast-feeding) is then no longer the sole source of nutrition. In severe cases, particularly those with multiple food allergies, a small number of infants require continuation of extensively hydrolyzed formulas or amino acid–based formulas as an exclusive source of nutrition, or as a major part of their diet. Most of these formulas are nutritionally designed to meet this purpose. In these infants, the goal is to reintroduce the offending foods in hope that with time they become increasingly tolerant. Most children will likely outgrow food allergies to milk, egg, soy, and wheat in the first two to three years. Food allergies to peanut, tree nuts, fish, and crustacean shellfish take longer and are less likely to be outgrown. In those with particularly severe symptoms, follow-up testing may be helpful, and the results can guide decision making regarding whether it is safe to reintroduce the allergenic food into the diet. Unfortunately, there is no consensus on the timing for retesting or food reintroduction. Whether testing is done annually or at other intervals depends on the food in question, the age of the child, and the intervening clinical history [40].

The avoidance diet needs to be thorough and carefully defined. Avoidance of other potential allergens than those identified in the diagnosis has not been shown to reduce the severity or accelerate resolution of food allergy in unselected cases of related AD [40,66]. The family and the patient must be taught how to read food labels to avoid potential sources of allergen contamination. In addition, patients and/or their parents need to be instructed to treat a potential reaction after accidental ingestion, and need to be equipped with an emergency treatment kit for anaphylaxis (antihistamines and self-injectable epinephrine) if there is a risk for systemic reaction. To date, treatment of food allergy by food-specific immunotherapy has not yet been proven to be safe and effective in well-designed trials, although oral desensitization trials are currently ongoing.

Nutritional advice needs to be thorough and complete, as deficiencies are not uncommon in children on significantly restrictive diets [67]. Children with two or more specific food allergies, following avoidance diets, have been documented to have lower height-for-age. Those with cow's milk allergy or multiple food allergies were found to consume lower then recommended dietary calcium and vitamin D [68]. Adequate supplementation should be considered in these situations.

DIET IN THE PREVENTION OF ATOPIC DERMATITIS

Given the rising incidence and worldwide distribution of the disease, the primary prevention of AD continues to be an important but elusive goal.

MATERNAL DIET IN PREGNANCY AND LACTATION

Although there are obvious methodological limitations to studying fetal immune systems, two large birth cohort studies have shown no measurable specific food IgE in cord blood, even in those children who subsequently developed clinical or immunologic food sensitization [37,69]. Thus, there is little support for the hypothesis that allergic sensitization can occur in utero [70]. There is insufficient evidence that maternal diet during pregnancy or lactation affects the development or clinical course of food allergy. Most consensus statements today do not recommend restricting maternal diet during pregnancy or lactation as a strategy for preventing the development or clinical course of AD or food allergies in general [40].

Breast-Feeding

The evidence for the preventive role of exclusive breast-feeding in allergic conditions (especially for the first six months of age) has been equivocal. Positive studies [71,72] have been countered by negative ones [57,73]. These results may, in part, be related to the populations studied and the methodologies applied. Many are retrospective, or done in general populations—rather than in those at higher allergic risk, and the specific infant formulas used in the nonexclusively breast-fed infants are not specified.

However, in the largest, well-designed cohort study of infants with a positive family history of allergy, who were part of an interventional cohort examining the effect of breast-feeding and specific infant formulas, exclusive breast-feeding through four months of age significantly reduced cow's milk sensitization and AD by approximately 50% [74]. A more recent report on the study of this patient cohort, of close to 4000 infants, documented that exclusive breast-feeding was not associated with risk reduction of AD in infants in the observational subgroup. However, in the group participating in a randomized prospective intervention, comparing it to specific infant formulas, breast-feeding showed a significant protective effect (approximately 40% risk reduction) on AD, up to three years of age, when compared with conventional intact cow's milk protein formulas. The study's authors concluded that observational studies might not be able to effectively control for selection bias and reverse causation and that exclusive breast-feeding is AD protective when compared with conventional intact cow's milk protein formulas. The findings did not apply to hydrolyzed protein formulas [75].

Independent of the potential benefits of breast-feeding on AD, due to its multiple positive effects on child and maternal health, it is recommended that all infants, including those with a family history of atopic disease, be exclusively breast-fed until four to six months of age, unless breast-feeding is contraindicated for medical reasons.

INFANT FORMULAS AND ATOPIC DERMATITIS

Today, standardized and well-regulated infant formulas are the only appropriate nutritional alternative for infants who are not exclusively breast-fed in the first year of life. Most AD occurs in the first year of life, and is associated with early allergen sensitization, mostly to cow's milk protein formulas, and the vast majority of infant formulas, which are the only source of proteins outside breast milk, are made with cow's milk. Thus, the potential for prevention by modifying intact cow's milk protein formulas to reduce their allergenicity is significant. In fact, given these factors, infant formula choice may be the only significant risk-reduction strategy today to minimize AD risk in infants.

Routinely used cow's milk protein based infant formulas are nutritionally designed for healthy term infants through the first year of life. Two types of routine formulas are commercially available: intact cow's milk protein formulas, containing intact bovine casein and whey fractions (with a median molecular weight of 10,000 Daltons), and partially hydrolyzed formulas made with 100% whey proteins (hydrolyzed to peptides of a median molecular weight of 1000 Daltons). In addition, formulas with extensively hydrolyzed 100% casein proteins are also commercially available (with a median molecular weight of 500 Daltons). These extensively hydrolyzed formulas, generally classified as therapeutic formulas, are designed for the dietary management of infants with documented cow's milk protein allergies and digestive disorders. They have significantly less desirable taste and higher cost than intact protein and partially hydrolyzed formulas. Nevertheless, they can support adequate growth of infants and have also been studied in trials addressing prevention of AD.

A number of studies over the last two decades have examined the potential of hydrolyzed formulas for reducing the risk of AD and other allergies. A systematic review by Hays [76], and two meta-analyses [77,78] concluded that both extensively hydrolyzed, 100% casein formulas and 100% partially hydrolyzed whey formulas are appropriate alternatives to breast milk for allergy prevention, and specifically AD, in infants with a family history of allergy. The degree of reduction in the risk of developing any atopic manifestation has varied in these trials, ranging between 32 to 88%. Most recently, an additional meta-analysis [58] concluded that a reduction of approximately 50% risk of AD was attained, regardless of study design, infant population, follow-up time, or study location, with the use of a 100% whey based partially hydrolyzed routine infant formula, compared to intact casein-whey based infant formulas.

The largest study assessing the effect of these hydrolyzed formulas, the German Infant Nutrition Intervention (GINI) study, documented a preventive effect of extensively hydrolyzed casein and partially hydrolyzed whey formulas through six years of age. Children with a family history of allergy had a twofold higher risk of eczema than children without a familial predisposition. The results clearly show that use of these specific hydrolyzed formulas compensated for the enhanced risk of AD due to familial predisposition [59].

The American Academy of Allergy, Asthma, and Immunology, in its recommendations to parents, advocates exclusive breast-feeding for the first four to six months of age, and if not possible, use of an extensively hydrolyzed casein formula, or a partially hydrolyzed whey formula instead of cow's milk or soy formulas [79].

The Expert Panel convened by NIAID, in its recent guidelines stated that the evidence indicates that extensively and partially hydrolyzed infant formulas reduce the development of food allergy in infants at risk and that "exclusive use of extensively or partially hydrolyzed infant formulas be considered for infants who are not exclusively breast-fed and are at risk for developing atopic disease."

Because extensively hydrolyzed infant formulas have a less desirable taste, and are more costly, the Expert Panel added, "Cost or availability of extensively hydrolyzed infant formulas may be weighed as prohibitive factors." In addition, the panel concluded that it does not recommend using soy infant formula instead of cow's milk infant formula as a strategy for preventing the development of food allergy or for modifying its clinical course in at-risk infants [40].

In summary, specific infant formulas made with 100% casein extensively hydrolyzed, or 100% whey partially hydrolyzed can significantly reduce the risk of AD in infants, particularly those with a family history of allergy, when compared to infant formulas made with intact cow casein and whey proteins. The reduction of risk reported is consistent with the degree of risk reduction expected, given the fact that 30–50% of patients with AD are typically sensitized to cow's milk proteins. Given the rising incidence of AD and inadequate means to predict individual risk, the use of partially hydrolyzed whey protein formulas in the general population of infants who are not exclusively breast-fed has been proposed [58].

INTRODUCTION OF SOLID FOODS

Introduction of weaning foods to breast-fed or formula-fed infants varies tremendously by geographic area and cultural and ethnic background. In developed countries, recommendations have changed significantly over the years from extremely delayed introduction (until after one year) in the 1920s, to the first three months in the 1950s [80], to around four to six months in the 1980s [81]. The increased awareness of food allergies in the 1990s led to increasingly delayed introduction recommendations—such as delaying introduction of cow's milk until after one year, and egg and nuts until after two years of age, for infants with a family history of allergy [82]. But in fact, there are no data to support these recommendations. In fact, delaying introduction may increase risk of allergy. As an example, a study specifically assessing the timing of introduction of egg and risk of egg allergy showed that those introduced to egg after 10 months of age were more likely to be egg allergic at one year than those introduced to egg at four to six months, even after controlling for family and personal history of allergy [83]. Large prospective cohort studies have now shown that delaying introduction of potentially allergenic foods is not beneficial and may actually increase risk of AD. Delaying introduction of dairy foods beyond six months and of other foods beyond three to four months was found to increase the risk of AD [84,85]. The GINI study, which followed more than 4000 infants through six years of age, found no evidence that delayed introduction of solids beyond the fourth month of life, or of most potentially allergenic solids beyond the sixth month of life, prevented AD [86].

The guidelines from the NIAID Expert Panel recommend that the introduction of solid foods should not be delayed beyond four to six months of age. Potentially allergenic foods may be introduced at this time as well. While the data for mechanisms to explain this are not yet strong, some have suggested that delayed introduction of allergenic foods may actually prevent the development of normal oral tolerance that occurs when foods are introduced, leading to the concept of a window of opportunity for development of tolerance to potential allergens in early infancy—not before three to four months of age, and not after 10–12 months of age [87].

PROBIOTICS

Probiotics are generally defined as live microorganisms, added to the diet, which may confer a benefit to the host. Various species of lactobacilli and bifidobacteria have been studied for their potential benefits. Over the last two decades, and in part as a response to the hygiene hypothesis, the idea of increasing or reintroducing a richer microbial experience, particularly in developed areas of the world, has bolstered the notion that probiotics could be helpful in atopic disorders.

Intestinal microbes (gut microbiota) are an essential factor in the development of the host immune response. The intestine of a newborn is essentially sterile. During the birthing process, and during the first few days of life, the gut is inoculated with bacteria. Children born vaginally are this way exposed very early to maternal flora. The microflora develops rapidly after birth and is markedly dependent on genetic factors, mode of delivery (vaginal vs. C section), the mother's flora, type of feeding, and early environmental surroundings.

The fact that approximately 80% of all immunologically active cells of the body are in the gut associated lymphoid tissue (GALT) is an affirmation of the importance of microbe—gut immune system interaction. It is now clear that normal microbial flora is necessary for the development of gut associated lymphoid tissue. Thus, gut luminal microbes are responsible for mucosal immune system development in healthy infants. There is now abundant evidence that signaling through specific receptors, particularly toll-like receptors, intestinal bacteria affect epithelium cell function, which determines T-cell differentiation and antibody responses to T-cell–dependent antigens, regulating immune gut response. Colonization is thus apparently responsible for IgA responses to luminal antigens. Secretory IgA is amongst the most important component of antibody response to gut lumen protein, including food, and pathogen antigens. Colonization also indices modulation of the ratio of T helper type 2 (Th2—pro allergic) to T helper type 1 (Th1—suppressive) responses, which could decrease the chances for allergic disease [88].

Lower counts of bifidobacteria have been reported in atopic compared to nonatopic children preceding allergen sensitization, and bifidobacteria are hypothesized to more effectively promote tolerance to nonbacterial antigens, primarily by inhibiting the development of a Th2 (pro-allergic) type response. Some bifidobacteria and lactobacilli given orally may enhance the production of a balanced T helper cell response, and stimulate production of IL-10 and transforming growth factor-β, both of which have a role in the development of immunologic tolerance to antigens and can decrease allergic type immune responses [89,90].

In a small study, infants with atopic dermatitis who received hydrolyzed whey formula supplemented with *L. rhamnosus* (GG) showed greater clinical improvement than those who received the hydrolyzed formula alone. They also excreted less TNF-alpha and alpha-1-antitrypsin in their stool, suggesting that the probiotics decreased gut inflammation [91]. Atopic infants, treated with extensively hydrolyzed whey-based formula with *L. rhamnosus* (GG) or *B. lactis* showed greater improvement in severity of skin manifestations than with hydrolysate formula alone. The probiotic-supplemented group also demonstrated a reduction in serum soluble CD4 (a marker of T-cell activation) and an increase in serum TGF-β 1 (involved in suppressing the inflammatory response via IgA production and oral tolerance induction) [92]. These studies suggest that regular probiotic supplementation may stabilize intestinal barrier function, and play a role in modulating allergic responses leading to a decreased severity of atopic symptoms, particularly atopic dermatitis associated with cow's milk protein [88].

Feeding probiotics to pregnant mothers and newborn infants resulted in significantly reduced AD at two years (23% in intervention group versus 46% in placebo group). This protective effect was also seen at a four-year follow-up study [93]. While these and other results [94,95] are promising, additional work may be necessary to better define the specific species, timing, and duration of probiotic use for the management of AD [96].

CONCLUSIONS AND CLINICAL SUMMARY

Atopic Dermatitis and Diet

Atopic dermatitis affects about 20% of infants in developed countries, and its prevalence is increasing globally. It is a chronic and intensely pruritic skin inflammation with characteristic patterns of distribution, and the diagnosis is based on specific clinical criteria. There are no specific confirmatory diagnostic tests for AD. While it may occur or persist into adulthood, it is primarily a disease of infancy; and can have profound effects on quality of life of the infant and child, as well as on the physical, social, and emotional function of parents and the entire family.

The pathophysiology of AD has just begun to be unraveled. Deficiencies in innate and adaptive immunity associated with genetic predisposition result in skin barrier dysfunction, with heightened immune reactivity to environmental stimuli, including food proteins, which influence the development, course, and severity of the disease. The reasons for the higher prevalence of AD, allergic rhinitis, asthma, and food allergies in developed countries are unclear.

AD and food allergens are inextricably bound. The great majority of patients with AD have elevated levels of IgE to specific food proteins; and using double-blind, placebo-controlled food challenges (the gold standard for diagnosis of food allergies), up to two-thirds of patients with AD will be diagnosed with food allergy. Ninety percent of food allergies can be accounted for by a small number of allergens: milk, soy, egg, wheat, peanut, tree nuts, and fish. Although most food allergies are "outgrown" in late childhood, the occurrence of AD predisposes individuals to allergic rhinitis, and asthma, a phenomenon called the atopic march.

Treatment

The standard treatment of AD is directed principally to diminishing pruritus and improving the skin barrier with topical and systemic medications. The only currently available treatment for patients with AD associated with food allergens is strict dietary avoidance of the causative food. In infants, cow's milk proteins are the most common offender, and the use of extensively hydrolyzed casein infant formulas, or in resistant cases, amino acid–based formulas, are effective. For infants and children on table foods, the avoidance diet needs to be thorough and carefully defined, based on the specific allergenic foods identified. The family and the patient must be taught how to read food labels to avoid potential sources of allergen contamination. Nutritional counseling is often necessary to avoid unnecessary restrictions as well as nutritional deficiencies.

Prevention

Breast-feeding has preventive potential on the development of AD. While some studies are equivocal, large cohort studies demonstrate that exclusive breast-feeding for the first four months of age can reduce the risk of AD, when compared to infants feeding intact cow's milk protein formulas, particularly when there is a family history of allergy.

Most AD occurs in infancy, and most infant formulas are made with cow's milk. Thus, cow's milk is the most common allergenic food in this age group. Specific infant formulas—made with 100% casein extensively—hydrolyzed, or 100% whey partially hydrolyzed, can significantly reduce the risk of AD in infants, particularly those with a family history of allergy, when compared to infant formulas made with intact cow casein and whey proteins. Given the rising incidence of atopic disease and inadequate means to predict individual risk, the use of specific and cost-effective hydrolyzed protein formulas in the general population of infants who are not exclusively breast-fed should be considered a practical and potentially effective public health measure.

Previously, the delayed introduction of other potentially allergenic foods in infant diets was an approach to allergy prevention. There is no evidence that this is effective. In fact, delaying introduction of potential allergens beyond a year of age may actually increase risk of atopic manifestations in susceptible individuals. The dietary use of probiotics as a potential prophylactic and therapeutic measure is promising, but additional confirmatory studies will be necessary for clear recommendations.

REFERENCES

1. U.S. Department of Health and Human Services and National Institutes of Health. Atopic dermatitis (a type of eczema). 2003. NIH Publication No. 03–4272.
2. Simpson EL, Hanifin JM. Atopic dermatitis. Med Clin North Am 2006;90:149–67.
3. Caubet JC, Eigenmann PA. Allergic triggers in atopic dermatitis. Immunol Allergy Clin North Am 2010;30:289–307.

4. Johansson SG, Bieber T, Dahl R et al. Revised nomenclature for allergy for global use: Report of the Nomenclature Review Committee of the World Allergy Organization, October 2003. J Allergy Clin Immunol 2004;113:832–6.

5. Schmid-Grendelmeier P, Simon D, Simon HU, Akdis CA, Wuthrich B. Epidemiology, clinical features, and immunology of the "intrinsic" (non-IgE-mediated) type of atopic dermatitis (constitutional dermatitis). Allergy 2001;56:841–9.

6. Kay J, Gawkrodger DJ, Mortimer MJ, Jaron AG. The prevalence of childhood atopic eczema in a general population. J Am Acad Dermatol 1994;30:35–9.

7. Eichenfield LF, Hanifin JM, Luger TA, Stevens SR, Pride HB. Consensus conference on pediatric atopic dermatitis. J Am Acad Dermatol 2003;49:1088–95.

8. Williams HC, Burney PG, Strachan D, Hay RJ. The U.K. Working Party's Diagnostic Criteria for Atopic Dermatitis. II. Observer variation of clinical diagnosis and signs of atopic dermatitis. Br J Dermatol 1994;131:397–405.

9. Chamlin SL, Frieden IJ, Williams ML, Chren MM. Effects of atopic dermatitis on young American children and their families. Pediatrics 2004;114:607–11.

10. Chamlin SL, Chren MM. Quality-of-life outcomes and measurement in childhood atopic dermatitis. Immunol Allergy Clin North Am 2010;30:281–8.

11. Schmitt J, Apfelbacher C, Chen CM et al. Infant-onset eczema in relation to mental health problems at age 10 years: Results from a prospective birth cohort study (German Infant Nutrition Intervention plus). J Allergy Clin Immunol 2010;125:404–10.

12. Schultz LF. Epidemiology of atopic dermatitis. Immunol Allergy Clin North Am 2002;22:1–24.

13. Horii KA, Simon SD, Liu DY, Sharma V. Atopic dermatitis in children in the United States, 1997–2004: visit trends, patient and provider characteristics, and prescribing patterns. Pediatrics 2007;120:e527–e534.

14. Moore MM, Rifas-Shiman SL, Rich-Edwards JW et al. Perinatal predictors of atopic dermatitis occurring in the first six months of life. Pediatrics 2004;113:468–74.

15. Carroll CL, Balkrishnan R, Feldman SR, Fleischer AB, Jr., Manuel JC. The burden of atopic dermatitis: Impact on the patient, family, and society. Pediatr Dermatol 2005;22:192–9.

16. Mancini AJ, Kaulback K, Chamlin SL. The socioeconomic impact of atopic dermatitis in the United States: A systematic review. Pediatr Dermatol 2008;25:1–6.

17. Spergel JM, Paller AS. Atopic dermatitis and the atopic march. J Allergy Clin Immunol 2003;112:S118–S27.

18. Brim SN, Rudd RA, Funk RH, Callahan DB. Asthma prevalence among US children in underrepresented minority populations: American Indian/Alaska Native, Chinese, Filipino, and Asian Indian. Pediatrics 2008;122:e217–e22.

19. Jyonouchi S, Brown-Whitehorn TA, Spergel JM. Association of eosinophilic gastrointestinal disorders with other atopic disorders. Immunol Allergy Clin North Am 2009;29:85–97.

20. Pratt CA, Demain JG, Rathkopf MM. Food allergy and eosinophilic gastrointestinal disorders: Guiding our diagnosis and treatment. Curr Probl Pediatr Adolesc Health Care 2008;38:170–88.

21. Cherian S, Smith NM, Forbes DA. Rapidly increasing prevalence of eosinophilic oesophagitis in Western Australia. Arch Dis Child 2006;91:1000–4.

22. Liacouras CA, Spergel JM, Ruchelli E et al. Eosinophilic esophagitis: A 10-year experience in 381 children. Clin Gastroenterol Hepatol 2005;3:1198–206.

23. Strachan DP. Hay fever, hygiene, and household size. BMJ 1989;299:1259–60.

24. Williams HC, Pembroke AC, Forsdyke H, Boodoo G, Hay RJ, Burney PG. London-born black Caribbean children are at increased risk of atopic dermatitis. J Am Acad Dermatol 1995;32:212–7.

25. Jancin B. Antibiotics in infancy up atopic dermatitis risk. Skin Allergy News 2008;39:15.

26. Schaub B, Lauener R, von ME. The many faces of the hygiene hypothesis. J Allergy Clin Immunol 2006;117:969–77.

27. Bufford JD, Gern JE. The hygiene hypothesis revisited. Immunol Allergy Clin North Am 2005;25:247–63.

28. Leung DY, Boguniewicz M, Howell MD, Nomura I, Hamid QA. New insights into atopic dermatitis. J Clin Invest 2004;113:651–7.

29. Kang KF, Tian RM. Atopic dermatitis. An evaluation of clinical and laboratory findings. Int J Dermatol 1987;26:27–32.

30. Larsen FS, Holm NV, Henningsen K. Atopic dermatitis. A genetic-epidemiologic study in a population-based twin sample. J Am Acad Dermatol 1986;15:487–94.

31. Nichols KM, Cook-Bolden FE. Allergic skin disease: Major highlights and recent advances. Med Clin North Am 2009;93:1211–24.

32. Elias PM, Schmuth M. Abnormal skin barrier in the etiopathogenesis of atopic dermatitis. Curr Allergy Asthma Rep 2009;9:265–72.

33. Ong PY, Boguniewicz M. Atopic dermatitis. Prim Care 2008;35:105–17.
34. Hoffjan S, Stemmler S. On the role of the epidermal differentiation complex in ichthyosis vulgaris, atopic dermatitis and psoriasis. Br J Dermatol 2007;157:441–9.
35. Hudson TJ. Skin barrier function and allergic risk. Nat Genet 2006;38:399–400.
36. Osawa R, Akiyama M, Shimizu H. Filaggrin gene defects and the risk of developing allergic disorders. Allergol Int 2011;60:1–9.
37. Lack G, Fox D, Northstone K, Golding J. Factors associated with the development of peanut allergy in childhood. N Engl J Med 2003;348:977–85.
38. Maintz L, Novak N. Getting more and more complex: The pathophysiology of atopic eczema. Eur J Dermatol 2007;17:267–83.
39. Sampson HA. Food sensitivity and the pathogenesis of atopic dermatitis. J R Soc Med 1997;90 Suppl 30:2–8.
40. National Institute of Allergy and Infectious Disease. Guidelines for the diagnosis and management of food allergy in the United States: Report of the NIAID-sponsored Expert Panel. The Journal of Allergy and Clinical Immunology 2010;126(6):S1–S58.
41. Sicherer A, Sampson HA. Food allergy. J Allergy Clin Immunol 2010;125:S116–25.
42. Atherton DJ, Sewell M, Soothill JF, Wells RS, Chilvers CE. A double-blind controlled crossover trial of an antigen-avoidance diet in atopic eczema. Lancet 1978;1:401–3.
43. Juto P, Engberg S, Winberg J. Treatment of infantile atopic dermatitis with a strict elimination diet. Clin Allergy 1978;8:493–500.
44. Lever R, MacDonald C, Waugh P, Aitchison T. Randomised controlled trial of advice on an egg exclusion diet in young children with atopic eczema and sensitivity to eggs. Pediatr Allergy Immunol 1998;9:13–9.
45. Neild VS, Marsden RA, Bailes JA, Bland JM. Egg and milk exclusion diets in atopic eczema. Br J Dermatol 1986;114:117–23.
46. Bock SA, Lee WY, Remigio L, Holst A, May CD. Appraisal of skin tests with food extracts for diagnosis of food hypersensitivity. Clin Allergy 1978;8:559–64.
47. Sampson HA. Role of immediate food hypersensitivity in the pathogenesis of atopic dermatitis. J Allergy Clin Immunol 1983;71:473–80.
48. Sampson HA, McCaskill CC. Food hypersensitivity and atopic dermatitis: Evaluation of 113 patients. J Pediatr 1985;107:669–75.
49. Sampson HA. Atopic dermatitis. Ann Allergy 1992;69:469–79.
50. Brockow I, Zutavern A, Hoffmann U et al. Early allergic sensitizations and their relevance to atopic diseases in children aged 6 years: Results of the GINI study. J Investig Allergol Clin Immunol 2009;19:180–7.
51. Sampson HA. The evaluation and management of food allergy in atopic dermatitis. Clin Dermatol 2003;21:183–92.
52. Woods RK, Thien F, Raven J, Walters EH, Abramson M. Prevalence of food allergies in young adults and their relationship to asthma, nasal allergies, and eczema. Ann Allergy Asthma Immunol 2002;88:183–9.
53. Breuer K, Wulf A, Constien A, Tetau D, Kapp A, Werfel T. Birch pollen-related food as a provocation factor of allergic symptoms in children with atopic eczema/dermatitis syndrome. Allergy 2004;59:988–94.
54. Sampson HA, Scanlon SM. Natural history of food hypersensitivity in children with atopic dermatitis. J Pediatr 1989;115:23–7.
55. Fergusson DM, Horwood LJ, Shannon FT. Early solid feeding and recurrent childhood eczema: A 10-year longitudinal study. Pediatrics 1990;86:541–6.
56. Kajosaari M. Atopy prophylaxis in high-risk infants. Prospective 5-year follow-up study of children with six months exclusive breastfeeding and solid food elimination. Adv Exp Med Biol 1991;310:453–8.
57. Kramer MS, Kakuma R. Maternal dietary antigen avoidance during pregnancy or lactation, or both, for preventing or treating atopic disease in the child. Cochrane Database Syst Rev 2006, Issue 3. Art. No.: CD000133. DOI: 10.1002/14651858.CD000133.pub2.
58. Alexander DD, Cabana MD. Partially hydrolyzed 100% whey protein infant formula and reduced risk of atopic dermatitis: A meta-analysis. J Pediatr Gastroenterol Nutr 2010;50:422–30.
59. von Berg A., Filipiak-Pittroff B, Kramer U et al. Preventive effect of hydrolyzed infant formulas persists until age 6 years: Long-term results from the German Infant Nutritional Intervention Study (GINI). J Allergy Clin Immunol 2008;121:1442–7.
60. Bohme M, Wickman M, Lennart NS, Svartengren M, Wahlgren CF. Family history and risk of atopic dermatitis in children up to 4 years. Clin Exp Allergy 2003;33:1226–31.
61. Cabon N, Ducombs G, Mortureux P, Perromat M, Taieb A. Contact allergy to aeroallergens in children with atopic dermatitis: Comparison with allergic contact dermatitis. Contact Dermatitis 1996;35:27–32.

62. Breuer K, Heratizadeh A, Wulf A et al. Late eczematous reactions to food in children with atopic dermatitis. Clin Exp Allergy 2004;34:817–24.

63. Celik-Bilgili S, Mehl A, Verstege A et al. The predictive value of specific immunoglobulin E levels in serum for the outcome of oral food challenges. Clin Exp Allergy 2005;35:268–73.

64. Ho MH, Wong WH, Heine RG, Hosking CS, Hill DJ, Allen KJ. Early clinical predictors of remission of peanut allergy in children. J Allergy Clin Immunol 2008;121:731–6.

65. Sampson HA. Food allergy. Part 1: Immunopathogenesis and clinical disorders. J Allergy Clin Immunol 1999;103:717–28.

66. Bath-Hextall F, Delamere FM, Williams HC. Dietary exclusions for established atopic eczema. Cochrane Database Syst Rev 2008, Issue 1. Art. No.: CD005203. DOI: 10.1002/14651858.CD005203.pub2.

67. Kirby M, Danner E. Nutritional deficiencies in children on restricted diets. Pediatr Clin North Am 2009;56:1085–103.

68. Christie L, Hine RJ, Parker JG, Burks W. Food allergies in children affect nutrient intake and growth. J Am Diet Assoc 2002;102:1648–51.

69. Hide DW, Matthews S, Tariq S, Arshad SH. Allergen avoidance in infancy and allergy at 4 years of age. Allergy 1996;51:89–93.

70. Du TG, Lack G. Can food allergy be prevented? The current evidence. Pediatr Clin North Am 2011;58:481–509.

71. Grulee CG, Sanford HN. The influence of breast and artificial feeding oninfantile eczema. Journal of Pediatrics 1936;9:223–5 (abstr).

72. Hide DW, Guyer BM. Clinical manifestations of allergy related to breast and cows' milk feeding. Arch Dis Child 1981;56:172–5.

73. Van Asperen PP, Kemp AS, Mellis CM. Relationship of diet in the development of atopy in infancy. Clin Allergy 1984;14:525–32.

74. Schoetzau A, Filipiak-Pittroff B, Franke K et al. Effect of exclusive breast-feeding and early solid food avoidance on the incidence of atopic dermatitis in high-risk infants at 1 year of age. Pediatr Allergy Immunol 2002;13:234–42.

75. Laubereau B, Brockow I, Zirngibl A et al. Effect of breast-feeding on the development of atopic dermatitis during the first 3 years of life—results from the GINI-birth cohort study. J Pediatr 2004;144:602–7.

76. Hays T, Wood RA. A systematic review of the role of hydrolyzed infant formulas in allergy prevention. Arch Pediatr Adolesc Med 2005;159:810–6.

77. Osborn DA, Sinn J. Formulas containing hydrolysed protein for prevention of allergy and food intolerance in infants. Cochrane Database Syst Rev 2006, Issue 4. Art. No.: CD003664. DOI: 10.1002/14651858.CD003664.pub3.

78. Szajewska H, Horvath A. Meta-analysis of the evidence for a partially hydrolyzed 100% whey formula for the prevention of allergic diseases. Curr Med Res Opin 2010;26:423–37.

79. American Academy of Allergy Asthma & Immunology. Prevention of Allergies and Asthma in Children. 2009.

80. Committee on Nutrition. On the feeding of solid foods to infants. Pediatrics 1958;21:685–92.

81. Barness LA, Dallman PR, Anderson H et al. On the feeding of supplemental foods to infants. Pediatrics 1980;65:1178–81.

82. Committe on Nutrition. Hypoallergenic infant formulas. Pediatrics 2000;106:346–9.

83. Koplin JJ, Osborne NJ, Wake M et al. Can early introduction of egg prevent egg allergy in infants? A population-based study. J Allergy Clin Immunol 2010;126:807–13.

84. Snijders BE, Thijs C, van RR, van den Brandt PA. Age at first introduction of cow milk products and other food products in relation to infant atopic manifestations in the first 2 years of life: The KOALA Birth Cohort Study. Pediatrics 2008;122:e115–e22.

85. Zutavern A, Brockow I, Schaaf B et al. Timing of solid food introduction in relation to eczema, asthma, allergic rhinitis, and food and inhalant sensitization at the age of 6 years: Results from the prospective birth cohort study LISA. Pediatrics 2008;121:e44–e52.

86. Filipiak B, Zutavern A, Koletzko S et al. Solid food introduction in relation to eczema: Results from a four-year prospective birth cohort study. J Pediatr 2007;151:352–8.

87. Prescott SL, Smith P, Tang M et al. The importance of early complementary feeding in the development of oral tolerance: Concerns and controversies. Pediatr Allergy Immunol 2008;19:375–80.

88. Saavedra JM. Use of probiotics in pediatrics: Rationale, mechanisms of action, and practical aspects. Nutr Clin Pract 2007;22:351–65.

89. Arunachalam K, Gill HS, Chandra RK. Enhancement of natural immune function by dietary consumption of bifidobacterium lactis (HN019). Eur J Clin Nutr 2000;54:263–7.

90. Isolauri E, Arvola T, Sutas Y, Moilanen E, Salminen S. Probiotics in the management of atopic eczema. Clin Exp Allergy 2000;30:1604–10.
91. Majamaa H, Isolauri E. Probiotics: A novel approach in the management of food allergy. J Allergy Clin Immunol 1997;99:179–85.
92. Kalliomaki M, Salminen S, Poussa T, Arvilommi H, Isolauri E. Probiotics and prevention of atopic disease: 4-year follow-up of a randomised placebo-controlled trial. Lancet 2003;361:1869–71.
93. Pessi T, Sutas Y, Hurme M, Isolauri E. Interleukin-10 generation in atopic children following oral Lactobacillus rhamnosus GG. Clin Exp Allergy 2000;30:1804–8.
94. Kirjavainen PV, Salminen SJ, Isolauri E. Probiotic bacteria in the management of atopic disease: Underscoring the importance of viability. J Pediatr Gastroenterol Nutr 2003;36:223–7.
95. Rosenfeldt V, Benfeldt E, Valerius NH, Paerregaard A, Michaelsen KF. Effect of probiotics on gastrointestinal symptoms and small intestinal permeability in children with atopic dermatitis. J Pediatr 2004;145:612–6.
96. Tang ML, Lahtinen SJ, Boyle RJ. Probiotics and prebiotics: Clinical effects in allergic disease. Curr Opin Pediatr 2010;22:626–34.

Section V

Kidney Disorders

24 Kidney Stones

Preventing Recurrence with Diet and Nutrients

Lynda Frassetto, M.D., and Ingrid Kohlstadt, M.D., M.P.H.

INTRODUCTION

Nephrolithiasis incidence is rising in the United States and worldwide, and in populations formerly at lower risk for kidney stones, women and young adolescents. Preventing recurrence is largely specific to the type of stone. Even when the stone cannot be retrieved, urine pH and 24-hour urine assessment can guide prevention. Medications such as the HIV protease inhibitors, antibiotics, and some diuretics elevate the risk of forming specific types of kidney stones; anticipating the increased risk imposed by medications allows clinicians to counsel at-risk patients accordingly. This chapter explains how to leverage diet, medication, and nutrient intakes to prevent calcium oxalate, calcium phosphate, uric acid, struvite (ammonium urate), and cystine stones. The recommendations are correlated with the strength of clinical evidence and the biologic rationale.

EPIDEMIOLOGY

The prevalence of kidney stone disease is increasing in women and across the age spectrum, starting in childhood. The current risk for Americans to ever develop kidney stones is 10–15% [1] and trending higher. Contributing risk factors are obesity, insulin resistance, gastrointestinal pathology, food, nutrient and dietary supplement selection, dietary patterns, increasing population age, rising use of associated medications, and warmer climates [2,3]. As the prevalence of risk factors change, the distribution of kidney stones will shift as well. Table 24.1 reflects the distribution of kidney stones as reported in the medical literature.

PATHOPHYSIOLOGY

ANATOMIC FACTORS

There are several proposed mechanisms of kidney stone formation. Crystals can form from supersaturation of urine. Crystalline deposits may also begin in the interstitium following loss of the normal uroepithelial lining [4]. Interstitial deposits containing calcium oxalate [5] are known as Randall's plaques and are visible on uroscopy as whitish deposits (Figure 24.1) [6]. Plaque formation increases with increased urinary calcium excretion and decreased urine pH. Stones may also form in the tubules at sites of luminal injury such as the opening of the ducts of Bellini. Calcium phosphate stones, often seen in those with renal tubular acidifying abnormalities, are found protruding from the ducts of Bellini [6].

453

TABLE 24.1

Distribution of Kidney Stone Types by Age

Type of Stones	Children %	Adult %
Calcium Oxalate	45–65	56–61
Calcium Phosphate	24–30	8–18*
Cystine	5–8	1
Struvite	7–13	2–4
Uric Acid	2–4	9–17
Other	4	2

*up to 75% incidence in pregnant women [14]
Source: Adapted from [2,10,11,12,13].

Urine Specific Gravity

High fluid intake is the cornerstone of the treatment for most types of nephrolithiasis [7,8]. Supersaturation of mineral crystals can be prevented by increasing the amount of water in solution; this is the historical basis for the recommendation to drink 8–10 glasses of water a day during episodes of nephrolithiasis. Urine specific gravity measures the weight of solution compared to an equal volume of distilled water. The urine specific gravity of plasma is 1.008–1.010. The higher the solute load, the higher the specific gravity of urine, which has a normal range of 1.005–1.035 [9].

Urine pH

Urine pH is an important biochemical factor in the production of kidney stones. Renal function, dietary intake of acid- and base-forming precursors, some dietary supplements, and medication determine the amount of acid excreted. Calcium oxalate and uric acid stones tend to form in acidic

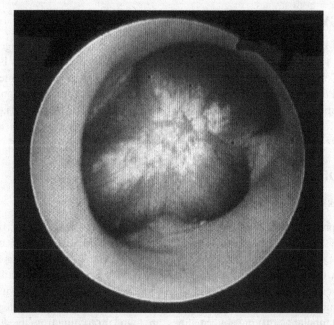

FIGURE 24.1   Endoscopic view of Randall's plaque and yellowish crystal deposits at the opening of the duct of Bellini.

urine. Treatment and prevention therefore include dietary modification and supplementation with potassium citrate or bicarbonate to provide alkali substrate [15]. Sodium citrate raises urine pH, but does not lower urinary calcium excretion to the same extent as the potassium salt [16]. Calcium phosphate and struvite stones form in alkaline urine. High dietary acid loads and ammonium sulfate can lower urine pH and potentially help prevent these kinds of stones [17]. Carbonic anhydrase inhibitors, such as acetazolamide and topiramate, contribute to calcium phosphate stone formation by inhibiting renal tubular reabsorption of bicarbonate with resultant high urine pH, hypercalciuria, and low urine citrate [18,19,20].

FRUCTOSE INTAKE

The National Health and Nutrition Examination Survey (NHANES) and Health Professionals Follow-up Study databases associate high dietary fructose with an increased risk for stone disease by as much as 38% [21]. In magnesium deficient animals and humans, high fructose intake increases urinary calcium excretion [22]. Fructose is the only dietary carbohydrate known to increase uric acid levels, which has led to a potential causal role for sugar-sweetened soda and orange juice in uric acid nephrolithiasis. Epidemiologic studies have linked both beverages with gout, the clinical manifestation of extracellular fluid supersaturated with urate crystals [23].

OBESITY AND WEIGHT LOSS

Several mechanisms link obesity and stone disease, some of which a patient is less able to modify than dietary indiscretion. The associated changes in body composition pose the biophysical challenges of disturbed thermogenesis and dehydration. Since body fat is hydrophobic, the proportion of body water decreases with increasing adiposity, predisposing to dehydration [24]. The decrease in surface area to body volume additionally complicates heat exchange and metabolic rate [25]. Obesity is a proinflammatory state associated with electrolyte imbalances and altered urine chemistry. Obesity predisposes stone formers to have hyperuricemia, gout, hypocitraturia, hyperuricosuria, and uric acid stones [26]. A recent retrospective analysis found that kidney stone formers with diabetes excrete more oxalate and have lower urine pH. This is due in part to higher urinary sulfate excretion and lower ammonium ion excretion [27,28]. Stone formers with obesity and diabetes may have less genetic predisposition, and more responsiveness to environmental modification such as diet and hydration.

The rise in kidney stone rates in post–World War II Europe corresponds to the shift toward a Western diet and the increasing incidence of obesity that occurred concomitantly. However, this powerful epidemiologic data is difficult to buttress with clinical evidence that an individual who eats a more healthful diet will lower the risk of stone recurrence. Weight loss may improve or undermine stone management, depending on how it is achieved. Weight loss could undermine prevention of renal stone formation if associated with a high animal protein intake, laxative abuse, rapid loss of lean tissue, or poor hydration. High acid diets, such as the Atkins diet and the ketogenic diet, increase the risk for uric acid stones [29,30]. Therefore, diet advice should be tailored to each individual's stone type. Surgical weight reduction is associated with high incidence of kidney stones attributed to low urine volume, citrate concentrations, and hyperoxaluria [31]. The biochemistry underlying the hyperoxaluria is unknown, possibly from reduced colonization and activity of *Oxalobacter formigenes* (discussed in the following paragraph) and fat malabsorption.

BACTERIAL EFFECTS

Bacteria exert both pathogenic and protective roles. Struvite (magnesium ammonium phosphate) stones are associated with recurrent infections due to high urinary pH levels from urease-splitting bacteria and the body's inability to rid the urinary tract of bacteria that become embedded in the stones [32]. *Oxalobacter formigenes* is an anaerobic bacterium that colonizes the intestinal tract where it metabolizes oxalate to formate and carbon dioxide. Absence of colonization with *O. formigenes* predisposes to oxalate stones [33]. Preliminary studies of ingestion of these bacteria in normal human volunteers fed a high oxalate diet [33] and in subjects with primary hyperoxaluria demonstrated decreases in urinary oxalate levels by as much as 90% [34]. However, one study of subjects with mild hyperoxaluria demonstrated that urinary oxalate levels decreased with dietary reduction of oxalate, but not with supplemental probiotics [35].

MEDICATIONS

Medications contribute to kidney stone formation through various mechanisms (Table 24.2) [36–42]. Some medications crystallize in urine and others contribute to stone formation due to their effects on urine pH, volume, and composition. Several antibiotics have been associated with kidney stones through unspecified mechanisms. Antibiotics can alter gastrointestinal microbiota, reducing *O. formigenes* concentrations. Laxatives, especially when taken in excess (laxative abuse), are associated with ammonium urate stones. The laxatives lead to primarily gastrointestinal loss of potassium and bicarbonate; through a compensatory mechanism, the kidneys excrete ammonium. The Food and Drug Administration (FDA) has been able to draw on its drug safety databases to assess a medication's potential to lower the threshold for kidney stones, whether or not it will affect clinical decision making (Table 24.2) [43].

PUBLIC HEALTH CASES

Since the previous edition of this book, case clusters of otherwise rare melamine stones and death from acute kidney failure in infants occurred as a result of a breach in food safety [44]. Manufacturers of infant formula contaminated their product with melamine for economic gain; the high nitrogen

---

TABLE 24.2
Medications Associated with Kidney Stone Formation

Mechanism of Action and/or Class	Examples of Drugs in Class
Agents that decrease uric acid production	Allopurinol
Agents that contain ammonium or promote GI potassium losses (specific to ammonium urate stones)	Laxatives, especially if abused
Antibiotics across mechanisms of action	Sulfamides, ampicillin, amoxicillin, ceftriaxone, quinolones, furans, pyridines
Carbonic anhydrase inhibitors	Acetazolamide; topiramate
Ephedra alkaloids (historically, prior to ban)	Illegally imported herbal products used as stimulants and appetite suppressants; use has been associated with drug and alcohol abuse
Potassium channel blockers	Amiodarone, sotalol, ampyra (multiple sclerosis therapy)
Potassium-channel sparing diuretics	Triamterene
Reverse transcriptase inhibitors and protease inhibitors	Highly active antiretroviral therapy (HAART)
Sulfonylureas	Various for treatment of type 2 diabetes
New Mechanisms with Urolithiasis Potential	
Chemokine CXCR2 (IL-8 B receptors) antagonists	Under development for HIV-1 and cancer
Drugs acting on cannabinoid receptors	Under development for various indications such as appetite suppression and pain management
Gamma-secretase inhibitors	Under development for Alzheimer's disease

Source: Adapted from [36–42].

content of melamine allowed diluted formula to pass the protein assay [45]. Melamine levels in contaminated formula were up to 100 times the FDA guidelines of 2.5 mg/day or 3.3 ppm. The incidence of melamine cyanurate stones expanded with increasing exposure [42,43]. The epidemic was primarily in China, while a parallel outbreak caused by contaminated, Chinese-imported, pet food sickened animals in the United States.

GENETICS

Kidney stones run in families and some heritable predispositions have been identified. Improving our understanding of cell transporter abnormalities and genetic linkages should lead to new drug targets and specific dietary recommendations. Monogenetic causes of nephrolithiasis are relatively uncommon and usually identified in childhood. Most links are polygenic with variable penetrance [46]. Urinary excretion of calcium is one such trait. In animals and humans, polymorphic genes have been found that affect intestinal calcium uptake as well as renal calcium excretion [47,48]. Many mutations are in the transporters that move ions and compounds into and out of cells. Mutations in the pathway associated with renal phosphate transport raise 1,25-OH vitamin D and thereby increase intestinal calcium uptake [49]. Mutations in oxalate (SLC26A6) [50] and urate (hURAT1) [51] transporters increase nephrolithiasis risk and urinary citrate concentrations [52]. From a nutrigenomics perspective, new genetic tools allow the study of how diet, foods, and individual nutrients can modify kidney stone risk.

PATIENT EVALUATION

Beyond the advances in acute diagnosis and management of kidney stones recently reviewed by the authors [53], renal stone evaluation involves identifying modifiable risk factors and guiding individualized treatment and prevention.

A family medical history remains a simplified genetic test for kidney stones. Examples include many types of stones associated with high urinary excretion of calcium, which are likely polygenic with variable effects on phenotype. Children who are homozygous for mutations in dibasic amino acid transporters form cystine calculi.

History taking identifies medical problems associated with increased kidney stone risk: inflammatory bowel disease or bowel surgery, gout, diabetes, obesity or recent changes in weight, metabolic syndromes, hyperparathyroidism-associated conditions, frequent urinary tract infections, and chronic kidney disease [54]. A thorough medication history establishes temporal associations, records medications recently discontinued, including off-label uses of medications, herbal preparations, and supplements for weight loss, and screens for illicit drug use.

With the increasing incidence and prevalence of stone disease and chronic kidney disease, some reviewers now recommend studying all patients after their first episode of kidney stones [10]. We concur with this approach since most nutritional strategies to treatment and prevention are type specific. Stones are usually collected by straining the urine. However, some stones pass without being retrieved even when urine is strained. Sometimes stone type can be inferred when retrieval for analysis is not possible. For example, struvite stones are readily detected on X-ray. Uroscopy usually allows for stone retrieval and in addition may demonstrate characteristics such as Randall's plaques, which point to a specific stone type. Results of a prior stone analysis are highly relevant since stone recurrences are rarely of a different type.

Even when a stone is not retrieved for analysis and family and medical history do not point to a specific stone type, laboratory analysis can guide clinical decision making. Stone forming predilections can often be assessed even after the stone has passed, through blood and urine analysis:

- Elevated serum uric acid suggests uric acids stones, especially when combined with a history of gout and fructose ingestion.

- Elevated serum calcium can suggest primary hyperparathyroidism associated with calcium phosphate stones. Approximately 5% of patients with nephrolithiasis have elevated parathyroid hormone levels [55].
- Serum 25-hydroxy vitamin D is valuable because both high and low levels promote stone formation. Low levels are associated with secondary hyperparathyroidism. High levels increase calcium uptake.
- Urine pH is an important biochemical factor in the production of kidney stones; uric acid, cystine, and calcium oxalate stones tend to form in acid urine, while struvite and calcium phosphate stones form in alkaline urine.
- A 24-hour urine collection can be analyzed for calcium, phosphorus, magnesium, uric acid, oxalate, and the stone-inhibiting factors citrate and phytate. In the absence of the actual stone analysis, these 24-hour urine parameters help indicate potentially abnormal or treatable conditions such as low urinary citrate.
- Twenty-four-hour urine creatinine should be measured to evaluate the adequacy of the collection. The creatinine index is defined as 24-hour urine creatinine in grams divided by body weight in kilograms. The normal range is from 8–20 g/kg depending on the muscle mass of the person being tested.
- An elevated urine calcium excretion is another important stone-forming risk factor. Elevation can occur with increased diet acid loads, increased salt intake, and both inadequate and excessive vitamin D levels.

Because kidney stones predispose to chronic kidney disease (CKD), even small amounts of protein in the urine should be noted. Random urine samples may test positive for microalbumin due to recent exercise, trauma, or elevations in blood pressure. Before starting a workup for microalbuminuria, retest the urine to be sure the results remain positive. Since some of the problems that lead to progression of CKD are partly responsive to nutritional interventions, evaluating for CKD in patients with nephrolithiasis risk factors may be effective prevention. Additional tests to evaluate kidney function include serum creatinine or the estimated glomerular filtration rate (eGFR), hemoglobin A1c for blood sugar control, and urinalysis with microscopy.

Referral to a nephrologist is sometimes appropriate, since kidney stones are a risk factor for CKD and progression to end stage renal disease [56]. Stone formers are more likely to have both traditional risk factors of hypertension, preexisting kidney disease, diabetes, proteinuria or albuminuria, and nontraditional factors such as interstitial nephritis or recurrent pyelonephritis [57]. The American Society of Nephrology suggests referral to a nephrologist if the eGFR is 60 ml/min or below (Stage 3 CKD) or earlier if macroalbuminuria is present [58].

SPECIAL POPULATIONS: CHILDREN AND PREGNANT WOMEN

There are special considerations for pediatric and pregnant patients. More children are developing kidney stones, which is attributed to the corresponding rise in diabetes, obesity, and hypertension in children. Because increasing age is a risk factor for stone disease, adolescents are more likely to form stones than younger children. The underlying stone types (see Table 24.1), causes, and resulting treatments differ in children and adults. Children with kidney stones are more likely to have anatomic and metabolic abnormalities [11,59], increased urinary calcium excretion, decreased urinary oxalate and citrate excretion, and much higher urinary calcium oxalate saturations than children with no history of stone disease [2]. Patients with cystinuria and other hereditary forms of nephrolithiasis are at increased risk for renal functional decline compared to age-matched controls, although progression to end-stage renal disease is uncommon. Children of aboriginal Australians and Pacific Islanders appear to have genetic factors that predispose them to kidney stones and a higher incidence of acute kidney injury from post-streptococcal glomerulonephritis and hemolytic-uremic syndrome [60]. Low birth weight in these children* is associated with low nephron number and glomerulomegaly, and seems to predispose them to albuminuria and hypertension in later life [61].

Pregnant women are twice as likely to have calcium phosphate stones compared to nonpregnant age-matched controls and are two to three times more likely to have calcium phosphate stones than oxalate stones [62]. Stone incidence increases in the second and third trimesters. Pregnant women have an increased glomerular filtration rate and higher urinary calcium excretion throughout pregnancy, with higher urine pH in the second and third trimesters, which may predispose them to calcium phosphate stones.

Ultrasound is considered the imaging modality of choice. Maternal kidney stones are significantly associated with several pregnancy complications, including recurrent abortions, hypertensive disorders, gestational diabetes, and cesarean deliveries [63]. Pregnant stone formers are more likely to develop urinary tract infections, and pregnant women with renal colic have nearly double the risk of preterm delivery compared to women without stones [64]. One meta-analysis suggests that ureteroscopy in pregnant stone formers has the same complication rate as in nonpregnant stone formers [65].

TREATMENT AND PREVENTION

FLUID INTAKE AND HYDRATION

How one increases fluid intake and maintains hydration matters:

- Fluid intake should not be a significant source of calories. Drinking calories is associated with excess weight gain, since calories consumed in beverages are not as satiating as calories that are eaten. Water, fruit tea, green tea, and coffee are suitable noncaloric beverages.
- Water is effective and for some stone types (Table 24.3). Added lemon and carbonation are additionally beneficial, because of their effects on pH.
- Bottled water can be a hidden source of sodium.
- For athletes replacing fluid and salt loss, salts and spices more diverse than table salt are recommended. A 2% glucose solution (WHO oral rehydration salts) optimizes gastrointestinal uptake of salt and water. Most sports drinks are excessively sweet and salty.
- Fructose, especially high fructose corn syrup added to sodas, should be avoided.
- Most high-intensity (artificial) sweeteners create an osmotic load, thereby reducing gastrointestinal fluid absorption. Most lower urine pH.
- Preliminary studies suggest that unique phytonutrients found in cranberry juice and green tea may exert yet uncharacterized anti-lithogenic properties for some stone types [70,71].
- Hydrating isn't limited to beverages. Eating hydrous foods and humidifying a room may be helpful.

RAISING URINE pH (ALKALINIZING)

Since Western diets are characteristically high in acid-producing foods such as grains, dairy products, legumes, and meat, alkalinizing the urine involves eating a high fruit and vegetable diet, taking supplemental or prescription citrate, or drinking alkaline mineral waters. How much citrate or alkaline mineral water to take will depend in part on how much acid is being ingested and produced by the body. Testing urine pH on a regular basis throughout the day will give some indication of the body's total acid load; the lower the urine pH, the more exogenous alkali needs

---

* Spencer et al. suggested parental age, but not hypertension or proteinuria, as a risk factor for decreased nephron number in the infant [61]; other authors disagree [60].

TABLE 24.3

Diet and Medication Recommendations for Stone Type and Urinary Properties

Stone Type	Diagnostic Test	Interventions	Specifics	Comments
All stone types	Urine specific gravity > 1.015	Fluid intake, mostly water	Drink at least two liters/24 hours; consider mineral water, depending on the type of stone.	www.mineralwaters.org lists mineral content of thousands of mineral waters globally.
	Body Mass Index > 18 or < 25 kg/m², fasting blood sugar > 105, random glucose > 140 mg/dL, serum Ca > 10 mg/dL	Optimal weight; Suggestive of insulin resistance or early diabetes; Consider primary hyperparathyroidism: check intact parathyroid hormone level.	Promote diet and exercise. Promote low glycemic diet. (Normal range is laboratory dependent.)	
	Urine pH (either dipstick or from 24-hour urine)	Urine alkalinizing measures (i.e., raising urine pH) ~6.5–7 with dietary changes (see text), oral base supplementation, or until 24-hr urine citrate levels are in the normal range; Urine acidifying measures (lower urine pH) ≤ 7 with dietary changes (see text) or oral acid supplements	Potassium citrate 10–20 mEq PO with meals (prescription required); Calcium citrate 500 mg (= 120 mg Ca, 6 mEq HCO_3/tab), two tabs with meals; Cranberry juice (at least 16 oz/day); Betaine hydrochloride 650 mg PO TID with meals	
Calcium oxalate (CaOx)	Stone analysis	Appropriate protein intake; Take calcium supplements with meals: calcium citrate is preferred if also trying to raise urine citrate levels. Check serum 25-Vitamin D levels. Medications:	Maintain at ≤ 30% of total caloric intake. Take at least 250 mg/dose or total calcium > 850 mg/day. LOW < 30 ng/mL. Thiazide diuretics; e.g., HCTZ 25–50 mg/day	Vitamin D increases intestinal calcium absorption and renal calcium and phosphate absorption.
	24-hour urine oxalate (HIGH > 40 mg/day)	Moderate fruits and vegetables; do not restrict calcium. Consider magnesium potassium citrate supplementation. Encourage moderate vitamin C intake by dietary sources rather than supplements.	Restrict high oxalate foods (> 6 mg/serving): beans, spinach, rhubarb, chocolate, wheat, nuts, berries. Each tab: (Mg 3 mEq, K 7 mEq, citrate 10 mEq) 2 tabs TID with meals; Limit total < 1 g/day	Oxalate restriction is minimally effective and probably applies primarily to those few with genetic mutations in the oxalate transporters.
	24-hour urine calcium (HIGH; mg Ca/g Cr; children (1 mo–17 yr) > 0.8; adult male, > 210; adult female, > 275	Sodium restriction to 2gms/day or less; Do not restrict calcium intake below recommendations for age and gender.	Do not add salt to food, avoid foods high in salt (e.g., canned or processed foods, cheese, pickles, dried meats).	Urinary values may vary by laboratory; the values cited come from Quest Diagnostics (San Jose, CA).

Type	Diagnostic criteria	Treatment approach	Dietary / medication details	Comments
	24-hour urine magnesium (LOW <70 mg/day)	Increase dietary sources of magnesium. Consider magnesium potassium citrate supplementation.	Eat fish, nuts, grains, yogurt. Each tab: (Mg 3 mEq, K 7 mEq, citrate 10 mEq) 2 tabs TID with meals	Urinary values come from the UCSF clinical lab.
	24-hour urine citrate LOW: Adult male, <450 mg/day Adult female, <550 mg/day	Citrate is available as a potassium, calcium or sodium salt. Lemon or lime juice in water is encouraged.	Potassium citrate 10-20 mEq PO with meals (prescription required) Calcium citrate 500 mg (= 120 mg Ca, 6 mEq HCO_3/tab), 2 tabs with meals Put 1 cup concentrated juice in 7 cups water.	Sodium salts can increase urinary calcium excretion.
Calcium phosphate (CaP)	24-hour urine phytates LOW: (PPi < 3.8 mg/L; IP6 < 0.4 mg/L)[1] Stone analysis	Consider increased intake of fiber.	Eat whole grains, legumes, seeds, nuts.	Phytate levels depend on methodology used; increasing phytates may also increase oxalate intake
	Stone analysis	If female, check if pregnant. Urine acidifying measures Lower diet phosphate intake?	Urine or serum pregnancy test See urine pH. Decrease dairy products, legumes, chocolate, nuts by ~1/3.	Minimal human data; decreases the formation of CaP stones in genetically predisposed rats
Cystine	Stone analysis 24-hour urine cystine levels (HIGH >250 mg/day)	Urine alkalinizing measures Decrease methionine (sulfur) intake. Medications: cystine-binding agents	See urine pH. Avoid dairy products, eggs, legumes, greens. Tiopronin (dose divided TID) Children—15 mg/kg Adults—800-1000 mg/day Penicillamine: 20-40 mg/kg/day	Dose adjusted to maintain urine free cystine concentration <250 mg/day if possible
Struvite	Stone analysis or characteristic radiologic appearance	Urine acidifying measures Avoid supplemental magnesium based on animal studies. Medication for subjects who cannot tolerate surgical intervention.	See urine pH. Acetohydroxamine (urease inhibitor) 15 mg/kg in divided doses 3–4 times/day	
Uric Acid	Stone analysis, 24-hour urine uric acid levels (HIGH >800 mg/day); prior history of gout	Decrease protein intake. Reduce or eliminate beer and alcohol intake. Increase coffee, tea, decaffeinated coffee. Urine alkalinizing measures Medication	Maintain <30% of total caloric intake. See urine pH. Allopurinol 300 mg PO daily (dose reduction for low eGFR)	Increased caffeine intake may reduce stones in diabetics.

[1] PPi stands for inorganic phosphate, IP6 stands for inositol phosphate-6, HCO_3 is bicarbonate also called hydrogen carbonate.

Source: Adapted from [3,7,8,66–69].

to be ingested. Typical Western diets produce 40–50 millimoles of acid daily, yielding urine pH in 5–6 range.

The Dietary Approaches to Stop Hypertension (DASH) diet is associated with reduction in kidney stone risk. It is an alkalinizing diet; 24-hour urine analysis suggests that the risk reduction is due in part to increasing urinary citrate and volume. The additional risk reduction not accounted for in the 24-hour urine analysis suggests that unidentified components of dairy or the phytonutrients from plants consumed in the DASH diet may inhibit stone formation [72]. The recommendation to patients here is not necessarily to use the DASH diet to prevent kidney stones, but that if they have been prescribed in the diet to manage hypertension, a beneficial side effect is reduced risk of the most common types of kidney stones.

Lowering Urine pH (Acidifying)

Cranberry juice or betaine hydrochloride can lower urine pH without some of the adverse effects associated with the acid-producing foods in typical Western diets. Table salt (NaCl) will also lower urine pH but can increase blood pressure, insulin excretion, and urine calcium excretion, which may not be appropriate in many patients.

Herbal Therapies

Phytonutrients in green tea, turmeric, and berries reduce associated infection risk, and parsley promotes diuresis. The traditional herb *Agropyron repens* helps achieve flushing of the urinary tract according to a recent European Medicines Agency monograph. Herbs have been used in acute kidney stone treatment since antiquity, but many challenges surround their contemporary use—quality and safety of dietary supplements, interactions with medications, interactions with anesthesia if surgical intervention is needed, and lack of stone-specific efficacy data.

Prudent Weight Reduction

See Chapter 18: Obesity, for weight-reduction strategies. This is specifically important for uric acid stones [14] and when blood glucose or inflammatory markers are elevated.

CLINICAL SUMMARY

- Increase fluid intake to at least 2 liters/day.
- Identify stone type when possible, even on initial stone occurrence.
- Obtain urine characteristics to guide treatment and prevention.
- Counsel patients on stone-specific dietary interventions.
- Assess for risk of chronic kidney disease.
- Modify medication-related stone risk when applicable.

REFERENCES

1. Long LO, Park S. Update on nephrolithiasis management. *Minerva Urol Nefrol*. 2007;59(3):317–25.
2. Acar B, Inci Arikan F, Emeksiz S, Dallar Y. Risk factors for nephrolithiasis in children. *World J Urol*. 2008;26(6):627–30.
3. Pietrow PK, Karellas ME. Medical management of common urinary calculi. *Am Fam Physician*. 2006;74(1):86–94.
4. Coe FL, Evan AP, Worcester EM, Lingeman JE. Three pathways for human kidney stone formation. *Urol Res*. 2010;38(3):147–60.
5. Matlaga BR, Williams JC Jr, Kim SC, Kuo RL, et al. Endoscopic evidence of calculus attachment to Randall's plaque. *J Urol*. 2006;175(5):1720–24.

6. Evan AP. Physiopathology and etiology of stone formation in the kidney and urinary tract. *Pediatr Nephrol*. 2010;25:831–41.

7. Marangella M, Bagnis C, Bruno M, Vitale C, Petrarulo M, Ramello A. Crystallization inhibitors in the pathophysiology and treatment of nephrolithiasis. *Urol Int*. 2004;72Sl 1:6–10.

8. Borghi L, Meschi T, Amato F, Briganti A, Novarini A, Giannini A. Urinary volume, water and recurrences in idiopathic calcium nephrolithiasis: A 5-year randomized prospective study. *J Urol*. 1996;155(3):839–43.

9. Rose, BD. Meaning and application of urine chemistries. In *Clinical Physiology of Acid-Base and Electrolyte Disturbances*, McGraw-Hill, Inc, 4th Ed., 284–86.

10. Curhan GC. Epidemiology of stone disease. *Urol Clin North Am*. 2007;34(3):287–93.

11. Sas DJ, Hulsey TC, Shatat IF, Orak JK. Increasing incidence of kidney stones in children evaluated in the emergency department. *J Pediatr*. 2010;157(1):132–37.

12. Milliner, DS, Murphy, ME. Urolithiasis in pediatric patients. *Mayo Clin Proc*. 1993;68:241–48.

13. Ross AE, Handa S, Lingeman JE, Matlaga BR. Kidney stones during pregnancy: An investigation into stone composition. *Urol Res*. 2008;36(2):99–102.

14. Taylor EN, Curhan GC. Body size and 24-hour urine composition. Am J Kidney Dis. 2006 Dec;48(6):905–15.

15. Trinchieri A, Esposito N, Castelnuovo C. Dissolution of radiolucent renal stones by oral alkalinization with potassium citrate/potassium bicarbonate. *Arch Ital Urol Androl*. 2009;81(3):188–91.

16. Sakhaee K, Nicar M, Hill K, Pak CY. Contrasting effects of potassium citrate and sodium citrate therapies on urinary chemistries and crystallization of stone-forming salts. *Kidney Int*. 1983;24(3):348–52.

17. Pizzarelli F, Peacock M. Effect of chronic administration of ammonium sulfate on phosphatic stone recurrence. *Nephron*. 1987;46(3):247–52.

18. Sterrett SP, Penniston KL, Wolf JS Jr, Nakada SY. Acetazolamide is an effective adjunct for urinary alkalization in patients with uric acid and cystine stone formation recalcitrant to potassium citrate. *Urology*. 2008;72(2):278–81.

19. Welch BJ, Graybeal D, Moe OW, Maalouf NM, Sakhaee K. Biochemical and stone-risk profiles with topiramate treatment. *Am J Kidney Dis*. 2006;48(4):555–63.

20. Reid G, Bruce AW. Probiotics to prevent urinary tract infections: The rationale and evidence. *World J Urol*. 2006;24(1):28–32.

21. Taylor EN, Curhan GC. Fructose consumption and the risk of kidney stones. *Kidney Int*. 2008;73(2):207–12.

22. Koh ET, Reiser S, Fields M. Dietary fructose as compared to glucose and starch increases the calcium content of kidney of magnesium-deficient rats. *J Nutr*. 1989;119:1173–78.

23. Choi HK, Willett W, Curhan G. Fructose-rich beverages and risk of gout in women. *J Am Med Assoc*. 2010;304(20):2270–78.

24. Batmanghelidj FW. A driving force in the musculoskeletal system. In *Scientific Evidence for Musculoskeletal, Bariatric and Sports Nutrition*, I. Kohlstadt, ed., Boca Raton, FL: CRC Press, 2006, 127–35.

25. Livingston EH, Kohlstadt I. Simplified resting metabolic rate-predicting formulas for normal-sized and obese individuals. *Obes Res*. 2005;13(7):1255–62.

26. Ekeruo WO, Tan YH, Young MD, Dahm P, et al. Metabolic risk factors and the impact of medical therapy on the management of nephrolithiasis in obese patients. *J Urol*. 2004;172(1):159–63.

27. Eisner BH, Porten SP, Bechis SK, Stoller ML. Diabetic kidney stone formers excrete more oxalate and have lower urine pH than nondiabetic stone formers. *J Urol*. 2010;183(6):2244–48.

28. Maalouf NM, Cameron MA, Moe OW, Sakhaee K. Metabolic basis for low urine pH in type 2 diabetes. *Clin J Am Soc Nephrol*. 2010;5(7):1277–81.

29. Breslau NA, Brinkley L, Hill KD, Pak CY. Relationship of animal protein-rich diet to kidney stone formation and calcium metabolism. *J Clin Endocrinol Metab*. 1988;66(1):140–46.

30. Sampath A, Kossoff EH, Furth SL, Pyzik PL, Vining EP. Kidney stones and the ketogenic diet: Risk factors and prevention. *J Child Neurol*. 2007 Apr;22(4):375–78.

31. Lieske JC, Kumar R, Collazo-Clavell ML. Nephrolithiasis after bariatric surgery for obesity. *Semin Nephrol*. 2008 Mar;28(2):163–73.

32. Jarrar K, Boedeker RH, Weidner W. Struvite stones: Long term follow up under metaphylaxis. *Ann Urol (Paris)*. 1996;30(3):112–17.

33. Siva S, Barrack ER, Reddy GP, Thamilselvan V, et al. A critical analysis of the role of gut Oxalobacter formigenes in oxalate stone disease. *BJU Int*. 2009;103(1):18–21.

34. Hoppe B, Beck B, Gatter N, von Unruh G, et al. Oxalobacter formigenes: A potential tool for the treatment of primary hyperoxaluria type 1. *Kidney Int*. 2006;70(7):1305–11.

35. Lieske JC, Tremaine WJ, De Simone C, O'Connor HM, Li X, Bergstralh EJ, Goldfarb DS. Diet, but not oral probiotics, effectively reduces urinary oxalate excretion and calcium oxalate supersaturation. *Kidney Int*. 2010;78(11):1178–85.

36. Saltel E, Angel JB, Futter NG, Walsh WG, O'Rourke K, Mahoney JE. Increased prevalence and analysis of risk factors for indinavir nephrolithiasis. *J Urol.* 2000;164(6):1895–97.

37. Kohan AD, Armenakas NA, Fracchia JA. Indinavir urolithiasis: An emerging cause of renal colic in patients with human immunodeficiency virus. *J Urol.* 1999;161(6):1765–68.

38. Sörgel F, Ettinger B, Benet LZ. The true composition of kidney stones passed during triamterene therapy. *J Urol.* 1985;134(5):871–73.

39. Topamax (topiramate) drug label section "Description." Accessed on 12/30/10 through http://dailymed.nlm .nih.gov/dailymed/drugInfo.cfm?id=7412 (dailymed.nkm.nih.gov).

40. Chopra N, Fine PL, Price B, Atlas I. Bilateral hydronephrosis from ciprofloxacin induced crystalluria and stone formation. *J Urol.* 2000;164(2):438.

41. Siegel WH. Unusual complication of therapy with sulfamethoxazole-trimethoprim. *J Urol.* 1977;117(3): 397.

42. Dick WH, Lingeman JE, Preminger GM, Smith LH, Wilson DM, Shirrell WL. Laxative abuse as a cause for ammonium urate renal calculi. *J Urol.* 1990;143(2):244–47.

43. Matthews EJ, Kruhlak NL, Benz RD, Aragonés Sabaté D, Marchant CA, Contrera JF. Identification of structure-activity relationships for adverse effects of pharmaceuticals in humans: Part C: Use of QSAR and an expert system for the estimation of the mechanism of action of drug-induced hepatobiliary and urinary tract toxicities. *Regul Toxicol Pharmacol.* 2009;54(1):43–65.

44. Guan N, Fan Q, Ding J, Zhao Y, et al. Melamine-contaminated powdered formula and urolithiasis in young children. *N Engl J Med.* 2009;360(11):1067–74.

45. http://www.who.int/foodsafety/fs_management/infosan_events/en/ (accessed 1/17/12).

46. Attanasio M. The genetic components of idiopathic nephrolithiasis. *Pediatr Nephrol.* 2011;26(3):337–46.

47. Bushinsky DA, Frick KK, Nehrke K. Genetic hypercalciuric stone-forming rats. *Curr Opin Nephrol Hypertens.* 2006;15(4):403–18.

48. Worcester EM, Coe FL. Evidence for altered renal tubule function in idiopathic calcium stone formers. *Urol Res.* 2010;38(4):263–69.

49. Karim Z, Gérard B, Bakouh N, Alili R, et al. NHERF1 mutations and responsiveness of renal parathyroid hormone. *N Engl J Med.* 2008;359(11):1128–35.

50. Clark JS, Vandorpe DH, Chernova MN, Heneghan JF, Stewart AK, Alper SL. Species differences in Cl- affinity and in electrogenicity of SLC26A6-mediated oxalate/Cl- exchange correlate with the distinct human and mouse susceptibilities to nephrolithiasis. *J Physiol.* 2008;586(5):1291–306.

51. Capasso G, Jaeger P, Robertson WG, Unwin RJ. Uric acid and the kidney: Urate transport, stone disease and progressive renal failure. *Curr Pharm Des.* 2005;11(32):4153–59.

52. Shah O, Assimos DG, Holmes RP. Genetic and dietary factors in urinary citrate excretion. *J Endourol.* 2005;19(2):177–82.

53. Frassetto L, Kohlstadt I. Treatment and prevention of kidney stones: An update. *Am Fam Physician.* 2011;84(11):1234–42.

54. Paige NM, Nagami GT. The top 10 things nephrologists wish every primary care physician knew. *Mayo Clin Proc.* 2009;84(2):180–6.

55. Parks J, Coe F, Favus M. Hyperparathyroidism in nephrolithiasis. *Arch Intern Med.* 1980;140(11): 1479–81.

56. Rule AD, Bergstralh EJ, Melton LJ 3rd, Li X, Weaver AL, Lieske JC. Kidney stones and the risk for chronic kidney disease. *Clin J Am Soc Nephrol.* 2009;4(4):804–11.

57. Gambaro G, Favaro S, D'Angelo A. Risk for renal failure in nephrolithiasis. *Am J Kidney Dis.* 2001;37(2):233–43.

58. http://www.asn-online.org/policy_and_public_affairs/patient-care.aspx (accessed 1/17/12).

59. Cochat P, Pichault V, Bacchetta J et al. Nephrolithiasis related to inborn metabolic diseases. *Pediatr Nephrol.* 2010;25(3):415–24.

60. White A, Wong W, Sureshkumur P, Singh G. The burden of kidney disease in indigenous children of Australia and New Zealand, epidemiology, antecedent factors and progression to chronic kidney disease. *J Paediatr Child Health.* 2010;46(9):504–9.

61. Spencer J, Wang Z, Hoy W. Low birth weight and reduced renal volume in Aboriginal children. *Am J Kidney Dis.* 2001;37:915–20.

62. Ross AE, Handa S, Lingeman JE, Matlaga BR. Kidney stones during pregnancy: An investigation into stone composition. *Urol Res.* 2008; 36(2):99–102.

63. Rosenberg E, Sergienko R, Abu-Ghanem S, Wiznitzer A, Romanowsky I, Neulander EZ, Sheiner E. Nephrolithiasis during pregnancy: Characteristics, complications, and pregnancy outcome. *World J Urol.* 2011;29(6):743–47.

64. Swartz MA, Lydon-Rochelle MT, Simon D, Wright JL, Porter MP. Admission for nephrolithiasis in pregnancy and risk of adverse birth outcomes. *Obstet Gynecol.* 2007;109(5):1099–104.

65. Semins MJ, Trock BJ, Matlaga BR. The safety of ureteroscopy during pregnancy: A systematic review and meta-analysis. *J Urol.* 2009;181(1):139–43.

66. Hesse A, Siener R, Heynck H, Jahnen A. The influence of dietary factors on the risk of urinary stone formation. *Scanning Microsc.* 1993;7(3):1119–27.

67. Serio A, Fraioli A. An observational and longitudinal study on patients with kidney stones treated with Fiuggi mineral water. *Clin Ter.* 1999;150(3):215–19.

68. Parks JH, Coe FL. Evidence for durable kidney stone prevention over several decades. *BJU Int.* 2009;103(9):1238–46.

69. Reddy ST, Wang CY, Sakhaee K, Brinkley L, Pak CY. Effect of low-carbohydrate high-protein diets on acid-base balance, stone-forming propensity, and calcium metabolism. *Am J Kidney Dis.* 2002;40(2):265–74.

70. Jeong, B.C., et al., Effects of green tea on urinary stone formation: An in vivo and in vitro study. *J Endourol.* 2006;20(5):356–61.

71. McHarg, T., A. Rodgers, and K. Charlton, Influence of cranberry juice on the urinary risk factors for calcium oxalate kidney stone formation. *BJU Int.* 2003;92(7):765–68.

72. Taylor EN, Stampfer MJ, Mount DB, Curhan GC. DASH-style diet and 24-hour urine composition. *Clin J Am Soc Nephrol.* 2010 Dec;5(12):2315–22.

25 Chronic Kidney Disease

Overview and Nutritional Interventions

Shideh Pouria, M.B.B.S., Ph.D.

INTRODUCTION

The incidence of chronic kidney disease is increasing. Established kidney failure is a major burden on the patient, health care providers, and society alike. Fundamental changes in lifestyle predispose Western societies to compromised renal integrity and progressive deterioration of kidney function. It is important to include the evaluation of renal status and its diverse etiologies in the health assessment of patients. Prompt diagnosis, exploration, and alteration of modifiable lifestyle, nutritional, and environmental risk factors provide an opportunity to reduce the risk of kidney disease and its incident and pervasive complications.

EPIDEMIOLOGY

At present, more than 10% of the U.S. adult population has chronic kidney disease (CKD) [1]. In 2007, the Centers for Disease Control analyzed the most recent data from the National Health and Nutrition Examination Survey (NHANES) [2]. By disease stage, the prevalence of CKD was found to be: stage 1, 5.7%; stage 2, 5.4%; stage 3, 5.4%; and stages 4/5, 0.4%. This is more than 20 million people in the United States alone, where over half a million people currently receive dialysis for established kidney failure, and that number is increasing by 7% per annum [3]. Hemodialysis, peritoneal dialysis, and kidney transplantation are the methods of treatment for established kidney failure.

The major causes of end-stage kidney disease are diabetes mellitus, accounting for 45% of cases, and hypertension, accounting for 27% [4] (Table 25.1). Since the majority of cases of diabetes and hypertension are preventable, and nearly all can be mitigated, optimal clinical, dietary, and lifestyle management would greatly reduce the prevalence of end-stage kidney disease. Table 25.2 lists the underlying causes of CKD and kidney failure.

PATHOPHYSIOLOGY

The kidneys have myriad functions, the loss of which impact every system in the body. The compensatory and adaptive mechanisms in the body are able to maintain life until the glomerular filtration rate (GFR) is below 15 ml/min and life-sustaining renal excretory and homeostatic functions continue at GFRs of above 5 ml/min. The homeostatic functions of the kidneys are summarized here.

TABLE 25.1

Prevalence of the Most Common Causes of Established Kidney Failure in the United States in 2010

Disease	Prevalence
Diabetes	205,724
Hypertension	133,537
Primary Glomerular Disease	83,268
Cystic Kidney Disease	26,094
Urological Disease	13,065
All Others	86,294

Source: Adapted from [4].

---

1. Water homeostasis: The inability to conserve urine in the presence of dehydration is one of the signs of renal failure manifesting as nocturia, polyuria, and thirst. Diluting capacity is conserved until the GFR drops below 30 ml/min and eventually the urinary osmolality becomes fixed at around 300 mosmol/kg. Defective urine concentration is due to increased solute load in the surviving nephrons. In late kidney failure, large water loads will be excreted more slowly and excessive fluid intake results in hyponatremia, cognitive disturbances, and even convulsions.

2. Electrolyte homeostasis: Patients with renal failure have disturbances of electrolytes— namely hyponatremia, hyperkalemia, hypocalcemia, hyperphosphatemia, hypermagnesemia, and their complications. Sodium conservation is lost at GFRs below 10 ml/min, whereas potassium homeostasis is lost at GFRs less than 5 ml/min.

3. Acid base balance: The kidneys are the principal organs of acid base homeostasis through reabsorption of filtered bicarbonate, acidification of urinary buffers, and excretion of ammonia. As renal failure advances at GFRs of less than 20 ml/min metabolic acidosis and impaired organ function develops leading to growth retardation, renal osteodystrophy, and acceleration of renal impairment.

4. Waste product excretion: Accumulation of water-soluble toxins normally excreted by the kidneys may cause anorexia, nausea, loss of muscle, cachexia, neurological dysfunction,

---

TABLE 25.2

Causes of Chronic Kidney Disease

- Diabetes
- Hypertension
- Primary glomerular disease such as IgA nephropathy
- Cystic kidney disease
- Obstructive nephropathy
- Vascular causes such as reno-vascular disease, vasculitis, and hemolytic uremic syndrome
- Secondary glomerular disease such as systemic lupus erythematosus
- Tubulo-interstitial diseases such as pyelonephritis and analgesic nephropathy
- Kidney stone disease
- Secondary damage from other systemic diseases such as sickle cell anemia and amyloidosis
- Toxic metals and chemicals—cadmium, mercury, lead, perfluoroalkyls, diamino dyes, toluene, and trichloroethane
- Infectious diseases such as HIV nephropathy, renal tuberculosis, and post-streptococcal infection syndrome
- Hematologic causes such as multiple myeloma
- Hereditary kidney diseases such as Alport's syndrome
- Metabolic diseases such as gouty nephropathy and oxalosis

metabolic bone disease, and soft tissue deposition of oxalates, beta2-microglobulin, and phosphates.

5. Blood pressure regulation: Development of hypertension is one of the early complications of kidney dysfunction, which in turn accelerates the progress of kidney disease.

6. Endocrine mediators:
   - Reduced production of erythropoietin at GFRs below 60 ml/min, leading to renal anemia and its complications
   - Renin angiotensin system activation, leading to hypertension and endothelial damage
   - Impaired conversion of vitamin D precursors to 1,25 OH_2 vitamin D, leading to renal bone disease, immune dysfunction, increased cardiovascular risk, and increased rate of progression of renal failure
   - Secondary hyperparathyroidism at GFRs below 60ml/min, leading to metabolic bone disease and disseminated soft tissue calcification
   - Prolonged half-life of peptide hormones due to reduced degradation, including insulin, glucagon, growth hormone, parathyroid hormone, prolactin, gastrin, and follicle-stimulating hormone

PATIENT EVALUATION

The symptoms and signs of chronic kidney failure often develop insidiously and late; it is unusual for the diagnosis to be reached due to symptomatic presentation. Abnormalities are often found in the course of routine medical checks or in the assessment of patients with other medical conditions associated with kidney disease. It is therefore important to detect abnormalities prior to the onset of irreversible damage. The progression of renal disease can be modified, but in most cases it is not possible to restore kidney function once lost. It is in the aforementioned group of patients that a specific diagnosis may be made and interventions meant to preserve kidney function put into place; some of which could be based on lifestyle changes and nutritional interventions. Given the multitude of causes leading to kidney failure, the most important part of the initial evaluation of the patient is a careful medical history to pinpoint the factors potentially involved in inducing kidney damage. Underlying conditions such as systemic diseases affecting the kidneys should be sought and treated. Primary renal inflammatory diseases must be diagnosed and possible underlying infectious, environmental, or dietary factors identified and modulated. The following factors contribute to the initiation and progression of kidney disease.

HYPERTENSION AND VASCULAR DISEASE

Hypertension is not only a major cause of kidney disease, but also determines the rate of progression of kidney failure [5]. The target blood pressure for CKD patients is less than 130/80. Patients with greater proteinuria were shown to derive more benefit from tighter blood pressure control in a National Institutes of Health–funded study of 840 adults with CKD of various origins entitled Modification of Diet in Renal Disease [6]. Nutritional and lifestyle modifications included restrictions in dietary sodium and alcohol intake, along with exercise and weight loss. After 10 years, the incidence of kidney failure in the low blood pressure group was only 0.68, the incidence in the usual blood pressure group. The type of medication used to lower blood pressure did not influence the results.

UNCONTROLLED DIABETES MELLITUS AND METABOLIC SYNDROME

The metabolic syndrome is defined as three or more of the following factors: elevated blood sugar, low HDL cholesterol, high triglycerides, elevated blood pressure, and abdominal obesity. The metabolic syndrome has long been recognized as a significant risk factor for heart disease, stroke, and diabetes. In a study by Chen et al. that identified metabolic syndrome as a risk factor for the development of chronic renal disease, the odds ratio of chronic kidney disease (GFR less than 60) was 2.6 in persons with metabolic syndrome compared to normal [7]. The odds ratio of kidney disease for individuals with four components of the metabolic syndrome was 4.2, and for those with five components it was 5.8. The risk for microalbuminuria (urinary albumin-creatinine ratio of 30–300 mg/gm) increased in a similar fashion. Individually and collectively, low HDL and high triglycerides, obesity, high blood pressure, and glucose intolerance correlated strongly with the development of renal disease. There is a direct association between obesity, glomerular hyper-filtration, and development of proteinuria and kidney damage. Lifestyle measures addressing obesity will reduce the risk of established renal failure in morbid obesity [8].

URINARY OUTFLOW TRACT OBSTRUCTION

Patients with CKD must be assessed to rule out obstruction to the flow of urine from the urinary tract.

NEPHROTOXIC MEDICINES AND REMEDIES

Prescription and nonprescription drugs frequently damage renal function. A variety of drugs such as different classes of antibiotics, antiviral agents, diuretics, nonsteroidal anti-inflammatory drugs (NSAIDs), xanthine oxidase inhibitors, anticonvulsants, immunosuppresants, and chemotherapeutic agents are known to cause acute or chronic renal problems.

The use of statin drugs (HMG-CoA reductase inhibitors) is controversial in kidney disease. Statins may cause rhabdomyolysis-causing tubular toxicity [9]. Recent studies have revealed no significant reduction of cardiovascular events in dialysis patients receiving statins, despite the lowering of cholesterol [10].

Radio-contrast dyes are a frequent cause of acute renal toxicity but may lead to permanent damage in advanced cases of CKD. Prevention of contrast-induced nephropathy requires adequate hydration with intravenous saline and N-acetylcysteine before and the day after the procedure [11]. The magnetic resonance imaging contrast injectable gadolinium may cause a severe systemic reaction in people with pre-existing renal disease causing nephrogenic systemic fibrosis [12]. The condition is progressive and usually irreversible, having no effective treatment. It is crucial to measure serum creatinine prior to injecting gadolinium in any patient.

Aristolochic acid, a Chinese herb used primarily for weight loss, may cause chronic interstitial nephritis. It also causes urological malignancies and was responsible for the deaths of more than 60 people in China and several cases of renal failure in Belgium, England, and other European countries [13].

EXPOSURE TO ENVIRONMENTAL AND OCCUPATIONAL TOXINS

Several studies have pointed to the role of environmental toxins in the development of renal disease [14–16]. Owing to its diverse function and small mass in relation to the high percentage of cardiac output that it handles, the kidney is a target for both toxic and pharmacologically active chemicals. Avoidance of exposure to heavy metals and volatile hydrocarbons and their derivatives, mainly in individuals with diagnosed renal disorders, remains the best approach toward a substantial reduction in the burden of renal diseases. However, it is possible to use nutrients such as phospholipids, glutathione, and methylation factors as well as treatment with appropriate chelating agents to reduce the total body burden of these toxins.

There are numerous reports on the toxic effects of heavy metals on the kidney [17]. These include lead, cadmium, mercury, arsenic, industrial chromium, beryllium, germanium, gold, aluminum, and uranium [18,19]. Whilst the body burden of some of these metals such as lead may be reduced with treatments such as chelation, others such as cadmium appear resistant to such interventions.

Solvents have also been associated with kidney damage. These include perfluoroalkyl chemicals that are highly prevalent in the population. A recent study by Shankar et al. showed that in the United States there was a significant association between PFC exposure and CKD [20]. There have been cases of kidney failure reported in the literature with substance abuse (naphthalene, paradicholoro-benzene from mothballs), toluene, trichloroethane [21], and other volatile organic compounds. One study has shown a high prevalence of renal impairment, proteinuria, and hematuria in hairdressers exposed to paraphenyldiamine dyes as well as bromates used in hairdressing salons [22].

ALLERGIES AND INTOLERANCES

Despite well-established studies of immune mechanisms in glomerular pathology, there has been only marginal interest in the role of allergens in particular foods as immune sensitizers in kidney disease. Some studies have demonstrated a higher incidence of atopy in patients with glomerulo-nephritis although other studies have not replicated these findings. There are also clear published reports linking food allergy to renal disease—in particular reports by both Matsumura's and Sandberg's groups looking at patients with childhood nephrotic syndrome due to minimal change disease, membranous glomerulopathy, and anaphylactoid purpura [23–25]. They published results of clinical studies of large number of children as well as adults with nephrosis in whom prolonged remission was achieved through implementing exclusion diets [26,27]. Foods identified as allergens included cow's milk, chicken egg, wheat, beef, and pork. Human basophil degranulation tests were used to confirm a role for food antigens [27].

A few reports of aeroallergens triggering relapses in patients with minimal change disease have also been reported. These report relapses of nephrosis on exposure to dust mites, seasonal pollens, and animal dander [28,29]. Such cases demonstrate a potential role for IgE-mediated reaction within the kidney. Interestingly, treatment with the antihistamine sodium cromoglycate has been effective in preventing relapses in some cases of nephrotic syndrome [27].

IgA nephropathy (IgAN) is the most common type of glomerulonephritis and leads to kidney failure in about 25% of patients. Disease recurs in transplanted kidneys, and causes graft failure in a significant proportion of transplants. In IgAN patients, treatments have been implemented to eliminate antigens. These include the use of antibiotics, tonsillectomy, and gluten- and antigen-free diets. There appears to be a close association between IgAN and inflammatory bowel disease and celiac disease [30]. Gluten-free diets in these patients have lead to reduced proteinuria [31]. Coppo et al. have experi-mentally induced IgAN by oral immunization with alimentary antigens. Likewise, her group showed that exclusion of gluten reduced circulatory IgA immune complexes. High levels of IgA antigliadin, glutenin, glyc-gli, bovine serum albumin, casein, soya bean protein, rice protein, and ovalbumin spe-cific antibodies have been identified in patients with IgAN [32]. Two studies have shown the presence of mesangial deposition of food antigens bound to IgA antibodies [33]. A low-antigen diet reduced the degree of proteinuria and reduced the IgA, complement, and fibrinogen deposits on repeat biopsy [34].

Patients with IgAN are known to have alterations in the IgA glycosylation. It may be that food and bacterial antigens determine the pattern of glycosylation, which may in turn lead to increased mesangial deposition and inflammation.

Patients with gastrointestinal candidiasis appear to be prone to increased hypersensitivity reac-tions both to foods and perhaps also to the fungal antigens themselves. In this context, a recent small-scale pilot study by Ranganathan et al. showed a renoprotective effect from the use of a pro-biotic preparation in patients with chronic kidney disease [35].

OTHER FACTORS CONTRIBUTING TO PROGRESSION OF KIDNEY DISEASE

These include uncontrolled proteinuria, inflammation, deposition of crystals (which act both as a complication and a risk factor of kidney disease) and proteins such as amyloid, metabolic abnor-malities such as hyperuricemia, acidemia, and high-protein/high-phosphorus diets.

DIAGNOSTICS

Investigations aim to stage the degree of renal dysfunction, characterize the type of renal injury, and elucidate the underlying causes of kidney disease. A wide range of laboratory, radiological, and histological tools are available to this end.

The five stages of kidney disease, as classified by the United States Kidney Disease Outcome Quality Initiative (US KDOQI) group are based on the level of estimated glomerular filtration rate:

Stage 1: Normal GFR; (GFR > 90 mL/min/1.73 m^2) with other evidence of CKD*
Stage 2: Mild loss of kidney function (GFR 60–89) with other evidence of CKD*
Stage 3: Moderate loss of kidney function (GFR 30–59)
Stage 4: Severe loss of kidney function (GFR 15–29)
Stage 5: Established kidney failure (GFR < 15 or on dialysis)

* The other evidence of chronic kidney disease may be one of the following:

- Persistent microalbuminuria
- Persistent proteinuria
- Persistent hematuria (after exclusion of other causes, e.g., urological disease)
- Structural abnormalities of the kidneys
- Biopsy proven chronic glomerulonephritis

Two measurements of kidney function should be made—glomerular filtration rate (GFR) and the degree of albuminuria. A routine chemistry panel provides the level of creatinine. Utilizing this number along with age, weight, and sex in the Cockroft-Gault equation calculates the GFR: GFR in ml/min = (140–age) × (weight in kg) × (0.85 for women and 1 for men)/72 × creatinine.

Albuminuria, or protein loss through the kidneys, is a marker for the degree of renal damage. Microalbuminuria, especially in diabetics, occurs prior to the rise of serum creatinine. This may be assessed using special urine dipsticks or by measuring the ratio of albumin to creatinine, in an early morning urine sample. Monitoring albuminuria offers information on the degree of glomerular damage and rate of loss of renal function, since the rate of loss of GFR increases with the rate of protein loss. Additionally, the degree of albuminuria correlates with the risk of other complications, including myocardial infarction, stroke, and congestive heart failure. Controlling proteinuria is the key to preservation of kidney function. This may be achieved in a number of ways including medication, dietary manipulations, and specific nutrient supplementation.

NUTRITIONAL INTERVENTIONS

These may be considered in two parts, those to treat the causes of kidney disease and prevent progression of kidney failure and those to support the patient in preventing complications of advanced and end-stage kidney disease.

PREVENTION OF PROGRESSIVE KIDNEY DISEASE

Treating comorbid conditions is important in prevention especially hypertension, diabetes, and glomerulonephritis.

Hypertension

The single most important intervention is to establish a normotensive state. In general, angiotensin-converting enzyme (ACE) inhibitors and angiotensin II receptor blockers (ARBs) are used for blood pressure control in patients with renal impairment because of their superior effects on proteinuria.

Protein intake also influences blood pressure. The International Study of Macronutrients and Blood Pressure confirmed that more vegetable protein, but not animal protein, was associated with lower blood pressure [36]. The Dietary Approaches to Stop Hypertension (DASH) study revealed that salt restriction and an increase in protein intake from 14% to 18% of calories reduced systolic and diastolic blood pressure in both hypertensive and nonhypertensive subjects [37]. Primitive populations eating unprocessed foods have an intake of potassium greater than 150 mmol per day, a sodium intake of 20–40 mmol per day, and a ratio of dietary potassium to sodium of 3–10/1. By contrast, industrialized societies ingest foods with a potassium-to-sodium ratio of less than 0.4. The long-term effect of potassium depletion is to further promote sodium retention creating a vicious cycle of hypertension and vascular disease. The forms of potassium not containing chloride, such as those found in fruits and vegetables, allow more effective cellular exchange of sodium for potassium and a better antihypertensive effect [38]. Finally, in our practice we have had several cases of hypertension associated with food intolerance. Exclusion of the sensitizing food (often grains) results in a significant diuresis, weight loss, and correction of previously intractable hypertension. Nutrients that support optimal blood pressure control are discussed in detail in the chapter on hypertension.

Diabetes and Metabolic Syndrome

The medical literature indicates that more than 50% of diabetes type 2 is preventable using lifestyle changes in cases of impaired glucose tolerance [39]. Metabolic syndrome and diabetic nephropathy can be effectively controlled on a diet devoid of refined carbohydrates and with adequate nutrient density. Compared with a low-fat diet, such a diet has superior effects on systolic blood pressure, glucose levels, and cholesterol/HDL ratio [40]. A comprehensive approach to the management of diabetes and insulin resistance does not stop with pharmacotherapy. The chapter on diabetes presents food, nutrient, and other lifestyle interventions. Nutrients that may be used for optimizing glycemic control safely in the presence of pre-existing kidney disease include:

1. Chromium—up to 1000 mcg/day in divided doses. Facilitates glucose uptake into cells [41]. There are a few reports of acute tubular necrosis in patients who have taken chromium supplements in excessive doses.
2. Vanadium—50 mg/day enhances insulin action with no evidence of toxicity at this dose [42].
3. Alpha-lipoic acid—300-1800 mg/day. Improves insulin sensitivity, also effective in treating diabetic neuropathy. It is a strong antioxidant and detoxifier, regenerates vitamins C and E, and glutathione [43].
4. Biotin—3000 mcg/day. Improves both insulin sensitivity and diabetic neuropathy [44].
5. Oil of evening primrose—2–4 g daily according to red blood cell (RBC) fatty acid analysis,
6. Cinnamon—as a spice and in supplemental doses of cinnaminic acid 150 mg/day.

GLOMERULONEPHRITIS

The mainstay of management of glomerulonephritis has been the use of immunosuppression regimens. A subset of patients responds to formal exclusion diets and antigen avoidance. We have reported an unpublished case of a patient with recurrence of end-stage focal and segmental glomerulosclerosis in the transplanted kidney whose severe proteinuria was curbed and the need for thrice weekly plasma exchange reduced to monthly by identification of allergy to a number of aeroallergens and desensitization using low-dose immunotherapy.

Fish oils may reduce proteinuria and protect kidney function through a reducing vasoconstriction and proinflammatory eicosanoids and decreasing cytokine release [45]. Donadio et al. found omega-3 fatty acids were effective in slowing the rate of renal dysfunction in high-risk patients with IgA nephropathy, particularly those with moderately advanced disease. In another study, 10 g/day of EPA and DHA was given to 10 patients with focal sclerosis or membranous glomerulonephritis [46]. Proteinuria declined from 3.7 g/day to 2.6 g/day at week six, when treatment was stopped. The decline in proteinuria persisted for another 12 weeks, and then returned to prior levels.

Dietary protein restriction as a therapeutic means in chronic renal failure has been in and out of favor amongst nephrologists. When animals with renal injury were fed a high-protein diet, renal failure ensued, while a low-protein diet slowed the progression. High-protein diets may aggravate renal disease by stimulating cellular hypertrophy and proliferation, glomerular scarring, increasing reactive oxygen species, creating an acid load causing ammonium production and complement formation, increasing urea formation, causing hypertrophy of renal tubules, and generating aldosterone and angiotensin. On the other hand, renal patients often suffer from renal cachexia and are in a catabolic state; therefore, restriction of protein intake results in a further negative nitrogen balance. There is currently no consensus on the role of low-protein diets in renal disease amongst nephrologists.

Food and Nutrients in Delaying Progression of Chronic Kidney Disease Apart from Any Comorbidity

Vitamin D deficiency is widely associated with chronic kidney disease and cardiovascular disease. There is increasing evidence that it may also accelerate renal disease progression [47]. Dysregulation of vitamin D metabolism caused by renal insufficiency causes low vitamin D status. A number of studies have demonstrated impressive therapeutic outcome with both vitamin D supplementation and low-calcemic vitamin D analogues in renal and cardiovascular disease. The mechanism underlying the renal and cardiovascular protection involves regulation of multiple signaling pathways by vitamin D including nuclear factor κB, Wnt/β-catenin, FGF-23, Klotho, and the renin angiotensin aldosterone system (RAAS) [48,49]. Vitamin D is known to act as a transcription factor to suppress the renin gene leading to RAAS blockade, reduction in proteinuria, and fibrosis. This signifies a cross-conversation between the kidney and the cardiovascular system and marks a simple path for reducing both renal and cardiovascular risk.

Vitamin A levels are elevated in CKD. However, a study by Ayazi and coworkers demonstrated the protective role for prevention of renal scarring in patients with pyelonephritis [50]. Fifty children with first-time pyelonephritis verified by an uptake defect on dimercaptosuccinic acid (DMSA) scan were randomly allocated to the case or control groups. All were given antibiotics. Cases in addition were given a single intramuscular dose of vitamin A, 25,000 IU for infants below one year of age and 50,000 IU for older children. Repeat DMSA scan after three months, showed five of 25 cases (20%) and 17 of 25 controls (68%) had renal scarring (p = 0.001). They concluded that administration of vitamin A was associated with a significantly lower rate of renal damage.

Increased oxidative stress and reduced antioxidant activity are associated with declining renal function. In this respect, the use of dietary selenium supplementation in renal transplant recipients has shown beneficial effects in reducing plasma and LDL lipid peroxidation via activation of the glutathione system, thus reducing atherogenesis and the potential for transplant vasculopathy [51].

Other antioxidants: A number of compounds with known potent antioxidant properties have been investigated in animal models of renal ischaemic reperfusion injury and acute renal failure. These include curcumin and curcuminoids, flavagenol proanthocyanidins, gingerol, ginsenoside, and buckwheat. They have all shown the capacity to reduce oxidative damage in their respective experimental models but whether these may be extrapolated into clinical scenarios is unclear. Certainly future studies to assess any protective role in the context of progression to end-stage kidney disease are necessary.

Lifestyle changes: Cigarette smoking has been shown to effect the rate of progression of kidney disease. In studies looking at the effect of smoking, cessation of smoking reduced the rate of disease progression. Tobacco smoke is a major source of exposure to cadmium (Cd). Urine Cd levels (CdU) above 1.0, 0.7, and 0.5 µgCd/g creatinine have been associated with increased rates of microproteinuria and reduction in glomerular filtration rate. Mortensen et al. have reported cigarette smoking greatly increases the relative risk of exceeding renal risk–associated CdU, which increased with age in current smokers [52].

Chelation therapy with Ethylenediaminetetraacetic acid (EDTA) has been offered as a treatment for cardiovascular disease and more recent evidence indicates that it may also delay the progression of renal disease. Investigators in Taiwan studied patients with chronic renal insufficiency (creatinine 1.5–3.9 mg/dl) [53]. One gram of calcium disodium EDTA was infused over two hours, and urine lead was measured in a 72-hour collection. Patients with urinary lead excretion over 80 mcg were assigned to either weekly chelation therapy or placebo. Chelation therapy was provided weekly for 24 months. GFR increased by 11.9% in the chelation therapy group, while declining in the control group. The body lead burden prior to therapy was similar to that in the general population. Results suggest that chronic low-level environmental lead exposure may aggravate the progression of chronic renal disease and that chelation therapy may delay progression in patients with chronic renal disease.

Phospholipids: Early studies by Szymanski and Jacyszyn reported favorable results from the treatment of nephrotic syndrome with infusions of phosphatidylcholine [54]. In a further study, Jacyszyn also found significant reduction in serum creatinine in a group of patients with moderate renal insufficiency with intravenous infusion followed by oral phosphatidylcholine. Other studies have looked at the effect of phosphatidylcholine on proteinuria in nephrotic children and found a significant improvement in a subset of patients [55].

ADVANCED AND END-STAGE KIDNEY DISEASE

Cardiovascular mortality in dialysis patients is extremely high, 25% per year, somewhat related to pre-existing disease. Homocysteine levels are markedly elevated. Treatment with high doses of folic acid, vitamin B12, and vitamin B6, while reducing homocysteine levels, has not affected cardiovascular complications significantly [56]. Cholesterol levels are also often elevated in dialysis patients, but treatment with statin drugs has not improved survival [57]. The results suggest a different pathophysiology of cardiovascular disease in dialysis patients, perhaps related to the dialysis process itself or vascular calcification. Vitamin D is believed to significantly reduce the cardiovascular complications of renal disease. Furthermore, a study on antioxidant treat- ment in patients on hemodialysis has shown that the use of silymarin and vitamin E reduced the levels of malondialdehyde, but significantly increased the levels of glutathione peroxidase and hemoglobin [58].

Amino acid metabolism changes: Taurine and L-carnitine levels are depressed in dialysis patients, impairing the beta-oxidation of long chain fatty acids in mitochondria and peroxisomes, thus affect- ing energy production. L-carnitine supplementation is often provided either intravenously or orally, mainly to patients with muscle weakness, cramps, cardiomyopathy, anemia, and hypotension. The oral dose is 0.5 grams per day.

Phosphorus levels rise in chronic renal failure, lowering serum calcium and leading to hyper- parathyroidism. This causes increased morbidity and mortality. Reduced phosphorus intake plus calcium carbonate, citrate, or acetate supplementation can effectively lower phosphorus levels.

Calcium requirements increase in renal failure because of impaired renal production of 1,25-dihydroxyvitamin D and resistance to vitamin D actions. Further, the low-protein and low-phosphorus diet is also low in calcium. Most renal failure patients on low-protein diets require supplemental calcium of 1000–1400 mg/day. All patients with CKD should be supplemented with 1,25 dihydroxy vitamin D (calcitriol) or a related compound such as alpha-calcidol or paricalcitol.

Patients with advanced renal disease or on dialysis may be depleted of water-soluble vitamins and certain minerals. Anorexia, poor food intake, and the protein-limited diet cause these defi- ciencies, along with altered metabolism, prescribed medications, and the dialysis process itself. Vitamin B6, vitamin C, and folic acid are most often deficient. Vitamin C should not be given in doses higher than 60 mg/day. Ascorbic acid may be converted to oxalate, which is highly insoluble and may be deposited in tissues, thus aggravating renal insufficiency. Vitamin A levels are elevated in uremia, and vitamin A should not be supplemented. Doses above 7500 IU/day may cause bone toxicity.

A number of studies have looked at interventions to support renal patients on dialysis. Many studies have examined ways of improving the overall health of these patients through optimizing erythropoeisis. Nutritional factors that contribute to renal anemia include low iron stores, uncontrolled tertiary hyperparathyroidism, and B vitamin deficiencies—in particular vitamin B12 and folic acid, and aluminum intoxication. These may be corrected by appropriate supplementation for any identified deficiencies as well as avoidance of exposure to aluminum. Treatment with pulsed vitamin D will also help control hyperparathyroidism. Vitamin C has also been identified as an adjuvant in treating erythropoeitin resistant renal anemia. It is thought that Vitamin C improves hemoglobin levels through mobilization of iron stores for the synthesis of heme. Many patients on hemodialysis have features of scurvy such as bleeding gums, fatigue, increased susceptibility to infection, as well as increased bone resorption. Low doses of vitamin C supplementation may help with these complications and will avoid the complications of oxalosis.

By scavenging reactive oxygen species, antioxidant compounds can attenuate oxidative stress and lipid peroxidation. Several animal and human studies have suggested that antioxidant vitamins such as vitamins C and E might reduce oxidative stress caused by reperfusion injury and calcineurin inhibitor nephrotoxicity in renal transplant recipients. In one study, five patients supplemented with vitamin C (500 mg per day), vitamin E (500 mg per day), or both in the first three months after kidney transplantation exhibited more than 20% reduction in serum creatinine levels. The serum creatinine levels increased by more than 50% on discontinuing the vitamins [59].

Phospholipids have been shown to have a positive effect on ultra-filtration rates in patients on continuous ambulatory peritoneal dialysis (CAPD). Peritoneal mesothelial cells normally secrete a surfactant-like substance consisting mainly of phosphatidylcholine. It lowers the surface tension, repels water, and acts as a lubricant. The phospholipid content in the dialysis effluent of CAPD patients decreased with time especially in those with low ultra-filtration or peritonitis. Di Paolo and coworkers found that addition of phosphatidylcholine into the CAPD bags resulted in significant increase in ultra-filtration and creatinine and urea clearance [60].

CLINICAL SUMMARY

Kidney disease is largely a consequence of hypertension, obesity, diabetes, metabolic syndrome, renal inflammation, drugs, and environmental toxicities. Correction and prevention of these conditions will reduce the incidence of renal failure at a population level.

At the patient care level early diagnosis is critical for subsequent treatment. Kidney disease is often not discovered until it is advanced, when the opportunity to reverse the damage has become remote. To facilitate prompt diagnosis, physicians may want to be vigilant for the following:

- Increasing serum creatinine, even within the normal range.
- Proteinuria correlating with advancing kidney disease.
- Increasing hypertension.
- Possible drug toxicities, especially in patients taking one or more drugs, such as nonsteroidal anti-inflammatory drugs and antibiotics, known to cause kidney damage.
- Possible environmental/occupational exposure to xenobiotics and biotoxins.
- Possible role for allergies and intolerances.

If renal impairment is detected early, and corrective measures are implemented, it need not progress. An example of a comprehensive approach incorporating food and nutrients is presented in Table 25.3.

TABLE 25.3
Therapeutic Options

Approaches to Preventing Progression of Kidney Disease and Its Associated Complications

Lifestyle, Dietary, and Environmental Therapies
- Stop smoking cigarettes (cadmium exposure is of particular concern)
- Exercise
- Avoid excessive caloric intake
- Moderate alcohol intake, among those who drink at all
- Maintain adequate hydration
- Avoid refined carbohydrates
- Choose a nutrient-dense diet with a balance of protein, complex carbohydrates, and fatty acids
- Consume foods rich in bioflavinoids, curcuminoids, and other antioxidants
- Restrict processed foods containing high levels of salts
- Consider a trial of a food allergy elimination diet, possibly adding low-dose antigen-specific immunotherapy for food hypersensitivity
- Avoid nephrotoxic exposures through occupation and recreation
- Avoid aeroallergens, possibly using adjunct low-dose antigen-specific immunotherapy

Nutrient Supplementation
- Vitamin D3 according to blood vitamin D, parathyroid hormone, calcium, and phosphate levels
- Calcium 1.4–1.6 g/day
- Magnesium 200 mg daily but check red cell magnesium levels to avoid hypermagnesemia in advanced kidney disease
- Iron, folic acid, vitamin B12 according to levels and serum hemoglobin
- Antioxidants: vitamin E 400 IU daily, vitamin C 500 mg daily whilst monitoring levels, selenium 200 ug daily as required and according to plasma levels
- Zinc, copper, and manganese to support superoxide dismutase function as necessary according to plasma levels
- Support for sulphation pathways using branched chain amino acids, N-acetylcysteine 500 mg BD, and molybdenum in the presence of detectable urinary sulphites
- Essential fatty acids: gamma-linolenic acid 2–6 g/day and omega-3 EFAs according to results of red cell fatty acid analyses
- Phospholipids: oral or intravenous phosphatidylcholine for cell membrane regeneration and reduction in total body burden of xenobiotics

Medical Interventions That May Slow the Progression of Kidney Disease
- Control of proteinuria using ACE inhibitors
- Have patients with diabetes maintain tight glycemic control using dietary measures, oral hypoglycemics, and nutrient supplements carefully; adjust doses for CKD: biotin, GLA, vanadium, α lipoic acid, chromium, and cinnamic acid
- Have patients adhere to tight blood pressure control, incorporating food and nutrient interventions where possible
- Consider immunosuppression therapy in patients with glomerulonephritis or vasculitis
- Avoid nephrotoxic medications
- Prescribe EDTA chelation therapy in patients with concomitant cardiovascular disease or high burden of heavy metals such as lead. Dose adjustment is needed according to GFR
- Treat dysbiosis or other chronic infections, by addressing the predisposing factors such as chronic use of antibiotics, steroids, or hormonal exposures. Use a diet devoid of refined carbohydrates, sugar, and fermented foods to redress any disturbances in the microflora. Add intra-luminal antifungals such as Nystatin where indicated and consider supplemental probiotics

REFERENCES

1. CDC National Chronic Kidney Disease Fact Sheet: General information and national estimates on chronic kidney disease in the United States, 2010.
2. Saydah S, Eberhardt M, Rios-Burrows N et al. Prevalence of chronic kidney disease and associated risk factors in U.S.A. 1999–2004. MMWR. 2007;56(08):161–5.
3. Goldman L, et al. *Cecil Medicine*. 23rd edition, Saunders Elsevier. 2008;922.

4. *USRDS 2010 Annual Report*, United States Renal Data System Website. November 2010. http://www.urds.org/atlas10.aspx.

5. Initiative KDOQ: K/DOQI clinical practice guidelines on hypertension and antihypertensive agents in chronic kidney disease. Am J Kidney Dis. 2004;43:S1–S290.

6. Sarnak M, Greene T, Wang X, et al. The effect of a lower target blood pressure on the progression of kidney disease: Long-term follow-up of the Modification of Diet in Renal Disease Study. Ann Intern Med. 2005;142:342–51.

7. Chen J, Munter P, Hamm L, et al. The metabolic syndrome and chronic kidney disease in U.S. adults. Ann Intern Med. 2004;140:167–74.

8. Morales E, Valero MA, Leon M, et al. Beneficial effects of weight loss in overweight patients with chronic proteinuric nephropathies. Am J Kidney Dis 2003;41(2):319–27.

9. Goldman L, et al. *Cecil Medicine*. 23rd edition, Saunders Elsevier. 2008;863.

10. Fellström B, Holdaas H, Jardine AG et al. Effect of Rosuvastatin on outcomes in chronic haemodialysis patient: Baseline data from the AURORA Study. Kidney Blood Press Res. 2007; Sep;30(5): 314–22.

11. Kelly A, Dwamena B, Cronin P et al. Meta-analysis: Effectiveness of drugs for preventing contrast-induced nephropathy. Ann Intern Med. 2008;148:284–94.

12. Broome DR. Nephrogenic systemic fibrosis associated with gadolinium based contrast agents: A summary of the medical literature reporting. Eur J Radiol. 2008 May;66(2):230–4.

13. Debelle FD, Vanherweghem JL, Nortier JL. Aristolochic acid nephropathy: A worldwide problem. Kidney Int. 2008;Jul;74(2):158–69.

14. Franchini I, Alinovi R, Bergamaschi E et al. Contribution of studies on renal effects of heavy metals and selected organic compounds to our understanding of the progression of chronic nephropathies towards renal failure. ACTA BIOMED. 2005;Suppl 2; 58–67.

15. Wedeen RP. Occupational and environmental renal disease. Semin Nephrol. 1997;Jan;17(1):46–53.

16. Staessen JA, Nawrot T, Hond ED et al. Renal function, cytogenetic measurements, and sexual development in adolescents in relation to environmental pollutants: A feasibility study of biomarkers. Lancet. 2001;May;26;357(9269):1660–9.

17. Fowler BA. Mechanisms of kidney cell injury from metals. Environ Health Perspectives. 1992;100:57–63.

18. Vacca CV, Hines JD, Hall PW, III. The proteinuria of industrial lead intoxication. Environ Res. 1986; Dec;41(2):440–6.

19. Ding X, Zhang Q, Wei H, Zhang Z. Cadmium-induced renal tubular dysfunction in a group of welders. Occup Med (Lond). 2011;Jun;61(4):277–9.

20. Shankar A, Xiao J, Ducatman A. Perfluoroalkyl chemicals and chronic kidney disease in US adults. Am J Epidemiol. 2011;Oct;15;174(8):893–900.

21. Bruning T, Sundberg AG, Birner G et al. Glutathione transferase alpha as a marker for tubular damage after trichloroethylene exposure. Arch Toxicol. 1999;Jun–Jul;73(4–5):246–54.

22. Hamdouk M, Abdelraheem M, Taha A et al. The association between prolonged occupational exposure to paraphenylenediamine (hair-dye) and renal impairment. Arab J Nephrol Transplant. 2011;Jan;4(1):21–5.

23. Matsumura T, Koroume T, Fukushima I. The role of allergy in the pathogenesis of nephrotic syndrome. Jpn J Pediatr. 1961;14:921.

24. Sandberg DH, McLeod TF, Strauss J. Renal disease related to hypersensitivity to foods. In *Food Allergy: New Perspectives*. Gerrard JW, ed. Springfield: Charles C Thomas, 1980;144.

25. Sandberg DH, McIntosh RM, Bernstein CW et al. Severe steroid-responsive nephrosis associated with hypersensitivity. Lancet. 1977;I:388.

26. Laurent J, Rostoker G, Robeva R et al. Is adult nephrotic syndrome food allergy? Nephron. 1987;47:7–11.

27. Lagrue G, Heslan JM, Belghiti D et al. Basophil sensitisation for food allergens in idiopathic nephrotic syndrome. Nephron. 1986;42:123–7.

28. Reeves WG, Cameron JS, Johansson SGO et al. Seasonal nephrotic syndrome. Clin Allergy. 1975; 5:121–37.

29. Williams DG. Allergy and the kidney. In: *Allergy: Immunological and Clinical Aspects,* Lessof MH, ed. New York: Wiley, 1984:373.

30. Collin P, Syrjänen J, Partanen J et al. Celiac disease and HLADQ in patients with IgA nephropathy. Am J Gastroenterol. 2002;Oct;97(10):2572–6.

31. Takemura T, Okada M, Yagi K, et al. An adolescent with IgA nephropathy and Crohn's disease: Pathogenetic implications. Pediatr Nephrol. 2002;17(10):863–6.

32. Coppo R, Roccatello D, Amore A, Quattrocchio G, et al. Effects of a gluten-free diet in primary IgA nephropathy. Clin Nephrol. 1990;Feb;33(2):72–86.

33. Sato M, Kojima H, Takayama K et al. Glomerular deposition of food antigens in IgA nephropathy. Clin Exp Immunol. 1988;73:295–9.

34. Ferri C, Puccini R, Longombardo G et al. Low-antigen-content diet in the treatment of patients with IgA nephropathy. Nephro Dial Transplant. 1993;8(11):1193–8.

35. Ranganathan N, Ranganathan P, Friedman EA et al. Pilot study of probiotic dietary supplementation for promoting healthy kidney function in patients with chronic kidney disease. Adv Ther. 2010; Sep;27(9):634–47.

36. Elliot P, Stamler J, Dyer A, et al. Association between protein intake and blood pressure: The INTERMAP study. Arch Intern Med. 2006;166:79–87.

37. Sacks F, Svetkey L, Vollmer W, et al. Effects on blood pressure of reduced dietary sodium and the Dietary Approaches to Stop Hypertension (DASH) diet. NEJM. 2001;344:3–10.

38. Sinai A, Strazzullo P, Giacco A, et al. Increasing the dietary potassium intake reduces the need for antihypertensive medication. Ann Intern Med. 1991;115:753–9.

39. Tuomilehto J, Lindstrom J, Eriksson J, et al. Prevention of type 2 diabetes mellitus by changes in lifestyle among subjects with impaired glucose tolerance. NEJM. 2001;344:1343–50.

40. Estruch R, Martínez-Gonzalez MA, Corella D, et al. Effects of a Mediterranean-style diet on cardiovascular risk factors: A randomized trial. Ann Intern Med. 2006;145:1–11.

41. Anderson RA, Cheng N, Bryden NA, et al. Elevated intakes of supplemental chromium improve glucose and insulin variables in individuals with type 2 diabetes. Diabetes. 1997;46:1786–91.

42. Boden G, Chen X, Ruiz, et al. Effects of vanadyl sulfate on carbohydrate and lipid metabolism in patients with non-insulin-dependent diabetes mellitus. Metabolism. 1996;45:1130–5.

43. Jacob S, Russ P, Hermann R, et al. Oral administration of RAC-alpha-lipoic acid modulates insulin sensitivity in patients with type-2 diabetes mellitus: A placebo controlled pilot trial. Free Radic Biol Med. 1999;27:309–14.

44. Koutsikos D, Agroyannis B, Tazanatos-Exarchou. Biotin for diabetic peripheral neuropathy. Biomed Pharmacother. 1990;44:511–14.

45. De Caterina R, Caprioli R, Giannessi D, et al. N-3 fatty acids reduce proteinuria in patients with chronic glomerular disease. Kidney International. 1993;44:843–50.

46. Donadio JV, Larson TS, Bergstralh, EJ, et al. A randomized trial of high dose compared with low dose omega-3 fatty acids in severe IgA nephropathy. J Am Soc Nephrol. 2001;12(4):791–9.

47. LiYC. Vitamin D: Roles in renal and cardiovascular protection. Curr Opin Nephrol Hypertens. 2012; Jan;21(1):72–9.

48. De Borst MH, Vervloet MG, ter Wee PM et al. Cross talk between the renin-angiotensin-aldosterone system and vitamin D-FGF-23-klotho in chronic kidney disease. J Am Soc Nephrol. 2011;Sep;22(9):1603–9.

49. Shroff R, Wan M, Rees L. Can vitamin D slow down the progression of chronic kidney disease? Pediatr Nephrol. 2011;Dec 10. [epub ahead of print]

50. Ayazi P, Moshiri SA, Mahyar A et al. The effect of vitamin A on renal damage following acute pyelonephritis in children. Eur J Pediatr. 2011;170:347–50.

51. Nafar M, Sahraei Z, Salamzadeh J et al. Oxidative stress in kidney transplantation: Causes, consequences, and potential treatment. Iranian J of Kidney Dis. 2011;5(6):358–72.

52. Mortensen ME, Wong LY, Osterloh JD. Smoking status and urine cadmium above levels associated with subclinical renal effects in U.S. adults without chronic kidney disease. Int J Hyg Environ Health. 2011; Jul;214(4):305–10.

53. Lin J, Lin-Tan D, Hsu K, et al. Environmental lead exposure and progression of chronic renal disease in patients without diabetes. NEJM. 2003;348:277–86.

54. Jacyszyn K and Szymanski R. Phospholide in der Therapie der chronischen Glomerulonephritis mit nephrotischem syndrom. Med Monatsschr. 1961;15:819–22.

55. Petrushina AD, Krylov VJ, Moreva GB et al. Essentiale forte in comprehensive treatment of Glomerulonephritis in children. Pediatriya (Russ.). 1987;52–5.

56. Jamison R, Hartigan P, Kaufman J, et al. Effect of homocysteine lowering on mortality and vascular disease in advanced chronic kidney disease and end-stage renal disease. JAMA. 2007;298:1163–70.

57. Wanner C, Krane V, März W, et al. Atorvastatin in patients with type 2 diabetes mellitu undergoing hemodialysis. NEJM. 2005;353:238–48.

58. Roozbeh J, Akmali M, Vessal G et al. Comparative effects of silymarin and vitamin E supplementation on oxidative stress markers and levels of haemoglobin among patients on hemodialysis. Ren Fail. 2011; 33(2):118–23.

59. Loong CC, Chang YH, Wu TH, et al. Antioxidant supplementation may improve renal transplant function: A preliminary report. Transplant Proc. 2004;36:2438–9.

60. Di Paolo N, Buoncristiani U, Capotondo L et al. Phosphatidylcholine and peritoneal transport during peritoneal dialysis. Nephron. 1986;365–70.

Section VI

Neurologic and Psychiatric Disorders

26 Cognitive Decline

Prevention through Delay

Daniel G. Amen, M.D.

INTRODUCTION

The phrase Alzheimer's disease and related disorders (ADRD) is used to define a group of diseases that have one thing in common: each is a cause of mild cognitive impairment (MCI) or dementia. Dementia is a progressive condition with two or more impairments in mental skills that interfere with a person's ability to function in his usual manner in his social, family, personal, or professional life. Just as delayed diagnosis and treatment of high blood pressure, diabetes, heart disease, stroke, and most other diseases lead to less effective treatment results, the same holds for delayed diagnosis and treatment of ADRD.

Alzheimer's disease (AD) begins an average of 30 years before the first symptoms. The accumulation of beta amyloid plaques in the brain, the major mechanism thought to cause Alzheimer's disease, can even be seen in young adult brains. Half of U.S. families have a member with Alzheimer's disease. It affects approximately five million people in our country and the chance of developing AD doubles every five years after the age of 65. By age 85, there is a 50% chance of developing AD. The average cost to the family with a member with AD is $200,000–$400,000 over the average eight- to 10-year course of the illness. The average cost to the United States is estimated to be $100 billion annually. Beyond the financial cost, and potentially more devastating, is the severe psychological and social pain many families suffer. Losing a loved one's mind, even though they seem to have a healthy body, coupled with the chronic stress of having to caretake an adult every minute, can exact a heavy toll.

Despite how awful Alzheimer's can be, many people remain in denial because they don't believe anything can be done about it or that early awareness can lead to positive action. Contrary to popular belief, with current medical and scientific knowledge, the onset and progression of AD can be delayed by an average of six years. That delay can reduce by half the total number of people who develop the symptoms of AD. These remarkable medical and scientific advances in ADRD research allow the benefit of prevention through delay. Namely, if you can delay the onset and progression of the symptoms of a disease long enough, you will live out your natural life without suffering from that disease.

The concept of prevention through delay is very useful in preventing the disability that occurs with many diseases of aging. At 40 years of age, both men and women have more-or-less fulfilled the evolutionary purpose of perpetuating the species. After that, from a biologic perspective, the daily repair to the cells of the brain and body can no longer keep up with the daily damage, and function begins to decline. Based on what one does to protect against the variety of mechanisms that cause cell, tissue, and organ damage, the onset and progression of diseases associated with aging can be delayed. Through simple prevention strategies, there is evidence that the risk of ADRD can be cut by up to 50% [1].

PATHOPHYSIOLOGY

New Information Leads to New Prevention and Treatment Strategies

As knowledge about dementia and aging accumulate, certain patterns are becoming clear. Unlike most diseases of the young, diseases of aging involve multiple factors. When damage exceeds the brain's ability to repair itself, the first symptoms begin. For example, we now know that memory loss begins in Alzheimer's disease when the entorhinal cortex, an area involved in building new memories, loses neurons faster than they are being replaced.

It was previously thought that we have all of the brain cells we will ever have at birth. In the 1990s, together with his colleagues, William Shankle discovered that the human brain can generate new nerve cells or neurons after birth [2,3]. Subsequent discoveries by Drs. Gage, Gould, and others, demonstrated that the human and primate brain continue to make neurons in the cerebral cortex throughout the lifespan [4]. Because the numbers of neurons in each brain area tends to stay relatively constant, it was discovered that the number of new neurons produced matches the number of neurons lost in each area. However, when the production of new neurons in a brain region does not keep up with the number of neurons that are dying or being removed, then that brain region's function begins to decline. In the case of Alzheimer's disease, short-term memory begins to fail when the number of neurons in the entorhinal cortex is reduced by about one-third.

Understanding the causes of brain cell loss is relevant to understanding how to effectively prevent diseases of aging in the brain. In Alzheimer's disease, there are a number of ways brain cells die.

1. Excessive formation of free radicals, which can be toxic to brain cells. A lack of antioxidants that protect the brain from free-radical formation may be partially to blame.
2. Too much of a neurotransmitter called glutamate, which is released in large quantities when we are stressed. The right amount of glutamate helps the brain function properly, too much is toxic to brain cells.
3. An accumulation of a toxic plaque-like substance called beta amyloid (ßA) that disrupts brain cell pathways and causes short circuits in the brain.
4. Inflammation of brain tissue, although the inflammation may be a process to clear amyloid.
5. Twisting and damage to the backbone of brain cells caused by a protein called tau.

Degenerative diseases directly damage certain brain areas by destroying neurons or their supporting cells. Up to a point, the brain's repair processes can keep up with this damage. Eventually, degenerative diseases will cause more damage than can be repaired and the numbers of neurons begin to decline. However, the symptoms related to a damaged brain area do not appear until its number of neurons declines by about one-third [5]. For example, it takes between 10 and 50 years of damage to the entorhinal cortex— the first brain area affected by Alzheimer's disease— before the first symptom, memory loss for recent events, appears. At this time, between 30% and 60% of the neurons in the entorhinal cortex are lost [6].

When a symptom first appears, it may only be occasional, such as under pressure or stress. A patient may go somewhere and not remember having been there before even though it was memorable. They may not remember a conversation a few days ago that was important to them. Over time, as the disease continues to destroy brain cells, the symptom will appear more consistently.

All types of degenerative diseases usually begin after 40 years old because cells are then more susceptible to damage and death. After 40 years old, the body produces less energy due to slower metabolism. Consequently, cells are less able to produce antioxidants, which soak up free radicals (a waste product of cell activity) and prevent them from killing cells.

Programmed cell death, or apoptosis, is one important mechanism by which free radicals kill cells. Free radicals can turn on specific proteins in cells that activate death genes, which instruct cells to literally commit suicide. Apoptosis is known to occur in Alzheimer's disease, Parkinson's disease, Lewy body disease, frontal temporal lobe disease, Huntington's disease, stroke, epilepsy, and many other disorders.

Degenerative brain diseases are often due to a combination of genetic and behavioral factors. Changing behavioral patterns can change risk. The most dramatic example of this gene-behavior interaction is with Alzheimer's disease in Africans. The E4 version (allele) of the apolipoprotein E gene is the major genetic risk factor for inheriting Alzheimer's disease. Africans living in the United States who have the apolipoprotein E4 allele have an expected increased risk of Alzheimer's disease. However, Africans living below the Sahara desert who have the apolipoprotein E4 allele actually have a reduced risk of developing Alzheimer's disease [7]. One major difference between these two groups of Africans is that those living in sub-Saharan Africa eat low-fat diets and have increased exercise. The apolipoprotein E4 allele also increases risk for heart disease and stroke due to hardening of the arteries by increasing levels of low-density lipoprotein. Thus, exercise and diet may protect against the increased risk of Alzheimer's disease among those with genetic vulnerability.

The brain is classically divided into four main lobes or regions: frontal, temporal, parietal, and occipital. A useful generalization about how the brain functions is that the back half—the parietal, occipital, and back part of the temporal lobes—takes in and perceives the world. The front half of the brain integrates this information, analyzes it, decides what to do, then plans and executes the decision. All four lobes can be involved in dementia, as overviewed in Table 26.1.

Dementing diseases start by affecting a very small amount of brain, usually in just one location. Each dementing disease tends to start in its own distinctive location and can take years before enough brain damage has amassed to produce the first symptom. The specific symptom produced depends upon which brain area is damaged. As long as only one symptom exists, the condition is classified as MCI. MCI is the stage at which ADRD diseases are most easily distinguished from each other. If the disease causing MCI is not diagnosed and treated effectively, it will progress and affect other brain areas. Once enough damage accumulates in these other brain areas, additional symptoms will appear, and the dementia syndrome has begun. With further progression of the dementia, ADRD diseases share more and more of the same symptoms. Their brains also start to look the same when they are imaged. By the time dementia has become moderate or severe, diagnosing its cause is much more difficult.

DIAGNOSIS

Ninety-five percent of persons with ADRD are diagnosed years after the first symptoms appear [8]. By that time, they are moderately demented and completely dependent upon others for their care. Detecting ADRD this late is equivalent to diagnosing diabetes when the patient loses vision, has kidney failure, or can no longer feel their limbs. Annual screening for diabetes, hypertension, heart disease, cancer, and other chronic diseases facilitates early detection and effective treatment. Given that we can detect ADRD early and that early treatment can improve function, why should detecting ADRD late be acceptable to anyone, given its devastating consequences?

Unfortunately, 95% of mild dementia and 75% of moderate dementia is not detected in the primary care setting. Neither are standardized screening and diagnostic criteria currently incorporated into the practices of 75% of primary care physicians.

The following case scenario highlights the importance of early detection.

TABLE 26.1

Summary of Brain Functions by Region

Prefrontal Cortex	Temporal Lobes	Parietal Lobes	Occipital Lobes
Functions			
Judgment	Hearing/listening	Direction sense	Sight
Impulse control	Reading	Sensory perception	Color perception
Attention span	Reading social cues, including speech tone	Spatial processing, seeing motion	Lines
Organization	Short-term memory	Visual guidance, such as to grab objects	Depth
Self-monitoring	Long-term memory	Recognizing objects by touch	
Problem solving	Recognizing objects by sight	Ability to know where you are in space	
Critical thinking	Mood stability	Know right from left	
Empathy	Naming things	Reading and creating maps	
Problems			
Poor judgment	Memory problems	Impaired direction sense	Deficits in vision
Impulsivity	Reading problems	Trouble dressing or putting objects together	Deficits in perception
Short attention	Word finding problems	Left-right confusion	Visual hallucination
Disorganization	Trouble reading social cues	Denial of illness	Visual illusions
Trouble learning from experience	Mood instability	Impaired position sense	Blindsight
Confusion	Poor visual recognition	Trouble with math or writing	Functional blindness
Poor time management	Abnormal sensory perceptions	Neglect or unawareness of what you see	
Repeated mistakes	Religious or moral preoccupation	Impaired copying, drawing, or cutting	
Lack of empathy			

CASE 1

S was a 54-year-old schoolteacher who was brought in by her husband for evaluation. S had been having trouble teaching her usual classes, had angry outbursts for seemingly trivial problems, and was starting to alienate her children and colleagues. She also forgot meetings with her other teachers, was late paying bills (very unlike her), and got lost twice in a town she had lived in for 32 years. She attributed these problems to a lifelong history of anxiety combined with stress due to the loss of her father who had recently died of Alzheimer's disease. Her family doctor agreed that stress was the cause of her problems. S's husband and daughter were more concerned about her behavior than she was.

S was evaluated with a computerized screening battery, a standardized set of blood tests to diagnose treatable conditions that mimic AD, and underwent a brain single photon emotion computed tomography (SPECT) scan. The computerized screening battery and SPECT scan showed early signs of a serious problem. The SPECT scan (see Figure 26.1) showed decreased activity in the temporal and parietal lobes, a hallmark finding for AD.

S was started on a cholinesterase inhibitor, fish oil, intense daily physical exercise, a diet high in vegetables and free of processed food, and increased structure in her daily schedule. Within two months, she improved her ability to teach her classes, remember recent events, and no longer had problems driving. Her children were counseled on their risk factors for AD and given a plan on the best ways to fend off and delay AD.

Healthy (SPECT) scan:

Image 1: View from the top

Image 2: Underside view

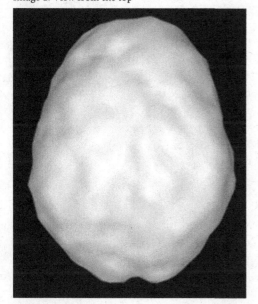

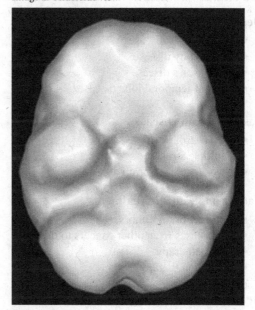

full, symmetrical activity

full, symmetrical activity

S's SPECT scan demonstrating mild cognitive impairment:

Image 3: View from the top

Image 4: Underside view

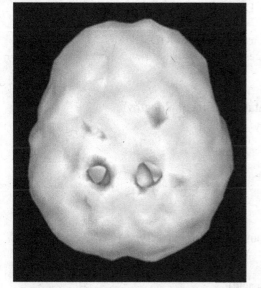

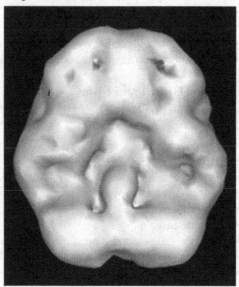

mild decreased parietal lobe activity

decreased temporal lobe activity

FIGURE 26.1 Single photon emission computed tomography (SPECT) scans images of normal brain function and mild cognitive impairment.

The Most Common Causes of Mild Cognitive Impairment and Alzheimer's Disease and Related Disorders

Degenerative Brain Diseases

- Alzheimer's disease
- Lewy body disease
- Parkinson's disease
- Frontal-temporal lobe diseases

Vascular Brain Diseases

- Large strokes
- Multiple strokes
- Strokes in deep brain areas

Cancer and Cancer Treatments

- Primary brain tumors
- Metastases from other cancers to the brain
- Chemotherapy
- Radiation therapy

Head Trauma

Infectious and Immunological Diseases

- Multiple sclerosis (MS)
- Chronic fatigue immunodeficiency syndrome (CFIDS)
- Chreutzfeld-Jakob disease (CJD or "Mad Cow Disease")
- Herpes viruses
- Human immunodeficiency viruses (HIV, the virus that causes AIDS)
- Brain infections (meningitis, encephalitis, abscess)

Alcohol and Other Brain Toxins

Disorders Affecting Nerve Cell Metabolism (Metabolic Encephalopathy)

- Depression
- Thyroid diseases
- Diabetes
- Hypoglycemia
- Kidney diseases
- Liver diseases
- Lung diseases
- Hydrocephalus (normal pressure, obstructive, and non-obstructive Types)
- Seizures (epilepsy)
- Hypoxia
- B vitamin deficiencies (B12, thiamine, or folic acid)
- High calcium levels
- High homocysteine levels
- High or low cortisol levels
- Sleep apnea (most common reversible cause of dementia)

The most common of the degenerative brain diseases that cause MCI and dementia are the following four: Alzheimer's disease, Lewy body disease, Parkinson's disease, and the frontal temporal lobe diseases.

Diagnosing Cognitive Decline

A proper diagnosis begins with a careful history, including family members, physical exam, mental status examination, cognitive testing, genetic and laboratory testing, and neuroimaging. Standard lab tests usually include: urinalysis, CBC, liver function tests, folate, homocysteine, vitamin B12, electrolyte and blood glucose, thyroid function tests, syphilis screening, HIV, erythrocyte sedimentation, apolipoprotein E genotype, fasting lipid panel, testosterone level (for men and women), and—if sleep problems are present—a sleep study to rule out sleep apnea.

GENETIC TESTING IN ALZHEIMER'S DISEASE

JAY LOMBARD, D.O.

To date, genetic studies have identified several genes associated with dementia, including apolipoprotein E (ApoE), which is the strongest and most common genetic risk factor for Alzheimer's disease (AD). There appears to be a dose-dependency of ApoE-4, such that two ApoE-alleles, (the 4/4 genotype), confer a substantially greater risk for developing Alzheimer's in comparison to those with only a single copy of the ApoE gene (3/4), who in turn are at greater risk than those without a 4 allele. [9] The presence of an ApoE 4 allele is associated with earlier symptom onset and a more rapid clinical decline [10,11] as well as with greater hippocampal atrophy [12], and cerebral hypometabolism [13].

ApoE is involved in lipid transfer, cell metabolism, repair of neuronal injury due to oxidative stress, ischemia, inflammation, amyloid-β peptide accumulation, and the aging process [14]. Although ApoE4 is over represented in AD patients, APOE4 is not a determinant of the disease; there are clearly other genetic and environmental factors which influence risk. In addition to ApoE, recent large genome-wide association studies (GWAS) have identified several other genes/loci including CR1, MS4A4, CD2AP, CD33, and ABCA7 for late-onset Alzheimer's disease [15].

The results of GWAS in Alzheimer's suggest a possible interaction of genes encoding proteins that underlie disease susceptibility. In particular, abnormal expression of these genes may be interconnected through multiple immune and lipid based pathways. For instance, The ATP-binding cassette transporter A7 gene is highly expressed in the brain and mediates the transport of a variety of physiologic lipid compounds across membrane barriers [16]. Polymorphisms of this gene may reduce amyloid efflux across the blood brain barrier. Inflammatory processes involving all components of the immune system have been implicated in the pathogenesis of AD and several gene variants support these observations. Failure of molecular and cellular mechanisms related to amyloid handling via brain-immune mechanisms may be, at least in part, a cause of AD. Genes associated with AD risk related to immune based pathways include CR1, CD33, and MS4A. CR1 encodes complement pathways which may be critical for clearance of amyloid based immune complexes [17]. The CD33 gene encodes a membrane receptor expressed by monocytes, and reduced expression of CD33 correlates with augmented production of inflammatory cytokines. It is interesting to note that CD33 expression is significantly decreased in monocytes from patients with type-2 diabetes [18]. MS4A is involved in regulatory T cell function, which helps the immune system distinguish self from non-self [19]. Genetic polymorphisms in this gene suggest an autoimmune process involved in AD pathogenesis.

Thus, gene testing in individuals offers the potential opportunity to stratify risk but even more importantly, to provide insight about disease pathogenesis and preventive treatment strategies.

NEUROIMAGING

Neuroimaging, including structural imaging (MRI and CT) and functional imaging such as SPECT, PET, and quantitative EE (QEEG) can be especially helpful in complex cases. Neuroimaging approaches are changing rapidly with technical progress. This chapter details how imaging may guide prevention of cognitive decline.

ALZHEIMER'S DISEASE

Alzheimer's disease was first described in 1906 by the German physician Alois Alzheimer after evaluating, treating, and eventually autopsying a 50-year-old woman. Her husband had complained that his wife had serious memory problems and that she relentlessly (and inaccurately) accused him of being unfaithful. Dr. Alzheimer found that the patient could recognize and describe common objects, but their names eluded her. When she was shown a cup, for instance, she described it as a milk jug. And then, several minutes later, she did not remember seeing the cup at all. Because of the naming problem, she frequently stopped mid-sentence, unable to find the right words to express herself. Upon her death, Dr. Alzheimer examined her brain using a newly developed, high-resolution microscope. He found "peculiar formations" outside of neurons and "dense tangled bundles" within them. These lesions are now known to be the signature neuritic plaques (outside neurons) and neurofiblillary tangles (within neurons) of Alzheimer's disease [20].

It is thought that there are two primary processes that cause AD: the accumulation of toxic beta amyloid plaques and the formation of neurofibrillary tangles inside neurons. Amyloid precursor protein (APP) is a normal protein (a protein is a string of amino acids) necessary for brain development and repair. After it is used, APP gets broken down into a harmless 37 amino acid fragment, which is then recycled into APP. People with Alzheimer's disease, though, have significantly higher levels of one of two enzymes, the beta and gamma secretases, which break down APP into a 40 or 42 amino acid fragment, both of which are called beta amyloid. This 42 amino acid fragment (BA42) is believed to be a major cause of the disease process in AD. BA42 fragments combine with salt and water in the brain to create a sticky mess of crisscrossing proteins (BA42 complexes). BA42 complexes damage the brain in two ways. First, normal plaques, which consist of harmless breakdown products that accumulate with age (like aging spots on your skin) are invaded by BA42 complexes to convert them into deadly neuritic plaques (Figure 26.2). Neuritic plaques disrupt the brain's normal repair process to cause short circuits to accumulate, resulting in brain dysfunction.

Image with no neuritic plaques   Image loaded with neuritic plaques

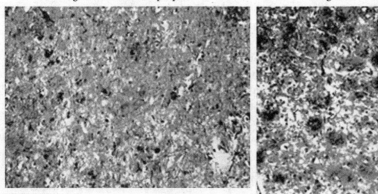 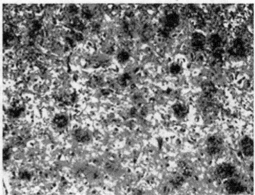

FIGURE 26.2   Microscopic images.

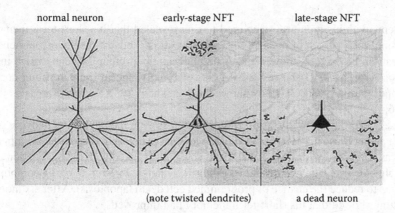

normal neuron   early-stage NFT   late-stage NFT

(note twisted dendrites)   a dead neuron

FIGURE 26.3 Neurofibrillary tangle progression.

Second, BA42 complexes cause too much calcium to enter neurons, which overexcites them and turns on death genes that program neurons to commit suicide (apoptosis).

Recently, an in vivo function for beta amyloid as an antimicrobial peptide (AMP) has been discovered. Experiments established in vitro assays to compare antimicrobial activities of beta amyloid have surprisingly revealed that it exerts antimicrobial activity against microorganisms, suggesting that it may function as an innate immune response. There is anectodal and limited evidence for infection and AD. Recently Alzheimer's disease has been associated with serological evidence of exposure to periodontal organisms and systemic inflammation. Individuals with the highest P gingivalis IgG (> 119 ELISA units (EU) were more likely to have poor delayed verbal recall and impaired subtraction. Antibodies against periodontal bacteria are elevated in AD patients and independently associated with AD. The level of positive IgG to periodontal bacteria is significantly elevated in dementia patients.

The second primary process occurs within the cells themselves. Proteins called "tau" normally form the neuron's basic shape and backbone. Microscopically, they look like steel girders that give the neuron its characteristic shape. Mutations of a gene on chromosome 17 have been found to cause the tau protein to twist, blocking the flow of molecules from the cell body to the outer regions, causing the cell to wither and die (Figure 26.3). With AD, there is a significant increase in these tangled filaments, or neurofibrillary tangles, which accumulate inside the neuron and block healthy activity.

The first symptoms of Alzheimer's almost always arise because the person has trouble encoding new information or experiences. Most frequently, this manifests as forgetting appointments, names, taking your medication on time (particularly ones the doctor changed), significant family events or holidays, or locations you have recently visited. Short-term memory loss can present itself in many other forms. One may find it hard to perform complex tasks, get lost when trying to visit a new place, or have trouble following directions about how to do something. Of all the eventual symptoms of Alzheimer's disease, short-term memory loss is usually the earliest, because the entorhinal cortex—the main bridge for getting memory into storage—is disrupted.

The following is a clinical case from our practice where AD was diagnosed before the patient experienced symptoms, which allowed for effective prevention.

CASE 2

T was a 59-year-old successful shopkeeper. He had no symptoms of his own and was not concerned about his own memory per se, but his mother had recently died of AD and he wanted to find out about prevention in case he was at risk. Although neither T nor his wife perceived any problems with his memory, structured testing revealed that his short-term memory was below normal for a person of his age, sex, and education. The test results recommended further evaluation. Blood tests showed that T had one apolipoprotein E4 gene, which increased his risk for AD. His MRI showed a 25% loss of brain tissue in the entorhinal cortex and hippocampus. A brain SPECT study showed reduced activity in the same areas as the MRI (Figure 26.4).

Because T's testing showed short-term memory loss even though he and his wife were not aware of it and because his MRI showed tissue loss in the entorhinal cortex and hippocampus only, he was diagnosed with stage 2 AD. He is now being treated with the medication rivastigmine to help block neuritic plaque and neurofibrillary tangle formation, plus a combination of antioxidants to reduce the chance of programmed cell death (apoptosis). After six months, T's repeat testing showed that his short-term memory had improved.

LEWY BODY DISEASE

Lewy body disease (LBD), initially described by neurologist F. H. Lewy in 1912, accounts for 10–20% of MCI and dementia in older adults, usually over 70 years of age. It is a degenerative disorder associated with abnormal deposits (Lewy bodies) found in certain areas of the brain. Lewy bodies contain deposits of a protein called alpha-synuclein that is also linked to Parkinson's disease. Early symptoms include those involving movement, visual perception, level of consciousness, and memory loss. Early LBD symptoms affecting movement are similar to Parkinson's disease symptoms. Early LBD symptoms affecting visual perception are usually visual hallucinations due to Lewy bodies accumulating in the visual cortex in the occipital lobes of the brain. Dwarf-like people are often described, and are quite vivid, but not necessarily frightening. Another early symptom that is often diagnostic of LBD is the response to medications that block the neurotransmitter dopamine. Neuroleptics are used to treat hallucinations in persons with schizophrenia but are also given to older individuals who have hallucinations. However, people with LBD have markedly reduced

Underside view

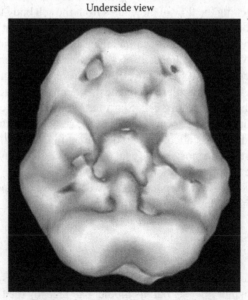

Decreased activity in the temporal lobes

FIGURE 26.4 T's SPECT study.

dopamine levels in their brains, which is the cause of their difficulty with movement. Giving a medication to an LBD person that further reduces dopamine can cause a marked worsening of their symptoms, making them rigid as a board, and sometimes putting them into coma.

LBD first affects the frontal, parietal, and occipital lobes, all of which can be seen with a SPECT or PET scans. Only later, after neurons die off, can an MRI detect atrophy in these brain areas.

PARKINSON'S DISEASE AND DEMENTIA

Parkinson's disease is caused by loss of neurons that make the neurotransmitter dopamine in a part of the brain that balances muscle movements, such as walking, reaching, grasping, standing, crouching, speaking, eating, and so on. The chances of experiencing dementia increase 5% for every year the person has PD. In fact, people with PD are from three to six times more likely to develop dementia than those in the general population.

PD starts as a physical movement disorder. The hallmark features of Parkinson's disease are: difficulty starting a movement, reduced eye blinking (which looks like a stare), trouble slowing down movement, muscles feeling stiff and resisting movement, a rhythmic shaking of the hands or head when doing nothing (called a resting tremor), and walking with quick, stuttering, short little baby steps. Dementia associated with PD always comes later, three or more years after the movement-related symptoms appear.

FRONTAL TEMPORAL LOBE DEMENTIA

Frontal temporal lobe dementia (FTLD), as its name implies, is a series of diseases that affect the frontal lobes and temporal lobes. These disorders are also associated with damage to deep areas of the brain (also called subcortical), including the basal ganglia (which controls movements), and the hypothalamus (which regulates hormone release into the blood stream to regulate the body's organs). FTLD accounts for 10% of all cases of dementia and often begins in people who are under 65. This stands in contrast to AD, where people usually first experience symptoms after age 60 (except for rare early-onset genetic forms of AD). FTLD usually causes progressive and irreversible decline in a person's abilities during a period of two to 15 years.

The most common causes of FTLD involve abnormalities of the tau protein, the structural backbone of the neuron. These FTLD diseases produce overlapping symptom groups that fall into four syndromes:

1. Frontal lobe dementia: uninhibited behavior with virtually no insight about how it affects others (social disinhibition), apathy, disinterest, or disengagement from activities that used to be enjoyable.
2. Primary progressive aphasia: mainly affects the left temporal lobe, and there is a progressive loss of language, beginning about two years before the dementia symptoms develop
3. Corticobasal degeneration syndrome: the inability to perform complex tasks, paralysis of voluntary eye movements, lightning-like muscle jerks in response to various stimuli such as bright lights or loud noises, and a failure to recognize a part of one's own body
4. Amyotrophic lateral sclerosis (ALS or Lou Gehrig's disease): spontaneous twitching of specific muscles at rest followed by a wasting away of these muscles, difficulties with swallowing, difficulty speaking or a change in voice pitch, and respiratory distress

For many families, the most devastating aspect of FTLD is often the individual's lack of insight. FTLD persons simply do not see themselves as impaired and cannot be reasoned with when they make reckless decisions. Eldercare attorneys specialize in establishing a legal conservator to keep FTLD persons from bringing financial ruin to themselves and their loved ones. (Contact the local bar association for attorneys who specialize in eldercare.) The course of FTLD is usually progressive deterioration over two to 15 years, with most living between six and 12 years.

TREATMENT APPROACHES

ADRD PREVENTION PROGRAM

Decreasing Alzheimer's disease and related disorders is a worthy goal that requires forethought, a well-researched scientific plan, and a good prefrontal cortex so that patients will follow through on the plan. Here is our five-step plan to decrease AD and keep the brain healthy with age.

PATIENT GUIDE FOR PREVENTION

Step 1. Know Your Risk for Alzheimer's Disease and Related Disorders

The following is a list of risk factors. The number in parentheses is a loading factor on the importance of each risk factor. For example, 2 = twice the risk of the general population; 3.4 = 3.4 times the risk of the general population.

Elevated Risk	Risk Factor
3.5	One family member with Alzheimer's disease or other cause of dementia
7.5	More than one family member with Alzheimer's disease or other dementia
2.0	A single head injury with loss of consciousness for more than a few minutes
2.0	Several head injuries without loss of consciousness
4.4	Alcohol dependence or drug dependence in past or present
2.0	Major depression diagnosed by a physician in past or present
10	Stroke
2.5	Heart (coronary artery) disease or heart attack (myocardial infarction or MI)
2.1	High cholesterol (hyperlipidemia)
2.3	High blood pressure (hypertension)
2.0	High homocysteine levels
3.4	Diabetes
3.0	History of cancer or cancer treatment
1.5	Seizures in past or present
2.0	Obesity
2.0	Sleep apnea
2.0	Limited exercise (less than twice a week or less than 30 minutes per session)
2.0	Less than a high school education
2.0	Jobs that do not require periodically learning new information
2.0	Within the age range, 65 to 74 years old
7.0	Within the age range, 75 to 84 years old
38.0	Over 85 years old
2.3	Smoking cigarettes for 10 years or longer
2.5	Has one apolipoprotein E4 gene, (if known)
5.0	Has two apolipoprotein E4 genes, (if known)

Step 2. Reduce Your Risk

Once you have an idea of what risk factors you or your patients may have, what can you do about it? Here is a list of recommendations:

Risk: Family member with Alzheimer's disease or related disorder or you have the Apo E4 gene
Reduce: Early screening and take prevention very seriously.

Risk: Single head injury with loss of consciousness for more than a few minutes
Reduce: Prevent further head injuries.

Risk: Several head injuries without loss of consciousness
Reduce: Prevent further head injuries and start prevention strategies early.

Risk: Alcohol dependence, drug dependence, or smoking in past or present
Reduce: Get treatment to stop and look for underlying causes; start prevention strategies early.

Risk: Major depression diagnosed by a physician in past or present. People with depression are at higher risk of cognitive impairment. Depression has been associated with hippocampal volume loss, neuron dendrite shrinkage, and glial cell loss, suggesting that mood disorders may have a degenerative component. Untreated depression may increase extracellular levels of glutamate in the amygdala, which may contribute to the increased risk of developing visible and measurable structural brain changes and dementia in patients with intractable mood disorders.
Reduce: Get treatment and start prevention strategies early.

Risk: Stroke, heart disease, high cholesterol, hypertension, diabetes, history of cancer treatment, seizures in past or present
Reduce: Get treatment and start prevention strategies early.

Risk: Limited exercise (less than twice a week or less than 30 minutes per session)
Reduce: Exercise three times a week or more. There is mounting evidence that regular physical conditioning protects the brain.

Risk: Less than a high school education or job that does not require periodically learning new information
Reduce: Engage in lifelong learning.

Risk: Obesity and insulin resistance. There is also a growing body of work that suggests a direct link between insulin and AD pathology. Insulin receptors, located in astrocytes and neuronal synapses, are highly concentrated in the cerebral cortex, hippocampus, and hypothalamus, consistent with the notion that insulin influences memory. Furthermore, reduced brain insulin signaling is associated with increased tau phosphorylation and Aβ levels, the pathological hallmarks of Alzheimer's disease
Reduce: Get to a healthy weight and maintain it.

Risk: Sleep apnea
Reduce: Evaluation and treatment for sleep apnea

Risk: High homocysteine levels
Reduce: Take B vitamins, especially folic acid, 1 milligram a day.

Risk: Parkinson's disease
Reduce: CoQ10 and other prevention strategies

Step 3. Keep Your Body and Brain Active

Exercise, which decreases with age for many, has many helpful effects on the brain. It increases the levels of nerve growth factors in the brain, which has been seen in young animals to stimulate new brain cell formation and helps strengthen connections between brain cells (the synapses). Exercise also improves the strength of the heart muscle so that the deep areas of the brain receive better blood flow. It is these deep areas of the brain that are the most susceptible to reduced blood flow and cellular starvation as we age. The well-designed Canadian Study of Health and Aging, which followed 4615 cognitively normal Canadians over 65 years old for five years, found that regular physical exercise doubled the chance of remaining cognitively normal [21].

Several mechanisms may explain the association between physical activity levels and lower risk for dementia. Active laboratory animals have been found to have more hippocampal neurons than inactive controls. Cardiovascular fitness is associated with greater volumes of parietal, temporal, and frontal cortical tissue, which are key cognitive areas [22]. Controlled studies of older people on aerobic or cardiovascular conditioning programs show that aerobic conditioning has broad effects on cognition. Benefit accrues to neural networks that support attention and short-term memory and to the frontal, temporal, and parietal brain regions.

Step 4. Consider Supplementing

There is a lot of information and misinformation about supplements. Table 26.2 contains a list of supplements where evidence is fair to good and may merit use.

Essential Fatty Acids

As major constituents of neuronal lipids, n-3 polyunsaturated fatty acids are of particular interest in the prevention of cognitive decline as valuable dietary ingredients whose neuroprotective properties exert beneficial effects on neurodegenerative processes. More than a dozen epidemiological studies have reported that reduced levels or intake of omega-3 fatty acids or fish consumption is associated with increased risk for age-related cognitive decline or ADRD. Docosahexaenoic acid (DHA), a component of the omega-3 fatty acids, is broadly neuroprotective via mechanisms that include downregulation of excitotoxic glutamate neurotransmission, reduced arachidonic acid metabolites, and reduction in amyloid oligomers. Increased dietary consumption or blood levels of DHA appear protective for ADRD in multiple epidemiological studies; however, three studies suggest that the ApoE4 genotype limits protection. A subgroup analysis of populations with and without the APOE

TABLE 26.2

Recommended Prevention Strategies

Prevention Agent	Risks Reduced	Dosage
Alpha-lipoic acid	Diabetes, stroke, solid cancers	300 mg twice a day
Coenzyme Q10 (CoQ10)	Parkinson's disease, possibly Lewy Body disease	1200 mg/day if symptoms; 100–400 mg/day if no symptoms
Diet, calorie restricted, high in fish/antioxidants	ADRD, cancer, vascular disease, diabetes	
Nonsteroidal anti-inflammatory medications (NSAIDs)	AD, heart attack, stroke, peripheral vascular disease	100–200 mg a day
Omega-3 fatty acids	Depression, ADHD, heart disease, dementia	1–4 grams a day
Vitamins B6, B12, and folate	AD, heart disease, especially if high homocysteine levels	100% RDA
Vitamin C (ascorbic acid)	AD (with vitamin E), CAD, stroke	1000 mg twice a day
Vitamin D	AD, diabetes, heart disease, cancer, MS, depression	Strive for a mid-range to high-normal level

ε4 allele was performed and while there was no DHA treatment effect on any outcome measure in the APOE ε4–positive group, those receiving DHA in the APOE ε4–negative group had a significantly lower decline in mean change in ADAS-cog score over 18 months (6.23 points [4.08 to 8.38 points] for 61 participants in the DHA group vs 10.11 points [7.12 to 13.10 points] for 48 participants in the placebo group). This differential DHA effect was also evident for the MMSE score (−3.36 in the DHA group vs −5.12 in the placebo group).

B Vitamins

B vitamins appear to slow cognitive and clinical decline in people with MCI, in particular those with elevated homocysteine. In a double-blind, placebo-controlled study, individuals with MCI were randomized to receive 0.8 mg folic acid, 0.5 mg vitamin B12, and 20 mg vitamin B6 (133 participants) or placebo (133 participants). There was significant benefit of B-vitamin treatment among participants with baseline homocysteine above the median (11.3 μmol/L) in global cognition (mini mental state examination), episodic memory, and semantic memory. Clinical benefit occurred in the B-vitamin group for those in the upper quartile of homocysteine at baseline in global clinical dementia rating score.

Bacteria in our intestinal tract synthesize several B vitamins. Emerging research suggests that gut microbes mediate risk of cognitive decline through this and other mechanisms. A healthful diet can favorably influence gut microbes.

Vitamin D

Physiological roles for vitamin D metabolism in the brain that suggest a potential neuroprotective effect include regulation of calcium homeostasis via downregulation of calcium channel expression in neurons or by induction of calcium binding proteins. Low levels of serum 25-hydroxy-vitamin D (25[OH]D) have been associated with an increased risk of substantial cognitive decline in several population-based studies. Individuals who are severely serum 25(OH)D deficient (levels < 25 nmol/L) have been associated with substantial cognitive decline, which raises important new possibilities for treatment and prevention. Vitamin D is lower with excess body fat, staying inside, and applying long-acting sunscreen. In this way, several lifestyle choices can alter risk of MCI.

Step 5. Start with Our Children

Many of the risks for AD occur in childhood. If we are sincere about preventing ADRD we must start with our children. The ApoE4 gene increases the risk of AD. Having this gene plus a head injury dramatically increases the risk further. Many head injuries occur in childhood, especially when playing contact sports or doing other high-risk activities. If children are allowed to engage in these activities, we think they should first be screened for the ApoE4 gene. If they have it, we should be more cautious with their heads. Children with ADHD and learning problems often drop out of school, leaving them at higher risk for dementia. Making sure we properly diagnose and help these children is essential to helping them become lifelong learners. The seeds for depression occur in childhood. Depression often is a result of persistent negative thinking patterns. School programs should be developed to teach children how to correct these patterns, which could help decrease depression. Childhood obesity leads to adult obesity. Educating children on nutrition and exercise can have lifelong benefits.

CONCUSSION AS AN EXAMPLE OF A MODIFIABLE RISK FOR COGNITIVE DECLINE

Does playing professional football put players at risk for long-term damage to the brain? The potential lasting brain damage suffered by National Football League (NFL) players due to the thousands of helmet-to-helmet blows over a career has been the subject of much recent controversy. For years, the NFL said that it did not know if playing professional football caused long-term brain damage, even though they started their concussion committee in 1994. Our research suggest the NFL brain seemed to have its own pattern, with damage typically affected the prefrontal cortex (called the executive part of the brain that controls judgment, impulse control, attention span, organization, and planning), temporal lobes (mood stability and memory), and cerebellum [23].

The players tended to score poorly on the neuropsychological tests except for reaction time and spatial processing. Forty-eight percent of our players had problems with obesity and nearly 30% suffered with or had been treated for depression. The incidence of memory problems and dementia were significantly higher than the rate in the general population. A concurrent study, from the University of Pittsburgh, reported as a person's weight went up the actual physical size of their brain goes down [24].

Is it possible through nutrient strategies to rehabilitate brains that have been damaged by chronic trauma? This question became part 2 of our study. Players were on a brain healthy program that included a weight-loss group, regular exercise, mental exercises, and nutritional supplements that support brain health, including fish oil; a multiple vitamin with high dose B6, B12, and folate; and a formula including huperzine A, vinpocetine, acetyl-l-carntine, among others. Among the follow-up results [25] on 55 players, 80% have shown improvement on either their neuropsychological testing, SPECT scans, or both. Memory-enhancing medications, antidepressants, hyperbaric oxygen treatment, and neurofeedback were administered on a personal basis, often with measurable improvement on clinical and imaging parameters.

The following is a clinical example.

CASE 3

At 34, CC was one of the younger retired NFL players. He volunteered for the study because he was struggling with problems of depression, irritability, frustration, high stress, obsessive thinking, memory problems, and marital problems. He had been diagnosed with a total of eight concussions— three in college and five in the pros. CC's SPECT scan showed clear brain damage and his Microcog showed significant decreases in general cognitive functioning, information processing speed, attention, memory, and spatial processing. After eight months on the brain rehabilitation program, he reported feeling much better and noticed significant improvements in his attention, mental clarity, memory, mood, motivation, and anxiety level. He felt his anger was under better control and he was getting along better with his small children.

His SPECT scan showed improvement in the areas of his temporal lobes (memory and mood stability), prefrontal cortex (attention and judgment), and cerebellum (processing speed). His Microcog showed significant improvement as well.

SUMMARY

ARDS are progressive conditions with two or more impairments in mental skills that interfere with a person's ability to function in his usual manner in his social, family, personal, or professional life. Just as delayed diagnosis and treatment of high blood pressure, diabetes, heart disease, stroke, and most other diseases leads to less effective treatment results, the same holds for delayed diagnosis and treatment of any ARDS. Given that Alzheimer's disease starts an average of 30 years before people have symptoms, it is essential to disseminate the information about delaying these devastating diseases. As we presented, the best way to accomplish this is to prevent or decrease all of the illnesses that are associated with them. Going forward, the use of neuroimaging, nutrients, and genetic markers are essential pieces of the puzzle to be able to individualize or personalize treatment, together with appropriate lifestyle changes.

REFERENCES

1. Barnes DE, Yaffe K. The projected effect of risk factor reduction on Alzheimer's disease prevalence. *Lancet Neurol* 2011;10(9):819–28. Epub Jul 19, 2011.

2. Shankle R, Rafii MS, Landing BH. Functional relationships associated with pattern of development in developing human cerebral cortex. *Concepts in Neuroscience* 1993;4(1):77–87.

3. Shankle WR, Landing BH, Rafii MS, Schiano AVR, Chen JM, Hara J. Numbers of neurons per column in the developing human cerebral cortex from birth to 72 months: Evidence for an apparent post-natal increase in neuron numbers. *J Theor Biol* 1998;191:115–40.

4. Eriksson PS, Bjork-Eriksson T, Alborn AM, Nordborg C, Peterson DA, Gage FH, Perfilieva E. Neurogenesis in the adult human hippocampus. *Nat Med* 1998;4:1313–17.

5. Landing BH, Shankle WR. Considerations of quantitative data on organ sizes and cell numbers and sizes in Down syndrome. *Progress in Clinical and Biological Research* 1995;393:177–91.

6. Hansen LA, et al. Neocortical morphometry, lesion counts, and choline acetyltransferase levels in the age spectrum of Alzheimer's disease. *Neurology* 1998;38:48–54.

7. Shankle WR, Amen DG. *Preventing Alzheimer's: Ways to Help Prevent, Delay, Detect, and Even Halt Alzheimer's Disease and Other Forms of Memory Loss*. New York: Perigee, 2004.

8. Fillit H, Hill J. Economics of dementia and pharmacoeconomics of dementia therapy. *Am J Geriatr Pharmacother* 2005;3(1):39–49.

9. Bookheimer S, Burggren AAPOE-4 genotype and neurophysiological vulnerability to Alzheimer's and cognitive aging. *Annu Rev Clin Psychol* 2009;5:343–62.

10. Cosentino S, Scarmeas N, Helzner E, Glymour MM, Brandt J, Albert M, et al. APOE epsilon 4 allele predicts faster cognitive decline in mild Alzheimer disease. *Neurology* 2008;70:1842–49.

11. Craft S, Teri L, Edland SD, Kukull WA, Schellenberg G, McCormick WC, et al. Accelerated decline in apolipoprotein E-epsilon4 homozygotes with Alzheimer's disease. *Neurology* 1998;51:149–53.

12. Mori E, Lee K, Yasuda M, Hashimoto M, Kazui H, Hirono N, Matsui M. Accelerated hippocampal atrophy in Alzheimer's disease with apolipoprotein E epsilon 4 allele. *Neurology* 2002;51:209–14.

13. Drzezga A, Riemenschneider M, Strassner B, Grimmer T, Peller M, Knoll A, et al. Cerebral glucose metabolism in patients with AD and different APOE genotypes. *Neurology* 2005;64:102–7.

14. Mahley RW, Weisgraber KH, Huang Y. Apolipoprotein E4: A causative factor and therapeutic target in neuropathology, including Alzheimer's disease. *Proc Natl Acad Sci U S A* 2006;103(15):5644–51.

15. Kamboh MI, Demirci FY, Wang X. Genome-wide association study of Alzheimer's disease. *Transl Psychiatry* 2012;May;15;2:e117.

16. Meurs I, Calpe-Berdiel L, Habets KL. Effects of deletion of macrophage ABCA7 on lipid metabolism and the development of atherosclerosis in the presence and absence of ABCA1. *PLoS One* 2012;7(3).

17. Brouwers N, Van Cauwenberghe C, Engelborghs S. Alzheimer risk associated with a copy number variation in the complement receptor 1 increasing C3b/C4b binding sites. *Mol Psychiatry* 2012;17(2):223–33.

18. Gonzalez Y, Herrera MT, Soldevila G. High glucose concentrations induce TNF-α production through the down-regulation of CD33 in primary human monocytes. *BMC Immunol* 2012;14;13:19.

19. Howie D, Nolan KF, Daley S, Butterfield E. MS4A4B is a GITR-associated membrane adapter, expressed by regulatory T cells, which modulates T cell activation. *J Immunol* 2009;183(7):4197–204.

20. Braak E, Griffing K, Arai K, Bohl J, Bratzke H, Braak H. Neuropathology of Alzheimer's disease: What is new since A. Alzheimer? *Eur Arch Psychiatry Clin Neurosci* 1999;249;Suppl 3:14–22.

21. Laurin D, Verreault R, Lindsay J, MacPherson K, Rockwood K. Physical activity and risk of cognitive impairment and dementia in elderly persons. *Arch Neurol* 2001;58:498–504.

22. Bonte FJ, Weiner MF, Bigio EH, White CL. Brain blood flow in the dementias: SPECT with histopathologic correlation in 54 patients. *Radiology* 1997;202:793–97.

23. Amen DG, Newberg A, Thatcher R, Jin Y, Wu J, Keator D, Willeumier K. Impact of playing professional American football on long term brain function. *J Neuropsychiatry Clin Neurosci* 2001;23(1):98–106.

24. Raji CA, Ho AJ, Parikshak NN, Becker JT, Lopez OL, Kuller LH, Hua X, Leow AD, Toga AW, Thompson PM. Brain structure and obesity. *Hum Brain Mapp* 2010;Mar;31(3):353–64.

25. Amen DG, Wu JC, Taylor D, Willeumier K. Reversing brain damage in former NFL players: Implications for TBI and substance abuse rehabilitation. *Journal of Psychoactive Drugs* 2011;43(1); Online publication date April 08, 2011.

27 Parkinson's Disease

Nutrient Interventions Targeting Disease Progression

David Perlmutter, M.D.

INTRODUCTION

Most authoritative texts attribute the first description of Parkinson's disease to James Parkinson who discussed the disease in 1817 in his *Essay on the Shaking Palsy*. However, exploring medical literature beyond those of Western cultures reveals descriptions of this disease predating that of James Parkinson's by more than 2000 years. The *Yellow Emperor's Internal Classic of International Medicine*, considered the first Chinese medical masterwork, written around 425–221 B.C. recounts:

> A person appears with crouching of the head and with staring eyes, bending the trunk with shoulders drooped, with difficulty turning and rocking the low back, inability of the knees to flex and extend, with the back bowed, failure to stand for long periods, and tremor while walking [1].

This description represents what would more than 2000 years later be called Parkinson's disease.

Even more prescient, however is that the text describes Parkinson's disease as a consequence of liver dysfunction. Western science is only recently recognizing the association of genetic polymorphisms related to hepatic detoxification and Parkinson's risk [2], linking the disease with the body's ability to decrease toxicant burden, which is salient to disease treatment and therefore supportive of the critical role of food and nutrients.

EPIDEMIOLOGY

Parkinson's disease is the second most common neurodegenerative disorder after Alzheimer's disease [3]. In the United States, Parkinson's afflicts approximately one million people with more than 50,000 new cases being diagnosed each year [3]. The incidence of the disease increases steadily with age, possibly as a consequence of progressive decline in antioxidant functionality leading to an overall increasing prevalence of the disease as our population ages.

PHARMACOLOGY

The physical manifestations of Parkinson's disease—including tremor, bradykinesia, rigidity, loss of automatic movements, and impaired balance—are thought to represent downstream effects of a primary brain biochemical abnormality, the loss of dopamine production as a consequence of neuronal degeneration in the pars compacta of the substantia nigra. Projection of dopamine from the substantia nigra to other brain centers including the caudate nucleus and the putamen plays a pivotal role in initiating and coordinating motor activity. When the dopaminergic transmission is compromised, these motor activities deteriorate.

For the most part, pharmaceutical approaches to the treatment of Parkinson's disease target this dopaminergic deficiency in an attempt to ameliorate the various motor manifestations described here. These approaches include the use of dopamine-based preparations designed to directly stimulate the dopaminergic receptor including: Sinemet®, Sinemet CR®, Stalevo®, and Parcopa®, as well as a newer group of nondopamine-based agents that nevertheless also stimulate the dopamine receptor—the dopamine agonists including: Mirapex® and Requip®. Other agents including anticholinergic (used for controlling tremor) and medications designed to enhance the activity of the dopaminergic drugs are also commonly prescribed.

When patients have exhausted the benefits of pharmacotherapy, an increasing number of surgical options are becoming available. These procedures include ablative surgery targeting inhibitory brain centers as well as deep brain stimulator (DBS) implantation technology designed to activate deep brain structures rendered dormant by dopamine deficiency [4].

The horizon holds promise for surgical interventions that do more than treat symptoms. Future restorative treatment modalities include gene therapy and neural transplantation [5].

Important to underscore is that food and nutrient interventions have also been shown to be more than palliative. They restore function and delay disease progression, possibly long enough for patients to benefit from surgical restorative treatments as they become available. In other words, nutrition focuses on the fire, not just the smoke.

Further, pharmaceutical interventions may compromise health as a consequence of specific nutritional deficiencies they induce. For example, the metabolism of levodopa consumes pyridoxine (vitamin B6), which may lead to a functional deficiency of this nutrient and may enhance the risk for homocysteine elevation. Laboratory assessments of pyridoxine and homocysteine levels are available in standard clinical laboratories and should be routinely performed when patients are treated with levodopa. Other nutritional considerations include decreased absorption of Mirapex® when taken with food, while it is recommended that Requip® be taken with a meal to reduce the risk of nausea.

PATHOPHYSIOLOGY

Treating the fire, the underlying predisposing conditions, requires addressing oxidative damage to mitochondria and whole body inflammation. Out of this pathophysiology meaningful clinical interventions emerge.

MITOCHONDRIAL DYSFUNCTION AND OXIDATIVE STRESS

Mitochondrial dysfunction of dopaminergic neurons in the substantia nigra is now looked upon as having a pivotal role in the pathogenesis of Parkinson's disease [6]. Specifically, complex I of the electron transport chain involved in the process of oxidative phosphorylation has been demonstrated to be compromised in Parkinson's patients [7]. Interestingly, this deficiency is not confined to the substantia nigra, or even to the brain, having been observed systemically in platelets, fibroblasts, and muscle cells. The impairment of complex I activity ranges from 16–54% with the degree of impairment correlating with the severity of the disease [6,8]. A fundamental consequence of impaired mitochondrial energy production is an increase in endogenous oxidative burden. That is, as mitochondrial function is compromised, there is a consequent increase in the production of damaging oxyradicals. This heightened condition of increased oxidative stress damages neurons and is thought to underlie the progressive decline in dopamine production from substantia nigra neurons in Parkinson's disease.

The specific initiating factor leading to mitochondrial function in Parkinson's disease remains unclear. Multiple studies have demonstrated a strong epidemiological relationship between exposure to various environmental mitochondrial toxins including herbicides, pesticides, industrial chemicals, heavy metals, and Parkinson's disease risk [9–12]. Further, specific genetic polymorphisms are now identified which may enhance susceptibility of an individual to Parkinson's disease by conferring deficiency of detoxification or antioxidant function emphasizing the potential significance of gene-environment interactions [13]. Testing for genetic susceptibility for hepatic detoxification flaws, which may predispose an individual to the development of Parkinson's disease, is now widely available [14]. Beyond family members of Parkinson's patients, who could be at increased risk for carrying these genetic polymorphisms, screening all individuals for this predisposition represents a new threshold in preventive medicine.

Ultimately, a feed-forward cycle is produced whereby excessive oxyradicals produced as a consequence of mitochondrial complex I dysfunction further damage mitochondrial function, enhancing oxyradical production. This situation is exacerbated by a deficiency of antioxidant protection of substantia nigra neurons. Multiple studies have described a dramatic deficiency of neuron protective reduced glutathione in the substantia nigra of Parkinson's disease patients; the degree of glutathione depletion correlates directly with disease severity [15–17]. Based upon the understanding of the protective role of glutathione as a neuronal antioxidant, its pivotal role in detoxification processes related to potentially neurotoxic environmental exposures, and the finding of deficiency in the Parkinson's brain, Sechi and colleagues at the University of Sassari, Italy, administered reduced glutathione intravenously to a group of Parkinson's patients twice daily for 30 days. The subjects were then evaluated at one-month intervals for the following six months. Their published report indicated, "All patients improved significantly with a 42% decline in disability. Once glutathione was stopped, the therapeutic effect lasted 2–4 months." They concluded that "glutathione has symptomatic efficacy and possibly retards the progression of the disease" [18]. Our experience with intravenous reduced glutathione has been similar, and we recently concluded a double-blind, placebo-controlled trial, the objective of which was to evaluate the safety, tolerability, and preliminary efficacy of intravenous glutathione in Parkinson's disease (PD) patients. This was a randomized, placebo-controlled, double-blind, clinical trial in subjects with PD whose motor symptoms were not adequately controlled with their current medication regimen. Subjects were randomly assigned to receive intravenous glutathione 1400 mg or placebo administered three times a week for four weeks. Twenty-one subjects were randomly assigned, 11 to glutathione and 10 to placebo. One subject who was assigned to glutathione withdrew from the study for personal reasons prior to undergoing any postrandomization efficacy assessments. Glutathione was well tolerated and there were no withdrawals because of adverse events in either group. Reported adverse events were similar in the two groups. There were no significant differences in changes in Unified Parkinson's Disease Rating Scale (UPDRS) scores. Over the four weeks of study medication administration, UPDRS activities of daily living (ADL) + motor scores improved by a mean of 2.8 units more in the glutathione group ($P = 0.32$ and over the subsequent four weeks worsened by a mean of 3.5 units in the glutathione group after the glutathione was discontinued [$P = 0.54$]) [19].

Coenzyme Q10 serves a critical role as an electron acceptor for complex I in oxidative phosphorylation. In addition, it also has potent antioxidant activity [20]. And like glutathione, deficiency of coenzyme Q10 is also noted in the mitochondria of platelets from Parkinson's when compared to controls [21]. These attributes have placed coenzyme Q10 in the spotlight as a candidate to effect disease progression in Parkinson's patients.

In a landmark study, Dr. Clifford Shults and coworkers at the University of California, San Diego, evaluated the effectiveness of mitochondrial therapy on the progression of Parkinson's disease using coenzyme Q10. Their large, multicenter, randomized, placebo-controlled, double-blind study demonstrated that high dosage coenzyme Q10 (1200 mg per day) slowed the functional decline in Parkinson's patients by a remarkable 44% when compared to the placebo group as measured by the UPDRS. The effect on total UPDRS was due to slowed decline in all three components of this widely used scale—mental function, activities of daily living, and motor function [20].

Oxidative stress plays a central role in the progression and possibly the initiation of nigral metabolic compromise ultimately manifesting in the clinical picture of Parkinson's disease, prompting in-depth investigation of the role of antioxidants [22]. Studies evaluating risk for the disease as well as disease progression in relation to dietary intake of antioxidants date back at least two decades. These reports have included both retrospective epidemiological studies correlating dietary habits with risk for the disease as well as actual interventional studies wherein the administration of one or more specific antioxidant(s) is evaluated in terms of effectiveness on disease progression. In 1988, a report entitled, "Case-Controlled Study of Early Life Dietary Factors in Parkinson's Disease" was published in *Archives of Neurology*. This early report paved the way to the current understanding that dietary choices may offer protection against a neurodegenerative condition. The researchers found that simple dietary sources of vitamin E profoundly reduced the risk of Parkinson's disease. Risk was reduced to 39% in those reporting the highest consumption of nuts, while consumers of seed-based salad dressing had a risk of 30%, and those who regularly consumed plums, a rich source of water-soluble antioxidants, demonstrated risk for the disease of only 24% in comparison to those not engaged in this dietary preference [23].

More recently, German researchers published a report evaluating the retrospective specific micronutrient and macronutrient intake of 342 Parkinson's patients in comparison to 342 control individuals from the same neighborhood or region [24]. This study provides strong evidence that dietary choices play a meaningful role in risk determination for the disease. Risk for Parkinson's disease was markedly reduced in those individuals whose dietary choices provided the highest levels of certain antioxidants. Disease risk was reduced by 33% in those having the highest consumption of beta-carotene, with those consuming the most vitamin C having a risk 40% less than those reporting the least consumption. High levels of monosaccharide as well as total energy consumption were very strongly associated with disease risk. While the authors did not specifically comment on this finding, research published subsequent to their report may help explain this relationship. Increased caloric consumption of total calories, especially monosaccharides, favors the formation of advanced glycosylation end products (AGEs). AGEs are formed when monosaccharides react nonenzymatically with the terminal amino group of proteins. This post-translational change imparts pathophysiological activity stimulating inflammation and its many downstream effects.

As a consequence, AGEs are thought to play an important role in neurodegeneration and aging [25]. Risk for Parkinson's disease was reduced by 51% in those with the highest riboflavin consumption compared to the lowest quartile. In human metabolism, riboflavin plays a role in diverse redox reactions through the coenzyme electron carriers flavin adenine dinucleotide (FAD) and flavin mononucleotide (FMN) [26]. FAD is part of the electron transport chain, and as such it is a requisite participant in mitochondrial function. Further, glutathione reductase is an FAD-dependent enzyme that participates in the regeneration of glutathione, a fundamentally important brain protective antioxidant that is deficient in Parkinson's patients (as noted earlier). Perhaps because of the role of riboflavin in glutathione production, deficiency of riboflavin is associated with increased oxidative stress [27]. In an interventional trial, researchers at the University of Sao Paulo provided oral riboflavin 30 mg every eight hours to a group of 31 advanced-stage Parkinson's patients. Interestingly, blood levels of riboflavin were depressed in all participants. After six months, motor capacity improved from 44% to 71% (Hoehn and Yahr scale) with improvements noted in nighttime sleep, reasoning, motivation, as well as reduced depression. These improvements were correlated with increased blood levels of riboflavin [28]. The highest quartile of folic acid consumption showed a reduced risk for Parkinson's disease of 49%, compared to the lowest quartile. Folate coenzymes are required for the metabolism of several important amino acids including the synthesis of methionine from homocysteine. Thus, folate deficiency is strongly associated with elevation of homocysteine and elevation of homocysteine levels are common in Parkinson's patients [29]. Germaine to the aforementioned pathophysiological model of Parkinson's disease, homocysteine enhances oxidative stress, compromises mitochondrial function, and ultimately leads to neuronal apoptosis [30]. See Table 27.1.

Nuclear factor-erythroid 2 p45-related factor 2 (Nrf2) is a transcription factor that regulates the expression of many cytoprotective genes. Cytoprotective downstream effects of Nrf2 activated target genes to activate powerful antioxidant and detoxification mediators and, as such, the Nrf2 pathway is being aggressively studied as a "valuable target" in neurodegenerative conditions [31,32]. Cellular protective antioxidants and phase 2 detoxification enzymes readily activated by Nrf2 include catalase, reduced glutathione (GSH), glutathione reductase (GR), GSH S-transferase (GST), and superoxide dismutase (SOD) [33]. Several lines of evidence including postmortem studies of PD brains, as well as genetic association studies of patients, indicate a link between Nrf2 dysregulation and PD pathogenesis. In light of both the understanding of the pivotal role of toxicant-induced oxidative stress in the pathogenesis of Parkinson's disease, and the potent neuronal protective activity of the Nrf2 pathway, researchers now indicate that Nrf2 should be "emphasized as a promising therapeutic approach" in Parkinson's treatment [34].

Several potent upregulators of Nrf2 include sulforaphane, an organosulfur compound found in cruciferous vegetables; curcumin, a member of the ginger family found in the popular Indian spice turmeric; and resveratrol, a polyphenol found in the skin of red grapes and other fruits [35].

TABLE 27.1

Adjusted Odds Ratios for Parkinson's Disease by Quartiles of Macronutrient and Micronutrient Intakes With "1" Representing the Lowest Quartile and "4" the Highest

Variable	Quartile	Adjusted Odds Ratio
Beta-carotene	1	1.00
	2	1.13
	3	0.85
	4	0.67
Ascorbic acid	1	1.00
	2	1.19
	3	0.97
	4	0.60
Riboflavin	1	1.00
	2	0.65
	3	0.67
	4	0.49
Folic Acid	1	1.00
	2	0.86
	3	0.62
	4	0.51
Monosaccharides	1	1.00
	2	1.67
	3	1.57
	4	2.59
Total energy intake	1	1.00
	2	2.19
	3	2.91
	4	3.25

Source: [27].

These Nrf2 activators are each the subject of intensive research specifically with respect to their roles in Parkinson's disease treatment with sulforaphane being described as serving as a "potential candidate for development of treatment and/or prevention of PD" [36], curcumin as a "potential candidate for inhibiting the oxidative damage that leads to Parkinson's disease," and resveratrol as exerting "a neuroprotective effect on the Parkinson's disease rat model" [37].

Our protocol for enhancing Nrf2 activity in Parkinson's disease treatment incorporates sulforaphane glucosinolate, 30 mg twice daily; curcumin as turmeric rhizome extract, 200 mg twice daily; and organic resveratrol 50 mg twice daily.

INFLAMMATION

A fundamental pathophysiologic feature of this disease is the finding of enhanced parameters of inflammation [38]. Areas of maximal degeneration within the substantia nigra demonstrate robust increases in the number of activated immune mediating microglial cells along with elevated levels of cytokines including interleukin-1β, tumor necrosis factor-alpha and interferon-γ that are increased by seven- to 15-fold in the substantia nigra of Parkinson's patients [38,39]. Cyclooxygenase-2 (COX-2) is also significantly elevated in the Parkinson's brain. COX-2 converts arachidonic acid to proinflammatory prostanoid prostaglandin E2, with research by Dr. Peter Teismann and coworkers demonstrating "a critical role for COX-2 in both the pathogenesis and selectivity of the Parkinson's disease neurodegenerative process [40].

Epidemiological studies also support the relationship between Parkinson's disease and inflammation with research demonstrating an overall risk reduction for the disease by 45% in regular users of over-the-counter nonsteroidal anti-inflammatory medications (NSAIDS) [41]. Further, glial cell–mediated inflammation is not unique to Parkinson's disease and implicated in a variety of other common neurodegenerative conditions including Alzheimer's disease and amyotrophic lateral sclerosis [42,43].

One important mechanism by which NSAIDs suppress inflammation is by activation of peroxisome proliferator-activated receptor-γ (PPARγ). This finding has led researchers to explore more fully the role of PPARγ in reducing inflammation in neurodegenerative disorders including Parkinson's disease [44]. In what has now become the standard animal model of Parkinson's disease, researchers are able to mimic human neuropathological changes in animals treated with the neurotoxin 1-methyl-4-phenyl-1,2,3,6-tetrahydropyridine (MPTP). MPTP-treated mice demonstrate mitochondrial dysfunction and consequent dramatic enhancement in the generation of reactive oxygen species, excitotoxicity, and apoptosis specifically in dopaminergic cells of the pars compacta of the substantia nigra. Further, these changes are accompanied by marked neuroinflammatory changes including microglial activation [45].

To more fully elucidate the role of PPARγ in the Parkinson's disease animal model, Dr. Tilo Breidert and colleagues evaluated the neuroprotective effects of specific PPARγ ligands in MPTP-treated mice. Their research demonstrated significant reduction of neuronal death in substantia nigra dopaminergic neurons in animals treated with the PPARγ ligand pioglitazone (Actos®) [46].

The profound activity of PPARγ ligand–mediated activation in terms of modulating inflammation is now a major focus of research in several important neurodegenerative conditions including Alzheimer's disease, multiple sclerosis, amyotrophic lateral sclerosis, and cerebral ischemia [44]. One would anticipate that the outcome of the basic science and ultimately interventional trials might lead to the development of an effective pharmaceutical agent. This could provide meaningful interventions for these and other devastating neurological conditions, but is many years hence. Further, pharmaceutical manipulation of PPARγ is not without risk as has been noted with the recent finding of a marked increase in risk of cardiovascular death in individuals using the diabetes medication rosiglitazone (Avandia®) [47].

What naturally serves as a ligand for PPARγ? How can biochemistry, perhaps the body's own biochemistry made from food and nutrients, affect the role of PPARγ in modulating inflammation?

Docosahexaenoic acid (DHA) is known to have beneficial effects in a variety of human diseases including atherosclerosis, asthma, cardiovascular disease, cancer, and depression [48]. These benefits are presumably derived from the anti-inflammatory activity of this fatty acid that demonstrates potent inhibition of COX-2 [49]. In a recent publication entitled, "Identification of Putative Metabolites of Docosahexaenoic Acid as Potent PPARγ Agonists and Antidiabetic Agents," Japanese researchers discovered potent PPARγ ligand activity from several metabolites of DHA with one metabolite demonstrating almost twice the potency compared to pioglitazone (Actos®) [50]. This new information adds to the understanding of the mechanisms underlying the potent anti-inflammatory effects of DHA and further helps explain why, for example, people with the highest blood levels of DHA have been shown to have a 47% lower risk of developing dementia and a 39% lower risk of developing Alzheimer's disease, compared with those with lower DHA levels [51].

While no study has as yet been undertaken to assess risk for Parkinson's disease in relation to DHA levels, based upon the understanding of its role in modulating PPARγ, it seems reasonable to consider adequate dietary supplementation of this important nutrient. Further, with the unique sensitivity of dopaminergic neurons in genetically sensitive individuals to neurotoxins that may concentrate higher in the food chain, DHA derived from marine algae may provide a greater net benefit.

While the concept of preventive medicine has taken root in such disciplines as cardiology and women's health, precious little attention is paid to applying evidence-based information to health recommendations related to neurodegenerative conditions. Science supports the contention that modifiable lifestyle factors are important considerations in relation to risk and progression of conditions like Parkinson's disease. Understanding the central roles of oxidative stress and inflammation in this disease should serve as motivation for dietary changes enhancing antioxidant protection while reducing the propensity for inflammation. Such dietary recommendations form the basis of the Mediterranean diet, now well described as having a marked effect in terms of reducing inflammation [52]. Key components of the Mediterranean diet [53] include:

- Generous intake of vegetables grown aboveground
- Consuming minimally processed fats such as olive oil and coconut oil
- Eating raw nuts and seeds
- Drinking red wine in moderation (for adults where not otherwise contraindicated)
- Sparingly consuming red meat from grass-fed livestock or wild game (without high-heat cooking)
- Eating wild, not farm-raised, fish on a regular basis

Further, specific supplementation with DHA provides a powerful nonpharmaceutical approach to inflammation as mediated through both COX-2 inhibition as well as through PPARγ. In our clinic, we generally recommend a daily consumption of DHA as a supplement in a dosage of 800–1000 mg for Parkinson's disease.

COMORBID CONDITIONS

Obesity is a cause of mitochondrial dysfunction that is readily modifiable and shows strong relationship to Parkinson's disease risk. In a study entitled, "Midlife Adiposity and the Future Risk of Parkinson's Disease," researchers determined adiposity using measurements of triceps skinfold thickness in a group of 7990 men aged 45–68 years between the years 1965 and 1968. Surviving participants were then examined an average of 30 years later. Comparing the incidence of Parkinson's disease in those originally in the highest quartile of triceps skinfold thickness to those with the lowest found an increased risk of developing Parkinson's disease of 300% associated with the thickest triceps skinfold [54].

Body fat may act as a reservoir for lipid-soluble neurotoxins that selectively damage dopamine-producing neurons in the substantia nigra. Several persistent organic pollutants such as pesticides are lipid soluble and act as neurotoxins as a consequence of their ability to disrupt mitochondrial function. In addition, excessive body fat is associated with upregulation of inflammatory cytokines that in turn act to increase the production of mitochondria damaging oxyradicals.

CONCLUSION

Modern therapeutic interventions for Parkinson's disease are effective in symptom management but provide very little in terms of modulating disease progression. However, food and nutrient interventions have been shown to treat the underlying pathophysiology. The following interventions and studies can be incorporated into medical practice:

- Understanding and correcting nutrient-drug interactions
- Optimizing antioxidant function to include—coenzyme Q10, 200 mg per day, vitamin C 1000 mg per day, vitamin E 400 IU per day, alpha-lipoic acid 200 mg per day, N-acetyl cysteine 800 mg per day, acetyl-L-carnitine 800 mg per day, vitamin D dosage required to achieve blood level of 70–90 ng/ml, beta-carotene 25,000 IU per day, sulforaphane gluco-sinolate, 30 mg twice daily, curcumin as turmeric rhizome extract, 200 mg twice daily, and resveratrol (preferably organic) 50 mg twice daily
- Blood tests for nutrient optimizations to include measurements of antioxidant function (lipid peroxide profile) as well as levels of specific nutrients including pyridoxine, beta-carotene, riboflavin, folate, vitamin B12, and coenzyme Q10
- Reducing inflammation with DHA—800–1000 mg per day as a supplement
- Attention to lifestyle issues including exercise and weight management

REFERENCES

1. Zhang ZX, Dong ZH, Román GC. Early descriptions of Parkinson's disease in ancient China. *Arch Neurol.* 2006;63:782–784.
2. Elbaz A, Levecque C, Clavel J, Vidal JS, Richard F, Amouyel P, Alpérovitch A, Chartier-Harlin MC, Tzourio C. CYP2D6 polymorphism, pesticide exposure, and Parkinson's disease. *Ann Neurol.* 2004 Mar;55(3):430–434.
3. Saunders CD. *Parkinson's Disease: A New Hope.* Boston, MA: Harvard Health Publications; 2000.
4. Krack P, Poepping M, Weinert D, et al. Thalamic, pallidal, or subthalamic surgery for Parkinson's disease? *J Neurol.* 2000;247 Suppl. 2:122–134.
5. Erlick, A. C., et al. Surgical insights into Parkinson's disease. *J R Soc Med.* 2006;99:238–244.
6. Reichmann H, Janetsky B. Mitochondrial dysfunction—a pathogenetic factor in Parkinson's disease. *J Neurol.* 2000;247 Suppl. 2:63–68.
7. Haas RH, Nasirian F, Nakano K, et al. Low platelet mitochondrial complex I and complex II/III activity in early untreated Parkinson's disease. *Ann Neurol.* 1995;37:714–722.
8. Swerdlow RH, Parks JK, Miller SW, et al. Origin and functional consequences of the complex I defect in Parkinson's disease. *Ann Neurol.* 1996;40:663–671.
9. Hirsch EC, Brandel JP, Galle P, et al. Iron and aluminum increase in the substantia nigra of patients with Parkinson's disease: An x-ray microanalysis. *J Neurochem.* 1991;56:446–451.
10. Bocchetta A, Corsini GU. Parkinson's disease and pesticides. *Lancet* 1986;2:1163.
11. Tanner CM, Langston JW. Do environmental toxins cause Parkinson's disease? A critical review. *Neurology* 1990;40 Suppl.3:17–31.
12. Stephenson J. Exposure to home pesticides linked to Parkinson's disease. *JAMA* 2000;283:3055–3056.
13. Checkoway H, Farin FM, Costa-Mallen P, Kirchner SC, Costa LG. Neurotoxicology. Genetic polymorphisms in Parkinson's disease. 1998 Aug–Oct;19(4–5):635–643.
14. Genovations™ Genova Diagnostics, 63 Zillicoa Street, Asheville, NC 2880-074 Tel. 800-522-4762.
15. Perry TL, Godin DV, Hansen S. Parkinson's disease: A disorder due to nigral glutathione deficiency? *Neurosci Lett.* 1982;33:305–310.

16. Jenner P. Oxidative mechanisms in nigral cell death in Parkinson's disease. *Mov Disord.* 1998;13:S24–S34.

17. Riederer P, Sofic E, Rausch W, et al. Transition metals, ferritin, glutathione, and ascorbic acid in Parkinsonian brains. *J Neurochem.* 1989;52:515–520.

18. Sechi G, Deledda MG, Bua G, et al. Reduced intravenous glutathione in the treatment of early Parkinson's disease. *Progr Neuropsychopharmacol Biol Psychiatry* 1996;20:1159–1170.

19. Hauser, RA, Lyons, KE, McClain, T., Carter, S. and Perlmutter, D. Randomized, double-blind, pilot evaluation of intravenous glutathione in Parkinson's disease. *Movement Disorders* 2009;24:979–983.

20. Shults, C.W. et al. Effects of coenzyme Q10 in early Parkinson's disease—Evidence of slowing of the functional decline. *Arch Neurol.* 2002;59:1541–1550.

21. Matsubara, T.A., et al. Serum coenzyme Q10 level in Parkinson syndrome. In Folkers K., et al. eds. *Biomedical and Clinical Aspects of Coenzyme Q10.* New York, NY: Elsevier Science Publishers, 1991:159–166.

22. Hellenbrand W, Seidler A, Boeing H, Robra B-P, Vieregge P, Nischan P, Joerg J, Oertel WH, Schneider E, Ulm G, Diet and Parkinson's disease I: A possible role for the past intake of specific foods and food groups: Results from a self-administered food-frequency questionnaire in a case-control study. *Neurology* 1996;47:636–643.

23. Golbe LI, Farrell TM, David PH. Case-controlled study of early life dietary factors in Parkinson's disease. *Arch Neurol.* 1988;45(12):1350–1353.

24. Hellenbrand W, Boeing H, Robra B-P, Seidler A, Vieregge P, Nischan P, Joerg J, Oertel WH, Schneider E, Ulm G. Diet and Parkinson's disease 11: A possible role for the past intake of specific nutrients. Results from a self-administered food-frequency questionnaire in a case-control study. *Neurology* 1996;47:644–650.

25. Ramasamy R, Vannucci SJ, Yan SSD, Herold K, Yan SF, Schmidt AM. Advanced glycation end products and RAGE: A common thread in aging, diabetes, neurodegeneration, and inflammation. *Glycobiology* 2005;15(7):16R–28R.

26. McCormick DB, Innis WSA, Merrill AH Jr, Bowers-Komro DM, Oka M, Chastain JL. An update on flavin metabolism in rats and humans. In Edmondson DE, McCormick DB, eds. *Flavin and Flavoproteins.* New York: Walter de Gruyter, 1988:459–471.

27. Powers HJ. Current knowledge concerning optimum nutritional status of riboflavin, niacin and pyridoxine. *Proc Nutr Soc.* 1999;58(2):435–440.

28. Coimbra CG, Junqueira, VBC. High doses of riboflavin and the elimination of dietary red meat promote the recovery of some motor functions in Parkinson's disease patients. *Brazilian Journal of Medical and Biological Research* 2003;36:1409–1417.

29. Religa D, Czyzewski K, Styczynska M, Peplonska B, Lokk J, Chodakowska-Zebrowska M, Stepien K, Winblad B, Barcikowska M. Hyperhomocysteinemia and methylenetetrahydrofolate reductase polymorphism in patients with Parkinson's disease. *Neurosci Lett.* 2006 Aug 14;404(1–2):56–60.

30. Mattson MP, Kruman II, Duan W. Folic acid and homocysteine in age-related disease. *Ageing Research Reviews* 2002;1:95–111.

31. Lee J-M, Johnson JA. An important role of Nrf2-ARE pathway in the cellular defense mechanism. *Journal of Biochemistry and Molecular Biology* 2004;37(2):139–143.

32. Calkins MJ, Johnson DA, Townsend JA, Vargas MR, Dowell JA, Williamson TP, Kraft AD, Lee J-M, Li J, Johnson JA. The Nrf2/ARE pathway as a potential therapeutic target in neurodegenerative disease. *Antioxid Redox Signal.* 2009;11(3):497–508.

33. Zhu H, Itoh K, Yamamoto M, Zweier JL, Li Y. Role of Nrf2 signaling in regulation of antioxidants and phase 2 enzymes in cardiac fibroblasts: protection against reactive oxygen and nitrogen species-induced cell injury. *FEBS Lett.* 2005 Jun 6;579(14):3029–3036.

34. Tufekci KU, Bayin EC, Genc S, Genc K. The Nrf2/ARE pathway: A promising target to counteract mitochondrial dysfunction in Parkinson's disease. *Parkinson's Disease* 2011; Article ID 314082, 14 pages. doi:10.4061/2011/314082 http://www.hindawi.com/journals/pd/2011/314082/.

35. Maulik N, Mauli G. *Nutrition, Epigenetic Mechanisms, and Human Disease.* CRC Press: Boca Raton, 2010:199.

36. Han JM, Lee YJ, Lee SY, Kim EM, Moon Y, Kim HW, Hwang O. Protective effect of sulforaphane against dopaminergic cell death. *Journal of Pharmacology and Experimental Therapeutics*; 2007, 249, 321.

37. Jin F, Wu Q, Lu YF, Gong QH, Shi JS. Neuroprotective effect of resveratrol on 6-OHDA-induced Parkinson's disease in rats. *Eur J Pharmacol.* 2008;Dec 14;600(1-3):78–82. Epub 2008 Oct 10.

38. Hirsch EC, Hunot S, Damier P, Brugg B, Faucheux BA, Michel PP, Ruberg M, Muriel MP, Mouatt-Prigent A, Agid Y. Glia cells and inflammation in Parkinson's disease: A role in neurodegeneration. *Ann Neurol.* 1998;44[Suppl 1]:S115–S120.

39. Mogi M, Harada M, Narabayashi H, Inogaki H, Minami M, Nagatsu TInterleukin (IL)-1 beta, IL-2, IL-4, IL-6 and transforming growth factor-alpha levels are elevated in ventricular cerebrospinal fluid in juvenile parkinsonism and Parkinson's disease. *Neurosci Lett*. 1996;211:13–16.
40. Teismann P, Tieu K, Choi DK, Wu DC, Naini A, Hunot S, Vila M, Jackson-Lewis V, Przedborski S. Cyclooxygenase-2 is instrumental in Parkinson's disease neurodegeneration. *Proc Natl Acad Sci*. USA 2003 Apr 29;100(9):5473–5478.
41. Chen H, Zhang SM, Hernán MA, Schwarzschild MA, Willett WC, Colditz GA, Speizer FE, Ascherio A. Nonsteroidal anti-inflammatory drugs and the risk of Parkinson's disease. *Arch Neurol*. 2003;60:1059–1064.
42. Klegeris A, McGeer PL. Cyclooxygenase and 3-lipoxygenase inhibitors protect against mononuclear phagocyte neurotoxicity. *Neurobiol Aging* 2002;23:787–794.
43. In t' Veld BA, Ruitenberg A, Hofman A, et al. Nonsteroidal antiinflammatory drugs and the risk of Alzheimer's disease. *N Engl J Med*. 2001;345:1515–1521.
44. Heneka MT, Landreth GE, Hüll M. Drug insight: Effects mediated by peroxisome proliferator-activated receptor-gamma in CNS disorders. *Nat Clin Pract Neurol*. 2007 Sep;3(9):496–504.
45. Liberatore GT et al. Inducible nitric oxide synthase stimulates dopaminergic neurodegeneration in the MPTP model of Parkinson disease. *Nat Med*. 1999;5:1403–1409.
46. Breidert T et al. Protective action of the peroxisome proliferator-activated receptor-gamma agonist pioglitazone in a mouse model of Parkinson's disease. *J Neurochem*. 2002;82:615–624.
47. Nissen SE, Wolski K. Effect of rosiglitazone on the risk of myocardial infarction and death from cardiovascular causes. *N Engl J Med*. 2007;356:2457–2471.
48. Horrocks LA, Yeo YK. Health benefits of docosahexaenoic acid (DHA). *Pharmacol Res*. 1999; Sep;40(3):211–225.
49. Massaro M, Habib A, Lubrano L, Del Turco S, Lazzerini G, Bourcier T, Weksler BB, De Caterina R. The omega-3 fatty acid docosahexaenoate attenuates endothelial cyclooxygenase-2 induction through both NADP(H) oxidase and PKCε inhibition. Proc. *Natl. Acad. Sci*. USA 2006;103:15184–15189.
50. Yamamoto K, Itoh T, Abe D, Shimizu M, Kanda T, Koyama T, Nishikawa M, Tamai T, Ooizumi H, Yamada S. Identification of putative metabolites of docosahexaenoic acid as potent PPARγ agonists and antidiabetic agents. *Bioorganic & Medicinal Chemistry Letters* 15. 2005;517–522.
51. Schaefer EJ, Bongard V, Beiser AS, Lamon-Fava S, Robins SJ, Au R, Tucker KL, Kyle DJ, Wilson PWF, Wolf PA. Plasma phosphatidylcholine docosahexaenoic acid content and risk of dementia and alzheimer disease: The Framingham Heart Study. *Arch Neurol*. 2006;63:1545–1550.
52. Trichopoulou A, Costacou T, Bamia C, Trichopoulos D. Adherence to a Mediterranean diet and survival in a Greek population. *NEJM* 2003;348:2600–2608.
53. Mediterranean diet for heart health. www.mayoclinic.com/health/mediterranean-diet/CL00011.
54. Abbott RD, Ross GW, White LR et al. Midlife adiposity and the future risk of Parkinson's disease. *Neurology* 2002;59:1051–1057.

28 Migraine Headache

New Understanding of Mechanisms and Therapies

Damien Downing, M.B.B.S., M.S.B., Joseph E.
Pizzorno, N.D., and Maya Shetreat-Klein, M.D.

INTRODUCTION

Migraine headaches take an extraordinary toll in terms of cost as well as the burden of pain and suffering. In 2010, it is estimated that the healthcare costs associated with migraine were $4.3 billion, not including drug costs or indirect costs, such as loss of productivity [1]. Affecting 17.1% of women and 5.6% of men, roughly half of those with migraines have never been diagnosed, and only a surprising 12% use preventive treatments for their headaches [2].

Current research highlights a neuronal pathophysiology rather than a primarily vascular one. Recent theories also point to evidence that there may be evolutionarily conserved, genetically conferred responses shaped by past environment. Part of the complexity of migraines may be due to the individual differences in both triggers and underlying pathophysiology. Said another way, by grouping all migraines together, we may have lost sight of the cause of migraines in the individual and in the process overlooked the value of individualized treatments.

The natural therapies reviewed in this chapter have been proven effective for migraines, particularly for use as prophylactic agents, and when used in the context of an individualized approach they not only reduce headaches but restore the underlying abnormalities for which migraine is just one manifestation.

OVERVIEW: UNDERSTANDING MIGRAINES

Migraine is a constellation of symptoms rather than one specific etiology, or even one specific sequence of physiological dysfunction. Clinically diagnosed, the criteria for a migraine per the International Headaches Society include: headaches lasting 4–72 hours, usually unilateral, of pulsating quality, of moderate to severe pain intensity, made worse by activity, and accompanied by nausea and/or vomiting, and often phonophobia and/or photophobia [3]. Not all of these symptoms need to be present, and none of them are unique only to migraine. In other words, the definition of migraine is one agreed upon by convention and may not be reflective of the biochemical diversity driving symptoms.

Some commonalities among migraineurs do exist though. For example, it is thought that most if not all migraines have a trigger, some endogenous or exogenous event that initiates the reversible dysfunction known as a migraine attack. The trigger induces a neurological event, considered central to migraine pathology per the current neuronal theory of migraine. This then triggers downstream events, some of which are vascular changes, as well as sensitization and activation of the trigeminal nerve. Recurrent and maladaptive activation of the trigeminocervical pain apparatus, in turn, activates meningeal nociceptors and stimulates the release of neuropeptides such as substance P, calcitonin gene-related peptide (CGRP), and neurokinin A, which dilate the meningeal arteries [4]. Migraineurs appear to have increased cortical excitability, rendering them more susceptible to migraine triggers [5].

One recent review summarizes the multifactorial nature of migraine thus: "Taken together, virtually all aspects of life have been suspected to trigger migraine or tension-type headache, but scientific evidence for many of these triggers is poor" [6]. In a questionnaire survey of 1207 migraineurs [7], the frequencies for a range of factors as triggers were reported as in Table 28.1.

It is interesting to note that many of these migraine triggers affect the brain directly and may thus be perceived as internal or environmental threats to the brain [8]. If this theory proves accurate, it casts a different light on migraine as an attempt to maintain homeostasis or control an excessive allostatic load that may have a genetically favorable basis and shifts away from a disease-based perspective.

While it is not completely clear what predisposes an individual to that primary neuronal event, a number of nutritional factors appear to modulate this sensitivity through related mechanisms, including impaired neuronal mitochondrial function, polymorphisms in methyltetrahydrofolate reductase (MTHFR) and ion channel genes, abnormal histamine metabolism, food allergies, imbalances in neurotransmitter activity, and even insulin resistance. Migraineurs are also likely exposed to increased levels of oxidative stress, as evidenced by the association of migraine onset with shorter telomere length [9]. By considering each of the following potential dysfunctions, clinicians may be able to tailor treatments to address the specific predisposing factors in each individual patient.

ALTERED HISTAMINE, IGE, AND MAST CELL PHYSIOLOGY

Abnormalities in histamine metabolism and an allergy component have long been suspected to play a role in migraine, and have contributed to earlier theories postulating a primary vascular etiology.

TABLE 28.1
Frequency of Self-Identified Triggers for Migraines

Factor	Frequency %
Stress	80
Menstrual Cycle	65
Hunger	57
Weather	53
Insomnia	50
Odors	44
Light	38
Alcohol	38
Smoke	36
Food	27
Exercise	22
Sex	5

Source: From [7].

There are well-established comorbidities of migraine and other allergic conditions that support this link. Migraine incidence in a population with allergic rhinitis was documented to be over 14-fold greater than in a control population [10]. Individuals with asthma, asthma-related symptoms, and other respiratory disorders, as well as children with atopic disease also have an increased likelihood of migraine [11,12]. Forty percent of children with migraine have had positive IgE allergy tests [13], and an increase in both total IgE and histamine levels has also been found in adults [14].

The release of histamine by mast cells after IgE binding seems to be the shared feature of these conditions and is a well-established trigger of vasodilation. Histamine also increases vascular permeability, a commonality among migraineurs, as well as local neurogenic inflammation. Additionally, histamine stimulates the release of nitric oxide, to be discussed in detail here [10]. In addition to histamine elevation among migraineurs, some studies have also shown that symptoms can be induced after histamine administration, and H1 receptor antagonists can relieve headaches in some individuals, providing further evidence for this common dysfunction. Treatments that prevent mast cell degranulation are thus good candidates for migraine prevention.

BUTTERBUR

Butterbur extract was first used clinically to treat allergic rhinitis, as its components have demonstrated the ability to stabilize mast cells, and initial trials show comparable efficacy to standard allergy medications [15–17]. When used for migraine prophylaxis, 45% of adults in a small clinical trial were responders (i.e., they experienced a 50% reduction in migraine frequency, a standard gauge of effectiveness) versus only 15% receiving placebo [18]. Trials in both adults and children have typically shown benefit, with the percentage of patients responding approximately equal to those with elevated IgE antibodies [15], suggesting this is the mechanism of action (although not confirmed). Butterbur also may act as a calcium-channel blocker or an anti-inflammatory agent [19].

OTHER HISTAMINE BASED TREATMENTS

Dietary interventions, including those based upon IgE or IgG antibody testing, an elimination diet, reduced fat intake, and low inflammation, have also been used with great clinical success for migraine prophylaxis, but this will not be reviewed here. In one small study, children utilizing relaxation techniques were able to both reduce their migraine frequency as well as urinary tryptase levels, highlighting a potential mechanism by which stress may trigger migraines [20]. Lastly, in a recent prospective study, individualized allergen-specific sublingual immunotherapy was shown to both reduce migraine frequency as well as C-reactive protein levels (and rhinitis symptoms if present), suggesting that identifying and treating specific causes of excessive histamine release is warranted, particularly among those with signs of this abnormality [21].

MITOCHONDRIAL DYSFUNCTION

Mitochondrial dysfunction may be a relatively common component of migraineurs and has been documented by several avenues of investigation, including morphological, biochemical, and neuroradiological studies, and more recently by phosphorus magnetic resonance spectroscopy analyses (P-MRS). P-MRS monitors ATP production and in vivo brain energy metabolism, which were indicative of an "unstable metabolic state of the brain and a decreased ability to cope with further energy demand" among migraineurs [22]. Excessive lactic acid in the cerebrospinal fluid and reduced activity of enzymes necessary for oxidative phosphorylation, such as succinate-dehydrogenase and NADH-cytochrome-c-reductase, have been documented among migraineurs, and a small number also appear to have a carnitine palmitoyltransferase II deficiency, responsive to carnitine supplementation [23].

A growing number of studies have identified genetic risk factors for migraine, some related to mitochondrial function. Although there do not yet appear to be mutations common among migraineurs, one study among individuals with cyclic vomiting syndrome (CVS), often considered a migraine equivalent condition, along with those who had migraine with no aura compared their entire mitochondrial genome to controls. Two polymorphisms of mitochondrial DNA were found at a very high rate: a 16519C→T polymorphism was found in 70% of CVS patients (OR 6.2) and in 52% of migraineurs (OR 3.6), compared to only 27% of controls, and a 3010G→A polymorphism in 29% of CVS patients (OR 17.0) and 26% of migraineurs (OR 15.0) compared to only 1.6% of controls [24].

The involvement of mitochondrial dysfunction in migraine pathology is also indirectly supported by the clinical benefit of nutrients that enhance oxidative phosphorylation, namely riboflavin and CoQ10. Their effectiveness, or at least that of riboflavin, also appears to depend somewhat on an individual's haplotype, a term that indicates a common ancestor marked by some shared mitochondrial DNA mutations, further supporting the link between mitochondrial function and migraine.

RIBOFLAVIN

Riboflavin is the precursor of flavin mononucleotide and flavin adenine dinucleotide, cofactors for enzymes in the electron transport chain, particularly Complex I [25]. In controlled trials, riboflavin has been shown to halve migraine frequency in 60–70% of migraineurs (vs. 15% placebo) at a dose of 200–400 mg per day [26,27]. Similarly, almost 70% of children and adolescents were considered responders and also experienced a decrease in migraine intensity [28].

A study published in 2000 highlights both the efficacy of riboflavin, as well as what may be an additive potential for preventing migraine through multiple mechanisms of action. In a randomized trial, participants were given either riboflavin (400 mg per day) or beta blockers (metoprolol, 200 mg per day; bisoprolol 10 mg per day). In addition to measuring clinical response, researchers measured what is known as auditory-invoked cortical potentials, a marker for cortical excitability. Both treatments had the same percentage of responders (53% and 55%) and thus were clinically equivalent. However, beta blockers were only effective in those individuals who experienced a reduction in the intensity dependence of cortical potentials (i.e., their cortical hyperexcitability was decreased). Because riboflavin had no effect on this parameter, this suggests different mechanisms of action, as well as the potential for an additive prophylactic effect and for the alternation of treatments if one becomes intolerable [29].

As mentioned earlier, an individual's haplogroup appears to influence the effectiveness of riboflavin [30]. Indeed, the responder rate in patients with haplogroup H (European ancestry) was 44.8% compared to 77% in non-H haplogroups, with an overall responder rate of 62.5%, a combined rate comparable to previous controlled trials. Several interpretations may explain these differences: riboflavin may be more effective for those with non-H haplogroups, perhaps because complex I activity is impaired and/or improved to a greater degree with riboflavin therapy, a likely explanation [31]. This finding also suggests that those with haplogroup H have inefficiencies in other mitochondrial complexes, such as II, III, or IV, which would be improved by therapies targeting those steps in the electron transport chain. Haplotype H is found at the same frequency in those with and without migraine, but appears to increase the risk for conditions with likely mitochondrial dysfunction, such as Alzheimer's and Parkinson's diseases [32,33]. Greater understanding of the specific abnormalities associated with each haplotype is likely to improve treatment specificity.

The MTHFR genotype may be a potential indicator of riboflavin's effectiveness. Although no clinical trials have evaluated MTHFR genotype as a predictor of efficacy in migraine, because the T677 allele results in a lower affinity for FAD (flavin adenine dinucleotide), a riboflavin derivative, supplementation in these individuals seems warranted and has shown proof of concept in other conditions [34].

CoQ10

CoQ10 transports electrons between complex I and complex II, and functions as a cellular anti-oxidant, and a regenerator of both vitamins C and E. Reduced levels of CoQ10 have been documented among migraineurs, as has the benefit of CoQ10 supplementation for migraine prophylaxis. In an open-label trial, a 13% mean reduction in frequency occurred at one month, and a 55% at three months [35]. In a more recent placebo-controlled trial, a 50% response rate occurred at three months compared to a 15% among the placebo group. It was shown to reduce headache frequency and nausea, with no effect on headache severity or duration [36].

Serum CoQ10 levels of more than 1500 children and adolescents with migraine were measured, with a surprising 32.9% of participants found to have a total CoQ10 level below the reference range (< 0.5 µg/mL), and a total of 74.6% with suboptimal levels (< 0.7 µg/mL) [37]. Those with a deficiency given supplemental CoQ10 (1–3 mg/kg/day) had a response rate of nearly 50%. This prevalence of either deficiency or suboptimal levels is thought to reflect increased utilization due to oxidative or mitochondrial stress or possibly vascular inflammation.

THIOCTIC ACID

Thioctic acid, also known as alpha-lipoic acid, was shown (at 600 mg per day) to reduce headache frequency, the number of headache days, and severity compared to placebo, although no difference was found in the number of responders [38]. It is thought to have antioxidant effects, as well as mitochondrial benefit.

MTHFR POLYMORPHISMS AND ALTERED HOMOCYSTEINE AND FOLATE METABOLISM

Although the neuronal theory of migraine is now widely accepted, it does not explain all features of migraine, and there is still considerable evidence for a primary or at least secondary vascular component. One aspect of migraine-associated vasculopathy is an abnormality in homocysteine metabolism, at least partly due to polymorphisms in the MTHFR gene. MTHFR is responsible for converting 5,10-methylenetetrahydrofolate into 5-methylenetetrahydrofolate, a cofactor for the re-methylation of homocysteine to methionine, and the primary circulating form of folate. One common variant of this gene is the C677T polymorphism, shown to result in reduced enzymatic activity and, as a consequence, increased serum homocysteine levels. Homocysteine has direct vascular toxicity. The TT genotype as well as hyperhomocysteinemia are risk factors for peripheral and central cardiovascular disease [39,40]

Hyperhomocysteinemia and the TT genotype are associated with an increased risk of migraine, particularly migraine with aura [41,42]. Oterino et al. [43] found that elevated homocysteine levels were associated with as high as a sixfold increased risk for migraine with aura in those with levels > 15.0 microM, and the greatest predictor of homocysteine levels was the number of T alleles. The cerebrospinal fluid of migraineurs also contains higher homocysteine levels compared to controls: 41% higher in those without aura and a remarkable 376% higher in those with aura [44]. This may be an important causative factor for the heightened risk of cardiovascular disease among migraineurs with aura; an increase in both all-cause and cardiovascular mortality has been found, as well as pre-eclampsia and both hemorrhagic and ischemic stroke [45–47].

Homocysteine may contribute to a systemic vasculopathy by causing cerebral microvascular changes and may directly cause endothelial dysfunction [48]. It is also possible that homocysteic acid (HCA), a metabolite of homocysteine that mimics the neurotransmitter glutamate, has an excitatory effect [44]. HCA may activate N-methyl-D-aspartate receptors that are implicated in the cortical spreading depression of migraineurs, induce neuronal apoptosis, deplete glutathione levels, and generate reactive oxygen species stress [49,50]

B Vitamins

In a randomized, double-blinded and placebo-controlled trial, folic acid, B6, and B12 were given to 52 patients who had migraine with aura. This intervention caused a reduction in Migraine Disability Assessment (MIDAS) scores from 60% to 30% after six months, with no change in placebo, along with a 39% reduction in homocysteine levels [51]. (The MIDAS score is used to monitor health-related quality of life.) It is worth noting that it also reduced pain severity, an uncommon benefit for prophylactic therapies, and had a greater response among those with the C allele for the MTHFR C677T polymorphism. This may indicate a need for higher doses for those with the T allele.

Folic acid alone (5 mg per day) has also been used in an open-label trial among children with hyperhomocysteinemia, migraine without aura, and a variant in the MTHFR gene. It was associated with complete resolution in 62%, a 75% reduction in an additional 31%, and a 50% reduction in the remaining children, as well as homocysteine normalization in 100% of participants [52].

The MTHFR 677T allele results in reduced FAD binding, and riboflavin may be at least as relevant to its enzymatic activity as folic acid, though the status of each appears to influence the effect of the other. Although no clinical trials in migraine have been performed, it is likely that migraineurs with this allele, particularly homozygotes, would benefit from riboflavin supplementation. As reviewed by Ames et al. in the *American Journal of Clinical Nutrition*, riboflavin status is an important determinant of homocysteine and methylation metabolism, especially among those with the 677CT mutation who are highly susceptible to low dietary consumption [53]. Interactions between riboflavin intake and MTHFR status have been shown to modulate risk for a number of diseases, including risk of fracture [54] and in the treatment of hyperhomocysteinemia [34] and hypertension [55], suggesting that they are highly relevant to migraine as well.

Variants in the MTHFR gene appear to predict the actual symptoms that migraineurs have, suggesting that migraine symptoms are not random, but reflective of underlying metabolomics and pathophysiology. The TT genotype of the C677T polymorphism was associated with a diagnosis of migraine with aura and unilateral head pain, and the CT genotype was linked to stress as a trigger and discomfort with physical activity [56]. This marks the potential for the use of migraine symptomatology as providing keys to underlying pathology, rather than the limited understanding of an amorphous classification of migraine based upon a checklist of criteria. It should also be noted that treating the underlying metabolic aberrations may reduce risk for migraine comorbidities, most notably stroke.

NITRIC OXIDE HYPOTHESIS

Also implicated in the pathophysiology of migraine is excessive nitric oxide (NO) production and/or sensitivity. Not only does nitric oxide facilitate cranial blood flow, it affects nociceptor processing. In healthy individuals, it can initiate a migraine attack and is involved for the duration of an attack [57,58]. A recent genetic analysis comparing 200 women with migraine to 142 controls found that polymorphisms in the inducible nitric oxide synthase (iNOS) gene contribute both to susceptibility to migraine with aura and the susceptibility to aura in migraine patients [59]. Although regulation of iNOS is thought to be primarily transcriptional, some evidence indicates that the implicated polymorphisms are associated with much higher enzyme activity. Furthermore, nonselective NOS inhibitors such as L-NMMA are effective in reducing migraine frequency, but adverse effects prevent their use clinically. The herb feverfew, which will be discussed later in this chapter, has recently been shown to downregulate both eNOS and iNOS at the translational and/or post-translational level [60].

Some data also point to compounds scavenging of NO as a possible therapeutic strategy. One example that suggests this possibility is the increase in headaches at high elevations. Lower availability of the superoxide radical, a known scavenger of NO, may account for excessive NO availability. Similarly, L-arginine increases exhaled NO and headaches at high altitude and may precipitate migraine attacks [61]. Triptan overuse among migraineurs may also lead to an increase in headache frequency, possibly due to induction of neuronal nitric oxide synthase [62].

VITAMIN B12

After in vitro data documented the ability of vitamin B12 to act as a nitric oxide scavenger [63], a small open-label trial of intranasal hydroxocobalamin (1 mg per day) reported a 53% responder rate among migraineurs and 63% had a 30% or greater decrease in frequency [64]. Although a placebo is not likely to have had such a potent effect, no subsequent trials have been done. It is not clear if any markers of vitamin B12 status, such as methylmalonic acid, would help predict response to treatment.

FEVERFEW

As mentioned previously, feverfew may have inhibitory effects on iNOS activity. It is also thought to inhibit prostaglandin production and reduce blood vessel reactivity and the secretion of serotonin from platelets. In one double-blinded and randomized trial, an extract of feverfew had greatest efficacy at a dose of 6.25 mg three times per day, but only in a small subset of migraineurs [65]. A second study at this dose reduced migraine frequency by 1.9 per month compared to 1.3 in the placebo group (from an initial 4.76) [66].

NEUROTRANSMITTERS AND RECEPTORS

An increase in cortical synaptic excitability seems to be a feature of migraine, although the mechanisms are not well established. Glutamate, the major excitatory neurotransmitter in the central nervous system, has been implicated as a principal factor in this phenomenon [67], along with an imbalance between glutamate and GABA (gamma aminobutyric acid), the major inhibitory transmitter, in the brain of migraineurs.

In 2010, the first evidence was produced for an association between genetic variations. Polymorphisms in the glutamate receptor genes GRIA1 and GRIA3 (GRI standing for glutamate receptor ionotropic) have been found to be strongly associated with migraine, both with and without aura; different polymorphisms were associated with each migraine type [68]. Drug development is now underway to develop glutamate receptor antagonists [69].

Dopamine is likely to be responsible for some nonheadache symptoms of migraine, including nausea/vomiting and hypotension. Dopamine agonists increase the number of yawns over time in migraineurs compared to controls, indicating a likely hypersensitivity [70]. Given that tyrosine hydroxylase converts tyrosine to L-dopa, an increase in trace amines may induce dopaminergic activity. Genetic evidence for this link was established in 2009, when polymorphisms in dopamine-beta hydroxylase (which converts dopamine to norepinephrine) and dopamine transporter genes were found in migraineurs with aura [71].

MELATONIN

The hormone melatonin has been shown to reduce the sensitivity of central dopamine receptors in animal studies and to inhibit dopamine release [72,73], suggesting it may have a beneficial role in migraine. Additionally, a urinary metabolite of melatonin was found to be decreased in individuals with chronic migraine compared to controls [74], and inhibition of melatonin production appears to be much more sensitive to light in migraineurs versus controls [75].

Two clinical trials without controls found excellent results for migraine prevention. A dose of 3 mg immediate-release melatonin had a responder rate of 80%, and after three months no migraines occurred in 25% of participants [76]. The second trial in children had a responder rate of 66%, with 20% experiencing complete resolution [77].

The first controlled trial of melatonin in migraine was published in *Neurology* in 2010; after eight weeks of 2 mg prolonged-release melatonin before bedtime, no difference was seen compared to placebo. Although migraine frequency was significantly reduced by melatonin, a similar benefit was observed with the (undefined) placebo. Limitations of this study include the short time frame, crossover format, an unexpectedly high placebo effect, and possibly the use of prolonged-release versus immediate-release melatonin, as was used in the open-label trials. As mentioned by the authors, previous studies of jet lag found 0.5 mg immediate-release to have superior benefit to 2 mg prolonged-release melatonin [78].

In 2010, an analysis linking an increase with latitude in migraine and in tension type headache prevalence was released [79], suggesting a possible light-mediated connection with melatonin and/ or vitamin D.

MAGNESIUM

Magnesium has been examined in a number of clinical trials for migraine, with mixed results, yet a significant benefit emerges from the data. Levels have been shown to be reduced in the brains of migraineurs, especially during an attack, and magnesium influences multiple mechanisms likely to have benefitted, including serotonin receptors, NO synthesis, NMDA (n-methyl d-aspartate) receptors, and the ability to block glutamate-dependent spreading depression [80,81]. In a randomized and placebo-controlled trial that enrolled migraineurs without aura, 600 mg magnesium citrate per day was given daily for three months. This produced reductions in both attack frequency and severity compared to placebo, and the researchers documented changes in cortical blood flow (by computed tomography) likely to be associated with benefit [82]. It is notable that the citrate form of magnesium was used in this study, as the use of other less absorbable forms may help to explain negative findings of previous trials. When given intravenously, magnesium sulfate (1000 mg) was found to reduce pain and other migraine symptoms in patients with aura, compared to controls, and relieved related symptoms such as phonophobia/photophobia [83,84].

BIOGENIC AMINES

Tyramine is produced from the amino acid tyrosine in a slow process during fermentation. It is rarely present in fresh food but any food that has spent time being fermented, matured, or cured may contain it. Foods known to contain tyramine include matured cheeses, cured meats, hung game, nonfresh fish, overripe fruits, fermented vegetable products (e.g., sauerkraut), and fermented soya products.

It has long been suspected that tyramine, along with other trace amines such as octopamine, synephrine, and phenylethylamine (in chocolate) modulate cortical hyperexcitability by acting as false neurotransmitters; they displace neurotransmitters such as norepinephrine and glutamate from their storage vesicles and can act as both neurotransmitters and neuromodulators at dopamine and norepinephrine synaptic clefts [85].

Elevations in these amines have now been documented in primary headaches [86], with different profiles in migraineurs with and without aura [87], perhaps thus explaining some of the autonomic disturbances, behavioral changes, and premonitory migraine symptoms [88].

Tyramine can replace norepinephrine in presynaptic vesicles of nerves. Normally, this substitution has little effect, but as it is metabolized by the enzyme monoamine oxidase A (MAO), in persons taking monoamine oxidase inhibitors (MAOIs) tyramine may not be cleared and may accumulate in higher concentrations. The effect is mediated by action on peripheral, autonomic nerve endings and may involve hypertension, tachycardia, and severe headache. If severe, this can amount to hypertensive crisis.

The tyramine hypothesis for migraine arose when it was noted that the list of foods causing severe headaches in patients on MAOIs was similar to that reported as suspected dietary triggers by some migraine sufferers. In a pilot study, capsules of 100 mg tyramine were given to four migraineurs with a definite dietary history and provoked migraines in all cases; placebo capsules of 100 mg lactose did not. In four migraineurs without known or suspected dietary triggers, neither tyramine nor lactose provoked symptoms [89].

Since that time, the amine hypothesis has been repeatedly studied clinically, and the results have repeatedly disappointed. In 2003, a systematic review [90] of randomized, controlled trials (RCTs) of biogenic amines' effects identified 13 oral challenge studies, of which only five were positive in outcome. Of the 13 total studies, three were deemed ineligible for the meta-analysis and six yielded inconclusive findings. The remaining four conclusive studies (two on tyramine and migraine, one on phenylethylamine from chocolate and headaches, and one on amines in red wine and symptoms) all reported no effect. Moreover, in the open study of elimination diets conducted by Grant [91], while 85% of subjects became migraine free on the allergen elimination diet, only 13% did so on the amine-free diet.

Despite this overall negative finding, the scientific plausibility of the amine hypothesis remains unrefuted, given the MAOI experience in particular. It has been hypothesized that only a subgroup of migraineurs are susceptible to tyramine. Some scientists have estimated that these individuals represent 10% of the total migraine-affected population (unconfirmed news report).

Genomics offers a possible mechanism for such a susceptibility, based around the sulfotransferases. This large family of enzymes adds sulfate groups to a range of molecules. The addition has a predominantly inactivating effect; steroid hormones, for example, are mainly transported in the inactive, sulfated form but can then be reactivated by sulfatase enzymes on cell surfaces.

Sulfotransferase enzymes coded for by the genes SULT1A1 and SULT1A3 are mainly present in platelets, and enable sulfation of phenolic compounds such as biogenic amines. SULT1A1 enzyme activity is reduced by approximately 50% in migraineurs compared to patients with tension headache or controls [92], and SULT1A3 has also been found to be lowered in at least one study [93].

Current understanding of epigenetics suggests that polymorphisms of the two genes might alter the response to inhibitors and inducers of gene expression. In common with several other enzyme genes, the SULT genes are inhibited (in some cases by 100%) by sulforaphane, present in most vegetables but found in significant quantities only in the cruciferi: broccoli, cabbage, and cauliflower. The result of inhibiting the SULT gene is less production of the enzyme for which it encodes and so less enzyme activity. This epigenetic effect may mean that foods can alter an individual's predisposition to migraine by altering the amine pathway, either instead of or as well as by triggering intolerance reactions.

Recent advances in the detection of these amines, as well as the discovery of a new class of G-protein coupled receptors (trace amine receptors, TAARs) that have a high affinity for these amines, have also stimulated a renewal of interest in this area.

CAFFEINE

Caffeine is a vasopressor and stimulant found in coffee, tea, cocoa, mate, and guarana, and is the most widely used psychoactive agent worldwide. The caffeine withdrawal syndrome is consequently well recognized and described. It involves some or all of the following symptoms, the overlap of which with migraine is evident [94]: headache, fatigue, drowsiness, loss of concentration, irritability, anxiety, depression, nausea and vomiting, and motor performance impairment.

Although the typical headache of caffeine withdrawal is described as diffuse and not hemicranial, it is associated with considerable comorbidity of different types of headache including migraines, and many migraineurs report both caffeine consumption and caffeine avoidance/cessation as risk factors. One case-control study (n = 713) found caffeine consumption to be a modest risk factor for headaches regardless of type [95]. Caffeine is also widely used as an adjuvant in analgesic medications for headache, even though a nonsystematic review did not find a significant adjuvant effect with its inclusion [96].

The CYP1A2 gene codes for a major cytochrome P450 enzyme of the same name, which is responsible for 90% of caffeine metabolism—specifically, converting it into other dimethylxanthines. Known polymorphisms in this enzyme could well account for substantial variability in caffeine sensitivity. One of the most common of these polymorphisms, CYP1A2*1F, also known more simply as F allele (nucleotide change 164A → C, U.K. prevalence of the allele approximately 33%), is a highly inducible variant; inducers include cruciferous vegetables, chargrilled meat, and insulin (in diabetics). Exposure to these products can increase enzyme activity much more in persons with the variant form of the gene.

One population study [97] found that homozygosity for the F allele was significantly more common in migraineurs. No subtype analysis for caffeine sensitivity was performed, so this association is merely suggestive at present.

ALCOHOL

Hannington (1967) observed that alcohol was often reported as a trigger for migraines, and this finding has been confirmed by most surveys since then [89]. For example, one survey [98] noted that 22 of 126 questionnaire responders (17%) found alcohol to be a trigger; none of them said alcohol triggered 50% or more of their attacks. Another by Kelman [7] found that 37.8% of 1307 migraineurs, and Garcia-Martín et al. [99] 32% of 197 migraineurs, reported alcohol as a trigger.

Garcia-Martín et al. went on to examine polymorphisms of the genes for the enzyme alcohol dehydrogenase, in particular ADH2. One polymorphism of this gene, rs1229984, causes the substitution of the amino acid histidine for arginine at location 48. Having the ADH2His allele appears to protect against alcohol abuse and alcoholism [100]. The same study revealed that the ADH2His allele was significantly more common in migraineurs who reported alcohol as a trigger than in those who did not. However, the allele frequency was 7.1% versus 2.4%, respectively, while the frequency of the same allele in nonmigraineurs was 7.6%, so it is difficult to see what this proves.

FOODS

In 1930, Albert Rowe described a case series of 86 patients with migraine triggered by specific foods [101]. He reported a comorbidity of migraines with allergic toxemia, a term no longer in common medical use, which encompasses drowsiness, confusion, slowness of thought, mood changes, and fatigue (no statistics given), together with gastrointestinal symptoms such as bloating, discomfort, and change of bowel habit (occurring in 64% of the migraine group), as well as skin reactions (43%).

In 1979, in an open study of 126 patients attending a London hospital migraine clinic, Ellen Grant examined the effect of elimination diets [91]. For the first five days subjects ate only two foods considered to be low risks for triggering migraine and drank only bottled spring water. Most had migraines or headaches in the first three days, but were free of them by the fifth day. They were then instructed to introduce common foods into their diet one by one, to record their symptoms, and to avoid any foods associated with the onset of symptoms. Ninety-one patients completed the process and continued afterward to avoid identified triggers. The first 60 consecutive patients to complete the trial were included in the analysis (52 were females). All patients improved; of the 60, only 9 (15%) still had headaches or migraines at follow-up. The most frequent triggers were: wheat (78%), orange (39%), egg (45%), tea and coffee (40%), chocolate (37%), milk (37%), beef (35%), corn and cane sugar (33%), yeast (33%), mushrooms (30%), and peas (28%).

This study provides a proof of concept for food triggers of migraine. Another group of researchers [102,103] concluded that two-thirds of severe migraineurs are allergic to foods. Both studies used therapeutic response to cromoglycate to argue that the mechanism in migraine is allergic.

Randomized controlled trials (RCTs) are scarce in this area. However, a key study in children, part of a series conducted at Great Ormond St. Children's Hospital in London, was an RCT [104]. In this investigation, 88 children with severe frequent migraines underwent oligoantigenic diets and

78 of them (88%) recovered completely. In a second phase, 40 of the patients then underwent further double-blinded, placebo-controlled challenge testing to confirm the triggering foods. Twenty-six (65%) developed headaches after active challenge, but not after placebo challenge.

Researchers noted improvements in comorbidities of abdominal and central nervous symptoms and allergic disorders such as asthma and eczema. Nondietary triggers such as stroboscopic effects and exertion no longer caused migraines when the children were on the diet. These findings were broadly confirmed in a subsequent RCT of an oligoantigenic diet in hyperkinesis; headaches including migraines also improved when patients were on the diet [105].

GLUCOSE DYSREGULATION

Hunger was reported as a trigger by 57% of responders in a survey [7]. Three-quarters of migraineurs in another study [106] had extended glucose tolerance tests that were consistent with reactive hypoglycemia.

The role of body mass index and insulin resistance in migraine pathogenesis is beginning to grow. Insulin resistance has recently been correlated with the duration of migraine attacks, and the metabolic syndrome with multiple migraine triggers [107]. Recent reports also suggest that obesity may be related to migraine progression [108], and weight loss may help reduce headaches among obese patients [109]. BMI has been associated with headache severity and frequency, as well as migraine symptoms such as photophobia and phonophobia [110].

OTHER DIETARY INTERVENTIONS

Clinical benefit has also been described for natural therapies without a clear mechanism of action. For example, in a randomized trial of individuals with recurrent headaches and a total fluid intake less than 2.5 L per day, instructions to increase water intake by 1.5 L resulted in significant improvement on the Migraine-Specific Quality of Life (MSQOL) scale [111]. Similar to hydration, exercise improves circulation. A controlled trial of exercise compared to both relaxation and medication use found similar efficacy for migraine prophylaxis [112].

Given the role neuronal inflammation and mitochondrial dysfunction are thought to play in migraine, the use of EPA (eicosapentaenoic acid) and DHA (docosahexaenoic acid) seem likely candidates for a prophylactic effect. Two placebo-controlled studies have been published, both of which reported no benefit compared to placebo, yet a marked improvement from baseline. Both trials used olive oil as placebo, raising questions about the potential for a benefit from the olive oil to be obscuring the data [113,114].

Lipoprotein(a) elevations, perhaps beginning in childhood, have also emerged as a risk factor for migraine, and may contribute to the increased risk of stroke [115]. Therapies such as niacin may be warranted to address this abnormality.

MENSTRUAL MIGRAINES

Menstrual migraines also represent unique migraine physiology, with changes in sex hormones thought to modulate CGRP levels, cortical excitability, norepinephrine and serotonin synthesis, as well as magnesium status [116]. Iron deficiency anemia has also emerged as a potential contributor to menstrual migraines [117].

Clinically, phytoestrogens have had impressive results in a double-blind trial (60 mg soy isoflavones, 100 mg dong quai, and 50 mg black cohosh) [118], as has magnesium supplementation, which also improved premenstrual complaints [119]. Magnesium levels are at their lowest during menstrually related attacks, and response to therapy may best be predicted by serum ionized magnesium [120]. Lastly, although much data was unreported, results of a double-blind, controlled trial with 400 IU vitamin E for five days (two before menstruation and three after) was shown to reduce pain severity, disability, and need for additional medications [121].

PEDIATRIC MIGRAINE

THE EPIDEMIOLOGY OF PEDIATRIC MIGRAINE

The estimated prevalence of headache in children is as high as 50–70%. Incidence has increased over the past 30 years. For example, a 1996 study of migraine showed a prevalence of 51.5% among seven-year-olds in 1992 as compared to 14.4% in 1974 [122]. In a Cleveland study, the researchers found that 8.6% of school children met the International Headache Society (IHS) criteria for migraine. Yet only 20% of these children had been diagnosed by a physician as having migraines and most of those had not received treatment [123]. Until age 12, the incidence of migraine is equal in both genders. After puberty, females have an increased incidence of migraine over males [124].

DIAGNOSTIC EVALUATION

After extensive but fruitless gastrointestinal work-up, some children present with gastrointestinal variants of migraine such as abdominal migraines or cyclic vomiting [125]. Imaging with magnetic resonance imaging (MRI) of the brain or computed tomography (CT) is necessary either if the neurological exam is abnormal or if headache presentation is atypical with new or sudden onset, or with an increase in frequency, duration, or intensity.

ACUTE PHARMACOLOGICAL TREATMENT

Medications, used successfully in many adults, are less effective in children. In particular, children under the age of six have been shown to do better with conservative, nonpharmacological treatment for their migraines [126]. Ergotamine, a vasoconstrictor of the external carotid artery, is often given during the aura phase in order to prevent the vasodilatation that causes migraine pain. However, it is less successful in younger children because at high doses it causes nausea and vomiting [127]. Other side effects include ergotamine-induced headache and potential dependence on the medication. However, when other treatments fail, intravenous dihydroergotamine has been shown to be successful in children over six. Oral metoclopramide was given 30 minutes prior to the dihydroergotamine. This was repeated every 20 minutes for up to three doses in outpatients and every six hours for up to eight doses in inpatients. Eighty percent responded with minimal side effects [123]. Although nasal sumatriptan has been shown to have some efficacy in children, oral sumatriptan in the pediatric population shows no benefit over placebo [128].

Prophylactic treatment is generally considered if the child has three to four attacks per month, the headaches are severe and school attendance is disrupted, or acute therapies are ineffective or have significant side effects. Propranolol is the most common beta blocker prescribed for migraines in children. The drug has a short half-life and therefore must be administered in a three-times-a-day schedule beginning at 1 mg/kg. However, beta blockers are contraindicated in asthma and certain cardiac conditions. In children with frequent migraines, tricyclic antidepressants are used. Clinical effectiveness may be delayed by weeks after treatment has begun. Tricyclic antidepressants are contraindicated in the presence of cardiac disease. Other choices include antiepileptic medications such as valproic acid and topirimate [123].

NONPHARMACOLOGICAL TREATMENT

Nearly a quarter of children with migraine are considered to be refractory to pharmaceutical approaches [129]. Migraines are a clinical manifestation of a body and nervous system in distress. As such, successful therapy for children requires a multipronged approach. A regimen of normal sleep, regular eating schedules, and preferably, exercise, is imperative [130]

However, migraine in children has well-known connections to food and drink. Food additives of all types may trigger migraine, including artificial sweeteners, monosodium glutamate, and preservatives, which disrupt normal neurochemistry by triggering aberrant metabolic processes in the neuron such as excitotoxicity [131]. In addition, allergy plays a significant role. Increased Th2 immune response and associated abnormal inflammatory cytokine levels in pediatric migraineurs support the role of immune dysfunction in the etiology of childhood migraine [132,133]. Further, high prevalence of red-ear syndrome in children with migraine as well as in allergy further supports the allergic-migraine connection [134–135]. In one large-scale double-blind trial involving 88 patients treated with an oligoantigenic diet, eliminating all but a few sensitizing food antigens, 93% with severe frequent migraine were free of headaches [111]. The diet consisted of lamb or chicken, rice or potato, banana or apple, cruciferous vegetables, water, and vitamin supplements. Of the 82 patients who improved on the diet, all but eight patients relapsed upon the reintroduction of one or more foods. A remarkable fondness for migraine-provoking foods was a common finding, with some patients craving them and eating them in large amounts. These cravings for foods that provoke neurological or other problematic symptoms is an often observed hallmark of food sensitivities or allergies. Cow's milk and cheese caused headaches in most of the patients in the study, but none of the patients complained of headaches after substituting goat's milk cheese. Another double-blind, placebo-controlled provocation study by the same group found that 89% of children (n = 36) who had comorbid migraines and refractory epilepsy experienced statistically significant reduction in migraine and seizure symptoms on the oligoantigenic diet [136]. Gluten sensitivity or celiac, too, can be a significant trigger for pediatric migraine. Children with migraine have also been shown to have a slightly higher risk of celiac disease than controls as measured by tissue transglutaminase antibodies [137]. Children with celiac disease are more likely to have neurological symptoms such as migraines, than is the general population [138].

Despite impressive evidence supporting the role of food in migraine, the concept of food removal remains controversial. In part due to lack of education in nutrition, many neurologists and allergists are skeptical of the use of restrictive diets in treatment. However, by recording events in a headache diary, children and adolescents are able to compare headache frequency and intensity before and after diet to objectively assess improvement. Foods can then be reintroduced one at a time in order to assess for exacerbation of headaches. Though this process can be inconvenient, many families find that changing diet is far less difficult than having a child with refractory headaches who misses school frequently and is often in pain. This option should be one that is offered to patients with appropriate support from a physician or nutritionist.

By any standard, elimination diet is the gold-standard approach to elucidating which foods, if any, impact the child's health. A headache diary, including daily meals, may be helpful in the process of identifying triggers. While it is worthwhile to measure IgE and IgG panels of common allergens, these panels represent an inexact science—a negative result should never take priority over the observations of food reactivity from parents or from the children themselves. Skin testing identifies food allergies less effectively than blood testing, as noted in studies on eosinophilic esophagitis [139]. Conversely, even low or equivocal positivity should trigger investigation due to the limitations of testing for food allergens in skin or blood.

The practitioner must monitor for and address specific nutrient deficiencies when applicable. Before considering the elimination of a broad array of foods, careful logging of diet and symptoms can often identify specific triggers. Often, one or two triggers can be identified without the induction of the oligoantigenic diet. Common food allergens to investigate include dairy, egg, soy, wheat, corn, citrus, peanut, tree nuts, and shellfish.

Children with migraine have been shown to have increased vulnerability to oxidative stress [140], lipid peroxidation [141], as well as mitochondrial dysfunction [142]. In addition, those with childhood migraine are more likely to have MTHFR polymorphisms [143,144], and elevated stroke-associated hypercoagulability markers such as homocysteine and lipoprotein(a) [145]. Supplemental nutrients and botanicals target these areas of vulnerability.

High-dose riboflavin (200 mg or 400 mg) alone may contribute to decreased frequency of pediatric headaches, with better response to abortive therapy than placebo [146,147]. Although riboflavin has not been shown to effectively prevent pediatric migraine in some studies at doses of 50–200 mg [148,149], these studies were complicated by unprecedented response to placebo treatments. In general, riboflavin may improve the cumulative effect of combination therapy in pediatric migraine, as seen further in studies outlined here.

Intracellular magnesium levels have been found to be reduced in populations with migraines [150,151]. Ongoing oral repletion of magnesium reduces frequency and intensity of events [152]. In a randomized, double-blind, placebo-controlled trial, magnesium oxide supplements led to significant reduction in headache days in children who suffered from migraine [153]. Doses were 9 mg/kg daily, though significantly higher doses can be used in smaller children. Furthermore, magnesium oxide is less well absorbed than magnesium glycinate or chelated magnesium, which may have shown increased efficacy at lower doses.

Children and adolescents with migraine commonly have deficiency in CoQ10 levels and show improvement in headache frequency and intensity with repletion [154]. In a randomized, double-blind, placebo-controlled, cross-over trial of pediatric and adolescent migraine, CoQ10 was shown to improve frequency significantly in the first four weeks of treatment, though both groups showed benefit by the last four weeks [155]. Other studies support this finding; 75% of children with refractory cyclic vomiting syndrome, also thought to stem in part from mitochondrial dysfunction, improved or resolved with a combination of CoQ10, L-carnitine, and amitryptiline [156].

An open-label, prospective trial investigating Gingkolide B in 30 children showed benefit as a preventive treatment with few side effects. Treatment was well tolerated, and compliance was good, indicating that gingko may be considered as a prophylactic treatment in pediatric migraine [157]. Gingko has been effective in reducing migraine frequency as part of a combination supplement as well.

In a double-blind, placebo-controlled study of 60 subjects, 208 attacks of migraine were treated with either sublingual feverfew/ginger or a sublingual placebo preparation [158]. At two hours, 32% of subjects receiving active medication and 16% of subjects receiving placebo were pain free (P = .02). At two hours, 63% of subjects receiving feverfew/ginger found pain relief (pain free or mild headache) versus 39% for placebo (P = .002). Though well tolerated, oral numbness and nausea were the most frequently occurring adverse event.

Butterbur (*Petasites hybridus*) has repeatedly been shown to be safe, effective, and well tolerated in the prevention of adult and pediatric migraine [147,159,160]. In a four-week, placebo-controlled trial, migraine frequency improved by 50% or more in subjects. In a four-month trial, 75 mg of butterbur decreased migraine frequency by greater than 50%, with occasional side effects only of burping [161].

Two open trials have explored the impact of some combination of the following: gingkolide B, coenzyme Q10, riboflavin, B12, and magnesium. A 50% reduction in migraine frequency was seen after three months of treatment [162,163].

Folic acid is known to play a role in decreasing elevated homocysteine levels [164]. Di Rosa et al. examined 16 children with polymorphisms of the MTHFR enzyme and elevated homocysteine. When replete with folic acid, homocysteine levels dropped significantly with events decreasing over 75% in 15 out of 16 children [52]. While larger studies are needed, the level of response indicates that child migraineurs with a history or family history of stroke or hypercoagulability should undergo full evaluation for these polymorphisms and markers. Those with positive findings may well benefit from a trial of B complex vitamins including 5-methylene tetrahydrofolate (5-MTHF) supplementation.

CSF phospholipase C activity is elevated in migraineurs during episodes [165], which affects phospholipid concentration and activity of cell membrane. Dimyristoylphosphatidylcholine experimentally has been shown to prevent cleavage of the apoB conformation on the LDL surface that inhibits lipoprotein (a) assembly [166].

Phosphatidylcholine administration may have a role in treatment of underlying pathophysiology of migraine, as well as mitigating stroke risk factors [167] related to elevated lipoprotein(a) in children with migraine. Further studies are warranted.

CLINICAL SUMMARY

More than 300 million people across the globe suffer from migraine, driving intensive research in recent years to more deeply understand the pathophysiology behind this complex neurological disorder. As our understanding of the unique triggers and individualized factors behind migraine advances, our therapies can expand from just pain relief to selecting therapies that address root causes, and thereby provide an authentic healing response rather than mere suppression of symptoms.

Clinical key points can be summarized as follows:

- Migraine is multifactorial; most sufferers report multiple triggers.
- Stress is a trigger for most sufferers.
- Amines such as tyramine cannot be more than minor triggers.
- Food can trigger migraine.
- Absent controlled trials, two-thirds of migraineurs (and more of child sufferers) respond to elimination diets.
- Hunger or low blood sugar is a trigger in at least one-half of sufferers.
- Two-thirds of sufferers benefit from high-dose riboflavin supplements.
- At least one-half benefit from vitamin B12.
- Nearly one-half respond to prophylactic butterbur.

REFERENCES

1. Insinga RP, et al. Costs associated with outpatient, emergency room and inpatient care for migraine in the USA. *Cephalalgia*. 2011 Nov 31(15):1570–75.
2. Diamond S, et al. Patterns of diagnosis and acute and preventive treatment for migraine in the United States: Results from the American Migraine Prevalence and Prevention study. *Headache*. 2007 Mar 47(3):355–63.
3. Mueller LL. Diagnosing and managing migraine headache. *J Am Osteopath Assoc*. 2007 Nov 107(10 Suppl 6):ES10–16.
4. Cutrer FM. Pathophysiology of migraine. *Semin Neurol*. 2010 Apr 30(2):120–30.
5. Mathew NT. Pathophysiology of chronic migraine and mode of action of preventive medications. *Headache*. 2011 Jul–Aug 51 Suppl 2:84–92.
6. Wöber C, Wöber-Bingöl C. Triggers of migraine and tension-type headache. *Handb Clin Neurol*. 2010 97:161–72.
7. Kelman L. The triggers or precipitants of the acute migraine attack. *Cephalalgia*. 2007 27:394–402.
8. Cortelli P, Pierangeli G, Montagna P. Is migraine a disease? *Neurol Sci*. 2010 Jun 31 Suppl 1:S29–31.
9. Ren H, et al. Shorter telomere length in peripheral blood cells associated with migraine in women. *Headache*. 2010 Jun 50(6):965–72.
10. Ku M, et al. Prevalence of migraine headaches in patients with allergic rhinitis. *Ann Allergy Asthma Immunol*. 2006 Aug 97(2):226–30.
11. Aamodt AH, et al., Is headache related to asthma, hay fever, and chronic bronchitis? The Head-HUNT Study. *Headache*. 2007 Feb 47(2):204–12.
12. Mortimer MJ, et al. The prevalence of headache and migraine in atopic children: An epidemiological study in general practice. *Headache*. 1993 Sep 33(8):427–31.
13. Wendorff J, et al. Allergy effect on migraine course in older children and adolescents. *Neurol Neurochir Pol*. 1999 33 Suppl 5:55–65.
14. Gazerani P, et al. A correlation between migraine, histamine and immunoglobulin E. *Scand J Immunol*. 2003 Mar 57(3):286–90.
15. Agosti R, et al. Effectiveness of Petasites hybridus preparations in the prophylaxis of migraine: A systematic review. *Phytomedicine*. 2006 Nov 13(9–10):743–46.

16. Schapowal A, Petasites Study Group. Butterbur Ze339 for the treatment of intermittent allergic rhinitis: Dose-dependent efficacy in a prospective, randomized, double-blind, placebo-controlled study. *Arch Otolaryngol Head Neck Surg.* 2004 Dec 130(12):1381–86.

17. Schapowal A, Study Group. Treating intermittent allergic rhinitis: A prospective, randomized, placebo and antihistamine-controlled study of Butterbur extract Ze 339. *Phytother Res.* 2005 Jun 19(6):530–37.

18. Diener HC, et al. The first placebo-controlled trial of a special butterbur root extract for the prevention of migraine: Reanalysis of efficacy criteria. *Eur Neurol.* 2004 51(2):89–97.

19. Horak S, et al. Use-dependent block of voltage-gated Cav2.1 Ca2+ channels by petasins and eudesmol isomers. *J Pharmacol Exp Ther.* 2009 Jul 330(1):220–26.

20. Olness K, et al. Mast cell activation in children with migraine before and after training in self-regulation. *Headache.* 1999 Feb 39(2):101–7.

21. Theodoropoulos DS, et al. Allergen-specific sublingual immunotherapy in the treatment of migraines: A prospective study. *Eur Rev Med Pharmacol Sci.* 2011 Oct 15(10):1117–21.

22. Sparaco M, et al. Mitochondrial dysfunction and migraine: Evidence and hypotheses. *Cephalalgia.* 2006 Apr 26(4):361–72.

23. Kabbouche MA, et al. Carnitine palmityltransferase II (CPT2) deficiency and migraine headache: Two case reports. *Headache.* 2003 May 43(5):490–95.

24. Zaki EA, et al. Two common mitochondrial DNA polymorphisms are highly associated with migraine headache and cyclic vomiting syndrome. *Cephalalgia.* 2009 Jul 29(7):719–28.

25. Scholte HR, et al. Riboflavin-responsive complex I deficiency. *Biochim Biophys Acta.* 1995 May 24 1271(1):75–83.

26. Schoenen J, et al. High-dose riboflavin as a prophylactic treatment of migraine: Results of an open pilot study. *Cephalalgia.* 1994 Oct 14(5):328–29.

27. Schoenen J, et al. Effectiveness of high-dose riboflavin in migraine prophylaxis. A randomized controlled trial. *Neurology.* 1998 Feb 50(2):466–70.

28. Condò M, et al. Riboflavin prophylaxis in pediatric and adolescent migraine. *J Headache Pain.* 2009 Oct 10(5):361–65.

29. Sándor PS, et al. Prophylactic treatment of migraine with beta-blockers and riboflavin: Differential effects on the intensity dependence of auditory evoked cortical potentials. *Headache.* 2000 Jan 40(1):30–35.

30. Di Lorenzo C, et al. Mitochondrial DNA haplogroups influence the therapeutic response to riboflavin in migraineurs. *Neurology.* 2009 May 5 72(18):1588–94.

31. Ruiz-Pesini E, et al. Human mtDNA haplogroups associated with high or reduced spermatozoa motility. *Am J Hum Genet.* 2000 Sep 67(3):682–96.

32. Fesahat F, et al. Do haplogroups H and U act to increase the penetrance of Alzheimer's disease? *Cell Mol Neurobiol.* 2007 May 27(3):329–34.

33. Pyle A, et al. Mitochondrial DNA haplogroup cluster UKJT reduces the risk of PD. *Ann Neurol.* 2005 Apr 57(4):564–67.

34. McNulty H, et al. Riboflavin lowers homocysteine in individuals homozygous for the MTHFR 677C→T polymorphism. *Circulation.* 2006 Jan 3 113(1):74–80.

35. Rozen TD. Open label trial of coenzyme Q10 as a migraine preventive. *Cephalalgia.* 2002 Mar 22(2):137–41.

36. Sándor PS, et al. Efficacy of coenzyme Q10 in migraine prophylaxis: A randomized controlled trial. *Neurology.* 2005 Feb 22 64(4):713–15.

37. Hershey AD, et al. Coenzyme Q10 deficiency and response to supplementation in pediatric and adolescent migraine. *Headache.* 2007 Jan 47(1):73–80.

38. Magis D, et al. A randomized double-blind placebo-controlled trial of thioctic acid in migraine prophylaxis. *Headache.* 2007 Jan 47(1):52–57.

39. Khandanpour N, et al. Peripheral arterial disease and methylenetetrahydrofolate reductase (MTHFR) C677T mutations: A case-control study and meta-analysis. *J Vasc Surg.* 2009 Mar 49(3):711–18.

40. Durga J, et al. Homocysteine and carotid intima-media thickness: A critical appraisal of the evidence. *Atherosclerosis.* 2004 Sep 176(1):1–19.

41. Pizza V, et al. Migraine and coronary artery disease: An open study on the genetic polymorphism of the 5, 10 methylenetetrahydrofolate (MTHFR) and angiotensin I-converting enzyme (ACE) genes. *Cent Nerv Syst Agents Med Chem.* 2010 Jun 1 10(2):91–96.

42. Schürks M, et al. MTHFR 677C>T and ACE D/I polymorphisms in migraine: A systematic review and meta-analysis. *Headache.* 2010 Apr 50(4):588–99.

43. Oterino A, et al. The relationship between homocysteine and genes of folate-related enzymes in migraine patients. *Headache.* 2010 Jan 50(1):99–168.

44. Isobe C, et al. A remarkable increase in total homocysteine concentrations in the CSF of migraine patients with aura. *Headache.* 2010 Nov 50(10):1561–69.

45. Gudmundsson LS. Migraine with aura and risk of cardiovascular and all cause mortality in men and women: Prospective cohort study. *BMJ.* 2010 Aug 24 341:c3966.

46. Kurth T, et al. Migraine and risk of haemorrhagic stroke in women: Prospective cohort study. *BMJ.* 2010 Aug 24 341:c3659.

47. Schürks M, et al. Migraine and cardiovascular disease: Systematic review and meta-analysis. *BMJ.* 2009 Oct 27 339:b3914.

48. Tietjen GE. Migraine as a systemic vasculopathy. *Cephalalgia.* 2009 Sep 29(9):987–96.

49. Ratan RR. Oxidative stress induces apoptosis in embryonic cortical neurons. *J Neurochem.* 1994 Jan 62(1):376–79.

50. Ratan RR, et al. Macromolecular synthesis inhibitors prevent oxidative stress-induced apoptosis in embryonic cortical neurons by shunting cysteine from protein synthesis to glutathione. *J Neurosci.* 1994 Jul 14(7):4385–92.

51. Lea R, et al. The effects of vitamin supplementation and MTHFR (C677T) genotype on homocysteine-lowering and migraine disability. *Pharmacogenet Genomics.* 2009 Jun 19(6):422–28.

52. Di Rosa G, et al. Efficacy of folic acid in children with migraine, hyperhomocysteinemia and MTHFR polymorphisms. *Headache.* 2007 Oct 47(9):1342–44.

53. Ames BN, Elson-Schwab I, Silver EA. High-dose vitamin therapy stimulates variant enzymes with decreased coenzyme binding affinity (increased K(m)): Relevance to genetic disease and polymorphisms. *Am J Clin Nutr.* 2002 Apr 75(4):616–58.

54. Yazdanpanah N, et al. Low dietary riboflavin but not folate predicts increased fracture risk in postmenopausal women homozygous for the MTHFR 677 T allele. *J Bone Miner Res.* 2008 Jan 23(1):86–94.

55. Wilson CP, et al. Riboflavin offers a targeted strategy for managing hypertension in patients with the MTHFR 677TT genotype: A 4-yr follow-up. *Am J Clin Nutr.* 2012 95(3):766–72.

56. Liu A, et al. Analysis of the MTHFR C677T variant with migraine phenotypes. *BMC Res Notes.* 2010 Jul 28 3:213.

57. Olesen J, et al. Nitric oxide is a key molecule in migraine and other vascular headaches. *Trends Pharmacol Sci.* 1994 May 15(5):149–53.

58. Olesen J. The role of nitric oxide (NO) in migraine, tension-type headache and cluster headache. *Pharmacol Ther.* 2008 Nov 120(2):157–71.

59. de O S Mansur T, et al. Inducible nitric oxide synthase haplotype associated with migraine and aura. *Mol Cell Biochem.* 2012 364(1–2):303–8.

60. Aviram A, et al. Inhibition of nitric oxide synthesis in mouse macrophage cells by feverfew Supercritical Extract. *Phytother Res.* 2011 26(4):541–45.

61. Mansoor JK, et al. L-arginine supplementation enhances exhaled NO, breath condensate VEGF, and headache at 4,342 m. *High Alt Med Biol.* 2005 Winter 6(4):289–300.

62. De Felice M, et al. Triptan-induced enhancement of neuronal nitric oxide synthase in trigeminal ganglion dural afferents underlies increased responsiveness to potential migraine triggers. *Brain.* 2010 Jul 13.

63. Brouwer M, et al. Nitric oxide interactions with cobalamins: Biochemical and functional consequences. *Blood.* 1996 Sep 1 88(5):1857–64.

64. van der Kuy PH, et al. Hydroxocobalamin, a nitric oxide scavenger, in the prophylaxis of migraine: An open, pilot study. *Cephalalgia.* 2002 Sep 22(7):513–19.

65. Pfaffenrath V, et al. The efficacy and safety of tanacetum parthenium (feverfew) in migraine prophylaxis—a double-blind, multicentre, randomized placebo-controlled dose-response study. *Cephalalgia.* 2002 Sep 22(7):523–32.

66. Diener HC, et al. Efficacy and safety of 6.25 mg t.i.d. feverfew CO2-extract (MIG-99) in migraine prevention—a randomized, double-blind, multicentre, placebo-controlled study. *Cephalalgia.* 2005 Nov 25(11):1031–41.

67. Ramadan NM. The link between glutamate and migraine. *CNS Spectr.* 2003 Jun 8(6):446–49.

68. Formicola D, et al. Common variants in the regulative regions of GRIA1 and GRIA3 receptor genes are associated with migraine susceptibility. *BMC Med Genet.* 2010 Jun 25 11:103.

69. Raddant AC, Russo AF. Calcitonin gene-related peptide in migraine: Intersection of peripheral inflammation and central modulation. *Expert Rev Mol Med.* 2011 Nov 29 13:e36.

70. Blin O, et al. Apomorphine-induced yawning in migraine patients: Enhanced responsiveness. *Clin Neuropharmacol.* 1991 Feb 14(1):91–95.

71. Todt U, et al. New genetic evidence for involvement of the dopamine system in migraine with aura. *Hum Genet.* 2009 Apr 125(3):265–79.
72. Abílio VC, et al. Effects of melatonin on behavioural dopaminergic supersensitivity. *Life Sci.* 2003 May 16 72(26):3003–15.
73. Zisapel N. Melatonin-dopamine interactions: From basic neurochemistry to a clinical setting. *Cell Mol Neurobiol.* 2001 Dec 21(6):605–16.
74. Masruha MR, et al. Urinary 6-sulphatoxymelatonin levels are depressed in chronic migraine and several comorbidities. *Headache.* 2010 Mar 50(3):413–19.
75. Claustrat B, et al. Melatonin secretion is supersensitive to light in migraine. *Cephalalgia.* 2004 Feb 24(2):128–33.
76. Peres MF, et al. Melatonin, 3 mg, is effective for migraine prevention. *Neurology.* 2004 Aug 24 63(4):757.
77. Miano S, et al. Melatonin to prevent migraine or tension-type headache in children. *Neurol Sci.* 2008 Sep 29(4):285–87.
78. Alstadhaug KB, et al. Prophylaxis of migraine with melatonin: A randomized controlled trial. *Neurology.* 2010 Oct 26 75(17):1527–32.
79. Prakash S, et al. The prevalence of headache may be related with the latitude: A possible role of vitamin D insufficiency? *J Headache Pain.* 2010 Aug 11(4):301–7.
80. D'Andrea G, et al. Pathogenesis of migraine: From neurotransmitters to neuromodulators and beyond. *Neurol Sci.* 2010 Jun 31 Suppl 1:S1–7.
81. Mauskop A, et al. Role of magnesium in the pathogenesis and treatment of migraines. *Clin Neurosci.* 1998 5(1):24–27.
82. Köseoglu E, et al. The effects of magnesium prophylaxis in migraine without aura. *Magnes Res.* 2008 Jun 21(2):101–8.
83. Bigal ME, et al. Intravenous magnesium sulphate in the acute treatment of migraine without aura and migraine with aura. A randomized, double-blind, placebo-controlled study. *Cephalalgia.* 2002 Jun 22(5):345–53.
84. Mauskop A, et al. Intravenous magnesium sulfate rapidly alleviates headaches of various types. *Headache.* 1996 Mar 36(3):154–60.
85. Berry MD. Mammalian central nervous system trace amines. Pharmacologic amphetamines, physiologic neuromodulators. *J Neurochem.* 2004 Jul 90(2):257–71.
86. D'Andrea G, et al. Elevated levels of circulating trace amines in primary headaches. Elevated levels of circulating trace amines in primary headaches. *Neurology.* 2004 May 25 62(10):1701–5.
87. D'Andrea G, et al. Abnormal platelet trace amine profiles in migraine with and without aura. *Cephalalgia.* 2006 Aug 26(8):968–72.
88. D'Andrea G, et al. Biochemistry of neuromodulation in primary headaches: Focus on anomalies of tyrosine metabolism. *Neurol Sci.* 2007 May 28 Suppl 2:S94–6.
89. Hannington E. Preliminary report on tyramine headache. *Brit Med J.* 1967 2:550–51.
90. Jansen SC, van Dusseldorp M, Bottema KC, Dubois AE. Intolerance to dietary biogenic amines: A review. *Ann Allergy Asthma Immunol.* 2003 91:233–40.
91. Grant EC. Food allergies and migraine. *Lancet.* 1979 1(8123):966–69.
92. Alam Z, et al. Platelet sulphotransferase activity, plasma sulphate levels and sulphation capacity in patients with migraine and tension headache. *Cephalalgia.* 1997 17:761–64.
93. Marazzitti D, et al. Platelet 3H-imipramine binding and sulphotransferase activity in primary headache. *Cephalalgia.* 1994 14:210–14.
94. Griffiths RR, Juliano LM, Chausmer AL. Caffeine pharmacology and clinical effects. In: Graham AW, Schultz TK, Mayo-Smith MF, et al., eds. Principles of Addiction Medicine (3rd ed.). Chevy Chase, MD: American Society of Addiction; 2003
95. Scher AI, Stewart WF, Lipton RB. Caffeine as a risk factor for chronic daily headache: A population-based study. *Neurology.* 2004 63:2022–27.
96. Gray RN, et al. *Self-Administered Drug Treatments for Acute Migraine Headache.* AHRQ Technical Reviews and Summaries. Rockville, MD: Agency for Health Care Policy and Research 1999.
97. Gentile G, et al. Frequencies of genetic polymorphisms related to triptans metabolism in chronic migraine. *J Headache Pain.* 2010 11:151–56.
98. Hauge AW, Kirchmann M, Olesen J. Characterization of consistent triggers of migraine with aura. *Cephalalgia.* 2011 31:416–38.
99. García-Martín E, et al. Alcohol dehydrogenase 2 genotype and risk for migraine. *Headache.* 2010 50:85–91.
100. Eriksson CJ, et al. Functional relevance of human ADH polymorphism. *Alcohol Clin Exp Res.* 2001 25:157S–63S.

101. Rowe AH. Allergic toxaemia and migraine due to food allergy. *Calif West Med*. 1930 33:785.
102. Monro J, Brostoff J, Carini C, Zilkha K. Food allergy in migraine: Study of dietary exclusion and RAST. *Lancet*. 1980 2(8184):1–4.
103. Monro J, Carini C, Brostoff J. Migraine is a food-allergic disease. *Lancet*. 1984 2(8405):719–21.
104. Egger J, et al. Is migraine food allergy? A double-blind controlled trial of oligoantigenic diet treatment. *Lancet*. 1983 2(8355):865–69.
105. Egger J, et al. Controlled trial of oligo-antigenic treatment in the hyperkinetic syndrome. *Lancet*. 1985 1(8428):540–45.
106. Dexter JD, et al. The five-hour glucose tolerance test and effect of low sucrose diet in migraine. *Headache*. 1978 18:91–94.
107. Bhoi SK, Kalita J, Misra UK. Metabolic syndrome and insulin resistance in migraine. *J Headache Pain*. 2012 13(4):321–26.
108. Bigal ME, Rapoport AM. Obesity and chronic daily headache. *Curr Pain Headache Rep*. 2012 Feb 16(1):101–9.
109. Bond DS, et al. Migraine and obesity: Epidemiology, possible mechanisms and the potential role of weight loss treatment. *Obes Rev*. 2011 12(5):e362–71.
110. Bigal ME, et al. Obesity and migraine: A population study. *Neurology*. 2006 Feb 28 66(4):545–50.
111. Spigt M, et al. A randomized trial on the effects of regular water intake in patients with recurrent headaches. *Fam Pract*. 2011 29(4):370–75.
112. Varkey E, et al. Exercise as migraine prophylaxis: a randomized study using relaxation and topiramate as controls. *Cephalalgia*. 2011 Oct 31(14):1428–38.
113. Pradalier A, et al. Failure of omega-3 polyunsaturated fatty acids in prevention of migraine: A double-blind study versus placebo. *Cephalalgia*. 2001 Oct 21(8):818–22.
114. Harel Z, et al. Supplementation with omega-3 polyunsaturated fatty acids in the management of recurrent migraines in adolescents. *J Adolesc Health*. 2002 Aug 31(2):154–61.
115. Gouni-Berthold I, Berthold HK. Lipoprotein(a): Current perspectives. *Curr Vasc Pharmacol*. 2011 Nov 9(6):682–92.
116. Gupta S, et al. Potential role of female sex hormones in the pathophysiology of migraine. *Pharmacol Ther*. 2007 Feb 113(2):321–40.
117. Vuković-Cvetković V, et al. Is iron deficiency anemia related to menstrual migraine? Post hoc analysis of an observational study evaluating clinical characteristics of patients with menstrual migraine. *Acta Clin Croat*. 2010 Dec 49(4):389–94.
118. Burke BE, et al. Randomized, controlled trial of phytoestrogen in the prophylactic treatment of menstrual migraine. *Biomed Pharmacother*. 2002 Aug 56(6):283–88.
119. Facchinetti F, et al. Magnesium prophylaxis of menstrual migraine: Effects on intracellular magnesium. *Headache*. 1991 May 31(5):298–301.
120. Mauskop A, et al. Serum ionized magnesium levels and serum ionized calcium/ionized magnesium ratios in women with menstrual migraine. *Headache*. 2002 Apr 42(4):242–48.
121. Ziaei S, et al. The effect of vitamin E on the treatment of menstrual migraine. *Med Sci Monit*. 2009 Jan 15(1):CR16–19.
122. Sillanpaća, M, Anttila P. Increasing prevalence of headache in 7-year-old schoolchildren. *Headache*. 1996 36: 466–70.
123. Jacobs H, Gladstein J. Pediatric headache: A clinical review. *Headache*. 2012 52(2):333–39.
124. Moriarty-Sheehan, ibid.
125. Carson L, Lewis D, Tsou M, McGuire E, Surran B, Miller C, Vu TA. Abdominal migraine: An under-diagnosed cause of recurrent abdominal pain in children. *Headache*. 2011 May 51(5):707–12.
126. Eidlitz-Markus T, Haimi-Cohen Y, Steier D, Zeharia A. Effectiveness of nonpharmacologic treatment for migraine in young children. *Headache*. 2010 Feb 50(2):219–23.
127. Termine C, Ozge A, Antonaci F, Natriashvili S, Guidetti V, Wöber-Bingöl C. Overview of diagnosis and management of paediatric headache. Part II: therapeutic management. *J Headache Pain*. 2011 Feb 12(1):25–34.
128. Eiland LS, Hunt MO. The use of triptans for pediatric migraines. *Paediatr Drugs*. 2010 Dec 12(6):379–89.
129. Kung TA, Totonchi A, Eshraghi Y, Scher MS, Gosain AK. Review of pediatric migraine headaches refractory to medical management. *J Craniofac Surg*. 2009 Jan 20(1):125–28.
130. Powers SW, Mitchell MJ, Byars KC, Bentti A-L, LeCates SL, Hershey AD. A pilot study of one-session biofeedback training in pediatric headache. *Neurology*. 2000 56:133.
131. Millichap JG, Yee MM. The diet factor in pediatric and adolescent migraine. *Pediatr Neurol*. 2003 Jan 28(1):9–15.

132. Boćkowski L, Smigielska-Kuzia J, Sobaniec W, Zelazowska-Rutkowska B, Kułak W, Sendrowski K. Anti-inflammatory plasma cytokines in children and adolescents with migraine headaches. *Pharmacol Rep*. 2010 Mar–Apr 62(2):287–91.

133. Boćkowski L, Sobaniec W, Zelazowska-Rutkowska B. Proinflammatory plasma cytokines in children with migraine. *Pediatr Neurol*. 2009 Jul 41(1):17–21.

134. Raieli V, Compagno A, Brighina F, La Franca G, Puma D, Ragusa D, Savettieri G, D'Amelio M. Prevalence of red ear syndrome in juvenile primary headaches. *Cephalalgia*. 2011 Apr 31(5):597–602.

135. Raieli V, Monastero R, Santangelo G, Eliseo GL, Eliseo M, Camarda R. Red ear syndrome and migraine: Report of eight cases. *Headache*. 2002 Feb 42(2):147–51.

136. Egger J, Carter CM, Soothill JF, Wilson J. Oligoantigenic diet treatment of children with epilepsy and migraine. *J Pediatr*. 1989 114:51–58.

137. Alehan F, Ozçay F, Erol I, Canan O, Cemil T. Increased risk for celiac disease in paediatric patients with migraine. *Cephalalgia*. 2008 Sep 28(9):945–49.

138. Zelnik N, Pacht A, Obeid R, Lerner A. Range of neurologic disorders in patients with celiac disease. *Pediatrics*. 2004 Jun 113(6):1672–76.

139. Erwin EA, et al. Serum IgE measurement and detection of food allergy in pediatric patients with eosinophilic esophagitis. *Ann Allergy Asthma Immunol*. 2010 Jun 104(6): 496–502.

140. Erol I, Alehan F, Aldemir D, Ogus E. Increased vulnerability to oxidative stress in pediatric migraine patients. *Pediatr Neurol*. 2010 Jul 43(1):21–24.

141. Boćkowski L, Sobaniec W, Kułak W, Smigielska-Kuzia. Serum and intraerythrocyte antioxidant enzymes and lipid peroxides in children with migraine. *J. Pharmacol Rep*. 2008 Jul–Aug 60(4):542–48.

142. Zaki EA, Freilinger T, Klopstock T, Baldwin EE, Heisner KR, Adams K, Dichgans M, Wagler S, Boles RG. Two common mitochondrial DNA polymorphisms are highly associated with migraine headache and cyclic vomiting syndrome. *Cephalalgia*. 2009 Jul 29(7):719–28.

143. Alsayouf H, Zamel KM, Heyer GL, Khuhro AL, Kahwash SB, de los Reyes EC. Role of methylenetetrahydrofolate reductase gene (MTHFR) 677C>T polymorphism in pediatric cerebrovascular disorders. *J Child Neurol*. 2011 Mar 26(3):318–21.

144. Bottini F, et al. Metabolic and genetic risk factors for migraine in children. *Cephalalgia*. 2006 26:731–37.

145. Teber S, Bektas Ö, Yılmaz A, Aksoy E, Akar N, Deda G. Lipoprotein a levels in pediatric migraine. *Pediatr Neurol*. 2011 Oct 45(4):225–28.

146. Condò M, Posar A, Arbizzani A, Parmeggiani A.J Riboflavin prophylaxis in pediatric and adolescent migraine. *Headache Pain*. 2009 Oct 10(5):361–65.

147. Schiapparelli P, Allais G, Castagnoli Gabellari I, Rolando S, Terzi MG, Benedetto C. Non-pharmacological approach to migraine prophylaxis: Part II. *Neurol Sci*. 2010 Jun 31 Suppl 1:S137–39.

148. MacLennan SC, Wade FM, Forrest KM, Ratanayake PD, Fagan E, Antony J. High-dose riboflavin for migraine prophylaxis in children: a double-blind, randomized, placebo-controlled trial. *J Child Neurol*. 2008 Nov 23(11):1300–1304.

149. Bruijn J, Duivenvoorden H, Passchier J, Locher H, Dijkstra N, Arts WF. Medium-dose riboflavin as a prophylactic agent in children with migraine: a preliminary placebo-controlled, randomised, double-blind, cross-over trial. *Cephalalgia*. 2010 Dec 30(12):1426–34.

150. Smeets MC, Vernooy CB, Souverijn JH, Ferrari MD. Intracellular and plasma magnesium in familial hemiplegic migraine and migraine with and without aura. *Cephalalgia*. 1994 Feb 14(1):29–32.

151. Talebi M, Savadi-Oskouei D, Farhoudi M, Mohammadzade S, Ghaemmaghamihezaveh S, Hasani A, Hamdi A. Relation between serum magnesium level and migraine attacks. *Neurosciences* (Riyadh). 2011 Oct 16(4):320–23.

152. Sun-Edelstein C, Mauskop A. Foods and supplements in the management of migraine headaches. *Clin J Pain*. 2009 Jun 25(5):446–52.

153. Wang F, Van Den Eeden SK, Ackerson LM, Salk SE, Reince RH, Elin RJ. Oral magnesium oxide prophylaxis of frequent migrainous headache in children: A randomized, double-blind, placebo-controlled trial. *Headache*. 2003 Jun 43(6):601–10.

154. Hershey AD, Powers SW, Vockell AL, Lecates SL, Ellinor PL, Segers A, Burdine D, Manning P, Kabbouche MA. Coenzyme Q10 deficiency and response to supplementation in pediatric and adolescent migraine. *Headache*. 2007 Jan 47(1):73–80.

155. Slater SK, Nelson TD, Kabbouche MA, LeCates SL, Horn P, Segers A, Manning P, Powers SW, Hershey AD. A randomized, double-blinded, placebo-controlled, crossover, add-on study of CoEnzyme Q10 in the prevention of pediatric and adolescent migraine. *Cephalalgia*. 2011 Jun 31(8):897–905.

156. Boles RG. High degree of efficacy in the treatment of cyclic vomiting syndrome with combined coenzyme Q10, L-carnitine and amitriptyline, a case series. *BMC Neurol*. 2011 Aug 16 11:102.

157. Usai S, Grazzi L, Bussone G. Gingkolide B as migraine preventive treatment in young age: Results at 1-year follow-up. *Neurol Sci.* 2011 May 32 Suppl 1:S197–99.

158. Cady RK, Goldstein J, Nett R, Mitchell R, Beach ME, Browning R. A double-blind placebo-controlled pilot study of sublingual feverfew and ginger (LipiGesic™ M) in the treatment of migraine. *Headache.* 2011 Jul–Aug 51(7):1078–86.

159. Pothmann R, Danesch U. Migraine prevention in children and adolescents: Results of an open study with a special butterbur root extract. *Headache.* 2005 Mar 45(3):196–203.

160. Danesch U, Rittinghausen R. Safety of a patented special butterbur root extract for migraine prevention. *Headache.* 2003 Jan 43(1):76–78.

161. Lipton RB, Göbel H, Einhäupl KM, Wilks K, Mauskop A. Petasites hybridus root (butterbur) is an effective preventive treatment for migraine. *Neurology.* 2004 Dec 28 63(12):2240–44.

162. Esposito M, Carotenuto M. Ginkgolide B complex efficacy for brief prophylaxis of migraine in school-aged children: An open-label study. *Neurol Sci.* 2011 Feb 32(1):79–81.

163. Bianchi A, Salomone S, Caraci F, Pizza V, Bernardini R, D'Amato CC. Role of magnesium, coenzyme Q10, riboflavin, and vitamin B12 in migraine prophylaxis. *Vitam Horm.* 2004 69:297–312.

164. de Bree A, et al. Effect of the methylenetetrahydrofolate reductase 677C–<T mutation on the relations among folate intake and plasma folate and homocysteine concentrations in a general population sample. *Am J Clin Nutr.* 2003 77:687–93.

165. Fonteh AN, Chung R, Sharma TL, Fisher RD, Pogoda JM, Cowan R, Harrington MG. Cerebrospinal fluid phospholipase C activity increases in migraine. *Cephalalgia.* 2011 Mar 31(4):456–62.

166. Wang YT, von Zychlinski A, McCormick SP. Dimyristoylphosphotidylcholine induces conformational changes in apoB that lowers lipoprotein(a). *J Lipid Res.* 2009 May 50(5):846–53.

167. Cho HJ, Kim YJ. Efficacy and safety of oral citicoline in acute ischemic stroke: Drug surveillance study in 4,191 cases. *Methods Find Exp Clin Pharmacol.* 2009 Apr 31(3):171–76.

29 Attention Deficit Hyperactivity Disorder

Valencia Booth Porter, M.D., M.P.H.,
and Kelly L. Olson, Ph.D.

INTRODUCTION

Attention deficit hyperactivity disorder (ADHD) is the most common behavioral disorder in children, affecting approximately four to five million children in the United States and with prevalence increasing over the last 10 years [1]. Behavioral measures and pharmacotherapy are the cornerstones of medical management of ADHD, with stimulant drugs the mainstay of treatment for more than 60 years. Newer, nonstimulant medications have also shown benefit in ameliorating symptoms of ADHD and comorbid disorders. However, with approximately 65% to 70% of patients reporting medication side effects [2,3] and up to 30% of children who may not respond to medication [4], many families and physicians alike look to diet and nutrient interventions as an adjunct in long-term management of the disorder [5].

A number of studies have shown the importance of various nutrients in brain development and function including omega-3 fatty acids, carbohydrates, and proteins. Specific vitamins and minerals serve as cofactors to create these building blocks. In addition, food components can negatively impact behavior in certain children who are prone to these sensitivities. Food colorings, flavorings, preservatives, and refined sugars have been linked to ADHD, with parents and other observers frequently reporting dramatic improvements in hyperactive children on a variety of defined diets [6–8].

BACKGROUND

In the United States, the prevalence of ADHD in school-age children is estimated between 3% and 10% [1]. Onset is typically between age four and seven years, with boys affected six times more than girls. ADHD may persist into adulthood in 40% to 60%. Although clinically heterogeneous, those suffering from ADHD have core features including developmentally inappropriate inattention, impulsivity, and hyperactivity. Currently recognized subtypes include predominantly inattentive, predominantly hyperactive and impulsive, or combined type [1]. Comorbid conditions include oppositional defiant disorder, conduct disorder, both unipolar and bipolar mood disorders, anxiety disorders, and learning disorders [9,10]. Traditional treatment includes behavior modification, educational techniques, psychotherapy, and pharmacotherapy, most commonly with stimulant medications. In the United States and United Kingdom, use of stimulant medication for this condition has dramatically increased since the 1990s.

While the precise cause of ADHD remains unknown, it appears to have a multifactorial etiology including genetic, biologic, and environmental and epigenetic contributors. Evidence points toward a dysfunction in dopaminergic and adrenergic systems as well as fatty acid metabolism [11]. Environmental exposures may play a role in the development of ADHD, with associations found between exposure to lead, organohalide pollutants, and prenatal exposure to maternal cigarette smoking and alcohol use [12,13].

Thyroid problems such as hyperthyroidism are often included in the differential diagnosis, but studies have not shown a clear association between thyroid function and ADHD. Abnormal thyroid function has been found to occur more often in children with ADHD than in the general population [14,15]. Some children with generalized resistance to thyroid hormone (GRTH), where target tissues are less responsive to thyroid hormone, have also been found to have ADHD [16,17]. It is also possible that environmental thyrotoxicants such as PCBs may play a role in the etiology of ADHD [18]. In utero, maternal hypothyroxinemia has known neurodevelopmental consequences, and it has also been hypothesized that maternal exposure to environmental antithyroid and goitrogenic agents and insufficient dietary iodine intake can result in fetal brain changes [19].

PATHOPHYSIOLOGY AND PHARMACOLOGY

Evidence from pharmacological effects and brain imaging studies highlight frontal lobe and subcortical regions of the brain as being affected in ADHD. The dopaminergic anterior system is thought to be related to behavioral inhibition and executive functioning, whereas the noradrenergic posterior system may play a role in selective attention [10,20]. Stimulant drugs that modulate dopaminergic and noradrenergic systems, such as methylphenidate, have been the mainstay of pharmacological treatment [10,21]. Other medications used in treatment include amoxetine (which inhibits norepinephrine transport), tricyclic antidepressants (TCA), non-TCA antidepressants, clonidine, and buproprion [22,23]. Despite interaction between serotonin and dopamine systems, the serotonergic drugs have demonstrated little effect in treatment of ADHD [24].

Numerous studies of stimulant medication for ADHD have demonstrated increased attention span, improved concentration, decreased excessive motor behavior, and improved social behavior when used alone or in conjunction with behavioral and cognitive interventions. Despite these robust benefits, however, long-term academic performance does not appear to be improved [25]. Approximately 70% of patients will respond to the first stimulant taken, with at least 80% responding if medications are tried systematically.

Up to 30% may not respond to stimulants and side effects are common, including appetite suppression, headache, sleep disturbance, mood difficulties, or exacerbation of tic disorders [26]. In a study examining attitudes of 40 students on medication ages 11 to 18 years regarding ADHD medications, 64% reported some side effects [2]. Reports of sudden death with stimulant use generated understandable concern, but the majority of reported cases occurred in children with pre-existing structural cardiac abnormalities.

As some of the drugs used to treat ADHD are dopamine and norepinephrine reuptake inhibitors, chronic use of these medications may lead to increase in dopamine and norepinephrine metabolism.

DIET AND FOOD SENSITIVITIES

Food and nutrients from early childhood and on are thought to play a role in the pathophysiology of this condition. In early life, children given soy-based formula due to food reactivities may be at added risk due to the goitrogenic properties of soy isoflavones as well as high levels of manganese [27,28]. In addition to nutrients affecting thyroid function, over the last century, dietary patterns have included dramatic changes in the ratio of essential fatty acids and a shift toward low-protein/high-carbohydrate diets [29–31]. A recent prospective observational study tracking 2868 live births in Australia to age 14 years indicated that a Western diet may be associated with ADHD [32]. Another longitudinal study found that children eating more junk food, described as high-fat processed foods and snack foods high in fat and/or sugar at an early age had increased hyperactivity at age seven [33]. Food additives with the potential for reactivities in the diet have also drastically increased, with more than 2300 now approved for use.

In the diet, exposure to food additives and other substances has been commented on extensively in the literature. Differences and inadequacies in controlled trials make analysis difficult, but studies do indicate a limited positive association between defined diets and decrease in hyperactivity. A 1983 NIH consensus panel on defined diets and childhood hyperactivity stated that "defined diets should not be universally used in the treatment of childhood hyperactivity at this time. However, the Panel recognizes that initiation of a trial of dietary treatment or continuation of a diet may be warranted in patients whose family and physicians perceive benefits" [34].

FOOD ADDITIVES

With domestic production of food dyes increasing fourfold between 1955 and 1998, more than 2000 food additives are approved by the Food and Drug Administration (FDA) [35]. While preservatives such as benzoates serve to increase shelf life of food, artificial food colorings have no nutritional value or other benefits to consumers and are mainly used for cosmetic purposes, often to make non-nutritious foods more appealing to children. An unpublished 1976 study by the FDA noted that the average American child consumed 27 mg of artificial food colors daily [36]. These substances are generally regarded as safe, but hypersensitivity responses or idiosyncratic reactions could have effects on central nervous system functioning.

A 2007 study reignited interest in the influence of food additives on children's behavior. Replicating an earlier study showing that ingestion of usual amounts of food colorings and additives may significantly increase hyperactivity in some 3-year-old children, McCann and colleagues showed similar effects in 8- to 9-year-old children [8]. In the first study, 3-year-old children from the general population given a diet free of artificial dyes and benzoate preservatives had reduction in hyperactive behavior. When challenged with a mix containing commonly used additives sodium benzoate and sunset yellow, carmoisine, tartrazine, and Ponceau 4R, hyperactivity increased [37].

The repeat study evaluated both 3-year-olds and 8- to 9-year-olds from the general population initially placed on an elimination diet free of challenge elements for 6 weeks [8]. Elements tested included those in the original study (mix A) and mix B containing sodium benzoate plus the dyes sunset yellow, carmoisine, quinolone yellow, and allura red AC. These elements were typical of the artificial food colors and additives found in some children's foods and were given in amounts representative of average daily intake of these additives by young children in the United Kingdom. In both age groups, small but significant increases in hyperactivity as assessed by parents, teachers, and trained observers were seen with mix A. Mix B was also associated with a small significant increase in hyperactivity in the older children, but not in the three-year-olds, who exhibited a wider range of responses. These findings are consistent with a 2004 meta-analysis of 15 double-blind, placebo-controlled trials of artificial food colorings that showed increase in hyperactivity as measured by behavioral rating scales in hyperactive children [38].

The results of this study correspond to the clinical observation that some hyperactive children are highly sensitive to food colorings and additives, while other children are not. On the basis of this study, the British Food Standards Agency advised parents of hyperactive children to consider eliminating the additives used in the study from their diets. Individual differences in response may have a genetic component and a recent study has shown a relationship of histamine degradation gene polymorphisms and the adverse effect of food additives [39]. Further study is needed to evaluate the influence of genetics on environmental factors, such as diet, and the relationship to ADHD symptoms.

As one hypothesis for these reactions is a potential hypersensitivity to these compounds, additional studies have looked at children with ADHD who were also atopic. One study looking at behavioral improvement in children with ADHD placed on an elimination diet showed more response to the diet in atopic children versus those who were not atopic [40]. In addition, a dose-response effect of the food coloring tartrazine was observed in some hyperactive children and all of those who reacted to tartrazine were also found to have atopy [41].

FEINGOLD DIET

In the 1970s, Dr. Benjamin Feingold, a pediatrician and allergist, popularized the idea of diet affecting children's hyperactive behavior. He originally hypothesized that hyperactivity was a symptom of salicylate intolerance in genetically predisposed individuals and because many of these people also had hypersensitivity to tartrazine (yellow dye no. 5) he suggested that this additive as well as several artificial flavors similar in structure to salicylates were involved.

The original Feingold Diet, also known as Kaiser-Permanente or K-P diet, eliminates all foods containing artificial (synthetic) colors and/or flavors and all foods high in naturally occurring salicylates, a category that includes almonds, cucumbers, tomatoes, berries, apples, oranges, and several other fruits. The role of salicylates was later diminished and preservatives sodium benzoate, butylated hydroxyanisole (BHA), and butylated hydroxytoluene (BHT) were added to the exclusion list [42–44]. After several weeks on the elimination diet, salicylate-containing foods are gradually reintroduced, looking for adverse reactions. Feingold reported anecdotally that 40% to 70% of children who strictly adhered to the diet had a marked reduction in hyperactive behavior and suggested that younger children tended to respond more rapidly and more completely [44].

For the most part, other researchers evaluating the Feingold hypothesis yielded inconclusive results and suffered from small sample sizes and methodological deficiencies [36]. However, a subgroup of hyperactive children may show improvement on the diet, although it is uncertain what component of the dietary change is responsible, be it lack of additives, salicylate avoidance, placebo effect, change in nutrient status, or other variables including family dynamics [36,45]. It is possible that salicylates accounted for more cases in the 1970s than in current times in which the intake of sugar and other additives is much higher and ADHD has reached epidemic levels. While the potential for food reactivities is great, with thousands of artificial compounds in use, the amount of testing needed to assess the role in ADHD would likely take decades. On the other hand, motivated parents may find that their child benefits from this approach and the Feingold Association* provides ample resources to support them in this endeavor.

ELIMINATION/OLIGOANTIGENIC/FEW FOODS DIET

In addition to food additives and salicylates, common foods including milk, soy, eggs, wheat, corn, legumes, sugar, and chocolate have also been implicated as factors responsible for behavioral problems in ADHD. In 1981, Dr. William Crook, an allergist and pediatrician, reported parent-noted food triggers in 70% of 182 hyperactive patients; with dietary elimination of these substances, an excellent or good response was reported by nearly 80% [46].

Similar to the Feingold Diet, the rationale behind the very restrictive oligoantigenic or few foods diet is to eliminate foods and ingredients that may provoke adverse behavioral reactions, including additives and artificial colorings as well as other substances assumed to be antigenic such as cereal proteins and citrus fruits. As first described by Egger, this diet consists of two types of meats (lamb, turkey/chicken), two carbohydrate sources (rice, potatoes), two types of vegetables (Brassica, carrots), and two fruits (apple, banana). For preparing the meals, oil, margarine, salt, and water are allowed. Beverages include apple juice and mineral water and calcium and multivitamins are given as supplements [47].

In the original study of 76 children, 62 improved, with the behavior of 21 normalizing. Other symptoms such as headaches and abdominal pain often improved as well. When re-exposed in a double-blind, crossover, placebo-controlled trial, symptoms returned or were exacerbated within two to three days. Artificial colorings (tartrazine) and preservatives (benzoates) were the most common provoking substances, but all children had multiple sensitivities [47]. Other studies of children with ADHD or hyperactivity have shown that at least in some children, hyperactivity may be a

---

* Feingold Association of the United States, http://www.feingold.org (accessed Jan. 5, 2012).

manifestation of food intolerance and behavior may improve with an oligoantigenic or few foods diet [48–51]. Elimination diets may be helpful to determine if symptoms are influenced by food [52–53].

SUGAR

It is commonly believed that foods high in refined sugar exacerbate behavioral problems in children [54]. Anecdotal and observational studies have supported this belief, showing deteriorations in attention or behavior after sucrose challenge versus placebo in children with and without ADHD [55,56].

Interestingly, it may not only be the sugar, but the relationship to other food components. Changes in behavior have been correlated with the amount of sugar ingested, with the ratio of sugar products to other foods, and with the ratio of carbohydrate to protein in the diet. In a challenge study, behavioral deteriorations in normal and hyperactive children were seen when sucrose was given after a breakfast consisting of mostly carbohydrates, but not after fasting or a high-protein breakfast [57]. Another study showed that declines in attention and memory seen in children in a fasting condition or given a glucose drink were not seen when a breakfast of complex carbohydrates was given [58]. Indeed, a higher ratio of sugar to total energy has been found to be associated with increases in activity, off-task behaviors, and attention problems [59]. As drops in blood sugar can trigger sympathetic nervous system response, it is hypothesized that altering the carbohydrate:protein ratio might influence neurotransmitters, leading to these behavioral symptoms [60]. Serum levels of precursor amino acids (tyrosine, phenylalanine, and tryptophan) for neurotransmitters affected in hyperactivity are increased by dietary consumption and lowered by carbohydrate load.

A number of controlled studies in the literature do not support the notion that sugar intake leads to increase in activity [54,59–64]. Some even reported a decrease in activity levels after sucrose or glucose ingestion [64,65]. One should note, however, that many of these negative studies use another sweetener such as aspartame or saccharin as the placebo challenge, with unknown behavioral effects in general and some associations emerging that food reactivities and these synthetic compounds may be linked [66–70]. With a link to dopamine reward signals in the brain, Johnson et al. recently hypothesized that chronic excessive sugar intake may lead to changes in dopamine signaling, which influences behavior in ADHD. Further studies are needed to evaluate this potential relationship [71].

SPECIFIC NUTRIENTS

ESSENTIAL FATTY ACIDS

Fatty acids have fundamental structural and functional roles in the central nervous system, comprising key components of neuronal membranes, neurotransmitter receptor sites, as well as second messenger systems [72,73]. Essential fatty acids (EFAs) cannot be synthesized by the body and therefore must be provided in the diet. Sometimes dietary intake is inadequate; however, other times further metabolic processing of EFAs is impaired. The conversion is dependent on precursor levels and can also be influenced by environmental factors [74,75]. The omega-6 linoleic acid (LA) and omega-3 alpha-linolenic acid (ALA) undergo desaturation and elongation to become the omega-6s arachidonic acid (AA) and dihomo-gamma-linolenic acid (DGLA), a metabolite of gamma-linolenic acid (GLA), and omega-3s eicosapentaenoic acid (EPA) and docosahexaenoic acid (DHA) [76]. AA and DHA are key components of neuronal membranes, and AA additionally plays a role in cellular processes underlying learning and memory. DGLA, AA, and EPA are also important eicosanoid precursors affecting many other biochemical processes [76].

While both the omega-3s and omega-6s are crucial to brain development and function, the omega-3s in particular are often lacking in diets of developed countries where dramatic increases in consumption of processed foods have led to relative deficiencies in certain EFAs and a change in the omega-6:omega-3 ratio from approximately 3:1 to more than 20:1 in some cases [72,77]. These dietary changes may have contributed to the increased incidence of many diseases including neurodevelopmental disorders [72]. Dietary omega-3 sources include fish and shellfish, as well as plant sources such as flax oil, hemp oil, soy oil, canola oil, pumpkin seeds, sunflower seeds, leafy vegetables, and walnuts, which do not contain EPA or DHA.

Various behavioral and developmental problems including ADHD have been linked to deficiencies or imbalances of fatty acids [78]. Hyperactive and ADHD children have been noted to have symptoms of EFA deficiency such as dry hair and skin, excessive thirst and urination, and other findings including follicular keratoses, brittle nails, and symptoms of eczema, asthma, and other atopic conditions [78,79]. In addition to physical signs of fatty acid deficiency, plasma and erythrocyte fatty acid levels, particularly omega-3s, have been found to be decreased in subjects with ADHD [80–82]. Recent studies have shown that genes involved in fatty acid metabolism can influence tissue concentrations and these may have a potential role in ADHD [83]. A deficiency in omega-3s can further disrupt the dopaminergic mesocorticolimbic pathway by reducing dopamine vesicle density [74].

ESSENTIAL FATTY ACID SUPPLEMENTATION

Supplementation with omega-3s changes blood levels and can lead to changes in mood and behavior. A 4:1 ratio of omega-6:omega-3 has been found to be optimal for neuronal membrane functioning although this has not yet been applied specifically to ADHD [84].

A recent meta-analysis of ten trials involving 699 children concluded that omega-3 fatty acid supplementation, particularly with higher doses of EPA, was modestly effective in the treatment of ADHD [85]. Early intervention studies of supplementation with evening primrose oil (primarily GLA) in children with ADHD had mixed, but unsatisfactory outcomes [86,87]. Further studies of DHA supplementation alone also failed to demonstrate improvement in ADHD symptoms [88,89].

A study of children with ADHD also having symptoms suggestive of fatty acid deficiency (thirst and skin problems) were randomized to receive four months of either olive oil or a mixture of 480 mg DHA, 80 mg EPA, 40 mg AA, 96 mg GLA, and 24 mg alpha-tocopherol acetate [90]. Changes in plasma and erythrocyte EFA composition as well as improvements in ADHD behaviors were consistently observed for the treatment group more than the control group, with significant changes on parent-rated conduct problems and teacher-rated attention symptoms. Also, more children had improvement in oppositional defiant behaviors with the EFA mixture compared with olive oil. For both groups, biochemical changes were related to improvements in behavior. Significant correlations were found for increasing erythrocyte EPA levels and decreasing parent-rated disruptive behavior, and for erythrocyte EPA and DHA levels and teacher-rated attention. Interestingly, significant correlations were also observed between a decrease in scores for all four teacher subscales (hyperactivity, attention, conduct, and oppositional/defiant disorder) and increase in erythrocyte alpha-tocopherol concentrations, suggesting an additional role for vitamin E. This supports prior trials of supplementation with EFAs that have shown improvements based on parent-rating scales [91,92].

Children may use an omega-3 supplement that has roughly equal amounts of DHA and EPA with a dose of 500 mg to 1000 mg per day for children four to six years of age and one to two grams per day for children seven years and older. Side effects may include gastrointestinal upset, nausea, and loose stool. Avoid fish oil–based supplements in those with fish allergy.

L-CARNITINE

Both L-carnitine and its esterified form, acetyl-L-carnitine, have potential neuroprotective, neuromodulatory, and neurotrophic properties and have demonstrated improvements in cognitive processes such as memory and learning [93]. Frank carnitine deficiency is known to have major deleterious effects on the central nervous system as well as other organ systems. L-carnitine has an important role in fatty acid metabolism and regulation [93,94]. Acetyl-L-carnitine is more efficiently incorporated into PUFA and is an important constituent of brain phospholipids.

Looking at this potential, L-carnitine was given to 26 boys with ADHD in an eight-week double-blind, placebo-controlled, double-crossover study [94]. Doses of 100 mg/kg daily were given twice after meals with a maximum of four grams daily. Improvements of 30% or more on two objective measures were seen in approximately half of the children. Of note, plasma-free carnitine and acetyl-L-carnitine levels were significantly different between responders and nonresponders after treatment. A study of 40 children with ADHD on methylphenidate who received 500 to 1500 mg/day of acetyl-L-carnitine or placebo, however, failed to show a difference between groups although plasma levels were not evaluated in this study [95].

Most people obtain enough carnitine from their diet, but some may have dietary deficiencies or cannot properly absorb it from food. Common food sources include red meat (particularly lamb) and dairy products. Carnitine is also found in fish, poultry, tempeh (fermented soybeans), wheat, asparagus, avocados, and peanut butter. Certain medications and low dietary levels of the amino acids lysine and methionine may cause deficiencies. Dietary supplementation of L-carnitine does not appear to cause significant side effects. Nausea, vomiting, diarrhea, and body odor have been reported in higher doses above 3 g/day.

IRON

Iron plays a role in regulation of dopaminergic activity and may therefore contribute to ADHD [96]. Children with ADHD have been shown to have lower mean serum ferritin levels than age- and sex-matched controls [97]. In addition, low serum ferritin levels corresponded to more severe behavioral symptoms [98,99]. Even in the absence of anemia, iron supplementation may have an impact on ADHD symptoms. A pilot study of 14 boys with ADHD showed that administration of an iron preparation (Ferrocal) 5 mg/kg/day for 30 days had significant increase in serum ferritin levels and significant decreases on parent- but not teacher-rating scores [100]. A 12-week placebo-controlled study of oral ferrous sulfate 80 mg/day in nonanemic children with low serum ferritin levels (< 30 ng/mL) showed improvement on parent- but not teacher-rated ADHD behavior on iron versus placebo [101].

Restless legs syndrome (RLS) frequently occurs with iron deficiency anemia and improves with iron supplementation [102]. Pharmacologic and PET studies show that RLS is related to impaired dopaminergic transmission, in which iron plays a role. Given that RLS and ADHD may share common pathophysiological mechanisms, it is not surprising that up to 26% of subjects with RLS have been found to have ADHD or ADHD symptoms and up to 44% of subjects with ADHD have been found to have RLS or RLS symptoms [103]. In a small study of seven children with both ADHD and RLS, four of whom failed prior stimulant therapy, treatment with dopaminergic mono-therapy improved RLS symptoms as well as behavior and neuropsychological assessments [104].

ZINC

Zinc (Zn) is an important cofactor for metabolism related to neurotransmitters such as dopamine, fatty acids, prostaglandins, and melatonin [105,106]. With a role in synthesis of complex omega-3 and omega-6 FAs, zinc deficiency may further exacerbate problems related to these EFAs in children with ADHD.

In a population study, nearly one-third of children with ADHD had significantly lower serum zinc levels than age- and sex-matched controls [107]. This could not be explained by obvious factors concerning diet, health, or medication status. Another study also found significantly lower mean serum EFA and mean serum zinc levels in 48 children with ADHD versus 45 children without ADHD [108].

Other evidence suggests that zinc deficiencies may also reduce the treatment response to stimulants such as methylphenidate [106]. A small study looking at 18 ADHD subjects by zinc status, showed a linear relationship with response to d-amphetamine whereas response to evening primrose oil yielded benefit only in those with borderline zinc status [106]. With mild zinc deficiency, effect size for both treatments was diminished. Zinc sulfate may be useful as an adjunct to treatment with methylphenidate as shown in a double-blind, placebo-controlled trial with significant differences in both parent- and teacher-rated behaviors [109]. A recent study evaluating zinc supplementation at doses of 15 to 30 mg/day versus placebo monotherapy and then with added d-amphetamine showed equivocal clinical outcomes except for a reduction in amphetamine optimal dose with supplementation of 30 mg/day of zinc [110].

Dietary zinc can be found in high-protein foods such as organ meats, seafood, especially shellfish, whole grains, and legumes.

MAGNESIUM

Magnesium (Mg) has a role in both neuronal function and fatty acid enzyme activity. In Poland, children with ADHD were commonly found to have deficiency of magnesium in the hair, erythrocytes, and less often in plasma [111]. Magnesium deficiency also occurred more often among hyperactive children than among healthy children [112]. When children with hyperactivity who were found to have magnesium deficiency were given magnesium supplementation 200 mg/day for six months, a decrease in hyperactivity was seen in those supplemented versus those who did not receive supplementation [113]. In another study, children with ADHD showed significantly lower erythrocyte Mg levels than controls [114]. When given 6 mg/kg/d Mg with 0.6 mg/kg/d vitamin B6 (pyridoxine) for eight weeks, hyperactivity and aggressiveness were significantly reduced and school attention increased along with an increase in erythrocyte Mg levels. Within a few weeks of stopping treatment, symptoms returned and Mg levels again decreased. Blood levels of magnesium may be increased with use of dextroamphetamine, therefore, monitoring of magnesium as well as calcium during treatment is advised and corrected with supplementation if necessary [115].

AMINO ACIDS AS NEUROTRANSMITTER PRECURSORS

Imbalances and relative deficiencies in neurotransmitters are implicated in ADHD pathophysiology [116] and are the target of pharmacotherapies. As mentioned, ADHD is most commonly associated with a dysregulation in catecholamine neurotransmission through the noradrenergic and dopaminergic systems [117,118]. Low catecholamine levels are associated with ADHD [116,119], and clinical findings have demonstrated an inverse relationship between catecholamine excretion and inattentive/restless behavior [120,121].

The synthesis of neurotransmitters in the CNS is partly dependent on the availability of precursor amino acids presented in Figure 29.1, thus supplementation has been evaluated as monotherapy or in combination to support pharmaceutical interventions [122,123,124]. Research only recently possible with molecular and imaging tools supports the hypothesis that increasing the metabolic precursors to the catecholamines (epinephrine, norepinephrine and dopamine) through dietary supplementation may therapeutically raise catecholamine levels in the central nervous system. The theory further posits that tachyphylaxis of ADHD medications may be in part the result of depleted precursors.

Most pharmaceuticals used in the treatment of ADHD target dopamine and norepinephrine transmission; however, there is a growing body of research pointing to several neurotransmitter pathways being involved, suggesting that constant cross-talk and balance are critical. In support of this, prior published trials using L-dopa alone, DL-phenylalanine alone, and L-tyrosine alone did not result in lasting therapeutic effects [126–128].

It is generally known that decreased neurotransmission of serotonin is linked to impulsive and aggressive behavior [129]. Tryptophan and 5-hydroxytryptophan (5-HTP) are amino acid precursors to serotonin (see Figure 29.1). Serotonin support may be considered in addition to catecholamine support to avoid depletion of neurotransmitter stores potentially caused by a number of physiological

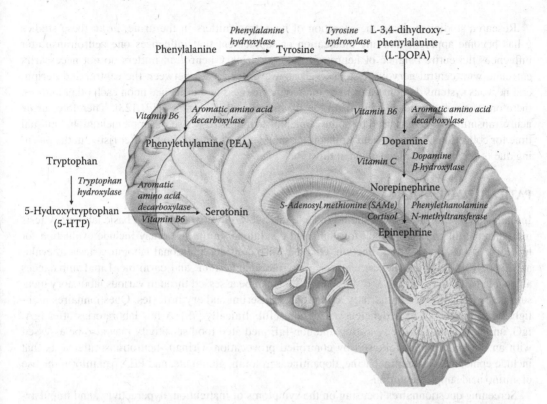

FIGURE 29.1 Amino acids such as phenylalanine, tyrosine, tryptophan, 5-hydroxytryptophan (5-HTP), and L-3,4-dihydroxyphenylalanine (L-DOPA) act as precursors to important neurotransmitters. Following ingestion, these amino acids can cross the blood brain barrier where they are synthesized into their respective neurotransmitters in the brain. The precursors that are illustrated as outside the brain are those that can cross the blood brain barrier. (This material was reprinted with permission from NeuroScience, Inc., 2012.)

methods including pathologically upregulated enzymatic processes. A recently published retrospective study of 85 children aged 4 to 18 years with ADHD given serotonin and dopamine amino acid precursors and other cofactors for a period of eight to 10 weeks showed a significant decrease in symptoms [130]. Further clinical study looking at responders and nonresponders with respect to urinary levels of neurotransmitters and their precursors would be important.

Additionally, research has suggested that abnormally high levels of glutamate release can result in symptoms associated with ADHD such as inattention [131,132]. Glutamate can also be linked to the discharge of other excitatory neurotransmitters as it plays a role in stimulating catecholamine release at the somatic level [133]. The degree to which glutamate contributes to ADHD is still unknown, and further study is needed.

Kusaga et al. demonstrated that subjects diagnosed with ADHD tended to have decreased urinary beta-phenylethylamine (PEA) levels [134]. In this study, PEA levels were significantly increased in patients that responded to treatment with methylphenidate but were not increased in nonresponders [134]. Supplementation with an amino acid precursor, such as L-phenylalanine, may be another target aimed at increasing PEA neurotransmission, although increased PEA levels out of balance with other neurotransmitters can become stimulatory. To address the potential of excitatory stimulation, gamma amino-butyric acid (GABA) has been broadly examined. The clinical interconnectedness between GABA and ADHD, however, is still mostly unknown. Nevertheless, GABA is the primary inhibitory neurotransmitter found in the brain principally responsible for providing a more sedative response. The recognition of the important role GABA plays in reducing anxiety may make this a key agent to help lessen anxiousness in children [135].

Research studies evaluate the excretion of neurotransmitters in the urine. From these studies it has become apparent that any medication or supplement that influences one neurotransmitter influences the entire balance of neurotransmitters. Urinary neurotransmitters do not necessarily correlate with central nervous system levels; however, crosstalk between the central and peripheral nervous systems demonstrates their interconnectedness and influence upon each other and can therefore show response to administration of amino acid precursors [121,123]. Therefore, urine neurotransmitter testing is used by some clinicians to assess response to supplementation. Optimal time for collection of urinary neurotransmitter samples is one to two hours after rising in the morning due to the low diurnal variation at this time.

PATIENT EVALUATION

Initial evaluation of the patient should include interview, physical exam, and basic laboratory tests to assure the diagnosis and look for comorbid conditions. Initial tests may include evaluation for lead, iron status, and thyroid function. One may also consider additional laboratory tests to evaluate for potential nutrient deficiencies such as zinc, magnesium, and carnitine. Lipid imbalances amenable to dietary changes and supplementation can be assessed through various laboratory measurements evaluating essential fatty acid profiles in serum and erythrocytes. Questionnaires highlighting symptoms of EFA deficiency may be useful clinically [79]. A few laboratories offer IgA, IgG, and IgM food sensitivity testing and non-IgE mediated food sensitivity may also be assessed with an elimination diet followed by controlled provocation. Urinary neurotransmitter tests that include epinephrine, norepinephrine, dopamine, serotonin, glutamate, and PEA can inform the use of amino acid supplementation.

Screening questionnaires focusing on the symptoms of inattention, hyperactivity, and impulsivity are useful in the initial evaluation as well as in following treatment effects. A large number of rating scales are available for assessment of ADHD, with each having unique characteristics [136].

TREATMENT RECOMMENDATIONS

Dietary recommendations should be addressed in the primary treatment plan. Many parents are ready to adopt diet as a treatment for their child's behavior although adherence to a strict and demanding diet is a burden to the family. To prevent the child from feeling different, to reduce temptation, and to provide motivation, the whole family should be encouraged to participate. Initial dietary recommendations include eating a well-balanced, whole-foods diet, with minimal processed and artificial foods. A consultation with a nutritionist or integrative practitioner may be helpful in reinforcing nutrient needs: complex carbohydrates as brain fuel; proteins for amino acids and neurotransmitters; vitamins and minerals as cofactors; healthful (non-trans), balanced (omega-3:6) fats; and water.

Encouraging families to pay attention to foods rich in the EFAs has the potential for a multitude of health benefits. The omega-3 fats should be emphasized and they are found in coldwater fish such as salmon, herring, sardines, and rainbow trout. It is important, however, to avoid contamination of fish and fish oil products by methyl-mercury, polychlorinated biphenyls, and dioxin. ALA is also found in green vegetables and some nuts and seeds including flax and walnuts, but conversion to EPA and DHA is limited in some individuals. Algal sources of DHA are also available. Omega-6 fats are generally abundant in the standard American diet with most vegetable oils rich in LA and dairy and meat products providing AA.

If food reactivities are suspected, an elimination diet or few foods diet may be employed as both a diagnostic and therapeutic tool. Such an approach takes dedication from the parent and child, and eating out such as in a school cafeteria or restaurant is extremely difficult. Practical information on implementing the *Feingold Diet is available.

---

* Feingold Association of the United States, http://www.feingold.org (Jan. 5, 2012).

SUMMARY

- Initial workup should address possible underlying medical conditions, considering the potential for lead toxicity and thyroid disorders as well as evaluation of iron status.
- Reinforce eating a well-balanced, whole foods–based diet, with minimal processed and artificial foods.
- When making dietary changes, do not single out the child unless there are specific allergies. Instead, encourage the whole family to eat healthier.
- Reduce sugary foods and beverage, being careful also of sugar substitutes. Breakfast with complex carbohydrates and protein can help maintain steady blood sugar levels.
- If potential food reactivities are suspected, consider an elimination diet that is both diagnostic and therapeutic. Diagnostic testing to evaluate patients for celiac disease and gluten sensitivity is now widely available.
- Consider supplementation with omega-3 fatty acids with approximately equal amounts of EPA and DHA and/or encourage eating fatty fish three times a week. The dose for children four to six years of age is 500 mg to 1000 mg per day; for children seven years and older one to two grams per day.
- A trial of acetyl-L-carnitine 100 mg/kg daily with a maximum of 4 g daily may be helpful, particularly if plasma carnitine is low.
- Zinc and erythrocyte magnesium levels can be checked or add a high-quality multivitamin with trace minerals especially if diet is poor.
- The amino acids that are the metabolic precursors of neurotransmitters can be supplemented to facilitate a balance of neurotransmitters. Monitoring with urinary metabolite testing may be indicated especially if used in conjunction with pharmacotherapy. Equally important is the recognition among clinicians that an amino acid or medication directed at one neurotransmitter will, over time, alter the inherent balance of all neurotransmitters.
- Consider supplementation with B complex vitamins as essential cofactors for neurotransmitter production, which are especially depleted in stress.
- Behavioral therapy and mind-body approaches can be employed. Evaluate sleep quality and quantity, with the added concern that pharmacotherapy and neurotransmitter imbalances associated with ADHD can interfere with sleep.

All of the aforementioned may be used in combination with pharmacologic management. Physicians may also wish to utilize online patient resources and laboratory testing information.

REFERENCES

1. Visser SN, Bitsko RH, Danielson ML, Perou R, Blumberg SJ. Increasing prevalence of parent-reported attention-deficit/hyperactivity disorder among children—United States, 2003 and 2007. *MMWR,* 2010; 59:1439–1443.
2. Moline S, Frankenberger W. Use of stimulant medication for treatment of attention-deficit/hyperactivity disorder: A survey of middle and high school students' attitudes. *PsycholSch,* 2001; 38:569–584.
3. Kemper KJ. Dietary supplements for attention-deficit/hyperactivity disorder—a fishy business? *JPediatr,* 2001; 139:173–174.
4. Garber SW, Garber MD, Spizman RF. *Beyond Ritalin.* 1997. New York: Harper Collins.
5. Sinha D, Efron D. Complementary and alternative medicine use in children with attention deficit hyperactivity disorder. *J Paediatr Child Health,* 2005; 41:23–126.
6. Schnoll R, Burshteyn D, Cea-Aravena J. Nutrition in the treatment of attention-deficit hyperactivity disorder: A neglected but important aspect. *Appl Psychophysiol Biofeedback,* 2003; 28:63–75.
7. Stevenson J. Dietary influences on cognitive development and behaviour in children. *Proc Nutr Soc,* 2006; 65:361–365.
8. McCann A, Barrett A, Cooper A, et al. Food additives and hyperactive behaviour in 3-year-old and 8/9-year-old children in the community: A randomised, double-blinded, placebo-controlled trial. *Lancet,* 2007; 370:1560–1567.

9. Spencer T, Biederman J, Wilens T. Attention-deficit/hyperactivity disorder and comorbidity. *Pediatr Clin North Am,* 1999; 46:915–927.
10. Pliszka SR, McCRacken JT, Maas JW. Catecholamines in attention-deficit/hyperactivity disorder: Current perspectives. *J Am Acad Child Adolesc Psychiatry,* 1996; 35:264–272.
11. Comings DE. Clinical and molecular genetics of ADHD and Tourette syndrome. Two related polygenic disorders. *Ann NY Acad Sci,* 2001; 931:50–83.
12. Biederman J. Attention-deficit/hyperactivity disorder: A selective overview. *Biol Psychiatry,* 2005; 57:1215–1220.
13. Rowland AS, Lesesne CA, Abramowitz AJ. The epidemiology of attention-deficit/hyperactivity disorder (ADHD): A public health view. *Ment Retard Dev Disabil Res Rev,* 2002; 8:162–170.
14. Braun JM, Kahn RS, Froehlich TM, Auinger P, Lanphear BP. Exposures to environmental toxicants and attention deficit hyperactivity disorder in U.S. children. *Environ Health Perspect,* 114:1904–1909.
15. Toren P, Karasik A, Eldar S, et al. Thyroid function in attention deficit and hyperactivity disorder. *J Psychiatr Res,* 1997; 3e1:359–363.
16. Hauser P, Zametkin AJ, Martinez P, et al. Attention deficit-hyperactivity disorder in people with generalized resistance to thyroid hormone. *N Engl J Med,* 1993; 328:997–1001.
17. Refetoff S, Weiss RE, Usala SJ. The syndromes of resistance to thyroid hormone. *Endocrine Rev,* 1993; 14:348–399.
18. Schettler T. Toxic threats to neurologic development of children. *Environ Health Perspect,* 2001; 109(Suppl 6):813–816.
19. Roman GC. Autism: Transient in utero hypothyroxinemia related to maternal flavonoid ingestion during pregnancy and to other environmental antithyroid agents. *J Neurol Sci,* 2007; 262:15–26.
20. Barkley RA. Behavioral inhibition, sustained attention, and executive functions: Constructing a unifying theory of ADHD. *Psychol Bull,* 1997; 121:65–94.
21. Zametkin AJ, Liotta W. The neurobiology of attention-deficit/hyperactivity disorder. *J Clin Psychiatry,* 1998; 59(suppl 7)1986:17–23.
22. Michelson D, Adler L, Spencer T, et al. Atomoxetine in adults with ADHD: Two randomized, placebo-controlled studies. *Biol Psychiatry,* 2003; 53:112–120.
23. Spencer T, Biederman J, Wilens T et al. Pharmacotherapy of attention-deficit hyperactivity disorder across the life cycles. *J Am Acad Child Adolesc Psychiatry,* 1996; 35:409–432.
24. Zametkin AJ, Rapoport JL. Noradrenergic hypothesis of attention deficit disorder with hyperactivity: A critical review. In: *Psychopharmacology: The Third Generation of Progress.* 1987. Meltzer HY, ed. New York: Raven, 837–842.
25. Jadad AR, Boyle M, Cunningham C, Kim M, Schachar R. Treatment of attention-deficit/hyperactivity disorder. Evidence report/technology assessment, 1999; 11 (AHCPR Publication No.99-E01). Rockville, MD: Agency for Health Care Policy and Research.
26. Banaschewski T, Roessner V, Dittmann RW, Santosh PJ, Rothernberger A. Non-stimulant medications in the treatment of ADHD. *Eur Child Adolesc Psychiatry,* 2004; 13, 102–116.
27. Doerge DR, Sheehan DM. Goitrogenic and estrogenic activity of soy isoflavones. *Environ Health Perspect,* 2002; 101:349–353.
28. Crinella FM. Does soy-based infant formula cause ADHD? Expert Rev. *Neurotherapeutics,* 2003; 3:145–148.
29. Simopoulos AP. Evolutionary aspects of diet, the omega-6/omega-3 ratio and genetic variation: Nutritional implications for chronic diseases. *Biomed & Pharmacotherapy,* 2006; 60:502–507.
30. Kidd PM. Attention deficit/hyperactivity disorder (ADHD) in children: Rationale for its integrative management. *Altern Med Rev,* 2000; 5:401, 402–428.
31. Harding KL, Judah RD, Gant C. Outcome-based comparison of Ritalin versus food-supplement treated children with AD/HD. *Altern Med Rev,* 2003; 8:319–330.
32. Howard AL, Robinson M, Smith GJ, Abrosini GL, Peik JP, Oddy WH. ADHD is associated with a "Western" dietary pattern in adolescents. *J Atten Disord,* 2011;15: 403–411.
33. Wiles NJ, Northstone K, Emmett P, Lewis G. "Junk food" diet and childhood behavioural problems: Results from the ALSPAC cohort. *Eur J Clin Nutr,* 2009; 63:491–498.
34. National Institutes of Health. NIH Consensus Development Conference: Defined Diets and Childhood Hyperactivity. NIH Consensus Statement. *Clinical Pediatrics,* 1982; 21;627.
35. Jacobson MF, Schardt MS. Diet, ADHD & Behavior: A Quarter-Century Review. Center for Science in the Public Interest. Accessed February 8, 2007, at: www.cspinet.org.
36. Stare FJ, Whelan EM, Sheridan M. Diet and hyperactivity: Is there a relationship? *Pediatrics,* 1980; 66:521–525.

37. Bateman B, Warner JO, Hutchinson E, Dean T, Rowlandson P, Gant C, Grundy J, Fitzgerald C, Stevenson J. The effects of a double blind, placebo controlled, artificial food colourings and benzoate preservative challenge on hyperactivity in a general population sample of preschool children. *Arch Dis Child,* 2004; 89:506–511.

38. Schab DW, Trinh N-HT. Do artificial food colors promote hyperactivity in children with hyperactive syndromes? A meta-analysis of double-blind placebo-controlled trials. *Dev Behav Peds,* 2004; 25:423–434.

39. Stevenson J, Sonuga-Barke E, McCann D, Grimshaw K, Parker KM, Rose-Serilli MJ, Holloway JW, Warner JO. The role of histamine degradation gene polymorphisms in moderating the effects of food additives on children's ADHD symptoms. *Am J Psychiatry,* 2010; 167:1108–1115.

40. Boris M, Mandel FS. Foods and additives are common causes of the attention deficit hyperactive disorder in children. *Ann Allergy,* 1994; 72:462–468.

41. Rowe KS, Rowe JK. Synthetic food coloring and behavior: A dose response effect in a double-blind, placebo-controlled, repeated-measures study. *J Pediatrics,* 1994; 125:691–698.

42. Feingold BF. *Why Your Child Is Hyperactive.* 1975. New York: Random House.

43. Feingold BF. Hyperkinesis and learning disabilities linked to artificial food flavors and colors. *Am J Nurs,* 1975; 75:797.

44. Feingold BF. Hyperkinesis and learning disabilities linked to the ingestion of artificial food colors and flavors. *J Learn Disabil,* 1976; 9:19.

45. Klassen AF, Miller A, Fine S. Health-related quality of life in children and adolescents who have a diagnosis of attention-deficit/hyperactivity disorder. *Pediatrics,* 2004; 114:e541–547.

46. Crook WG. Diet and hyperactivity. *Pediatrics,* 1981; 68:300–301.

47. Egger J, Carter CM, Graham PJ, Gumley D, Soothill. Controlled trial of oligoantigenic treatment in the hyperkinetic syndrome. *Lancet,* 1985; 540–545.

48. Carter CM, Urbanowicz M, Hemsley R, Mantilla L, Strobel S, Graham PJ, Taylor E. Effects of a few food diet in attention deficit disorder. *Arch Dis Child,* 1993; 69:564–568.

49. Schulte-Korne G, Deimel W, Gutenbrunner C, Hennighausen K, Blank R, Rieger C, Remschmidt H. Effect of an oligo-antigen diet on the behavior of hyperkinetic children. *Zeitschrift fur Kinder-und Jugendpsychiatrie und Psychotherapie,* 1996; 24:176–183.

50. Pelsser LM, Buitelaar JK. Favourable effect of a standard elimination diet on the behavior of young children with attention deficit hyperactivity disorder (ADHD): A pilot study. *Nederlands Tijdschrift voor Geneeskunde,* 2002; 146:2543–2547.

51. Pelsser LM, Frankena K, Toorman J, Savelkoul HF, Pereira RR, Buitelaar JK. A randomised controlled trial into the effects of food on ADHD. *Eur Child Adolesc Psychiatry,* 2009;18:12–19.

52. Pellser LM, Frankena K, Toorman J, Savelkout HF, Dubois AE, Pereira RR, Haagen TA, Rommelse NN, Buitelaar JK. Effects of a restricted elimination diet on the behaviour of children with attention-deficit hyperactivity disorder (INCA study): A randomised controlled trial. *Lancet,* 2011; 377:494–503.

53. Nigg JT, Lewis K, Edinger T, Falk M. Meta-analysis of attention-deficit/hyperactivity disorder or attention-deficit/hyperactivity disorder symptoms, restriction diet, and synthetic food color additives. *J Am Acad Child Adolesc Psychiatry,* 2012; 51:86–97.

54. Wender EH, Solanto MV. Effects of sugar on aggressive and inattentive behavior in children with attention deficit disorder with hyperactivity and normal children. *Pediatrics,* 1991; 88:960–966.

55. Goldman JA, Lerman RH, Contois JH, et al. Behavioral effects of sucrose on preschool children. *J Abnorm Child Psychol,* 1986; 14:565–577.

56. Prinz RJ, Riddle DB. Association between nutrition and behavior. *Nutr Rev,* 1986; 44(Suppl):151–158.

57. Conners CK, Glasgow A, Raiten D, et al. Hyperactives differ from normals in blood sugar and hormonal response to sucrose. Presented at Annual Meeting, American Psychological Association; August 1987; New York, NY.

58. Wesnes KA, Pincock C, Richardson D, Helm G, Hails S. Breakfast reduces declines in attention and memory over the morning in schoolchildren. *Appetite,* 2003; 41:329–331.

59. Wolraich M, Stumbo P, Milich R, Chenard C, Schultz F. Dietary characteristics of hyperactive and controls boys and their behavioural correlates. *J Am Diet Assoc,* 1986; 84:500–504.

60. Benton D. The impact of the supply of glucose to the brain on mood and memory. *Nutr Rev,* 2001; 59: S20–21.

61. Wolraich M, Milich R, Stumbo P, Schultz F. Effects of sucrose ingestion on the behavior of hyperactive boys. *J Pediatr,* 1985; 106:675.

62. Ferguson HB, Stoddart C, Simeon PG. Double blind challenge studies of behavioural and cognitive effets of sucrose-aspartame ingestion in normal children. *Nutr Rev,* 1986; 44(Suppl):144–150.

63. Roshon MS, Hagen RL. Sugar consumption, locomotion, task orientation, and learning in preschool children. *J Abnorm Child Psychol,* 1989; 17:349–357.

64. Mahan LK, Chase M, Furukawa CT, Sulzacher S, Shapiro GG, Pierson W, Bierman CW. Sugar "allergy" and children's behavior. *Ann Allergy,* 1988; 61:453–458.
65. Behar D, Rapoport JL, Adams AA, Berg CK, Cornblath M. Sugar challenge testing with children considered behaviorally "sugar reactive." *Nutr Behav,* 1984; 1:277–288.
66. Saravis S, Schachar R, Zlotkin S, Leiber LA, Anderson GH. Aspartame: Effects on learning, behavior and mood. *Pediatrics,* 1990; 86:75–80.
67. Garriga MM, Metcalfe DD. Aspartame intolerance. *Ann Allergy,* 1988; 61:63–69.
68. Maher TJ, Wurtman RJ. Possible neurologic effects of aspartame, a widely used food additive. *Environ Health Perspect,* 1987; 75:53–57.
69. Coulombe RA, Sharma RP. Neurobiological alterations induced by the artificial sweetener aspartame (NutraSweet). *Toxicol Appl Pharmacol,* 1986; 83:79–85.
70. Craig ML, Hollis KL, Dess NK. The bitter truth: Sensitivity to saccharin's bitterness predicts overactivity in highly arousable female dieters. *Int J Eat Disord,* 2003; 34:71–82.
71. Johnson RJ, Gold MS, Johnson DR, Ishimoto T, Lanaspa MA, Zahniser NR, Avena NM. Attention-deficit/hyperactivity disorder: Is it time to reappraise the role of sugar consumption? *Postgrad Med,* 2011; 123:39–49.
72. Richardson AJ, Puri BK. The potential role of fatty acids in attention-deficit hyperactivity disorder. *Prostaglandins Leukot Essent Fatty Acids,* 2000; 63:79–87.
73. Yehuda S, Rabinovitz S, Mostofsky DI. Essential fatty acids and the brain: From infancy to aging. *Neurobio of Aging,* 2005; 26S:S98–102.
74. Yehuda S, Rabonivitz S, Mostofsky DI. Essential fatty acids are mediators of brain biochemistry and cognitive functions. *J Neurosci Re,* 1999; 56:565–570.
75. Attar-Bashi NM, Frydenberg M, Li D, Sinclair AJ. Docosahexaenoic acid (DHA) accumulation is regulated by the polyunsaturated fat content of the diet. *Asia Pac J Clin Nutr,* 2004; 13(Suppl):S78.
76. Richardson AJ. Long-chain polyunsaturated fatty acids in childhood developmental and psychiatric disorders. *Lipids,* 2004; 39:1215–1222.
77. Simopoulos AP. The importance of the ratio of omega-6/omega-3 essential fatty acids. *Biomed Pharmacother,* 2002; 56:365–379.
78. Colquhoun I, Bunday S. A lack of essential fatty acids as a possible cause of hyperactivity in children. *Med Hypotheses,* 1981; 7:673–679.
79. Mitchell EA, Aman MG, Turbott SH, Manku M. Clinical characteristics and serum fatty acid levels in hyperactive children. *Clin Pediatr,* 1987; 26:406–411.
80. Stevens LJ, Zental SS, Deck JL, Abate ML, Lipp SR, Burgess JR. Essential fatty acid metabolism in boys with attention-deficit hyperactivity disorder. *Am J Clin Nutr,* 1995; 62:761–768.
81. Chen JR, Hsu SF, Hsu CD, Hwang LH, Yang SC. Dietary patterns and blood fatty acid composition in children with attention-deficit hyperactivity disorder in Taiwan. *J Nutr Biochem,* 2004; 15:467–472.
82. Young GS, Maharaj NJ, Conquer JA. Blood phospholipids fatty acid analysis of adults with and without attention deficit/hyperactivity disorder. *Lipids,* 2004; 39:117–123.
83. Brookes KJ, Chen W, Xu X, Taylor E, Asherson P. Association of fatty acid desaturase genes with attention-deficit/hyperactivity disorder. *Biol Psychiatry,* 2006; 60:1053–1061.
84. Yehuda S. N-6/n-3 ratio and brain-related functions. *World Rev Nutr Diet,* 2003; 92:37–56.
85. Bloch MK, Qawasmi A. Omega-3 fatty acid supplementation for the treatment of children with attention-deficit/hyperactivity disorder symptomatology: Systematic review and meta-analysis. *J Am Acad Child Adolesc Psychiatry,* 2011; 50:991–1000.
86. Aman MG, Mitchell EA, Turbott SH. The effects of essential fatty acid supplementation by Efamol in hyperactive children. *J Abnorm Child Psychol,* 1987; 15:75–90.
87. Arnold LE, Kleykamp D, Votolato NA, Taylor WA, Kontras SB, Tobin K. Gamma-linolenic acid for attention-deficit hyperactivity disorder: Placebo-controlled comparison to D-amphetamine. *Biol Psychiatry,* 1989; 25:222–228.
88. Voigt RG, Llorente A, Jensen CL, Fraley JK, Berretta MC, Heird WC. A randomized, double-blind, placebo-controlled trial of docosahexaenoic acid supplementation in children with attention-deficit/hyperactivity disorder. *J Pediat,* 2001; 139:189–196.
89. Hirayama S, Hamazaki T, Terasawa K. Effect of docosahexaenoic acid-containing food administration on symptoms of attention-deficit/hyperactivity disorder—a placebo-controlled double-blind study. *Eur J Clin Nutr,* 2004; 58:467–473.
90. Stevens L, Zhang W, Peck L, Kuczek T, Grevstad N, Mahon A, Zentall SS, Arnold LE, Burgess JR. EFA supplementation in children with inattention, hyperactivity, and other disruptive behaviors. *Lipids,* 2003; 38:1007–1021.

91. Sinn N, Bryan J. Effect of supplementation with polyunsaturated fatty acids and micronutrients on learning and behavior problems associated with child ADHD. *J Dev Behav Pediatr,* 2007; 28:82–91.

92. Joshi K, Lad S, Kale M, Patwardhan B, Mahadik SP, Patni B, Chaudhary A, Bhave S, Pandit A. Supplementation with flax oil and vitamin C improves the outcome of attention deficit hyperactivity disorder (ADHD). *Prostaglandins Leukot Essent Fatty Acids,* 2006; 74:17–21.

93. Virmani A, Binienda Z. Role of carnitine esters in brain neuropathology. *Mol Aspects Med,* 2004; 25:533–549.

94. Van Oudheusden LJ, Scholte HR. Efficacy of carnitine in the treatment of children with attention-deficit hyperactivity disorder. *Prostaglandins Leukot Essent Fatty Acids,* 2002; 67:33–38.

95. Abbasi SH, Heidari S, Mohammadi MR, Tabrizi M, Ghaleiha A, Akhondzadeh S. Acetyl-L-carnitine as an adjunctive therapy in the treatment of attention-deficit/hyperactivity disorder in children and adolescents: A placebo-controlled trial. *Child Psychiatry Hum Dev,* 2011; 42:367–375.

96. Youdim MB, Ben-Shachar D, Yehuda S. Putative biological mechanisms of the effect of iron deficiency on brain biochemistry and behavior. *AmJClinNutr,* 1989; 50(3 Suppl):607–615.

97. Konofal E, Cortese S, Marchand M, Mouren M-C, Arnulf I, Lecendreux M. Impact of restless legs syndrome and iron deficiency on attention-deficit/hyperactivity disorder in children. *Sleep Medicine,* 2007; 8:711–715.

98. Konofal E, Lecendreux M, Arnulf I, Mouren MC. Iron deficiency in children with attention-deficit/hyperactivity disorder. *Arch Pediatr Adolesc Med,* 2004; 158:1113–1115.

99. Oner O, Alkar OY, Oner P. Relation of ferritin levels with symptom ratings and cognitive performance in children with attention deficit-hyperactivity disorder. *Pediatr Int,* 2008; 50:40–44.

100. Sever Y, Ashkenazi A, Tyano S, Weizman A. Iron treatment in children with attention deficit hyperactivity disorder. A preliminary report. *Neuropsychobiology,* 1997; 35:178–180.

101. Konofal E, Lecendreux M, Deron J, Marchand M, Cortese S, Zaïm M, Mouren Mc Arnulf I. Effects of iron supplementation on attention deficit hyperactivity disorder in children. *Pediatr Neurol,* 2008; 38:20–26.

102. Konofal E, Cortese S. Restless legs syndrome and attention-deficit/hyperactivity disorder. *Ann Neurol,* 2005; 58:341–342.

103. Cortese S, Konofal E, Lecendreux M, et al. Restless legs syndrome and attention-deficit/hyperactivity disorder: A review of the literature. *Sleep,* 2005; 28:1007–1013.

104. Walters AS, Mandelbaum DE, Lewin DS, et al. Dopaminergic therapy in children with restless legs/periodic limb movements in sleep and ADHD. *Pediatric Neurology,* 2000; 22:182–186.

105. Black MM. Zinc deficiency and child development. *J Clin Nutr,* 1998; 8(suppl):464S–469S.

106. Arnold LE, Pinkham SM, Votolato N. Does zinc moderate essential fatty acid and amphetamine treatment of attention-deficit/hyperactivity disorder? *J Child Adolesc Psychopharmacol,* 2000; 10:111–117.

107. Toren P, Eldar S, Sela BA, Wolmer L, Weitz R, Inbar D, Koren S, Reiss A, Weizman R, Laor N. Zinc deficiency in attention-deficit hyperactivity disorder. *Biol Psychiatry,* 1996; 40:1308–1310.

108. Bekaroglu M, Aslan Y, Gedik Y, Deger O, Mocan H, Erduran E, Karahan C. Relationships between serum free fatty acids and zinc, and attention deficit hyperactivity disorder: A research note. *J Child Psychol Psychiatry,* 1996; 37:225–227.

109. Akhondzadeh S, Mohammadi M-R, Khademi M. Zinc sulfate as an adjunct to methylphenidate for the treatment of attention deficit hyperactivity disorder in children: A double blind and randomized trial. *BMC Psychiatry,* 2004; 4:9.

110. Arnold LE, Disilvestro RA, Bozzolo D, et al. Zinc for attention-deficit/hyperactivity disorder: Placebo-controlled double-blind pilot trial alone and combined with amphetamine. *J Child Adolesc Psychopharmacol,* 2001; 21:1–19.

111. Kozielec T, Starobrat-Hermelin B. Assessment of magnesium levels in children with attention deficit hyperactivity disorder (ADHD). *Magnes Res,* 1997; 10:143–148.

112. Starobrat-Hermelin B. The effect of deficiency of selected bioelements on hyperactivity in children with certain specified mental disorders. *Annales Academiae Medicae Stetinensis,* 1998; 44:297–314.

113. Starobrat-Hermelin B, Kozielec T. The effects of magnesium physiological supplementation on hyperactivity in children with attention deficit hyperactivity disorder (ADHD). Positive response to magnesium oral loading test. *Magnesium Res,* 1997; 10:149–156.

114. Monsain-Bosc M, Roche M, Polge A, Pradal-Prat D, Rapin J, Bali JP. Improvement of neurobehavioral disorders in children supplemented with magnesium-vitamin B6. I. Attention deficit hyperactivity disorders. *Magnesium Res,* 2006; 19:46–52.

115. Schmidt ME, Kruesi MJ, Elia J, Borcherding BG, Elin RJ, Hosseini JM, McFarlin KE, Hamburger S. Effect of dextroamphetamine and methylphenidate on calcium and magnesium concentration in hyperactive boys. *Psychiatry Res,* 1994; 54:199–210.

116. Oades RD. Dopamine–serotonin interactions in attention-deficit hyperactivity disorder (ADHD). *Progress Brain Res*, 2008; 172:543–565.

117. Harding KL, Judah RD, Gant CE. Outcome-based comparison of ritalin versus food-supplement treated children with AD/HD. *Alt Med Rev*, 8200, 8:319-330.

118. Ludolph AG, Kassube J, Schmeck K, Glaser C, Wunderlich A, Buck AK, Reske S N, Fegert JM, Mottaghy FM. Dopaminergic dysfunction in attention deficit hyperactivity disorder (ADHD), differences between pharmacologically treated and never treated young adults: A 3,4-dihdroxy-6-[18F]fluorophenyl-l-alanine PET study. *Neuroimage*, 2008; 41:718–727.

119 Anderson GM, Dover MA, Yang BP, Holahan JM, Shaywitz SE, Marchione KE, Hall LM, Fletcher JM, Shaywitz BA. Adrenomedullary function during cognitive testing in attention-deficit/hyperactivity disorder. *J Am Acad Child Adolesc Psychiatry*, 2000; 39:635–643.

120. Hanna GL, Ornitz EM, Hariharan M. Urinary catecholamine excretion and behavioral differences in ADHD and normal boys. *J Child Adolesc Psychopharmacol*, 1996; 6:63–73.

121. Dvorakova M, Jezova D, Blazicek P, Trebaticka J, Skodacek I, Suba J, Iveta W, Rohdewaki P, Durackova Z. Urinary catecholamines in children with attention deficit hyperactivity disorder (ADHD): Modulation by a polyphenolic extract from pine park (pycnogenol). *Nutr Neurosci*, 2007; 10:151–157.

122. Wurtman RJ, Fernstrom JD. Control of brain neurotransmitter synthesis by precursor availability. *Biochem Pharmacol*, 1976; 25:1691–1696.

123. Lechin F, van der Dijs B. Cross talk between the autonomic and central nervous systems: Mechanistic and therapeutic considerations for neuronal, immune, vascular, and somatic-based diseases. In K. Maiese (Ed.), *Neurovascular Medicine: Pursuing Cellular Longevity for Healthy Aging*. 2009. USA: Oxford University Press.

124. Johansson J, Landgren M, Fernell E, Vumma R, Ahlin A, Bjerkensted L, Venizelos N. Altered tryptophan and alanine transport in fibroblasts from boys with attention-deficit/hyperactivity disorder (ADHD): An in vitro study. *Behav Brain Funct*, 2011; 7: 40.

125. Fan X, Xu M, Hess EJ. D2 dopamine receptor subtype-mediated hyperactivity and amphetamine responses in a model of ADHD. *Neurobiol Dis*, 2010; 37:228–236.

126. Wood D, Reimherr F, Wender PH. Effects of levodopa on attention deficit disorder, residual type. *Psychiatry Res*, 1982; 6:13–20.

127. Wood DR, Reimherr FW, Wender PH. Treatment of attention deficit disorder with dl-phenylalanine. *Psychiatry Res*, 1985; 16:21–26.

128. Reimherr FW, Wender PH, Wood DR, Ward M. An open trial of l-tyrosine in the treatment of attention deficit disorder, residual type. *Am J Psychiatry*, 1987; 144:1071–1073.

129. Zepf FD, Holtmann M, Stadler C, Demisch L, Schmitt M, Wöckel L, Poustka F. Diminished serotonergic functioning in hostile children with ADHD: Tryptophan depletion increases behavioural inhibition. *Pharmacopsychiatry*, 2008; 4:60–65.

130. Hinz M, Stein A, Neff R, Weinberg R, Uncini T. Treatment of attention deficit hyperactivity disorder with monoamine amino acid precursors and organic cation transporter assay interpretation. *Neuropsyh Dis Treat*, 2011; 7:31–38.

131. Ludolph AG, Udvardi PT, Schaz U, Henes C, Adolph O, Weigt HU, Fegert JM, Boeckers TM, Föhr KJ. Atomoxetine acts as an NMDA receptor blocker in clinically relevant concentrations. *Br J Pharmacol*, 2010; 160:283–291.

132. Pozzi L, Baviera M, Sacchetti G, Calcagno E, Balducci C, Invernizzi RW, Carli M. Attention deficit induced by blockade of N-methyl D-aspartate receptors in the prefrontal cortex is associated with enhanced glutamate release and cAMP response element binding protein phosphorylation: Role of metabotropic glutamate receptors 2/3. *Neuroscience*, 2011; 176:336–348.

133. Russell VA. Dopamine hypofunction possibly results from a deficit in glutamate-stimulated release of dopamine in the nucleus accumbens shell of a rat model for attention deficit hyperactivity disorder—the spontaneously hypertensive rat. *Neurosci Biobehav Rev*, 2003; 27:671–682.

134. Kusaga A, Yamashita Y, Koeda T, Hiratani M, Kaneko M, Yamada S, Matsuishi T. Increased urine phenylethylamine after methylphenidate treatment in children with ADHD. *Ann Neurol*, 2002; 52:372–374.

135. Nemeroff CB. Anxiolytics: Past, present, and future agents. *J Clin Psychiatry*, 2003; 64 Suppl 3:3–6.

136. DeMaray MK, Elting J, Schaefer K. Assessment of Attention-Deficit/Hyperactivity Disorder (ADHD): A comparative evaluation of five, commonly used, published rating scales. *Psychol Sch*, 2003; 40:341–361.

30 Sleep Disturbance

Jyotsna Sahni, M.D.

INTRODUCTION

Fifty to 70 million Americans have chronic problems with sleep [1]. Adequate, quality sleep is crucial to good health yet there are many medical barriers to achieving it. The biologic basis of these disturbances may be influenced by nutrition. This chapter presents diet, food, and nutrient strategies as adjunct interventions in a primary care setting.

PHYSIOLOGY OF SLEEP

Sleep has four stages known as sleep architecture. Each stage lasts roughly 90 minutes. Stages 1 and 2 are light, while stage 3 is deep and restorative. During deep sleep, the body synthesizes growth hormone, testosterone, thyroid hormone, and immune mediators. Stages 1 through 3 are followed by the fourth stage known as rapid eye movement (REM) sleep. REM accounts for approximately 25% of sleep. It is the dream cycle, the lightest sleep, during which time we consolidate memories [2].

NUTRITION-RELATED CONSEQUENCES OF POOR SLEEP

Sleep deprivation is associated with weight gain. In a study of 924 participants between the ages of 18 and 91, researchers found that people who slept the least weighed the most [3]. Sleep deprivation may also lead to poor food choices that affect weight gain. In a study of 1203 individuals in the rural Midwest, the participants with less sleep ate more, chose fewer fruits and vegetables, and were less physically active [4]. The Wisconsin Sleep Cohort Study showed that participants with less sleep had reduced leptin and elevated ghrelin [5]. Since leptin signals satiety and ghrelin mediates hunger, the higher rates of obesity were attributed to excess caloric intake. Additionally, the choice of calories ingested during fatigued states tends to be calorie-dense foods with a high carbohydrate content [6]. In an epidemiological study of 2494 individuals born from 1981 to 1983 in Australia, sleeping problems at ages two to four years increased the odds of being obese in young adulthood by 90% [7]. A 13-year prospective trial of young adults in the United States also showed an association of short sleep duration and obesity [8]. The association between less sleep and body weight spans age groups but the underlying mechanisms remain poorly characterized.

Sleep duration and quality have emerged as predictors of levels of hemoglobin A1c [9]. The Massachusetts Male Aging Study, a large prospective trial of 1564 men followed for 16 years, reported that those whose sleep duration was less than or equal to five and six hours were twice as likely to develop diabetes. Men reporting sleep duration greater than eight hours were more than three times as likely to develop diabetes. Since this was a self-report, overall sleep time in this latter group is likely to represent duration in bed and could have represented men with obstructive sleep apnea (OSA), who may spend more time in bed sleeping poorly. The authors suggest that the effects of sleep on diabetes could be mediated via changes in endogenous testosterone levels. The relative ratios of risk remained significant when adjusted for testosterone levels [10]. Short- and long-duration sleep times were associated with type 2 diabetes and impaired glucose tolerance in both men and women [11]. Collectively, these studies suggest a novel approach to optimizing glycemic control: optimize sleep quantity and quality.

MEDICAL CONDITIONS THAT DISRUPT SLEEP

INSOMNIA

Trouble sleeping is a common complaint of patients and is often a symptom of another medical problem. By working on the root problem, the insomnia is usually improved. There are two main kinds of insomnia. The first is called sleep onset insomnia where the onset of sleep is delayed beyond the average 5- to 20-minute sleep latency. Behavioral evaluation and techniques are often successful in treating sleep onset insomnia. The second form of insomnia, sleep maintenance insomnia, involves difficulty staying asleep. Frequent awakenings usually require medical evaluation and treatment. Many patients suffer from both types of insomnia. Women have more trouble with insomnia than men.

There are multiple reasons for both types of insomnia. Many medications, prescribed or over the counter (OTC), affect sleep. Avoiding these drugs, using them sparingly, or finding substitutes that do not have sleep side effects can help. The treatments throughout this book can decrease or eliminate the need for many medications (see Table 30.1).

ANXIETY AND DEPRESSION

Sleep, diet, and anxiety affect one another. Anxiety makes restful sleep difficult to achieve while difficulty sleeping can increase anxiety. Increased anxiety can lead to food cravings that can interfere with sleep. Stimulants including foods with caffeine and high glycemic index carbohydrates should be avoided. Psychological and/or nutritional counseling can help many people reduce

TABLE 30.1

Substances That Keep People Awake

Alcohol

Nicotine

Cocaine

Caffeine

Decongestants like Sudafed™ (pseudophedrine)

Ritalin™ (methylphenidate), diet pills, or other stimulants

Ginkgo

Guarana

Siberian ginseng

Ephedrine, ephedra, and ma huang

Bitter orange

Yohimbe

Kola nut

Beta blockers

Albuterol

Theophylline

Wellbutrin™ (bupropion)

Selective serotonin reuptake inhibitors

Prednisone and other steroids

anxiety. Natural mind-body relaxation techniques such as meditation, yoga, and yogic breathing are shown to be effective at reducing anxiety [12–14].

Depression and poor sleep are linked, but it is not always clear which comes first. It is interesting to note that sad mood, irritability, difficulty making decisions, and a sense of hopelessness and helplessness can be part of a diagnosis of clinical depression as well as of sleep deprivation. While early morning awakening can signal depression, insomnia itself can cause depression. Common antidepressants such as Prozac or Wellbutrin may have a negative impact on sleep. A study in patients with obstructive sleep apnea showed that treatment with continuous positive airway pressure (CPAP) caused symptoms of depression to abate [15]. Nutritional strategies for treating depression including vitamin D, omega-3 fats, and neurotransmitter precursors such as L-tryptophan may also improve sleep quality [16].

PAIN

Pain from arthritis, headaches, gastroesophageal reflux disease, and fibromyalgia can make it hard to fall asleep and stay asleep. Sleep deprivation exacerbates pain [17]. Medications and nutritional therapies targeted at the cause of pain can be employed to reduce pain and maximize good sleep.

BLADDER PROBLEMS

Patients commonly complain that frequent trips to the bathroom during the night disturb their sleep. A multiple sclerosis patient may have a neurogenic bladder. A urinary tract infection may cause urinary frequency, urgency, and dysuria. Prostatic hypertrophy can cause urinary frequency. Taking prescription diuretics before bed such as hydrochlorothiazide or Lasix for blood pressure or heart issues, or drinking a diuretic dieter's tea such as dandelion root may cause a patient to have urinary urgency during the night. Simply overdoing fluids before going to bed will result in a necessary and appropriate diuresis. Caffeinated beverages exacerbate this problem because the caffeine acts as a stimulant and also a mild diuretic. However, most patients misperceive that they're getting up to urinate when in fact they are awakening for another reason. It is therefore important for a physician to consider alternative explanations and treatable diagnoses.

GASTROESOPHAGEAL REFLUX

Consuming too much food close to bedtime can disturb sleep. Symptoms of gastroesophageal reflux disease (GERD) can significantly diminish sleep quality and quantity [18,19]. Shorter dinner-to-bed time has been associated with an increased risk of GERD. Ideally, a gap of 4 hours between eating and sleeping is recommended [20].

FOOD REACTIVITIES

Infants with cow milk intolerance may present with a disturbed sleep pattern, along with the more usual cutaneous, gastrointestinal, and respiratory problems [21]. Sleep disturbance secondary to food allergies has a broad biologic basis, but its prevalence and pathophysiology are understudied.

MENOPAUSAL SYMPTOMS

Sleep problems increase with age in both sexes, but women are more susceptible to sleep problems at all ages. Menopause is an especially important milestone, as falls in both estrogen and progesterone reduce sleep quality [22]. Elevated beta EEG activity on polysomnogram suggests that arousal level during sleep is higher in menopausal women [23]. Mood symptoms and weight gain at midlife may exacerbate sleep pathology [24].

Insomnia is considered a primary symptom of menopause [25]. The classic sleep disturbance of menopause involves falling asleep easily, but then being troubled with multiple awakenings throughout the night. The arousals may occur in isolation or be followed by a hot flash [26]. Severe hot flashes are significantly associated with symptoms and a diagnosis of chronic insomnia, leading to poor health, chronic pain, and depression [27,28]. Interestingly, most hot flashes occur during the first half of the night, as REM sleep suppresses hot flashes and associated arousals and awakening. REM periods lengthen as the night goes on with the greatest amount of REM occurring in the early morning hours [29].

As aforementioned, depression is more common in women than men and in those women with menopause-associated depression, improvement in depression is predicted by improved sleep [30]. Menopause-related sleep disturbance also has a measured impact on healthcare utilization and its associated costs, health-related quality of life, and work productivity [31]. Menopausal women with sleep disturbance used massage and other forms of body work fourfold more often than those patients with undisturbed sleep. In the same study, sleep disturbance led to a threefold increase in the use of stress management and more than doubled the use of dietary soy products to manage menopausal symptoms [32] The frequent disturbances make other sleep problems such as restless leg syndrome worse [33], and lead to periodic limb movement disorder as well as obstructive sleep apnea [34].

Sleep disturbances in menopausal women should not be assumed to be merely a consequence of falling levels of hormones. There is a threefold increase in obstructive sleep apnea in women immediately following the onset of menopause. In a study evaluating the impact of menopause on the prevalence and severity of sleep apnea, there were proportionately more postmenopausal than premenopausal women in all ranges of apnea severity. Even after adjusting for body mass index (BMI) and neck circumference, the postmenopausal women had a significantly higher mean Apnea-Hyponea Index, suggesting that functional rather than anatomic differences in the upper airway of both groups of women accounted for the difference in apnea prevalence and severity [35]. Women, unlike men, may complain of insomnia rather than daytime fatigue as their presenting sign of obstructive sleep apnea, thereby delaying accurate diagnosis and treatment [36]. Diagnostic evaluation with a polysomnogram may be warranted.

Independent of sleep-disordered breathing, postmenopausal women may experience a blunting of the normal drop in blood pressure from day to night, which may contribute to increased cardiovascular morbidity and mortality. A racial difference was also observed because this increase in both systolic and diastolic blood pressure during the night was more pronounced in African American women compared to white women [37]. Decreased heart rate variability is another cardiovascular risk factor that is observed in menopausal women suffering hot flashes during sleep. It is thought to be caused by elevated sympathetic activation, which consequently triggers hot flashes [38].

Given the results of the Women's Health Initiative, many women are reluctant to use hormone replacement therapy to treat their hot flashes and other menopausal symptoms and have therefore sought more natural alternatives such as botanicals and dietary supplements [39]. While controlled studies are limited, treatment with isoflavones [40] from soy foods [41] and supplemental use of the herb black cohosh (*Cimicifuga racemosa*) may be helpful [42–48]. Sometimes hormone replacement therapy is necessary and efficacious [49], but it may be that naturopathy may be even more effective than pharmacotherapy: women utilizing naturopathy were approximately seven times more likely than conventionally treated patients to report improvement for insomnia, but also improvements in anxiety, hot flashes, menstrual changes, and vaginal dryness [50].

Dong quai, one of the most commonly prescribed Chinese herbs for women has been used as a "female tonic" for menstrual problems for centuries [51]. A medicinal herb extract preparation of dong quai (*Angelica sinensis*) and chamomile (*Matricaria chamomilla*) (Climex) also showed marked alleviation of sleep disturbances and fatigue as well as hot flashes [52]. Another combination product, Phyto-Female Complex, containing standardized extracts of black cohosh, dong quai, milk thistle, red clover, American ginseng, and chastetree berry, showed a 73% decrease in hot flashes and a 69% reduction of night sweats, accompanied by a decrease in their intensity and a significant benefit in terms of sleep quality [53]. Femal, an herbal remedy made from bee pollen, showed a 72% reduction in hot flashes by three months of use [54]. *Hericium erinaceus*, a well-known edible mushroom, was used in a Japanese study to show improvements in the Pittsburgh Sleep Quality Index as well as in depression and other menopausal symptoms in four weeks by stimulating nerve growth factor synthesis to affect autonomic nervous system function [55]. Another combination, isoflavones plus *Lactobacillus sporoagenes* and magnolia bark extract, targeted improvements on symptoms of insomnia, anxiety, and irritability [56]. An earlier study utilized the same ingredients along with the addition of calcium, magnesium, and vitamin D showing similar results: improvements on psycho-affective and sleep disturbances in menopause, along with reduction of vasomotor symptoms [57]. Valerian improves the quality of sleep in women with menopause who are experiencing insomnia [58].

Melatonin levels were found to be significantly lower in postmenopausal women with insomnia, suggesting that supplementation may be efficacious [59]. Chastetree (*Vitex agnus castus*) has been approved for PMS, breast tenderness, and irregular menses by European regulators [60]. Its progesterone-like effect has been verified by endometrial biopsy, blood hormone levels, and examination of vaginal secretions; therefore, it has been recommended for women in early menopause with irregular menstrual cycles [61]. A single study has been performed on chastetree alone and, while it did show improvement in mood and hot flashes, there was no placebo or comparison group [62].

St. John's wort (*Hypericuum perforatum*) has been heavily studied for its role in treating depression. In one nonplacebo-controlled clinical trial conducted among women experiencing menopausal symptoms, 900 mg of St. John's wort, taken for 12 weeks, showed significant improved psychological, psychosomatic, and sexual parameters [63]. Used in combination with black cohosh, a synergistic effect was seen improving insomnia, depression, mood swings, and irritability [64]. Unfortunately, herb-drug interactions are common with St. John's wort. It decreases the blood levels of anticoagulants, cyclosporine, digoxin, and protease inhibitors for HIV. In addition, breakthrough bleeding and unplanned pregnancies have been seen in women using both St. John's wort and oral contraceptives [65].

Kava (*Piper methysticum*) is an herb from the South Pacific that has been used for the treatment of anxiety and has shown significant improvement in insomnia and irritability compared with placebo in menopausal women [66]. However, due to its potential hepatoxicity, its use is discouraged.

Wild yam (*Dioscorea villosa*) has been used for postpartum pain as well as menstrual cramps. There was no difference seen in either menopausal symptoms or serum/salivary hormone levels compared to placebo in a randomized placebo-controlled trial. Apparently, wild yam does not convert to progesterone when taken internally or applied topically; not surprisingly, no benefit was gained [67].

Hops (*Humulus lupulus*) have been evaluated by European regulators for sleep disruptions and anxiety. It was shown in a randomized, double-blind, placebo-controlled study of 67 menopausal women to decrease menopausal symptoms, especially hot flashes, at either 100 mg or 250 mg compared to placebo at six weeks, but not at 12 weeks [68].

Maca (*Lepidium peruvianum*), a plant native to the high Andes of Peru and Bolivia, was studied in 169 postmenopausal women and found to reduce insomnia, hot flashes, and depression, as well as improve memory, concentration, energy, lipids, blood pressure, body mass index, and bone density. Increased estradiol and lowered levels of luteinizing hormone, cortisol, and adrenocorticotropic hormone (ACTH) were noted. The commonly recommended dose of maca extract is 2000 mg/day [69].

Evening primrose oil contains gamolenic acid, which is believed to reduce vasomotor symptoms of menopause, but the only randomized controlled trial for menopausal symptoms showed no difference with placebo [70].

While many herbs have been looked at in the treatment of menopause, unfortunately evidence supporting the use of alternative and complementary treatments for menopausal symptoms and sleep disturbance is limited, and larger and better controlled studies are necessary [71].

OBSTRUCTIVE SLEEP APNEA (OSA)

OSA is characterized by disordered breathing during sleep. To make the diagnosis, apnea must last for at least 10 seconds five times in one hour of sleep. Patients may be unaware of their frequent arousals or may awake with an obvious resuscitative snort. Although 5% of the population has OSA, both physicians and patients alike are poorly aware of this common disorder. People with OSA are at higher risk for hypertension, heart attacks, arrhythmias, diabetes [72], strokes [73], and motor vehicle accidents. Most of the time, OSA is easy to identify and to treat. The most frequent symptom is excessive daytime sleepiness, the severity of which can be determined by the Epworth Sleepiness Scale, a simple questionnaire that can be administered to the patient in the waiting room before the doctor's appointment (see Figure 30.1). A score greater than 10 is associated with significant disability and should prompt referral to a sleep specialist or directly to a polysomnogram.

The diagnosis of OSA is made by taking a good history of the patient's sleepiness and snoring. A bed partner can be interviewed or patients can videotape themselves sleeping. Physical exam may identify obesity, neck girth greater than 17 inches in men or 16 inches in women, a small chin, and large tonsils. Patients with risk factors can be referred for a polysomnogram. This entails an overnight stay at a hospital or independent sleep lab where a patient can be monitored for abnormalities in respiration, EKG, EEG, and limb movement. CPAP (continuous positive airway pressure), a mechanical device, which blows air into the nose and/or oral cavity to keep the soft tissues from collapsing, can be adjusted during the sleep study. Often, diagnosis and treatment can be accomplished on the same visit.

Weight loss is usually necessary to improve, if not cure, OSA. This has prompted some physicians to emphasize weight reduction without diagnosing and treating OSA. However, for many patients, weight loss can only be achieved once the OSA is appropriately treated with CPAP [74]. OSA promotes insulin resistance and sleep deprivation, creating a vicious cycle of weight gain and worsening OSA. CPAP should therefore be viewed as a primary care intervention for obesity as well as a treatment for OSA.

RESTLESS LEG SYNDROME

Restless leg syndrome (RLS) is a disorder that is characterized by an uncomfortable, creepy, crawling feeling in the legs, feet, or thighs that is temporarily relieved by movement. Sometimes patients describe a pins-and-needles sensation and try to rub their legs or walk it off to relieve the discomfort. It can make falling asleep and staying asleep difficult. It can also occur during the day when one has to sit still at a desk or in a movie. Afflicting about 10% of the population, it tends to begin in

Use the following scale to choose the most appropriate number for each situation:
- *0 = no chance of dozing*
- *1 = slight chance of dozing*
- *2 = moderate chance of dozing*
- *3 = high chance of dozing*

Situation	Chance of dozing
Sitting and reading	
Watching TV	
Sitting inactive in a public place (e.g., a theater or a meeting)	
As a passenger in a car for an hour without a break	
Lying down to rest in the afternoon when circumstances permit	
Sitting and talking to someone	
Sitting quietly after a lunch without alcohol	
In a car, while stopped for a few minutes in traffic	

FIGURE 30.1 Epworth Sleepiness Scale.

the third decade of life and get worse over time. It is about 60% genetic and occurs more in women than men. RLS is thought to be due to abnormal iron metabolism and dopaminergic systems in the brain. It can be a primary disorder or secondary to iron deficiency. Of individuals with conditions associated with iron-deficiency states, including pregnancy, renal failure, and anemia, 25% to 30% may develop RLS [75]. Caffeine, nicotine, saccharine [76], several prescription medications, fatigue, and extreme temperatures of either hot or cold can exacerbate this condition. RLS can cause periodic limb movements, insomnia, sleepiness, and phase delay. It is associated with attention deficit hyperactivity disorder and depression. RLS is under-diagnosed.

Adequate doses of iron may help treat restless leg syndrome and give relief to the patients who suffer from it [77]. Iron repletion improved sleep disturbance in children with autism [78]. Iron-rich foods, cooking in iron pots, and iron supplements have been shown to be effective in normalizing serum ferritin levels to at least 40 ng/mL. Minerals influence the central nervous system in poorly understood ways. Food cravings stemming from iron deficiency were identified in the 1950s and given the name pica, although the mechanism is still not understood. Folate [79] and magnesium supplements [80] may help. Nutritional analysis using red blood cell levels are available to quantify deficiencies of these and other minerals. Typically these tests give a retrospective look at the three months prior to testing as that is the lifespan of the typical red cell. As nutritional deficits are identified, specific diet and supplement recommendations can be made by the clinician. Sedating herbs such as kava, valerian, and hops also have a helpful role in promotion of sleep.

Gamma aminobutyric acid (GABA) is the most abundant inhibitory neurotransmitter in the mammalian brain. Barbiturates, benzodiazepines, nonbenzodiazepine hypnotics, and alcohol all affect the GABA receptor [81]. GABA is produced from glutamate with the aid of vitamin B6. GABA is available as an over-the-counter supplement. It has shown efficacy as a relaxant and anxiolytic [82]. Dopamine agonists such as Mirapex (pramipexole) and Requip (ropinirole) are considered first-line pharmacologic treatments for RLS; however gabapentin and opioids do have a role in refractory cases [83]. L-tryptophan is an amino acid precursor of monoamines and has been shown to increase dopamine levels and may be beneficial in symptomatic relief of RLS.

PERIODIC LIMB MOVEMENT DISORDER

Periodic limb movement disorder (PLMD) causes the legs to twitch during the night, causing a brief awakening. The twitching typically occurs every 20 to 40 seconds and lasts between half a second to five seconds. PLMD can involve the big toe, ankle, knee, or hip. It can occur in one leg, both, or alternate legs and occasionally the arms. Since PLMD usually occurs during light sleep, stages 1 and 2, it may be difficult to fall asleep. Some patients are unaware of their kicking, but know they have trouble falling asleep; others feel that their feet are extremely cold; some report excessive daytime sleepiness. Bed partners are often aware of the kicking behavior and may sleep elsewhere to avoid being kicked all night. The diagnosis is made by a polysomnogram and is defined by five or more kicks in each hour of sleep that cause an awakening. The underlying cause of periodic limb movement disorder is not well understood, but it does seem to have a genetic component and worsens with age. Similar to RLS, iron supplementation may improve severity of symptoms [84] as may magnesium therapy [85]. Dopaminergic medications are the first line of pharmacologic treatment. Medications that interfere with neurotransmitter balance such as selective serotonin reuptake inhibitors, most antipsychotic drugs, and anti-dopaminergics like metoclopramide can precipitate PLMD.

NOCTURNAL LEG CRAMPS

Nocturnal leg cramps are common in both adults and children. They are present in nearly half of the population over the age of 50 years, have an increased prevalence with age, and are equally seen in men and women. Leg cramps are characterized by sudden painful muscle tightness, most commonly in the foot, calf, or thigh. The cramp may last for seconds to minutes and is relieved by stretching of the affected muscles. Most cramps only occur at night and lead to pain and sleep disturbance. They are often idiopathic or associated with structural disorders such as flat feet or hypermobility syndrome. Often there is a family history in these cases. Prolonged sitting, inappropriate leg position while sedentary, or excessive time walking on hard flooring such as concrete may increase the occurrence of leg cramps. Medications, exercise, as well as neurological and metabolic disorders can also cause leg cramps. Leg cramps may also result from volume depletion due to excessive sweating without adequate hydration and salt replacement, diuretic use, or fluid removal during dialysis or dialysis disequilibrium syndrome. Pregnancy-related leg cramps may be due to low serum magnesium, which may improve with magnesium repletion [86]. In addition to magnesium supplementation, other nutritional treatments include adequate hydration, calcium, iron (in patients with iron-deficiency anemia), vitamin E, and vitamin B6 [87].

Desynchronosis

There are differences in circadian rhythms based on stages of life and also among individuals. For example, teenagers prefer going to bed late and waking up late. They also need closer to nine hours of sleep, a little more than the typical adult. This tendency is known as delayed phase disorder. While most outgrow this pattern eventually, many continue to prefer the night when they are most alert and energetic. With age, many shift to an early-to-bed, early-to-rise routine. If bedtime has become unreasonably early (i.e., 7 p.m.), this is known as advanced phase disorder. Treatment for both delayed and advanced phase disorders includes consistency of wake and bedtimes, phototherapy, and possibly melatonin replacement.

Abnormal patterns and production of cortisol can be seen in disorders of desynchronosis. Cortisol levels are easily and reliably measured by saliva testing at intervals throughout the day [88]. In a normal individual, cortisol levels are high in the morning, upon awakening, giving alertness and energy during the day. Levels should wane in the evening, allowing for sleep. At times, this pattern is reversed, resulting in both sleep onset and/or sleep maintenance insomnia. If cortisol levels are abnormally high suggesting some degree of adrenal hyperreactivity, dietary intervention with high-potency multivitamins with extra vitamin C, vitamin B5, vitamin B6, zinc, and phosphatidyl serine may be beneficial. Conversely, low cortisol levels suggest some degree of adrenal insufficiency and may lead to nonrestorative sleep and daytime fatigue. This situation may be served by a higher protein, balanced blood sugar with lower carbohydrate diet [89], with ample fiber and complex carbohydrates along with the above-mentioned supplements. In both hyper- or hypocortisolemia, herbs, glandular formulas, and hormone replacement may be helpful. If cortisol patterns are significantly disturbed, this may prompt investigation into the diurnal variation of melatonin levels, which may also be abnormal. Hypercortisolemia is associated with decreased melatonin levels, disrupting circadian rhythms (Figure 30.2) [90]. It is the tendency for patients with desynchronosis from whatever cause to choose stimulant foods high in sugar, fat [91], salt, and caffeine. In addition to poor food choices, patients may also time their meals poorly. Abnormal cortisol production may be both a cause and consequence of poor sleep as well as excess weight. In a British study, blunted cortisol profiles were associated with significantly poorer sleep quality and significantly greater waist-hip ratio, as well as a tendency to exhibit a less favorable metabolic profile [92].

Magnesium may have an important role in maintaining a healthy circadian rhythm (see related section in this chapter).

According to the National Sleep Foundation, 17% of Americans are shift workers and their sleep problems are compounded. As a group, they tend to be more sleep deprived than people working traditional hours. It is very difficult to reset internal circadian clocks. The body's urge to sleep is strongest between 12 midnight and 6 a.m. This is why 10% to 20% of shift workers report falling asleep on the job, especially on the second half of the shift. This also accounts for why it may be hard for shift workers to sleep during the day, despite being tired. Sleep deprivation increases the

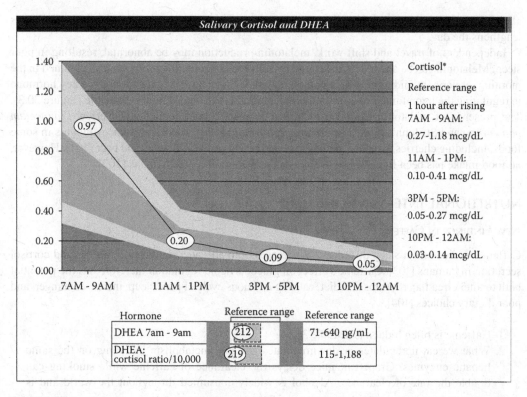

FIGURE 30.2 Salivary cortisol and DHEA sample lab report. (From Genova Diagnostics Labs. With permission.)

probability of having other health problems, particularly indigestion, colds, flu, weight gain, cardiac problems, and higher blood pressure. Female shift workers also suffer irregular menstrual cycles, difficulty getting pregnant, higher rates of miscarriages, premature births, and low birth-weight babies. The risk of workplace accidents and automobile crashes rises for shift workers, especially on the drive to and from work.

To combat jet lag, a few days before traveling, a gradual shift to the sleep and wake times of the destination will help. Upon arriving at the destination, adopting the prevailing sleep/wake time as soon as possible also is beneficial. In the morning, natural light in the eyes sends messages to the pineal gland, the area of the brain that makes melatonin. Melatonin is a chronobiotic hormone that is synthesized from tryptophan. It affects the circadian rhythm, duping the brain into thinking it is dark and therefore time to go to sleep. This resets the internal clock and has sleep-promoting effects, both shortening sleep latency and lengthening sleep duration. Levels of melatonin are highest prior to bedtime. When traveling west to east, melatonin supplements, which are sold over the counter, may diminish sleep latency and reduce the number of days necessary to establish a normal sleep pattern, improve alertness, and reduce daytime sleepiness [93–95]. Melatonin supplementation should be started on the day of travel (close to the target bedtime at the destination) and continued for several days [96]. Doses range from 0.5 to 5 mg; above 5 mg there seems to be no added benefit. In one study, the smaller and larger doses had similar efficacy, although the larger dose did afford an earlier sleep onset [97]. In a study of 100 children with sleep problems, over 80% benefited from supplementation with melatonin, which proved to be effective, inexpensive, and safe [98]. Ramelteon is a prescription agonist that works only on melatonin MT(1) and MT(2) receptors and decreases sleep latency and increases total sleep time and sleep efficiency, without causing hangover, addiction, or withdrawal, at least for short-term application [99]. Conversely, if traveling east to west, taking Benadryl (diphenhydramine), which tends to prolong the night and allows longer sleep, is a better choice. In general, it is easier to travel east to west because this lengthens the day.

Independent of travel and shift work, melatonin production may be abnormal, resulting in poor sleep. Melatonin can be accurately measured by saliva measurement with specimens obtained in the morning, at noon, at midnight, over a complete dark-light cycle. Since melatonin is a key hormone in regulating the hyopituitary axis and supplementation is safe, evaluation is valuable (Figure 30.3). The presence of melatonin has been identified in many plants including Feverfew (*Tanacetum pathenium*) and St. John's wort (*Hypericum perforatum*) [100]. It occurs in trace amounts in some foods, including cherries, bananas, grapes, rice and cereals, olive oil, wine, and beer [101]. However, no food intake has been found to elevate plasma melatonin levels in humans [102].

NUTRITIONAL INTERVENTIONS

NEW FINDINGS IN CAFFEINE

Caffeine worsens most sleep disorders. It increases both adrenocorticotropin (ACTH) and cortisol secretion in humans [103]. Caffeine's effect on glucocorticoid regulation therefore has the potential both to alter circadian rhythms and diet, causing a vicious cycle of poor sleep, increased hunger, and poor dietary choices [104].

1. Caffeine is often hidden (see Table 30.2).
2. What we eat upregulates or downregulates caffeine metabolism by acting on the same hepatic enzymes. Grapefruit juice delays the clearance of caffeine while smoking can double the rate of clearance. Alcohol is widely consumed throughout the world and is

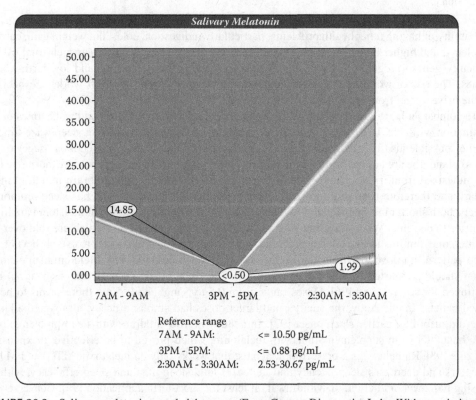

FIGURE 30.3   Salivary melatonin sample lab report. (From Genova Diagnostics Labs. With permission.)

TABLE 30.2
Caffeine Content of Food and Drugs

Coffees	Serving Size (oz)	Caffeine (mg)
Coffee, generic brewed	8	133 (range: 102–200)
	16	266
Starbucks brewed coffee (grande)	16	320
Einstein Bros. regular coffee	16	300
Dunkin' Donuts regular coffee	16	206
Starbucks Vanilla Latte (grande)	16	150
Coffee, generic instant	8	93 (range: 27–173)
Coffee, generic decaffeinated	8	5 (range: 3–12)
Starbucks Espresso, doppio	6.5	150
Starbucks Frappuccino blended coffee beverages, average	9.5	115
Starbucks Espresso, solo	1	75
Einstein Bros. Espresso	1	75
Espresso, generic	1	40 (range: 30–90)
Starbucks Espresso, decaffeinated	1	4

Teas	Serving Size (oz)	Caffeine (mg)
Tea, brewed	8	53 (range: 40–120)
Starbucks Tazo Chai Tea Latte (grande)	16	100
Snapple Lemon (and diet version)	16	42
Snapple Peach (and diet version)	16	42
Snapple Raspberry (and diet version)	16	42
Arizona Iced Tea black	16	32
Nestea	12	26
Snapple, Just Plain, unsweetened	16	18
Arizona Iced Tea, green	16	15
Snapple, Kiwi Teawi	16	10

Soft Drinks	Serving Size (oz)	Caffeine (mg)
FDA official limit for cola and pepper soft drinks	12	71
Vault	12	71 (20 = 118)
Jolt Cola	12	72
Mountain Dew MDX, regular or diet	12	71 (20 = 118)
Coke Black	12	69 (20 = 115)
Coke Red, regular or diet	12	54 (20 = 90)
Mountain Dew, regular or diet	12	54 (20 = 90)
Pepsi One	12	54 (20 = 90)
Mello Yello	12	53
Diet Coke	12	47 (20 = 78)
Diet Coke Lime	12	47 (20 = 78)
Tab	12	46.5
Pibb Xtra, Diet Mr. Pibb, Pibb Zero	12	41 (20 = 68)
Dr. Pepper	12	42 (20 = 68)
Dr. Pepper, diet	12	44 (20 = 68)
Pepsi	12	38 (20 = 63)
Pepsi Lime, regular or diet	12	38 (20 = 63)
Pepsi Vanilla	12	37
Pepsi Twist	12	38 (20 = 63)
Pepsi Wild Cherry, regular or diet	12	38 (20 = 63)
Diet Pepsi	12	36 (20 = 60)

continued

TABLE 30.2 (*continued*)
Caffeine Content of Food and Drugs

Soft Drinks	Serving Size (oz)	Caffeine (mg)
Pepsi Twist, diet	12	36 (20 = 60)
Coca-Cola Classic	12	35 (20 = 58)
Coke Black Cherry Vanilla, regular ordiet	12	35 (20 = 58)
Coke C2	12	35 (20 = 58)
Coke Cherry, regular or diet	12	35 (20 = 58)
Coke Lime	12	35 (20 = 58)
Coke Vanilla	12	35 (20 = 58)
Coke Zero	12	35 (20 = 58)
Barq's Diet Root Beer	12	23 (20 = 38)
Barq's Root Beer	12	23 (20 = 38)
7Up, regular or diet	12	0
Fanta, all flavors	12	0
Fresca, all flavors	12	0
Mug Root Beer, regular or diet	12	0
Sierra Mist, regular or free	12	0
Sprite, regular or diet	12	0

Energy Drinks	Serving Size (oz)	Caffeine (mg)
Spike Shooter	8.4	300
Cocaine	8.4	280
Monster Energy	16	160
Full Throttle	16	144
Rip It, all varieties	8	100
Enviga	12	100
Tab Energy	10.5	95
SoBe No Fear	8	83
Red Bull	8.3	80
Red Bull Sugarfree	8.3	80
Rockstar Energy Drink	8	80
SoBe Adrenaline Rush	8.3	79
Amp Energy	8.4	74
Glaceau Vitamin Water, Energy Tropical Citrus	20	50
SoBe Essential Energy, Berry Pomegranate/Orange	8	48

Frozen Desserts	Serving Size (fl. oz)	Caffeine (mg)
Ben & Jerry's Coffee Heath Bar Crunch	8	84
Ben & Jerry's coffee flavored ice cream	8	68
Häagen-Dazs coffee ice cream	8	58
Häagen-Dazs coffee light ice cream	8	58
Häagen-Dazs Frozen Yogurt, Coffee	8	58
Häagen-Dazs Coffee & Almond Crunch ice cream bar	8	58
Starbucks Coffee Ice Cream	8	50–60

Chocolates/Candies/Other	Serving Size	Caffeine (mg)
Jolt caffeinated gum	1 stick	33
Hershey's Special Dark chocolate bar	1:45 oz	31
Hershey's Milk Chocolate bar	1.55 oz	9
Hershey's Kisses	41g (9 pieces)	9
Hot cocoa	8 oz	9 (range: 3–13)

a known inducer of P450 (CYP2E1). Like smoking, chronic alcohol use may lead to increased clearance of caffeine [105].

3. Many common drugs interfere with the metabolism of caffeine. This may result both in an increase in caffeine blood levels and also may enhance caffeine's diuretic effect. Unlike the other fluoroquinolones, ciprofloxacin inhibits the metabolism of caffeine, resulting in increased effects of caffeine. Cimetidine also increases caffeine levels, thereby a different H_2 antagonist (e.g., ranitidine, famotidine) should be administered to chronic caffeine users. Oral contraceptives and prednisone also increase caffeine levels due to the inhibition of caffeine metabolism [106]. Conversely, caffeine inhibits the metabolism of theophylline, which shares a similar chemical structure with caffeine, and can increase the serum concentrations of theophylline [107]. A synergistic effect of increased stimulation can occur in patients taking theophylline and caffeine-containing foods and beverages.

4. Caffeine metabolism varies widely based on genetics. That means medications that are hepatically metabolized influence people differently. Medication can make one person more sensitive to their daily cup of coffee and not affect someone else's metabolism of three cups of coffee. If a patient notices difficulty in sleep at the time they began a medication, they may benefit from reevaluating their caffeine intake, even if it has not changed; their metabolism of caffeine may have changed due to the introduction of the new medication increasing their caffeine sensitivity, thereby disturbing their sleep.

FOOD AS A SOURCE OF NEUROTRANSMITTER PRECURSORS

Going to bed hungry interrupts sleep. Hypoglycemia can cause multiple awakenings. Later in the night, hormonal counter-regulatory mechanisms are less effective [108]. This study suggests that the composition and timing of meals affect sleep quality [109].

Nutritional rehabilitation of infants with protein-energy malnutrition measurably improved sleep quality. Disturbed serotonin levels were postulated to affect the sleep-wake cycle [110]. Protein malnutrition is an extreme situation with inadequate substrate to synthesize the neurotransmitters required to mediate sleep. The principle, however, appears more broadly applicable. In a crossover design study, healthy infants given milk enhanced with tryptophan, a serotonin precursor, showed improvements in sleep parameters compared to when they were given standard milk [111]. A study of Horlicks™, a malted milk hot drink popular in the United Kingdom, was shown to promote sleep and reduce bodily movements when consumed at bedtime [112]. A diet low in carbohydrates and high in dairy intake, intended to generate ketosis in children with epilepsy, also improved sleep quality [113]. In a small study of elderly Japanese men and women given 100 g of fermented milk that contained *Lactobacillus helveticus*, there were significant improvements in both sleep efficiency and number of wakening episodes [114].

Here is another reason "breast is best." Parents of infants who were breast-fed in the evening and/or at night slept an average of 40 to 45 minutes more than parents of infants given formula. Since this held true for fathers as well as mothers parental sleep was interpreted as a marker for the infant's sleep, rather than due to a mother's need for additional rest while breastfeeding [115].

FOOD AS A SOURCE OF MICRONUTRIENTS

Information that treating iron deficiency improves sleep is likely to be one of many findings on how nutrient components of food influence brain function. Neuroimaging techniques are just now becoming available to study this. Long considered folklore, choices of food intake before bed may influence dream content, as seen in a small interesting study showing differing effects of micronutrient-rich organic food versus nutrient-poor junk foods [118].

HERBS AND NUTRIENTS FOR SLEEP

Use of natural products for sleep is very common. In a study of 997 adults of which 60% were women, 18.5% reported the use of natural products as sleep aids in the previous 12 months, with chamomile being the most popular. These products may have side effects, safety concerns, and herb-drug interactions with broader relevance to a patient's health [119].

Chamomile is used broadly in the Western world for ameliorating insomnia, anxiety, digestive problems, skin conditions, and infection, among other indications. German chamomile (*Matricaria recutita*) is more commonly used than Roman or English chamomile (*Chamaemelum nobile*). Both are utilized as teas, ointments, capsules, tinctures, and extracts. Chamomile showed a significant decrease in sleep latency at a dose of 300 mg/kg, which was reversed by the administration of a flumazenil, a benzodiazepine receptor antagonist, thereby suggesting that chamomile has a benzodiazepine-like hypnotic activity [120]. In a small randomized, double-blind, placebo-controlled pilot trial, modest benefits were seen in daytime functioning and mixed benefits on sleep diary measures were observed [121]. While considered generally safe, chamomile may make asthma worse in people allergic to ragweed, asters, daisies, and chrysanthemums. It may have estrogenic effects, so women with a history of hormone-sensitive cancers, such as breast or uterine cancers, may want to avoid it. It may be synergistic with sedating drugs such as alcohol, tricyclic antidepressants, anticonvulsants, barbiturates, benzodiazepines, and other sedative hypnotics. It may also affect hepatic metabolism of cytochrome P450, causing herb-drug interactions with fexofenadine, statins, oral contraceptives, some anti-fungal agents, and others. It may mildly lower both blood pressure and blood sugar, as well increase bleeding risk [122,123].

Lemon balm (*Melissa officinalis*) is a member of the mint family and has been used since the Middle Ages as a calming herb. It grows all over the world. It is used in capsules, teas, tinctures, and topically. For the purposes of insomnia and anxiety, it is most often used in combination with valerian, hops, and chamomile. However, a recent small pilot study showed full remission of insomnia in 85% of subjects with mild-to-moderate sleep disturbance and anxiety disorders with administration of a standardized *Melissa officinalis* leaf extract (Cyracos) for 15 days. The mechanism of action is thought to be inhibition of GABA catabolism [124]. Lemon balm may interact with medications for the thyroid and HIV as well exacerbate the effects of sedatives [125].

Kava (*Piper methysticum*) is a plant native to the South Pacific. It has been a popular over-the-counter treatment for both insomnia and anxiety as well as fibromyalgia, which is almost universally accompanied by sleep disturbance. It is claimed to induce relaxation without impairment in memory or motor function; it may even improve cognitive function and sharpen awareness. It has a rapid onset of action, adequate duration of action, and minimal morning-after effects [126]. It seems to work through a unique mechanism by acting on the amygdala in the limbic system, which moderates many emotional processes. Unlike benzodiazepines or barbiturates, it does not bind significantly to GABA receptors. It is available as capsules or in teas. Unfortunately, due to concerns of serious hepatoxicity, it has been banned in most countries worldwide, making its use limited. Additionally, it is contraindicated in pregnancy, lactation, Parkinson's disease, and with concurrent use of antianxiety, antidepressant, antipsychotic medications or sedative/hypnotics [127,128].

Valerian root (*Valeriana officinalis*) has a long history as a sedative and anxiolytic, dating back to the time of Hippocrates (ca. 460–377 BCE) and has been reported to help with sleep quality as well as improve restless leg syndrome. It comes in various forms including teas, tinctures, capsules, and tablets. It has a distinctive, noxious odor, likened to the smell of dirty socks. Like many of the herbs mentioned here, valerian is often combined with other sedating herbs such as hops, passionflower, lemon balm, chamomile, and lavender. In a study of 918 children less than 12 years old, in combination with lemon balm, there was success in the treatment of restlessness and dyssomnia [129]. In a RCDB study with hops, patients suffering from nonorganic sleep disorder had significantly shorter sleep latency, but valerian without hops was not superior to placebo [130]. In two meta-analyses, results regarding efficacy were conflicting [131,132]. Valerian is considered generally safe and appears to cause little or no residual morning sleepiness, unlike benzodiazepines, but is believed to have a benzodiazepine-like mechanism of action. Adverse effects may rarely include headache and stomach upset. Like many herbal supplements, more rigorous study is needed.

Hops (*Humulus lupulus*) has been used for centuries in brewing (it is what makes beer taste bitter) and as a tonic for insomnia and nervous tension. It is often combined with valerian [133] and passionflower. Its constituents may have a central nervous system depressant activity and have exhibited an estrogenic effect (see earlier section on menopause), although its mechanism of actions are not fully understood. It may exacerbate the sedating effect of sedating medications and, due to the presence of phytoestrogens in hops, may exert either estrogen receptor agonist or antagonist properties.

Magnesium, a mineral found in multiple common food sources, has many effects on sleep by a variety of disparate mechanisms. It has been shown to be important in regulation of the circadian rhythm by maintaining optimal efficacy of the suprachiasmatic nuclei (the location of the body's "biological clock") and the pineal gland that produces melatonin. With magnesium depletion, there is decreased production of melatonin, thereby resulting in delayed phase disorder, but it also may contribute to the development of fibromyalgia, migraine headaches, chronic fatigue syndrome, and other symptoms [134]. In a small Italian study of 43 patients with primary insomnia in a long-term care facility, those given a combination of 225 mg of magnesium, 5 mg of melatonin, and 11.25 mg zinc, showed improvement in both the quality of their sleep and quality of life, as quantified by the Pittsburgh Sleep Quality Index, Epworth sleepiness scale, the Leeds Sleep evaluation questionnaire, the Short Insomnia questionnaire, and a validated quality of life instrument [135]. Oral magnesium supplementation may also reverse the age-related neuroendocrine and sleep EEG changes in humans [136]. Magnesium levels were lower in both acute and chronic sleep deprived men, leading to decreased heart rate variability and exercise tolerance due to a hypersensitivity to sympathetic nervous stimulation, suggesting that magnesium depletion occurs as a consequence of sleep deprivation [137]. Magnesium supplementation with 320 mg of magnesium citrate was found to improve the inflammatory marker, C-reactive protein, in 100 patients with poor quality sleep as determined by the Pittsburgh Sleep Quality Index [138]. As mentioned earlier in the section on restless legs syndrome, magnesium sulfate repletion may relieve restless legs syndrome in some pregnant women [139] and some patients with mild-to-moderate RLS- or PLMS-related insomnia [140]. Since magnesium deficiency promotes muscle weakness, it has been postulated that magnesium deficiency is at least one major unifying factor that explains increased Sudden Infant Death Syndrome (SIDS) in prone sleeping infants [141].

L-tryptophan and 5-HTP are marketed as sleep aids because they are considered "melatonin prescursors." L-tryptophan is converted to 5-HTP, which is converted to serotonin and then melatonin. While this is a biologically plausible scenario, data is limited as to the effectiveness of these substances for insomnia, and they are linked to the rare, but dangerous, development of eosinophilimyalgia syndrome [142].

Relaxation drinks are being marketed, especially to adolescents, to help reduce stress; they often contain melatonin, valerian, kava, and tryptophan, among other ingredients. Studies of efficacy and safety are limited [143].

ALCOHOL

Alcohol and sleep disturbance are closely linked. Alcohol use can create sleep disturbance; sleep disturbance can promote the use of alcohol. Self-reported use of alcohol to facilitate sleep in a survey of 1699 patients was strongly associated with hazardous drinking with an odds ratio of 4:5 [144]. Alcohol is a commonly used soporific because of its effect as a central nervous system depressant. After an initial disinhibition, one becomes sleepy. But for each drink, this early sedation is then followed by an equal amount of arousal. The sedation lasts roughly one hour and the hyperadrenergic stimulation lasts for roughly one hour. Therefore, it takes the liver about two hours to clear each drink. Excess alcohol intake leads to a restless sleep, night sweats, and headaches [145,146]. In terms of sleep architecture, low doses of alcohol (one alcoholic beverage) reduce sleep latency, increase total sleep time, and reduce awakenings during the night. Stage 1 sleep and REM sleep are suppressed with alcohol use during the first half of the night. However, moderate and higher doses (two or three alcoholic beverages) disrupt sleep by causing a rebound of stage 1 and REM sleep during the second half of the night, causing restlessness, vivid dreams and nightmares [147]. Essentially, the body is experiencing a miniature alcohol withdrawal. There is a predominance of sympathetic activation interfering with the restorative functions of sleep [148]. This sets the stage for a vicious cycle of excess caffeine use in the morning to help with daytime alertness, but then the excess use of alcohol at night to help promote sleep onset.

Sleep and hormonal disruptions following withdrawal from chronic alcohol use are the greatest predictors of relapse [149–151]. Recovering alcoholics who are abstaining from alcohol use have delayed sleep latency due to attenuation of melatonin secretion and circadian clock timing [152]. In addition, elevation of cortisol levels and core body temperature during sleep contribute to poor sleep maintenance [153,154]. Substance abusers are more than five to 10 times likely to have sleep disorders [155]. Depressed mood and substance abuse are greatly linked: in a Polish study of 304 patients in an addiction treatment program, insomnia severity was associated with suicidal ideation [156].

Persistent trouble sleeping from childhood to adolescence predicts the future use of alcohol [157]. Pubertal development in 431 subjects (mean age: 13.66 years) is associated with sleep problems and preference for later bedtimes, which in turn are related to alcohol use [158]. But for many adolescents, alcohol is just the tip of the iceberg: those adolescents with sleep problems were more likely to use alcohol, tobacco, methamphetamine, cannabis, inhalants, cocaine, ecstasy, and any other illegal drug in a study of 427 adolescents in Cape Town, South Africa. Unfortunately, all these substances exacerbate sleep issues, setting up a downward spiral of unhealthy behaviors [159].

Restricting quantity of alcohol, drinking it earlier in the evening, and slowing its absorption by eating food will help reduce the deleterious effects on sleep. Adequate hydration can also help. Alcohol, like any sedating drug, can worsen snoring and OSA [160,161].

CONCLUSION

Sleep disturbance is exceedingly common and is associated with many medical problems such as obesity, diabetes, cognitive challenges, pain, hypertension, and mood disorders. Primary care physicians should be able to diagnose common sleep disorders, understand their clinical consequences, and prescribe appropriate interventions that include diet and nutrient recommendations.

REFERENCES

1. National Sleep Foundation. Survey: *Sleep in America*. Washington, DC: National Sleep Foundation, 2000.
2. Ancoli-Israel S. *All I Want Is a Good Night's Sleep*. St. Louis: Mosby-Year Book, 1996.
3. Vorona RD, Winn MP, Babineau TW et al. *Overweight and obese patients in a primary care population report less sleep than patients with a normal body mass Index*. Arch Intern Med. 2005; 165:25–30.
4. Stamatakis KA, Brownson RC. *Sleep duration and obesity-related risk factors in the rural midwest*. Prev Med. 2007 Nov 22 [Epub ahead of print].
5. Taheri S, Lin L, Austin D et al. *Short sleep duration is associated with reduced leptin, elevated ghrelin, and increased body mass index*. PLoS Med. 2004 Dec; 1(3):e62.
6. Spiegel K, Tasali E, Penev P, et al. *Brief communication: Sleep curtailment in healthy young men is associated with decreased leptin levels, elevated ghrelin levels, and increased hunger and appetite*. Ann Intern Med. 2004; 141:846.
7. Al Mamun A, Lawlor DA, Cramb S et al. *Do childhood sleeping problems predict obesity in young adulthood? Evidence from a prospective birth cohort study*. Am. J. Epidemiol. 2007; 166:1368–73.
8. Hasler G, Buysse DJ, Klaghofer R et al. *The association between short sleep duration and obesity In young adults: A 13-year prospective study*. Sleep. 2004 Jun 15; 27(4):661–66.

9. Knutson KL, Ryden AM, Mander VA, Van Cauter E. *Role of sleep duration and quality in the risk and severity of type 2 diabetes mellitus.* Arch Intern Med. 2006; 166:1768–64.

10. Yaggi HK, Araujo AB, McKinlay JB. *Sleep duration as a risk factor for the development of type 2 diabetes.* Diabetes Care. 2006 Mar; 29(3):657–61.

11. Chaput JP, Després JP, Bouchard C, Tremblay A. *Association of sleep duration with type 2 diabetes and impaired glucose tolerance.* Diabetologia. 2007 Nov; 50(11):2298–2304.

12. Brown RP, Gerbarg PL, and Muskin PR. *Complementary and alternative treatments in psychiatry.* In Tosman A, Kay J, Lieberman J (Eds.), *Psychiatry,* 2nd ed. (Chapter 104). New York: Wiley, 2003.

13. Jerath R, Edry JW, Barnes VA, Jerath V. *Physiology of long pranayamic breathing.* Medical Hypotheses. 2006; 67:566–71.

14. Naga Venkatesha Murthy PJ, Janakiramaiah N, Gangadhar BN, Subbakrishna DK. *P300 amplitude and antidepressant response to Sudarshan Kriya Yoga (SKY).* J Affect Disord. 1998 Jul; 50(1):45–48.

15. Schwartz DJ, Kohler WC, Karatinos G. *Symptoms of depression in individuals with obstructive sleep apnea may be amenable to treatment with continuous positive airway pressure.* Chest. 2005; 128:1304–6.

16. Conklin SM, Manuck SB et al. *High omega-6 and low omega-3 fatty acids are associated with depressive symptoms and neuroticism.* Psychosom Med. 2007 Dec; 69(9):932–34.

17. Roth T, Krystal AD, Lieberman JA, III. *Long-term issues in the treatment of sleep disorders.* CNS Spectr. 2007 Jul; 12(7 Suppl 10):1–13.

18. Dickman R, Green C et al. *Relationships between sleep quality and pH monitoring findings in persons with gastroesophageal reflux disease.* J Clin Sleep Med. 2007 Aug 15; 3(5):505–13.

19. Chen CL, Robert JJ et al. *Sleep symptoms and gastroesophageal reflux.* J Clin Gastroenterol. 2008 Jan; 42(1):13–17.

20. Fujiwara Y, Machida A, Watanabe Y et al. *Association between dinner-to-bed time and gastro-esophageal reflux disease.* Am J Gastroenterol. 2005 Dec; 100(12):2633–36.

21. Jamison JR, Davie NJ. *Chiropractic management of cow's milk protein intolerance in infants with sleep dysfunction syndrome: A therapeutic trial.* J Manipulative Physiol Ther. 2006 Jul–Aug; 29(6):469–74.

22. Minarik PA. *Sleep disturbance in midlife women.* J Obstet Gynecol Neonatal Nurs. 2009 May-Jun; 38(3):333–43.

23. Campbell G, Bromberger JT, Buysee DJ, et al. *Evaluation of the association of menopausal status with delta and beta EEG activity during sleep.* Sleep. Nov 1;34(11):1561–68.

24. Polo-Kantola P. *Sleep problems in midlife and beyond.* Maturitas. 2011 Mar; 68(3):224–32.

25. Xu M, Belanger L, Ivers H, et al. *Comparison of subjective and objective sleep quality in menopausal and non-menopausal women with insomnia.* Sleep Med. 2011 Jan; 12(1):65–69.

26. Eichling PS, Sahni, J. *Menopause related sleep disorders.* Journal of Clinical Sleep Medicine. 2005; 1(3):291–300.

27. Ohayon MM. *Severe hot flashes are associated with chronic insomnia.* Arch Intern Med. 2006 Jun 26; 166(12):1262–68.

28. Woods NF, Mitchell ES. *Sleep symptoms during the menopausal transition and early postmenopause: Observations from the Seattle Midlife Women's Health Study.* Sleep 2010 Apr; 33(4):539–49.

29. Freedman RR, Roehrs TA. *Effects of REM sleep and ambient temperature on hot flash-induced sleep disturbance.* Menopause. 2006 Jul-Aug; 13(4):576–83.

30. Joffe H, Petrillo LF, Kouskopoulos A, et al. *Increased estradiol and improved sleep, but not hot flashes, predict enhanced mood during the menopausal transition.* J Clin Endocrinol Metab. 2011 Jul; 96(7):R1044–54.

31. Bolge SC, Balkrishnan R, Kannan H, et al. *Burden associated with chronic sleep maintenance insomnia characterized by nighttime awakenings among women with menopausal symptoms.* Menopause. 2010 Jan-Feb; 17(1):80–86.

32. Newton KM, Buist DS, Keenan NL, et al. *Use of alternative therapies for menopause symptoms: Results of a population-based survey.* Obstet Gynecol. 2002 Jul; 100(1):18–25.

33. Polo-Kantola P. *Sleep problems in midlife and beyond.* Maturitas. 2011 Mar; 68(3):224–32.

34. Joffe H, Massler A, Sharkey KM. *Evaluation and management of sleep disturbance during the menopause transition.* Semin Reprod Med 2010 Sep; 28(5):404–21.

35. Dancey DR, Hanly PJ, Soong C, et al. *Impact of menopause on the prevalence and severity of sleep apnea.* Chest. 2001 Jul; 120(1):151–55.

36. Pavlova M, Shiekh LS. *Sleep in women.* Semin Neurol. 2011 Sep; 31(4):397–403.

37. Sherwood A, Thurston R, Steffen P, et al. *Blunted nighttime blood pressure dipping in postmenopausal women.* Am J Hypertens. 2001 Aug; 14(6 Pt 1):749–54.

38. Freedman RR, Kruger ML, Wasson SL. *Heart rate variability in menopausal hot flashes during sleep.* Menopause. 2011 Aug; 18(8):897–900.

39. McKee J, Warber SL. *Integrative therapies for menopause.* South Med J. 2005 Mar; 98(3):319–26.

40. Hachul H, Brandao LC, D'Almeida V, et al. *Isoflavones decrease insomnia in postmenopause.* Menopause. 2011 Feb; 18(2):178–84.

41. Bolanos R, Del Castillo A, Francia J. *Soy isoflavones versus placebo in the treatment of climacteric vaso-motor symptoms: Systematic review and meta-analysis.* Menopause. 210 May–Jun;. 17(3);660–66.

42. Jacobson JS, Troxel AB, Evans J et al. *Randomized trial of black cohosh for the treatment of hot flashes among women with a history of breast cancer.* J Clin Oncol. 2001; 19:2739–45.

43. Tice JA, Ettinger B, Ensrud K, et al. *Phytoestrogen supplements for the treatment of hot flashes: The Isoflavone Clove Extract Study: A randomized controlled trial.* JAMA. 2003; 290:207–14.

44. Kronenberg F, Fugh-Berman A. *Complementary and alternative medicine for menopausal symptoms: A review of randomized, controlled trials.* Ann Intern Med. 2002 Nov 19; 137(10):805–13.

45. Borrelli F, Ernst E. *Alternative and complementary therapies for the menopause.* Maturitas. 2010 Aug; 66(4):333–43.

46. Palacio C, Masri G, Mooradian AD. *Black cohosh for the management of menopausal symptoms:Aa systematic review of clinical trials.* Drugs Aging. 2009; 26(1):23–36.

47. Ross SM. *Menopause: A standardized isopropanolic black cohosh extract (remifemin) is found to be safe and effective for menopausal symptoms.* Holist Nurs Pract. 201 Jan; 26(1):58–61.

48. Rostock M, Fischer J, Mumm A. *Black cohosh (Cimicifuga racemosa) in tamoxifen-treated breast can-cer patients with climacteric complaints—a prospective observational study.* Gynecol Endocinol. 2011 Oct; 27(10):844–48.

49. Tranah GJ, Parimi N, Blackwell T, et al. *Postmenopausal hormones and sleep quality in the elderly: A population based study.* BMC Womens Health. 2010 May 4; 10–15.

50. Cramer EH, Jones P, Keenan NL, et al. *Is naturopathy as effective as conventional therapy for treatment of menopausal symptoms?* J Altern Complement Med. 2003 Aug; 9(4):529–38.

51. *Radix Angelicae Sinensis. WHO monographs on selected medicinal plants.* Geneva, Switzerland : WHO, 2001.

52. Kupfersztain C, Rotem C, Fagot R, et al. *The immediate effect of natural plant extract, Angelica sinensis and Matricaria chamomill (Climex) for the treatment of hot flushes during menopause. A preliminary report.* Clin Exp Obstet Gynecol. 2003; 30(4):203–6.

53. Rotem C, Kaplan B. *Phyto-Female Complex for the relief of hot flushes, night sweats and qual-ity of sleep: Randomized, controlled, double-blind pilot study.* Gynecol Endocinol. 2007 Feb; 23(2):117–22.

54. Winther K, Rein E, Hedman C. *Femal, a herbal remedy made from pollen extracts, reduces hot flushes and improves quality of life in menopausal women: A randomized, placebo-controlled parallel study.* Climacteric. 2005 Jun; 8(2):162–70.

55. Nagano M, Shimizu K, Kondo R, et al. *Reduction of depression and anxiety by 4 weeks Hericium eri-naceus intake.* Biomed Res. 2010 Aug; 31(4):231–37.

56. Agosta C, Altante M, Benvenuti C. *Randomized controlled study on clinical efficacy of isoflavones plus Lactobacillus sporogenes, associated or not with a natural anxiolytic agent in menopause.* Minerva Ginecol. 2011 Feb; 63(1):11–17.

57. Mucci M, Carraro C, Mancino P, et al. *Soy isoflavones, Lactobacilli, Magnolia bark extract, Vitamin D3 and calcium. Controlled clinical study in menopause.* Minerva Ginecol. 2006 Aug; 58(4):323–34.

58. Taavoni S, Ekbatani N, Kashaniyan M, et al. *Effect of valerian on sleep quality in postmenopausal women: A randomized placebo-controlled clinical trial.* Menopause. 2011 Sep; 18(9):951–55.

59. Blaicher W, Speck E, Imhof MH, et al. *Melatonin in postmenopausal females.* Arch Gynecol Obstet. 200 Feb; 263(3):116–18.

60. Blumenthal M. *Herbal Medicine: Expanded Commision E Monographs.* Newton, MA: Integrative Medicine Communications, 2003.

61. Brown D. *The use of Vitex agnus castus for hyperprolactinemia.* Quarterly Review of Natural Medicine. 1997; Spring:19–21.

62. Lucks BC, Sorensen J, Veal L. *Vitex agnus-castur essential oil and menopausal balance: A self-care survey.* Complement Ther Nurs Midwifery. 2002; 8:148–54.

63. Grube B, Walper A, Wheately D. *St John's wort extract: Efficacy for menopausal symptoms of psycho-logical origin.* Adv Ther. 1999; 16:177–86.

64. Liske E. *Therapeutic efficacy and safety of* Cimicifuga racemosa *for gynecologic disorders.* Adv Ther. 1998;15:45–53.

65. Zhou S, Chan E, Pan SQ, et al. *Pharmacokinetic interactions of drugs with St John's wort.* J Psychopharmacol. 2004; 18:262–76.

66. Warnecke G. *Psychosomatic dysfunctions in the female climacteric. Clinical effectiveness and tolerance of Kava extract WS 1490.* Fortschr Med. 1991; 109:119–22.

67. Komesaroff PA, Black CV, Cable V, et al. *Effects of wild yam extract on menopausal symptoms, lipids, and sex hormones in healthy menopausal women.* Climacteric. 2001; 4:144–50.

68. Heyerick A, Vervarke S, Depypere H, et al. *A first prospective, randomized, double-blind, placebo-controlled study on the use of a standardized hop extract to alleviate menopausal discomforts.* Maturitas. 2006; 54:164–75.

69. Meisner H, et al. *Hormone-balancing effect of pre-gelatinized organic Maca* (Lepidium peruvianum *Chacon): (III) Clinical responses of early-postmenopausal women to Maca in double blind, randomized, placebo-controlled, crossover configuration, outpatient study.* Int J Biomed Sci. 2006; 2(4):375–94.

70. Chenoy R, Hussain S, Tayob Y, et al. *Effect of oral gamolenic acid from evening primrose oil on menopausal flushing.* BMJ. 1994; 308:501–3.

71. Shou C, Li J, Liu Z. *Complementary and alternative medicine in the treatment of menopausal symptoms.* Chin J Integr Med. 2011 Dec; 17(12):883–88.

72. Punjabi NM, Polotsky VY. *Disorders of glucose metabolism in sleep apnea.* J Appl Physiol. 2005; 99(5):1998–2007.

73. Kasasbeh E, Chi DS, Krishnaswamy G. *Inflammatory aspects of sleep apnea and their cardiovascular consequences.* South Med J. 2006; 99:58–67.

74. Trenell, MI et al. *Influence of constant positive airway pressure therapy on lipid storage, muscle metabolism and insulin action in obese patients with severe obstructive sleep apnoea syndrome.* Diabes Obes Metab. 2007; (5):679–87.

75. Ryan M, Slevin JT. *Restless leg syndrome.* Am J Health Syst Pharm. 2006 Sept; 1p63(17): 1599–1612.

76. Tijdschr Tandheelkd N. *Restless legs due to ingestion of "light" beverages containing saccharine. Results of an N-of-1 trial.* 2007 Jun; 114(6):263–66.

77. Earley CJ, Connor JR, et al. *Abnormalities in CSF concentrations of ferritin and transferrin in restless legs syndrome.* Neurology. 2000; 54:1698–1700.

78. Dosman CF, Brian JA, Drmic IE, Senthilselvan A, Harford MM, Smith RW, Sharieff W, Zlotkin SH, Moldofsky H, Roberts SW. *Children with autism: Effect of iron supplementation on sleep and ferritin.* Pediatr Neurol. 2007 Mar; 36(3):152–58.

79. Patrick LR. *Restless legs syndrome: Pathophysiology and the role of iron and folate.* Altern Med Rev. 2007 Jun; 12(2):101–12.

80. Bartell S, Zallek S. *Intravenous magnesium sulfate may relieve restless legs syndrome in pregnancy.* J Clin Sleep Med. 2006; 2:187–88.

81. Harrison NL. *Mechanisms of sleep induction by GABA(A) receptor agonists.* J Clin Psychiatry. 2007; 68 Suppl 5:6–12.

82. Abdou AM, Higashiguchi S, Horie K, Kim M, Hatta H, Yokogoshi H. *Relaxation and immunity enhancement effects of gamma-aminobutyric acid (GABA) administration in humans.* Biofactors. 2006; 26(3):201–8.

83. Winkelman JW, Allen RP, Tenzer P, Hening W. *Restless legs syndrome: Nonpharmacologic and pharmacologic treatments.* Geriatrics. 2007 Oct; 62(10):13–16.

84. Simakajornboon N, Gozal D et al. *Periodic limb movements in sleep and iron status in children.* Sleep. 2003 Sep; 26(6):735–38.

85. Hornyak M, Vodrholzer U, Hohagen F, et al. *Magnesium therapy for periodic leg movements-related insomnia and restless legs syndrome: An open pilot study.* Sleep. 1998 Aug 1; 21(5):501–5.

86. Dahle Lo, Berg G, Hammar M, et al. *The effect of oral magnesium substitution on pregnancy-induced leg cramps.* Am J Obstet Gynecol. 1995; 173–75.

87. Chan P, Huang TY, Chen YJ, et al. *Randomized, double-blind, placebo-controlled study of the safety and efficacy of vitamin B complex in the treatment of nocturnal leg cramps in elderly patients with hypertension.* J Clin Pharmacol. 1998; 38:1151.

88. Gozansky WS, Lynn JS, Laudenslager ML, Kohrt WM. *Salivary cortisol determined by enzyme immunoassay is preferable to serum total cortisol for assessment of dynamic hypothalamic—pituitary—adrenal axis activity.* Clin Endocrinol (Oxf). 2005 Sep; 63(3):336–41.

89. Anderson KE, Rosner W, Khan MS et al. *Diet-hormone interactions: Protein-carbohydrate ratio alters reciprocally the plasma levels of testosterone and cortisol and their respective binding globulins in man.* Life Sci. 1987; 40:1761–68.

90. Soszyinski P, Stowinsk-Stednicka J, Kasperlik-Zatuska A et al. *Decreased melatonin in Cushing Syndrome*. Horm Metab Res. 1989; 21:673–74.

91. Torres SJ, Nowson CA. *Relationship between stress, eating behavior, and obesity*. Nutrition. 2007 Nov–Dec; 23(11–12):887–94.

92. Lasikiewicz N, Hendrickx et al. *Exploration of basal diurnal salivary cortisol profiles in middle-aged adults: Associations with sleep quality and metabolic parameters*. Psychoneuroendocrinology. 2008 Feb; 33(2):143–51.

93. Mishima K, Satoh K, Shimizu T et al. *Hypnotic and hypothermic action of daytime-administered melatonin*. Psychopharmacology (Berl). 1997; 133:168–71.

94. Haimov I, Lavie P, Laudon M et al. *Melatonin replacement therapy of elderly insomniacs*. Sleep. 1995; 18:598–603.

95. Hughes RJ, Sack RL, Lewy AJ. *The role of melatonin and circadian phase in age-related sleep maintenance insomnia: Assessment in a clinical trial of melatonin replacement*. Sleep. 1998; 21:52–68.

96. Almeida Montes LG, Ontiveros Uribe MP, Cortes Sotres J et al. *Treatment of primary insomnia with melatonin: A double-blind, placebo-controlled, crossover study*. J Psychiatry Neurosci. 2003; 28(3):191–96.

97. Herxheimer A, Petrie KJ. *Melatonin for the prevention and treatment of jet lag*. Cochrane Database Syst Rev. 2002; (2):CD001520.

98. Jan EJ, O'Donnell ME. *Use of melatonin in the treatment of paediatric sleep disorders*. J Pineal Res. 1996; (21):193–99.

99. Pandi-Perumal SR, Srinivasan V et al. *Insight: The use of melatonergic agonists for the treatment of insomnia-focus on ramelteon*. Nat Clin Pract Neurol. 2007 Apr; 3(4):221–28.

100. Paredes SD, Korkmaz A, Manchester LC, et al. *Phytomelatonin: A review*. Journal of Experimental Botany. 2008; 60(1):57–69.

101. Burkahardt, S, Tan, DX, Manchester LC, et al. *Detection and quantification of the antioxidant melatonin in Montmorency and Balaton art cherries (Prunus cerasus)*. Journal of Agricultural and Food Chemistry. 2001; 49(10):4898–902.

102. Coates, PM. *Encyclopedia of Dietary Supplements*. CRC Press, 2005. 457–66 .

103. Lovallo WR, al'Absi M et al. *Stress-like adrenocorticotropin responses to caffeine in young healthy men*. Pharmacol Biochem Behav. 1996; 55:365–69.

104. Lovallo, WR, Whitsett, TL et al. *Caffeine stimulation of cortisol secretion across the waking hours in relation to caffeine intake levels*. Psychosomatic Medicine. 2005; 67:734–39.

105. Djordjevi´c D, Nikoli´c J, Stefanovi´c V . *Ethanol interactions with other cytochrome P450 substrates including drugs, xenobiotics, and carcinogens*. Pathol Biol (Paris). 1998 Dec; 46(10):760–70.

106. Lacy CF, Armstrong LL, Goldman MP, Lance LL. *Lexi-Drugs Comprehensive and Specialty Fields*. Hudson, OH: Lexi-Comp, Inc; 2006.

107. Leibovich ER, Deamer RL, Sanserson LA. *Food-drug interactions: Careful drug selection and patient counseling can reduce the risk in older patients*. Geriatrics. 2004; 59:19–33.

108. Jauch-Chara K, Hallschmid M et al. *Awakening and counter regulatory response to hypoglycemia during early and late sleep*. Diabetes. 2007 Jul; 56(7):1938–42.

109. Sato-Mito N, Sasaki S, Murakami K, et al. *The midpoint of sleep is associated with dietary intake and dietary behavior among young Japanese women*. Sleep Med. 2011 Mar; 12(3):289–94.

110. Shaaban SY, Ei-Saved HL, Nassar MF et al. *Sleep-wake cycle disturbances in protein-energy malnutrition: Effect of nutritional rehabilitation*. East Mediterr Health J. 2007 May–June; 13(3): 633–45.

111. Aparicio S, Garau C, Estèban S et al. *Chrononutrition: Use of dissociated day/night infant milk formulas to improve the development of the wake-sleep rhythms. Effects of tryptophan*. Nutr Neurosci. 2007 Jun–Aug; 10(3–4):137–43.

112. Southwell PR, Evans CR et al. *Effect of a hot milk drink on movements during sleep*. Br Med J. 1972 May 20; 2(5811):429–31.

113. Hallböök T, Lundgren J, Rosén I. *Ketogenic diet improves sleep quality in children with therapy-resistant epilepsy*. Epilepsia. 2007 Jan; 48(1):59–65.

114. Yamamura S, Morishima H, Kumano-Go T et al. *The effect of Lactobacillus helveticus fermented milk on sleep and health perception in elderly subjects*. Eur J Clin Nutr. 2007 Sep 12 [Epub ahead of print].

115. Doan T, Gardiner A, Gay CL, Lee KA. *Breast-feeding increases sleep duration of new parents*. J Perinat Neonatal Nurs. 2007 Jul–Sep; 21(3):200–206.

116. Center for Science in the Public Interest. *Nutrition Action Health Letter*. September 2007. Available: www.cspinet.org.

117. Juliano LM, Griffiths RR. Caffeine. In Lowinson, JH, Ruiz, P, Millman, RB, Langrod, JG. (Eds.). *Substance Abuse: A Comprehensive Textbook*, 4th ed. (pp.403–21). Baltimore: Lippincott, Williams, & Wilkins, 2005.

118. Kroth J, Briggs A, Cummings M, Rodriguez G, Martin E. *Retrospective reports of dream characteristics and preferences for organic vs. junk foods.* 2007 Aug; 101(1):335–38.

119. Sanchez-Ortuno MM, Bgelanger L, Ivers H, et al. *The use of natural products for sleep: A common practice?* Sleep Med. 2009 Oct; 10(9):982–87.

120. Shinomiya K, Inoue T, Utsu Y, et al. *Hypnotic activities of chamomile and passiflora extracts in sleep disturbed rats.* Biol Pharm Bull. 2005 May; 28(5):808–10.

121. Zick SM, Wright BD, Sen A, et al. *Preliminary examination of the efficacy and safety of a standardized chamomile extract for chronic primary insomnia: A randomized placebo-controlled pilot study.* BMC Complement Altern Med. 2011 Sep 22; 11:78.

122. McKay DL, Blumber JB. *A review of the bioactivity and potential health benefits of chamomile tea (Matricaria rectutia L).* Phytother Res. 200 Jul; 20(7):519–30.

123. Miller L. *Herbal medicinals: Selected clinical considerations focusing on know or potential drug-herb interactions.* Arch Intern Med. 1998;158(20);2200–2211.

124. Cases J, Ibarra A, FeuillAre N, et al. *Pilot trial of Melissa officinalis L. Leaf extract in the treatment of volunteers suffering from mild-to-moderate anxiety disorders and sleep disturbances.* Med J Nutrition Metab. 2011 Dec; 4(3):211–18.

125. Gruenwald J, Brendler T, Jaenicke C. *PDR for Herbal Medicines*, 4th ed. Montvalie, NJ: Thomson Healthcare, 2007. 514–15.

126. Wheatley D. *Medicinal plants for insomnia: A review of their pharmacology, efficacy and tolerability.* J Psychopharmacol. 2005 Jul; 19(4):414–21.

127. Schelosky L, Raffauf C, Jendroska K, et al. *Kava and dopamine antagonism.* J Neurol Neurosug Psychiatry. 1995; 58(5):639–40.

128. Almeida JC, Grimslely EW. *Coma from the health food store: Interaction between kava and alpazolam.* Ann Intern Med. 1996; 125(11):940–41.

129. Muller SF, Klement S. *A combination of valerian and lemon balm is effective in the treatment of restlessness and dyssomnia in children.* Phytomedicine. 2006 June; 13(6):383–87.

130. Koetter U, Schrader E, Kaufeler R, et al. *A randomized, double blind, placebo-controlled, prospective clinical study to demonstrate clinical efficacy of a fixed valerian hops entract combination (Ze 91019) in patients suffering from non-organic sleep disorder.* Phytother Res. 20007 Sep; 21(9):847–51.

131. Bent S, Padul A, Moore D, et al. *Valerian for sleep: A systematic review and meta-analysis.* Am J Med. 2006 Dec; 119(12):1005–12.

132. Fernandez-San-Martin MI, Masa-Font R, Palacios-Soler L, et al. *Effectiveness of Valerian on insomnia: A meta-analysis of randomized placebo-controlled trials.* Sleep Med. 2010 Jun; 11(6):505–11.

133. Morin CM, Koetter U, Bastien C, et al. *Valerian-hops combination and diphenhydramine for treating insomnia: A randomized placebo-controlled clinical trial, Sleep.* 2005; 28(11):1465–71.

134. Durlach J, Pages N, Bac P, et al. *Biorhythms and possible central regulation of magnesium status, phototherapy, darkness therapy and chronopathological forms of magnesium depletion.* Magnes Res. 2002 Mar; 15(1-2):49–66.

135. Rondanelli M, Opizzi A, Monteferrario F, et al. *The effect of melatonin, magnesium, and zinc on primary insomnia in long-term facility residents in Italy: A double-blind, placebo-controlled clinical trial.* J Am Geriatr Soc. 2011 Jan; 59(1):82–90.

136. Held K, Antonijevic IA, Kunzel H, et al. *Oral Mg(2+) supplementation reverses age-related neuroendocrine and sleep EEG changes in humans.* Pharmacopsychiatry. 2002 Jul; 35(4):135–43.

137. Omiya K, Akashi YJ, Yoneyama K, et al. *Heart-rate response to sympathetic nervous stimulation, exercise, and magnesium concentration in various sleep conditions.* Int J Sport Nutr Exerc Metab. 2009 Apr; 19(2):127–35.

138. Nielsen FH, Johnson LK, Zeng H. *Magnesium supplementation improves indicators of low magnesium status and inflammatory stress in adults older than 51 years with poor quality sleep.* Magnes Res. 2010 Dec; 23(4):158–68.

139. Bartell S, Zallek S. *Intravenous magnesium sulfate may relieve restless legs syndrome in pregnancy.* J Clin Sleep Med. 2006 Apr 15; 2(2):187–88.

140. Hornyak M, Vodrholzer U, Hohagen F, et al. *Magnesium therapy for periodic leg movements-related insomnia and restless legs syndrome: An open pilot study.* Sleep. 1998 Aug 1; 21(5):501–5.

141. Caddell JL. *Magnesium deficiency promotes muscle weakness, contributing to the risk of sudden infant death (SIDS) in infants sleeping prone.* Magnes Res. 2001 Mar; 14(1–2):39–50.

142. *Information paper on L-tryptophan and 5-hydroxy-L-tryptophan*. US Food and Drug Administration, Center for Food Safety and Applied Nutrition Website. Accessed at http://www.cfsan.fda.gov/-dms/ds-tryp1.html.

143. Stacy S. *Relaxation drinks and their use in adolescents*. J Child Adolesc Pscychopharmacol. 2011 Dec; 21(6):605–10.

144. Vinson D, Manning B, Galliher J, et al. *Alcohol and sleep problems in primary care patients: A report from the AAFP National Research Network*. Ann Fam Med. 2010 Nov; 8(6):484–92.

145. Yules RB, Lippman ME, Freedman DX. *Alcohol administration prior to sleep; the effect on EEG sleep stages*. Arch Gen Psychiatry. 1967; 16:94–97.

146. Madsen BW, Rossi L. *Sleep and Michaelis-Menten elimination of ethanol*. Clin Pharmacol Ther. 1980; 27:114–19.

147. Roehrs T, Roth T. *Sleep, sleepiness, and alcohol use*. Alcohol Research & Health. 2001; 25(2):101–9.

148. Sagawa Y, Kondo H, Matsubuchi N, et al. *Alcohol has a dose-related effect on parasympathetic nerve activity during sleep*. Alcohol Clin Exp Res. 2011 Nov; 35(11):2093–100.

149. Feige B, Scaal, Hornyak M, et al. *Sleep electroencephalographic spectral power after withdrawal from alcohol in alcohol-dependent patients*. Alcoholism: Clinical and Experimental Research. 2007 Jan; 31(1):19–27.

150. Brower KJ. *Insomnia, alcoholism, and relapse*. Sleep Med Rev. 2003; 7:523–39.

151. Brower KJ, Krentzman A, Robinson E. *Persistent insomnia, abstinence, and moderate drinking in alcohol-dependent individuals*. Am J Addict. 2011 Sep; 20(5):435–40.

152. Brager AJ, Ruby CL, Prosser RA, et al. *Acute ethanol disrupts photic and serotonergic circadian clock phase-resetting in the mouse*. Alcohol Clin Exp Res. 2011 Aug; 35(8):1467–74.

153. Kuhlwein E, Hauger RL, Irwin MR. *Abnormal nocturnal melatonin secretion and disordered sleep in abstinent alcoholics*. Biol Psychiatry. 2003; 54:1437–43.

154. Danel T, Libersa C, Touitou Y. *The effect of alcohol consumption on the circadian control of human core body temperature is time dependent*. Am J Physiol Regulatory Integrative Comp Physiol. 2001; 281:R52–55.

155. Youssef M, Talih F, Streem D, et al. *Sleep disorders in substance abusers: How common are they?* Psychiatry. 2009 Sep; 6(9):38–42.

156. Klimkiewicz A, Bohnert AS, Jakubczyk A, et al. *The association between insomnia and suicidal thought in adults treated for alcohol dependence in Poland*. Durg Alcohol Depend. 2011 Oct 11.

157. Wong MM, Brower KJ, Nigg JT, et al. *Childhood sleep problems, response inhibition, and alcohol and drug outcomes in adolescence and young adulthood*. Alcohol Clin Exp Res. 2010 June; 34(6):1033–44.

158. Pieters S, Van Der Vorst H, Burk WJ, et al. *Puberty-dependent sleep regulation and alcohol use in early adolescents*. Alcohol Clin Exp Res. 2010 Sep 1; 34(9):1512–18.

159. Fakier N, Wild LG. *Associations among sleep problems, learning difficulties and substance use in adolescence*. J Adolesc. 2011 Aug; 34(4):717–26.

160. Scanlan MF, Roebuck T, Little PJ et al. *Effect of moderate alcohol upon obstructive sleep apnea*. Eur Respir J. 2000; 16:909–13.

161. Riemann R, Volk R, Muller A, et al. *The influence of nocturnal alcohol ingestion on snoring*. Eur Arch Otorhinolaryngol. 201 Jul; 267(7):1147–56.

31 Alcohol and Drug Addiction

Using Nutrition as the Foundation of Recovery

Patricia Mulready, M.D.

INTRODUCTION

For centuries, humans have sought ways to make life more pleasurable. Alcohol and drugs figure prominently in this quest. Unfortunately, some people become harmfully involved. Research has been pointing to addictions as the blend of brain dysfunction combined with environmental factors and learning. The brain dysfunction of addictions is often managed by pharmaceutical medications that have their place in treatment. However, this chapter focuses on the powerful impact that nutrition may have on reregulating the brain. It is the fundamental stabilizing force in the early days of recovery and beyond. Through nutrient strategies, relapse may be prevented and medications may not be needed. With a stable brain, learning new ways to live a drug-free life is possible and pleasurable [1–3].

EPIDEMIOLOGY

Biology may play a key role in whether someone progresses from experimentation to social use into harmful use of substances. Some people have bodies that are more vulnerable to addiction due to genetics, metabolic abnormalities, co-occurring mental illness, or biochemical changes from trauma.

When people who use alcohol and drugs are born with a biochemistry that makes them vulnerable to addiction, they will not necessarily become harmfully involved with substances. Vulnerability increases significantly when alcohol and drugs are used as the primary way to change feelings and cope with life. In addition, addiction usually requires interaction with unhealthful forces in the environment to activate the weakened biology that eventually results in disease. What is required to move along the path to addiction seems to be:

- Poor nutrition to stir up biology
- Experimentation with alcohol and drugs to teach they are dependable ways to change feelings and cope with life
- Negative environment that does not promote healthy psycho-social development, especially healthy role models and relationships, achievements, positive view of the future, and inner resources
- Reliance on alcohol and drugs to change feelings to the exclusion of other healthier ways
- The drug of choice since some drugs have a higher addiction potential and cause more harm than others

- Significant use of alcohol and drugs to interact with activated biology to change brain chemistry
- Poorly developed spiritual life so there is little meaning to life, low interconnectedness, helplessness, and hopelessness [1]

One environmental factor that stands out as a contributor to addictions is the strong association between addictions and malnutrition. Drug abuse contributes to malnutrition because abusers place their time and energy into getting high and finding drugs. Food is not a major consideration in an addicted person's life. Additionally, the food choices tend to be whatever is easy and affordable. This typically translates into fast food and junk food, especially sweets. Some abusers take their meals at shelters and soup kitchens that feed many people and are unable to provide meals tailored to enhance recovery. Biochemically, drugs of abuse are able to stimulate the reward center much more strongly than food so drugs take precedence over food as a way to feel good. In a cross-sectional prospective study, comparing hospital admitted drug addicted patients with healthy subjects, 92.4% were identified as underweight compared to the general population [4].

It has been known for many years that heavy consumption of alcohol results in the loss of vitamins, minerals, and antioxidants. Alcohol contributes calories that provide energy but have no other useful ingredients since the calories are devoid of vitamins, minerals, amino acids, and fatty acids. When 30% of calories of a normal diet are replaced with alcohol, it results in diagnosable malnutrition. Despite the caloric intake, the patient may not be able to maintain weight because alcohol interferes with digestive functions that process food including peristalsis, pancreatic release of digestive enzymes, and absorption. However, alcohol may promote abdominal fat because alcohol interferes with glucose dispersal while it increases insulin release. The result is insulin resistance, which is a prelude to diabetes type 2 [5–7].

Malnutrition is compounded by loss of appetite and, therefore, less consumption of food, because alcohol satisfies the hunger-satiety center. Further, alcohol and food share common pathways to the reward center. When the reward center is excessively stimulated by alcohol, food runs a distant second in its ability to stimulate pleasure [8,9].

Studies have demonstrated that 75% of opiate (narcotic) abusers are vitamin deficient. Of these, 50% were low in vitamin B6, which is an essential cofactor in many biochemical reactions. They were also deficit in folic acid, which is involved in one of the pathways that reduces homocysteine. Another 13–19% of abusers were deficient in vitamin B2, which is involved in energy production and in vitamin B3, which is an essential cofactor in many important biochemical reactions [10].

Stimulants such as cocaine, amphetamines, and methamphetamine create malnutrition by sending inappropriate messages to the hunger-satiety center. The center receives false feedback that causes it to reduce hunger signals. Though the body needs food, the stimulant abuser feels no hunger and has no desire to eat. Muscle protein is sacrificed to sustain life [11].

Stimulants create malnutrition and a serious health situation by the action of norepinephrine and epinephrine. These chemical signals impact carbohydrate metabolism and raise the level of glucose in the blood via an increase in gluconeogenesis, glycogenolysis, and lipolysis. They increase glucagon release, which works in opposition to insulin. Additionally, these drugs interfere with pancreatic secretion of insulin. The result is high blood glucose with reduced insulin capacity to place glucose into cells. In severe enough cases, ketogenesis is activated with increased risk of ketoacidosis [3,12,13].

Tobacco smoke contains millions of free radicals in every puff. This overtaxes the body's antioxidant capability to neutralize them, setting up vulnerability to disease. Research has found that smokers are particularly deficit in the antioxidants glutathione and vitamin C. Smokers are also deficient in folic acid, which reduces their capacity to convert homocysteine into harmless products. This contributes to heart disease as does tobacco's tendency to raise cholesterol [9].

To provide a sense of the magnitude of the substance abuse problem in the United States, the Substance Abuse and Mental Health Services Administration (SAMHSA), a division of the National

Institutes of Health, collected data in 2010 on people 12 years and older. It is becoming unusual to find substance abusers who use only one drug. Many combine alcohol with cocaine, heroin with cocaine, or alcohol, marijuana, and cocaine. Drugs are combined to synergistically enhance the high such as with methadone and benzodiazepines. Or drugs will be combined to create a different high as with cocaine and heroin in speedballing. The cocaine gives a euphoric rush that lasts no more than 30 minutes while the heroin eases down into a dreamy relaxed high that lasts for several hours. Abusers will also substitute drugs when the drug of choice is not available [14,15].

ALCOHOL

Almost 50% of Americans, or 131.3 million people age 12 years and older, drank alcohol in the past month. Of these drinkers, almost 25% or 58.6 million people participated in binge drinking, which the National Institute on Alcohol Abuse and Alcoholism (NIAAA) has defined as the number of drinks needed to raise the blood alcohol content (BAC) to at least 0.08%. Typically, it takes five drinks for men and four drinks for women within a two-hour timeframe to reach this BAC. For many people who binge drink, the purpose is to get drunk. The U.S. Department of Education prefers the broader term "high risk drinking" to focus on the negative consequences of drinking rather than the amount consumed. High-risk drinking includes binge drinking, drunk driving, and underage drinking, which is another concern because almost 10 million drinkers were young people (26%) under 21 years old [15,16].

Heavy drinkers were reported at 6.7%, or 16.9 million people. The NIAAA defines heavy drinking as consistently drinking more than two drinks for men and more than one drink for women per day. Another assessment measure is 15 drinks or more in a week for men and 12 drinks or more for women. Drinking five drinks in one event one or more times in a week is considered heavy drinking [15,17,18].

People who drank alcohol were more likely than nondrinkers to use illegal drugs: 32% of drinkers vs. 4% of nondrinkers. Young people under the age of 21 were more likely to use illegal drugs within two hours of drinking. The drug of choice was marijuana. Alcohol use was also associated with cigarette and cigar smoking. Heavy drinkers smoked the most tobacco (55%) vs. nondrinkers (2%) [15,16].

DRUGS

There were three million persons aged 12 or older introduced to illicit drugs in 2010, which is 9% of the American population. This means that 8100 people per day began using drugs with more than 50% under the age of 18. Marijuana was the most commonly used drug with 17.4 million users (77%). Nonmedical use of prescription medications was the next category of use with seven million people (3%) abusing prescription medications. The most abused medications were narcotics, followed by sedatives and stimulants used to treat attention deficit hyperactivity disorder. Inhalants, such as items in spray cans, paint thinner, gasoline, and magic markers, were abused more often by young people who do not have easy access to other drugs—0.7% (1.4 million). Other drugs of abuse include: hallucinogens: 0.5% = 1.2 million, cocaine: 0.6% = 1.5 million, ecstasy: 0.3% = 695,000, and methamphetamine: 0.1% = 353,000. Almost 70 million (25%) used tobacco products, which are the most commonly abused drugs worldwide [15,16].

To bring it closer to home, at least 8–12% of physicians were estimated to be harmfully using drugs, especially opiates and benzodiazepines. Emergency medicine physicians and anesthesiologists are most vulnerable [15,19].

In one study of nurses, 32% were involved in inappropriate use of drugs. The drugs of choice included marijuana, alcohol, cocaine, prescription medications (opiates, benzodiazepines), and nicotine. Emergency department nurses were 3.5 times more likely to use drugs than other specialties. Nurses in oncology and administration tended to binge drink 50% more than other nurses [15,20].

TREATMENT

In 2010, an estimated 22.1 million persons (9%) were classified with substance abuse or dependence in the past year. Of these, 4.1 million received treatment (1.6% of the population). Alcohol was by far the most commonly treated substance. It was followed in decreasing order by marijuana, narcotic pain relievers, cocaine, heroin, tranquilizers, stimulants, and hallucinogens.

Self-help groups provided assistance to 2.3 million people. Private physicians treated 653,000 people. Women more commonly seek treatment from a primary care physician, psychiatrist, or therapist. They are less likely to become involved in facilities that specialize in addiction treatment [15,16].

SUMMARY OF DRUG INFORMATION

Table 31.1 provides a brief overview of drugs based on their primary action on the brain. It is not possible to provide details and nuances in this chapter.

ROLE OF NUTRITION IN ADDICTION MEDICINE

Nutrition is an important part of recovery from the harmful use of alcohol and drugs. As discussed in the section on epidemiology, using alcohol and drugs drains the body of essential nutrients such as vitamins, minerals, amino acids, and fatty acids. This makes it difficult for the brain to re-establish normal function necessary for recovery. Three important functions that are vital to recovery are the capacity to make decisions, use appropriate judgment, and project consequences for actions. When these functions are lacking, other parts of the brain take control and promote the drive back to drug use. Giving the brain proper food and nutrients helps the whole brain work better so it can guide recovery.

When people stop using alcohol and drugs, their bodies are significantly malnourished. The typical diet in early recovery does not promote the reduction of this malnourishment. The diet is loaded with refined carbohydrates and does not include protein in sufficient amounts to replace neurotransmitters diminished by drugs. It does not include healthful fats needed to make prostaglandins and endocannabinoids. This leaves people vulnerable to relapse in the early days of abstinence and recovery [23–25].

POST ACUTE WITHDRAWAL SYNDROME

Post acute withdrawal syndrome (PAWS) is the name given to problems commonly found during early recovery. These problems include: difficulty with emotional control with either lability or numbness, making decisions, being motivated, memory issues, extra sensitivity to stress, and clumsiness. PAWS can last up to two years or longer. Proper nutrition has helped some people shorten this time as their brains received the ingredients needed to stabilize and rebuild function. For many people, healthful eating is ongoing and necessary to maintain recovery. Returning to poor eating habits that include large amounts of sugar and caffeine can reactivate dormant neurotransmitter pathways contributing to relapse. Additionally, some forms of depression and anxiety that frequently accompany alcohol and drug use have their roots in poor nutrition [26–32].

THE ABSTINENCE TRIAD™

People in early recovery seek the abstinence triad: sugar, caffeine, and nicotine. Consuming these items is an effort to manage brain dysfunction and cravings that result from the absence of their drug of choice. These substances bind to some of the same receptors as drugs of abuse, which, in turn, activate the drug-using pathways. This eases cravings and assists in brain stabilization.

TABLE 31.1

Overview of Drugs

Depressants	Stimulants	Hallucinogens
Alcohol	Amphetamines	Dextromethorphan
Anesthetics	Methamphetamine	Ecstasy
Ketamine	Amphetamine Derivatives	GHB
GHB	Ecstasy	Ketamine
PCP	Bath Salts	K2 ~ Spice
Barbiturates	Caffeine	LSD
Benzodiazepines	Cocaine	Marijuana—high THC content
Dextromethorphan	Crack	Mescaline
Inhalants	Dextromethorphan	PCP
Aerosol Sprays	Khat	Peyote
Hair spray	Nicotine	Psilocybin
Deodorant	Yaba	Salvia divinorum
Paint		
Insecticides		
Solvents		
Gasoline		
Model cement		
White out		
Paint thinner		
Marijuana—low THC content		
Narcotics		

Desired Effects	**Desired Effects**	**Desired Effects**
Well being	Euphoria	Hallucinations
Relaxation	Energy	Mystical experiences
Decreased inhibitions	Alertness	
Hallucinations		
Amnesia: Date Rape		

Negative Effects	**Negative Effects**	**Negative Effects**
Disorientation	Agitation	Anxiety
Poor judgment	Paranoia	Panic
Reduced memory	Increased heart rate	Dangerous behavior
Reduced coordination	Arrhythmia	

Withdrawal	**Withdrawal**	**Withdrawal**
Activate SNS: fight-flight	Depression	Depression, anxiety, poor judgment, fatigue,
	Anxiety	appetite and sleep changes

Overdose	**Overdose**	**Overdose**
Decreased respiration	Panic attack	Symptoms range from discomfort to death
Decreased heart rate	Cerebral vascular accident	depending on the drug
Coma	Myocardial infarction	
Death		

Addiction Potential	**Addiction Potential**	**Addiction Potential**
Tolerance	Tolerance	**Psychological Dependence**
Dependence	Dependence	Ecstasy, LSD, mescaline, peyote, psilocybin, salvia
		divinorum

Source: [21].

> **Sugar**
> • Binds to opioid receptors → Euphoria
> • Binds to dopamine receptors → Pleasure
>
> **Caffeine**
> • Binds to dopamine receptors → Pleasure
> • Binds to norepinephrine receptors → Alertness
>
> **Nicotine**
> • Binds to acetylcholine receptors → Dopamine → Pleasure
> • Binds to norepinephrine receptors → Alertness
> • Activates cortisol → Glucose → Energy

FIGURE 31.1　Abstinence triad. (From [26].)

However, these substances also keep the pathways primed so relapse to the drug of choice occurs more easily. See Figure 31.1.

All drugs of abuse lead to the release of dopamine, which activates the pleasure center. The legal substances, sugar, caffeine, and nicotine, cause the release of some dopamine, which provides pleasure.

Refined carbohydrates rapidly break down into sugar. This sugar binds to opioid receptors as does alcohol, narcotics, cocaine, marijuana, and PCP. Stimulation by sugar provides mild euphoria.

Caffeine binds to norepinephrine receptors as do all stimulants including cocaine, methamphetamine, khat, and bath salts. This provides alertness and energy.

Nicotine increases energy by binding to norepinephrine receptors. It also binds to cortisol receptors that cause the release of glucose, a major fuel source, leading to more energy production. Nicotine binds to acetylcholine receptors, which indirectly causes the release of dopamine resulting in pleasure [26].

DIGESTION PEARLS

Poor eating habits frequently lead to digestive and malabsorption disorders in early recovery. Consuming large amounts of refined carbohydrates and sugar tends to feed the pathological bacteria and yeast in the large intestine, leading to symptoms of bloating, flatulence, malodorous stool, and malabsorption leading to fatigue. These colonies can overgrow so significantly that they can invade the small intestine and disrupt normal intestinal flora. Treatment with antibiotics may bring initial relief but compounds the issue by further killing the guardian bacteria that promote health. One of the longer lasting solutions is to provide a probiotic that contains multiple strains of bacteria. There are products on the market that contain 10–12 different strains. These products should contain billions of units. They should be either purchased refrigerated or be designed for refrigeration upon opening the bottle. Some of the products contain inulin or fructooligosaccharides (FOS) that act as nourishment for the probiotics. Some sensitive patients have difficulty with FOS so these products should be used with caution with such patients.

An additional solution is to educate patients to choose whole grain products instead of refined grains. Grains that retain the husk contain vitamins, minerals, and oils that are removed with refining. Whole grains tend to nourish the guardian bacteria that keep pathological bacteria and yeast within bounds.

People in early recovery need to consume more protein in order to rebuild neurotransmitters diminished by drug use. However, for the body to make use of protein, it has to be unraveled from its tightly coiled state by the breaking of bonds. This is accomplished by hydrochloric acid (HCl) in the stomach. With the aging process and poor nutrition, the level of HCl may be too low to perform adequately. Symptoms of low acid are unfortunately similar to those of high acid including indigestion, abdominal fullness, gas, and bloating. Many hypochlorhydric patients have worsened when mistakenly placed on antacids. It is important to be sure there are no underlying conditions such as hypothyroidism, hypoadrenalism, helicobacter pylori, or intestinal candidiasis infection that may provide similar symptoms [33].

The Heidelberg gastrogram is a gastric pH study that provides an indication of the status of stomach acid. It is an ideal test to perform, yet finding practitioners with the necessary equipment is more difficult than years ago. Instead, many physicians rely on home testing. The test consists of using 10 mg HCl tablets at meals. The patient takes increasing amounts of HCl tablets until digestive symptoms resolve or heartburn occurs. Again, it is difficult to find HCl tablets in 10 mg [34].

As a practical option, many physicians use apple cider vinegar for testing. Depending on the sensitivity of the patient, starting dose is one teaspoon to one tablespoon mixed in a shot glass with water. It is taken at the beginning of the meal. The dose can be increased every day or so until resolution of symptoms or heartburn. If heartburn occurs immediately, there is no need for acid supplementation. When heartburn occurs after increasing the dose several times, the needed amount of acid has been surpassed. Reduce the dose to the previous level. Always emphasize to patients before beginning the test to have available fresh bicarbonate of soda to mix with water to neutralize heartburn. If the amount of vinegar needed is low but helpful, the physician may choose to use vinegar as the acidifying agent. When the level of vinegar is high, switching to HCl tablets may be more convenient. It is important to remember that as health is restored the need for acidification may decrease or cease. Monitoring clinical symptoms is important. If a gastrogram is available, it can be used for monitoring [33].

An appropriately acidic stomach is also needed for the absorption of some vitamins and minerals. It is difficult to absorb zinc with low stomach acid. Some physicians will test for low zinc by having the patient swish one to two teaspoons of aqueous zinc in the mouth for 10 seconds and spit it out. After 30 seconds, if zinc tastes like water or has minimal taste, there is considered to be a zinc deficiency. When zinc tastes metallic, there is no deficiency. Many physicians treat with aqueous zinc (1.15 mg per teaspoon) for severely deficient patients at three to six teaspoons per day until taste improves, then four tablets of 15 mg each (gluconate, citrate) for two months. Severely zinc-deficient patients may also be deficit in vitamin B6 and magnesium. Many physicians supplement vitamin B6 with the activated version P-5-P at 20 mg tid and 400 mg magnesium citrate or gluconate (not magnesium oxalate) in the evening. While this test is widely used, it is criticized for its subjective nature and varying accuracy [35,36].

Poor digestion can also be the result of insufficient pancreatic digestive enzymes. Some physicians supplement with digestive enzymes. Products that measure enzymes in units of activity such as protease HUT (Hemoglobin Unit Tyrosine) or lactase ALU (acid lactase units) are often preferred over products that simply measure enzymes by weight in milligrams. Activity units reflect enzyme activity that is guaranteed by the manufacturer. The weight of an enzyme does not guarantee enzyme activity [33].

UNDERLYING PATHOPHYSIOLOGICAL CONDITIONS AND TREATMENT

NEUROTRANSMITTER DEPLETION FROM ALCOHOL AND DRUG USE

Most neurotransmitters are protein based since they are built from amino acids. The typical patient diet is very deficit in protein because protein does not satisfy the cravings for sweets.

The diet preferred by patients is high in refined carbohydrates, which is also deficit in vitamins and minerals needed as cofactors in the making of neurotransmitters. These cofactors assist enzymes to process amino acids into specific neurotransmitters. A deficit in cofactors contributes to a deficit in neurotransmitters [37].

Acetylcholine

Acetylcholine is necessary for the creation and retrieval of memories. It is also active during REM sleep. Acetylcholine action causes muscles to relax. This contributes to the sensation of drug-induced relaxation and to the ongoing issue of constipation when narcotics interfere with this neurotransmitter action. Users of marijuana experience the antinausea effect of acetylcholine in the gastrointestinal tract. They also have difficulty placing and retrieving information from long-term memory. Acetylcholine is produced from protein such as eggs and chicken. It combines with Acetyl Co-A, which is a by-product from many metabolic reactions via the enzyme choline acetyltransferase. Pantothenic acid (vitamin B5) is a required cofactor in this process of producing acetylcholine [38–40].

Endorphins

The amino acid phenylalanine is converted into the amino acid tyrosine. This is a major player in the production of neurotransmitters that are affected by alcohol and drugs. Endorphins are produced from tyrosine when there are sufficient cofactors available: vitamin B6, vitamin C, folic acid, zinc, copper, magnesium, iron, and manganese. Endorphins are involved in pain management and in creating a sense of well-being. Marijuana, cocaine, narcotics, and alcohol bind to endorphin receptors, which contributes to the euphoria created by these drugs [38,39,41].

Dopamine, Norepinephrine, Epinephrine

Tyrosine converts to dopamine. All drugs of abuse cause the release of dopamine, which stimulates the reward center. Dopamine is also involved in managing executive functions. The conversion from tyrosine to dopamine requires the cofactors of vitamin B6, vitamin C, folic acid, zinc, copper, magnesium, iron, and manganese. From dopamine, norepinephrine and epinephrine are produced in the presence of vitamin B3, vitamin B12, vitamin C, and folic acid. These neurotransmitters participate in the activation of the sympathetic nervous system to manage fight-flight. Norepinephrine is also involved in alertness, memory, good mood, and pain management. Stimulants such as cocaine and amphetamines cause increased norepinephrine action as does the depressant marijuana. Excessive norepinephrine action causes anxiety and paranoia in some people using stimulants or marijuana [38–40,42].

Serotonin

The amino acid tryptophan converts into niacin (vitamin B3) or serotonin depending on which substance the body needs more and the availability of cofactors. To convert tryptophan to serotonin requires the presence of vitamin B6, B12, folic acid, and magnesium.

Serotonin is necessary for good mood, proper perception, and a sense of calm. It is involved in the hunger-satiety center. As darkness falls, serotonin converts into the hormone melatonin, which induces sleep.

Narcotics bind to serotonin receptors contributing to relaxation, dreaminess, nodding, and lack of concern. They also bind to serotonin receptors in the gastrointestinal tract, which inhibits acetylcholine contributing to constipation by decreasing peristalsis. Marijuana binds to serotonin receptors in the hunger-satiety center producing the "munchies." It also causes an increase in norepinephrine action that in some people provokes anxiety and paranoia. Cocaine and amphetamines bind to serotonin receptors producing the excessive self-confidence associated with these drugs [38,39,43,44].

Glutamate and GABA

Glutamic acid is the amino acid that converts into glutamate. This is the major excitatory neurotransmitter of the brain. It is activated during learning to increase neuronal plasticity. This places information into long-term memory. Drug-using behavior is learned behavior. Every episode of drug use is another learning experience that uses glutamate, leading to potential deficit. Low levels of glutamate contribute to cravings that often continue into early days of abstinence.

Gamma-aminobutyric acid (GABA) is produced from glutamate when the cofactor vitamin B6 is available in sufficient amounts. GABA is the major inhibitory neurotransmitter of the brain. Under normal circumstances, GABA inhibits the release of dopamine to the reward center to promote survival. Walking around blissful and unaware of one's surroundings is dangerous. However, GABA allows dopamine to be released in small amounts during pleasurable activities to enhance the quality of life [38,39,45–48].

When the inhibitory action of GABA is impacted by other inhibitory neurotransmitters such as endorphins or cannabinoids, it nullifies GABA's prohibition on dopamine release. This allows higher amounts than normal of dopamine to flood the reward center creating a high. Many drugs of abuse, including alcohol, marijuana, cocaine, and narcotics, involve this process of "inhibit the inhibitor" as a way to enhance the release of dopamine to the reward center [38].

Endocannabinoids

Endocannabinoids, such as anandamide and 2-arachidonylglycerol, are fat-based neurotransmitters. They begin production in the cell membrane. Endocannabinoids are involved in relaxation, memory, and the prevention of nausea. Marijuana and alcohol bind to cannabinoid receptors [38,49,50].

Eating affordable, healthful food helps to restore levels of neurotransmitters depleted by drug use. The author and a substance abuse treatment program in Rhode Island, CODAC, are collaborating on a nutrition research project with opiate-addicted women in methadone treatment. The patients are being taught about healthy eating through a curriculum created by the author. The hypothesis of the study is to assess how good nutrition will impact recovery and whether incentives increase participation and learning. Preliminary results are positive.

Fatty Acid Deficiency

Prostaglandin E_1 (PGE_1) is necessary for good mood. Deficits result in chronic depression. Normally, fat-oriented protein products such as beef or dairy are converted into an omega-6 fatty acid, gamma-linoleic acid (GLA), that in turn convert to di-homo-gamma-linolenic acid (DGLA). In the presence of the proper cofactors of vitamins B3, B6, C, zinc, and magnesium, PGE_1 is produced. However, poor diet, lack of proper cofactors, insulin dysregulation, alcohol, and opiate use can interfere with this multistep conversion [51].

In addition, there is a genetic abnormality that prevents the conversion of dietary fat to PGE_1. These people have been chronically depressed since childhood. Their family history shows generations of depression, suicide, and alcoholism. The ethnic groups most strongly affected are Irish, Welsh, Scottish, Scandinavian, and Native American. See Figure 31.2.

Alcoholism runs rampant in these families because alcohol raises the blood histamine level that, in turn, activates the conversion of di-homo-gamma-linolenic acid (DGLA) to a limited amount of PGE_1. The depression lifts temporarily, so initially, alcohol seems to be the solution to the life-long depression. However, fairly quickly there comes the need for increasingly higher levels of alcohol to resolve the depression. These people are caught in a trap: alcohol relieves the depression, but they have become addicted to alcohol, so if they stop drinking, the depression returns. The depression is often so severe that suicide is contemplated.

A way to intervene in this alcohol-depression cycle is to give gamma-linoleic acid along with the cofactors. This bypasses the genetic glitch so that PGE_1 can be made. Depression resolves and the option to genuinely treat the alcohol issue is possible. Gamma-linoleic acid (GLA) is found in evening primrose oil. It is a lifetime supplement. The typical dose of GLA needed to correct this condition is up to 1500 mg per day in divided doses. For sensitive patients who may not need the full dose, it may be wise to start with 500 mg and add an additional 500 mg after four days if there is no resolution or onset of new symptoms. Less sensitive patients may be able to begin with 1500 mg. It is best to take evening primrose oil with a meal that contains healthful fat to insure proper processing [52–54].

Glutamate: Friend or Foe

Glutamate is an excitatory neurotransmitter when it binds to the AMPA and NMDA receptors. This promotes plasticity of nerves so that learning takes place and information is placed into long-term

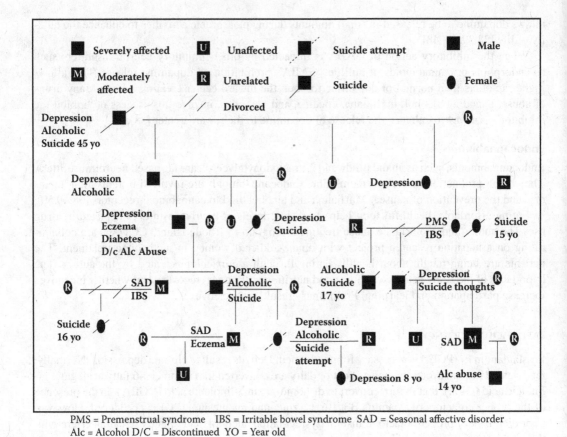

FIGURE 31.2 Genogram of a fatty acid deficit Irish family. (From [52].)

memory. Every episode of drug use is a learning experience that affects neuronal plasticity. With significant drug use, there appears to be glutamate drug-induced neuronal plasticity that seems to increase excitatory signaling at AMPA receptors in the corticostriatal pathway. This is associated with drug cravings.

There is another glutamate receptor called the metrobamate receptor that is inhibitory. For this receptor to function there must be sufficient glutamate available to activate the cysteine-glutamate exchanger. Glutamate resides within the nerve. Cysteine rests outside the nerve. When the exchanger functions, cysteine enters the nerve and glutamate is forced out of the nerve where it binds to the metrobamate receptor. This slows the release of glutamate to the excitatory AMPA and NMDA receptors. Unfortunately, in addicted persons, the cysteine-glutamate exchanger does not function well because glutamate is being channeled to the excitatory AMPA receptors in the corticostriatal pathway. Cravings continue [55].

National Institute on Drug Addiction (NIDA) funded studies on cocaine use in rats. Researchers used a product called n-acetyl-cysteine (NAC) to overload cysteine and prime the cysteine-glutamate exchanger to work. When glutamate was forced out of the nerve, it bound to the metro-bamate receptor. Cravings diminished in rats and fewer rats returned to cocaine use. Studies were repeated with humans addicted to cocaine. See Figure 31.3.

Human studies used varying amounts of NAC. In one study (LaRowe), a total of 2400 mg per day in divided doses of 600 mg were given for three days. Another study (Amen) provided 1200–2400 mg

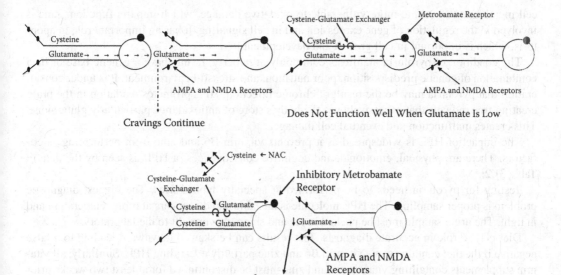

FIGURE 31.3   Cysteine-glutamate exchanger reduces cravings. (From [67].)
AMPA Receptor = Alpha-amino-3-hydroxy-5methyl-4-isoxazole- propionic acid Receptor
NMDA Receptor = N-methyl-D-Aspartate Receptor
NAC = N-Acetyl-Cysteine

of NAC in divided doses daily over four days. The outcome of these studies demonstrated reduced withdrawal symptoms and decreased cravings. NAC at these doses was well tolerated [56–60].

These results suggest that NAC is well tolerated in healthy, cocaine-dependent individuals and may reduce cocaine-related withdrawal symptoms and cravings potentially resulting in relapse reduction. NAC does not change the high induced by cocaine but seems to alter the pathogenic drug-induced plasticity by returning the pathways closer to normal. NAC has been studied with good results in tobacco abuse, pathological gambling, and other compulsive behaviors such as trichotillomania [61–67].

PYROLURIA

Importance of Identifying Pyroluria

A by-product of hemoglobin synthesis is a substance known as pyrrole. In most people, pyrroles are harmlessly excreted. For people with the condition known as pyroluria, a particular pyrrole, 3-ethyl-5-hydroxy-4,5-dimethyl-delta-3-pyrroline-2-one, known as HPL, remains in the blood longer and binds to vitamin B6 and zinc. This results in functional deficits of these key cofactors needed in many biochemical reactions [68].

Vitamin B6 is needed as a cofactor to convert glycogen into glucose; generate glucose from amino acids via gluconeogenesis; synthesize serotonin, dopamine, norepinephrine, and GABA; synthesize heme and vitamin B3; reduce the impact of estrogen, progesterone, testosterone, and other steroid hormones by binding to their receptors; mobilize single-carbon functional groups in the synthesis of nucleic acids; and improve immunity by increasing production of lymphocytes and interleukin-2.

Zinc is needed as a cofactor in over 100 reactions. It is important in the structure of proteins. Zinc is also important in the structure and function of cell membranes. Low zinc levels cause the cell membrane to become more vulnerable to oxidative damage, which impairs function. Zinc is involved in the regulation of gene expression and in cell signaling. It has an important role in apoptosis, which is important in cell growth and development [69].

The condition of pyroluria manifests commonly at puberty. It may have a genetic base or be a combination of genetic predisposition, poor nutrition, and stressful environment. It is under consideration that pyroluria may be the result of chronic infection. HPL promotes oxidation in the brain creating free radicals that excessively use the body's store of antioxidants, particularly glutathione. This creates malfunction and eventual cell damage.

The impact of HPL is widespread as it prevents vitamin B6 and zinc from performing as cofactors. There are physical, emotional, and cognitive consequences of HPL as seen by the data in Table 31.2.

Testing for pyroluria needs to be performed at specialty laboratories. The biggest diagnostic problem is proper sampling. The HPL molecule is unstable and disappears at room temperature and in light. The urine sample must be packed in ice and shipped overnight to the laboratory.

Diet plays a role in accurate diagnosis. Test results can be skewed downward leading to a false negative if the diet contains some vitamin B6 and zinc partially overriding HPL. Similarly, all vitamin supplements containing vitamin B6 and zinc must be discontinued for at least two weeks prior to testing for more accurate results.

It is important to identify people suffering from pyroluria who struggle with addictions. The chances of recovery are slim when this metabolic condition continually dysregulates the brain [68,70,71].

Treatment

Treatment consists of vitamin B6 and zinc supplementation. The dose recommendations are variable. Typically daily supplementation of 200–800 mg of vitamin B6 is sufficient for most patients. Severe cases of pyroluria may need to take higher doses for resolution of symptoms. The caution of not taking more than 100 mg of vitamin B6 to prevent peripheral neuropathy seems to be unwarranted with these patients. However, some patients may develop reversible median nerve paresthesia with long-term, high-dose treatment. Using the activated version of vitamin B6, P-5-P, does not seem to cause any of these nerve problems. Monitoring vitamin B6 via pyridoxine blood levels has not been considered useful.

The typical daily dose for zinc replacement ranges from 25–100 mg. Caution needs to be taken with zinc supplementation since excessive amounts can suppress both copper and manganese. Adults taking more than 50 mg of elemental zinc daily should be followed with cellular or plasma zinc and copper levels. Zinc levels should not exceed the upper limit of normal. Copper levels should not fall below normal range. Manganese can be monitored via serum or red cell levels. The results should be within the normal range. If the manganese is low, consider supplementing 5 mg for every 30 mg of zinc.

Symptoms in mild cases of pyroluria begin to resolve within several days. It may take weeks to months for resolution of severe cases, or when patients are compromised with several metabolic disorders. Treatment is considered a life-time regime. However, initial treatment doses may be higher than subsequent maintenance doses. Many patients who stop their supplements begin deteriorating within 48 hours and are significantly impaired within three months [70,71].

HYPOGLYCEMIA

Pathophysiology

Maintaining normal blood sugar levels is the balance between the action of two hormones, insulin and glucagon. Insulin is released from the pancreas in response to and in proportion to the presence of glucose in the digestive tract. Insulin transports and transfers glucose into cells where it is oxidized in the mitochondria to produce adenosine-5'-triphosphate (ATP).

TABLE 31.2

Signs and Symptoms of Pyroluria

Physical Appearance and Symptoms

- Pale skin
- Reduced eyebrows, eyelashes, hair
- Overcrowded upper teeth
- Poor quality tooth enamel
- White marks on fingernails
- Thin finger nails
- Acne
- Eczema
- Inability to tan
- Sensitive to light and sound
- Fatigue
- Inability to tolerate alcohol and drugs

Emotional and Cognitive Symptoms

Emotions

- Nervousness
- Severe inner tension
- Anxiety
- Depression
- Mood swings
- Episodic anger
- Loner
- Poor stress management

Cognition

- Racing thoughts
- Hallucinations
- Poor memory
- Poor concentration
- Poor dream recall

Pyroluria: Often Misdiagnosed As

- Anxiety disorder
- Schizophrenia
- Bipolar disorder
- Neurotransmitter-based depression
- Malingering

Source: [68].

As insulin removes glucose from the blood, the level of glucose declines. If glucose levels dip too low for normal function, glucagon is released from the pancreas. It stimulates gluconeogenesis and glycogenolysis in the liver. When glucose is released into the blood, glucose levels are restored. See Figure 31.4.

Postprandial reactive hypoglycemia (PRH) is a malfunction of this insulin-glucagon mechanism that normally maintains the balance between glucose supply and utilization. Symptoms frequently appear two to four hours after a meal, particularly a high carbohydrate meal. In PRH, the body's ability to maintain proper blood glucose levels is impaired by three known defects:

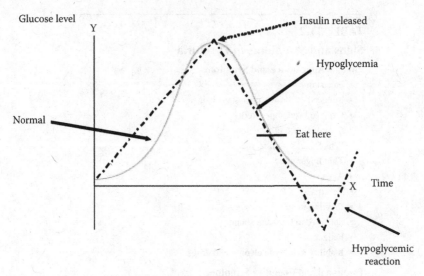

FIGURE 31.4   Postprandial reactive hypoglycemia blood sugar curve. (From [73].)

1. Insulin binds to its receptors in a very efficient manner that is called high insulin sensitivity. This results in glucose being more rapidly removed from the blood.
2. Inability of glucagon to generate enough glucose to replace the removed glucose in a timely manner.
3. Increased sensitivity to norepinephrine and epinephrine so that the body responds quickly and excessively to the release of these chemicals. As the brain detects a drop in its glucose supply, it sends SOS signals to the adrenal glands. They engage with the sympathetic nervous system's (SNS) fight-flight response with the release of norepinephrine and epinephrine. Simultaneously, the adrenal glands release cortisol, which signals the liver to release glucose. Some symptoms of PRH are related to the presence of these emergency hormones in the blood. The level of glucose in the blood is often normalized by these hormones making it difficult to catch the lowered blood glucose level unless glucose and insulin are properly tested [72]. (See Figure 31.5.)

The symptoms of postprandial reactive hypoglycemia can be divided into two types. Neuroglucopenic signs are due to the body's reaction to low glucose in the brain. Sympathetic signs are due to the different hormones, especially norepinephrine and epinephrine, attempting to re-regulate and normalize blood sugar [73,74]. (See Table 31.3.)

Testing

The five- to six-hour glucose tolerance test (GTT) is rarely used today to identify PRH because it has been found to have excessive false positives. The 3-hour GTT can be helpful to identify the pattern of insulin activity. Blood sugar may be normal but the pattern of insulin is often abnormal indicating excessive sensitivity.

The hyperglucidic breakfast test has become a more frequently used test. It consists of a high carbohydrate meal: bread/toast (80 g), butter (10 g), jelly, condensed skim milk (80 ml), sugar (10 g), and instant coffee (2.5 g). This meal is composed of 9.1% protein, 27.5% fat, and 63.4% carbohydrates, which is similar to the breakfast consumed by many people. Blood glucose levels are drawn at several intervals after the meal. It is a good idea to also draw insulin levels to identify the insulin pattern.

Another common test is ambulatory glucose sampling performed at home. Carbohydrates are consumed and the patient uses a glucometer to assess blood sugar whenever s/he experiences

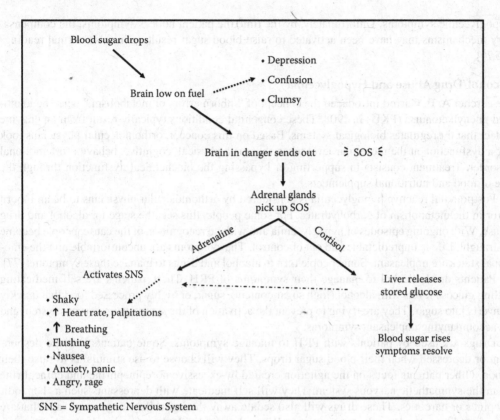

FIGURE 31.5 Process of postprandial reactive hypoglycemia: Patients turn to alcohol and drugs to manage symptoms. (From [73].)

TABLE 31.3

Signs and Symptoms of Postprandial Reactive Hypoglycemia

Neuroglucopenic Signs	Sympathetic Signs
Headache	Increased heart rate
Dizziness	Palpitations
Confusion	Hyperventilation
Impaired judgment	Tremors
Blurred vision	Sweating
Fatigue	Flushing
Depression	Cold waves
Anxiety	Irritability
Anger	Anxiety

Source: [73].

hypoglycemic symptoms. Unfortunately, by the time the patient notices symptoms, the compensatory mechanisms may have been activated to raise blood sugar resulting in false normal readings [75,76].

Alcohol/Drug Abuse and Hypoglycemia

Researcher A. E. Garrod introduced the concept of "inborn errors of metabolism," when he identified phenylketonuria (PKU) in 1908. These congenital conditions typically result from an enzyme defect that dysregulates biological systems. Based on this concept, orthomolecular physicians look for a dysfunction at the molecular level when there is a physical, cognitive, behavior, or emotional disorder. Treatment consists in supporting or bypassing the biochemical dysfunction through the use of food and nutritional supplements.

Postprandial reactive hypoglycemia is considered by orthomolecular physicians to be an inborn error in the metabolism of carbohydrates. For some people, this sets the stage for alcohol and drug abuse. With ongoing episodes of hypoglycemia and with no recognition of the cause, people become distraught. Life is unpredictable and out of control. The symptoms are uncomfortable and the emotional states are unpleasant. Some people turn to alcohol and drugs to manage these symptoms [77].

Patients drink alcohol to manage their symptoms of PRH. These patients are self medicating falling glucose levels with alcohol (high sugar content), sugar, or highly processed food that quickly converts into sugar. They are trying to prevent the activation of the sympathetic nervous system and its accompanying unpleasant symptoms.

Drugs are used by patients with PRH to manage symptoms. Some patients become despondent or depressed when their blood sugar drops. They will choose to use stimulants to raise their mood. Other patients focus on the agitation created by excessive norepinephrine and epinephrine from the sympathetic nervous system. They will self medicate with depressants such as benzodiazepines or narcotics. These drugs will also sedate away the irritability, anger, and rage that are manifested by some hypoglycemic patients. When these individuals stop using drugs, they are left with unmasked imbalanced chemistry. If left untreated, imbalanced blood sugar will drive many people to relapse [78].

Treatment

Most people respond well to dietary change. Eating by the clock is the first step. It is important to notice when the symptoms begin and eat 15–30 minutes before their onset. The purpose is to catch the declining blood sugar before it enters the danger zone and activates the sympathetic nervous system.

Eating a balanced diet is the treatment for postprandial reactive hypoglycemia. The purpose is to supply steady fuel over several hours to compensate for a faulty fuel delivery system. Complex carbohydrates supply the immediate fuel. Protein supplies the intermediate fuel, while fat provides the long-range fuel. Half the plate should be covered with a variety of vegetables, one quarter of the plate with protein, and one quarter whole grains, legumes, or starchy vegetables. Healthful fat is used as a condiment, adding flavor and taste as well as health benefits. Fruit is used modestly because fructose converts to glucose and to belly fat if eaten excessively. Pastries and sweets are reserved for special occasions and eaten as part of a meal to buffer fluctuating blood sugar. Caffeinated beverages are used very modestly because they stimulate the adrenal glands with the release of norepinephrine and epinephrine. Water intake is encouraged. All of these dietary suggestions may need to be modified if there are other health conditions [73,79–81].

DIAGNOSIS OF ALCOHOL AND DRUG ABUSE AND ADDICTION

Patients with alcohol and drug problems are found in all medical specialties. Their addiction issues may be masked by other diagnoses such as hypertension, diabetes, infertility, and sexual concerns. Gastrointestinal issues may present as gastritis, pancreatitis, liver disease, malabsorption, and weight loss/gain. Psychiatric issues of depression, anxiety, sleep disorders, and suicidal attempts are found in pediatrics, primary care, and psychiatry. Accidents, commonly associated with substance use, are treated by many specialties.

As physicians, we need to do a better job of identifying substance-abusing patients because of the cost to the patient, family, and society. One study typifies the need to improve our diagnostic skills. This study investigated resident physicians' capacity to identify patients with substance abuse issues. Of the 20% of patients with addiction issues, residents only identified 5%. By history, 22% of alcohol-dependent and 23% of drug-dependent patients were identified [82].

LABORATORY TESTS

There are no definitive tests to diagnose alcohol or drug addiction. Tests can suggest but cannot diagnose. However, they may be part of accumulated evidence to break through the denial of a substance-abusing patient.

Alcohol

It has been common practice to use laboratory tests to diagnose alcoholism: liver enzymes gamma-glutamyl transferase (GGT) and aspartate transaminase (AST), mean corpuscular volume (MCV), and levels of magnesium and folate. Studies have found the sensitivity and specificity of these tests to be poor because other health conditions may give similar abnormal test results. These tests may be helpful for screening at-risk populations with the intention of more intensive follow-up [83]. See Table 31.4.

Drug Toxicology Screens

Toxicology screenings provide evidence of drug use under certain conditions: 1) the suspected drug is included in the test panel, 2) the drug was used within the specific detectable time frame, 3) the collection and processing was performed accurately. Random testing produces more accurate results because a drug user will not be able to schedule the test at a time when s/he has temporarily stopped using drugs. Toxicology screens provide evidence of use but do not allow a diagnosis of substance abuse or addiction.

A urine sample will provide information about the presence or absence of the drug in the body while a blood sample will also provide quantitative information. However, blood screens typically have a shorter window of time to determine the presence of a drug. Urine drug concentration doses do not correlate well to blood concentrations.

Urine screens are more commonly used because they are less expensive, provide more rapid results, and are quite accurate. In order to have accurate results, the collection and processing must

TABLE 31.4
Common Laboratory Tests Used to Identify Heavy Alcohol Use

Test	Acronym	Results with Heavy Alcohol Use
Gamma-glutamyl transferase	GGT	Liver enzyme increases
Aspartate transaminase	AST	Liver enzyme increases
Mean corpuscular volume	MCV	Size of RBC increases
Magnesium level		Low due to poor dietary intake
Folate level		Low due to poor absorption & increased excretion
Vitamin B12 level		Low due to poor absorption & increased excretion

Source: [87].

be performed according to strict guidelines. The individual must be positively identified, usually with a state or federally issued photo identification card. The full chain of custody procedures must be followed as outlined in the drug testing kit. The temperature of the urine sample must be determined upon acceptance of the sample to prevent adulteration or substituted samples. The acceptable temperature range is 96–99 degrees Fahrenheit. Temperatures below this range are suspect for a substituted sample. For accuracy, use a digital thermometer instead of the temperature strips included in the kit. When this procedure is followed, it is not necessary to collect the sample under observation.

An abnormal screening result should be confirmed by gas chromatography–mass spectrometry to insure no false positives. [84,85]

Types of Tests

There are two types of tests: cut off and limit of detection. In a cut-off type of test, a limit has been set that will be used as the cut-off point to identify an abnormal result. This increases false negatives. There may be drugs in the system, but they are reported as normal because the amount is below what the test has been set to identify as abnormal. In contrast, limit of detection tests, also known as zero-tolerance tests, will identify any amount of drug in the system within the capacity of the laboratory. When it is necessary to have extremely accurate information because the test results will significantly impact a patient's life, consider sending the sample to a laboratory that performs zero-tolerance testing [85].

Drugs Included in Tests

The drugs included in the test depend on the laboratory. As an example, take two laboratories that provide drug testing and the types of testing included in a panel as a sample of what to expect. One company includes the following drugs in their standard screen: amphetamines, benzodiazepines, cocaine, cannabinoid, methadone, and opiates. Additional tests can be added for a greater cost including buprenorphine, methadone, ketamine, and LSD. Another company has two standard panels. The five panel includes marijuana (THC), methamphetamine, amphetamine, cocaine, opiates, and phencyclidine (PCP). The 10 panel includes marijuana (THC), methamphetamine, amphetamine, cocaine, opiates, phencyclidine (PCP), propoxyphene (Darvon), methadone, barbiturates, and benzodiazepines. More tests can be added for additional cost [85,86].

Different companies list varying times that drugs can be detected in the system. Table 31.5 provides a composite of several companies. The duration is the number of days or weeks that the drug may be detected from the time the drug or metabolic initially arrives in the urine [84, 86–88].

DIAGNOSIS: *DIAGNOSTIC AND STATISTICAL MANUAL OF MENTAL DISORDERS*

The standard for diagnosing addictions by criteria is the use of American Psychiatric Association's *Diagnostic and Statistical Manual of Mental Disorders* (DSM). The fourth edition of the DSM of 2000 is being replaced in 2013 with the fifth edition DSM (or DSM-V).

The proposed DSM-V (2013) creates a category of substance use and addictive disorders that includes substances and behavioral addictions such as gambling. A significant change from DSM-IV TR is the removal of the distinction between abuse and dependence. In its place is a severity scale that ranges from no diagnosis to severe substance use disorder based on the number of criteria the patient meets. The disorders are listed by substance abuse type: alcohol-related disorders, caffeine-related disorders, cannabis-related disorders, hallucinogen-related disorders, inhalant-related disorders, opioid-related disorders, sedative/hypnotic-related disorders, stimulant-related disorders, tobacco-related disorders, unknown substance disorders, gambling disorder, and substance-induced disorders including psychosis, bipolar, depression, anxiety, obsessive-compulsive, sleep, sexual dysfunction, delirium, and neurocognitive disorders.

TABLE 31.5

Duration of Drugs Detected in Urine

Drug	Detected in Urine
Alcohol	Up to 24 hours
Barbiturates	1–3 days; chronic: up to 3–6 weeks
Benzodiazepines	1–3 days; chronic: up to 3–6 weeks
Heroin	1–2 days
Morphine	1–2 days
Codeine	1–5 days
Oxycodone	1–4 days
Methadone	2–3 days
Cocaine	1–4 days; heavy use 10–22 days
Amphetamine	1–3 days
Methamphetamine	1–4 days
Marijuana	2–7 days; heavy use: up to 4–6 weeks
PCP	2–8 days
Ecstasy	1–4 days

Source: [84,86,87,88].

To receive a diagnosis of addiction, two criteria must be met over a 12-month period:

- Not meeting important role obligations
- Continued use despite disruption of interpersonal relationships
- Reduced involvement in important life activities because of substances
- Continued use regardless of the negative impact
- Craving or strong desire to use the substance
- Persistent desire to stop but cannot
- Considerable time and effort used to obtain, consume, and recover from substances
- Taken in larger amounts or for longer period than intended
- Continued use in dangerous situations such as driving
- Tolerance
- Withdrawal

Also noted in the DSM-V are the issues of tolerance and withdrawal. All drugs of addiction do not create these physiological states. To prevent the erroneous thinking that addiction cannot be diagnosed if tolerance or withdrawal are not present, the DSM-V adds this modifier:

- With physiological dependence: has symptoms of tolerance, withdrawal
- Without physiological dependence—no symptoms of tolerance, withdrawal

The DSM-V is a work in progress. As the work group receives feedback from the field, the material is amended. At the time of this writing, this information is accurate. However, the final version of the DSM-V may show variation from the information included in this chapter [89].

QUESTIONNAIRES

Addiction is commonly diagnosed via screening surveys and interviews. These instruments can be administered by nurses or medical assistants. Some questionnaires are self-administered either with

TABLE 31.6

Sample of Alcohol and Drug Questionnaires

Title	Acronym	Purpose	Method	Comments
CAGE Alcohol Screening	CAGE	Identify alcoholism	Four questions	
Rapid Alcohol Problems Screen	RAPS4	Identify alcoholism in last year	Four questions	Valid across gender and ethnic groups
TWEAK Alcohol Screening	TWEAK	Identify high-risk drinking during pregnancy	Five questions	Can be used with men
Addiction Severity Index	ASI	Assesses seven areas: medical, legal, employment/support, drug and alcohol use, family/social, and psychiatric	Interview of 200 questions Information on life-time and last 30 days use	Original: 60 min Short: 30 minutes
Adolescent Drug Abuse Diagnosis	ADAD	Assesses eight areas: medical drug and alcohol use, legal, family, school and employment, social activities, peer relations, and psychological status	Interview of 150 questions	45 minutes
Cannabis Use Disorders Identification Test	CUDIT	Assess cannabis abuse and dependence	10 questions Information on current and last 6 months use	
Why Do You Smoke?	WDS	Identify primary motivations for smoking	24 questions	

Source: [87,90,91,92].

paper and pencil or online. There are many instruments available. Some are purchased, while others are available at no cost. Several common screening questionnaires are in public domain [87,90–92]. See Table 31.6.

The diagnosis of substance abuse continues to be a blend of art and science. As the physician works with the scientific laboratory studies and instruments available, s/he will gain the experience and the intuition that is the hallmark of the seasoned diagnostician.

SUMMARY

Addiction frequently leads to malnutrition, which is not recognized as a major player in continuing to feel poorly in recovery and in causing relapse. Feeding the body what its needs to function will often allow it to respond with amazingly rapid healing. Identifying underlying metabolic conditions that drive the brain to relapse is vital for recovery. As the body recovers, so does the mind. Recovery is possible in body, mind, and spirit when nutrition is the foundation.

REFERENCES

1. Mulready, P.A. "Chapter 1: A Quick Overview of Addictions." *Drugs and the Brain*. Time To Live Better. com LLC. http://www.timetolivebetter.com. 4 July 2011. 7–8. E-book.

2. Mulready, P.A. "Chapter 1: Importance of Nutrition." *Nutrition: Feeding Your Body Right ~ Part 1*. Time To Live Better.com LLC. http://www.timetolivebetter.com. 4 July 2011. 6–7. E-book.

3. Nasser, J.A. Leitzsch, J.B. and Patel, K. "Addictive Disorders in Nutritional Diseases from a Nutritional Viewpoint." In *Addictive Disorders in Medical Populations*. West Sussex, UK: Wiley-Blackwell, 2010. 303–5. Print.

4. Santolaria-Fernández, F. Gómez-Sirvent, J. González-Reimers, C. et al. "Nutritional Assessment of Drug Addicts." *Drug and Alcohol Dependence* 38.1 (1995): 11–18. Print.

5. Feinman, L. and Lieber, C.S. "Nutrition and Diet in Alcoholism." In *Modern Nutrition in Health and Disease*. (eds. M Shils, J Olson, M Shike and A Ross) Lippincott Williams & Wilkins, 1999. 1523–42. Print.

6. Feinman, L. and Lieber, C.S. "Toxicity of Ethanol and Other Components of Alcoholic Beverages." *Alcohol Clin Exp Res* 12.1 (1988): 2–6. Print.

7. Hillers, V.N. and Massey, K.L. "Interrelationships of Moderate and High Alcohol Consumption with Diet and Health Status." *Am J Clin Nutr* 41.2 (1991): 356–62. Print.

8. Kleiner, K.D. Gold, M.S. Frost-Pineda, K. et al. "Body Mass Index and Alcohol Use." *J Addict Dis* 23.3 (2004): 105–18. Print.

9. Cocores, J.A. Graham, N.A. Gold, M.S. "Addictive Disorders in Nutritional Disease from an Addiction Viewpoint." In *Addictive Disorders in Medical Populations*. West Sussex, UK: John Wiley and Sons Ltd, 2010. 228–90. Print.

10. Nakah, A.E.L. Frank, O. Louria, D.B. et al. "A Vitamin Profile of Heroin Addiction." *AJPH* 69.10 (1979): 1058–60. Print.

11. Jean, A. Conductier, G. Manrique, C. et al "Anorexia Induced by Activation of Serotonin 5-HT4 Receptors Is Mediated by Increases in CART in the Nucleus Accumbens." *Proceedings of the National Academy of Sciences* 104.41 (2007): 16335–40. Print.

12. Vicentic, A. and Jones, D.C. "The CART (Cocaine-and Amphetamine-Regulated Transcript) System in Appetite and Drug Addiction." *J Pharmacol Exp Ther* 320.2 (2007): 499–506. Print.

13. Warner, E. A.Greene, G. S.Buchsbaum, M.S. et al. "Diabetic Ketoaciosis Associated with Cocaine Use." *Arch Intern Med* 158: 1799–802. Print.

14. Miller, N.S. Gold, M.S. "Addictive Disorders as an Integral Part of the Practice of Medicine" In *Addictive Disorders in Medical Populations*. West Sussex, UK: John Wiley & Sons Ltd, 2010. 7–11. Print.

15. Mulready, P.A. "Chapter 2: Epidemiology—What's The Data?" *Nutritional Pearls to Enhance Recovery*. Time To Live Better.com, http://www.timetolivebetter.com. July, 2011. 9–24. E-book.

16. SAMHSA: Center for Behavioral Health Statistics and Quality. *Results from the 2010 National Survey on Drug Use and Health: Summary of National Findings*. U.S. Department of Health and Human Services Substance Abuse and Mental Health Services Administration, Sept. 2011. Web. 12 Nov. 2011. http://www.samhsa.gov/data/NSDUH/2k10NSDUH/2k10Results.htm.

17. National Institute on Alcohol and Alcoholism (NIAAA). "What Is a Standard Drink?" *National Institute on Alcohol and Alcoholism*. Web. 2 Oct. 2011. http://pubs.niaaa.nih.gov/publications/practitioner/pocketguide/pocket_guide2.htm.

18. CDC. "Binge Drinking." *Alcohol and Public Health*. Centers for Disease Control and Prevention, 17 Dec. 2010. Web. 14 Dec. 2011. http://www.cdc.gov/alcohol/fact-sheets/binge-drinking.htm.

19. Cicala, R.S. "Substance Abuse among Physicians: What You Need to Know." *Hospital Physician* 39(7) (2003): 39–46. Print.

20. Trinkoff, A.M., and Storr, C.L. "Substance Use among Nurses: Differences between Specialties." *American Journal of Public Health* 88 (1998): 581–85. Print.

21. Mulready, P.A. "Classification: Drugs of Abuse." *Time To Live Better.com*. http://www.timetolivebetter .com. 4 July 2011. Web. 2 Oct. 2011.

22. NIDA. "Commonly Abused Drugs." *National Institute on Drug Abuse*. National Institutes of Health: National Institute on Drug Abuse. Web. 2 Oct. 2011. http://drugabuse.gov/DrugPages/DrugsofAbuse.html.

23. Mulready, P.A. "Importance of Nutrition in Recovery." Eating Your Way to Recovery. Civic Center, Augusta, ME. 2008–2011. Lecture.

24. Kaiser, S.K. Prendergast, K. and Ruter, T. "Nutritional Links to Addiction Recovery." *Journal of Addiction Nursing* 19.3 (2008): 125–29. Print.

25. Gawad, A.E. Hassan, S.A. Ghanem, AE-A. et al. "Effects of Drug Addiction on Antioxidant Vitamins and Nitric Oxide Levels." *J Basic Appl Sci Res* 1.6 (2011): 485–91. Print.

26. Mulready, P.A. "Chapter 4: Nutrition and Addictions." *Nutritional Pearls to Enhance Recovery*. Time To Live Better.com LLC. http://www.timetolivebetter.com. 4 July 2011. 28–31 E-book.

27. Rimondini, R. Sommer, W.H. Dall'Olio, R. Heilig, M "Long-Lasting Tolerance to Alcohol Following a History of Dependence." *Addict Biol* 13 (1) (March 2008): 26–30. Print.

28. De Soto, C.B. O'Donnell, W.E. Allred, L.J. Lopes, C.E. "Symptomatology in Alcoholics at Various Stages of Abstinence." *Alcohol Clin Exp Res* 9 (6) (December 1985): 505–12. Print.

29. Watanabe K.I. Ogihara-Hashizume, A. Kobayashi, Y. Mitsushio, H. Komiyama, T. "Impaired Sleep during the Post-Alcohol Withdrawal Period in Alcoholic Patients" *Addict Biol* 6 (2) (April 2001): 163–69. Print.

30. Vik, P.W. Cellucci, T. Jarchow, A. Hedt, J. "Cognitive Impairment in Substance Abuse." *Psychiatr Clin North Am* 27 (1) (March 2004): 97–109. Print.

31. Janiri, L. Martinotti, G. Dario, T. et al. "Anhedonia and Substance-Related Symptoms in Detoxified Substance-Dependent Subjects: A Correlation Study." *Neuropsychobiology* 2 (1) (June 3, 2005): 37–44. Print.

32. Mukherjee, S. Das, S.K. Vaidyanathan, K. and Vasudevan, D.M. "Consequences of Alcohol Consumption on Neurotransmitters—an Overview." *Curr Neurovasc Res* 5.4 (Nov 2008): 266–72. Print.

33. Golan, R. "Poor Digestion and Assimilation." *Optimal Wellness*. New York: Ballantine, 1995. 145–52. Print.

34. Biddle, J. "About the Gastrogram Study." *Asheville Integrative Medicine*. Web. 20 Dec. 2011. http://www.docbiddle.com/moreinfo/gastrogram.htm.

35. Myers, R.L. "The Zinc Taste Test." *The Zinc Taste Test*. 2004. Web. 22 Dec. 2011. http://www.funimky.com/downloads/The%20ZINC%20Taste%20Test.pdf.

36. "Biotic Research Corporation Products." *Pure Formulas*. 2007–2011. Web. 22 Dec. 2011. http://www.pureformulas.com.

37. Mukherjee, S. Das, S.K. Vaidyanathan, K. and Vasudevan, D.M. "Consequences of Alcohol Consumption on Neurotransmitters—an Overview." *Curr Neurovasc Res* 5.4 (Nov 2008): 266–72. Print.

38. Mulready, P.A. "Chapter 3: Introduction to the Brain and Nerves: Neurotransmitters." *Drugs and the Brain*. Time To Live Better.com LLC. 4 July 2011. 32–37. E-book. http://www.timetolivebetter.com.

39. Zimmerberg, B. "Uptake of Choline, a Precursor of Acetylcholine, Choline Acetyltransferase: The Binding of Choline and Acetate." *Synaptic Transmission: A Four Step Process*. Williams College, 2000. Web. 12 Dec. 2011. http://web.williams.edu/imput/synapse/pages/IA1.htm.

40. Vincenzi, E. "Acetylcholine as a Neurotransmitter." *CVANS: The Structure Function*. University of Washington School of Medicine, 2004. Web. 12 Dec. 2011. http://courses.washington.edu/chat543/cvans/sfp/acetylch.html.

41. Basbaum, A.I. and Fields, H.L. "Endogenous Pain Control Systems: Brainstem Spinal Pathways and Endorphin Circuitry." *Annual Review of Neuroscience* 7 (March 1984): 309–38. Print.

42. Volkow, N.D. Fowler, J.S. and Wang, G.J. "Role of Dopamine In Drug Reinforcement And Addiction In Humans: Results From Imaging Studies." *Behav Pharmacol* 13.5–6 (Sept 2002): 355–66. Print.

43. Andrews Research Group. "Serotonin and BDNF in Depression and Anxiety Disorders." *Andrews Research Group*. Huck Institute of the Life Sciences: Pennsylvania State University, 2006. Web. 12 Dec. 2011. http://www.brain.psu.edu/serotonin.htm.

44. Hyland, K. "Inherited Disorders Affecting Dopamine and Serotonin: Critical Neurotransmitters Derived from Aromatic Amino Acids." *Journal of Nutrition* 137 (2007): 1568S–72S. Print.

45. Hertz, L. Et Al. "Neuronal-Astrocytic Interactions in Metabolism of Transmitter Amino Acids of the Glutamate Family: Glutamate/GABA Synthesis and Metabolism." *Sigma-RBI Handbook of Receptor Classification and Signal Transduction,* 5th Edition. St. Louis, Missouri: Aldrich Publications, 2006. 114–15. Print.

46. Meldrum, B.S. "Glutamate as a Neurotransmitter in the Brain: Review of Physiology and Pathology." *J. Nutr* 4th ser. 130 (April 2000): 1007S–15S. Print.

47. Danbolt, N.C. "Glutamate Uptake." *Prog Neurobiol* 1st ser. 65 (Sep. 2001): 1–105. Print.

48. He, S. Ma, J. Liu, N. and Yu, X. "Early Enriched Environment Promotes Neonatal GABAergic Neurotransmission and Accelerates Synapse Maturation." *The Journal of Neuroscience* 30.23 (June 9, 2010): 7910–16. Print.

49. Lovinger D.M. "Presynaptic Modulation by Endocannabinoids." *Handb Exp Pharmacol* 184 (2008): 435–77. Print.

50. Kreitzer, A. "Neurotransmission: Emerging Roles of Endocannabinoids." *Current Biology* 15.14 (July 26, 2005): R549–51. Print.

51. Horrobin, D.F. and Manku, M.S. "Possible Role of Prostaglandin El in the Affective Disorders and Alcoholism." *Brit Med J* 280.6228 (June 7, 1980): 1363–66. Print.

52. Mulready, P.A. "Chapter 7: Fatty Acid Deficiency." *Nutritional Pearls To Enhance Recovery*. Time To Live Better.com LLC. 4 July 2011. 42–44. E-book. http://www.timetolivebetter.com

53. Larson, J.M "Week Five: Good Bye Depression." In *Seven Weeks to Sobriety*. NY: Fawcett Columbine, 1997. 227–30. Print.

54. Gant, C. and Lewis, G. "Stopping the Use of Marijuana." *End Your Addiction Now: The Proven Nutritional Supplement Program That Can Set You Free*. NY: Warner, 2002. 228–31. Print.

55. Mulready P.A. "Neurotransmitters." In *Knowing Drugs from The Inside Out*. Middletown, CT: P.A. Mulready Associates, LLC, 2006. 139–44. Print.

56. LaRowe, S.D. Myrick, H. Hedden, S. et al. "Cocaine Desire Reduced By N-Acetylcysteine." *Am J Psychiatry* 164.7 (Jul 2007): 1115–17. Print.

57. Amen, S.L. Piacentine, L.B. Ahmad, M.E. et al. "Repeated N-acetyl Cysteine Reduces Cocaine Seeking in Rodents and Craving in Cocaine-dependent Humans." *Neuropsychopharmacology* 6 (Mar 2011): 871–78. Print.

58. Reichel, C.M. and See, R.E. "Chronic N-Acetylcysteine after Cocaine Self-Administration Produces Enduring Reductions in Drug-Seeking." *Neuropsychopharmacology* 37 (Jan 2012): 298. Print.

59. Moussawi, K. Pacchioni, A. Moran, M. et al "N-Acetylcysteine Reverses Cocaine-Induced Metaplasticity." *Nat Neurosci* 12(2) (Feb 2009): 182–89. Print

60. Moussawi, K. Zhou, W. Shen, H. et al. "Reversing Cocaine-induced Synaptic Potentiation Provides Enduring Protection from Relapse." *Proc Natl Acad Sci U S A* 108.1 (Jan 4, 2011): 385–90. Print.

61. LaRowe, S.D. Mardikian, P. Malcolm, R. et al. "Safety And Tolerability of N-Acetylcysteine in Cocaine-Dependent Individuals." *Am J Addict* 15.1 (Jan/Feb 2006): 105–10. Print.

62. Baker, D.J. McFarland, K. Lake, R.W. et al. "Neuroadaptations in Cystine-Glutamate Exchange Underlie Cocaine Relapse." *Nature Neuroscience* 6.7 (2003): 743–49. Print.

63. Kalivas, P.W. "Glutamate Systems in Cocaine Addiction." *Current Opinion in Pharmacology* 4 (2004): 23–29. Print.

64. Grant, J. Kim, S. and Odlaug, B. "N-acetyl Cysteine, a Glutamate-modulating Agent, in the Treatment of Pathological Gambling: A Pilot Study." *Biol Psychiatry* 62.6 (Sep 15 2007): 652–57. Print.

65. Grant, J. Kim, S. and Odlaug, B. "N-acetylcysteine, a Glutamate Modulator, in the Treatment of Trichotillomania: A Double-blind, Placebo-controlled Study." *Arch Gen Psychiatry* 66.7 (Jul 2009): 756–63. Print.

66. Knackstedt, L. LaRowe, S.D. and Mardikian, P. "The Role of Cystine-Glutamate Exchange in Nicotine Dependence in Rats and Humans." *Biol Psychiatry* 65.10 (May 15 2009): 841–45. Print.

67. Mulready, P.A. "Chapter 8: Glutamate: Friend or Foe." *Nutritional Pearls To Enhance Recovery*. Time To Live Better.com LLC. 4 July 2011. 43–45. E-book. http://www.timetolivebetter.com.

68. Mulready, P.A. "Chapter 9: Pyroluria." *Nutritional Pearls To Enhance Recovery*. Time To Live Better. com LLC. 4 July 2011. 43–45. E-book. http://www.timetolivebetter.com.

69. Higdon, J. "Vitamins." *Micronutrient Information Center*. Oregon State University: Linus Pauling Institute, 2007. Web. 16 Oct. 2011. http://lpi.oregonstate.edu/infocenter/minerals/zinc/html.

70. McGinnis, W.R. Audhya, T. Walsh, W.J. et al. "Discerning the Mauve Factor, Part 1." *Alternative Therapies* 14.2 (Mar/Apr 2008): 40–50. Print.

71. McGinnis, W.R. Audhya, T. Walsh, W.J. et al. "Discerning the Mauve Factor, Part 2." *Alternative Therapies* 14.3 (May/Jun 2008): 50–56. Print.

72. Cryer, P.E. Axelrod, L. and Grossman, A.B. "Evaluation and Management of Adult Hypoglycemic Disorders: An Endocrine Society Clinical Practice Guideline." *Journal of Clinical Endocrinology & Metabolism* 94.3 (March 2009): 709–28. Print.

73. Mulready, P.A. "Chapter 10: Hypoglycemia." *Nutritional Pearls To Enhance Recovery*. Time To Live Better.com LLC. 4 July 2011. 49–54. E-book. http://www.timetolivebetter.com.

74. Harp, M.J. and Fox, L.W. "Correlations of the Physical Symptoms of Hypoglycemia with the Psychological Symptoms of Anxiety and Depression." *Journal of Orthomolecular Medicine* 5.1 (1990): 8–10. Print.

75. Brun, J.F. Fedou, C. Bouix, O. Raynaud, E. and Orsetti, A. "Evaluation of a Standardized Hyperglucidic Breakfast Test in Postprandial Reactive Hypoglycaemia." *Diabetologia* 38.4 (Apr 1995): 494–501. Print.

76. Brun, J.F. Fedou, C. and Mercier, J. "Postprandial Reactive Hypoglycemia." *Diabetes & Metabolism* 26 (2000): 337–51. Print.

77. Ross, H.M. "Hypoglycemia." *Orthomolecular Psychiatry* 3.4 (1974): 240–45. Print.

78. Petralli, G. "The HPA Axis: The 'Home' of Alcoholism." *Journal of Orthomolecular Medicine* 23.4 (2008): 187–90. Print.

79. Worden, M. and Rosellini, G. "Role of Diet in People-Work: Uses of Nutrition in Therapy with Substance Abusers." *Orthomolecular Psychiatry* 7.4 (1978): 249–57. Print.

80 Tintera, J.W. and Lovell, H.W. "Endocrine Treatment of Alcoholism." *Geriatrics* 4.5 (Sep/Oct 1949): 274–80. Print.

81. Lovell, H.W. and Tintera, J.W. "Hypoadrenocorticism in Alcoholism and Drug Addiction." *Geriatrics* 6.6 (Jan/Feb 1951): 1–11. Print.

82. Wyatt, A. and Dekker, M. "Improving Physician and Medical Education in Substance Abuse Disorders." *Journal of American Osteopathic Association* 1097.9 (2007): ES27–S28. Print.

83. Clark, P., Holder, R., Mullet M., Whitehead, T.P. "Sensitivity and Specificity of Laboratory Tests for Alcohol Abuse." *Alcohol and Alcoholism* 18 (3) (1983): 261–69. Print.

84. Transmetron. "Drug Test—How Long Do Drugs Stay In Your System?" *Drug Detection Window*. TransmetronDrugTest.com, 2010. Web. 5 Sept. 2011. http://www.drugdetectionwindow.com.

85. ExperTox. "Toxicology Tests: Frequently Asked Questions." *ExperTox: Drugs, Alcohol, Poisons Laboratory*. 2011. Web. 5 Sept. 2011. http://www.expertox.com/index.php.

86. West Midlands Toxicology Laboratory. "Drugs of Abuse Guidelines." *Drugs of Abuse Guidelines*. 2010. Web. 5 Sept. 2011. http://www.toxlab.co.uk/dasguide.htm.

87. Mulready, P.A. "Chapter 12: Diagnostic Tools." *Nutritional Pearls To Enhance Recovery*. Time To Live Better.com LLC. 4 July 2011. 57–62. E-book. http://www.timetolivebetter.com.

88. Heller, J.L. and Zieve, D. "Toxicology Screen." *Medline Plus*. National Institutes of Health: U.S. National Library of Medicine, 12 Jan. 2011. Web. 5 Sept. 2011. http://www.nlm.nih.gov/medlineplus/ency/article/003578.htm.

89. American Psychiatric Association. "DSM-5: The Future of Psychiatric Diagnosis." 2010. Web. 5 Sept. 2011. http://www.dsm5 .org/Pages/Default.aspx.

90. Alcohol and Drug Abuse Institute Library. "Screening and Assessment Instruments." University of Washington. Jan. 2011. Web. 5 Sept. 2011. http://lib.adai.washington.edu.

91. Center for Social Work Research. "Alcohol and Substance Abuse Measurement Instrument Collection." The Addiction Research Institute. The University of Texas at Austin. Web. 5 Sept. 2011. http://www.utexas.edu/research/cswr/nida/instrumentListing.html.

92. Cherpitel, C.J. "Screening for Alcohol Problems in the U.S. General Population: Comparison of the CAGE, RAPS4 and RAPS-QF by Gender, Ethnicity and Service Utilization." *Alcohol Clin Exp Res* 26.11 (2002): 1686–91. Print.

32 Bipolar Disorder

An Environmental and Nutritional Approach to Therapy

Alan R. Vinitsky, M.D., and Ronald R. Parks, M.D.

INTRODUCTION

Bipolar illness (BPI) is a major cause of pain and suffering for which conventional medical and psychiatric treatments provide but modest remediation. BPI is characterized by bouts of illness with relatively disease-free states in between and subclinical states as well. Therefore, BPI can be viewed as a continuum of disease, where it may be possible to consider underlying metabolic aberrations associated with the disease state. A continuum model of BPI further allows interconnected disciplines of psychophysiology, biochemistry, psychopharmacology, toxicology, genetics, psychology, sociology, as well as nutritional, environmental, and psychiatric medicine to inform treatment decisions. In this chapter, environmental and nutritional models offer insights into disease prognosis and prevention of relapse.

DEFINITION AND EPIDEMIOLOGY

The official nomenclature has been codified and defined in the fourth edition of the *Diagnostic and Statistical Manual of Mental Disorders* (*DSM-IV-TR*, with *DSM-V* anticipated) [1]. Bipolar I disorder describes a sufferer who experienced distinct periods of severe depression alternating with at least one episode of severe activation or mania, while bipolar II disorder had no distinct mania (see Table 32.1).

Both bipolar I and bipolar II can be devastating and severe. The difference between them is that by definition bipolar I must have had at least one manic episode, while bipolar II can present with hypomania. Mania may later present in a bipolar II individual, resulting in reclassification. Recurrent depression is characteristic of both conditions, and the depth of the depression usually determines overall severity. Some subtler bipolar I—more often bipolar II—present with irritability, anxiety, and moodiness, and alternating hard-to-define recurrent depression. Bipolar spectrum illness has been defined as recurrent depression with milder periods of activation (hypomania) and less dramatic symptoms [2].

Clinical presentations tend to vary. Diagnosed depression is often bipolar disorder misdiagnosed [3,4]. Additional clues to diagnosis include: poor response to treatments for depression, mania, psychosis, or induced rapid mood fluctuations triggered by antidepressants, family history of bipolar illness, onset of recurrent depression before the 20s, severe premenstrual syndrome (PMS) or premenstrual dysphoria syndrome (PMDS), postpartum depression, atypical depressions with a lot of irritability, sleep disturbance, and anxiety. Presentations of BPI in the older population (> 50 years) more often have comorbidities at the time of diagnosis, including cognitive changes [5].

TABLE 32.1
Bipolar Disorder I and II Characteristics

Bipolar Classification	Type I	Type II	Cyclothymia
Presentation	Distinct period of abnormal mood with at least one manic episode	Distinct period of mood change with no mania to date	Distinct periods of mood change less severe than type 1 or 2
Mood	1. Persistently elevated, expansive 2. Irritable mood 3. May include psychotic symptoms	At least one hypomanic episode	Fluctuation
Additional Symptoms 1. Unusually confident 2. Inflated self-esteem 3. Needs less sleep 4. Unusually talkative or pressure to keep talking 5. Racing thoughts or flight of ideas 6. Trouble concentrating 7. Distractibility 8. More goal-directed activity 9. Engages in pleasurable, high-risk activities, with painful consequences 10. Acts strangely	Three symptoms or four if irritable mood is present	Three symptoms or four if irritable mood is present	Symptoms are milder
Duration	At least seven days	At least four days	Fewer days
Depression	Usually one or more	One or more	Multiple cycles

Note: Based on *DSM IV-TR* criteria—the term bipolar spectrum disorder includes cyclothymia. Rapid cycling of any of the aforementioned applies to four or more mood changes in one year.

BPI is not uncommon. The epidemiology and lifetime prevalence estimates are 1.0% for bipolar I disorder, 1.1% for bipolar II disorder, and 2.4% to 4.7% for sub-threshold BPI [2,6]. Age at onset ranges from childhood to mid-20s and later, and BPI is unusual after the fourth decade. Recurrence rates of BPI over a five-year period are close to 100%, with periods of no symptoms, minor symptoms, or with more significant residual symptoms.

At its worst, it can lead to higher mortality from suicide and concurrent medical illness. Among psychiatric disorders, BPI has one of the highest rates of mortality from suicide—bipolar II is greater than bipolar I. Unrecognized co-occurrence of BPI and medical illness can lead to ineffectual treatment and poor outcomes. Six months after suffering myocardial infarction, victims with major depression (commonly seen in BPI) had six times the mortality of nondepressed patients [7].

Recurrence of bipolar episodes with depression, mania, or hypomania has adverse effects on family, social, and occupational functioning [8–13]. BPI disrupts normative functioning across spheres: social functioning such as failures of social relationships and work life, productivity, sleep disturbance, anxiety, depression, overactivation of mind or behavior (i.e., mania or hypomania), and irritability; cognitive functioning with impaired thinking and distraction; physical well-being with somatic pain and propensity for addictions; and emotional functioning evidenced by impulsivity, loss of interest or pleasure and of motivation, and suicidal thinking [14,15].

Appreciating the breadth of impairment adds urgency to diagnosis and initiation of treating any underlying metabolic dysfunction. Effectively treated, bipolar I sufferers—even those with recurrent hospitalizations for mania and depression—can become stable, functional, and productive for years.

PATHOGENESIS

GENETICS AND THE EARLY ENVIRONMENT

Epidemiologic studies support genetic risk factors in BPI. First-degree relatives of people with BPI are seven times more likely to develop bipolar I than the general population. Adopted children whose biologic parents have either BPI or a major depressive disorder remain at increased risk of developing an affective disorder. However, identical twins develop BPI at wide-ranging concordance rates of 33–90%, pointing to environmental factors affecting expression of susceptibility genes [16]. ANK3, CACNA1C, and CLOCK genes are identified in BPI, especially bipolar I [17–23].

Advanced parental age (APA) is an established risk factor for BPI [24]. APA is a summary marker because it reflects both elevated risk for genetic mutations and epigenetic factors.

Epigenetic factors also influence gene expression. The epigenome is a layer above the genetic code that regulates DNA depending on environmental inputs. Methylation of DNA, histones, and microsomal RNA is critical in suppressing or expressing certain genes that present as BPI or other neuropsychiatric disorders [25–29]. Examples include hypomethylation of serotonin type 2-A gene (HTR2A at T102C polymorphic site) [30], MB-COMT promoter [31], GAD1 promoter [32], and noncoding microRNA, which affects DISC1 and DISC2 [33] each of which increase the expression of BPI. In a postmortem brain tissue study, the hippocampus is a site of decreased mRNA expression of 43 mitochondrial oxidative phosphorylation and ATP-dependent processes [34]. Other loci of genetic change include the frontal and temporal lobes.

Epigenetic factors are of particular interest because methylation of DNA not only affects genetic expression in utero, it affects genetic expression throughout life, albeit to a much lesser extent, affording an opportunity to modify outcomes through facilitating impaired methylation.

EXTERNAL ENVIRONMENTAL FACTORS

BPI symptomatology is influenced by physical, chemical, and biologic factors in the external environment (Table 32.2). An example of a biologic factor is Pediatric Autoimmune Neuropsychiatric

---

TABLE 32.2
Environmental Factors

Biological	Chemical	Physical
Algae	Air pollutants	Desynchronosis resulting from travel across time zones or shift work
Bacteria	Heavy metals	Geographic latitude and elevation
Molds and Yeasts	Pesticides	Natural disasters
Parasites	Solvents and other volatile organic compounds	Particulates and other physical matter from construction
Viruses	Water pollutants	Radiation
Worms		Trauma

Many of these factors influence a person's health on a continuing basis. They must be considered in the context of explaining why (s)he is expressing symptoms, such as anxiety or depression. These factors are ordinarily ignored because they are so commonplace. For 15–30% of the population [79], environmental exposures are a source of stress on the autonomic nervous system and metabolic pathways. Inflammation may develop over time, resulting in symptoms such as anxiety or depression. In a chronic state, those symptoms may be indistinguishable from bipolar disorder. Multiple opportunities exist for extensive environmental exposure. Water damage in home, work, and school may promote a setting for microbes and generate particulates. Unexpected natural disasters and terrorist attacks could release radiation. Combustion of debris and fuel oil provide additional contaminations.

Disease Associated with Streptococcal infection (PANDAS). Since other infections and noninfectious environmental exposures can trigger a similar response, the term has been broadened to Pediatric Acute Onset Neuropsychiatric Syndrome (PANS). Metabolic effects of biotoxins including mycotoxins, and possible treatment approaches are detailed in this book (Chapter 44: Biotoxins and Chapter 43: Mycotoxin-Related Illness).

An example of a chemical factor is mercury exposure, giving rise to the expression "mad as a hatter." Haberdashers had an occupational exposure to mercury-cured furs.

An example of a physical factor is springtime in high-latitude environments, where changes in solar, barometric, and other factors in the physical environment exert effects significant enough to trigger BPI. Concurrent depletion of nutrients from diminished intake of fruits/vegetables in spring may also predispose, as can seasonal allergies [35]. Another physical factor may be exposure to ionizing and/or nonionizing radiation (Chapter 42: Electromagnetic Hypersensitivity).

Figure 32.1 [36] illustrates how diverse factors from our external environment alter the internal chemical environment, thereby predisposing us or protecting us from disease states to which we are vulnerable. Summary lab tests, more of which will be forthcoming from ongoing "omics" research, serve as biomarkers for the treatment-responsive underlying pathophysiology.

INTERNAL FACTORS, SPECIFICALLY METHYLATION

Methylation and aberrations in the methylation pathways are aspects of the internal chemical environment central to BPI pathophysiology. The rationale is as follows:

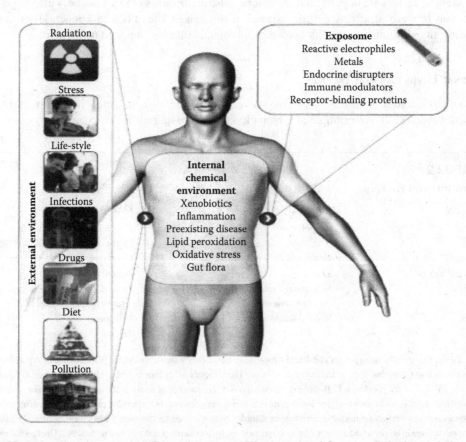

FIGURE 32.1   The exposome is influenced by external environmental factors and the internal chemical environment. Reproduced with permission from Rappoport 2010.

- An unknown but substantial portion of BPI expression results from the epigenomic effects of hypomethylation.
- Methylation generates adrenalin from norepinephrine and inactivates adrenalin, norepinephrine, and dopamine. Insufficient methylation can result in excess neurotransmitters that exacerbate anxiety.
- The first metabolite of acetylcholine includes the intrinsic production of formaldehyde, which raises sympathetic nervous system (SNS) activity, resulting in anxiety.
- Concurrent with inadequate methylation, protein destruction is ongoing, and synthesis of proteins and neurotransmitters is insufficient.
- Methylation is associated with reduction of bipolar gene expression, improvement in production and metabolism of neurotransmitters, stabilizing the autonomic nervous system (ANS), and improvement of comorbid conditions.

The production of S-adenosylmethionine (SAMe) is required for more than 50 methylation pathways present throughout the body [37]. SAMe is generated (Figure 32.2) by recycling methionine, an essential amino acid, through homocysteine, which is toxic at high levels.

Human biology has evolved a redundant pathway that bypasses the folate and hydroxocobalamin remethylation process of Figure 32.2. The redundant pathway is utilized when inadequate folate and hydroxocobalamin are available for the primary pathway and when methylation demands are excessive. The redundant pathway depends on betaine and zinc.

Methylation is a phase II detoxification pathway and as such influences neurohormonal and neurotransmitter balances. Methyl transferases use SAMe to methylate. Catechol-O-methyltransferase (COMT) processes adrenalin, norepinephrine, dopamine, l-dopa, methyldopa, and catechol estrogens. Vulnerability is in part genetic, since a single nucleotide polymorphism of COMT can lead to impaired metabolism of catechols and result in increased anxiety, which further potentiates the risk for BPI. Methylation inactivates histamine, serotonin, and converts melatonin from serotonin [38]. SAMe donates a methyl group to process estrogen, xenoestrogens, many heavy metals, and niacin, synthesize RNA, repair DNA, and create creatine.

OXIDATIVE STRESS AND METHYLATION

The primary methylation resources to ensure ample supply of SAMe are: folic acid, hydroxocobalamin, and reduced-glutathione. Their interaction is illustrated in Figures 32.3 and 32.4.

Oxidative stress increases malondialdehyde [39] and other aldehydes. Inflammation stress raises nitric oxide [40] and lowers glutathione. The degradation of glutathione (GSH) by increased gamma-glutamyl transaminase (GGT) further lowers GSH, while generating glutamate. Life stress also generates the same stress markers, and the concomitant need for increased ascorbate further depletes active reduced GSH.

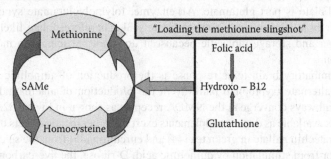

FIGURE 32.2 Loading the methionine slingshot: Methionine must ultimately be available to generate SAMe. In the simplest form of the "slingshot," hydroxocobalamin is activated by reduced glutathione. Activated folic acid then donates a methyl group to hydroxocobalamin yielding methylcobalamin.

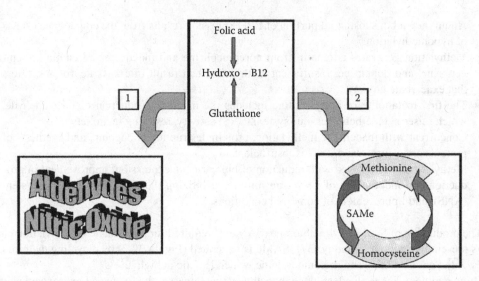

FIGURE 32.3 Stress marker cleanup is a necessary prerequisite to production of SAMe. 1) Folic acid (folate) scavenges for malondialdehyde and other aldehydes. Hydroxcobalamin (OH-B12) scavenges for nitric oxide, and reduced glutathione is depleted as it scavenges for toxins, such as mercury, pesticides, and solvents, or is oxidized while functioning as an antioxidant. 2) If one or more of these three scavengers is in short supply, methylation will be compromised for a lack of sufficient SAMe. Pharmacologic dosing of folate and hydroxy-cobalamine (OH-B12) in sufficient doses are required to clean up aldehydes and nitric oxide.

The enzyme paraoxonase is another place in the methylation pathways vulnerable to nutrient depletion and environmental toxicants, as shown in Figure 32.5.

INFLAMMATION AND METHYLATION

BPI has confirmed increased inflammation, separate from hypomethylation, yet with several inter-secting pathways, such as nitric oxide synthase (iNOS) [41]. Cleanup of inflammation begins with hydroxocobalamin (see Figure 32.4) scavenging for nitric oxide. As cortisol levels decrease when stress is reduced, inflammation may become more noticeable. As immune mechanisms strengthen, increased cellular, antibody, and cytokine inflammatory responses are observed. This transforma-tion permits detection of previously hidden etiologies for psychiatric and other symptoms as anti-body production may become more robust.

Another aspect of inflammation is the excitatory effect of glutamate on the N-Methyl-D-Aspartate (NMDA) receptor. An additional observation is that there is glutamate spillover in its regulation of synapses [42]. Glutamate rises in response to elevated cortisol and stimulates the NMDA receptor. Folate is part glutamate. An enzyme, folylpolyglutamate synthase, can attach multiple glutamate molecules one at a time to folate [43]. Therefore, folate likely functions as a glutamate scavenger and storage molecule because it does not participate in methylation in the polyglutamate form.

A notable inflammatory brain toxic response is the production of quinolinic acid, which is a metabolite of the alternate tryptophan pathway in the production of niacinamide (Figure 32.6). These metabolic pathways converge at the NMDA receptor as shown in Figure 32.7.

Several nutrients available as dietary supplements exert their therapeutic effects on the Figure 32.6 pathway. Epigallocatechin gallate in green tea [44] and curcumin [45] from the spice turmeric block the NMDA receptor from stimulation by quinolinic acid. D-ribose, the five-carbon sugar precursor to ATP, may further promote the conversion of quinolinic acid to niacinamide. Sufficiently high doses of niacinamide 500 mg administered twice daily can push back on quinolinic acid production, thereby reducing its neurotoxic effect. Other powerful anti-inflammatories include quercetin, which

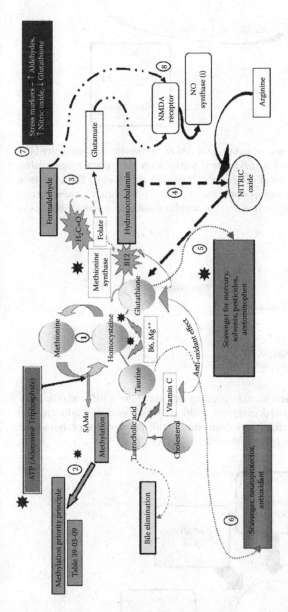

FIGURE 32.4 Sustaining methylation:

1. Methionine + Adenosine → S-Adenosyl Methionine (SAMe) → S-Adenosyl Homocysteine → Homocysteine → Methionine.

2. Methylation need is increased when an individual is stressed. Specific stressors requiring methylation further exacerbate the stressed state, thereby destabilizing the autonomic nervous system.

3. Folate scavenges for aldehydes and glutamate and recycles aldehydes through hydroxocobalamin (OH-B12) to homocysteine.

4. OH-B12 is reduced by glutathione but also scavenges for nitric oxide (NO) and peroxynitrite. OH-B12 can be inactivated by NO.

5. Glutathione (GSH) scavenges for mercury, pesticides, solvents, and acetominophen. GSH can be inactivated by NO, reduces vitamin C (ascorbate) or is reduced by it.

6. Taurine scavenges for hypochlorite and other chlorine-containing compounds. Taurine, magnesium, and vitamin B6 (pyridoxine) encourage the production of GSH, when homocysteine is converted to cysteine.

7. Oxidative physical and emotional stresses lead to increased aldehydes, nitric oxide, and oxidized glutathione (or less available reduced GSH).

8. Nitric oxide causes increased pain and inflammation through the inducible nitric oxide synthase (iNOS) pathway, which is potentiated by formaldehyde, glutamate, quinolinic acid (derived from tryptophan), carbon monoxide (from heme degradation via hemoxygenase), acidity, and solvents.

* indicates six pathways where mercury interrupts support of methylation: When nutrients are diverted for scavenging or are inactivated alone or in combination, methylation will become inadequate under stress. If OH-B12 is insufficient or dysfunctional, then methylation cannot adequately proceed. When GSH is insufficient or dysfunctional, OH-B12 is dysfunctional. In either instance, folate becomes functionally insufficient, even when levels are elevated, because it is saturated with methyl groups and aldehydes. This condition is called the folate trap [80].

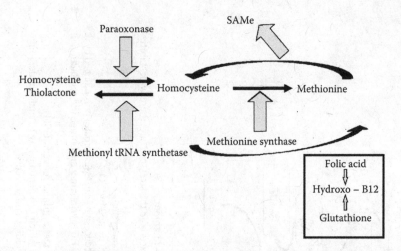

FIGURE 32.5   Thiolactone: Homocysteine thiolactone denatures proteins and promotes autoimmunity [46]. The tendency for this continuous destructive process is inevitable if methylation nutrients are unavailable. Paraoxonase draws thiolactone back into the loop. This enzyme is upregulated by methionine. Thus, this loop functions like a vortex. Paraoxonase is inhibited by mercury [47] and isoleucine [48]. Paraoxonase is carried by HDL protein. Thus, the association is drawn to hyperlipemias and insulin resistance, as comoribidities in elderly BPI.

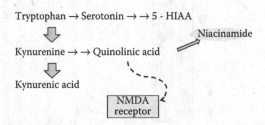

FIGURE 32.6   Quinolinic acid metabolism is critical to understanding inflammation in BPI and other neurologic conditions. Tryptophan shifts to the alternate kynurenine pathway, which provokes inflammation through quinolinic acid. Many neuropsychiatric conditions are dominated by this pathway. Excess quinolinic acid may be generated from the body as a whole—especially the liver.

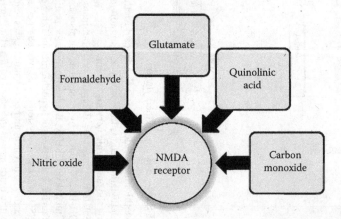

FIGURE 32.7.   NMDA stimulation: multiple agonists trigger inflammation at the NMDA receptor site. These include formaldehyde, nitric oxide, glutamate, quinolinic acid, carbon monoxide, acid (H+ ion), and solvents.

blocks NF-Kappa B, along with curcumin, vitamin D3 [49], and the proteolytic enzyme bromelain. The higher order omega-3 fatty acids exert anti-inflammatory effects, which may underlie their demonstrated benefit in BPI [50].

PATIENT EVALUATION

SCREENING FOR MODIFIABLE, EXTERNAL ENVIRONMENTAL FACTORS

Modifiable, external, environmental factors exert direct, measurable, demonstrated effects on methylation. Identifying some of the factors is a critical step to patient treatment, especially the factors of which the patient is not aware and can be easily removed or reduced. These factors are categorized in Table 32.2 and examples from the authors' clinics include:

- Low level, chronic carbon monoxide poisoning.
- Home, school, and office construction including renovation materials, carpeting, and glues and paints that generate aldehydes. Once inhaled, these demand additional aldehyde scavenging from folate.
- Alcohol consumption leads to increased acetaldehyde as a metabolite and increases folate demand.
- Tobacco smoke contains many toxins that use up folate, hydroxocobalamin, glutathione, and vitamin C.
- The stress of travel, injury, altitude, and work stress can, alone or in combination, raise adrenalin production and its inactivation, both of which require additional SAMe for methylation. Dehydration can raise histamine levels, which further increases methylation demands for its inactivation [51].
- Orthopedic injuries require increased protein production through RNA synthesis for bone production and muscle rebuilding.
- Lyme and other tick-borne coinfections are associated with neuroinflammation.
- Housecats are underestimated as a source of occult viral infections, toxoplasmosis, and bartonellosis.
- Food poisoning and dysbiosis are associated with biotoxin production and decreased nutrient absorption.
- Indoor water damage and the resulting remediation and renovation are major sources of exposure. Particulates, microbes, indoor mold, and biotoxins secondary to water-damage stresses genetically predisposed persons. Resulting neuroinflammation, autoimmunity, and hormonal disruptions—including hypothyroidism and antidiuretic hormone depletion—are potential consequences.
- Microbicides can affect some people and can be found in construction materials as well as food residues.
- Renovation materials—new wallboard, synthetic carpet, padding, and paint—contain formaldehyde and other volatile hydrocarbons.
- Recent dental work and amalgam fillings contribute mercury and other toxic metals, which impair methylation (Figure 32.4).

ASSESSMENT OF CONCURRENT MEDICAL CONDITIONS

Among the reasons BPI is associated with poor outcomes in concurrent medical conditions is common underlying metabolic dysfunction. Addressing the concurrent medical conditions can therefore correspondingly treat BPI. By way of illustration Table 32.3 lists the medical conditions concurrent in Vinitsky's patients with mood disorders.

TABLE 32.3
Concurrent Medical Diagnoses among Patients with Mood Disorders Presenting to Consultant Medical Practice

ICD	Diagnosis
270.8, 270.9	Amino Acid Deficiency
269.3	Mineral Deficiency (zinc, copper, selenium, magnesium, and others)
266.2	B12, B Vitamin Deficiency
080	Tick-borne: Lyme, Babesia, Ehrlichia, Bartonella
780	Fatigue
240–246	Thyroid Conditions
255	Adrenals (usually adrenal fatigue)
V83.89, V84	Genetic (polymorphisms)
780, 327.20	Sleep Apnea
337.1	Autonomic [includes all diagnoses or suspected]
279.9	Immune Disorder
401	Blood Pressure
985	Metals (mercury, cadmium, lead, arsenic, and others)
272	Cholesterol
281.0, 281.1	Pernicious Anemia & Other B12
470	Rhinitis
995.3	Environmental Sensitivities
337.1	Autonomic First Visit Only
493, 518.89, 786.09	Asthma, Restrictive, Short of Breath
082, 083, 135	Rickettsia, Q Fever, Sarcoid
250	Diabetes
075, 078, 483	EBV, CMV, Mycoplasma
008.47, 112.85	Dysbiosis
346	Migraine
288	Neutropenia
729	Fibromyalgia
136	Parasite
691	Eczema
790.6	Low Iron (Ferritin)
414	Coronary Artery Disease
710, 711, 714	Rheumatoid, Lupus, Arthropathy
530	GERD
780.93	Memory Loss
696	Psoriasis
784	Headache
079, 058	Coxsackie Virus, Parvovirus, Herpes
344.9	Mitral Valve Prolapse
728	Muscle Spasm
277.6, 708, 995.1	Urticaria
021, 023, 130	Tularemia, Brucella, Toxoplasmosis
440	Atherosclerosis

These diagnoses were included in the differential diagnoses at the time of presentation and are presented in the order of relative frequency. Over eight years, 399 patients with psychiatric conditions carried 540 diagnoses. Those codes ranging from 290–320 are not included. Of those, 63 mood disorders (11.7%) were identified, the majority of which were major depressive disorders. ICD-9 codes are American Medical Association derived, and these designations correspond to *DSM IV–TR* codes of the American Psychiatric Association.

Assessment of the Internal Chemical Environment for Nutrients and Toxicants

In patients with BPI, evaluation of serum vitamin B12, folate, and homocysteine require additional explanation. When these tests are within the normal laboratory range and a patient has symptomatic BPI, a likely scenario is that vitamin B12 and folate are functionally low [52], and methionine is depleted so that the vitamin B12 and folate are underutilized. Once these patients' stress markers are treated with simultaneous hydroxocobalamin and folate, previously normal levels of these vitamins will rise until methionine deficiency is recognized by a homocysteine level less than 6, and must also be treated. In patients with mood disorders, B12 levels of less than 500 are frequently associated with ANS dysfunction providing additional evidence that levels are inadequate for the metabolic demands [53–55].

A high normal mean cell volume (MCV) is a marker for inefficient vitamin B12 utilization and often suggests glutathione inadequacy. Low MCV implies iron deficiency, which is also associated with fatigue, and low MCV can also represent lead toxicity or B6 deficiency. Since ineffective vitamin B12 utilization can be concurrent with iron deficiency, inadequate vitamin B6 or lead toxicity, an MCV at a normal level may merely represent averages of metabolic dysfunction.

Another laboratory test, less often utilized, is a 24-hour urine collection for amino acids. In Vinitsky's clinic, patients with mood disorders prior to methylation support are consistently low in four amino acids: phosphoethanolamine, hydroxyproline, asparagine, and isoleucine. As treatment progresses, these amino acids may begin to normalize, even without amino acid supplementation. Additional considerations are as follows:

- Choline can be synthesized from phosphoethanolamine (the first of four amino acid deficiencies described earlier) in a series of steps that eventually requires three SAMe molecules. If it remains functional as phosphatidyl choline, it can be incorporated into cell membranes. As a precursor to acetylcholine, choline [37] is often deficient. When choline is assimilated into acetylcholine, that process heals; but choline, when metabolized, generates its first metabolite as formaldehyde, which is potently hypersympathetic and requires folate to scavenge. Carnitine (tri-methyl lysine) and betaine (tri-methyl glycine) also require SAMe for proper synthesis, and should therefore be supplemented only after methylation support is initiated.
- Asparagine facilitates oligosaccharide synthesis in the pituitary, such as thyroid stimulating hormone (TSH) [56]. Asparagine depletion functions to protect adrenal function, which supercedes thyroid function. Patients with BPI are among the many patients who have low body temperature, but whose TSH is normal, and among those patients with altered salivary cortisol levels, but who are not diagnosed as adrenally insufficient by standard synthetic ACTH stimulation. However, by applying methylation treatments as a foundation, asparagine levels improve without supplementation, and TSH levels begin to rise, leading to detection of a previously hidden hypothyroid state.
- Isoleucine is a precursor to methylmalonic acid (MMA) [57], which yields succinic acid. This second step requires vitamin B12. MMA is often used as a marker for vitamin B12 deficiency, since this pathway is the only one exclusive to vitamin B12. This form of B12 is actually adenosylcobalamin, which forms from adenosine + activated OH-B12 (which depends on glutathione). It is hypothesized that as MMA increases due to vitamin B12 deficiency, isoleucine is not needed, resulting in its depletion. Over time, MMA will return to normal. Note that isoleucine or glutathione deficiency can result in normal MMA, even when vitamin B12 is also deficient. Thus, MMA is not a reliable predictor of B12 deficiency in chronic illness. Isoleucine also inhibits paraoxonase (see Figure 32.5). It is possible that the loss of isoleucine will allow paraoxonase to remain more active, permitting thiolactone to return to the pathway that generates SAMe and serving as an adaptive mechanism. Isoleucine reduces hepatic gluconeogenesis and drives glucose into muscle when fed to fasting rats [58]. Hence, isoleucine depletion may over time contribute to rising glucose and lead to insulin resistance and type 2 diabetes comorbidity of BPI.

USING PHYSICAL EVALUATION OF THE AUTONOMIC NERVOUS SYSTEM AS AN APPROACH TO MONITOR IMPROVEMENT IN BPI

Typically, BPI criteria for improvement are reflected in stability of mood, functioning in different settings, and in clinical trials, a variety of administered screening scales. However, these parameters are focused on the disorder itself, not the broader ranging effects of methylation and other metabolic consequences. Stress manifests metabolically as increased malondialdehyde (oxidative stress), nitric oxide (inflammation stress), and the depletion of reduced glutathione. Glutathione may be measured, but at present, malondialdehyde and nitric oxide are not routinely measured, as these levels are in constant flux. However, the consequences of stress markers and their reduction can be observed through the autonomic nervous system [59–61].

Autonomic nervous system (ANS) dysfunction can be assessed in the review of symptoms, which include dizziness, especially on change of position, often presenting with cold hands and feet. When impaired, the ANS demonstrated a rigidity of function with the parasympathetic (PSNS) and sympathetic (SNS) systems not commensurate with physiologic demands (Table 32.4). Additional symptoms are balance disturbance in the dark (confirmed on physical exam with eyes closed), dry mucus membranes, lack or excess of secretions and sweating, unexplained shortness of breath and

---

TABLE 32.4
Neuropsychiatric and Behavioral Paradoxes May Manifest When the Autonomic Nervous System (ANS) Functions in a Rigid, Paradoxical Manner

Function	Sympathetic Overshoots or Parasympathetic Undershoots	Parasympathetic Overshoots or Sympathetic Undershoots
Sleep	Can't fall asleep, mid-sleep wakeups, early wakeups, phase shifts	Excessive sleepiness, daytime sleepiness
Behavior	Angry, impulsive, hyperactive, violent	Withdrawn, sluggish, lacking motivation
Concentration	Impaired	Impaired
Memory	Impaired	Impaired
Mood	Anxiety	Depression
Thinking	Altered	Altered
	Obsessive	Slowed
	Suicidal	Suicidal
Judgment	Impaired	Impaired
Movement	Tics, tremors, twitches, myoclonic jerks, hyperactivity	Not impaired
Electrical	Seizures	Not impaired
Coordination	Impaired	Impaired
Apraxia	Writing, speech–articulation	Not present
Balance	Dizziness	Impaired
Toe Balance	Impaired	Impaired
Heel-Toe Gait	Impaired	Impaired
Vertigo	Present	Not present
Socialization	Possible autistic spectrum	No consistent impairment

An "overshoot" represents the intrusion of an ANS branch into an organ system where it was not expected to be functioning. An "undershoot" means that one branch of the ANS does not perform as expected, thereby allowing its opposite to overperform. The more rigid the ANS, the wider are the swings and fluctuations. In the physical exam, balance disturbance with eyes closed reflects these gyrations. Contrast smooth efficient performance with overshoots/undershoots (overcompensation/ undercompensation) of slow performance, missteps, truncal wobble, breathing disturbance—rapid breathing or breath-holding, sweating, eyes tearing, and nervous laughter.

palpitations, increased urinary frequency and nocturia, and altered gastrointestinal patterns. As more systems are affected, the greater the ANS impairment. Organs other than the adrenal glands are under PSNS control.

ANS dysfunction and improvements in function can be observed on physical exam as follows:

- Alterations in blood pressure and heart rate can be assessed at rest and with short-term position change, and, when necessary, standing in one position with no movement for up to five minutes. Changes may occur from supine to standing, with an excessively brisk rise in heart rate (30 beats per minute from supine to stand) such as seen in postural orthostatic tachycardia syndrome (POTS). Twenty-beat increases usually reflect dehydration, while drops in blood pressure without compensating rise in heart rate may indicate neuropathy or adrenal dysfunction. In Vinitsky's experience, white coat hypertension is autonomic dysfunction, with hidden or obvious mercury burden.
- Cold hands and feet are sometimes present, and the patient may report this as a chronic symptom.
- Jaw clicking implies temporo-mandibular joint dysfunction. It may also suggest an under-lying impairment in ANS. The jaw is generally under PSNS control, as demonstrated by a yawn followed by a breath.
- Balance and coordination dysfunction can be present. The Romberg test is usually nega-tive. Finger-nose and finger-finger testing are sometimes abnormal. Fine tremor may be present with increased sympathetic nervous system activity and mercury burden. Single-foot balance, toe balance, tandem heel-toe, and static heel-toe are used to establish base-line ANS testing and monitor progress with treatment. Balance tests can be conducted first with the patient's eyes open and then with them closed. Standardizing these balance tests for 10-second trials helps the comparison. Toe-balance trials (heels raised off the floor) are repeated five times with eyes closed, for up to 10 seconds each, after one or more base-line eyes-open trial of 10 seconds. Repeat sets gather more information. Interpretations: Inability to balance with eyes open implies sensory neuropathy. Impaired toe balance with eyes closed reflects stressful breathing (increased SNS when PSNS should be domi-nant). Improvements identify a learning curve, while decline in performance on repeat sets reflects fatigue. A second successful eyes-open trial performed for 10 seconds con-firms the impairment during eyes closed. A second set of five, eyes closed, and third eyes open is confirmatory. For tandem heel-toe, 10 steps can be timed, forward and reverse. Errors are recorded. Normal in Vinitsky's clinic is 7–10 seconds without errors, eyes open or closed. Slower performance and more errors reflect greater ANS dysfunction. Static heel-toe substitutes for failure to complete tandem testing (when there is no physical dis-ability), and suggests greater ANS impairment. Place right foot in front of left, eyes open for 10 seconds, then close eyes for up to 10 seconds additional. Repeat the trial with feet reversed. Also record body language such as rapid breathing, breath holding, truncal wob-ble, nervous laughter, paradoxical tears, frustration, anger, and so on.

TREATMENT CONSIDERATIONS

DRUG NUTRIENT INTERACTIONS

Antidepressants

Antidepressants, such as citalopram or sertraline (selective serotonin reuptake inhibitors—SSRIs) raise serotonin levels by allowing serotonin to remain in the nerve synapses for a long period of time. Some patients may become paradoxically anxious if there are insufficient methylation resources available (see earlier discussion concerning methylation and quinolinic acid production).

A single-valent cation, lithium is a cousin of sodium and potassium in the Periodic Table of Elements. Lithium has been extensively studied and has been available by prescription since 1970, as lithium carbonate to treat BPI. Even though lithium is a prescription medication, lithium orotate and lithium aspartate are available without a prescription in the United States and are regulated in the category of dietary supplements. These forms of lithium are bioactive and are sometimes found in supplements claiming to boost mood.

The daily lithium dietary intake as estimated by the Environmental Protection Agency (EPA) in 1985 was 650–3100 µg for a 70-kg man. Per Schrauzer, 1000 µg (1 mg) is a daily recommended amount [62]. Dietary sources of lithium are grains and green vegetables. There are no reports of lithium deficiency, but it is reasonable to speculate that such is possible, given lithium's favorable neurological benefits, relative to reversal of dementia, mood stabilization, rise in neurotransmitter levels, neuronal signaling, and neuronal protection [63,64].

Extensive research is available on lithium's mechanism of action [63–68]. Substantial data suggests that lithium favorably influences methylation to modify glutamate metabolism or its effects on dopamine. Lithium has a modifying influence on glutamate by downregulating the NMDA receptor.

However, lithium appears to have opposite effects on methylation—both upregulating and downregulating, depending on site of action. By supporting methylation lithium is more biochemically available to exert its neuropsychiatric benefit. Lyoo et al. reported no change in psychiatric scales while treating with oral choline supplementation, yet there was reduction in purine residues of BPI patients treated with lithium [69]. This observation is important because there appears to be a reworking of signaling pathways and gene expression over time with lithium [64].

Divalproex, or valproate, is thought to decrease DNA methylation of histones—an epigenetic phenomenon—thereby turning off the manic phase of BPI [27]. Another potential site of action is demethylation of GAD67 and GAD1 (glutamic acid decarboxylase) GABAergic promoter site. GAD converts glutamate to GABA, and like all decarboxylases is vitamin B6 dependent. In this scenario, glutamate levels will increase and will act as a brake on dopamine-induced psychosis and mania. Valproate has an effect on chromatin remodeling over time [70]. By contrast, lamotrigine acts on the NMDA receptor to lower glutamate levels, thereby improving depressed mood [71].

Anxiolytics

Anxiolytics such as clonazepam and lorazepam are benzodiazepines, which function by increasing GABA affinity at the $GABA_a$ receptor [72]. These may help, when there is already sufficient GABA being generated from glutamate via GAD65 or GAD67. Lorazepam will not work for mania. Clonazepam does have a reasonable effect on hypomania and mania but may still aggravate or trigger mania [73].

Antipsychotic Medications

Antipsychotic medications' actions are several. Aripiprazole is a complex-functioning dopamine partial agonist/antagonist plus a partial serotonin antagonist for serotonin $5HT_{2A}$ and an agonist for $5HT_{1A}$. If dopamine levels are low, then aripiprazole is a dopamine partial agonist, but when levels are high, then it functions as an antagonist. Risperidone mechanisms are similar to aripiprazole, except that there is no partial agonism for $5HT_1a$. Response rates when compared to placebo are modest in these medications, and their side effects unfavorably influence appetite, inflammation, and blood sugar [74–76] among other metabolic processes shown to burden the body's methylation pathways.

Support of Methylation as Adjunct Treatment

An initial approach to nutritional support of methylation is presented in Table 32.5. Start with 5 mg of folic acid (folate) and 2 mg of hydroxocobalamin (OH-B12) administered sublingually or transbuccally and repeat as needed. Many patients begin treatment on their own. However, for initial dosing, monitor anxious or hesitant patients in the office, while instructing self-monitoring of blood pressure and pulse. Notably, patients with a vitamin B12 level of less than 500 are more likely to have an "adrenalin rush" reaction (BP and pulse increase, feeling cold, jittery, head rush, hungry)

TABLE 32.5
An Approach Using Supplemental Nutrients

Basic 6 Nutrients	Strength	Formulation	Means of Administration	Usual Starting Doses
1. Folic Acid*	5 mg	Liquid, capsules, and tablets	Sublingual or oral	1–2 doses, 3 times daily

Initiate folic acid dosing in a 5 to 2 ratio with hydroxocobalamin—take a fixed ratio of 5 parts folate:2 parts hydroxocobalamin. Target doses: Note that the dosing here may exceed that of recommended use for dietary supplements and should therefore be implemented under physician guidance with monitoring as described.

2. Hydroxocobalamin*	2 mg	Tablets	Sublingual or transbuccal	1–2 doses, 3 times daily
3. Vitamin C	1000 mg	Powder, tablets, (use buffered, ascorbic acid)	Oral (iv also available)	1–3 times daily

Target doses: Note that the dosing here exceeds that of recommended use for dietary supplements and should therefore be implemented under physician guidance.

4. Magnesium	100 mg	Glycinate, malate, aspartate	Oral	2–3 times daily

Target doses: 200 mg, 2–3 times daily. Magnesium malate helps muscles relax and is sometimes used to aid sleep, while aspartate is energizing and should be avoided in patients with anxiety.

5. Taurine	500 mg	Capsules	Oral	2–3 times daily

Target doses: 2 caps, 2–3 times daily. Note that taurine promotes homocysteine recycling and glutathione production.

6. Vitamin B6	50 mg	Pyridoxine, Pyridoxal 5-phosphate	Oral	1–2 twice daily

Target doses: 1–2 caps, 2 times daily. This can be achieved using a multivitamin or vitamin B complex supplement. Note that vitamin B6 promotes vitamin B3 and histamine production [51].

* **Folic acid and hydroxocobalamin should be taken simultaneously sublingually or transbuccally. The optimal ratio is 5:2. The number of doses daily depends on the extent of stress buildup, as reflected in stress markers.**

on their first one or two doses, and again, if they take doses too infrequently. It is thought that adrenals concentrate the first dose to make adrenalin, whereas subsequent doses distribute to tissues to inactivate adrenalin.

Multiple doses of folate/OH-B12 can be administered simultaneously, and patients should be encouraged to become flexible with doses, so long as they monitor and track their progress.

By contrast, intravenous hydroxocobalamin as a sole agent has been introduced to treat cyanide poisoning in 5 gm (5000 mg) doses with successful outcomes. In a study of 136 normal volunteers who received up to 10 gm hydroxocobalamin IV over 30 min, transient rise in blood pressure was observed in some healthy volunteers. Other side effects included "pustular/papular rash, headache, erythema at the injection site, decrease in lymphocyte percentage, nausea, pruritus, chest discomfort, and dysphagia". Two instances of allergy were observed [77].

Supporting nutrients are vitamin C (ascorbate), magnesium, taurine, and vitamin B6, which encourage production and sustained activity of reduced glutathione. Folate and hydroxocobalamin require reduced glutathione. Glutathione and vitamin C are paired antioxidants. The more powerful antioxidant molecule donates its electrons to the oxidized one. Therefore, presence of oxidized ascorbate will result in a shortage of reduced glutathione, since the latter will work to reduce ascorbate.

Glutathione (GSH) supplementation is required when supporting nutrients with additional N-acetyl cysteine (NAC) cannot improve the speed of dissolution of folate/OH-B12 combination in a nonresponding patient. A clue is a rising MCV in the face of current folate/OH-B12dosing. An explanation may include rapid degradation of GSH by gamma-glutamyl transaminase (GGT), releasing excess glutamate. Topical dosing is useful because the skin appears to function as a gate for the body's needs, just as the mucus membranes perform with folate/OH-B12. Sometimes even a small dose of GSH may suddenly speed up folate/OH-B12 dissolution, resulting in the aforementioned adrenalin rush.

Response can be monitored through laboratory testing and other parameters in several ways:

- During treatment at home, patients should keep a diary, recording BP and P, while tracking symptoms and other parameters. These may include the timing of sleep, diet, medications, supplements, relative to the doses of basic 6 nutrients. If BP becomes too low, adjustments of BP medications or hydration may be required. Normalization of methylation should be regarded as primary, as medication doses can often be reduced.
- Homocysteine should be monitored every three months. When it drops below 6 that implies methionine deficiency, which requires methionine supplementation to raise homocysteine back to 6. Such addition increases the power to make more SAMe as the patient needs it, which results in further repair and healing.
- MCV should be monitored every three months. MCV should move toward the middle of the reported lab normal range. Failure to do so reflects impaired B12 utilization, and adjustments in treatment are required.
- Urinary amino acids should begin to normalize phosphoethanolamine, asparagine, and isoleucine. Additional deficiencies may also correct. Timing of improvement may take three to six months, when testing is repeated. Further improvements of these require amino supplementation.
- Immune function improves and autoimmunity decreases, as methylation capacity improves.
- Parameters reflecting other medical conditions that were previously identified and environmental exposures that have been reduced, should improve. These may include metals, inflammation markers relative to mold biotoxins, and antibodies or other indicators relative to infections.
- Response to medications improves and over time need for medication doses reduces.
- Suspect or incorporate into testing any newly uncovered environmental exposure during review of a relapsed or nonresponsive patient.
- To date, genetic testing has not been repeated but may be appropriate over time to document if various polymorphisms have righted themselves through methylation treatment.

METABOLIC APPROACHES TO POOR INITIAL TREATMENT RESPONSE

Most often, responders begin to improve in days to weeks. Suspect nonresponders when treatments work intermittently or improvement simply stops. Also, suspect nonresponders when patient feels no change of daytime alertness, or sense of calm when doses are administered, or ease in preparing to sleep with absence of light. Another sign is the failure of BP and P to decrease after doses or to trend downward overtime.

In Vinitsky's approach, it is important to effectively clean up stress markers with folate/OH-B12 scavenger nutrients, after which methylation can proceed more effectively. Therefore, fixed daily doses is not the rule but a starting point in treatment. Quickly dissolving folate/OH-B12 in the presence of symptoms informs the patient to raise the doses at least in the short term.

Another common cause of poor response is that folate and hydroxocobalamin are dissolving slowly. Always inquire if hydroxocobalamin is used, since patients may substitute methylcobalamin or cyanocobalamin, thinking that these are equivalent. Infrequent dosing will result in a wear-off effect (i.e., return of symptoms), when there are abundant stress markers.

The primary underlying metabolism of nonresponse is that glutathione (GSH) is inactive, not present, not being created, or excessively metabolized. Nutrients to support glutathione can be beneficial.

Additional actions include the need to adjust medications, or re-evaluate recent adjustments. This may account for difficulties, when nutrients are added to an ongoing treatment regimen. At times, the previously dosed medication has become too powerful and should be titrated downward. Medication dosing can lead to thyroid and/or adrenal imbalances. Patients taking benzodiazepines for anxiety are more likely to be slow or nonresponders, based on the authors' clinical observations.

Occasionally, MTHFR–C677T, A1298C homozygous for either one, or heterozygous for both, will compromise folate activation. If homocysteine has always been close to normal, then this is not likely a viable issue, but active folate (methyltetrahydrofolate—800 mcg daily) can be added, while continuing folate and hydroxocobalamin at the same doses.

It may be appropriate to test for a COMT (C-O-Methyltransferase) SNP. Someone homozygous for a COMT polymorphism will have slowed utilization of SAMe for catechol metabolism. Mercury can compound this genetic susceptibility.

Hemopyrroluria, if present, has been shown to lead to loss of vitamin B6, zinc, and other nutrients [78] involved in methylation.

Underlying environmental factors and inflammation may be ongoing.

CLINICAL SUMMARY

Bipolar illness in its many forms is a serious, stubborn psychiatric condition. Methylation and other supportive treatments have the potential to positively influence the reduction in symptoms. Given the magnitude that hypomethylation plays in the expression of bipolar symptoms, methylation treatments should be strongly considered for their benefits in improving outcomes. Methylation is also relevant to physician awareness of drug-nutrient interactions in the treatment of BPI and is one possible underlying factor in medication tachyphylaxis. The authors' approach to methylation and correcting metabolic dysfunction are presented.

REFERENCES

1. American Psychiatric Association. *Diagnostic and Statistical Manual of Mental Disorders, Text Revision, DSM-IV-TR*. Fourth edition. Washington, DC: American Psychiatric Association, 2000.
2. Merikangas, KR, R Jin, JP He, et al. "Prevalence and correlates of bipolar spectrum disorder in the World Mental Health Survey Initiative." *Arch Gen Psychiatry* 68, no. 3 (2011): 241–51.
3. Wolkenstein, L, K Bruchmuller, P Schmid, and TD Meyer. "Misdiagnosing bipolar disorder—Do clinicians show heuristic biases?" *Journal of Affective Disorders* 130, no. 3 (2011): 405–12.
4. Frye, MA. "Diagnostic dilemmas and clinical correlates of mixed states in bipolar disorder." *J Clin Psychiatry* 69, no. 5 (2008): e13.
5. Chen, P, I Korobkova, K Busby, and M Sajatovic. "Managing late life bipolar disorder: An update." *Aging Health* 7, no. 4 (2011): 557–71.
6. Calabrese, JR. "Overview of patient care issues and treatment in bipolar spectrum and bipolar II disorder." *J Clin Psychiatry* 69, no. 6 (2008): e18.
7. McIntyre, RS, JK Soczynska, JL Beye, et al. "Medical comorbidity in bipolar disorder: Re-prioritizing unmet needs." *Curr Opin Psychiatry* 20, no. 4 (2007): 406–16.
8. Frasure-Smith, N F Lesperance, and M Talajic. "Depression following myocardial infarction. Impact on 6-month survival." *JAMA*, 270 (Oct 1993): 1819–25.
9. Garcia-Portilla, MP, et al. "Cardiovascular risk in patients with bipolar disorder." *Jl of Affective Disorders* 115, no. 3 (Jun 2009): 302–8.
10. Judd, LL, et al. "Residual symptom recovery from major affective episodes in bipolar disorders and rapid episode relapse/recurrence." *Arch Gen Psychiatry* 65, no. 4 (2008): 386–94.

11. Kessler, RC, P Berglund, O Demler, R Jin, KR Merikangas, and EE Walters. "Lifetime prevalence and age-of-onset distributions of DSM-IV disorders in the National Comorbidity Survey Replication." *Arch Gen Psychiatry* 62 (2005): 593–602.

12. Laursen, TM, T Munk-Olsen, E Agerbo, C Gasse, and PB Mortensen. "Somatic hospital contacts, invasive cardiac procedures, and mortality from heart disease in patients with severe mental disorder." *Arch Gen Psychiatry* 66 (July 2009): 713–20.

13. Crow, S. "Bipolar disorder: Part 1, recent advances in the treatment of bipolar disorder." *Audio Digest Psychiatry.* 39, no. 4 (Feb 21, 2010).

14. Judd, LL, HS Akiskal, PJ Schettler, et al. "A prospective investigation of the natural history of the long-term weekly symptomatic status of bipolar II disorder." *Arch Gen Psychiatry* 60–9 (2003): 261.

15. Judd, LL, HS Akiskal, PJ Schettler, et al. "The long-term natural history of the weekly symptomatic status of bipolar I disorder." *Arch Gen Psychiatry* 59 (2002): 530–37.

16. van der Schot, AC, R Vonk, RGH Brans, et al. "Influence of genes and environment on brain volumes in twin pairs concordant and discordant for bipolar disorder." *Arch Gen Psychiatry* 66, no. 2 (2009): 142–51.

17. Baum, AE, N Akula, M Cabanero, et al. "A genome-wide association study implicates diacylglycerol kinase eta (DGKH) and several other genes in the etiology of bipolar disorder." *Molecular Psychiatry* 13, no. 2 (Feb 2008): 197–207.

18. Wellcome Trust Case Control Consortium. "Genome-wide association study of 14,000 cases of seven common diseases and 3,000 shared controls." *Nature* 447, no. 7145 (Jun 2007): 661–78.

19. Sklar P, Smoller JW, Fan J, et al. "Whole-genome association study of bipolar disorder." *Molecular Psychiatry* 13, no. 6 (Jun 2008): 558–69.

20. Ferreira MA, O'Donovan MC, et al. "Collaborative genome-wide association analysis supports a role for ANK3 and CACNA1C in bipolar disorder." *Nature Genetics* 40, no. 9 (Sep 2008): 1056–58.

21. Sklar P, Ripke S, Scott LJ, et al. "Large-scale genome-wide association analysis of bipolar disorder identifies a new susceptibility locus near ODZ4." *Nature Genetics* 43, no. 10 (Sep 2011): 977–83.

22. Roybal K, Theobold D, Graham A, et al. "Mania-like behavior induced by disruption of CLOCK." *Proceedings of the National Academy of Sciences of the United States of America* 104, no. 15 (Apr 2007): 6406–11.

23. Bhagwagar, Z. "New findings in childhood bipolar disorder—Diagnostic issues in pediatric bipolar disorder." *Medscape.* July 15, 2008. http://www.medscape.org/viewarticle/577360.

24. Frans EM, S Sandin, A Reichenberg, et al. "Advancing paternal age and bipolar disorder." *Arch Gen Psychiatry* 65, no. 9 (Sep 2008): 1034–40.

25. Jirtle, R, A Bernal, and D Skaar. *Epigenetic Medicine.* Edited by Robert A. Meyers. Wiley-VCH Verlag Gmb H & Co. KGaA. October 2011. http://onlinelibrary.wiley.com/doi/10.1002/3527600906. mcb.201100010/pdf (accessed December 26, 2011).

26. Feng, J, S Fouse, and G Fan. "Epigenetic regulation of neural gene expression and neuronal function." *Pediatric Research* 61, no. 5, Pt 2 (2007): 58R–63R.

27. McGowan, PO, and T Kato. "Epigenetics in mood disorders." *Environ Health Prev Med* 13 (2008): 16–24.

28. Higuchi, F, S Uchida, Yamagata H, et al. "State-dependent changes in the expression of DNA of methyl-transferases in mood disorder patients." *Journal of Psychiatric Research* 45 (2011): 1295–1300.

29. Rodenhiser, D, and M Mann. "Epigenetics and human disease: Translating basic biology into clinical applications." *CMAJ* 174, no. 3 (2006): 341–48.

30. Ghadirivasfi, M, S Nohesara, H-R Ahmadkhaniha, et al. "Hypomethylation of the serotonin receptortype-2A gene (HTR2A) at T102C polymorphic site in DNA derived from the saliva of patients with schizophrenia and bipolar disorder." *American Journal of Medical Genetics Part B Neuropsychiatric Genetics* 156, no. 5 (2011): 536–45.

31. Nohesara, S, M Ghadirivasfi, S Mostafavi, et al. "DNA hypomethylation of MB-COMT promoter in the DNA derived from saliva in schizophrenia and bipolar disorder." *Journal of Psychiatric Research* 45, no. 11 (2011): 1432–38.

32. Chen, Y, E Dong, and DR Grayson. "Analysis of the GAD1 promoter: Trans-acting factors and DNA methylation converge on the 5′ untranslated region." *Neuropharmacology* 60 (2011): 1075–87.

33. Mehler, MF, and JS Mattick. "Non-coding RNAs in the nervous system." *J Physiol* 575, no. 2 (2006): 333–41.

34. Konradi C, M Eaton, M MacDonald, et al. 2004. "Molecular evidence for mitochondrial dysfunction in bipolar disorder." Source Archives of *Arch Gen Psychiatry* 61, no. 3 (2004): 300–308. [Erratum appears in *Arch Gen Psychiatry* 61, no. 6 (2004): 538.]

35. Shin, K, A Schaffer, AJ Levitt, and MH Boyle. "Seasonality in a community sample of bipolar, unipolar and control subjects." *Jl of Affective Disorders* 86, no. 1 (2005): 19–25.

36. Rappoport, SM and MT Smith. "Epidemiology: Environment and disease risks." *Science* 330, no. 6003 (Oct 2010): 460–61.

37. Debray, F-G, Y Boulanger, A Khiat, et al. "Reduced brain choline in homocystinuria." *Neurology* 71 (2008): 44–49.

38. Walsh, W. Dr. William Walsh on histamine levels at outreach 2010. 2010. http://www.biobalance.org.au/videos/post/21 (accessed January 30, 2012).

39. Onyango, AN, and N Baba. "New hypotheses on the formation of malondialdehyde and isofurans." *Free Radic Biol Med* 49, no. 10 (2010): 1594–1600.

40. Pall, ML, and JH Anderson. "The vanilloid receptor as a putative target of diverse chemicals in multiple chemical sensitivity." *Archives of Environmental Health* 59, no. 7 (2004): 363–75.

41. Rao, JS, JG Harry, SI Rapoport, and H-W Kim. "Increased excitoxicity and neuroinflammatory markers in postmortem frontal cortex from bipolar disorder patients." *Mol Psychiatry* 15, no. 4 (April 2010): 384–92.

42. Duguid, IC and TG Smart. Chapter 14, Presynaptic NMDA Receptors, in *Biology of the NMDA Receptor*, AM Van Dongen, ed. Boca Raton, FL: CRC Press, 2009.

43. Oppeneer, SJ, YA Ross, WP Koh, et al. "Genetic variationi in folylpolyglutamate synthase and gamma-glutamyl hydrolase and plasma homocysteine levels in the Singapore Chinese health study." *Molecular Genetics & Metabolism* 105, no. 1 (2012): 73–78.

44. Jang, S, HS Jeong, JS Park, et al. "Neuroprotective effects of (-)-epigallocatechin-3-gallate against quinolinic acid-induced excitotoxicity via PI3K pathway and NO inhibition." *Brain Research* 1313 (Feb 2010): 25–33.

45. Braidy, N, R Grant, S Adams, and GJ Guillemi. "Neuroprotective effects of naturally occurring polyphenols on quinolinic acid-induced excitoxocity in human neurons." *FEBS Journal*, (2010): 368–82.

46. Jakubowski, H. "Homocysteine-thiolactone: metabolic origin and protein homocysteinylation in humans." *J Nutr* 130 (2000): 377S–381S.

47. Houston, MC. "Role of Mercury Toxicity in Hypertension, Cardiovascular Disease, and Stroke." *Journal of Clinical Hypertension* 13 (2011): 621–27.

48. Jakubowski, H. "Calcium-dependent human serum homocysteine thiolactone hydrolase." *Jl Biological Chemistry* 275, no. 6 (2000): 3957–62.

49. Hoang, MTT, LF DeFina, BL Willis, et al. "Association between low 25-hydroxyvitamin D and depression in a large sample of healthy adults: The Cooper Center longitudinal study." *Mayo Clin Proc* 86, no. 11 (2011): 1050–55.

50. Adibhatia, RM, and JF Hatcher. "Altered lipid metabolism in brain injury and disorders." *Subcell Biochem* 49 (2008): 241–68.

51. Haas, HL, OA Sergeeva, and O Selbach. "Histamine in the nervous system." *Physiol Rev* 88 (2008): 1183–1241.

52. Lambie, DG, and RH Johnson. "Drugs and folate metabolism." *Drugs* 30, no. 2 (Aug 1985): 145–55.

53. Beitzke, M, P Pfister, J Fortin, and F Skrabal. "Autonomic dysfunction and hemodynamics in B12 deficiency." *Autonomic Neuroscience: Basic and Clinical* 97 (2002): 45–54.

54. Fine, EJ, and ED Soria. "Myths about vitamin B12 deficiency." *Southern Medical Journal* 84, no. 12 (1991): 1475–81.

55. Eisenhofer, G, DG Lambie, RH Johnson, EA Tan, and E Whiteside. "Deficient catecholamine release as the basis of orthostatic hypotension in pernicious anemia." *Journal of Neurology, Neurosurgery & Psychiatry* 45, no. 11 (1982): 1053–55.

56. Fares, FA, N Gruener, and Z Kraiem. "The role of the asparagine-linked oligosaccharides of the alpha-subunit in human thyrotropin bioactivity." *Endocrinology* 137, no. 2 (1996): 555–60.

57. Moelby L, K Rasmussen, MK Jensen, et al. "Serum methyl malonic acid before and after oral L-isoleucine loading in cobalamin-deficient patients. *Scand J Clin Lab Invest* 52, no. 4 (Jun 1992): 255–59.

58. Doi, M, I Yamaoka, M Nakayama, et al. "Hypoglycemic effect of isoleucine involves increased muscle glucose uptake and whole body glucose oxidation and decreased hepatic gluconeogenesis." *American Journal of Physiology, Endocrinology, and Metabolism* 292, no. 6 (Jun 2007): E1683–93.

59. Cetiner, M, G Sener, AO Sehirli, et al. "Taurine protects against methotrexate-induced toxicity and inhibits leukocyte death." *Toxicology & Applied Pharmacology* 209, no. 1 (Nov 2005): 39–50.

60. Surwit, RS, MS Schneider, and MN Feinglos. "Stress and Diabetes." *Diabetes Care* 15, no. 10 (Oct 1992): 1413–22.

61. Watson, WP, T Munter, and BT Golding. "A new role for glutathione: Protection of vitamin B12 from xenobiotics." *Chem Res Toxicol* 17, no. 12 (2004): 1562–67.

62. Schauzer, GN. "Lithium: Occurrence, dietary intakes, nutritional essentiality." *Journal of the American College of Nutrition* 21, no. 1 (Feb 2002): 14–21.

63. Jope, RS. "Anti-bipolar therapy: Mechanism of action of lithium." *Molecular Psychiatry* 4 (1999): 117–28.

64. Chiu, C and D Chuang. "Molecular actions and therapeutic potential of lithium in preclinical and clinical studies of CNS disorders." *Pharmacologic Therapy* 128, no. 2 (2010): 281–304.

65. D'Addario, C, B Dell'Osso, M Palazzo, et al. "Selective DNA methylation of BDNF promoter in bipolar disorder: Differences among patients with BD I and BD II." *Neuropsychopharmacology* 37, no. 7 (Jun 2012): 1647–55.

66. Popkie, AP, LC Zeidner, AM Albrecht, et al. "Phosphatidyl inositol 3-kinase (PI3K) signaling via glycogen synthase kinase-3 (gsk-3) regulates DNA methylation of imprinted loci." *Journal of Biological Chemistry* 285, no. 53 (2010): 41337–47.

67. Chen, C-L, CF Lin, CW Chiang, et al. "Lithium inhibits ceramide- and etoposide-induced protein phosphatase 2A methylaion, Bcl-2 dephosphorylation, caspase-2 activation, and apoptosis." *Mol Pharmacol*, 70 (2006): 510–17.

68. Bremer, T, C Diamond, R McKinney, et al. "The pharmacogenetics of lithium response depends upon clinical co-morbidity." *Molecular Diagnosis & Therapy* 11, no. 3 (2007): 161–70.

69. Lyoo, IK, CM Demopulos, F Hirashima, et al. "Oral choline decreases brain purine levels in lithium-treated subjects in rapid-cycling bipolar disorder: A double-blind trial using proton and lithium magnetic resonance spectroscopy." *Bipolar Disorders* 5, no. 4 (2003): 300–306.

70. Dong, E, DR Grayson, A Guidotti, and E Costa. "Antipsychotic drug types can be characterized by their ability to modify GABAergic promoter methylation." *Epigenomics* 1, no. 1 (2009): 201–11.

71. Tsapakis, EM, and MJ Travis. "Glutamate and psychiatric disorders." *Advances in Psychiatric Treatment* 8 (2002): 189–97.

72. Brambilla, P, G Perez, F Barale, et al. "GABAergic dysfunction in mood disorders." *Molecular Psychiatry* 8 (2003): 731–37.

73. Curtin, F, and P Schulz. "Clonazepam and lorazepam in acute mania: A Baynesian meta-analysis." *Journal of Affective Disorders* 78, no. 3 (2004): 201–8.

74. Potkin, SG, AR Saha, MK Kujawa, et al. "Aripiprazole, a novel anti-psychotic, and risperidone vs placebo in patients with schizophrenia and schizoaffective disorder." *Archives General Psychiatry* 60, no. 7 (2003): 681–90.

75. Fountoulakis, KN, and E Vieta. "Efficacy and safety of aripiprazole in the treatment of bipolar disorder: A systematic review." *Annals of General Psychiatry* 8, no. 16 (2009): 16–30.

76. Blanke, ML and AMJ VanDongen. Chapter 13, Activation Mechanisms of the NMDA Receptor, in *Biology of the NMDA Receptor*, AM Van Dongen, ed. Boca Raton, FL: CRC Press, 2009.

77. Uhl, W, Nolting, A. Golor, G, et al. "Safety of hydroxocobalamin in healthy volunteers in a randomized, placebo-controlled study." Clinical Toxicology: The Official Journal of the American Academy of Clinical Toxicology & European Association of Poisons Centres & Clinical Toxicologists, Suppl 44 (2006): 1:17–28.

78. Hoffer, A. "The discovery of kryptopyrrole and its importance in diagnosis of biochemical imbalances in schizophrenia and in criminal behavior." *J Orthomolecular Medicine* 10, no. 1 (1995): 3–7.

79. Bell IR, CM Baldwin, and GE Schwartz. "Sensitization studies in chemically intolerant individuals: Implications for individual difference research." *Annals of the New York Academy of Sciences* 933 (Mar 2001): 38–47.

80. Smulders YM, DEC Smith, RM Kok, et al. "Cellular folate vitamer distribution during and after correction of vitamin B12 deficiency: A case for the methylfolate trap." *British Journal of Haematology* 132, no. 5 (Mar 2006): 623–29.

Section VII

Soft Tissue and Musculoskeletal Disorders

33 Surgery

Nutrient Therapy to Optimize Outcomes

Frederick T. Sutter, M.D., M.B.A.

INTRODUCTION

This chapter provides the physician with specific oral nutrient strategies to support patients who have chosen to proceed with elective or nonemergent surgery. This timing allows for a more generous preoperative interval of a few weeks to several months to prepare a willing patient to achieve the best result possible. A recent study showed that physicians are personally using and recommending nutrients to their patients, with a majority in the orthopedic and cardiology specialties. It appears timely then, that physicians consider the abundant literature on this topic and begin prescribing specific diet, nutrient, and exercise regimens to benefit their patients [1].

Scientific literature [2] has made increasingly clear the interrelationship of nutritional status as a major determinant in achieving a successful surgical outcome. More recent surgical literature has recommended a preoperative nutritional history and assessment to include specific supplement use by the patient and considers nutrient intervention as a means of affecting the course of healing [3]. Most physicians have had little training in the use of nutrient therapies and the identification and treatment of sarcopenia and obesity, two significant surgical risk factors. They get questions almost daily about the use of dietary supplements and must routinely advise their patients to lose weight and exercise more. This combination of patient interest and an impending surgical event creates a superb opportunity for the treating physician to spark meaningful patient cooperation in a perioperative program.

The following offers a concise combination of current science and clinical experience outlining how busy physicians can effectively guide patients to improved surgical outcomes, even if there are no overt risk factors for negative outcomes. With this facilitation, the patient and treating physician can team up to achieve optimal results.

EPIDEMIOLOGY

With the trends of increased outpatient surgeries, shortened inpatient surgical stays, rising prevalence of obesity, bariatric procedures, published surgical results for hospitals, and a greater reliance on the primary physician for follow-up care, there is opportunity for the treating physician to expand their view beyond surgical technique to reduce perioperative risks in order to optimize outcomes.

The prevalence of obesity has more than doubled in the last 30 years. There has been a concurrent increase in total calories consumed primarily in the form of carbohydrates and a slight decrease in the amount of protein calories [4]. Obesity has increased the incidence of arthritic conditions requiring orthopedic procedures in younger adults, with greater complication rates of wound infection, deep venous thrombosis, cardiac events, and anesthesia risks [5–8]. Sarcopenic obesity increases these risks [9].

PATHOPHYSIOLOGY

The perioperative period creates many challenges for the patient. Even anticipation of the procedure increases stress, can interfere with sleep, and can prompt misguided attempts to lose weight. Mobility restriction due to the illness or orthopedic impairment commonly promotes deconditioning and poor appetite with secondary loss of lean body mass. Frequently, the patient has had limited sun exposure with an associated decline in vitamin D status. Restricting calories with inactivity decreases lean body mass and creates additional risk in the form of sarcopenia, which is associated with unfavorable outcomes [10]. Joint disease and subsequent surgery increases demand on the contralateral limb, thereby increasing risk of additional surgery [11]. The restriction of nutrients during the NPO period prior to surgery initiates catabolism of lean tissue and dehydration. Rapid elimination of caffeine can induce severe withdrawal headaches, complicating postoperative care and pain management. Eliminating anti-inflammatory medications and nutrients targeted for pain management prior to surgery in order to avoid surgical and anesthesia complications can increase pain, immobility, and the need for additional narcotic analgesics.

After surgery, postanesthesia nausea and vomiting and immobilization can advance catabolic wasting and limit nutrient intake. Major surgery is followed by a period of immunosuppression, increasing the risk of morbidity and mortality due to infections. Wound healing and blood loss increase demand for many nutrients well in excess of normal dietary intake, so for most elderly and sarcopenic surgical patients, consuming a "regular diet" is very unlikely to meet the metabolic demands for optimal healing.

PHARMACOLOGY

The use of nonsteroidal anti-inflammatory drugs (NSAIDs), cyclooxygenase-2 inhibitors, disease-modifying antirheumatic drugs (DMARDs), and biological response modifiers in the perioperative period needs some consideration given their impact on how inflammation contributes to the wound healing process. Potential complications include wound dehiscence, infection, and impaired collagen synthesis. There is no current consensus on the optimum time for withholding drug therapy prior to surgery other than that regarding antiplatelet effects [12]. Prudent limitation of NSAIDs in patients with proven stress fractures has been recommended in a more recent article [13]. For many of these medications, there are no human studies. The practitioner will need to consider disease severity, risk of exacerbation, and potential surgical risk factors in the context of the drug pharmacokinetics prior to making recommendations for cessation of therapy. In the case of some DMARD therapies, this would require a period of four weeks. Transitioning therapy to include chondroprotectants, such as glucosamine and chondroitin sulfates needs to be started one to three months in advance of weaning from pharmaceuticals to allow time for therapeutic benefit. These two nutrients have been demonstrated in randomized, double-blind, placebo-controlled trials to be effective not only with symptom management, but actually have been preventive for arthritis progression and can be a disease modifying agents in this light [14,15]. Treatment options for exacerbation of disease can combine alternative therapies for pain management that might include prescription analgesics and medical food products, supportive nutrients (such as glucosamine sulfate, chondroitin sulfate, and fish oils), specific diets for weight loss [16] and dysinflammation, acupuncture, and physical therapy, among other integrative approaches. Using a baseline symptom questionnaire can be very useful in the complex patient to monitor response to changes in therapy, for example, MOS SF-36 or MSQ [17,18]. Rakel's *Integrative Medicine* is an excellent reference source [19].

The orthopedic patient with months of chronic pain commonly has challenges with sleep. Frequently, the patient has concomitant myofascial pain, which several studies found to significantly impair sleep quality. Even without chronic pain, normal individuals who are sleep deprived or have disrupted sleep for a period of time will experience a lowered pain threshold and an increase in musculoskeletal discomfort and fatigue [20]. The majority of addictive, prescription sleep medications actually decrease time spent in the deep stages three and four, except for clonazepam and alprazolam.

PATIENT EVALUATION

PHYSICAL EXAM

The definition and significance of sarcopenia have been reviewed by Kohlstadt [9] and others. In general, sarcopenia can be defined as the age- or disuse-related loss of muscle and fat-free body mass, reducing muscle metabolism, strength, and mobility in older adults. Skeletal muscle mass is quantified as being less than or equal to two standard deviations (SD) below the mean. It begins in the fourth to fifth decade [21] and incidence in otherwise healthy individuals over the age of 60 years varies in reports from 8% to 25%. Then it increases dramatically in the very old, with a large increase over 80 years of 43% to 60%. Associated risk factors for sarcopenia are cigarette smoking, chronic illnesses, underweight, physical inactivity, and poorer sense of psychosocial well-being [22,23].

Waist and hip circumference used alone or in combination with BMI is an anthropometric indicator of health risk and is easily performed. The combination of both is a very sensitive metric to predict health risk. The National Institutes of Health [24] suggest abdominal obesity as a significant risk factor can be identified with waist circumference (measured at the umbilicus) in men $\geq$ 102 cm (40 inches) and in women $\geq$ 88 cm (35 inches). These individuals would be identified as having "high" abdominal fat, and therefore a "very high" health risk. The waist-to-hip ratio (WHR) is calculated by measuring the unclothed waist at the narrowest point between ribs and hips after exhaling when viewed from the front. The hip measurement is performed over light clothing at the level of the widest diameter around the buttocks. It is the preferred clinical measure of central obesity for predicting mortality, even in those regarded as very lean (BMI < 20), normal, and overweight (BMI > 25). Risk starts to rise significantly for cardiovascular mortality when the WHR goes beyond 0.8 for women and 0.9 for men. [25,26].

Clinical identification of sarcopenic obesity is more challenging. Features more suggestive of poor fat-free mass (FFM) in obese individuals can be appreciated as pendulous adiposity in the arms, abdomen, and even the thighs and legs. Gentle palpation over the triceps area, (as if performing a skin-fold fat measurement) and estimating the remaining muscle can also be revealing. This presentation would be opposed to the more stout or "solid" individual with considerable muscle mass, despite being identified as obese with a BMI in the Class I range of 30 to 34.9.

Individuals without sarcopenia have higher intakes of protein and antioxidant micronutrients than healthy individuals with sarcopenia [27]. Bench research on age-related sarcopenia and fatigability demonstrated the presence of enhanced reactive oxygen species, systemic inflammation, apoptotic susceptibility, and reduced mitochondrial biogenesis [28,29]. Therefore, consuming an antioxidant-rich diet or taking supplemental antioxidants may protect the individual who is exercising and consuming adequate protein from progression of sarcopenia.

Sarcopenic obesity in the frail elderly presents a great challenge. Simple interventions with nutrition, exercise, and weight loss have been demonstrated to ameliorate these risk factors over longer periods of time, such as six months [30].

RISK AND NUTRITION-SPECIFIC PREOPERATIVE LABORATORY EVALUATION

With the usual preoperative lab studies, several additional laboratory studies can be very useful in assessing potential nutritional deficiencies or surgical risks (see Table 33.1). Supplementing a low normal nutrient value prepares the patient for the catabolic stress of healing. Scientific literature has described metabolic therapy as that which involves the administration of a substance normally found in the body to enhance a metabolic reaction. This can be achieved in two ways: one, by giving a substance to achieve greater than normal levels in the body to drive a biochemical reaction in the desired direction; two, by using a substance to correct relative or absolute deficiency of a cellular component. This concept is useful in the context of prescribing nutrients to improve surgical outcomes.

High-sensitivity C-reactive protein has been associated with higher complications and greater length of stay for orthopedic patients. To address this, removing sugar, consuming low arachidonic acid food groups, targeting protein intake, and taking antioxidants are best (see Table 33.2A and 33.2B). Patients with low albumin were twice as likely to require prolonged hospitalization (> 15 days) for elective total hip replacement, compared with those in whom the albumin level was 3.9 g/dl or greater. Following transferrin and albumin levels perioperatively has also been used to predict delayed wound healing after total hip arthroplasty [31].

Prealbumin is a sensitive, cost-effective serum marker for protein malnutrition that responds quickly to increasing protein intake, particularly in the form of branched chain amino acids and can be monitored biweekly in acute situations. In critically ill patients, lower levels are associated with increased hospital length of stay, morbidity, and mortality [3].

Homocysteine (Hcy) is a cholesterol-independent risk factor for stroke, heart, bone, and thromboembolic disease [32]. Homocysteinemia is less common since fortification of grain products with folic acid began in 1998. B vitamins can safely lower elevation of Hcy. High Hcy levels have been associated with higher bone turnover, poor physical performance, and lower bone mineral density.

The incidence of healing complications was three times more frequent in individuals with lower preoperative total lymphocyte count (< 1500 cells/mm) compared with normals [33].

TREATMENT RECOMMENDATIONS

DIET

Adequate caloric intake is essential, especially in the form of protein. It is a key macronutrient in wound healing and managing complications related to sarcopenia, along with exercise [34]. Instruct the patient to target at least the recommended daily allowance of 0.8 g/kg body weight of protein intake, provided there is no concomitant liver or renal disease or a history of gout. Protein sources in the form of seafood and organ meats can be high in purines (some examples include: adenine, guanine, hypoxanthine, xanthine, theobromine, caffeine, uric acid, and isoguanine), usually restricted in treating gout. However, consumption of these in the presence of caffeinated or alcoholic beverages (especially beer) is more likely to precipitate a gouty attack at the RDA level for protein [35]. Higher dietary intakes (up to 1.6 g protein/kg/day or up to 30% of total caloric intake) can enhance response to resistance exercise in the elderly [34,36]. Protein intake will be metabolized best if consumed evenly throughout the day, particularly with the midday meal, or for convenience in the form of protein shakes. This should be continued as close to the NPO period as possible.

The anabolic response to increased protein intake is less robust in the elderly compared with younger individuals but can be improved with exercise and increased protein intake. Anabolic resistance to muscle protein synthesis (MPS) in age-related sarcopenia [37] can be addressed by using branched chain amino acids or leucine, along with specific exercise prescription (see Table 33.3). The notion of a "leucine threshold" has been postulated for the blunted response to MPS in elderly muscle. In addition, exercise is most effective with focus on structural appropriateness (e.g., arthritis or tendonitis in the area to be exercised) and intensity. In the elderly, low-load (30% of a

TABLE 33.1

Nutrition-Specific Preoperative Laboratory Assessment

Lab	Optimal Range	Indicator	Note	References
Albumin	3.9 g/dL or greater	↑ LOS and complication rates when low, associated with ↓ muscle mass in limbs	↑ dietary intake 0.8–1.4 g protein/kg body wt/day; divided doses	Del Savio et al. 1996 [72]
hs CRP	< 3 mg/L for orthopedic pts	If > 3 mg/L, associated with ↑ complication and LOS	Treat with anti-inflammatory diet; see Table 33.2	Ackland et al. 2007 [73]
DHEA-Sulfate	Women 150–180 µg/dL, men 350–400 µg/dL	Sarcopenia, precursor of testosterone	Mointor DHEA-S levels monthly with treatment	Teitelbaum 2006 [74]
Folate	> 5.4 ng/mL	Lowers Hcy	See Table 33.3	Theusinger et al. 2007 [75]
Iron, Ferritin	Per lab	Supports blood element formation	Support if < NL range; See Table 33.3	
Homocysteine (Hcy)	4–8 µM/L	↑ levels associated with ↑ risk of stroke, CAD, DVT	↑ risk 9–17 µM/L ↑↑ risk >17 µM/L; see Table 33.2	McCully 2007, Gerdhem et al. 2007, Selhub et al. 1993, Spence 2007 [76–79] 33.
Lymphocyte Count	> 1500 cells/mm3	3X ↑ in healing complications		Marin 2002 [32]
Magnesium	↑ NL range	Bone healing, ↓ in obesity, chronic pain	Rx depletion in combination with low intake in typical diet	Institute of Medicine 2006 [55]
Pre-Albumin	> 15 mg/dL	↓ cost, early marker for ↓ protein	Rapid response to correction	Kavalukas and Barbul 2011 [2]
Transferrin	> 200 mg/dL	Predictor of delayed wound healing in THA	Acute marker; may be ↑ in chronic Fe deficiency anemia	Gherini et al. 1993 [30]
Vitamin B6	> 50 nmol/L	↑ DVT <23 nmol/L	See Table 33.3	Hron et al. 2007 [56]
Vitamin B12	> 500 pg/mL	10%–15% over 60 years are deficient	IM injection typically not covered by insurances; patients usually willing to pay minor cost	Institute of Medicine 2006 [55]
Vitamin D (25-OH D3)	50–70 ng/dL	Bone healing, ↓ in obesity, chronic and nonspecific pain	See Table 33.3	Bischoff-Ferrari et al. 2004 [80]

CAD = Coronary Artery Disease; DVT = Deep Vein Thrombosis; hsCRP = High Sensitivity C-Reactive Protein; LOS = Length of Stay; Pts = Patients; THA = Total Hip Arthroplasty

TABLE 33.2A
Dietary Guidelines for the Management of Inflammation

Food Category	Serving Size	Svg/Day	Cal/Svg	Choices*
Concentrated Protein	3.5 oz (after cooking)	Aim to consume no more than 60 mg arachidonic acid (AA) daily.	150	Poultry (remove all skin); turkey breast and chicken. Lean meats: sliced boiled ham, pork tenderloin, beef flank steak, ground beef (5% fat). Fish (avoid farmed fish) (see Table 32.2B). Dairy: cottage cheese: 1%, ¾ cup; ricotta: reduced fat, ½ cup. Tofu products: tofu, 1 cup; tempeh, ½ cup; soy burger, 4 oz.
Vegetables	½ cup	5 to 7	10 to 25	All vegetables are allowed except:white potato, turnip, parsnip, rutabaga, and corn. Fresh vegetable juice or green beverages are allowed.
Fruits	Approx. 1 med.	3 to 4	80	All whole fruits except: banana, pineapple and papaya. Fruit juice not recommended.
Dairy	6 oz.	1–2 (if tolerated)	80 to 100	Plain yogurt (low-fat or nonfat), milk (nonfat, 1%, 2%), buttermilk, milk substitutes (soy, rice, nut).
Legumes	½ to 1 cup	1 to 2	100 to 200	All peas and beans, hummus, bean soups
Grains	½ cup	1 to 3	75 to 100	Whole grains such as 100% whole wheat bread and pasta, brown rice, whole oats, rye crackers, and pearled barley with at least 3 grams or more of fiber per serving.
Nuts/Seeds	1 small handful	1 per day	150 to 200	All nuts except cashews and macadamias; 1–2 tbsp of nut butter.
Oils	1 tsp	4 to 6	40	Olive and canola oils for cooking, flax seed (refrigerate) and walnut oils for salads, mayonnaise from canola oil (no egg or sugar added), avocado (1/8 of whole), green or black olives (8–10).
Beverages	Unlimited	Water intake recommended at ½ body wt, in oz.	0	Water, herbal tea, decaffeinated coffee or tea, mineral water, club soda or selzer, plain or flavored (no added artificial sweeteners).
Condiments	Unlimited, except salt	As desired	0	Cinnamon, carob, mustard, horseradish, vinegar, lemon, lime, flavored extracts, herbs/spices, stevia. No refined sugars or artificial sweeteners are allowed.

*Patients should be advised to avoid foods to which they have a history of reactivity.

one repetition maximum [1RM]), higher repetition (to fatigue or "shakiness") exercise has been demonstrated to produce MPS. Readers are referred to a more detailed review of exercise prescriptions [38].

General dietary guidelines to redirect the inflammatory cascade focus on fat content, arachidonic acid, refined carbohydrates, and simple sugars. Arachidonic acid is the physiologic precursor of pro-inflammatory eicosanoids such as prostaglandins and leukotrienes. These molecules can then go on to produce superoxide, which can play a role in a feed-forward, or propagated lipid peroxidation chain reaction, increasing antioxidant demand for the body. Many times, appreciable results occur

TABLE 33.2B
Arachidonic Acid Calculator

Concentrated Protein Food Meat and Poultry	Arachidonic Acid Content (mg/3.5 oz)†
Ham, sliced boiled	0
Pork tenderloin	30
Turkey breast, roast	40
Beef, flank steak	40
Ground beef, 5% fat	50
Chicken breast	60
Fish	
Mahi mahi	0
Pacific mackerel	10
Pink salmon	10
Pacific cod	20
Sockeye salmon	30
Atlantic cod	30
Haddock	40
Snapper	40
Yellowfin tuna	40
White tuna, canned in water	50
Flounder	50
Atlantic mackerel	50
Grouper	60
Eggs	70(per yolk)
Dairy	negligible
Soy	negligible

† 3.5 oz after cooking
Source: www.metagenics.com.

within 10 days, although the first five to seven days are more challenging if considerable sugar consumption has been habitual prior to initiating dietary changes. Here, the initial period of withdrawal can be associated with significant cravings, diuresis, cramps, and irritability for two to four days. Preparing the patient for this possibility is the most effective strategy for compliance and will support greater ease in transitioning through this period.

If the patient is consuming large amounts of caffeinated beverages, these should be tapered over two weeks prior to surgery. This can be done with minimal withdrawal headaches by reducing consumption of one serving every three to four days and replacing that serving with an equal volume of clean water; for example, if consuming four caffeinated beverages daily, day one of a taper would be three servings plus one serving of water, and so on until the last serving, which is cut in half and then eliminated in two to three days.

NUTRIENTS TO OPTIMIZE SURGICAL OUTCOMES

Self-directed use of supplemental nutrients, frequently unbeknownst to the treating physician is commonplace. A national study on the reasons patients use supplemental nutrients concluded patients are choosing supplemental nutrients not because they are dissatisfied with conventional medicine but because using supplemental nutrients is more congruent with their own values, beliefs, and philosophical orientations toward health and life [39,40]. Publications have effectively addressed many of the risks associated with the use of supplements in the preoperative period, and various surgical societies have recommended eliminating all supplements for some defined period prior to surgery. Given the safety profiles and short half-lives of most nutrient and herbal supplements, one week of abstinence prior to surgery appears to be a very safe guideline. Postoperatively, nutrients can be resumed in a similar time frame provided the patient is eating and there are no contraindications with newly prescribed medications (e.g., warfarin).

Discussion regarding the general classes of nutrients listed in Table 33.3 is worthwhile, as many of these applications pertain to metabolic therapy. Research is looking beyond the notion of treating or preventing deficiency disease states and moving to evaluate safe and economical nutrient applications in specific clinical environments that will promote a desired, measurable result. The simple recommendation of a high-quality multivitamin is the first step in optimizing surgical outcomes because it will enhance a broad spectrum of micronutrients with little effort. See Table 33.4.

AMINO ACIDS

Arginine and glutamine are semi-essential, or conditionally essential amino acids during critical illness and severe trauma. Arginine is considered to be a direct nitric oxide (NO) precursor. It induces nitric oxide release, which inhibits smooth muscle contraction, increases blood flow, and results in increased nutrient uptake and glucose utilization into muscle, particularly during exercise. Arginine stimulates collagen deposition in wound healing [41] and dramatically increases strength in trained men compared with controls [10]. It has also shown promise along with proper diet and exercise in patients with insulin resistance and obesity, while sparing lean body mass [42]. Use with caution and lower starting doses if the individual is diabetic, on blood pressure medicine, or has a history of herpes simplex virus (HSV) infections. History of HSV infection is a concern because arginine shares transport proteins with lysine, and relative deficiencies of lysine can be a trigger for an outbreak. High arginine foods such as cashews, peanuts, chocolate, and coffee can also limit lysine availability enough to induce HSV symptoms.

Leucine alone, or with the other branched-chain amino acids (BCAAs) of L-valine and L-isoleucine, has been shown to be more effective at stimulating MPS in the elderly compared with younger subjects. This may be an acceptable strategy for patients with renal impairment who cannot tolerate higher total protein intakes [2,44].

N-acetylcysteine (NAC) has been studied with attention to ischemia/reperfusion of orthopedically operated limbs. It appears to lessen the need for postoperative analgesics and can decrease hospital stay [45]. Along with other dietary amino acids such as glutamine and glycine, antioxidants such as vitamins C and E, selenium, phytonutrients, and lipoic acid, NAC provides cysteine as a substrate for the recycling of glutathione, which is frequently depleted in the presence of oxidative stress. Glutathione is recognized as the final pathway for the reduction of oxidants produced by ROS. L-carnitine may be important for vegetarians or those with metabolic syndrome and has been shown to enhance cardiac performance and increase exercise tolerance in humans with ischemic heart and peripheral vascular disease [46,47].

Creatine can also be useful in the frail elderly as an adjunctive support to increase muscle strength and mass with an exercise program. It can be mixed with the patient's favorite juice or nonalcoholic beverage and consumed one to two times per day. When taken along with caffeinated beverages, a stimulating effect may be experienced, so it is best taken earlier in the day.

A naturally occurring by-product of the amino acid methionine, s-adensosylmethionine (SAMe) is a methyl donor and inhibits synthesis of proinflammatory interleukens and TNF-alpha. It up-regulates proteoglycan synthesis and the proliferation rate of chondrocytes, promoting cartilage formation and repair in doses ranging from 400 to 1600 mg/day in divided doses. In a double-blind, crossover study at 1200 mg/day compared with celecoxib (200 mg), it had the same efficacy and a

continued

TABLE 33.3
Nutrients with Research Supporting Their Role(s) in Optimizing Surgical Outcomes

Nutrients (Listed alphabetically)	Dose	Support	Notes	Food Sources	Adult DRI	References
N-Acetyl Cysteine	500–600 mg bid	Antioxidant, ↓ LOS/pain mgt	Precursor to glutathione	ND	ND	Witte and Barbul 2003, Lucotti, Setola, Monti et al. 2006, Preli et al. 2002
L-Arginine	3–6 g bid, powder or time-release tabs	Collagen formation, supports synthesis of protein and mitochondria	Start at lower doses in diabetes and HTN, HSV infections	Dairy, beef, pork, nuts	ND	
Calcium	1200–1500 mg Ca Carbonate:800–1000 mg chelated MCHC products	Typical diet 500–600 mg day, supports bone healing	Monitor for constipation; citrate, malate best form Balance 2Ca:1 Mg	Dairy, kale, broccoli	800–2000 mg	
L-Carnitine	0.5–2 g bid	Sarcopenia, muscle/ cardiac support, ↑ mitochondrial efficiency	Can be low in vegans, helpful in DM wounds	Red meats	ND	L-carnitine Monograph 2005
Chondroitin Sulfate	400–600 mg bid	Improves pain in OA, may be disease modifying		Limited	ND	See text
Coenzyme Q10	50–1200 mg/day	Antioxidant, higher doses with CHF, monitor prothrombin time for warfarin pts	Reduced by statins, helps fatigue and muscle recovery	Insignificant amount in food	ND	Spigset 1994
Copper	1–4 mg/day	Collagen cross-linking	Use with zinc, dietary intake is low; avoid in cancer pts	Organ meats, seafood, nuts and seeds	0.9–10 mg	Berger and Shenkin 2007
Creatine	3–5 g	Sarcopenia in elderly	After exercise	n/a	ND	Candow and Chilibeck 2007
DHEA	10–15 mg/day women, 15–25 mg/ day men	Declines in elderly	Monitor levels q8 wks	n/a	ND	Valenti et al. 2004
EFA'S:EPA/ DHA	2000–2500 mg EPA+DHA	Reduces inflammation, prevents sarcopenia	Take with food; refrigeration helps "fish repeats"	Coldwater fish	ND	Robinson et al. 2007

TABLE 33.3 (continued)
Nutrients with Research Supporting Their Role(s) in Optimizing Surgical Outcomes

Nutrients	Dose	Support	Notes	Food Sources	Adult DRI	References
Folate	0.8–5 mg/day	lowers ↑ Hcy	Use with B6, B12	Dark greens, grains, beans	0.4–1.0 mg	
Flavocoxid	250–500mg q12h	Pain mgt OA, "medical food," anti-inflammatory, helps muscle recovery	Rx only. Can use with warfarin, monitor prothrombin time	Colored vegetables	ND	
Glucosamine Sulfate	750 mg bid	Pain management in OA, may be disease modifying	Use caution in shellfish allergy		ND	Reginster et al. 2007
Glutamine	5 g bid	Supports GI integrity, prevents loss of muscle mass	Constipation	"Conditionally essential" amino acid	ND	
Iron	Practitioner directed to tolerance at UL	Use gluconate, bis-glycinate chelate, vit C↑↑ absorption	GI upset; avoid in cancer patients	Meats, fish, poultry and dark greens	8–45 mg	
Leucine	4–5 g bid	Stimulates muscle protein synthesis in elderly > protein alone	Use if renal compromise prevents ↑ protein intake, substitute BCAA's 6–7g bid	Soy, lentils, beef, salmon	1–3 g (WHO)	Stohs and Dudrick 2011, Nicastro Artioli and Costa 2011
Lipoic Acid	300–600 mg bid	Diabetic neuropathy, ↓ damage ischemic reperfusion	May lower blood glucose levels, monitor diabetics Regen. Vit.C and E	Kidney, heart, liver, broccoli, spinach, potatoes	ND	See text
Magnesium	400–800 mg/day	Bone healing, use 2:1 Ca:Mg, Intake is generally inadequate	Can loosen stools	Leafy greens, grains, nuts	320–770 mg†	See text
Manganese	5–10 mg/day	Bone healing, enzyme and protein metabolism	Limit with liver disease/cholestasis	Grains, tea, greens	1.8–11 mg	Vaxman et al. 1996
Melatonin	0.5–3 mg 30 min before bedtime	Sleep and pain support	Studies done with lower doses, avoid in leukemia, Hodgkin's disease	Tart cherries	ND	Brzezinski et al. 2005
MSM	1000–3000 mg/day	Pain management in OA	GI intolerance		ND	Jacobs 1999

Name	Dose	Function	Notes	Food sources	RDA	References
Probiotics	1–10 B CFU's/day, Lacidophilus, B. bifidum, S.boulardii	Supports GI integrity, post antibiotic diarrhea	Flatulence Use 10–14 days pre- and post-op shown to reduce bacterial infection rates	Yogurt (Note: Food sources inadequate for therapeutic dose)	ND	Gionchetti et al. 2000, Rayes Soeters 2010
Protein	0.8–1.6 g/kg/day Equally divided doses	Poorly digested in hypochlor-hydric elderly, essential for wound healing, common deficiency worldwide	Use hydrolyzed protein shakes renal compromise	Meat, poultry, fish, eggs, milk, yogurt, nuts, legumes, seeds	0.66–1.52 g/kg/day	Campbell 2007, Helman 2006, Evans 2004
S-Adenosyl Methionine	400–600 mg bid	Pain mgt joint disease	GI intolerance may activate bipolar patients	Metabolite in the body	ND	Najm et al. 2004, Muller-Fassbender 1987, Vetter 1987
Selenium	50–400 µg/day	Antioxidant, supports healing, ↓ intake associated with sarcopenia	Hair loss, brittle nails in doses > 1 mg/day	Meat, seafood, grains, vegetables	55–400 µg/day	Chaput et al. 2007, Berger and Shenkin 2007
Silicon	5 mg bid	Deficiency leads to bone defects	Use caution in renal lithiasis, Best as orthosilicic acid	Cereal and unrefined grain products	ND	Jugdaohsingh et al. 2003
L-Theanine	50–200 mg	Improves mood, helps sleep	Well tolerated	Green tea (Camellia Sinensis)	ND	Juneja et al. 1999
L-Tryptophan	500 mg–3 g hs	Precursor of serotonin, supports sleep	Theoretical risk of serotonin syndrome if given with SSRI Rx	Chocolate, oats, dried dates, turkey, pumpkin seeds	ND	L-tryptophan Monograph 2006
Vitamin A	15,000–25,000IU/day	Antioxidant, wound healing, osteoporosis, sarcopenia	Use combination of mixed carotenoids	Retinol animal based foods, carotenoids vegetables, fruits	2310–9900 IU	Wicke et al. 2000
Vitamin B2 (Riboflavin)	10–100 mg/day	↑intake – ↓hip fx	Supplement sensitive to light exposure	Fortified cereals, organ meats	1.1–1.3 mg/day	Yazdanpanah et al. 2007
Vitamin B5 (Pantothenate)	500–750 mg bid	Wound healing	No toxicity	Chicken, beef, potatoes	5 mg/day	Vaxman et al. 1996
Vitamin B6	10–100 mg/day	Lowers ↑Hcy, low serum B6 assoc. w/DVT	Makes urine bright yellow	Cereals, beef liver, organ meats	1.3–100 mg/day	Yazdanpanah et al. 2007
Vitamin B12	500–5000 µg/day	Lowers ↑ Hcy, preferably As methylcobalamin, can improve sleep disruption	Well tolerated	Shellfish, organ meats, sardines	2.4 µg	Yazdanpanah et al. 2007

continued

TABLE 33.3 (continued)

Nutrients with Research Supporting Their Role(s) in Optimizing Surgical Outcomes

Nutrients	Dose	Support	Notes	Food Sources	Adult DRI	References
Vitamin C	1–2 g bid	Wound/bone healing prevents sarcopenia, ↑ need in smokers	If GI intolerance, use buffered or ester C	Citrus fruits, vegetables, tomatoes	75–2000 mg	Alcantara-Martos et al. 2007
Vitamin D3	800 IU daily to 50,000 IU weekly	Bone metabolism, low in chronic pain, may influence seasonal affective disorder	Well tolerated, hypercalcemia at 160–500 ng/dL, monitor levels q8–12 wks	Enriched food sources likely inadequate for surgical patients	600–4000 IU/ day††	See text
Vitamin E	100–200 IU/day mixed tocopherols	Prevents sarcopenia, supports high EFA intakes	Use caution in warfarin therapy or vitamin K deficiency	Vegetable oils, grains, vegetables, meats. nuts, avocados	12–15 mg (8–10 IU)	
Zinc	30–50 mg/day	Essential in wound healing	Take with copper, can cause GI upset	Seafood (oysters and sardines), organ meats, sunflower seeds	8–40 mg	Williams and Barbul 2003, Mahmood et al. 2007

Note: All DRIs were obtained from Dietary Reference Intakes, Institute of Medicine. (Institute of Medicine 2006) DRI = Dietary Reference Intakes, AI = Adequate Intakes, UL = Upper Limit, ND = Not Determined, CFU = colony Forming Units, Adult = 19 years and older. DRI presented as a range from RDA (Recommended Daily Allowance = average daily dietary nutrient intake level sufficient to meet requirements of 97% to 98% healthy individuals), or AI (Adequate Intake = recommended daily intake estimates when RDA cannot be determined) to UL (Tolerable Upper Limit = highest daily intake that is likely to pose no risk of adverse health effects to almost all individuals in the general population).

† 770 mg magnesium assumes maximum dietary intake of 420mg plus maximum supplemental intake of 350mg.

†† As cholecalciferol. Assumes minimal exposure to sunlight.

BCAA = branched chain amino acids; DM = Diabetes Mellitus; DVT = deep vein thrombosis; EFA = Essential Fatty Acids; Hcy = homocysteine; LOS = Length of Stay; OA = Osteoarthritis; MCHC = microcrystalline hydroxyapatite concentrate

TABLE 33.4

Better Quality Supplements

The product demonstrates:

Independent lab testing

Chelated minerals

Fish oils: label states free of heavy metals, PCBs

No artificial colors and limited fillers (e.g., glycols, sucrose, etc.)

Manufacturing guidelines:

cGMP (Current Good Manufacturing Practices)

NSF™ (NSF International, The Public Health and Safety Company™)

ISO 9000 or ISO 9001: 2000 (International Organization for Standardization)

lower incidence of side effects over a two-month period. It can also elevate mood and help with anxiety. Supportive nutrients such as B6, B12, folate, and trimethylgylcine should be given simultaneously. Hcy levels should be monitored if recommending higher doses of SAMe, which can theoretically drive serum levels above recommended normals.

ANTIOXIDANTS

Coenzyme Q10 (CoQ10) has been safely prescribed in daily doses of 400 to 1200 mg for individuals with congestive heart failure and severe neurological conditions.. In times of severe oxidative stress, CoQ10 along with lipoic acid can be viewed as conditionally essential nutrients because the body cannot make enough of them. There has been a case report of reduced effectiveness of warfarin drugs with CoQ10 use. Therefore, more frequent international normalized ratio (INR) testing is indicated when initiating therapy in this patient group. This coenzyme produces a favorable response in treating fatigue on a very consistent basis. For individuals taking statin prescription medications (as well as red yeast rice, the natural form of lovastatin), myopathy and the more common myalgias may be supported by the use of CoQ10 [48].

Alpha-lipoic acid is a potent, multifunctional antioxidant that improves tissue glutathione levels, reduces lipid peroxides, increases insulin sensitivity, and helps regenerate vitamins C and E. It has been used effectively in Germany for decades orally and intravenously for the treatment of diabetic polyneuropathy [49]. It can be a useful adjunct for improving insulin sensitivity and surgical recovery involving neural structures, especially in patients with diabetes. Alpha-lipoic acid was used in combination with CoQ10, magnesium, and omega-3 fatty acids preoperatively, up until the day of surgery and for one month thereafter, and was demonstrated to enhance several recovery parameters [50].

MINERALS

Minerals in the form of inorganic mineral salts such as carbonates, oxides, phosphates, and sulfates compete with one another for absorption in the gut. When minerals are consumed in this form they can also be blocked by the intake of natural fiber found in cereals and fruits [51]. While there are other considerations influencing absorption when patients are taking a specific mineral such as iron preoperatively, an important clinical application is to supplement calcium and magnesium together. Generally, a ratio of two parts calcium to one part magnesium is recommended. Apart from any pain medications that alter bowel motility, patients may find calcium to be constipating and magnesium to have a laxative effect. Calcium citrate and magnesium citrate may be better absorbed in patients with hypochlorhydria and can also confer an alkalinizing effect. Microcrystalline hydroxyapatite is a blend of minerals found in bone. Studies have shown magnesium levels and intake are strongly and independently associated with the anabolic hormones testosterone and IGF-1 [52].

Silicon can be helpful with bone healing and in supporting osteoporosis in men and premenopausal women. It is absorbed well as orthosilicic acid and is commonly available in multivitamin preparations in the form of silicon dioxide or magnesium trisilicate at about 2 mg, but higher doses are needed to influence bone density. It has been shown to stimulate collagen synthesis. Silica is often removed from food during processing.

Zinc carnosine is a preparation that has been helpful with relieving mild gastric upset, while supporting zinc levels. Dosage is 75 mg bid and provides 32 mg of zinc per dose [53].

HORMONES

Melatonin was a safe and effective sleep aid when studied as a preoperative anxiolytic in nine of 10 studies reviewed. Five studies showed opioid sparing or reduced pain scores and reduced pediatric emergence delirium. Its antioxidant properties are also being studied for use in sepsis and reperfusion injuries [54,55]. L-tryptophan is available again, cleared by the FDA for use after a decades-long ban related to contamination with an industrial chemical by one manufacturer, which resulted in hundreds of illnesses; 5-hydoxytryptophan is available and is a suitable substitute, although effective dosage is about one-fifth the effective dose of L-tryptophan. There is a theoretical risk of serotonin syndrome with nausea, vomiting, and excessive drowsiness if either is given in conjunction with selective serotonin reuptake inhibitors, so it is recommended to avoid this combination until further studies have been completed.

Dehydroepiandrosterone (DHEA) therapy to support low DHEA-sulfate levels in the elderly can be helpful with sarcopenia. Limit use to three to six months while following serum levels. Morning dosing is best as occasional activation can occur, and the dosage may be adjusted downward with this side effect.

VITAMINS

B12 absorption is inadequate in approximately 15% of individuals over 65 due to lack of gastric acidity, decreased intrinsic factor, and in *Helicobacter pylori* infections [56]. For individuals with low serum B12 levels where intramuscular dosing is not an option, doses of 5000 µg/day are acceptable in a sublingual form of methylcobalamin for shorter term use. Low serum B6 is associated with an increased risk of DVT [57,58] and is best supplemented in its activated form of pyridoxal-5'-phosphate. B5 (pantothenic acid) enhanced wound healing in a human study with a dosage of 200 to 900 mg/day [59]. There is a much higher incidence of heart disease and elevated Hcy levels compared with healthy controls for individuals with rheumatoid arthritis treated with methotrexate, which inhibits B6 metabolism. B6 therapy is frequently prescribed, however, when associated with elevated Hcy, the addition of B12 and folate is indicated.

Vitamin C therapy after distal radius fracture has been shown to reduce the incidence of complex regional pain syndrome (CRPS) from 10.1% to 2.4% studied in 427 fractures at doses of 500 mg/day, which is well above what can be consumed in a healthy diet of five vegetables and fruits per day [60].

General guidelines for treatment of 25-hydroxyvitamin D (25(OH) D3) deficiency/insufficiency with an effort to quickly optimize physiologic levels in the preoperative setting, are included in Table 33.5. The recommended form for treatment is cholecalciferol (D3) as opposed to ergocalciferol (D2), which has been shown in one calculation to have a relative potency of D3:D2 of 9.5:1; in another calculation, D2 was one-third that of D3 [61]. The guide is intentionally accelerated for achieving near term results, minimizing retesting expense [62–65], and represents this author's clinical approach based on experience. The targeted serum level for individuals with osteoporosis/-penia and sarcopenia is 50 to 70 ng/mL. Larger, obese patients will have a greater volume of distribution when "loading" vitamin D. If these target levels appear alarming, current data suggest that 25(OH) D3 concentrations must rise above 300 ng/ml to produce toxicity, and levels below 100

TABLE 33.5
Perioperative Treatment Guidelines for Low 25-Hydroxy Vitamin D3

Starting 25-OH D3 Levels (ng/mL)	Starting Dose	Testing Interval*	Next Dose	Retest	Maintenance
< 20	5000–10,000 IU/day	6–8 wks	3000–5000 IU/day	q 8–12 wks until level maintained	As indicated by lab values
20–32	5000 IU	6–8 wks	2000–5000 IU	16 wks	2000 IU
32–50	2000–5000 IU	q 3–4 mos until stable	2000 IU	q 6 mos	
50–75	800–2000 IU	Annually in winter			

*Retest 25-OH D3 and serum calcium

ng/ml will ensure a wide safety margin. Attention to timely lab studies and physician follow-up is recommended.

The Institute of Medicine has recently increased the RDA and UL for vitamin D; however, it has stated that the studies done on vitamin D "beyond bone health…provided often mixed and inconclusive results and could not be considered reliable" [66]. Despite this reporting, current peer review medical literature continues to demonstrate links of deficiency states to an expanding list of medical conditions, recommends laboratory assessment in the clinical guidelines for treating a growing number of diseases, and advises correction to optimal levels as a part of current medical therapy. The well-documented association of hypovitaminosis D with a long list of disease states [67] studied in very large cohorts (n > 300,000 men and women) should command the clinician's attention and, given its wide safety margin, dictate at least conservative intervention while monitoring serum 25(OH) D3 levels and calcium, as part of comprehensive medical therapy [68].

Patients with persistent, nonspecific musculoskeletal pain, particularly those with darker pigmented skin in more northern latitudes, have shown extraordinarily high incidences of severe hypovitaminosis D, even in younger individuals [69].

MACRONUTRIENTS

One fish oil study raises the possibility that the anti-inflammatory actions of omega-3 fatty acids may play a role in the prevention of sarcopenia [70]. Essential fatty acids in the form of eicosapentaenoic acid (EPA) and docosahexaenoic acid (DHA) at 1 g/day has been recommended by the American Heart Association in patients with documented atherosclerosis based on their anti-atherothrombotic effects. A review by Bays (2007) demonstrated that clinical trials have shown high-dose, omega-3 fatty acid consumption to be safe, even when concurrently administered with other agents that may increase bleeding, such as aspirin and warfarin [71]. In some animal studies, however, there have been mixed results regarding postoperative wound strength. For the management of preoperative pain, particularly before withdrawal of NSAIDs or other prescription drugs, this author suggests that patients use 2000 to 2500 mg of EPA and DHA (combined dose) for about three to four weeks prior to withdrawal of the prescription drugs. Following the precaution of one week abstinence from all added nutrients remains a safe margin until further studies are done in humans on wound healing.

PROBIOTICS

Simple use of pre- and postoperative probiotics in doses of 10 M to 10 B *lactobacillus* and *bifidobacter* species/day for one to two weeks before and after surgery in eight of 12 randomized controlled trials showed a significant reduction in bacterial infection rates in noncritically ill surgical patients [72].

SUMMARY AND CLINICAL RECOMMENDATIONS

Elective surgery has potential complications that are willingly assumed in order to improve the quality of life for patients. Many patients have inadequate levels of nutrients, which may have impaired various metabolic pathways and contributed to the development of their medical condition. The additional catabolic stressors of the perioperative period create further depletion of multiple nutrients that are essential for optimal recovery. The scientific literature demonstrates improved outcomes with targeted, metabolic nutrient therapies using individual nutrient interventions, particularly with antioxidants. New terms such as metabolic therapy, immunonutrition, and pharmaconutrition are the result of clinicians expanding their interest in nutrients intending to influence surgical results. There is great opportunity for rational, complex, and balanced nutrient therapy interventions to improve the surgical patient's preoperative experience and recovery. Many patients have already seized this opportunity using little professional advice and are eager to follow knowledgeable physician guidance. Surgeons and primary care physicians are well positioned to initiate effective nutrient therapies to optimize surgical outcomes, particularly orthopedists given the timing of elective total joint arthroplasty, through targeted diet, exercise, and nutrient therapies. The key points are:

- Nutrient therapy is safe and can measurably improve outcomes.
- Invite all, work with the willing and meet the rest with an invitation by sharing the opportunity of using nutrients to create better outcomes.
- The distinctive circumstance of impending surgical threat, combined with patient interest in nutrient therapy, creates a superb opportunity for the physician to spark motivated patient compliance in a preoperative program.
- The nutrient status of many surgical patients is surprisingly poor, particularly the obese elderly.
- Sarcopenia is underdiagnosed and treatable with professionally guided exercise and nutrient support. A first step to nutrient support is recommending unrefined, whole foods and high quality nutrients, starting with a multivitamin—better not higher quality preparations need to be taken as 1–2 caps/tabs twice daily. Physicians and their staff should become familiar with three or four quality preparations and where to direct patients to find them in their community or online.
- Three-day food diaries to measure protein content demonstrate inadequate protein intake with surprising frequency. Increase protein intake for six weeks before and after surgery and maintain intake as close as possible to the NPO period prior to surgery. Even three weeks of focused and directed intervention can make a difference in procedures that have a shorter preoperative interval.
- Protein shakes and amino acid formulas are convenient for the patient to support wound healing, even if changing the diet is not appealing.
- Limit or eliminate negative pharmaceutical and poor dietary influences on healing.
- Jump-start bone metabolism with focused treatment of vitamin D insufficiency/deficiency, and supplement with balanced, chelated minerals for orthopedic patients.
- For complex patients, establish a baseline symptoms reference to ease follow-up assessment, such as the validated MOS SF-36 [17] or the clinically useful Medical Symptoms Questionnaire [18].
- Dietary advice can be as simple as "Eat right!" followed by a few specifics:
  - No "white stuff" (refined flour or sugar) or soft drinks/juices; diabetics need to follow blood sugar closely
  - Lean meats with generous protein portions at every meal
  - Five half-cup servings of vegetables and one fruit/day
  - Drink only filtered water
  - Take a good quality multivitamin

REFERENCES

1. Dickinson A., et al., *Use of dietary supplements by cardiologists. dermatologists and orthopedists: Report of a survey,* Nutr J 2011; 10:20.
2. Stohs S., Dudrick S., *Nutritional supplements in the surgical patient.* Surg Clin N AM 2011;933–944.
3. Kavalukas S., Barbul A., *Nutrition and wound healing: An update.* Plast Reconstr Surg 2011 Jan;127 Suppl 1: 38S–43S.
4. Wright, J.D., et al., *Trends in intake of energy and macronutrients—United States, 1971–2000.* MMWR Feb 6, 2004;53(4):80–82.
5. Patel, N., et al., *Obesity and spine surgery: Relation to perioperative complications.* J Neruosurg Spine 2007 Apr;6(4):291–297.
6. Harms, S., et al., *Obesity increases the likelihood of total joint replacement surgery among younger adults.* Int Orthop 2007 Feb;31(1):23–26 Epub 2006 May 11.
7. Liu, B., et al., *Relationship of height, weight and body mass index to the risk of hip and knee replacements in middle-aged women.* Rheumatology (Oxford) 2007 May;46(5):861–867. Epub 2007 Feb 4.
8. Stürmer, T., et al., *Obesity, overweight and patterns of osteoarthritis: The Ulm Osteoarthritis Study.* J Clin Epidemiol 2000 Mar 1;53(3):307–313.
9. Kohlstadt, I., *Scientific Evidence for Musculoskeletal, Bariatric, and Sports Nutrition.* 2006, Boca Raton: CRC Taylor & Francis.
10. Cosqueric, G., et al., *Sarcopenia is predictive of nosocomial infection in care of the elderly.* Br J Nutr 2006 Nov;96(5):895–901.
11. McMahon, M., J.A. Block, *The risk of contralateral total knee arthroplasty after knee replacement for osteoarthritis.* J Rheumatol 2003 Aug;30(8):1822–1824.
12. Busti, A.J., et al., *Effects of perioperative anti-inflammatory and immunomodulating therapy on surgical wound healing.* Pharmacotherapy 2005 Nov;25(11):1566–1591.
13. Wheeler, P., *Do non-steroidal anti-inflammatory drugs adversely affect stress fracture healing?* Br J Sports Med 2005;39:65–69.
14. Kahan, A., et al., *Long term effects of chondroitins 4 and 6 sulfate on knee osteoarthritis. The study on Osteoarthritis progression, prevention, a two-year randomized, double-blind, placebo-controlled trial.* Arthritis Rheum 2009 Feb;60(2):524-533.
15. Reginster, J.Y., et al., *Current role of glucosamine in the treatment of osteoarthritis.* Rheumatology 2007;46:731–735.
16. Christensen, R., et al., *Effect of weight reduction in obese patients diagnosed with knee osteoarthritis: A systematic review and meta-analysis.* Ann Rheum Dis 2007;66:433–439.
17. Quality Metric Incorporated, 8/03/2012. www.sf-36.org.
18. Bland, J.S., Brailey, A. *Medical symptoms questionnaire.* Unpublished.
19. Rakel, D, *Integrative Medicine,* 2nd Edition. 2007, Philadelphia: Saunders, 1238p.
20. Lentz, M.J., et al., *Effects of selective slow wave sleep discruption on musculoskeletal pain and fatigue in middle aged women.* J Rheumatol 1999;26:1586–1592.
21. Janssen I., *Evolution of sarcopenia research.* Appl Physiol Nutr Metab 2010 Oct;35:707-712.
22. Petersen, A.M., et al, *Smoking impairs muscle protein synthesis and increases the expression of myostatin and MAFbx in muscle.* Am J Physiol Endocrinol Metab 2007 Sep;293(3):E943–948. Epub 2007 Jul 3.
23. Lee, J.S., et al., *Associated factors and health impact of sarcopenia in older Chinese men and women: A cross-sectional study.* Gerontol 2007 Aug 16;53(6):166–172.
24. National Institutes of Health National Heart Lung and Blood Institute, *Clinical guidelines on the identification, evaluation, and treatment of overweight and obesity in adults: The evidence report.* Obes Res 1998; 6:S51–S210.
25. Welborn, T.A., Dhaliwal, S.S., *Preferred clinical measures of central obesity for predicting mortality.* Eur J Clin Nutr 2007 Dec;61(12):1373–1379.
26. Yusuf, S., et al., *Obesity and the risk of myocardial infarction in 27,000 participants from 52 countries: A case-control study.* Lancet 2005;366:1640–1649.
27. Chaput, J.P., et al., *Relationship between antioxidant intakes and class I sarcopenia in elderly men and women.* J Nutr Health Aging 2007 Jul–Aug;11(4):363–369.
28. Chabi, B., et al., *Mitochondrial function and apoptotic susceptibility in aging skeletal muscle.* Aging Cell 2008 Jan; 7(1):2–12 [Epub Nov. 19, 2007].
29. Degens H., *The role of systemic inflammation in age-related muscle weakness and wasting.* Scand J Med Sci Sports 2010; 20:28–38.

30. Villareal, D.T., et al., *Effect of weight loss and exercise on frailty in obese older adults.* Arch Int Med 2006;166:860–866.

31. Gherini, S., et al., *Delayed wound healing and nutritional deficiencies after total hip arthroplasty.* Clin Orthop Relat Res 1993;293:188–195.

32. Cattaneo, M., *Hyperhomocysteinemia and venous thromboembolism.* Semin Thromb Hemost 2006 Oct;32(7):716–723.

33. Marin, L.A. et al., *Preoperative nutritional evaluation as a prognostic tool for wound healing.* Acta Orthop Scand 2002 Jan;73(1):2–5.

34. Campbell, W.W., *Synergistic use of higher-protein diets or nutritional supplements with resistance training to counter sarcopenia.* Nutr Rev 2007 Sep;65(9):416–422.

35. Helman, T. Gout. In: Kohlstadt, I. (ed.), *Scientific Evidence for Musculoskeletal, Bariatric, and Sports Nutrition.* 2006, Boca Raton, FL: CRC, Taylor & Francis, 427.

36. Evans, W.J., *Protein nutrition, exercise and aging.* J Am Coll Nutr. 2004 Dec;23(6Suppl):601S–609S.

37. Breen L., Phillips S., *Skeletal muscle protein metabolism in the elderly: Interventions to counteract the "anabolic resistance" of ageing.* Nutrition and Metabolism 2011;8:68.

38. Jonas, S., and E.M. Phillips. *ACSM's Exercise is Medicine™ A Clinician's Guide to Exercise Prescription.* 2009, Philadelphia: Lippincott Williams & Wilkins.

39. Astin, J.A., *Why patients use alternative medicine.* JAMA 1998;279(19):1548–1553.

40. Eisenberg, D.M., et al., *Unconventional medicine in the United States—prevalence, cost and patterns of use.* N Engl J Med 1993 Jan;328(4):246–252.

41. Witte M.B., Barbul A., *Arginine physiology and its implications for wound healing.* Wound Repair Regen 2003; 11:419–423.

42. Lucotti P., et al. *Beneficial effect of a long-term oral L-arginine treatment added to a hypocaloric diet and exercise training program in obese, insulin-resistant type 2 diabetic patients.* Am J Physiol Endocrinol Metab 2006;291:E906–E912.

43. Nicastro H., et al., *An overview of the therapeutic effects of leucine supplementation on skeletal muscle under atrophic conditions.* Amino Acids 2011 Feb;40(2):287–300.

44. Orban, J.C., et al., *Effects of acetylcysteine and ischaemic preconditioning on muscular function and postoperative pain after orthopaedic surgery using a pneumatic tourniquet.* Eur J Anaesthesiol 2006 Dec;23(12):1025–1030. Epub 2006 Jun 19.

45. Cherchi, A., et al., *Effects of L-carnitine on exercise tolerance in chronic stable angina: A multicenter, double-blind, randomized, placebo controlled crossover study.* Int J Clin Pharmacol Ther Toxicol 1985;23:569–572.

46. Brevetti, G., et al., *Increases in walking distance in patients with peripheral vascular disease treated with L-carnitine: a double-blind, cross-over study.* Circulation 1988;77:767–783.

47. Rundek, T., et al., *Atorvastatin decreases the coenzyme Q10 level in the blood of patients at risk for cardiovascular disease and stroke.* Arch Neurol 2004;61:889–892.

48. Ziegler, D., *Thioctic acid for patients with symptomatic diabetic polyneuropathy: A critical review.* Treat Endocrinol 2004;3(3):173–189.

49. Hadj, A., et al., *Pre-operative preparation for cardiac surgery utilizing a combination of metabolic, physical and mental therapy.* Heart Lung Circ 2006 Jun;15(3):172–181. Epub 2006 May 19.

50. Knudsen E, et al., *Zinc, copper and magnesium absorption from a fiber-rich diet.* J Trace Elem Med Biol 1996;2(10):68–76.

51. Maggio M., et al., *Magnesium and anabolic hormones in older men.* Int J Androl 2011 Jun 15; e594–e600.

52. Mahmood, A., et al., *Zinc carnosine, a health food supplement that stabilises small bowel integrity and stimulates gut repair processes.* Gut 2007 Feb;56(2):168–175. Epub 2006 Jun 15.

53. Yousaf, F., et al., *Efficacy and safety of melatonin as an anxiolytic and analgesic in the perioperative period: A qualitative systematic review of randomized trials.* Anesthesiology 2010 Oct:113(4):968–976.

54. Jarratt J., *Perioperative melatonin use.* Anaesth Intensive Care 2011 Mar;39(2):171–181.

55. Institute of Medicine, *Dietary Reference Intakes.* 2006, Washington, D.C.: National Academies Press, 343.

56. Hron, G., et al., *Low vitamin B6 levels and the risk of recurrent venous thromboembolism.* Haematologica 2007 Sep;92(9):1250–1253. Epub 2007 Aug 1.

57. Cattaneo, M., et al., *Low plasma levels of vitamin B(6) are independently associated with a heightened risk of deep-vein thrombosis.* Circulation 2001 Nov 13;104(20):2442–2446.

58. Vaxman, F., et al., *Can the wound healing process be improved by vitamin supplementations? Experimental study on humans.* Eur Surg Res 1996 Jul–Aug;28(4):306–314.

59. Shah A., et.al., *Use of oral vitamin C after fractures of the distal radius.* J Hand Surg AM 2009; Nov:34(9):1736–1738.
60. Armas, L.A., et al., *Vitamin D2 is much less effective than vitamin D3 in humans.* J Clin Endoncrinol Metab 2004 Nov:89(11):5387–5391.
61. Cannell, J.J., et al., *Diagnosis and treatment of vitamin D deficiency.* Expert Opin Pharmacother 2008 Jan;9(1):107–118.
62. Hollis, B.W., et al., *Circulating 25-hydroxyvitamin D levels indicative of vitamin D suffi ciency: implications for establishing a new effective dietary intake recommendation for vitamin D,* In *Symposium: Vitamin D Insufficiency: a significant risk factor in chronic diseases and potential disease-specific biomarkers of vitamin D suffi ciency.* J Nutr 2005 Feb;135(2):317–322.
63. Adams, J.S., et al., *Resolution of vitamin D insufficiency in osteopenic patients results in rapid recovery of bone mineral density.* J Clin Endocrinol Metab 1999 Aug;84(8):2729–2730.
64. Grant, W.B., Holick, M.F., *Benefits and requirements of vitamin D for optimal health: A review.* Altern Med Rev 2005 Jun;10(2):94–111.
65. Dietary Reference Intakes for Calcium and Vitamin D. November 30, 2010. Consensus Report. http://www.iom.edu/Reports/2010/Dietary-Reference-Intakes-for-Calcium-and-Vitamin-D.aspx (accessed 08/03/2012). Institute of Medicine, 2010.
66. Wei, Y., Giovannucci, E., *Vitamin D and multiple health outcomes in the Harvard cohorts.* Mol Nutr Food Res 2010 Aug:54(8):1114-1126.
67. Jones, G., *Pharmacokinetics of vitamin D toxicity.* Am J Clin Nutr 2008 Aug:88(2):582S–586S.
68. Plotnikoff, G.A. and Quigley, J.M., *Prevalence of severe hypovitaminosis D in patients with persistent, nonspecific musculoskeletal pain.* Mayo Clin Proc 2003 Dec;78(12):1463–1470.
69. Robinson, S.M., et al., *Diet and its relationship with grip strength in community dwelling older men and women: The Hertfordshire Cohort study.* J Am Geriatr Soc 2008 Jan;56(1):84–90. [Epub Nov 15, 2007].
70. Bays, H., *Safety considerations with omerga-3 fatty acid therapy.* Am J Card 2007;99(6A):35C–43C.
71. Rayes, N., Soeters P., *Probiotics in surgical and critically ill patients.* Ann Nutr Metab 2010;57(suppl 1):29–31.
72. Del Savio, G.C., et al., *Preoperative nutritional status and outcome of elective total hip replacement.* Clin Orthop Relat Res 1996 May;(326):153–161.
73. Ackland, G.L., et al., *Pre-operative high sensitivity C-reactive protein and postoperative outcome in patients undergoing elective orthopaedic surgery.* Anaesthesia 2007 Sep;62(9):888–894.
74. Teitelbaum, J. Fibromyalgia. In: Kohlstadt, I. (ed.), *Scientific Evidence for Musculoskeletal, Bariatric, and Sports Nutrition.* 2006, Boca Raton, FL: CRC, Taylor & Francis, 416.
75. Theusinger, O., et al., *Treatment of iron deficiency anemia in orthopedic surgery with intravenous iron: Effi cacy and limits: A prospective study.* Anesthesiology 2007 Dec;107(6):923–927.
76. McCully, K., *Homocysteine, vitamins, and vascular disease prevention.* Am J Clin Nutr 2007;86(suppl): 1563S–1568S.
77. Gerdhem, P., et al., *Associations between homocysteine, bone turnover, BMD, mortality and fracture risk in elderly women.* J Bone Miner Res 2007 Jan;22(1):127–134.
78. Selhub et al. "Vitamin status and intake as primary determinants of homocysteinemia in an elderly population." *JAMA* 1993 Dec;270(22):2693–98.
79. Spence, J.D., *Homocysteine-lowering therapy: A tale in stroke prevention?* Lancet Neurol 2007;6:830–838.
80. Bischoff-Ferrari, H.A., et al., *Higher 25-hydroxyvitamin D concentrations are associated with better lower-extremity function in both active and inactive persons aged = 60 y.* Am J Clin Nutr 2004;80:752–758.
81. Alcantara-Martos, T., et al., *Effect of vitamin C on fracture healing in elderly osteogenic disorder Shionogi rats.* J Bone Joint Surg Br 2007 Mar;89(3):402–407.
82. Berger, M.M., Shenkin, A., *Trace element requirements in critically ill burned patients.* J Trace Elem Med Biol 2007;21 Suppl 1:44–48. Epub 2007 Oct 31.
83. Brzezinski, A., et al., *Effects of exogenous melatonin on sleep; a meta-analysis.* Sleep Med Rev 2005 Feb;9(1):41–50.
84. Candow, D.G., Chilibeck, P.D. *Effect of creatine supplementation during resistance training on muscle accretion in the elderly.* J Nutr Health Aging 2007 Mar–Apr;11(2):185–188.
85. Gionchetti, P., et al., *Probiotics in infective diarrhea and inflammatory bowel diseases.* J Gastroenterol Hepatol 2000 May;15(5):489–493. Review.
86. Jacobs, S., *MSM.* The Arthritis Foundation's Guide to Alternative Therapies. Atlanta, Arthritis Foundation, 1999, p. 223.
87. Jugdaohsingh, R., et al., *Dietary silicon intake is positively associated with bone mineral density in men and premenopausal women of the Framingham Offspring cohort.* Bone 2003 May;32:S192.

88. Juneja, L.R., et al., *L-Theanine-a unique amino acid of green tea and its relaxation effect in humans.* Trends Food Sci Tech 1999;10:199–204.
89. *L-carnitine. Monograph.* Alter Med Rev 2005;10:42–50.
90. *L-Tryptophan. Monograph.* Altern Med Rev 2006 Mar;11(1):52–56.
91. Preli, R.B., et al., *Vascular effects of dietary L-arginine supplementation.* Atherosclerosis 2002;162:1–15.
92. Spigset, O., *Reduced effect of warfarin caused by ubidecarenone.* Lancet 1994;344:1372–1373.
93. Valenti, G., et al., *Effect of DHEAS on skeletal muscle over the life span: the InCHIANTI study.* J Gerontol A Biol Sci Med Sci 2004 May;59(5):466–472.
94. Vetter, G., *Double blind clinical trial with S-adenosylmethionine and indomethacin in the treatment of osteoarthritis.* Am J Med 1987;83(Suppl 5A):S78–S80.
95. Wicke, C., et al., *Effects of steroids and retinoids on wound healing.* Arch Surg 2000;135(11): 1265–1270.
96. Williams, J.Z., Barbul, A., *Nutrition and wound healing,* Surg Clin N Am 2003;83:571–596.
97. Yazdanpanah, N., et al., *Effect of dietary B vitamins on BMD and risk of fracture in elderly men and women: The Rotterdam Study.* Bone 2007;41:987–994.

34 Fibromyalgia

David M. Brady, N.D., D.C., Jacob Teitelbaum, M.D., and Alan Weiss, M.D.

INTRODUCTION

It is estimated that fibromyalgia syndrome (FMS) affects 6 to 12 million Americans, causing more disability than rheumatoid arthritis [1]. The prevalence is increasing, having risen by 200–400% in the last 10 years [2–5]. Fibromyalgia syndrome remains a condition without a fully understood etiology, in which patients report chronic widespread pain (allodynia or hyperalgesia) often accompanied by fatigue, sleep disorders, cognitive deficits, irritable bowel syndrome, headaches, and Raynaud's syndrome. This chapter presents a comprehensive approach to the care of patients with fibromyalgia. Food and nutrients are important in the care of patients with fibromyalgia in several ways. Nutrient strategies are demonstrated to improve overall well-being and reduce symptoms in patients with fibromyalgia. Many patients with chronic widespread pain have undiagnosed causes that may be directly responsive to nutrient strategies. In an effort to meet activities of daily living, people with fibromyalgia may have increased their intake of refined carbohydrates, caffeine, salt, and highly processed foods, forming unhealthful habits benefiting from lifestyle medicine. The comorbid and concurrent conditions experienced by many patients with fibromyalgia in our clinical practices improve with nutrient interventions resulting in overall improved well-being.

PATHOPHYSIOLOGY

Over the past decade, the formal FMS research and medical literature has significantly focused around the concept of central sensitization, often called central allodynia or classic fibromyalgia [6,7]. In this condition, there appears to be a change in the way the central nervous system processes sensory stimuli, resulting in the perception of stimuli that would not be painful in normal people, such as light touch, being perceived as painful. Hence, the term "central allodynia" (central = CNS and dynia = pain). This dysfunction of the central nervous system (CNS) is thought to result from significant acute or chronic stress, including pain, physical and psychological trauma, and other stressors, which can result in limbic system dysfunction and failure of the descending antinociceptive system (DANS). A lowering of pain threshold and increase in pain perception is generally present in these individuals, which is likely also related to the observed decrease in serotonin and increase in substance-P, a pain modulating peptide, in the CNS, and disordered catecholamine production [6–9]. Other alterations in neurotransmitter levels have been reported, such as decreases in dopamine, oxytocin, and acetylcholine levels, along with increased NMDA (*N*-methyl-D-aspartate) activity. Collectively, these changes have been found to be associated with a generalized state of hypervigilance (sympathetic overactivity), resulting in associated autonomic phenomenon such as irritable bowel/bladder syndrome, anxiety, depression, and disordered nonrestorative sleep, which are also commonly seen in hypervigilant patients with post-traumatic stress syndrome (PTSD) [10–12].

Hypothalamic dysfunction is also generally present in FMS [13]. The hypothalamus is a major control center for sleep, so that impaired function contributes to nonrestorative sleep. As a regulator of autonomic function, hypothalamic dysfunction contributes to the many symptoms of dysautonomia or somatic symptoms, including sweating and irritable bowel syndrome. The hypothalamus is also involved in hormonal regulation. Hormonal dysfunction, including hypothyroidism, is often present, as is poor sleep—which further decreases energy production, preventing resolution of the FMS [14,15].

Studies have shown differences in circadian cortisol release in FMS versus healthy controls, suggestive of initial overactivity followed by later exhaustion of the hypothalamic-pituitary-adrenal (HPA) axis [10,13]. This can include blunting of cortisol release in the morning, along with levels being too high in the evening, which may then disrupt sleep. Studies of a variety of thermal, mechanical, and electrical stimuli in FMS and healthy controls consistently show increase in reactivity in the FMS group suggestive of central sensitization [7]. PET scans and fMRI studies of the brain activity of FMS subjects versus healthy controls while they receive innocuous sensory stimulation have shown that FMS patients' limbic structures and CNS pain areas are activated by nonpainful stimuli that only activate the sensory cortex in healthy controls [8]. Genetic predisposition also seems to play a role.

PATIENT EVALUATION

DIAGNOSIS OF FIBROMYALGIA SYNDROME

The diagnosis of fibromyalgia syndrome (FMS) has been accompanied by a controversial history since its inception in 1990. The diagnosis has largely been based on American College of Rheumatology (ACR) criteria. The initial criteria required a tender point exam [16], which the large majority of physicians are not trained to do accurately. In part because of this, an ACR task force has come up with revised alternative diagnostic criteria no longer requiring a tender point exam [17]. Diagnosis is based on a total severity score that includes the number of painful areas, severity of fatigue, cognitive dysfunction, nonrestorative sleep, and the presence of other somatic symptoms (see Table 34.1). The ACR criteria suggest whether the patient has a pattern of physiologic responses that we may call fibromyalgia, but tell us little about its underlying cause or how it should be treated.

DIAGNOSES ASSOCIATED WITH CHRONIC WIDESPREAD PAIN

Making, or ruling out, a diagnosis of FMS begins the assessment process for chronic widespread pain (CWP). Whether or not a patient meets the diagnostic criteria for FMS, for treatment to be effective, clinicians still have to thoroughly evaluate the patient to determine the underlying cause(s) of their CWP and other symptoms. Examples of conditions often included, correctly or not, under the banner of an FMS diagnosis include central sensitization and amplification ("classic fibromyalgia"), myofascial pain syndrome, small fiber neuropathic pain, energy metabolism dysfunction with mitochondrial uncoupling, hypothyroidism, and other internal or musculoskeletal conditions previously undiagnosed, including many autoimmune conditions. Arachnoiditis is a less commonly recognized disorder that can be confused with FMS. Arachnoiditis results from inflammation of the arachnoid membranes surrounding the nerves of the spinal cord and can produce a variety of symptoms, including pain of various types, muscle cramps and spasms, bowel and bladder dysfunction, and lower extremity paralysis. Causes include infections, injury, direct compression by adhesions or scar tissue, and inflammatory processes. Multiple sclerosis, lupus, and rheumatoid arthritis are other common examples of illnesses that may present with widespread pain and FMS, but upon deeper questioning and examination other features pointing to these conditions also emerge to clarify the diagnosis.

TABLE 34.1

The American College of Rheumatology Preliminary Diagnostic Criteria for Fibromyalgia and Measurement of Symptom Severity

Criteria:

A patient satisfies diagnostic criteria for fibromyalgia if the following conditions are met:

1. Widespread pain index (WPI) ≥7 and symptom severity (SS) scale score ≥5 or WPI 3-6 and SS scale score ≥ 9
2. Symptoms have been present at a similar level for at least three months.
3. The patient does not have a disorder that would otherwise explain the pain.

Ascertainment:

1. WPI: Note the number of areas in which the patient has had pain over the last week. In how many areas has the patient had pain? (Score will be between 0 and 19).

Shoulder girdle, left	Hip (buttock, trochanter), left	Jaw, left	Upper back
Shoulder girdle, right	Hip (buttock, trochanter), right	Jaw, right	Lower back
Upper arm, left	Upper leg, left	Chest	Neck
Upper arm, right	Upper leg, right	Abdomen	
Lower arm, left	Lower leg, left		
Lower arm, right	Lower leg, right		

2. SS scale score: A) Fatigue, B) Waking unrefreshed, C) Cognitive symptoms

For each of the 3 symptoms above, indicate the level of severity over the past week using the following scale:

0 = No problem
1 = Slight or mild problems, generally mild or intermittent
2 = Moderate, considerable problems, often present and/or at a moderate level
3 = Severe, pervasive, continuous, life-disturbing problems

Considering somatic symptoms in general, indicate whether patient has:*

0 = No symptoms
1 = Few symptoms
2 = A moderate number of symptoms
3 = A great deal of symptoms

The SS scale score is the sum of the severity of the three symptoms (fatigue, waking unrefreshed, cognitive symptoms) plus the extent (severity) of the somatic symptoms in general. The final score is between 0 and 12.

*Somatic symptoms that might be considered: muscle pain, irritable bowel syndrome, fatigue/tiredness, thinking or remembering problem, muscle weakness, headache, pain/cramps in the abdomen, numbness/tingling, dizziness, insomnia, depression, constipation, pain in the upper abdomen, nausea, nervousness, chest pain, blurred vision, fever, diarrhea, dry mouth, itching, wheezing, Raynaud's phenomenon, hives/welts, ringing in ears, vomiting, heartburn, oral ulcers, loss of/changes in taste, seizures, dry eyes, shortness of breath, loss of appetite, rash, sun sensitivity, hearing difficulties, easy bruising, hair loss, frequent urination, painful urination, and bladder spasms.

From: American College of Rheumatology Web site. Available at: http://www.rheumatology.org/practice/clinical/classification/fibromyalgia/2010_Preliminary_Diagnostic_Criteria.pdf#search=%22Diagnostic%20Criteria%20for%20Fibromyalgia%22. Accessed January 12, 2011.

Fibromyalgia and widespread pain and fatigue represent heterogeneous syndromes with many different underlying triggers and pathologies, varying considerably from patient to patient. Different patterns can occur depending on whether the key symptoms and signs are peripheral (as with myofascial and neuropathic pain), central (with central sensitization), dysautonomic (including low blood pressure with neutally mediated hypotension [NMH] or postural orthostatic tachycardia syndrome [POTS], postexertional fatigue, spastic colon, etc.), structural, or some combination of these. These patterns, when recognized, can help the practitioner determine the perpetuating factors contributing to the patient's condition, so that they can create an effective individualized treatment protocol aimed at the specific cause of the patient's widespread pain and fatigue [18,19].

While there seems to be a distinct disorder involving altered processing of sensory information and increased perception of pain at the level of the central nervous system, which we have previously referred to as "classic" FMS, central sensitization, and central allodynia, this likely represents only a small percentage of patients who carry the diagnostic label of FMS [20]. Instead, the label FMS is likely not representative of this one CNS disorder, or one disease process, but rather it has become an umbrella term, accurately or not, under which a number of diagnostic subsets exist. It is likely that there are numerous medical causes for the symptoms of widespread pain and fatigue, and that a number of other diseases and conditions might inadvertently be labeled as FMS. An argument can be made over whether the single umbrella diagnosis causes more harm than good, unless it leads to a more thorough evaluation.

In order to facilitate diagnosis, the symptoms of chronic pain and fatigue in patients given the label FMS can be viewed in four distinct subsets: (1) classic FMS, which is hypothesized to be a CNS disorder of pain processing, (2) organic medical diseases, (3) more subtle metabolic and nutritional disorders, and (4) musculoskeletal disorders, with the latter three representing other causes of pain, fatigue and other symptoms that are commonly included under the FMS diagnostic umbrella (see Figure 34.1) [21,22]. Therefore, great care should be given to the initial work-up of patients presenting with symptoms suggestive of FMS. All potential causes, including more subtle metabolic and nutritional disorders, should be fully explored and ruled out as potential causes of the patient's complaints before a diagnosis of FMS is rendered.

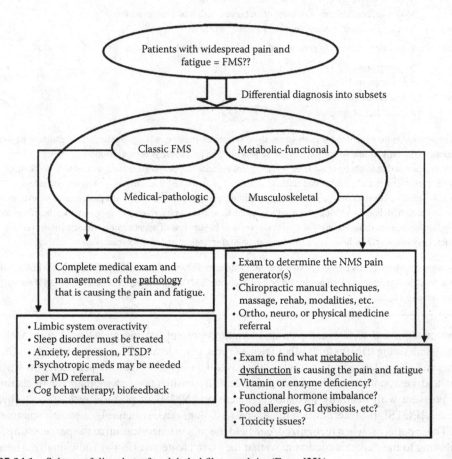

FIGURE 34.1   Subsets of disorders often labeled fibromyalgia. (From [22].)

Diagnosis of Associated Conditions, Comorbidities, and Underlying Causes (see Table 34.2)

Fatigue

Fatigue is a significant component of most cases of FMS and research studies have implicated mitochondrial and hypothalamic dysfunction as common denominators in these syndromes [13,23]. Dysfunction of hormonal, sleep [15], and autonomic control (all centered in the hypothalamus) and energy production centers (mitochondria) can explain the large number of symptoms and why most patients have a similar set of complaints.

Irritable Bowel Syndrome

Irritable bowel syndrome (IBS) affects approximately 11% to 14% of the population. It is a condition with multiple models of pathophysiology including altered motility, visceral hypersensitivity, abnormal brain-gut interaction, autonomic dysfunction, and immune activation [24]. This chronic functional bowel disorder, characterized by both visceral and somatic hyperalgesia, produces similar effects seen with the central hypersensitivity mechanisms in fibromyalgia (FMS) [25,26]. Many studies have demonstrated a common association or comorbidity between IBS and FMS ranging from 30% to over 80% [27–37]. Prevalence rates reported by Kurland et al. of IBS in FMS patients (n = 105) was 63% by Rome I and 81% by Rome II criteria, compared to the prevalence of IBS in controls (n = 62) of 15% by Rome I and 24% by Rome II criteria (FM vs. control; p < 0.001) [30].

Lubrano et al. reported a prevalence of FMS in approximately 20% of IBS patients [34]. However, since the commonly used diagnostic criteria of FMS includes IBS, the relationship of both syndromes is difficult to analyze [38]. A female predominance has been reported in both IBS and FMS. It has been suggested that the female predominance in IBS patients may result mainly from coexisting fibromyalgia [39].

Visceral hypersensitivity, measured by decreased pain thresholds to gut distension, is considered a biological marker of IBS. However, patients with IBS also have many extraintestinal symptoms consistent with hyperalgesic states; and they may also exhibit cutaneous hyperalgesia similar to that seen in other chronic and global pain disorders, including FMS [32]. This suggests not only comorbidity between IBS and FMS, but some shared mechanisms of central nociceptive pathophysiology.

Small Intestinal Bacterial Overgrowth

Patients with FMS frequently have nonspecific bowel complaints similar to those with small intestinal bacterial overgrowth (SIBO) [31]. SIBO is a condition where colonic aerobic and anaerobic bacteria are overrepresented in the small intestine. There is a growing body of evidence suggesting that SIBO may play a significant role in a wide range of gastrointestinal disorders, including Crohn's disease and IBS [40–43].

Pimentel et al., using lactulose hydrogen breath testing (LHBT), reported that of 123 subjects with FMS, 96 (78%) were found to have SIBO [44,45]. Of these 123 subjects with FMS, 87% also met the Rome I criteria for IBS. Of 25 subjects who returned for follow-up LHBT, 11 achieved complete eradication and 14 achieved incomplete eradication of their SIBO with antibiotic therapy. Improvement in GI symptoms, including bloating, gas, diarrhea, constipation, and abdominal pain, as well as general symptoms of pain, fatigue, and sleeplessness were also reported via follow-up patient questionnaires. Better clinical results were clearly observed with complete eradication. Rifaximin is a gut-selective antibiotic with negligible systemic absorption (< 0.4%), minimal side effects (similar to placebo), and broad-spectrum activity in vitro against gram-positive and gram-negative aerobes and anaerobes and results in effective eradication of SIBO in up to 70% of cases [46,47]. Rifaximin also has known activity against clostridium difficile [48]. Other options for treating SIBO are important to consider when rifaximin is not available or covered by insurance providers. These include the antibiotics neomycin (a low-cost nonabsorbable antibiotic that when used long term may rarely cause ototoxicity) and norfloxacin. Natural GI antimicrobials can be

TABLE 34.2

Common Associated Conditions, Comorbidities, and Underlying Causes in Fibromyalgia

Associated Conditions/ Comorbidities/Underlying Causes	Clinical Importance (1=very, 2= somewhat, 3=less frequent)	Diagnostic Tests (Optional- Diagnosis Can Very Often Be Made Based on Symptoms)	Is Treatment Likely to Improve Overall FMS Symptoms?
Adrenal dysfunction, both primary and secondary	1	ACTH stimulation test, salivary cortisol, DHEA-S, 24-hour urine cortisol, urine organic acids	Yes
Anxiety	2	Urinary neurotransmitters, urine organic acids	Yes
Bladder urgency and spasticity	3	Pelvic ultrasound, bladder residual volume, formal urological manometric testing	No
Depression	2	Urinary neurotransmitters, urine organic acids	Maybe
Disordered, nonrestorative sleep	1	Sleep questionnaire (Epworth), formal polysomnography	Yes
Dysautonomia	2	Tilt table testing, ANSARTM testing	Yes
Endometriosis	3	Pelvic imaging, laparoscopy	No
Hypothalamic/pituitary dysfunction	1	Adrenal/thyroid testing	Yes
Hypothyroidism both primary, secondary, peripheral T4→T3 conversion dysfunction, and T3 resistance	1	TSH, free and total T3, free and total T4, reverse T3, thyroid peroxidase/thyroglobulin antibodies, consider iodine sufficiency testing	Yes
Hypotension (POTS or neurally mediated)	3	Supine/standing blood pressures, tilt table testing	Maybe
Interstitial cystitis	3	Cystoscopy, urine culture to rule out other causes of pain	No
Irritable bowel syndrome/spastic colon	1	Colonoscopy, stool culture to rule out other causes of symptoms, use Rome questionnaire	Maybe
Migraines	2	Evaluation to rule out other causes of headaches	No
Polycystic ovary syndrome	3	Pelvic exam/ultrasound, serum testosterone, DHEA-S, and insulin, glucose tolerance testing	Maybe
Post-exertional fatigue	2	Evaluate adrenal/thyroid function	Yes
Restless leg syndrome	2	Polysomnogram	Yes
Sicca syndrome	3	Sjogren's screening	No
Sleep apnea/upper airways resistance syndrome	2	Polysomnogram	Yes
Small intestinal bacterial overgrowth	2	Hydrogen breath testing; rule out other causes of symptoms: endoscopy, colonoscopy, serology to rule out celiac, stool cultures	Maybe
Visceral hyperesthesia	2	None (history only)	Maybe

ACTH=Adrenocorticotropic Hormone, DHEA-S=Dehydroepiandrosterone Sulfate, TSH=Thyroid Stimulating Hormone, POTS=Postural Orthostatic Tachycardia Syndrome very effective in treating SIBO, as well as other gastrointestinal infections. These include oil of oregano, berberine-containing botanicals, *Juglans nigra* (black walnut), caprylic acid, grapefruit and other citrus seed extracts, and *Artemesia anuua* (wormwood) [49–56]. In addition, it is important to optimize thyroid function to restore compromised peristalsis, to decrease the recurrence of the SIBO.

Laboratory Diagnosis of Metabolic Disturbance

Laboratory testing can yield useful information that can direct proper treatment in FMS, such as the existence of suboptimal levels of vitamins and minerals that serve as critical enzyme cofactors, vitamin D insufficiency, as well as hormonal deficiency or excess.

A biomarker for uncovering metabolic, toxic, and infectious contributions to FMS is urinary organic acid testing (OAT) [57]. Comprehensive urinary OAT panels are now available from several commercial laboratories that commonly serve the integrative and nutritional medicine community. OAT inspects the levels of metabolic intermediates in pathways dependent on critical nutrients, as well as mitochondrial function and cellular energy (ATP) production (see Figure 34.2), detoxification, oxidative stress, neurotransmitter production and breakdown (see Figure 34.3), and metabolites produced by yeast or gastrointestinal bacteria (see Figure 34.4). Elevated levels of specific organic acids may indicate a functional block or inhibition of specific pathways due to inherited enzyme deficits, production of structurally aberrant enzymes, and/or nutrient deficiencies. Urinary OAT results may support the diagnosis and treatment of aberrant stress physiology, impaired detoxification metabolism, DNA damage resulting from excessive oxidative stress, suboptimal methylation, and intestinal dysbiosis and yeast overgrowth. It must be noted that any impairment in renal function may alter the accuracy and validity of timed urine studies, including organic acids.

OAT test results pertinent to treating FMS include the following:

- Elevated urinary levels of malate, fumarate, succinate, alpha-ketoglutarate, hydroxymethylglutarate, and other Krebs cycle intermediates may indicate co-enzyme Q10, B vitamins, lipoic acid, and/or magnesium deficiency, or other issues of mitochondrial function and energy production [58,59]. Clinical correlations include fatigue and muscle ache and intervention in such circumstances should include increased intake, through alteration of dietary intake and/or supplementation, of co-enzyme Q10, B vitamins, lipoic acid, and magnesium as discussed here in the nutrient-based treatment section of the SHINE protocol.
- Elevations in catecholamine metabolites, such as vanilmandelate (VMA) and/or homovanillate (HVA), can be indicative of the typical sympathetic compensation pattern and hypervigilence observed in classic FMS, IBS, and PTSD [60]. Clinical correlation would include anxiety, panic attack, insomnia, and overall signs of hypervigilance; intervention in such circumstances should include cognitive behavioral therapy, relaxation practices, and the administration of adaptogenic botanicals and calming neurotransmitter precursors as is discussed here in the hormonal (adrenal) section of the SHINE protocol.
- Deficiency of 5-hydroxyindoleacetate (5-HIAA) is indicative of reduction in total body serotonin (5-HT) production, which may correlate with increased pain perception, mild depression, IBS, and insomnia [61] and serves as a possible indicator for the use of prescription or natural serotonin modulators as outlined here in the treatment overview. Abnormalities of the kynurenin-quinolinate pathway of tryptophan metabolism can lead to alterations in pain perception via NMDA receptor activation (see Figure 34.5) [62]. Elevations in these markers may indicate the need for treatment of any underlying degenerative/inflammatory neurological condition. Reduction of systemic inflammation with omega-3 fatty acid (EPA-DHA from fish oil) therapy is also suggested.
- The status of B vitamins, lipoic acid, carnitine, and other nutrients critical to energy production can also be evaluated through OAT. Clinical correlations include fatigue and muscle ache; dietary modulation and/or supplementation can be initiated as required.

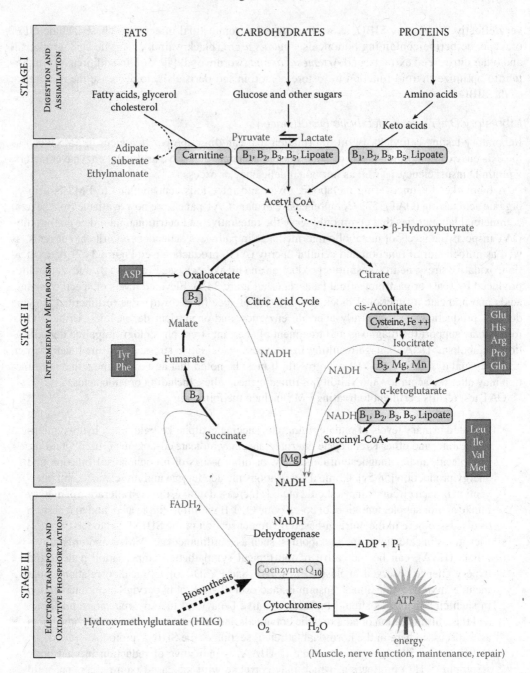

FIGURE 34.2 Urinary markers of nutrients involved in central energy pathways.
Note: Vitamin and mineral requirements for cofactors are shown in black boxes. Elevations of metabolites before these steps indicate functional deficit of the nutrients. (From [57]. Used with permission.)

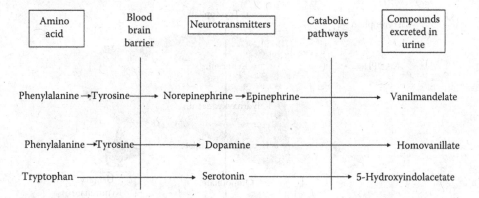

FIGURE 34.3 Urinary organic acid biomarkers of neurotransmitter synthesis. (From [57]. Used with permission.)

- Increased recovery of methylmalonate (MMA) and formiminoglutamate (FIGLU) indicates an insufficiency of vitamin B12 and folate, respectively, potentially resulting in suboptimal methylation and genetic expression. In subjects with elevations in either of these markers, increased intake of folate and/or B12 can be initiated through dietary modulation and/or supplementation.
- Elevated levels of various metabolic byproducts of opportunistic or pathogenic gastrointestinal organisms is indicative of a dysbiotic state of the microbiota and/or SIBO, with d-arabinitol specifically supporting a diagnosis of yeast overgrowth [63]. Clinical correlations include postprandial bloating, cramping, and excessive flatulence; interventions include prescription or natural antimicrobial therapy, as discussed previously in the section on SIBO.

OAT is generally repeated after one to three months to assess for improvement in metabolic function in areas found to be suboptimal on the initial testing and to help in refining any ongoing clinical intervention.

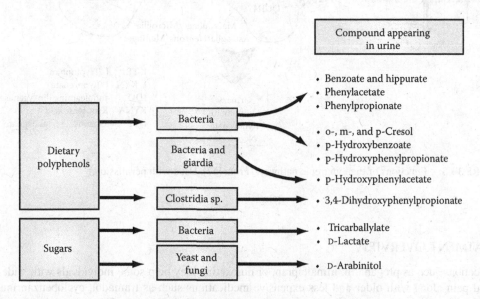

FIGURE 34.4 Urinary organic acid dysbiosis markers. (From [57]. Used with permission.)

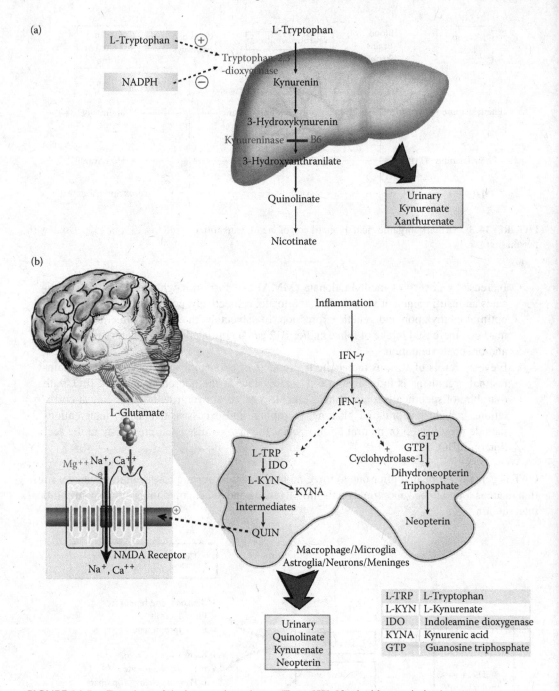

FIGURE 34.5. Functions of the kynurenic pathway. (From [57]. Used with permission.)

TREATMENT OVERVIEW

Medications such as pregabalin, minalcipran, or duloxetine may help some individuals with widespread pain along with older and less expensive medications such as tramadol, cyclobenzaprine, trazodone, and gabapentin. Medications may be particularly helpful in those patients with central sensitization but usually serve as no more than a way to give mild symptomatic pain relief without treating the underlying causes of the illness. If used this way, the medications may become an impediment to the clinician further exploring the underlying causes of the pain, as discussed earlier [19]. Pain is only one of many potentially disabling symptoms in FMS.

Treating central sensitization is the key focus of the three FDA-approved medications for FMS pain: pregabalin, duloxetine, and milnacipran. In 2007, pregabalin (Lyrica™), an alpha-2-delta (α2δ) ligand, became the first medication to gain FDA approval for treatment of FMS pain [64]. Although, as with each of the three approved FMS medications, the exact mechanism of pregabalin's antinociceptive action is not yet clear; it is currently believed to function via binding to the α2δ subunit of voltage-gated calcium channels in central nervous system neurons, reducing the release of glutamate and substance P and thus reducing neuronal hyperexcitability [65]. Pain reduction may also result from decreased calcium-dependent release of pronociceptive neurotransmitters in the ascending tracts of the spinal cord [66] and through interactions with descending noradrenergic and serotonergic pathways originating from the brainstem that modulate pain transmission in the spinal cord [67].

Pregabalin is structurally similar to gabapentin (Neurontin™), and both are often used for treatment of post-herpetic neuralgia, and as adjunctive therapy in adult epilepsy [66]. Off-label uses for both include treating sleep disorders and other pain syndromes [68]. While pregabalin is an analog of the inhibitory neurotransmitter gamma-aminobutyric acid (GABA), it does not bind directly to GABA or benzodiazepine receptors. However, GABA levels in the brain may be increased as an effect of these medications, which may be the reason for the improved sleep quality provided by pregabalin [69].

Though some pain relief may occur with lower doses of pregabalin, significant (> 30–50%) reduction in pain is more likely to occur at higher total daily dosages of 300–600 mg (dosed bid-tid) [70,71]. Note that FDA approval is only for doses up to 450 mg a day. Prescribers of pregabalin must take into account its wide range of side effects and consider slowly increasing the dosage to allow patients to tolerate higher amounts. Adverse effects include dizziness (38%), somnolence (20%), headache (12%), weight gain (11%), dry mouth (8%), blurred vision (8%), fatigue (7%), constipation (7%), euphoric mood (6%), and peripheral edema (6%) [64].

The other two medications approved for FMS pain are duloxetine (Cymbalta™) and milnacipran (Savella™), each of which is a serotonin-norepinephrine reuptake inhibitor. They are felt to provide benefit through amplifying serotonin and norephineprine modulation of descending pain-inhibitory pathways in the brain and spinal cord [72]. Neither of the medications have been tested head to head (or against pregabalin for that matter), which makes it difficult to assess relative efficacy.

Dosing of duloxetine ranges from 20–60 mg bid, and milnacipran from 25–100 mg qd-bid, with most of the benefits being seen by 60 mg and 100 mg qd respectively [73]. Tolerability seems to be more of an issue with milnacipran. Improving compliance and tolerance may be achieved through slow titration and taking the medications with meals to reduce nausea [74,75].

It is important to note that while these three medications do benefit substantial numbers of patients, a large percentage of FMS patients will not see significant lessening of their pain [73]. So other avenues clearly need to be explored, including other prescription medications and nonprescription supplements and modalities, which may effectively treat the underlying problems rather than simply masking pain.

Other medications may be indicated for managing conditions and symptoms associated with FMS. These include gabapentin (whose mechanism is similar to pregabalin) [68] and cyclobenzaprine, which has been shown to be helpful in FMS even at very low doses (e.g., 1–4 mg qhs) [76]. In addition, the tricyclic antidepressant medications amitriptyline and nortriptyline (at 10–25 mg qhs), and also trazodone (at 25–100 mg qhs), a unique medication that acts on multiple receptor types to reduce anxiety and improve mood, have been used widely and fairly successfully to reduce pain and improve sleep in patients with FMS. These medications are generally used in much lower amounts when treating FMS than when typically used in treating depression [77,78]. Fluoxetine or sertraline in combination with amitriptyline was found to be effective [79.80], as was fluoxetine in combination with cyclobenzaprine [81]. These findings attest to the multiple areas of dysfunction playing roles in the pathogenesis of FMS and that using low doses of different classes of medications can be effective. However, this often will need to be done on a trial and error basis with individual patients until an effective regimen is attained.

Benzodiazepines usually worsen sleep quality and are addictive, making them less effective than other sleep aids [77]. If needed, clonazepam may be less likely to worsen sleep quality and may also help the anxiety and restless leg syndrome sometimes associated with FMS.

Finally, a recent Stanford University study using very low doses (3–4.5mg qhs-higher doses are not effective) of naltrexone, an opiate antagonist, demonstrated a 30% reduction in pain for all 10 of the patients in this small study [82]. Further investigation is called for, especially given the low cost and benign side effects of this intervention, mostly regarding sleep disruption. Its mechanism of action is suspected to be via immune modulation, though this still is yet to be clarified.

There are potent nonprescription methods for improving the pain and sleep disturbance seen in FMS. Given that severity of FMS has been found by some researchers to correlate with a low serum serotonin level (which may correspond to low CSF levels), raising serotonin levels seems to be a logical course to try. And indeed 5-hydroxytryptophan (5-HTP), a downstream metabolite of the amino acid tryptophan and a serotonin precursor, has been shown to improve sleep, mood, and pain in FMS. Usual doses of 5-HTP are 50–300 mg [83]. Side effects are usually manageable and include gastrointestinal cramping, nausea, and increasingly vivid dreams. Caution should be used when using 5-HTP in combination with medications like SSRIs, SNRIs, or tramadol, which also raise serotonin levels and raise the specter of serotonin syndrome as a possible adverse reaction, although this is rare [84]. Long-term use of this single amino acid may lead to additional imbalances in the monoamine neurotransmitters (not unlike the well-established side effects of medications acting on this system), as this is a tightly regulated system.

Melatonin is secreted by the pineal gland and has a critical role in sleep initiation and maintaining circadian rhythm. Studies have also demonstrated its benefit in reducing pain, and improving GERD and IBS, both of which are common comorbidities in FMS. FMS patients have been demonstrated to have lower melatonin secretion during the hours of darkness than healthy subjects, which likely plays a role in impaired sleep at night, fatigue during the day, and altered pain perception. Treatment with melatonin in doses ranging from 0.5 mg to 9 mg, 30–60 minutes prior to bedtime, may help restore the circadian rhythm, decrease sleep latency (the time it takes to fall asleep), deepen sleep, and improve other parameters associated with FMS, including pain and IBS. Side effects include nausea or more vivid dreams [85,86].

Two receptors that have a role in pain sensation are the GABA (gamma-aminobutyric acid) and NMDA (N-methyl-D-aspartate) receptors [87]. Stimulation of the GABA receptors by medications (i.e., the benzodiazepines like alprazolam and clonazepam) or by supplementation (i.e., L-theanine, and the herbs valerian, passiflora, scutilaria, and kava) can reduce anxiety and muscle tension and improve sleep quality as well. Supplements containing GABA have been reported to provide calming benefits, though its ability to cross the blood-brain barrier is questionable [88].

Other modalities are useful in improving the overall health and well-being of people with FMS. Both yoga and tai-chi have been found to improve pain levels, mood, and sleep [89.90]. Beginning gentle, directed exercise can also be quite helpful [91], and the use of a pedometer with the ultimate goal of 10,000 steps each day can be effective [92]. However, one must recognize current limitations, and for some FMS patients three to five minutes of walking may be all that is possible at first. One of the pitfalls of beginning an exercise program is that people with FMS are often deconditioned due to the prolonged pain, immobility, and overall metabolic energy deficiency. As a result, they are prone to injury and fatigue, so starting slow and "leaving something in the tank" is essential. Pushing patients beyond their limit can result in what is called "post-exertional fatigue"—which is often enough to leave the patient in pain, exhausted, and bedridden for several days.

Research has provided support for the role of cognitive behavioral therapy and relaxation techniques in improving prospects for people with FMS [93]. Finding the right therapist to work with is critical, as working with someone who does not realize that FMS is a true physiological issue can leave the patient feeling guilt and self-blame for their condition. At the same time, there is a very real relationship between chronic stress and anxiety both proceeding and accompanying FMS. Being enabled to effectively deal with stress and anxiety and learning coping skills in the right therapeutic setting can go a long way to healing a person with FMS— or any severe chronic illness.

ONE COMPREHENSIVE THERAPEUTIC APPROACH

Few clinical trials are available evaluating patient benefit from a medical approach that integrates nutrient strategies and concurrent treatment of related comorbidities. An initial open study and a follow-up, double-blind RCT completed by Teitelbaum et al. showed that when this is done 91% of patients improve, with an average 90% improvement in quality of life; the majority of patients no longer qualified as having FMS by the end of three months (p < .0001 vs. placebo) [94,95]. Improving energy balance in the body was shown to improve quality of life an average of 90% in FMS (p < .0001 vs. placebo). The protocol used in these two studies included treating Sleep, Hormonal dysfunction, Infections, optimizing Nutritional support, and adding Exercise to the subject's tolerance, and is referred to as the **SHINE** protocol.

DISORDERED SLEEP

For patients to recover, it is critical that they get eight to nine hours of sleep per night. When one recognizes that many diagnosed with FMS have a hypothalamic sleep disorder—not poor sleep hygiene—this approach makes sense. Look for and treat restless leg syndrome (RLS), obstructive sleep apnea (OSA), and upper airway resistance syndrome (UARS) if clinically suspected, as these are more common in FMS. If the serum ferritin is under 60, iron supplementation is often very effective for treating RLS or periodic limb movement disorder (PLMD) [96]. Weight loss is also critical for OSA.

The use of 5-HTP (50–300 mg) and/or melatonin (0.5–9 mg) 30–60 minutes prior to bedtime is often helpful to improve sleep quality and possibly reduce pain perception [83–86].

HORMONAL DEFICIENCIES/DYSFUNCTION

The hypothalamus is the main control center for most of the glands in the body, through the hypothalamic-pituitary axis. When focusing on achieving hormonal balance, the standard laboratory testing alone is not sufficient for many reasons. For example, increased hormone binding to carrier proteins is often present in FMS. Because of this, total hormone levels are often normal while the active (free) hormone levels remain low, creating a functional deficiency in the patient. Also, most blood tests use two standard deviations from the mean to define blood test normal ranges. By definition, only the lowest or highest 2.5% of the population is in the abnormal (treatment) range. This does not work well if over 2.5% of the population has a problem. For example, 24% of patients with FMS have positive anti-TPO antibodies despite normal TSH levels, which is much higher than seen in healthy controls [97].

The goal in FMS management is to restore optimal function while keeping labs in the normal range for safety.

Thyroid

Many subjects labeled with FMS have thyroid dysfunctions (i.e., low T3 syndrome, T4 to T3 conversion disorder, thyroid hormone resistance syndrome, etc.) despite normal lab testing, and require some level of thyroid support. In these subjects, using natural prescription desiccated thyroid containing both thyroxine (T4) and triiodothyronine (T3), such as Armour Thyroid™ or NatureThroid™, often seem to work more effectively than synthetic thyroxine alone. In addition, correcting iodine deficiency may be helpful, as iodine intakes in the United States, where iodine deficiency has historically been a problem, dropped by 50% between 1971 and 1994 [98]. Optimizing iodine intake is especially important in those getting large amounts of soy in their diet (i.e., vegans who use it as a meat/milk substitute), as this can result in decreased thyroid hormone function in those with marginal iodine intakes [99]. Preventing selenium deficiency is also important, as selenium is needed for conversion of T4 to the more active T3.

Adrenal

Adrenal support is also important in many FMS patients as HPA axis dysfunction is present [13]. Natural adrenal support is helpful, including:

- Adaptogenic botanicals, particularly those that are not overtly stimulating, such as *Withania somnifera* (aswaganda), *Panex quinquifolia* (American ginseng), and *Rhodiola rosea* (rhodiola).
- Calming botanicals and nutrients, and neurotransmitter precursors, including *Valeriana officinalis* (valerian), *Passiflora incarnate* (passionflower), phosphatidylserine (PS), L-theanine, GABA, 5-HTP, and melatonin.
- Nutrients critical to adrenal function, including vitamin C, B vitamins (i.e., B2, B5, and B6), and tyrosine. Note: Use tyrosine and stimulating adaptogenic botanicals, such as Panex ginseng (Chinese or Korean ginseng), Eleutherococcus senticosus (eleuthero), and Glycyrrhiza glabra (licorice), with caution in those with elevated catecholamine metabolites on urinary organic acid testing, such as VMA and HVA, or clinical symptoms of anxiety and/or insomnia, as this may cause exacerbation.
- Adrenal glandulars, which contain most of the amino acid "building blocks" needed for adrenal repair.

Sex Hormones

Bioidentical estriol, estradiol, progesterone, and testosterone are also helpful in many cases based on individual need.

Unusual Infections

Many studies have shown immune system dysfunction with opportunistic infections in both FMS and chronic fatigue syndrome (CFS). Immune dysfunction can result in many unusual and opportunistic infections. These include reactivation of old viral infections (i.e., HHV-6, CMV, and EBV), parasites and other bowel infections, infections sensitive to long-term treatment with the antibiotics ciprofloxacin and doxycycline (i.e., mycoplasma, chlamydia, possibly Lyme and other tick-borne pathogens, etc.) and fungal infections. Although the latter is controversial, the research and extensive clinical experience of Teitelbaum et al. have found treating with an antifungal (i.e., probiotics and fluconazole at a dose of 200 mg qd for six weeks) to be very helpful with the many symptoms seen in these syndromes [94,95]. Avoiding sweets, with the exception of stevia, can also be very helpful.

Nutrition

Diet and Food-Based Treatment Approaches

It is recommended that patients eat those things that leave them feeling the best. They are also cautioned that what makes them feel best can be, and often is, different from what they crave.

The majority of FMS patients find that they do best with a high-protein, low-carbohydrate diet. The most critical advice is that the patient should avoid sugar and other noncaloric artificial sweeteners, excessive caffeine, and excess alcohol. Warn the patient that there may be a seven- to 10-day withdrawal period when coming off the sugar and caffeine. Stevia is an acceptable sweetener substitute. Another healthy sweetener is ribose, discussed later in this chapter. Ribose has a negative glycemic index, improves energy, is heat stable, and can be added to hot liquids and used in cooking.

If the patient has low blood pressure and/or orthostatic dizziness, increasing salt intake should also be considered, and even salt tablets may be needed during hot weather because of losses from sweat. Because of the low antidiuretic hormone production sometimes seen in FMS, these patients are often dehydrated despite drinking far more than most people. Do not have the patient counting glasses of water all day. Rather, have them keep a bottle or glass of water on hand and avoid dry mouth and lips.

Nutrient-Based Treatment

FMS patients are often nutritionally deficient because of malabsorption (in part likely from SIBO and chronic acid-blocker use), increased physiologic demand, and inadequate diet. Multiple nutrients are critical. B vitamins, ribose, magnesium, iron, coenzyme Q_{10}, malic acid, and carnitine are essential for mitochondrial function. These nutrients are also critical for many other processes. The following foundational nutritional regimen is often useful for patients diagnosed with FMS.

Multivitamin of High Quality

A multivitamin, or a multi in combination with other supplements, should contain at least 50 mg of B complex, 200 mg of lipoic acid, 150–200 mg of magnesium (glycinate or malate chelated forms), 900 mg of malic acid, 1000–2000 IU of vitamin D, 500 mg of vitamin C, 15–20 mg of zinc, 50 mcg of selenium, 200 mcg of chromium, and whey-based or free-form amino acids. A multivitamin should be taken long term.

Iron

If the serum ferritin is under 60 ng/ml, supplementation with iron should be considered for several reasons:

- Nonanemic women with chronic unexplained fatigue and a ferritin < 50 ng/ml benefit from iron supplementation [100].
- Ferritin levels will be in the normal range (over 12) in a dramatic 92% of anemic and chronically ill patients who have severe iron deficiency with absent iron stores documented on marrow testing [101].
- Anemia with normal hematocrit is the rule rather than the exception in FMS/CFS-related conditions because of a low red blood cell mass combined with fluid depletion [102].
- Iron is critical for immune function and dopamine production (both low in FMS) and as discussed earlier, the RLS common in FMS often continues to improve until ferritin is over 60 [96].
- Low iron impairs thyroid metabolism [103].

Iron supplementation of 30 mg, preferably in the iron-bis-glycinate form, plus vitamin C at 100 mg to enhance absorption, every other day for three to eight months is recommended as needed to bring ferritin levels over 60 [96]. Iron should be taken on an empty stomach, since food may decrease iron absorption. It should not be taken within six hours of thyroid hormone, since iron blocks absorption. As daily iron can cause decreased absorption, taking it three weeks each month or every other day is preferable to daily dosing. If ferritin levels are elevated initially, rule out hemochromatosis.

Vitamin B12

Problems with vitamin B12 deficiency, including low or even nondetectable levels in the brain in FMS patients, may occur even with normal blood levels [104–107]. If the serum B12 level is under 540 pg/ml, or there is an elevated MMA test, B12 injections may be recommended at 3000 micrograms IM three times a week for 10–15 weeks, then on an as needed basis depending on the patient's clinical response. Although controversial, this treatment is often both very helpful and very safe. Compounding pharmacies can make B12 at 3000 mcg/cc concentrations, available as hydroxycobalmin, and the preferred methylcobalamin forms. The use of a multivitamin that contains at least 500 micrograms of B12 daily is also recommended.

Coenzyme Q10

Coenzyme Q10 is a conditionally essential nutrient that improves energy production in patients with FMS. A daily supplemental dose of 200 mg is especially critical in patients on statin-family cholesterol treatments, which block endogenous coenzyme Q10 production and can actually cause widespread pain.

Acetyl-L-Carnitine

Carnitine plays many roles in the body. It has the critical function of preventing acetyl coenzyme-A from building up and shutting down the TCA cycle and the electron transport system, the cell's effective energy-burning systems. Also, without sufficient carnitine, the body cannot effectively burn fat and this may contribute to the weight gain often seen in FMS.

Acetyl-L-carnitine at 500 mg twice daily for four months is strongly recommended to help restore energy function. Muscle biopsies show CFS, and likely FMS, patient's intracellular levels to routinely be low. The acetyl-L-carnitine form, although more expensive, may be more effective [108], and has stronger antioxidant activity than L-carnitine.

D-Ribose

D-ribose should be administered at 5 gm tid for three weeks, then bid. D-ribose alone increased energy an average of ~60%, and decreased pain, in two studies of 298 FMS patients after three weeks of therapy [109,110].

D-ribose is a simple, 5-carbon (pentose) sugar, generally preserved for ATP synthesis and the production of DNA and RNA. Since fibromyalgia, for some, may represent a cellular energy crisis, it is critical that the patients have what is needed for optimal mitochondrial function. Two very interesting animal studies conducted by Terjung et al. showed how dramatic the effect of ribose could be on energy recovery in fatigued muscle [111]. Ribose administration in fatigued muscle increased the rate of energy recovery by 340% to 430%, depending on which type of muscle was tested. They also found that even very small amounts of ribose had the effect of helping the muscle cells preserve energy, a process known as energy salvage, and the higher the ribose dose, the more dramatic the effect on energy preservation [112].

EXERCISE

Daily exercise should be implemented as tolerated and as described previously.

SUMMARY

Fibromyalgia syndrome remains a condition without a fully understood etiology, in which patients report chronic widespread pain (allodynia or hyperalgesia) and a variety of other common complaints including fatigue, sleep disorders, cognitive deficits, irritable bowel syndrome, headaches, and a wide array of other symptom patterns that do not make sense unless one is familiar with the syndrome and its pathophysiology.

We use strategies in clinical practice that augment the medical model and provide additive benefit to the patients. Two studies, including an RCT by Teitelbaum et al., showed an average 90% improvement rate in FMS, along with a marked decrease in pain, when using the **SHINE** protocol: treating **S**leep, **H**ormonal support, **I**nfections, **N**utritional support, and **E**xercise (to patient tolerance) [94,95].

REFERENCES

1. F. Wolfe, K. Ross, J. Anderson, et al., The prevalence and characteristics of fibromyalgia in the general population. *Arthr Rheum* 1995 Jan;38(1):19–28.
2. Schmitt C, Spaeth M, André E, Caubere J, Taieb C . Fibromyalgia syndrome: A German epidemiological survey. *Annals Rheum Dis* 2006;65(Suppl 2):554.
3. Matucci Cerinic M, Zoppi M, Taieb C, Caubere J, Hamelin G, Schmitt C. Prevalence of fibromyalgia in Italy: Updated results. *Annals Rheum Dis* 2006;65(Suppl 2):555.
4. Guermazi M, Ghroubi S, Sellami M, Elleuch M, André E, Schmitt C, Taieb C, Damak J, Elleuch M. Epidemiology of fibromyalgia in Tunisia. *Annals Rheum Dis* 2006;65(Suppl 2):553.
5. Cobankara V, Ünal Ö, Öztürk M, Bozkurt A. The prevalence of fibromyalgia among textile workers in the City of Denizli in Turkey. *Annals Rheum Dis* 2006;65(Suppl 2):554.
6. Abeles AM, Pillinger MH, Solitar BM, Abeles M. The pathophysiology of fibromyalgia. *Ann Intern Med* 2007;146;726–34.
7. Desmeules J, Cedraschi C, Rapiti E, et al. Neurophysiologic evidence for a central sensitization in patients with fibromyalgia. *Arthr Rheum* 2003;48(5):1420–29.
8. Gracely RH, Petzke F, Wolf JM, Clauw DJ. Functional magnetic resonance imaging evidence of augmented pain processing in fibromyalgia. *Arthr Rheum* 2002;46(5):1333–43.
9. Juhl JH. Fibromyalgia and the serotonin pathway. *Altern Med Rev* 1998;3:367–75.
10. Crofford LJ, Young EA, Engleberg NC, et al. Basal circadian and pulsatile ACTH and cortisol secretion in patients with fibromyalgia and/or chronic fatigue syndrome. *Brain Behav Immun* 2004;18(4):314–25.
11. Garcia MD. Functional digestive disorders and fibromyalgia. *An R Acad Nac Med* (Madr) 2007; 124(3):479–90.
12. Raphael KG, et al. Psychiatric comorbidities in a community sample of women with fibromyalgia. *Pain* 2006;124:117–25.
13. Demitrack MA, Dale K, Straus SE, et al., Evidence for impaired activation of the hypothalamic-pituitary-adrenal axis in patients with chronic fatigue syndrome. *J Clin Endo Metabol* December 1991;73(6): 1223–34.
14. Lowe JC, Garrison RL, Reichman AJ, et al. Effectiveness and safety of T3 therapy for euthyroid fibromyalgia: A double-blind, placebo-controlled response driven crossover study. *Clin Bull Myofascial Ther* 1997;(2/3):91–124.
15. Roizenblatt S, Moldofsky H, Benedito-Silva AA, Tufik S. Alpha sleep characteristics in fibromyalgia. *Arthr Rheum* 2001;44(1):222–30.
16. Wolfe F, Smythe H, Yunus M, et al. The American College of Rheumatology 1990 criteria for the classification of fibromyalgia. *Arthritis Rheum* 1990;33(2):160–72.
17. Wolfe F, Clauw DJ, Fitzcharles M, et al., The American College of Rheumatology Preliminary Diagnostic Criteria for Fibromyalgia and Measurement of Symptom Severity. *Arthr Care Res* 2010;62(5):600–610.
18. Dadabhoy D, Clauw DJ. Fibromyalgia: Differential type of pain needing a different type of treatment. *Nature Clin Practice Rheumatol* 2006;2(7):364–72.
19. Arnold LM. New therapies in fibromyalgia. *Arth Res Ther* 2006;8:212.
20. Fitzcharles MA, Boulos P. Inaccuracy in the diagnosis of fibromyalgia syndrome: Analysis of referrals. *Rheumatology* (Oxford) 2003;42(2):263–67.
21. Schneider M, Brady DM. Fibromyaglia syndrome: A new paradigm for differential diagnosis and treatment. *J Manip Physiol Ther* 2001;24(8):529–41.
22. Schneider M, Brady DM, Perle SM. Differential diagnosis of fibromyalgia syndrome: Proposal of a model and algorithm for patients presenting with the primary symptom of widespread pain. *J Manip Physiol Ther* 2006;29(6):493–501.
23. Cordero MD, Moreno-Fernández AM, Carmona-López MI, et al., Mitochondrial dysfunction in skin biopsies and blood mononuclear cells from two cases of fibromyalgia patients. *Clin Biochem* 2010;43(13–14):1174–76. Epub 2010 Jul 1.
24. Lin HC. Small intestinal bacterial overgrowth: A framework for understanding irritable bowel syndrome. *JAMA* 2004;18;292(7):852–58.

25. Frissora CL, Koch KL. Symptom overlap and comorbidity of irritable bowel syndrome with other conditions. *Curr Gastroenterol Rep* 2005;7(4):264–71.
26. Moshiree B, Price DD, Robinson ME, Gaible R, Verne GN. Thermal and visceral hypersensitivity in irritable bowel syndrome. *Clin J Pain* 2007;23(4):323–30.
27. Riedl A, Schmidtmann M, Stengel A, et al. Somatic comorbidities of irritable bowel syndrome: A systematic analysis. *J Psychosom Res* 2008;64(6):573–82.
28. Garcia MD. Functional digestive disorders and fibromyalgia. *An R Acad Nac Med (Madr)* 2007; 124(3):479–90.
29. Cole JA, Rothman KJ, Cabral HJ, et al. Migraine, fobromyalgia, and depression among people with IBS: A prevalence study. BMC *Gastroenterol* 2006;28;6:26.
30. Kurland JE, Coyle WJ, Winkler A, Zable E. Prevalence of irritable bowel syndrome and depression in fibromyalgia. *Dig Dis Sci* 2006;51(3):454–60.
31. Wallace DJ, Hallegua DS. Fibromyalgia: The gastrointestinal link. *Curr Pain Headache Rep* 2004; 8(5):364–68.
32. Verne GN, Price DD. Irritable bowel syndrome as a common precipitant of central sensitization. *Curr Rheumatol Rep* 2002;4(4):322-28.
33. Whitehead WE, Palsson O, Jones KR. Systemic review of the comorbidity of irritable bowel syndrome with other disorders: What are the causes and implications? *Gastroenterology* 2002;122(4): 1140–56.
34. Lubrano E, Iovino P, Tremolaterra F, et al. Fibromyalgia in patients with irritable bowel syndrome association with the severity of the intestinal disorder. *Int J Colorectal Dis* 2001;16(4):211–15.
35. Sperber AD, Carmel S., Atzmon Y. Use of the Functional Bowel Severity Index (FBDSI) in a study of patients with irritable bowel syndrome and fibromyalgia. *Am J Gastroenterol* 2000;95(4):995–98.
36. Sperber AD, Atzmon Y, Neumann L, et al. Fibromyalgia in the irritable bowel syndrome: Studies of prevalence and clinical applications. *Am J Gastroenterol* 1999;94(12):3541–46.
37. Price DD, Zhou Q, Moshiree B, et al. Peripheral and central contribution to hyperalgesia in irritable bowel syndrome. *J Pain* 2006;7(8):529–35.
38. Azpiroz F, Dapoigny M, Pace F, et al. Nongastrointestinal disorders in the irritable bowel syndrome. *Digestion* 2000;62(1):66–72.
39. Akkus S, Senol A, Ayvacioglu NB, et al. Is female predominance in irritable bowel syndrome related to fibromyalgia? *Rheumatol Int* 2004;24(2):106–9.
40. Funayama Y, Sasaki I, Naito H, et al. Monitoring and antibacterial treatment for postoperative bacterial overgrowth in Crohn's disease. *Dis Colon Rectum* 1999;42(8):1072–77.
41. Pimentel M, Park S, Mirocha J, Kane SV, Kong Y. The effect of a non-absorbed oral antibiotic (rifaximin) on the symptoms of irritable bowel syndrome: A randomized trial. *Ann Inter Med* 2006;145(8):557–63.
42. Pimentel M. Chow EJ, Lin HC. Normalization of lactulose breath testing correlates with symptom improvements in irritable bowel syndrome. A double-blind, randomized, placebo-controlled study. *Am J Gastroenterol* 2003;98(2):412–19.
43. Sharara AI, Aoun E, Abdul-Baki H, et al. A randomized, double-blind, placebo-controlled trial of rifaximin in patients with abdominal bloating and flatulence. *Am J Gastroenterol* 2006;101(2):326–33.
44. Pimentel M, Chow EJ, Hallegua D, et al. Small intestinal bacterial overgrowth: A possible association with fibromyalgia. *J Musculoskel Pain* 2001;9(3):107–13.
45. Pimentel M, Wallace D, Hallegua D, et al. A link between irritable bowel syndrome and fibromyalgia may be related to findings on lactulose breath testing. *Ann Rheum Dis* 2004;63(4):450–52.
46. Jiang ZD, DuPont HL. Rifaximin in vitro and in vivo antibacterial activity—a review. *Chemotherapy* 2005;51 Suppl 1:67–72.
47. Di Stefano M, Malservisi S, Veneto G, Ferrieri A, Corazza GR. Rifaximin versus chlortetracycline in the short-term treatment of small bowel bacterial overgrowth. *Ailment Phramacol Ther* 2000;14:551–56.
48. Marchese A, Salerno A, Pesce A, Debbia EA, Schito GC. In vitro activity of rifaximin, metronidazole and vancomycin against clostridium difficile and the rate of selection of spontaneously resistant mutants against representative anaerobic and aerobic bacteria, including ammonia-producing species. *Chemotherapy* 2000;46;253–66.
49. Bacom A. *Incorporating Herbal Medicine Into Clinical Practice*. Philadelphia: F.A. Davis, 2002.
50. Chevallier A. *Encylopedia of Herbal Medicine*. London: Dorling Kindersley, 2000.
51. Fetrow C, Avila J. *Professional's Handbook of Complimentary & Alternative Medicines*. Springhouse, PA: Springhouse, 1999.
52. Pizzorno J, Murray M. *Textbook of Natural Medicine*. 2nd ed. Edinburgh: Churchill Livingstone, 1999.

53. Robbers J, Speedie M, Tyler V. *Pharmacognosy and Pharmacobiotechnology*. Philadelphia: Lippincott Williams & Wilkins, 1996.

54. Werbach M, Murray M. *Botanical Influences on Illness*. Tarzana, CA: Third Line Press, 1994.

55. Khin MU, Myo K, Nyunt NW, Aye K, Tin U. Clinical trial of berberine in acute watery diarrhoea. *Br Med J (Clin Res Ed)* 12-7-1985;291(6509):1601–5.

56. Rabbani GH, Butler T, Knight J, Sanyal SC, Alam K. Randomized controlled trial of berberine sulfate therapy for diarrhea due to enterotoxigenic Escherichia coli and Vibrio cholerae. *J Infect Dis* 1987;155(5):979–84.

57. Lord RS, Bralley JA (editors). *Laboratory Evaluations for Integrative and Functional Medicine*, 2nd ed. Duluth, GA: Metametrix Institute, 2008.

58. Kałużna-Czaplińska J. Noninvasive urinary organic acids test to assess biochemical and nutritional individuality in autistic children. *Clin Biochem* 2011;44:686–91.

59. Pieczenik S, Neustadt J. Mitochondrial dysfunction and molecular pathways of disease. *Exper Molec Path* 2007;83:84–92.

60. Martinez-Lavin M. Stress, the stress response system, and fibromyalgia. *Arthr Res Ther* 2007;9:216.

61. Jonnakuty C, Gragnoli C. What do we know about serotonin? *J Cellular Physiol* 2008;217:301–6.

62. Freese A, Swartz KJ, During MJ, Martin JB. Kynurenine metabolites of tryptophan: Implications for neurologic diseases. *Neurology* 1990;40(4):691–95.

63. Sigmundsdóttir G, Christensson B, Björklund LJ, Håkansson K, Pehrson C, Larsson L. Urine D-arabinitol/L-arabinitol ratio in diagnosis of invasive candidiasis in newborn infants. *J Clin Microbiol* 2000;38(8):3039–42.

64. Pregabalin (Lyrica) for fibromyalgia. *Med Lett Drugs Ther* 2007;49:77.

65. Field MJ, et al. Identification of the α2-δ-1 subunit of voltage-dependent calcium channels as a molecular target for pain mediating the analgesic actions of pregabalin. *Proc Natl Acad Sci USA* 2006;103(46):17537–42.

66. Kwan P, Schachter SC, Brodie MJ. Drug-resistant epilepsy. *N Engl J Med* 2011;365:919–26.

67. Mease PJ, et al. A randomized, double-blind, placebo-controlled, phase III trial of pregabalin in the treatment of patients with fibromyalgia. *J Rheumatol* 2008:35(3):502–14.

68. Arnold LM, Goldenberg DL, Stanford SB, et al. Gabapentin in the treatment of fibromyalgia: A randomized, double-blind, placebo-controlled, multicenter trial. *Arthritis Rheum* Apr 2007;56(4):1336–44.

69. Errante LD, Williamson A, Spencer DD, Petroff OA. Gabapentin and vigabatrin increase GABA in the human neocortical slice. *Epilepsy Res* 2002 May;49(3):203–10.

70. Crofford LJ, et al. Pregabalin for the treatment of fibromyalgia syndrome: Results of a randomized, double-blind, placebo-controlled trial. *Arthritis Rheum* 2005;52:1264.

71. Arnold L, et al. A 14-week, randomized, double-blind, placebocontrolled, monotherapy trial of pregabalin (BID) in patients with fibromyalgia syndrome (FMS). *J Pain* 2007;8 suppl:S24, abstract 695.

72. Kranzler JD, Gendreau RM. Role and rationale for the use of milnacipran in the management of fibromyalgia. *Neuropsychiatr Dis Treat* 2010 May 25;6:197–208.

73. Abeles M, Solitar B, Pillinger M, Abelesa A. Update on fibromyalgia therapy. *Amer J of Med* 2008 July 121;7:555–61.

74. Milnacipran (Savella) for fibromyalgia. *Med Lett Drugs Ther* 2009;51:45–46.

75. Duloxetine (Cymbalta) for fibromyalgia. *Med Lett Drugs Ther* 2008;50:57–58.

76. Tofferi JK, Jackson JL, O'Malley PG. Treatment of fibromyalgia with cyclobenzaprine: A meta-analysis. *Arthritis Rheum* 2004;51(1):9–13.

77. Goldenberg DL, Burckhardt C, Crofford L. Management of fibromyalgia syndrome. *JAMA* 2004; 292(19):2388–95.

78. Morillas-Arques P, et al. Trazodone for the treatment of fibromyalgia: An open-label, 12-week study. *BMC Musculoskel Dis* 2010;11:204.

79. Goldenberg D, Mayskiy M, Mossey CJ, Ruthazer R, Schmid CA. Randomized, double-blind crossover trial of fluoxetine and amitriptyline in the treatment of fibromyalgia. *Arthritis Rheum* 1996;39:1852.

80. Celiker R, Cagavi Z. Comparison of amitriptyline and sertraline in the treatment of fibromyalgia syndrome [abstract]. *Arthritis Rheum* 2000;43:S332.

81. Cantini F, Bellandi F, Niccolo L, et al. Fluoxetine combined with cyclobenzaprine in the treatment of fibromyalgia. *Minerva Med* 1994;85:97–100.

82. Younger J, Mackey S. Low-dose naltrexone reduces the primary symptoms of fibromyalgia. *Pain Med* 2009;10(4):663–72.

83. Birdsall T. 5-Hydroxytryptophan: A clinically-effective serotonin precursor. *Altern Med Rev* 1998; 3(4):271–80.

84. Boyer EW, Shannon M. The serotonin syndrome. *N Engl J Med* 2005;352:1112–20.
85. Hussain SA-R, Al-Khalifa II, Jasim N A, Gorial F. I. Adjuvant use of melatonin for treatment of fibromyalgia. *J Pineal Res* 2011;50:267–71.
86. Wikner J, Hirsch U, Wetterberg L, Röjdmark S. Fibromyalgia—a syndrome associated with decreased nocturnal melatonin secretion. *Clin Endo* 1998;49:179–83.
87. Staud R. Biology and therapy of fibromyalgia: Pain in fibromyalgia syndrome. *Arthr Res Ther* 2006, 8:208.
88. Randall S, Roehrs T, Roth T. Over-the-counter sleep aid medications and insomnia. *Prim Psychiatry* 2008;15(5):52–58.
89. Wang C, et al. A randomized trial of tai chi for fibromyalgia. *N Engl J Med* 2010;363:743–54.
90. Carson JW, Carson KM, Jones KD, Bennett RM, Wright CL, Mist SD. A pilot randomized controlled trial of the Yoga of Awareness program in the management of fibromyalgia. *Pain* 2010;151(2):530–39.
91. Etnier JL, Karper WB, Gapin JI, Barella LA, Chang YK, Murphy KJ. Exercise, fibromyalgia, and fibrofog: A pilot study. *J Phys Act Health* 2009 Mar;6(2):239–46.
92. Busch AJ, Barber KA, Overend TJ, Peloso PMJ, Schachter CL. Exercise for treating fibromyalgia syndrome. *Cochrane Database of Systematic Reviews* 2007.
93. Bernardy K, Füber N, Köllner V, Häuser W. Efficacy of cognitive-behavioral therapies in fibromyalgia syndrome—a systematic review and metaanalysis of randomized controlled trials. *J Rheumatol* 2010 Oct;37(10):1991–2005.
94. Teitelbaum JE, Bird B. Effective treatment of severe chronic fatigue: A report of a series of 64 patients. *J Musculoskel Pain* 1995;3(4):1–110.
95. Teitelbaum JE, Bird B, Weiss A, et al. Effective treatment of CFS and FMS: A randomized, double-blind placebo controlled study. *J Chron Fatigue Syn* 2001;8(2):3–24.
96. Wang J, O'Reilly B, Venkataraman R, Mysliwiec V, Mysliwiec A. Efficacy of oral iron in patients with restless legs syndrome and a low-normal ferritin: A randomized, double-blind, placebo-controlled study. *Sleep Med* 2009 Oct;10(9):973–75. Epub 2009 Feb 18.
97. Pamuk ON, Cakir N. The frequency of thyroid antibodies in fibromyalgia patients and their relationship with symptoms. *Clin Rheumatol* 2007;26:55–59.
98. Hollowell JG, Staehling NW, Hannon WH, et al. Iodine nutrition in the United States. Trends and public health implications: Iodine excretion data from National Health and Nutrition Examination Surveys I and III (1971–1974 and 1988–1994). *J Clin Endocrinol Metab* Oct 1998;83(10):3401–8.
99. Messina M, Redmond G. Effects of soy protein and soybean isoflavones on thyroid function in healthy adults and hypothyroid patients: A review of the relevant literature. *Thyroid* 2006 Mar;16(3):249–58.
100. Verdon F, Burnand B, Fallab-Stubi, et al. Iron supplementation for unexplained fatigue in non-anaemic women: Double blind randomised placebo controlled trial. *BMJ* 2003;326(24):1124–28.
101. Kis AM, Carnes M. Detecting iron deficiency in anemic patients with concomitant medical problems. *J Gen Intern Med* 1998 July;13(7):455–61.
102. Hurwitz BE, Coryell VT., Parker M, et al. Chronic fatigue syndrome: Illness severity, sedentary lifestyle, blood volume and evidence of diminished cardiac function. *Clinical Science* 2009;118(2):125–35.
103. Dillman E, Gale C, Green W, et al. Hypothermia in iron deficiency due to altered triiodothyronine metabolism. *Am J Physiol* 1980;239:R377–81.
104. Regland B, Andersson M, Abrahamsson L, et al. Increased concentrations of homocysteine in the cerebrospinal fluid in patients with fibromyalgia and chronic fatigue syndrome. *Scand J Rheumatol* 1997;26(4):301–7.
105. Lindenbaum J, Rosenberg IH, Wilson PW, et al. Prevalence of cobalamin deficiency in the Framingham elderly population. *Amer J Clin Nutr* July 1994;60(1):2–11.
106. Lindenbaum J, Healton EB, Savage DG, et al. Neuropsychiatric disorders caused by cobalamin deficiency in the absence of anemia or macrocytoses. *N Engl J Med* June 1988;318(26):1720–28.
107. Beck WS. Cobalmin and the nervous system (Editorial). *N Engl Medicine* 1988;318(26):1752–54.
108. Kuratsune H, Yamaguti K, Takahashi M, et al. Acylcarnitine deficiency in chronic fatigue syndrome. *Clin Infect Dis* Jan 1994;18(3) (Supplement 1):S62–67.
109. Teitelbaum JE, St. Cyr JA, Johnson C. The use of D-ribose in chronic fatigue syndrome and fibromyalgia: A pilot study. *J Altern Complem Med* 2006;12(9):857–62.
110. Teitelbaum J, Jandrain, J, et al. Effective treatment of fibromyalgia and CFS with d-ribose. A multi-center study. Scripps Integrative Medical Center's 7th Annual Natural Supplement Conference. La Jolla, CA. January 2010.
111. Tullson PC, Terjung RL. Adenine nucleotide synthesis in exercising and endurance-trained skeletal muscle. *Amer J Physiol* 1991;261:C342–47.
112. Brault JJ, Terjung RL. Purine salvage to adenine nucleotides in different skeletal muscle fiber types. *J Applied Physiol* 2001;91:231–38.

35 Osteoporosis

Joseph Lamb, M.D.

INTRODUCTION

Osteoporosis, literally "porous bone," is defined as a reduction in the mass and quality of bone and/or the presence of a fragility fracture. Osteoporosis can be a clinically silent systemic skeletal disease characterized by compromised bone strength predisposing to an increased risk of fracture. Osteoporosis is common, preventable when diagnosed early, and serious though treatable.

Given recent advances in our knowledge of the underlying pathophysiology and new therapeutic options, osteoporosis may be considered a lifestyle disease—that is, one that can be prevented or ameliorated by appropriate lifestyle choices. As such, bone health needs to be understood in the context of a broad clinical picture involving frailty (sarcopenia and osteoporosis) and metabolic syndromes [1]. This chapter presents the pathophysiology of osteoporosis to guide clinicians to early diagnosis and food and nutrient-based interventions.

EPIDEMIOLOGY

According to the International Osteoporosis Foundation [2], osteoporosis poses a major health threat. It is estimated currently that more than 200 million people worldwide have osteoporosis. The National Osteoporosis Foundation [3] estimates that for adults over age 50 one in two women and one in four men will suffer an osteoporotic fracture. Of those patients who suffer a hip fracture, only 40% fully regain their prefracture level of independence, leaving 60% who will experience chronic pain, disability, and a 10% to 20% excess mortality within one year [4]. And while osteoporosis is not simply estrogen deficiency, the recent decline in the prescribing of estrogen replacement therapies increases the number of women not actively involved in preserving bone health [5] and increases the risk for hip fracture (55%) in women who stopped hormone therapy [6]. It is therefore essential that early diagnosis and prevention/treatment strategies be designed and implemented in all patients at risk.

PHYSIOLOGY

Bone is a metabolically active endocrine organ with regulatory functions in calcium homeostasis, energy expenditure, and bone and muscle remodeling. The organic component of bone consists of a cellular component and the extracellular cartilage matrix that is the scaffolding for mineralization. The strength of bone is determined by both bone quality and bone density. Bone quality is a measure of the functional status of the organic matrix and is often a significant determinant of fracture risk [7]. Bone density is a function of the adequacy of mineralization.

Bone mineralization is regulated primarily by the activity of three cell types, osteoblasts, osteoclasts, and osteocytes, which are under both local and systemic control. These bone cells respond to changing environmental stimuli such as nutrient availability, hormonal messaging,

657

inflammation, and physiological demands. Mechanical loading is one such physiologic demand, modulated by the osteocyte through a complex array of cell signaling pathways. The mechanical message is transformed into altered gene expression resulting in proliferation and matrix synthesis. This message leads to upregulation of growth factors including insulin-like growth factor 1 (IGF-1), vascular endothelial growth factors, and bone morphogenetic proteins (BMP) 2 and 4 [8].

A broad range of cell surface receptors and intercellular skeletal structures including those in the extra-cellular matrix and the cellular cytoskeleton (integrins, cadherins, and Ca^{+2} channels), intracellular signaling kinases, prostaglandins, and nitric oxide are intimately involved in the regulation of matrix secretion and mineralization [8]. Many of the messengers involved in the mediating bone growth are intimately involved in inflammatory signaling pathways. The interplay of these messages is complex and bidirectional. Many growth factors influence osteoblast formation. Core binding Factor A1 (CBFA1) is a transcription factor expressed in osteoblast progenitors and stromal support cells that has been shown to be important in the control of osteoblast development. It regulates the expression of several osteoblast-specific genes including type 1 collagen, receptor-activator of NFKappaB (RANK) ligand also called osteoclast differentiation factor, osteocalcin, osteopontin, and bone sialoprotein. Osteoblasts, through secretion of RANK ligand (RANKL), actually promote differentiation and maturation of osteoclasts. Interestingly, when responding to different environmental signals, osteoblasts secrete osteoprotegerin (OPG), also called osteoclastogenesis inhibitory factor, which binds RANKL and acts as a receptor decoy to inhibit differentiation of osteoclasts [9]. Stromal support cells secrete macrophage colony stimulating factor and RANKL to promote osteoclast differentiation and maturation. Macrophages and adipocytes, residents of the bone marrow, play a role in this complex interplay, releasing locally produced growth factors and cytokines including gamma interferon, interleukins 1, 6, and 11 (IL-1, IL-6, IL-11), and tumor necrosis factor-α (TNF-α). These cytokines play an important role in osteoclast maturation process by stimulating secretion of RANKL.

In addition to the cell-mediated local control, several hormones provide system-wide oversight of bone metabolism. Both parathyroid hormone (PTH) and 1,25-dihydroxy-vitamin D_3 directly modulate osteoclastic activity to maintain appropriate serum calcium and phosphorus levels. Estrogen influences bone metabolism. Deficiency increases bone-remodeling intensity, which exacerbates propensity to bone resorption in functionally challenged bone and contributes to the development of primary osteoporosis in perimenopausal women. Testosterone deficiency has also been shown to be associated with osteoporosis [10]. Intervention trials have demonstrated that supplementation with estrogen in women, DHEA in men and women [11], and testosterone in hypogonadal men [12] is effective.

Interestingly, the medical literature has revealed that bone is intimately related to energy regulation and body composition. Research by Ducy [13], Karsenty [14], Fulzele [15], and Ferron [16] has demonstrated that osteocalcin (a protein secreted by osteoblasts as a linking site for minerals to the organic matrix) when carboxylated is intimately involved in insulin regulation. And Rosen, while having noted that osteoporosis may simply be obesity of bone [17], recently reviewed [18] the current state of the literature demonstrating the feed-forward cycle of insulin modulating bone turnover and of osteocalcin modulating insulin secretion. Thus bone, as a mechanoreceptor of muscular activity and mechanical stress, may be uniquely suited to convert mechanical messages to chemical signals active in energy regulation and body composition including preservation of muscle and skeletal mass. The osteoclast-associated receptor (OSCAR), a regulator of osteoclast differentiation, has also been identified on endothelial cells where stimulation by oxidized low-density lipoprotein—cholesterol may be involved in atherosclerosis-related cell activation and inflammation [19].

This interaction of local cells, communicating by growth factors and cytokines and modulated by systemic hormones, and simultaneously modulating basic energy regulation and body composition, is the healthy norm of bone metabolism. Osteoporosis is the pathophysiologic disturbance of this process.

Nutrients obtained primarily in our diet are biology's building blocks to erect strong bone. Table 35.2 lists these nutrients and the required intake in the absence of disease.

PATHOPHYSIOLOGY

As we explore the pathophysiology of osteoporosis, we find that underlying mechanisms rather than broad organ system classifications may cast more light on the underlying causes of osteoporosis. These broad mechanistic categories include diminished achievement of peak bone mass, decreased mineral availability, decreased osteoblast activity, increased osteoclast activity, abnormal protein metabolism, and systemic inflammation.

Indeed, much research over the last decade has demonstrated that inflammatory cytokines (RANKL, OPG, IL-6) and energy regulatory signaling (Insulin, IGF-1, and OC) are integral to the balance of bone resorption and formation. And while estrogen deficiency has been recognized as a cause of osteoporosis, it may do so not only as a deficiency of a growth factor, but as a consequence of increasing systemic inflammation associated with increased IL-6 levels [20–22]. RANKL and its downstream cytokines have important roles in bone, metabolic, and vascular disease [23].

In a clinical setting, it may be helpful to classify osteoporosis as primary or secondary. In a postmenopausal woman, estrogen deficiency results in primary osteoporosis. Whereas suppressed estrogen levels due to an adolescent girl receiving a GnRH agonist as contraception or a premenopausal woman receiving chemotherapy for breast cancer often lead to secondary osteoporosis. Secondary osteoporosis occurs in patients who are less likely to be screened for the disease because they may not present as a prototypic osteoporosis patient. Recognizing the pathophysiology of secondary osteoporosis (Table 35.2) increases "clinical suspicion" and offers the opportunity to intervene earlier.

DIMINISHED ACHIEVEMENT OF PEAK BONE MASS

Bone mass acquisition is largely genetically determined, with greater than 50% being attained during adolescence and peak mass typically achieved by the early 20s [3,24,25]. Emphasis needs to be placed on maximizing peak bone mass during adolescence or future bone mineral density (BMD) will be compromised as even relatively small incremental losses will have a proportionately greater effect on a lower peak bone mass. Acquisitional osteopenia is the failure to achieve the genetically determined peak bone mass and can be the result of chronic illness, use of certain medications, malnutrition, malabsorption, or disruption of key metabolic pathways [24,26,27]. Radioisotope studies have demonstrated turnovers of up to 18% of the calcium in adult bone per year—an indication of the significant persistent metabolic activity in postadolescent bone. Despite this, bone remodeling is a much slower process in adulthood than during adolescence. The primary purpose of adult bone remodeling is homeostasis during the ever-present processes of microdamage to repairs and skeletal strength maintenance.

Failure to attain peak bone mass can be caused by:

Early life nutrition, including in utero experiences, has been demonstrated to be associated with bone development. Breastfed children initially have lower bone mass than bottle-fed children. However, they attain higher peak bone mass [28]. Animal studies support these observations [29].

Adolescent eating disorders, including both anorexia and bulimia, are conditions associated with failure to achieve peak bone mass. In addition to decreased mineral and protein availability because of insufficient intake, contributing factors to osteoporosis include amenorrhea, calcium and vitamin D deficiency, increased endogenous steroid production, and low levels of growth factors including IGF. In these patients, nutritional rehabilitation with weight gain, adequate calcium and vitamin D intake, moderate weight-bearing exercise and resumption of normal menses has been shown to improve but not normalize bone mineral density [30,31].

TABLE 35.1
Key Bone Building Nutrients

Nutrient	Adult RDA or AI	Common Therapeutic Range for Bone Health	Dietary Considerations
Calcium	1000–1300 mg	1000–1500 mg	Typical diet is inadequate, averages 500–600 mg.[1,2]
Phosphorus	700 mg	700–1200 mg	Inadequate intake is rare except in elderly and malnourished; excessive intake common with use of processed foods and soft drinks.
Magnesium	420 mg men 320 mg women	400–800 mg	Intake generally inadequate: all ages, sexes, classes, except children less than five, fail to consume this RDA. 40% of population, 50% of adolescents consume less than two-thirds the RDA.[2,3,4,5]
Fluoride	4.0 mg men 3.0 mg women	—	Fluoride overdose has occurred through ingestion of fluoride toothpaste and high fluoride waters.[3]
Silica	No values yet set	5–20 mg	Intake is unknown. Silica is removed in food processing; current intake is suspected to be low.
Zinc	11 mg men 8 mg women	20–30 mg	Marginal zinc deficiency is common, especially among children.[3] Average intake was 46 to 63% of the RDA.[5]
Manganese	2.3 mg men 1.8 mg women	10–25 mg	Intakes are generally inadequate, 1.76 mg adolescent girls 2.05 mg women, 2.5 males.[6]
Copper	900 mcg men and women	2–3 mg	75% of diets fail to contain the RDA.[5,7] Average intake is below the RDA.[3]
Boron	No RDA established	3–4 mg	1/4 mg intake is common[8] to perhaps optimum of 3 mg.
Potassium	4700 mg men and women	4700–5000	Adult intake averages 2300 mg for women and 3100 mg for men.[9]
Vitamin D	600–until age 70; then 800 IU, men and women	1000–2000 IU & up as needed	Deficiency is common especially among the elderly, dark-skinned, and those with little UV sunlight exposure.
Vitamin C	90 mg men 75 mg women	Oral 500 mg–to bowel tolerance as needed	Average daily intake is about 95 mg for women and 107 mg for men.[10]
Vitamin A	2997 IU men 2331 IU adult women	5000 IU or less	31% consume less than 70% the RDA.[11] Current intake for women is about 2373 mcg/day.[12]
Vitamin B6	1.7 mg men 1.5 mg women	25–50 mg	Studies indicate widespread inadequate vitamin B6 consumption among all sectors of the population.[13]
Folic Acid	400 mcg men and women	800–1000 mcg	Inadequate intake was common among all age groups, but is improving with food fortification.[3]
Vitamin K	120 mcg men 90 mcg women	1000 mcg	Averages 45 to 150 mcg, which is well below the recommendation AI.[14]
Vitamin B12	2.4 mg men and women	100–1000 mcg	12% consume less than 70% RDA.[11] Older people and vegans are especially at risk.[3]

TABLE 35.1 (*continued*)
Key Bone Building Nutrients

Nutrient	Adult RDA or AI	Common Therapeutic Range for Bone Health	Dietary Considerations
Fats	Should comprise 7% of calories minimum, General recommendation is not to exceed 30% of calories.	20–30% of total calories is perhaps more ideal.	The average American consumes 33% of his/her calories in fat. The consumption of essential fatty acids, however, is frequently inadequate [26].[3]

Endnotes

[1] U.S. Department of Health and Human Services. *Bone Health and Osteoporosis: A Report of the Surgeon General.* Rockville, MD: U.S. Department of Health and Human Services, Office of the Surgeon General, 2004.

[2] Morgan K. Magnesium and calcium. *J American College Nutrition* 1985;4(2):195–206.

[3] Brown JE. *Nutrition Now.* 4th ed. Belmont, CA: Thomson Wadsworth, 2005.

[4] Lakshmanan F. Magnesium intakes, balances and blood levels of adults consuming self-selected diets. *The Amer Jrnl of Clinical Nutrition* 1984;40(Dec):1380–1389.

[5] Pennington J, Young B, Wilson D, Johnson R, Vanderveen J. Mineral content of food and total diets: The Selected Minerals in Foods Survey, 1982 to 1984. *J Am Diet Assoc* 1986;86:876–891.

[6] Freeland-Graves J. Manganese: An essential nutrient for humans. *Nutrition Today* 1988(Nov/Dec):13–19.

[7] Klevay L. Evidence of dietary copper and zinc deficiencies. *JAMA* 1979;241:1917–1918.

[8] Nielsen F, Hunt C, Mullen L. Effect of dietary boron on mineral, estrogen, and testosterone metabolism in postmenopausal women. *FASEB J* 1987;1:394–397.

[9] Hajjar IM, Grim CE, George V, Kotchen TA. Impact of diet on blood pressure and age-related changes in blood pressure in the US population: Analysis of NHANES III. *Arch Intern Med* 2001;161(4):589–593.

[10] http://www.pdrhealth.com/drug_info/nmdrugprofiles/nutsupdrugs/vit_0264.shtml.

[11] Pao E, Mickle S. Problem nutrients in the United States. *Food Technology* 1981:58–64.

[12] Feskanich D, Singh V, Willett WC, Colditz GA. Vitamin A intake and hip fractures among postmenopausal women. *Jama* 2002;287(1):47–54.

[13] Serfontein WJ, De Villiers LS, Ubbink J, Pitout MJ. Vitamin B6 revisited. Evidence of subclinical deficiencies in various segments of the population and possible consequences thereof. *S Afr Med J* 1984;66(12):437–441.

[14] Booth SL, Suttie JW. Dietary intake and adequacy of vitamin K. *J Nutr* 1998;128(5):785–788.

Use of **Depo-Provera as contraception** produces estrogen deficiency. Adolescent females who use Depo-Provera are at risk for low bone mass due to failure to achieve peak bone mass [31]. Calcium supplementation in adolescents has been shown to ameliorate only some of the potential loss.

A study in children with **high lead exposure** revealed significantly increased bone mineral density compared to normal controls. Despite the potential for heavy metals creating a false negative result in DXA scanning because of high X-ray absorption by lead, the investigators postulated that lead exposure may actually accelerate boney maturation by inhibition of parathyroid hormone (PTH). However, they concluded that the accelerated bone maturation results in a shorter period of mineralization and growth, resulting in decreased peak bone mass [32].

DECREASED MINERAL AVAILABILITY

Inflammatory bowel disease (IBD) activity strongly correlates with the severity of bone loss; therefore, effective disease management including calcium and vitamin D supplementation, risk factor reduction, and avoidance of glucocorticoids are equally important aspects of treatment [33]. And although appropriate diagnostic and therapeutic regimens addressing bone mineral density (BMD) in IBD patients are essential, a standard treatment strategy has yet to be defined [34,35].

Celiac enteropathy (discussed later in this chapter) causes marked mineral and calorie malabsorption (also see **Inflammation**, following).

Primary biliary cirrhosis (PBC) with its resultant underlying fat malabsorption has been shown to contribute to insufficiencies of fat-soluble vitamins, specifically vitamin D and vitamin K [36]. Additionally; PBC patients have attenuation of the liver's ability to adequately hydroxylate vitamin D.

Several studies have demonstrated a strong correlation with adult **lactase deficiency** and the development of osteoporosis. Patient avoidance of milk and other dairy products resulted in an increased incidence of osteoporosis and bone fracture [37].

Morbid obesity has historically been viewed as having a protective effect against the development of MBD. However, recent research has revealed that many obese individuals have inadequate nutrition status, vitamin D deficiency, elevated parathyroid hormone levels, and are at risk for low bone mass [38,39]. Studies attempting to define the pre-surgical prevalence of vitamin D deficiency have identified rates in excess of 60% among patients selected to undergo weight-loss surgery [38,40]. Similarly, the prevalence of preoperative elevated intact parathyroid hormone (PTH) in this population ranged from 25% to 48% [38].

Postoperatively, bariatric surgery patients experiencing significant weight loss, severely restricted oral intake, calcium malabsorption, and concomitant vitamin D deficiency are at extremely high risk for the development of MBD. Several factors are likely involved. Primarily, malabsorption plays a critical role with malabsorption of calcium, magnesium, fat-soluble vitamins including vitamin D, protein, B12, and folic acid all being reported. Essentially all **postgastrectomy patients** have an increased risk of fracture and should be routinely evaluated for the presence of MBD. The incidence of osteomalacia in this population is estimated to be 10% to 20% and although the incidence of osteoporosis in this patient population is not definitively known it is estimated to be as high as 32% to 42% [41].

Gastric hypoacidity because of atrophy, proton-pump inhibitors, and H_2 blockers is implicated in mineral malabsorption. Gastroesophageal reflux disease (GERD) does not share a causal relationship with MBD. Yet, chronic overuse of antacids containing aluminum hydroxide can lead to phosphorus deficiency and osteomalacia [42,43]. Calcium must be ionized to be optimally absorbed and ionization of calcium requires an acidic environment. Reduced gastric acidity contributes to the failure to ionize calcium in the small intestine and decreases the bioavailability of calcium. Calcium carbonate is much more vulnerable to being malabsorbed as opposed to other forms of calcium including citrate, lactate, and gluconate, as it is not already ionized. Although the effects of achlorhydria on the bioavailability of calcium are well documented, the relationship to MBD remains unclear. Advancing age combined with the growing use of H_2 blockers and proton-pump inhibitors now available over the counter for dyspepsia contribute to the magnitude of the problem. Adequate calcium absorption can be achieved by instructing the patient to take calcium supplements with meals or by switching to calcium citrate.

The evidence of a detrimental effect of **high-sodium diets and acid-load diets** on bone health is primarily limited to short-term effects of sodium on calcium metabolism. There is strong evidence in support of the fact that high salt intake produces a calciuretic effect but investigations attempting to define the association of sodium with bone loss and BMD have produced conflicting results [44]. The typical Western diet contains sodium far above evolutionary norms and potassium far below those norms. These changes associated with a decrease in fruit and vegetable intake creates a net acid-producing load. As a result of a need to excrete this acid load, renal calcium losses are increased [45].

Caffeine is known to increase urinary calcium losses and may have harmful effects on bone. A prospective study demonstrated that bone loss occurred in those women who had both low calcium intake and high caffeine intakes [46]. The deleterious effects of caffeine on bone can be negated by consuming adequate calcium [46,47].

Dietary protein is required to maintain bone structure; however, **high-protein diets** despite their potential to contain high amounts of calcium have shown a positive association between excess protein intake and urinary excretion of calcium, contributing to a negative calcium balance [48]. A link between high protein intake (regardless of whether it was of animal or vegetable origin) and an increased risk of fracture has also been demonstrated [48,49]. However, when high protein intake is coupled with adequate calcium intake, the potentially harmful effects of protein appear to be ameliorated [50–52] and evidence suggests that the recommended daily allowance of 0.8 grams of protein per kg body weight may be insufficient [53] (see **protein calorie malnutrition** in this chapter).

Phosphorus is plentiful in the food supply predominantly due to the increased use of phosphate salts in food additives and cola beverages. And although phosphorus is an essential nutrient, the current literature notes that both **phosphorus deficiency and excess intake** interfere with calcium absorption and lead to bone loss [54]. A large study examining carbonated beverages and incidence of fractures in school girls found a statistically significant increase in fractures in those girls who regularly consumed carbonated beverages, though it appeared that the fracture risk was the consequence of consuming beverages lacking in calcium [55].

Hypovitaminosis D interferes with absorption of calcium. Vitamin D plays a role both in intestinal adsorption of calcium as well as modifying the speed of bone turnover. Vitamin D is essential for calcium and phosphate absorption in the gut, stimulation of osteoblast activity, calcium reabsorption in the renal tubules, and normal bone mineralization throughout the life span. Absorption of vitamin D occurs mainly by passive diffusion in the proximal and mid small intestine and is highly dependent on bile salts [24].

DECREASED OSTEOBLAST ACTIVITY

Diabetes mellitus (DM) has been implicated as a cause of osteoporosis, but the causal relationship is still being defined. Advanced glycation end products have been implicated in the upregulation of RANKL (inducing increased osteoclastogenesis) and down regulation of alkaline phosphatase and osteocalcin (impairing matrix mineralization) [56,57]. Given the prevalence of DM, surveillance for osteoporosis in diabetics is of great importance [31].

Tobacco use has direct toxic effects on osteoblasts and also acts indirectly by modifying estrogen metabolism. Cigarette smokers on average reach menopause approximately one to two years earlier than nonsmokers. Tobacco abuse also leads to an increase in illnesses and earlier frailty by decreasing exercise capacity and increasing the likelihood of requiring corticosteroids for treatment of pulmonary diseases [58].

Excessive **alcohol use** has been shown to decrease osteoblast activity [59]. And yet several studies have shown that moderate consumption has positive impact on bone health [59]. Higher consumption, especially in men, however, increased the rate of fracture, perhaps related to increased falls or nutritional compromise related to alcohol abuse. Daily alcohol consumption of 50 grams (approximately three standard drinks) results in a dose-dependant decrease in osteoblast activity; daily consumption of greater than 100 grams eventually results in an osteopenic skeleton and increased risk for the development of osteoporosis [60]. One drink per day for women and two drinks per day for men is the recommended safe upper limit for consumption.

Corticosteroid excess, whether exogenous or endogenous can result in deleterious effects on healthy bone primarily due to decreasing osteoblast activity [61]. The profound effect of steroid excess is demonstrated by noting that it is the most common cause of secondary osteoporosis and is second only to menopause as a cause of osteoporosis. Glucocorticoid-induced bone loss occurs following the administration of pharmacologic doses of glucocorticoids for greater than a few days and is the result of uncoupling of the normal relationship between the resorption and formation phases of bone remodeling [24]. Glucocorticoids suppress 1-hydroxylase activity and function as a 1,25(OH)D antagonist thereby blunting calcium absorption [24,62]. Fifty percent of patients on chronic corticosteroid administration for six months or longer develop osteoporosis. In fact, a daily dose of 2.5 to 5.0 mg of prednisone may be sufficient to cause osteoporosis [63].

There is also evidence that potent inhaled glucocorticoids may have deleterious effects on the skeleton [64]. The cumulative dose of glucocorticoids correlates with the severity of the bone disease and the incidence of fracture. Of note, patients maintained on corticosteroid replacement due to adrenal insufficiency do not appear to be at increased risk [24]. The diagnosis of osteoporosis can be the presenting symptom of Cushing's disease. Subclinical hypercortisolism may be more common than generally recognized with an 11% prevalence among patients with low BMD and vertebral fractures [65]. Persistent physical and psychological stress can induce endogenous corticosteroids excess and increase BMD losses. Depression has been associated with elevated cortisol levels.

INCREASED OSTEOCLAST ACTIVITY

In **hyperparathyroidism**, parathyroid hormone (PTH) stimulates a release of calcium from bone by an increase in osteoclast activity. It does so by increasing activation of 25-hydroxy vitamin D3 to 1.25-dihydroxy vitamin D3, which increases bone resorption. Secondary hyperparathyroidism is the response to a lowered serum calcium level resulting in an increase in PTH levels and increased bone resorption. Intermittent exposure to PTH may lead to a net increase in BMD clinically, since bone formation due to increased calcium uptake may be greater than the resultant activation of osteoclasts [66].

Postmenopausal **estrogen deficiency** and other **hypogondal states**, both primary and secondary, are associated with osteoporosis. Estrogen deficiency increases the population of pre-B cells, a subset of bone marrow stromal cells, which in turn increase production of IL-1 and TNF-α. These cytokines induce cyclo-oxygenase 2 activity increasing prostaglandin E_2 production by osteoblasts and subsequent increase in RANKL expression and resultant osteoclastogenesis [67]. Many cancer therapies for breast, ovarian, and prostate cancer patients produce hypogonadal states. Tamoxifen has been shown to produce osteoporosis in premenopausal women. Aromatase inhibitors and GnRH agonists also produce estrogen deficiency. Estrogen deficiency may also be associated with the genetic hypogonadal states such as Turner's syndrome.

Several recent papers point to the need for appropriate balance of the metabolites of estrone and estradiol. Normal ratios of 2-hydroxy to 16α-hydroxy estrogens are associated with optimal bone health while imbalances marked by either an excess of 2-hydroxy or 16α-hydroxy estrogens are associated with osteoporosis [68,69].

Mature osteocytes, by sensing the mechanical forces exerted on bone by physical activity, directly influence bone remodeling. Conditions, including **inactivity, immobilization, paraplegia, and sarcopenia**, which decrease these forces, will have a negative effect on bone strength. Physical immobilization after trauma or due to neural damage from a cerebrovascular accident, poliomyelitis, and multiple sclerosis has been associated with osteoporosis. A reduction in compressive mechanical forces because of immobilization reduces the canalicular fluid flow in bone with resultant osteocyte hypoxemia and death leading to increased osteoclast activity [63].

Hyperthyroidism is associated with both increased osteoblastic and osteoclastic activities. Resorption is favored overall, however, as increased formation cannot keep pace with increased resorption. Treatment of thyrotoxicosis has been shown to increase bone density, but fails to restore BMD to healthy norms. The effect of exogenous subclinical hyperthyroidism on BMD in women is unclear with mixed reports of normal and decreased BMD [31]. However, a small uncontrolled case series, following women treated for thyroid hormone resistance with the development of exogenous subclinical hyperthyroidism manifested by modest suppression of TSH revealed increased BMD with thyroid hormone supplementation [70].

Low levels of chronic **cadmium exposure** have been associated with the development of osteoporosis [71].

IMPAIRED PROTEIN METABOLISM

Protein-calorie malnutrition (PCM) occurs as a result of many chronic diseases and left uncorrected, results in MBD. In the NHANES 1 study, hip fractures were associated with low energy intake, low serum albumin, and decreased muscle strength; all reflecting protein and caloric deficit [72]. A 10% decrease in body weight typically results in a 1% to 2% bone loss, and more severe weight loss and malnutrition are considered risk factors for osteoporosis, which is likely due to low protein intake [54]. High-protein diets have been shown to increase urinary calcium losses. However, there is growing evidence that a low-protein diet has a detrimental effect on bone. In two interventional trials examining graded levels of protein intake on calcium homeostasis, decreased calcium absorption and an acute rise in PTH were noted by day four of the 0.7 and 0.8 g/kg diets but not during the 0.9 or 1.0 g/kg diets [73,74]. This is particularly worrisome in that these studies suggest the current RDA of 0.8 g protein/kg is inadequate to promote calcium homeostasis.

Cushing's syndrome whether primary or secondary to exogenous long-term administration of glucocorticoids can cause decreased deposition of protein throughout the body in addition to increasing protein catabolism.

Increasing **age** is marked by decreasing levels of growth hormones and decreased protein anabolic activity.

Vitamin C deficiency, which is necessary for secretion of intercellular protein, interferes with formation of the matrix by osteoblasts [75].

Osteocalcin in bone matrix preferentially binds **lead** resulting in decreased calcium binding and failure to bind hydroxyapatite, resulting in decreased bone formation [76]. Serum lead levels increase by 25 to 30% due to mobilization as bone is resorbed in postmenopausal women with osteoporosis [77] contributing to lead toxicity and resultant illnesses late in life.

Liver disease: cholestatic disease, autoimmune hepatitis, chronic viral hepatitis, and alcoholic liver disease can result in osteoporosis. Vitamin D levels are typically low in patients with alcoholic liver disease, autoimmune hepatitis treated with glucocorticoids, and primary biliary cirrhosis; thereby increasing the risk of osteoporosis as well as osteomalacia [78.79]. Osteoporosis can be one of the first clinical manifestations of cholestatic disease [41]. Advanced chronic cholestatic disorders such as primary sclerosing cholangitis also place the patient at significant risk of developing low bone mass [79].

SYSTEMIC INFLAMMATION

Given the role of inflammatory messengers and cytokines in the cell-to-cell communication vital to the balanced remodeling process, systemic inflammatory diseases with resultant increases in proinflammatory messengers have direct effects on bone, leading to increased risk for the development of osteoporosis. These cytokines have been associated with increased osteoclastogenesis in multiple conditions including rheumatoid arthritis, periodontal disease, and multiple myeloma, for example. RANKL-induced osteoclastogenesis has been directly implicated in osteoporosis in cell-culture work [80] and clinical work [81]. Denosumab, recently approved by the Food and Drug Administration for the treatment of osteoporosis, is a monoclonal antibody to RANKL [82]. Evidence exists that protection against inflammation and oxidative stress offered by hydroxyl methylglutaryl CoA reductase inhibitors (the statin class of cholesterol-lowering agents) may also benefit bone health [83].

Inflammatory bowel disease: Patients with inflammatory bowel disease (IBD) have a high prevalence of decreased bone mineral density and an increased rate of vertebral fractures. Circulating proinflammatory cytokines increase osteoclast activity. Indeed, TNF-α decreases differentiation of osteoblasts, increases differentiation of osteoclasts, and increases osteoclast survival by decreasing apoptosis. High levels of IL-6 have been found in osteoporotic patients suffering from Crohn's disease compared to nonosteoporotic patients [84].

Gluten-sensitive enteropathy (celiac disease): Celiac disease is an autoimmune disorder of varying severity characterized by small bowel enteropathy resulting from exposure to wheat gluten in genetically susceptible individuals; it is frequently diagnosed in patients presenting with osteoporosis [27]. It is estimated that celiac disease affects 1% of the population and of those affected approximately 50% will not have clinically significant diarrhea [85]. Auto-antibodies to OPG have been identified in subjects with celiac disease [86].

Several **chronic diseases of aging** have been noted to be comorbid conditions with osteoporosis. These conditions, including atherosclerosis, osteoarthritis, and periodontal disease, share inflammation [87] as an underlying pathophysiological derangement.

UNCERTAIN ETIOLOGIES

Osteoporosis has been recognized as a complication of **parenteral nutrition** (PN) for more than 25 years and appears to be multifactorial. Early studies found intravenous nutrition solutions to contain excess aluminum, but despite newer formulations that limit this element, osteoporosis continues to occur [88]. A longitudinal study conducted in Denmark noted an absence of accelerated bone lost but found the BMD of many long-term PN patients substantially reduced, making them susceptible to fragility fractures and in need of preventive strategies [89].

Vitamin A (retinol) taken in excess can result in osteoporosis and can also lead to hypercalcemia. This noted toxic effect occurs in smaller doses as well and has been identified as a risk factor for hip fractures. Vitamin A as beta carotene does not appear to be associated with increased fracture risk; however, this fact is still being argued [47,90].

PATIENT EVALUATION

Risk factors for osteoporosis are present in susceptible patients prior to disease manifestation. Table 35.2 organizes these risk factors as often encountered in a patient's chart and **medical history**. Many commonly used medications including serotonin reuptake inhibitors [91], loop diuretics, amiodarone [92], heparin [31], thiazolidinediones [93,94], methotrexate [95], and antiepileptic drugs [96] have negative impacts on bone health. Bisphosphonates, though quite effective at increasing BMD

TABLE 35.2

Common Risk Factors for the Development of Metabolic Bone Disease

Diagnosis

Anorexia nervosa

Morbid obesity

    Crohn's disease

    Ulcerative colitis

Gluten-sensitive enteropathy (celiac disease)

Severe liver disease

Current or Previous Medical Interventions

Glucocorticoid use > 3 months or multiple courses

Antacids containing aluminum

Excess thyroid hormone

Methotrexate

Lithium

TABLE 35.2 (*continued*)

Common Risk Factors for the Development of Metabolic Bone Disease

Current or Previous Medical Interventions

Cholestyramine
Gonadotropin-releasing hormone (GnRH) and agonists
Anticonvulsants
Heparin–high dose
Parenteral nutrition > 6 months
Aromatase inhibitors
Calcinuerin inhibitors = cyclosporine, tacrolimus (FK 506), pinecrolimus

Medical History

Female > age 65; Male > age 70
Fragility fracture(s)
Postmenopausal
Early estrogen deficiency (< 45 years of age)
Hypogonadism
Chronic obstructive pulmonary disease
Significant weight loss

Surgical History

Gastrectomy
Bariatric surgery
Organ transplant

Family History

First degree relative with fragility fracture

Social History

Cigarette smoking
Alcohol in excess of two drinks daily
Little or no physical activity
Low calcium intake (lifelong)
Poor dietary habits or chronic dieting

Nutrition History

Insufficient intake or malabsorption
Protein-calorie malnutrition & weight loss
Calcium
Magnesium
Vitamin B12
Vitamin D
Vitamin K

Excess intake of:
Alcohol
Caffeine
Phosphorus
Protein
Sodium
Vitamin A (retinol)

[97], may have negative impacts on bone quality and an expanding literature documents increased risk for osteonecrosis [98] and atypical femoral fractures [99].

The **physical exam** also provides opportunities for early detection. Osteoporosis can be identified by using a stadiometer to measure height and monitor for height changes. When height is discordant with prior measured height or the patient's stated height by greater than one inch, this should prompt further evaluation. The FRAX® tool has been developed by the World Health Organization (WHO) to evaluate fracture risk of patients. Based on individual patient models that integrate the risks associated with clinical risk factors as well as bone mineral density (BMD) at the femoral neck, it can assist in making treatment choices for individual patients [100].

Laboratory diagnosis can point to modifiable risk factors for osteoporosis, particularly assays for gluten sensitivity and hypovitaminosis D. Gluten sensitivity may be a silent disease and it predisposes to calcium malabsorption. Celiac disease is estimated to be five- to tenfold more common among those with osteoporosis. Asking about bowel habits can provide clues, and utilizing common laboratory assays for gluten antibody (serum or stool antigliaden IgG and IgA, antitransglutaminase IgG and IgA, antiendomysial IgG and IgA) can lead to diagnosis of celiac disease. Screening for hypovitaminosis D by checking a serum 25-hydroxyvitamin D (25[OH]D) is indicated in the evaluation of osteoporosis and osteomalacia. Osteomalacia, an abnormal mineralization of cartilage and bone, is most commonly caused by vitamin D deficiency. Vitamin D deficiency can occur as a result of inadequate intake of vitamin D, inadequate exposure to sunlight, or malabsorption syndromes, and is frequently found in patients following gastrectomy, small bowel resection, and bariatric procedures [24,40,41]. Unlike osteoporosis, osteomalacia affects primarily cortical bone; therefore, bone densitometry testing (DXA) is unlikely to confirm the diagnosis. Clinically, these patients can present with bone pain and proximal muscle weakness; however, distinguishing osteomalacia from osteoporosis can be difficult. Diagnosis can be guided by clinical presentation and treatment can be guided by biochemical indices including 25(OH)D, calcium, phosphate, bone-specific alkaline phosphatase, parathyroid hormone; and urine calcium and phosphate [24,78].

Imaging studies are an important screening tool but are limited by evaluating bone density rather than bone strength. Bone strength is an integration of bone density and bone quality [101]. Central DXA is the most common study used to determine bone density and can be used to evaluate current bone status and risk stratification for future fractures. The WHO has defined normal bone density, osteopenia, and osteoporosis based on the T score. DXA results also quantify the standard deviation from that of an age and gender matched control, reported as the Z score. If bone loss is exclusively due to the normal process of aging, the Z score will be near zero; therefore, secondary disease should be suspected when there is a negative deviation of greater than –1.5 [26,102]. Despite the strengths of DXA as the gold standard radiographic study, screening seems to be most efficacious (cost effective) for white women aged 65 and older and for those women, though younger, who are at similar risk [103,104]. Given the slow change noted despite efficacious therapy on DXA scans, follow-up scans at two-year intervals are not unreasonable. Thus the use of biomarkers [105,106], including osteocalcin, urinary N-telopeptide of type 1 collagen (NTX), IGF-1, and N-terminal propeptide of type 1 procollagen (P1NP), can assist both in the diagnosis of osteoporosis [107,108] and overall bone quality [109] as well as providing important information about efficacy of interventions though variability on repeat testing can obscure the actual clinical picture.

TREATMENT

Nutrition and lifestyle changes should be considered as an integral first step in a therapeutic program for osteoporosis. A review of the patient's medical history and individual needs will identify at-risk behavioral, dietary, and nutritional choices. An individualized plan can then be created. Aerobic and resistance exercise are important constituents of a lifestyle program with beneficial changes on osteoporosis, sarcopenia, and insulin resistance [110].

Nutrients should be obtained primarily from a healthful diet. In a carefully crafted nutritional approach, supplements are reserved for nutrients whose level cannot be achieved in the diet either as a consequence of insufficiency in consumed foods or as a consequence of an individual's unique biochemical needs and underlying pathophysiology [111].

Calcium intake should be considered first when building a patient's individualized nutritional plan. Broccoli and leafy greens, such as kale, collards, parsley, and lettuce, are rich in calcium. However, calcium contained in dark leafy greens is often not biologically available due to the presence of phytates that irreversibly bind the calcium and vitamin K. Fruits and vegetables are also the primary dietary source of boron. Citrus fruits are a good source of vitamin C necessary for collagen formation and of potassium, which helps regulate calcium absorption. Eating five to nine servings of fruits and vegetable rich in potassium daily produces a net alkaline load and offsets the net calcium loss induced by the typical American diet's high sodium and acid load [112]. Other sources of potassium are seaweed, nuts and seeds, leafy greens, potatoes, and bananas. Seaweed, nuts and seeds, and some grains are good sources of magnesium, which also contributes to the formation of healthy bone. Dried plums have been shown to have a positive effect in animal models on bone density and a positive effect on bone formation biomarkers in human studies [59].

A frequently consumed food additive with negative implications for calcium metabolism and bone is caffeine. Caffeine, commonly found in coffee, tea, carbonated soft drinks, and chocolate, can also increase urinary excretion of calcium. However, tea drinkers have higher bone density compared to nondrinkers. Research demonstrates that the flavonoids found in tea may offset caffeine's effect and actually increase bone density. A recent prospective study demonstrated that bone loss occurred in those women who had both low calcium intake and high caffeine intakes [46]. The deleterious effects of caffeine on bone can be negated by consuming adequate calcium [46,47].

The evidence regarding the role of phosphoric acid in high-phosphate-containing carbonated beverages is mixed in regards to direct bone effects. Despite the lack of conclusive evidence for the role of phosphoric acid [55], soft drinks contain minimal calcium and displace calcium-containing beverages from the diet. This problem is expected to have significant impact on the prevalence of osteoporosis in the future as children raised with this habit reach adulthood with acquisitional osteopenia.

Calorie-restriction-induced weight loss has been associated with reductions in BMD while exercise-induced weight loss appears to minimize bone loss [113]. Fiber is an important component of the alkaline diet. Some forms of fiber can impair mineral absorption, but this is not uniformly the case and a diet high in fiber is recommended. One specific type of fiber found in fruits and vegetables is in the inulin-type fructans, a subclass of fructooligosaccharides, which have been shown to improve calcium absorption in adolescents and adults [114].

The bone-building nutrients presented in Table 35.1 provide a template for dietary nutrient needs. When patients are unable to achieve these goals through diet, especially when nutrient demands change with medications and underlying medical conditions, supplemental nutrients are an effective adjunct. There are numerous over-the-counter and over-the-internet supplements targeting bone health; while many are indeed beneficial, some may be ineffective or indeed detrimental. When choosing nutritional supplements, purchasing Good Manufacturing Practices–certified products reduces the risk of adulterated or contaminated products.

In general, chelated minerals, which are bound to organic acids, may be better absorbed than inorganic forms. Calcium citrate, for example, has been shown to attenuate the risk of calcium nephrolithiasis, is soluble in the presence of achlorhydria, and is absorbed as both ionic calcium and a calcium citrate complex [115]. Natural sources, including bone meal, dolomite, and oyster shell, are frequently contaminated with lead. Calcium hydroxyapatite has been shown in a few small studies to be superior to calcium carbonate in slowing trabecular bone loss [116,117]. Coral calcium is expensive and the extensive health claims made for this product have not been substantiated [118]. Dietary sources are still considered the best, though the standard diet of Western commerce generally falls far short of supplying adequate calcium. The Institute of Medicine recommends as the recommended dietary allowances 1300 mg daily for children ages nine to 18 years old; 1000 mg for men ages 19–70 years old and women ages 19–50 years old; and 1200 mg for men ages > 70 years old and women ages > 50 years old [119]. The literature supports up to 1800 mg daily for patients who are actively losing weight and for patients who have undergone bariatric surgery [120,121].

Epidemiological studies have shown a positive association of magnesium with bone density. Magnesium appears to affect bone remodeling and strength, has a positive association with hip BMD in both men and women and plays an important role in calcium and bone metabolism [47,54]. Hypomagnesemia blunts parathyroid hormone activity, resulting in altered calcium metabolism, hypocalcemia, vitamin D abnormalities, and further decreased jejunal magnesium absorption [54]. Studies have shown that women with osteoporosis have lower bone magnesium content than women without osteoporosis. One small trial demonstrated a modest improvement in the magnesium supplemented group compared to controls [122]. Other investigators have found no benefit for magnesium in addition to calcium supplementation [123,124].

In 222 consecutive hip-fracture patients evaluated for vitamin D deficiency, 60% were noted to be severely deficient with 25-hydroxy vitamin D levels below 12 ng/ml [125]. A recent meta-analysis of calcium supplementation or calcium and vitamin D supplementation revealed treatment was associated with a 12% reduction in overall fracture rates and a 24% rate in studies with a high compliance rate [126]. In addition to diminished outdoor time for vitamin D synthesis and low population-wide intake, common medications decrease the absorption of dietary vitamin D: cholestyramine, colestipol HCL, orlistat, mineral oil, and the fat substitute olestra [127].

Seniors and those diagnosed with osteopenia or osteoporosis should be evaluated with a 25-hydroxy vitamin D level and treated to optimize levels. Most experts agree that optimal levels of 25-hydroxy vitamin D levels are 40–65 ng/ml. Patients with vitamin D deficiency require immediate and aggressive therapy. Repletion with over-the-counter multivitamins is ineffective and not recommended due to the risk of concomitant vitamin A excess. Adequate tissue stores can be repleted by initially providing oral doses of 2000 to 5000 international units (IU) of vitamin D3 daily. Efficacy of the treatment should be determined by repeat serum levels. Maintenance dosing is recommended and should be based upon the Institute of Medicine recommendations: recommended dietary allowances of 600 IU daily for children and adults ages nine to 70 years old; and 800 IU daily for adults ages > 70 years old [119]. The tolerable upper intake level for vitamin D is 4000 IU daily. For patients, unable to tolerate or adequately absorb oral supplements, exposure to sunlight (UVB radiation) is an excellent source of vitamin D and is an effective alternative [128].

Increasingly, the medical literature demonstrates that botanicals modulate signaling pathways important to bone health. Berberine actively modulates protein kinases active in osteoclastogenesis [129,130]. Hops extracts—specifically rho-iso-alpha acids (RIAA)—also by modifying kinases, have been shown in vitro to inhibit osteoclastogenesis and in vivo animal models to reduce bone and cartilage degradation [131]. In a 12-week study of women with and without metabolic syndrome, biomarkers of bone turnover were favorably impacted by a combination of RIAA, berberine, and vitamins D and K [132,133].

Isoflavones, found in soy and red clover, have attracted the most research interest to date for the prevention and treatment of osteoporosis. Epidemiologic studies have demonstrated beneficial effects in premenopausal, perimenopausal, and postmenopausal women [134]. The research demonstrated a dose-dependent benefit curve. Despite these findings, soy isoflavones have been marketed in relatively high doses with resultant concerns regarding their safety noted. Specifically at higher than dietary levels, there are concerns that because of their estrogenic effects they may be procarcinogenic as well as goitrogenic. However, research has shown that across a broad range of hormonal parameters including thyroid function tests, follicle-stimulating hormone and luteinizing hormone levels, and total estrogen levels, one serving of soy food per day had no demonstrable negative effects [135,136]. Given the current data, soy supplementation as a food is considered an advantageous strategy [137,138], but supplementation with isolated isoflavones should be evaluated on a case-by-case basis.

CLINICAL SUMMARY

When, despite a healthful lifestyle, there remains an imbalance between bone formation and resorption, further dietary changes and targeted nutraceuticals are clinically assessed tools to address the unique needs of patients with osteopenia and osteoporosis.

REFERENCES

1. Matthews GDK et al. Translational musculoskeltal science: Is sarcopenia the next clinical target after osteoporsis? *Ann NY Acad Sci* 2011;1237:95–105.
2. International Osteoporosis Foundation website accessed 29 Jan 2012; http://www.iofbonehealth.org/health-professionals/about-osteoporosis/epidemiology.html.
3. National Osteoporosis Foundation website accessed 1 Jan 2012; http://www.nof.org/aboutosteoporosis/bonebasics/whybonehealth.
4. Lamb, JJ. Osteoporosis in Kohlstadt, I, ed., *Scientific Evidence for Musculoskeletal, Bariatric and Sports Nutrition.* Boca Raton: CRC Press–Taylor and Francis Group, 2006; 473–490.
5. Stevenson JC. Prevention of osteoporosis: One step forward, two steps back. *Menopause Int* 2011; 17(4):137–141.
6. Gambacciani M. HRT misuse and the osteoporosis epidemic. Epub *Climateric* 1 Dec 2011.
7. Seeman E. Bone quality: The material and structural basis of bone strength. *J Bone Mineral Metabolism* 2008;26:1–8.
8. Liedert A. et al. Signal transduction pathways involved in mechanotransduction in bone cells. *Biochemical and Biphysiological Research Communications* 2006;349:1–5.
9. Jilka, RL, Biology of the basic multicellular unit and the pathophysiology of osteoporosis, *Medical and Pediatric Oncology* 2003;41:182–185.
10. Meier C, Nguyen TV, Handelsman DJ, Schindler C, Kushnir MM, Rockwood Al, Meikle AW, Center JR, Eisman JA, Seibel MJ. Endogenous sex hormones and incident fracture risk in older men: The Dubbo Osteoporosis Epidemiology Study. *Arch Intern Med* 2008;168(1):47–54.
11. von Muhlen D, Laughlin GA, Kritz-Silveerstein D, Bergstrom J, Bettencourt R. Effect of dehydroepi-androsterone supplementation on bone mineral density, bone markers, and body composition in older adults: The DAWN Study. *Osteoporosis Int* 2008;19(5):699–707.
12. Armory JK et al. Exogenous testosterone or testosterone with finasteride increases bone mineral density in older men with low serum testosterone. *J Clin Endocrinol Metab* 2004;89:503–510.
13. Ducy P et al. Leptin inhibits bone formation through a hypothalamic relay: A central control of bone mass. *Cell* 2000;100(2):197–207.
14. Confavreux CB, Levine RL, Karsenty G. A paradigm of integrative physiology, the crosstalk between bone and energy metabolism. *Molecular Cell Endocrinol* 2009;310:21–29.
15. Fulzele K et al. Insulin receptor signaling in osteoblasts regulates postnatal bone acquisition and body composition. *Cell* 2010;142(2):309–319.
16. Ferron M et al. Insulin signalling in osteoblasts integrates bone remodeling and energy metabolism. *Cell* 2010;142(2):296–308.
17. Rosen CJ, Bouxesin ML. Mechanisms of disease: Is osteoporosis obesity of the bone? *Nat Clin Practice Rheumatology* 2006;2(1):35–43.
18. Rosen CJ, Motyl KJ. No bones about it: Insulin modulates skeletal remodeling. *Cell* 2010;142:198–200.
19. Goettsch C et al. The osteoclast-associated receptor (OSCAR) is a novel receptor regulated by oxidized low-densitylipoprotein in human endothelial cells. *Endocrinol* 2011;152(12):4915–4926.
20. Yasui T et al. Changes in serum cytokine concentrations during the menopausal transition, *Maturitas* 2007;56(4):396–403.
21. Kim OY et al. Effects of aging and menopause on serum interleukin-6 levels and peripheral blood mononuclear cell cytokine production in healthy nonobese women. Epub *Age* (Dordr)2012;34(2): 415–25.
22. Mundy GR. Osteoporosis and inflammation. *Nutrition reviews* 2007(II);65(12):S147–S151.

23. Hofbauer LC et al. Clinical implications of the osteoprotegerin/RANKL/RANK system for bone and vascular disease. *JAMA* 2004;292:490–495.

24. Shoback D, Marcus R, Bilke, D. Metabolic bone disease in Greenspan FS, Gardner DG, eds., *Basic and Clinical Endocrinology* (7th ed.). New York: McGraw-Hill, 2004; 295–361.

25. Styne D. Puberty in Greenspan FS, Gardner DG, eds., *Basic and Clinical Endocrinology* (7th ed.). New York; McGraw Hill, 2004; 608–636.

26. Dennisson E. "Osteoporosis." In Pinchera A, Bertagna X, Fischer J, eds., *Endocrinology and Metabolism*. London: McGraw-Hill International (UK) Ltd., 2001; 271–282.

27. Fiore CE et al. Altered osteoprotegerin/RANKL ratio and low bone mineral density in celiac patients on long-term treatment with gluten-free diet. *Horm Metab Res* 2006;38:417–422.

28. Jones G. Early life nutrition and bone development in children. *Nestle Nutr Workshop Ser Pediatr Program* 2011;68:227–233.

29. Lanham SA et al. Animal models of maternal nutrition and altered offspring bone structure—bone development across the lifetime. *Eur Cells Materials* 2011;22:321–332.

30. National Osteoporosis Foundation Osteoporosis Clinical Updates: *Osteoporosis in Children and Adolescents*. http://www.nof.org. Washington, DC, Fall 2005.

31. Stein E, Shane E. Secondary osteoporosis, *Endocrinology and Metabolism Clinics of North America* 2003;32:115–134.

32. Campbell JR, Rosier RN, Novotry L, Puzas JE. The association between environmental lead exposure and bone density in children, *Environmental Health Perspectives* 2004;12:1200–1203.

33. Lichtenstein GR, Sands BE, Paziansa M. Prevention and treatment of osteoporosis in inflammatory bowel disease. *Inflamm Bowel Dis* 2006;12(8):797–813.

34. von Tirpitz C, Reinshagen M. Management of osteoporosis in patients with gastrointestinal diseases. *Eur J Gastroenterol Hepatol* 2003;15(8):869–876.

35. Klaus J et al. High prevalence of vertebral fractures in patients with Crohn's disease. *Gut* 2002;51:654–658.

36. Levy, C. and Lindor, K.D., Management of primary biliary cirrhosis, *Current Treatment and Opinions in Gastroenterology* 2003;6:497–498.

37. Obermayer-Pietsch BM et al. Genetic predisposition for adult lactose intolerance and relation to diet, bone density, and bone fractures. *J Bone Miner Res* 2004;19(1):42–47.

38. Carlin AM et al. Prevalence of vitamin D depletion among morbidly obese patients seeking gastric bypass surgery. *Surg Obes Rel Dis* 2006;2(2):98–103.

39. Hamoui N, Anthone G, Crookes F. Calcium metabolism in the morbidly obese. *Obes Surg* 2004;14(1):9–12.

40. Mason EM, Jalagani H, Vinik AI. Metabolic complications of bariatric surgery: Diagnosis and management issues. *Gastroenterol Clin N Am* 2006;34:25–33.

41. Bernstein CN, Leslie WD, Leboff M. AGA Technical Review: Osteoporosis in gastrointestinal diseases. *Gastroenterology* 2003;124(3):795–841.

42. Chines A, Pacifici R. Antacid and sucralfate-induced hypophosphatemic osteomalacia: A case report and review of the literature. *Calcif Tissue Int* 1990;47(5):291–295.

43. Neumann L, Jensen BG. Osteomalacia from Al and Mg antacids. Report of a case of bilateral hip fracture. *Acta Orthop Scand* 1989;60(3):361–362.

44. Teucher B, Fairweather-Tait S. Dietary sodium as a risk factor for osteoporosis: Where is the evidence? *Proceedings of the Nutrition Society* 2003;62:859–866.

45. Frasseto LA et al. Adverse effects of sodium chloride on bone in the aging human population resulting from habitual consumption of typical American diets. *J Nutr* 2008;138:419S–422S.

46. Massey, LK. Is caffeine a risk factor for bone loss in the elderly? *Am J Clin Nutr* 2001;74:569–570.

47. National Osteoporosis Foundation. Osteoporosis Clinical Updates: *Over-the-Counter Products & Osteoporosis: Case discussions*. 2002; Vol III Issue 2. Washington, DC.

48. Munger RG, Cerhan JR, Chiu BC. Prospective study of dietary protein intake and risk of hip fracture in postmenopausal women. *Am J Clin Nutr* 1999;69:147–152.

49. Rizzoli R et al. Protein intake and bone disorders in the elderly. *Joint Bone Spine* 2001;68:383–392.

50. Weikert C et al. The relation between dietary protein, calcium and bone health in women: Results from the EPIC-Potsdam cohort. *Ann Nutr Metab* 2005;49:312–318.

51. Whiting SJ, Boyle JL, Thompson A. Dietary protein, phosphorus and potassium are beneficial to bone mineral density in adult men consuming adequate dietary calcium. *J Am Col Nutr* 2002;21: 402–409.

52. Teegarden D et al. Dietary calcium, protein, and phosphorus are related to bone mineral density and content in young women. *Am J Clin Nutr* 1998;68:749–754.

53. Bonjour JP. Protein Intake and Bone health. *Int J Vitamin Nutr Res* 2011;81(2):134–142.

54. Ilich JZ, Kerstetter JE. Nutrition in bone health revisited: A story beyond calcium. *J Am Coll Nutr* 2000;19(6):715–737.
55. Burckhardt P. "Mineral waters: Effects on bone and bone metabolism." In Burckhardt P, Dawson-Hughes B, Heaney RP, eds., *Nutritional Aspects of Osteoporosis* (2nd ed.). Boston: Elsevier, 2004; 439–447.
56. Franke S et al. Advanced glycation endproducts influence the mRNA expression of RAGE, RANKL, and various osteoblastic genes in human osteoblasts. *Arch Physiol Biochem* 2007;113(3):154–161.
57. Yamagishi S. Role of advanced glycation end products in osteoporosis in diabetes. *Curr Drug Targets* 2011;12:2096–2102.
58. Lindsay R, Cosman, F. "Osteoporosis." In Braunwald E, Fauci AS, Kasper DL, Hauser SL, Longo DL, Jameson JL, eds., *Harrison's Principles of Internal Medicine*, 15th ed. New York: McGraw-Hill, 2001: 2226–2237.
59. Shepherd, A.J., A review of osteoporosis, *Alternative Therapies in Health and Medicine* 2004;10: 26–33.
60. Chakkalakal DA. Alcohol-induced bone loss and deficient bone repair. *Alcohol Clin Exp Res* 2005;29(12):2077–2090.
61. Saag, K.G., Glucocorticoid-induced osteoporosis, *Endocrinology and Metabolism Clinics of North America* 2003;32:115–134.
62. National Osteoporosis Foundation. Osteoporosis Clinical Updates: *The Many Faces of Secondary Osteoporosis*. 2002; Vol III, Issue 3. Washington, DC.
63. Epstein S, Inzerillo AM, Caminis J, Zaidi M. Disorders associated with acute rapid and severe bone loss. *Journal of Bone and Mineral Research* 2003;18:2083–2094.
64. Lipworth BJ. Systemic adverse effects of inhaled corticosteroid therapy: A systematic review and meta analysis. *Arch Intern Med* 1999;159:941–955.
65. Chiodini I et al. Subclinical hypercortisolism among outpatients referred for osteoporosis. *Ann Intern Med* 2007;147:541–548.
66. Potts JT, Jr. "Diseases of the parathyroid gland and other hyper- and hypocalcemic disorders." In Braunwald E, Fauci AS, Kasper DL, Hauser SL, Longo DL, Jameson JL, eds., *Harrison's Principles of Internal Medicine*, 15th ed. New York: McGraw-Hill, 2001; 2205–2226.
67. Theriault RL. Pathophysiology and implications of cancer treatment—induced bone loss, *Oncology* 2004;18:11–15.
68. Napoli N et al. Increased 2-hydroxylation of estrogen in women with a family history of osteoporosis. *J Clin Endocrinol Metab* 2005;90:2035–2041.
69. Armamento-Villareal RC et al. The oxidative metabolism of estrogen modulates response to ERT/HRT in postmenopausal women. *Bone* 2004;35:682–688.
70. Hurlock, DG. Personal communication, June 2001.
71. Altuer T, Elinder CG, Carlsson MD, Grubb A, Hellstrom L, Persson B, Patterson C, Spang G, Schultz A, Jarup L. Low level chronic cadmium exposure and osteoporosis, *Journal of Bone and Mineral Research* 2000;5:1579–1586.
72. Huang Z, Himes JH, McGovern PG. Nutrition and subsequent hip fracture risk among a national cohort of white women. *Am J Epidemiol* 1996;144:124–234.
73. Kerstetter J et al. A threshold for low-protein-diet-induced elevations in parathyroid hormone. *Am J Clin Nutr* 2000;72:168–173.
74. Giannini S et al. Acute effects of moderate dietary protein restriction in patients with idiopathic hypercalciuria and calcium nephrolithiasis. *Am J Clin Nutr* 1999;69:267–271.
75. Guyton AC, Hall JE. Parathyroid hormone, calcitonin, calcium and phosphate metabolism, vitamin D, bone, and teeth in *Textbook of Medical Physiology*, 10th ed. Philadelphia: W.B. Saunders Co., 2000; 899–914.
76. Dowd TL, Rosen JF, Mirts L, Gundberg CM. The effect of Pb(2+) on the structure and hydroxyapatite binding properties of osteocalcin, *Biochimica Biophysica Acta* 2001;1535:153–163.
77. Nash D, Magder LS, Sherwin R, Rubin RT, Silbergeld EK. Bone density related predictors of blood lead levels among peri- and post-menopausal women in the United States, 3rd National Health Nutritional Examination Survey 1988–1994, *American Journal of Epidemiology* 2004;160:901–911.
78. Cijevschi C et al. Osteoporosis in liver cirrhosis. *Rom J Gastroenterol* 2005;14(4):337–341.
79. Sanchez AJ, Aranda-Michel J. Liver disease and osteoporosis. *Nutr Clin Prac* 2006;21:273–278.
80. To TT et al. Rankl-induced osteoclastogenesis leads to loss of mineralization in a medaka osteoporosis model. *Development* 2012;139(1):141–150.
81. Jabbar S et al. Osteoprotegerin, RANKL, and bone turnover in postmenopausal osteoporosis. *J Clin Pathol* 2011;64(4):354–357.

82. Cummings SR et al. Denosumab for prevention of fractures in postmenopausal women with osteoporosis. *NEJM* 2009;361(8):756–765.

83. Yin H et al. Protection against osteoporosis by statins is linked to a reduction of oxidative stress and restoration of nitric oxide formation in aged and ovariectomized rats. *Eur J Pharmacol* Epub 23 Nov 2011.

84. Siffledeen JS, Fedorak RN, Siminoski K, Jen H, Vaudan E, Abraham N, Seinhart H, Greenberg G. Bones and Crohn's: Risk factors associated with low bone mineral density in patients with Crohn's disease, *Inflammatory Bowel Disease* 2004;10:220–228.

85. Lee SK, Green PHR. Celiac sprue (the great modern-day imposter). *Curr Opin Rheumatol* 2006;18:101–107.

86. Riches PL et al. Osteoporosis associated with neutralizing autoantibodies against osteoprotegerin. *NEJM* 2009;361:1459–1465.

87. Serhan CN. Clues for new therapeutics in osteoporosis and periodontal disease: A new role for lipoxygenase. *Expert Opinion and Therapeutic Targets* 2004;8:643–654.

88. Seidner DL, Licata AA. Parenteral nutrition-associated metabolic bone disease: Pathophysiology, evaluation, and treatment. *Nutr Clin Prac* 2000;15:163–170.

89. Haderslev KV et al. Assessment of the longitudinal changes in bone mineral density in patients receiving home parenteral nutrition. *JPEN* 2004;28(5):289–294.

90 Maggio D, Polidori MC, Barabani M. Low levels of carotenoids and retinol in involutional osteoporosis. *Bone* 2006;38:244–248.

91. Richards JB et al. Effect of selective serotonin reuptake inhibitors on the risk of fracture. *Arch Intern Med* 2007;167(2):188–194.

92. Rejnmark L. Cardiovascular drugs and bone. *Curr Drug Saf* 2008;3(3):178–184.

93. Sardone LD et al. Effect of rosiglitazone on bone quality in a rat model of insulin resistance and osteoporosis. *Diabetes* 2011;60:3271.

94. Wan Y et al. PPAR-γ regulates osteoclastogenesis in mice. *Nature Med* 2007;13(12):1496–1503.

95. Pfeilschifter J, Diel IJ. Osteoporosis due to cancer treatment: Pathogenesis and management. *J Clin Oncology* 2000;28:1570–1593.

96. Pack AM, Gidal B, Vasquez B. Bone disease associated with antiepileptic drugs, *Cleveland Clinic Journal of Medicine* 2004;71:s42–s48.

97. Favus MJ. Bisphosphonate for osteoporosis. *NEJM* 2010;363(21):2027–2035.

98. Sedghizadeh PP et al. Oral bisphosphonate use and the prevalence of osteonecrosis of the jaw. *J Am Dental Assoc* 2009;140:61–66.

99. Park-Wyllie LY et al. Bisphosphonate use and the risk of subtrochanteric or femoral shaft fractures in older women. *JAMA* 2011;305(8):783–789.

100. Kanis JA et al. FRAX® and its applications to clinical practice. *Bone* 2009;44:734–743.

101. National Institutes of Health Consensus Conference: Osteoporosis prevention, diagnosis and therapy. *JAMA* 2001;285(6):785–795.

102. National Osteoporosis Foundation. *Physician's Guide to Prevention and Treatment of Osteoporosis*, 1998. http://www.nof.org/physguide. Washington, DC.

103. Nayak S et al. Cost-effectiveness of different screening strategies for osteoporosis in postmenopausal women. *Ann Intern Med* 2011;155(11):751–761.

104. Schousboe JT, Gourlay ML. Comparative effectiveness and cost-effectiveness of strategies to screen for osteoporosis in postmenopausal women. *Ann Intern Med* 2011;155(11):788–789.

105. Seibel MJ. Biochemical markers of bone turnover, part 1: Biochemistry and variability. *Clin Biochem Rev* 2005;26:97–122.

106. Devogelaer J et al. Is there a place for bone turnover markers in the assessment of osteoporosis and its treatment? *Rheum Dis Clin N Am* 2011;37:365–386.

107. Ravn P et al. High bone turnover is associated with low bone mass and spinal fracture in postmenopausal women. *Calcif Tissue Intl* 1997;60:255–260.

108. Schneider Dl, Barrett-Connor EL. Urinary N-telopeptide levels discriminate normal, osteopenic, and osteoporotic bone mineral density. *Arch Intern Med* 1997;157:1241–1245.

109. Eastell R, Hannon RA. Biomarkers of bone health and osteoporosis risk. *Proc Nutr Soc* 2008;67(2):157–162.

110. Sundell J. Resistance training is an effective tool against metabolic and frailty syndrome. *Adv Prev Med* 2011; 2011:984683.

111. Schulman RC, Weiss AJ, Mechanick JI. Nutrition, bone, and aging: An integrative physiology approach. *Curr Osteoporos Rep* 2011;9:184–195.

112. New SA. Intake of fruits and vegetables: Implications for bone health. *Proc Nutr Soc* 2003;62(4):889–899.

113. Villareal DT et al. Bone mineral density response to caloric restriction-induced weight loss or exercise-induced weight loss. *Arch Intern Med* 2006;166:2502–2510.

114. Coxam V. Current data with inulin-type fructans and calcium, targeting bone health in adults. *J Nutr* 2007;137:2527S-2533S.
115. Pak CY. Citrate and renal calculi: An update. *Miner Electrolyte Metab* 1994;20(6):371–377.
116. Ruegsegger P et al. Comparison of treatment effects of ossein-hydroxyapatite compound and calcium carbonate in osteoporotic females. *Osteoporosis Int* 1995;30:30–34.
117. Fernandez-Pareja A, Hernandez-Blanco E, Perez-Maceda JM, Rubio VJR, Palazuelos JH, Dalmau JM. Prevention of osteoporosis: Four-year follow-up of a cohort of postmenopausal women treated with an ossein-hydroxyapatite compound. *Can Drug Invest* 2007;27(4):227–232.
118. Weil, A., *Dr. Andrew Weil's Self Healing*, January 2003.
119. Food and Nutrition Board, Institute of Medicine, National Academies. *Dietary Reference Intakes for Calcium and Vitamin D* (2011). Accessed 10 January 2012: http://fnic.nal.usda.gov/nal_display/index .php?info_center=4&tax_level=3&tax_subject=256&topic_id=134.
120. Ricci TA et al. Calcium supplementation suppresses bone turnover during weight reduction in postmenopausal women. *J Bone Miner Res* 1998;13:1045–1050.
121. Jensen LB et al. Bone mineral changes in obese women during moderate weight loss with and without calcium supplementation. *J Bone Miner Res* 2001;16:141–147.
122. "Minerals." In Bland JS, Costarella L, Levin B, Liska D, Lukaczer D, Schiltz B, Schmidt MA, eds., *Clinical Nutrition: A Functional Approach*, Gig Harbor, WA: Institute for Functional Medicine, 1999.
123. Heaney RP. "Sodium, potassium, phosphorus, and magnesium." In Holick MF, Dawson-Hughes B, eds., *Nutrition and Bone Health*. Totown, NJ: Humana Press, 2004; 327–344.
124. Spencer H et al. Effect of magnesium on the intestinal absorption of calcium in man. *J Am Coll Nutr* 1994;13:483–492.
125. Bischoff-Ferrari HA et al. Severe vitamin D deficiency in Swiss hip fracture patients. *Bone* 2008, Mar;42(3):597–602. [Epub ahead of print].
126. Tang BMP et al. Use of calcium or calcium in combination with vitamin D supplementation to prevent fractures and bone loss in people aged 50 years and older—a meta-analysis. *Lancet* 2007;370:657–666.
127. Hendler SS, Rorvik DR, eds. *PDR for Nutritional Supplements*. Montvale: Medical Economics Company, Inc., 2001.
128. Rosen CJ. "Vitamin D and bone health in adults and the elderly." In Holick MF. *Vitamin D: Physiology, Molecular Biology, and Clinical Applications*. Totown, NJ: Humana Press, 1999;287–306.
129. Hu JP et al. Berberine inhibits RANKL-induced osteoclast formation and survival through suppressing the NF-kappaB and Akt pathways. *Eur J Pharmacol* 2008;580(1–2):70–79.
130. Lee YS et al. AMP kinase acts as a negative regulator of RANKL in the differentiation of osteoclasts. *Bone* 2010;47(5):926–937.
131. Konda VR et al. META060 inhibits osteoclastogenesis and matrix metalloproteinase in vitro and reduces bone and cartilage degradation in a mouse model of rheumatoid arthritis. *Arthritis Rheumatism* 2010;62(6):1683–1692.
132. Lamb JJ et al. Nutritional supplementation of hop rho iso-alpha acids, berberine, vitamin D_3, and vitamin K_1 produces a favorable bone biomarker profile supporting healthy bone metabolism in postmenopausal women with metabolic syndrome. *Nutr Res* 2011;31(5):347–355.
133. Holick MF et al. Hop rho iso-alpha acids, berberine, vitamin D3 and vitamin K1 favorably impact biomarkers of bone turnover in postmenopausal women in a 14-week trial. *J Bone Miner Metab* 2010;28(3):342–350.
134. Taku K et al. Soy isoflavones for osteoporosis: An evidence based approach. *Maturitas* 2011;70(4):333–338.
135. Kurzer MS. Hormonal effects of soy in premenopausal women and men. *J Nutr* 2003;132(3):570S–573S.
136. Persky VW, Turyk ME, Wang L, Freek S, Chatterton R Jr, Barmes S, Erdman J Jr, Sepkovic DW, Bradlow HL, Potter S. Effect of soy protein on endogenous hormone in postmenopausal women. *Am J Clin Nutr* 2002;75(1):145–153.
137. Matthews VL et al. Soy milk and dairy consumption is independently associated with ultrasound attenuation of the heel bone among postmenopausal women: The Adventist Health Study-2. *Nutr Res* 2011;31(10):766–775.
138. Reinwald S, Weaver CM. Soy components vs. whole soy: Are we betting our bones on a long shot? *J Nutr* 2010;140(12):2312S–2317S.

36 Osteoarthritis

David Musnick, M.D.

INTRODUCTION

Physicians in primary care practices have a significant number of patient visits in which the patient has complaints of musculoskeletal pain or joint dysfunction. A significant percent of these patient visits involve joints that are compromised by osteoarthritis (OA). Visits for OA-related pain are even more common in specialty practices such as physiatry, orthopedic surgery, rheumatology, and sports medicine. The usual approach of prescribing nonsteroidal anti-inflammatory drugs (NSAIDS) and pain medications does not adequately address the problems that most patients have in regard to dysfunction of their joints. It may also not adequately slow the breakdown of cartilage. NSAIDs and pain medication can have significant side-effect profiles. Nutritional approaches to OA can decrease pain and improve function. There is also evidence that the use of nutritional therapies may slow progression of OA. This chapter provides a clinical approach to this highly prevalent condition.

EPIDEMIOLOGY

Osteoarthritis is the most common type of arthritis. It can affect any joint of the body but most commonly involves the knees, hips, neck, low back, and hands. In early 2008, a study was published that estimated the prevalence of OA in the U.S. adult population to be approximately 27 million having clinically significant osteoarthritis [1].

This estimate has increased by six million from the 2005 figures, which shows a significant increase in the disease. This data is likely to underestimate the actual number of people with symptomatic OA in any one joint because the data was related to symptomatic OA of the knee, hand, or hip and did not include data on OA of the neck or low back for example.

PATHOPHYSIOLOGY

Osteoarthritis (OA) is characterized by progressive degeneration of articular cartilage with resultant joint space narrowing, cysts, and osteophyte formation. In addition, there can be subchondral bone changes. In the spine, OA is additionally characterized by disc dehydration, decreased disc space height and dysfunction, as well as facet joint hypertrophy and narrowing of the neuroforamen. OA of the knee may involve the articular cartilage of the patellofemoral, proximal tibia fibula, and tibia femur joints. OA of the knee commonly involves degeneration and tearing of meniscal cartilage on the medial or lateral meniscus, which increases risk of degeneration of the articular cartilage.

OA progresses when tissue regeneration cannot keep pace with the rate of cartilage loss. Joint damage may occur when the biomaterial properties of the articular cartilage are inadequate or the load on the joint is excessive [2,3]. Contributing factors related to the development or progression of

OA in a particular joint are: traumatic injury including sprains and contusion, malalignment including myofascial tightness and ligament laxity, prolonged muscle weakness in muscles stabilizing or moving the joint, genetic predisposition, aging, and nutritional factors. Additional insult on the total joint load can come from the extra weight burden associated with obesity and certain physical activities such as high-impact sports.

Osteoarthritis is characterized initially by irregularities of the articular cartilage surface, a thickening of subchondral bone, and formation of marginal osteophytes. Eventually changes include cartilage softening, ulceration, and focal disintegration within the joint with the most striking changes usually seen in load-bearing areas of the articular cartilage.

Chondrocytes comprise the entire cellular matrix of the joint capsule, whereas the substrate of the extracellular matrix is comprised of collagen and polysaccharides known as glucosaminoglycans (GAGs). Substantial GAGs in the extracellular matrix include hyaluronic acid, chondroitin-4-sulfate, chondroitin-6-sulfate, dermatan sulfate, and keratan sulfate. The primary roles of the extracellular matrix include absorbing shock, maintaining viscosity, and nourishing chondrocytes. The primary role of the chondrocytes is the ongoing synthesis of matrix components. In short, the health of the joint is dependent on the function and quality of the chondrocyte and the extracellular matrix.

Early in the course of the disease there is evidence of enhanced chondrocyte replication, suggestive of attempts at repair. In spite of accelerated metabolism within the chondrocyte, the synthesis of matrix substrates is insufficient and results in a decreased concentration of sulfur-containing proteoglycans within the extracellular space. The failure of chondrocytes to compensate for the proteoglycan loss results in a net loss of major matrix contents, including chondrocytes [4].

The loss of proteoglycan density causes an influx of water into the matrix. The influx of water weakens the chemical bonds within the matrix, decreasing the matrix viscosity as well as its capacity to absorb shock and nourish the chondrocytes. The hypertrophy and subsequent death of the chondrocytes causes hyaline cartilage to degenerate and the matrix begins to calcify [5,6].

The progressive depletion of sulfated proteoglycans from the extracellular matrix of articular cartilage, one of the earliest manifestations of osteoarthritis, is thought to be due to enhanced activity of the lysosomal enzymes arylsulfatases A and B [7].

There are inflammatory mediators in OA. Interleukin-1 (IL-1) is the prototypical inflammatory cytokine implicated in signaling the degradation of cartilage matrix in OA. IL-1 is synthesized by chondrocytes and mononuclear cells lining the synovium and it suppresses the synthesis of type 2 (articular) cartilage and promotes formation of type 1 (fibrous) cartilage. IL-1 induces catabolic enzymes such as stromelysin and collagenase and IL-1 upregulates the production of aggrecanases, which cleave proteoglycan. Intra-articular injection of IL-1 induces proteoglycan loss and an IL-1 receptor antagonist slows progression of cartilage loss in animal models of OA [8]. Given the role of IL-1 in promoting cartilage degradation, IL-1 inhibition is a logical treatment target in OA.

In addition to the production of aggrecanases, IL-1 triggers an entire cascade of proinflammatory and catabolic cytokines including tumor necrosis factor-α (TNF-α), IL-6, IL-8, and PGE$_2$, which act synergistically with IL-1 to perpetuate the proinflammatory cascade [8]. TNF-α induces cartilage degeneration by both sustaining cytokine production and increasing expression of collagenases and aggrecanases [9].

In response to IL-1, chondrocytes secrete neutral metalloproteinases (MMP) and active oxygen species that are directly implicated in the destruction of cartilage matrix. IL-1 is a potent inhibitor of proteoglycan and collagen synthesis [10].

There are other cytokines that may play a role in OA and these include IGF 1, transforming growth factor beta, and osteopontin. These cytokines may be primarily anabolic for cartilage.

A number of proteases including metalloproteinases can lead to degeneration of cartilage. These include collagenases, which are a family of enzymes known to cleave helical type 2 cartilage and have activity against type X cartilage. Connective tissue cells produce tissue inhibitors of metalloproteinases (TIMPs). There is likely an imbalance between the level of TIMPs and the metalloproteases that may lead to a catabolic effect and subsequent cartilage degradation [11].

Age is the risk factor most strongly correlated with OA, and some studies suggest that more than 80% of individuals over the age of 75 are affected [12,13]. Age-related tissue changes are believed to be due to a decrease in the repair mechanisms of chondrocytes. With age, chondrocytes are unable to maintain synthetic activity, exhibit decreased responsiveness to anabolic growth factors, and synthesize smaller and less uniform proteoglycans and fewer functional link proteins [13].

PATIENT EVALUATION

In general, severe degenerative joint disease (DJD) is associated with significant pain and disability. A patient may have mild to moderate OA of the knee and hip and not be very symptomatic. Patients can progress to becoming symptomatic and having significant dysfunction with progress of OA of the involved joint. OA appears to progress in perimenopause and menopause in women.

Given the vulnerability of aging joints to OA, it is advisable to include in a yearly physical exam visit a preventive history and physical examination directed at the knee and hip joints. In this exam:

- Evaluate lower extremity joint mechanics and alignment, looking especially for varus or valgus knee alignment and excessive pronation or supination of the feet.
- Evaluate and make suggestions on gait and footwear as many people (especially women) have footwear that does not support their feet well, especially against the pronation forces of gait; this could place abnormal forces on their knees and hips.
- Evaluate the spine and make suggestions to help patients sit in neutral spine posture to slow or prevent neck and low back OA.
- Evaluate and treat muscle weakness, muscle tightness, and age-related sarcopenia.

Assessing dysfunctional biomechanics of the knee and hip are essential for a complete treatment approach for OA. Osteoarthritis occurs more commonly in a number of areas of the body: the C5-7 areas of the cervical spine, the L4-S1 areas of the lumbar spine, the knees, hips, and the IP and DIP joints of the hands, as well as the CMC joint of the thumb. The hips and knees are weight-bearing joints and excessive or abnormal loads can contribute to the development and progression of OA. Dysfunctional mechanics at a joint can create excessive shearing and abnormal forces on articular cartilage contributing to the progression of DJD. Dysfunctional mechanics can result from alignment dysfunction from tight muscles (myofascial factors), loss of cartilage, gait dysfunction, weak muscles, poor posture, lax ligaments, and nonsupportive footwear. It is important to evaluate a patient that has OA for these factors and to suggest treatment. Biomechanical assessment also forms the basis of exercise recommendations to avoid excessive impact on the affected joints and to maximize the safe exercise in which patients will engage. A clinical exam can also evaluate the following comorbidities.

OVERWEIGHT AND OBESITY

Greater body mass index (BMI) in both women and men has been associated with an increased risk of knee OA. Obesity leads to abnormal alignment and loads at weight-bearing joints, especially the knee and hip. It may lead to altered posture (in standing, sitting, and sleeping), altered biomechanics of gait, and less physical activity, any or all of which may further contribute to altered joint biomechanics [14].

Obesity may also contribute to osteoarthritis because of the contribution of adipose cells of inflammatory cytokines. In any patient that has OA and is overweight or obese it is important to have a treatment plan to include weight loss that is concurrent with other OA recommendations. Obesity is an important comorbid condition to treat because of the increased relative risk of osteoarthritis in obese patients [15]. There is an increased relative risk of OA of the contralateral knee within two years of the onset of OA of a knee [16].

HYPERMOBILITY SYNDROMES

Patients that have ligament laxity in a single joint have a higher risk of developing OA in that joint. Patients that have joint laxity in numerous joints have a higher risk of developing OA in lower and upper extremity joints.

This is more common in patients that have the benign hypermobile joint syndrome (BHJS) [17]. Patients should be screened on history and physical exam for evidence of hypermobility. Patients with hypermobility of their hands are at higher risk of thumb OA at the first CMC joint. Patients with ligament laxity in the knee are at higher risk of progression of knee OA. Patient with BHJS should be given information regarding how to protect each hypermobile joint. They should be seen by a physical therapist trained in this disorder. It is also advisable for the patient to be on daily joint support such as glucosamine sulfate. Extraarticular ligament injections (prolotherapy) may be appropriate to stabilize hypermobile joints.

HEMOCHROMATOSIS

Hemochromatosis, an iron storage disease, is a comorbid condition as it can predispose to OA especially of the MCP joints of the hand. Serum ferritin, iron, and transferrin saturation should be checked in any patient with widespread OA or OA at an early age to rule out hemochromatosis.

TREATMENT

The primary treatment targets for OA include the reduction of pain and inflammation, improvement of joint function and joint biomechanical alignment, halting or slowing degeneration, and encouraging regeneration of cartilage. Nutritional therapies may be especially useful in the treatment of OA because they can provide the substrate for cartilage regeneration and have demonstrated efficacy in controlling pain and inflammation. Nutritional therapies are outlined in Table 36.1.

NUTRITIONAL THERAPIES CAN REDUCE THE SIDE EFFECTS OF MEDICATIONS

NSAIDS both over the counter (OTC) and prescription have been the primary treatment of OA. They appear to be moderately effective for pain control and in improving function. They are, unfortunately, associated with a significant side-effect profile. These side effects include stomach and duodenal ulcers and decreased renal blood flow along with potential decline in renal function.

While NSAIDs are effective in the reduction of pain, the long-term use of NSAIDs is not recommended in OA [18] due to the tremendous side-effect profile of these agents. Each year, as many as 7600 deaths and 76,000 hospitalizations in the United States, 2000 deaths in the United Kingdom, and 365 deaths and 3900 hospitalizations in Canada may be attributable to NSAIDs [19]. In addition to the inherent side effects of NSAIDs, there is evidence, both in animals with experimental OA and in humans, that administration of NSAIDs may actually accelerate joint destruction [20–23], but this is still debated in the literature [24]. Due to the high incidence of side effects from NSAIDS, clinicians are advised to avoid or minimize their use when possible and use on a short-term basis when necessary.

NSAIDs may lead to defects in the mucous lining of the gastric mucosa and the small or large intestine. They can lead to damage of the wall of the intestine. The former may be treated with nutritional support to improve the mucous lining. NSAIDs may also lead to an iron deficiency anemia that may be treated with supplemental iron. Prolonged NSAID use may increase the permeability of the small intestine and may predispose an individual to food allergies that may further aggravate joint pain. NSAIDs may be used topically three to four times per day to decrease pain at a particular joint. At the present time, Diclofenac is available as a topical in the United States and Canada.

TABLE 36.1
Mechanism of Action by Which Nutrients Protect against Osteoarthritis

Nutrient	Mechanism of Action	Reference
ANALGESIC		
Avocado/Soybean Unsaponifiable Residues (ASU)	Analgesic	Lequesne, Maheu et al. 2002
Chondroitin Sulfate	Analgesic	Morreale, Manopulo et al. 1996
Glucosamine Sulfate	Analgesic	Matheson and Perry 2003; Bruyere, Pavelka et al. 2004
SAMe	Analgesic	Najm, Reinsch et al. 2004
MODULATE INFLAMMATION		
Avocado/Soybean Unsaponifiable Residues (ASU)	Modulate inflammation by suppressing IL-1, PGE-2, IL-6, IL-8	Hauselmann 2001
Omega-3 Fatty Acids	Modulate inflammation by suppressing IL-1, TNF-alpha, PGE-2, 5-LOX, FLAP, COX-2	Curtis CL 2000
SAMe	Modulate inflammation by suppressing IL-1, TNF-alpha	Gloystein, Gillespie et al. 2003
Glucoasamine	Modulate inflammation by suppressing PGE-2	Nakamura, Shibakawa, et al. 2004
CARTILAGE REGENRATION		
Chondroitin Sulfate	Increase proteoglycan synthesis	Reginster JY 2003
Glucosamine Sulfate	Increase proteoglycan synthesis; increase chondrocyte matrix gene expression	Matheson and Perry 2003, Poustie, Carran et al. 2004
SAMe	Increase proteoglycan synthesis	Gloystein, Gillespie et al. 2003, Bottiglieri 2002
Vitamin C	Increase proteoglycan synthesis	Schwartz and Adamy 1977
Avocado/Soybean Unsaponifiable Residues (ASU)	Increase collagen synthesis; stimulate TGF-beta1; stimulate plasminogen activator inhibitor-1 expression	Boumediene, Felisaz et al. 1999; Hauselmann 2001
Vitamin C	Increase collagen synthesis; stabilization of the mature collagen fibril	Spanheimer, Bird et al. 1986; Peterkofsky 1991
DECREASE DEGRADATION		
Glucosamine Sulfate	Decrease collagen degradation	Christgau, Henrotin et al. 2004
N-3 PUFA	Decrease degradation by inhibiting ADAMTS-4, MMP-3, MMP-13, aggrecanase	Curtis CL 2000
Vitamin C	Decrease degradation by inhibiting aggrecanase	Schwartz & Adamy 1977
Avocado/Soybean Unsaponifiable Residues (ASU)	Decrease degradation by inhibiting metalloproteinase activity and collagenase synthesis	Henrotin, Labasse et al. 1998; Ernst 2003; Hauselmann 2001

Topical capsaicin, which depletes substance P, has been studied and appears to show efficacy topically in a high-strength preparation 0.25% applied to a joint area two times per day [25]. Narcotic pain-relieving medications are less frequently used for OA pain. These can slow intestinal motility and lead to constipation. These drugs may upset sleep and can even lead to pain sensitization.

Several nutritional supplements have been shown to be as effective as NSAIDs in reducing pain and improving functional limitation in patients with OA without adverse effects common to NSAIDs. These include glucosamine sulfate, lyprinol, and S-adenosyl l-methionine (SAMe). A 2004 study demonstrated SAMe (1200 mg/d) was as effective as a commonly prescribed COX-2 inhibitor but with a slower onset of action and a lower incidence of side effects [26].

Nutritional Therapies Can Reduce Inflammation

Inflammatory mediators are integral in the pathogenesis of OA. Human OA cartilage expresses modulators of inflammation (COX-2, 5-LOX, FLAP, IL-1α, TNFα) [27] that normal human cartilage does not.

Inhibition of inflammatory mediators may slow disease progression and has long been a target for treatment. The past decade has elucidated the mechanism by which several nutritional supplements reduce inflammation. Table 36.1 summarizes the mechanism by which avocado/soybean unsaponifiable residues, omega-3 fatty acids, SAMe, and glucosamine interfere with the inflammatory cascade. The clinician should also consider placing a patient on an anti-inflammatory, low-toxin diet rich in food-based antioxidants, as part of a long-term treatment program to reduce inflammatory mediators.

Nutritional Therapies Can Provide Substrates for Cartilage Repair and Regeneration

The regeneration of cartilage must be an emphasis of treatment to minimize disease progression. Substantial evidence, in vitro and in vivo, attests to the ability of nutritional agents to enhance proteoglycan synthesis, increase strength of collagen network, decrease proteinases that degrade collagen and proteoglycans (aggrecanase), and decrease IL-1 and subsequent proinflammatory cytokines that further perpetuate cartilage degradation.

Nourishment of the joint is complicated in that articular cartilage is neither vascularized nor supplied with nerves or lymphatic vessels. The outer one-third of the knee meniscus has a reasonable blood supply. Chondrocytes receive their nourishment from synovial fluid. The use of nutritional supplements to support joints with osteoarthritic changes makes sense primarily if there is cartilage surface remaining as opposed to bone on bone anatomy. It also makes sense as prevention for other joints in the setting of a joint that has minimal cartilage remaining or in one that has been replaced. Most of the studies regarding nutraceutical support have been done regarding osteoarthritis of the knee, but it is very reasonable to consider their use in other joints with OA.

Joint Support Nutrients

Glucosamine

The vast majority of published clinical research studies have demonstrated that glucosamine is effective for decreasing pain, improving range of motion, and improving function. A recent meta-analysis from 2010 [28] has brought the efficacy into question. The meta-analysis had strict criteria and indicated that many of the studies had problems in methodology. Outcome measures evaluated by the meta-analysis were decreasing pain and slowing joint space narrowing. It is also important to follow improvement in function, which many of the studies have used and have shown efficacy. A large multicenter prospective trial, the GAIT Trial, sponsored by the NIH [29] has released two-year data from its four-year trial. This data showed some benefit from glucosamine but not very much. One of the problems with this study was the use of glucosamine HCL instead of glucosamine sulfate. The studies that have showed efficacy with glucosamine have used glucosamine sulfate. Because of numerous studies that demonstrated efficacy of glucosamine sulfate, more detail regarding glucosamine is appropriate.

N-acetyl-D-glucosamine is a naturally occurring amino sugar found in all human tissues. It functions as a building block in the synthesis of structural substrates such as glycoproteins, glycolipids, GAGs, hyaluronate, and proteoglycans and is required to manufacture joint lubricants and protective agents such as mucin and mucous secretions [28].

Although glucosamine is not generally found in the human diet, it is easily obtained from the exoskeletons of shrimp, crabs, and lobsters for use in medical applications. As a supplement glucosamine is available as glucosamine sulfate, glucosamine hydrochloride, and N-acetyl glucosamine. Thus far, the majority of clinical research demonstrating efficacy in OA has been conducted with the sulfate form. Glucosamine sulfate is the recommended form at this time.

When administered orally, the absorption rate for glucosamine sulfate (GS) in the human gastrointestinal tract is approximately 87% [31]. In recent years, topical cream containing glucosamine and chondroitin sulfate has shown efficacy in relieving pain in OA of the knee [32]. Topical GS is reasonable to use for peripheral meniscus tears in patients with reasonable knee function, chondromalacia patella, and OA of the great toe, thumb, and fingers. It should be applied two to three times per day over the joint line areas.

Glucosamine sulfate has been shown in a number of studies to slow progression of joint space narrowing in the knee. One study compared GSA 1500 mg per day versus placebo and followed the patients for three years. It demonstrated a mean joint space narrowing of .04 mm in the GS group versus .19 mm in the placebo group [33]. These results were similar to another three-year study of GS versus placebo published in the *Lancet* in 2001 [34].

In 2004, a study was published documenting that glucosamine sulfate had the ability to reduce joint space narrowing in postmenopausal women with osteoarthritis of the knee [35]. The mechanism of action is purported to be the increased availability of substrate for proteoglycan synthesis as well as anti-inflammatory actions [23,27].

All of the aforementioned studies used a single daily dose of GS of 1500 mg. It is reasonable for the clinician to recommend that their patient use this dose and a dosing method as a minimum dose to achieve structure-modifying effects.

While studies of glucosamine and OA are largely positive, there are a few negative studies that raise several interesting questions about whether or not glucosamine may be more effective in OA subtypes. In a 2004 study, Christgau et al. explored using specific markers of collagen turnover to help classify patients at baseline. Using these markers, they were able to demonstrate that those patients who initially had high cartilage turnover were particularly responsive to glucosamine therapy [36]. Another question remaining for clinical investigation is the generalizability to glucosamine to treating OA of all joints, since the knee has been the most widely studied.

The one constant found in all studies reported in the medical literature is that glucosamine appears to be remarkably safe and well tolerated at 1500 mg per day given in either once daily or in divided doses. Side effects are significantly less common with glucosamine than either NSAIDs or placebo [37]. Recent studies have addressed concerns that glucosamine, a sugar, can have adverse effects on levels of plasma glucose and insulin but further research has found these concerns to be unfounded [37–40].

Glucosamine is often derived from shellfish and several authors have expressed concern that the supplement may cause allergic reactions in people who are sensitive to shellfish. Glucosamine is derived from the exoskeletons of shellfish but antibodies in individuals allergic to shellfish are targeted at antigens in the meat, not the shell. Thus far, there have been no documented reports of allergic reactions to glucosamine among shellfish-sensitive patients, but it is prudent to recommend the synthetically derived, generally corn-based form of the supplement be used in this population [41].

Most studies have concluded that patients taking glucosamine do not seem to notice much effect for at least six weeks. Patients need to be educated in regard to the duration of supplementation and how long it may take to notice an effect. Guidelines will be given at the end of this chapter for the duration of joint support supplementation.

Chondroitin Sulfate

Chondroitin sulfate (CS), a mucopolysaccharide, is a proteoglycan component that functions in the maintenance of cartilage elasticity, strength, and mass. In humans, chondroitin sulfate is made from glucosamine sulfate derivatives. Chondroitin sulfate, like glucosamine, is not present in significant amounts in the human diet. It is extracted from either bovine trachea or marine shell sources for use in OA.

The medical literature contains numerous studies, of varying quality, pertaining to the use of chondroitin as a therapy for OA. Many early studies have shown efficacy in relieving pain and improving function whereas some later studies and meta-analyses have not [42]. Chondroitin studies have often used combinations of chondroitin with glucosamine (often in the HCL form). CS has been shown in many studies to alleviate pain, decrease NSAID use, and improve joint mobility. A number of studies have shown that CS may be able to slow the progression of joint space narrowing with osteoarthritis of the knee [43–45]. A recent study demonstrated reduction in joint space narrowing of .1 mm compared to .24 mm in the placebo group [46].

Results of chondroitin supplementation typically take eight to 12 weeks to become apparent as in the glucosamine studies. The recommended dosage is 800–1200 mg per day given orally in one or two to three divided doses. Studies showing a reduction in joint space narrowing have evaluated single dosing at 800 mg per day [47–48].

There is not enough evidence to suggest an additive benefit of chondroitin when glucosamine sulfate is already being used in therapeutic doses but CS is generally relatively inexpensive and without side effects. Because of this, it is recommended that the clinician recommend glucosamine sulfate as a first-line agent; and make sure the patient is using glucosamine sulfate because of the research to support that formulation. One could then add 1200 mg per day of CS after a minimum of 12 weeks on GS to see if the patient improved in pain and function. It would also be reasonable to choose a different second agent other than CS based on a meta-analysis.

An important controversy in the medical literature as it pertains to the efficacy of chondroitin is whether or not clinically significant amounts are available to the body via oral dosing given the large size of the molecule. During the past few years, several studies have demonstrated a low oral absorption of chondroitin sulfate and shown absorption estimates across the gut mucosa range from 10–70% [49,50]. Low molecular weight CS was developed to improve absorption of CS.

Other than mild gastrointestinal distress, the incidence of adverse effects with chondroitin sulfate is extremely low. Chondroitin is typically extracted from bovine trachea and concern has been expressed about the potential risk of contamination by animals infected with bovine spongiform encephalopathy (BSE, mad cow disease). There are currently no documented cases of such contamination and risk of transmission is thought to be low. Low molecular weight CS is made from shellfish sources. Vegetarian patients should be informed of the bovine origin of chondroitin products.

S-Adenosyl Methionine

S-adenosyl methionine (SAMe) is synthesized endogenously from methionine and adenosine triphosphate (ATP). It is a methyl donor to numerous acceptor molecules and plays an essential role in many biochemical reactions involving enzymatic transmethylation. In addition, it has proved efficacious in treatment of OA in regard to treatment of inflammation and cartilage regeneration; its use is primarily limited by quality and cost factors.

SAMe has been shown to inhibit the synthesis and the activity of IL-1 and TNF-α at multiple locations in its signal transduction pathways. SAMe has demonstrated the ability to upregulate the proteoglycan synthesis and proliferation rate of chondrocytes, thereby promoting cartilage formation and repair. SAMe is an alternative to NSAIDs for treatment of joint inflammation and pain caused by trauma and disease states such as OA. It is a proven therapy for OA and has a low side-effect profile. The consensus among several published reviews is that SAMe appears to be of equivalent effectiveness to NSAIDs in reducing pain and improving functional limitations, with fewer side effects. One study suggested SAMe has a slower onset of action than NSAIDs with equivalent results at four weeks [51].

B12 and folate aid the body in using SAMe, and it may be useful to supplement with these nutrients as well. The amounts in a good multiple would usually be sufficient. SAMe can interact with tramadol as well as serotonergic antidepressants. One should try to use other agents when these drugs are prescribed or use SAMe with caution and monitor patients for a serotonergic syndrome. There appears to be some efficacy of SAMe in patients with fibromyalgia; therefore, it would be a good choice in a patient with OA and fibromyalgia [52].

SAMe is efficacious in depression so that its use would be indicated in a patient with OA and comorbid depression. One would then evaluate its efficacy on mood as well as its effect on joint pain and function.

There are a number of forms of SAMe available. Patients should be encouraged to use enteric coated SAMe. Most of the SAMe products available are in the tosylate form. The butanedisulfonate is more bioavailable and more stable although it is more expensive. The dosage of SAMe is typically 200 mg three times per day for OA and 800 mg per day if one is treating OA and fibromyalgia.

Methylsulfonylmethane

Methylsulfonylmethane (MSM) is a source of sulfur as well as a methyl donor. In one study MSM and glucosamine sulfate (GS) were used alone and in combination. Both agents were found to be efficacious in OA but the combination of 500 mg of MSM and 500 mg of GS were found to be more efficacious than the use of one of them alone. Also in this study, patents reported improvement in symptoms with less lag time than with the individual agents alone [53]. MSM has been shown at doses of 3 grams, two times per day in a placebo-controlled trial to decrease pain and function in activities of daily living [54]. MSM appears to have a minimal side-effect profile. Although there have only been two studies, MSM appears to show efficacy. Doses of 3000 mg twice a day are recommended if used alone, or 500 mg three times a day if used concurrently with GS.

Hyaluronic Acid

Hyaluronic acid (HA) is the main component of the extracellular matrix within the joint. It is a hydrophilic polysaccharide varying in length from 250 to 25,000 disaccharide units. The large size of this molecule and the water it holds give the matrix solution remarkable viscosity, tensile, and shock absorption properties. The oral form of hyaluronic acid is not well absorbed.

It is important to note that oral cartilage support supplements do not appear to have much effect in joints with little surface or meniscus cartilage remaining. Intra-articular hyaluronans (viscosupplementation) have been used extensively to treat pain and mechanical dysfunction associated with osteoarthritis of the knee. Many controlled clinical studies have demonstrated their efficacy and a low side effect profile for this indication and application [55–58].

Intra-articular injections of the knee are indicated if the patient has very little cartilage surface and wishes to avoid surgery. They are done one time per week for three to five weeks (depending on the viscosupplementation formulation used). An improvement in pain levels and in function appears to have clinical benefit lasting from six to nine months. The treatment often needs to be repeated after six to nine months. Side effects are minimal and may include swelling. It is of note that this treatment is usually given to patients in which there is little cartilage and joint space remaining. It can in fact be very beneficial in patients with mild to moderate joint space narrowing and in patients with chondromalacia patella.

Omega-3 Fatty Acids

Osteoarthritic cartilage expresses markers of inflammation that contribute to the dysregulation of chondrocyte function and the progressive degradation of the cartilage matrix. In vitro, when human

OA cartilage explants are exposed to omega-3 polyunsaturated fatty acids, the molecular modulators of inflammation are inhibited. Curtis et al. cultured human OA articular cartilage with various fatty acids and concluded omega-3 fatty acids, but not other fats, have the capacity to improve late-stage OA chondrocyte function. They found culture for 24 hours with omega-3 fatty acids resulted in a decrease loss of GAGs, reduced collagenase cleavage of type II collagen, a dose-dependent reduction in aggrecanases, and all studied modulators of inflammation (COX-2, 5-LOX, FLAP, IL-1α) and joint destruction (ADAMTS-4, MMP-3, MMP-13) were abrogated or reduced [59].

The concentration and distribution of fatty acids in the diet has long been known to exert influence over the inflammatory cascade. While no large-scale clinical studies have yet been done on the influence of omega-3 fatty acids on the symptoms or progression of OA, several clinical studies have demonstrated dietary supplementation with omega-3 fatty acids reduces the inflammatory symptoms of rheumatoid arthritis [60,61].

When treating patients with omega-3 fatty acids it is reasonable to use fish oil products consisting of EPA and DHA. It is reasonable to choose products that have been tested for purity and that are extremely low in contaminants of pesticides, mercury, and PCBs. It is reasonable to use approximately two to four grams of high-EPA fish oil per day. In patients with sluggish delta-6-desaturase enzymes, the omega-6 equivalent GLA may also need to be taken even though it is omega-6. This would be recommended for patients that are obese as well as for patients that have metabolic syndrome. Side effects of fish oil are minimal but caution should be used if a patient is on a medication such as Coumadin because of the platelet effects of fish oil.

Lyprinol is a patented extraction of New Zealand green-lipped mussel powder derived from *Perna canaliculus*. It has been shown to provide significant pain relief and improvement in joint function in 80% of subjects after eight weeks of treatment without adverse effect. The therapeutic value of Lyprinol has been attributed, in part, to its high concentration of omega-3 fatty acids [62].

There have been variable results in efficacy of trials using Lyprinol in patients with OA at the current starting dose of 900–1200 mg per day. It would not be a first line approach and EPA/DHA capsules or oil should be used first for their anti-inflammatory effect because of extensive research on safety and beneficial effects in joints and nonjoint systems. It appears that Lyprinol does not have the same adverse GI side effect profile as NSAIDS and therefore could be used as a safe anti-inflammatory for patients with OA.

Cetylated Fatty Acids

Cetylated fatty acids (CFA) have been used in studies both orally and topically. CFA have been marketed under the name of Celadrin and Cetyl Myristoleate and have minimal side effects. They have been demonstrated in short-term studies to improve range of motion and function of patients with knee OA [63,64]. A single short-term study has demonstrated efficacy of topical cetylated fatty acids on wrist and elbow function and endurance during exercise [65]. CFA may be taken orally in a dose of 350 mg or used topically to improve pain and function in OA of the knee, elbow, and wrist. One could extend this use to the thumb at the CMC joint.

Vitamin C/Ascorbic Acid

Ascorbic acid plays a role in the synthesis of joint components, encourages cartilage synthesis in vitro, and epidemiologic data suggests dietary intake of ascorbic acid is associated with a reduction of OA progression. Vitamin C is necessary for the synthesis of collagen and GAGs within the joint capsule. In collagen synthesis, ascorbic acid is a cofactor for enzymes essential for stabilization of the mature collagen fibril [66,67]. The role of vitamin C as a carrier of sulphate groups also makes it a requirement for GAG synthesis [7].

In vitro, addition of ascorbic acid to OA cultures results in a decreased level of aggrecanase, the primary enzyme responsible for the degradation of proteoglycan. Vitamin C has been shown to significantly increase the biosynthesis of proteoglycan in both normal and osteoarthritic tissues, suggesting it may be helpful in joint repair [7].

In the Framingham Osteoarthritis Cohort Study, a moderate intake of vitamin C (120–200 mg/d) was associated with a threefold lower risk of OA progression. The association was strong and highly significant and was consistent between sexes and among individuals with different severities of OA. The higher vitamin C intake also reduced the likelihood of development of knee pain [68].

Avocado/Soybean Unsaponifiable Residues

Avocado/soybean unsaponifiable residues (ASU) is a manufactured product, distributed in France as Piascledine, consisting of one-third avocado oil and two-thirds soybean unsaponifiables [69]. Three of four rigorous clinical trials suggest that ASU is an effective symptomatic treatment of OA. A dose of 300 mg ASU per day has demonstrated efficacy in both knee and hip OA but appears to have been studied more extensively for hip OA. Outcome measures have included a reduction in NSAID and analgesic intake, a reduction in pain, and an increase in function. ASU has been shown to have structure-modifying effects in the hip [70]. No serious side effects were reported in any of the published studies.

Based on in vitro research, the apparent mechanism of effect of ASU is via the attenuation of inflammatory mediators and the stimulation of anabolic processes within the cartilage. The anti-inflammatory effects of ASU include the inhibition of IL-1 and the inhibition of IL-1-stimulated PGE_2 and proinflammatory cytokines IL-6 and IL-8 in vitro and prevented the deleterious action of IL-1 on synovial cells and on articular chondrocytes of rabbits in vivo [10,71].

Several in vitro studies on cultured chondrocytes have demonstrated these unsaponifiable residues have an inhibitory action on collagenase synthesis, metalloproteinases, proinflammatory cytokines, IL-6 and IL-8, and the inducible form of nitric oxide synthase and PGE_2, all of which decrease inflammation. [16,72] The anabolic effects of ASU include the in vitro stimulation of collagen synthesis and transforming growth factor-β1 in articular chondrocyte cultures and the expression of plasminogen activator inhibitor-1 by articular chondrocytes [71]. ASU has also been found in a lab model to promote tissue inhibitors of metalloproteinases and limit MMP-3 production [73].

Niacinamide/Vitamin B3

Niacin, or vitamin B3, occurs in two forms, nicotinic acid (usually referred to as niacin) and nicotinamide (typically referred to as niacinamide). While both forms have many functions in the body and are crucial to cellular energy production as precursors of NAD and NADP, their therapeutic uses differ considerably.

Niacinamide has been in use as a therapy for osteoarthritis since the 1940s based on preliminary work by Kaufman [74,75]. In-office clinical research, reported by Kaufman on 455 patients receiving 1500–4000 mg/d niacinamide compared against untreated, age-matched controls suggested an increase in joint range index and subsequent reduction in pain in four to eight weeks. Recently investigators have examined efficacy and potential mechanism of action of niacinamide in OA more closely. Jonas et al. demonstrated in a 12-week randomized, double-blind, placebo-controlled trial (N = 72) that patients who took niacinamide (3000 mg daily) experienced an improvement in the global impact of their osteoarthritis, increased joint flexibility, reduced inflammation, and decreased use of anti-inflammatory medication, compared to controls [76].

While the mechanism of action of niacinamide in OA has yet to be fully elucidated, current theories suggest that niacinamide acts on chondrocytes to decrease cytokine-mediated inhibition of aggrecan and type II collagen synthesis. In addition, reduction in either production or effect of IL-1 on chondrocytes has been suggested as a plausible mechanism [77].

Adverse affects have not been widely reported with pharmaceutical-grade niacinamide [78]; however, nausea, heartburn, flatulence, and diarrhea have been reported. Elevated liver enzymes have been reported with the administration of niacinamide [79], and, for this reason, it is advisable to ensure niacinamide supplement quality and evaluate baseline liver function tests prior to, and periodically after, niacinamide administration. While large-scale safety, efficacy, and dosing studies are clearly lacking for the general recommendation of niacinamide treatment for osteo-arthritis, preliminary research suggests the nutrient has therapeutic value and warrants further investigation.

Strontium

Strontium ranelate is a nutrient that is being used in some European countries for the treatment of postmenopausal osteoporosis. A number of formulations of strontium have been used in the United States for the same purpose. Studies have provided a preclinical basis for the use of strontium ranelate in osteoarthritis. In OA and normal chondrocytes that are treated with or without interleu-kin 1β (IL-1β), strontium ranelate has been shown to stimulate the synthesis of type II collagen and proteoglycan [80]. In a three-year post-hoc analysis of the pool of Spinal Osteoporosis Therapeutic Intervention (SOTI) and Treatment of Peripheral Osteoporosis studies, strontium ranelate was shown to significantly decrease the levels of urinary C-terminal telopeptides of type II collagen (u-CTX-II), a cartilage degradation biomarker, compared with placebo [81].

A post-hoc analysis was done of pooled data on 1105 women with steoporosis and osteoar-thritis of the spine [82]. The data was from the Spinal Osteoporosis Therapeutic Intervention (SOTI) and Treatment Of Peripheral Osteoporosis (TROPOS) trials. In this study one group of women took two grams of strontium ranelate daily for three years and they were compared to a placebo group. The admission criteria for these studies were women age 50 and older that had been postmenopausal for at least five years and had osteoporosis documented by DEXA scan. The conclusions of the post-hoc study were "the proportion of patients with worsening overall spinal OA score was reduced by 42% in the strontium ranelate group compared to a placebo group" [82]. There appears to be a symptom- and structure-modifying effect of strontium in the spine. Studies have not looked at other joints. This study appears to indicate a role for strontium in patients that have spinal OA and osteoporosis. Because of the mechanism of action of stron-tium it is highly likely that it would be efficacious in women with osteoporosis and OA that were perimenopausal and or immediately postmenopausal as well as for women that were quite far out from the onset of menopause. Strontium ranelate at 2 grams per day would be the preferred form and delivers 680 mg of elemental strontium. Strontium chloride has not been adequately studied. Strontium ranelate appears to have interactions with calcium and vitamin D. There also may be a slight increased risk of venous thrombosis. The clinician should follow vitamin D levels and augment as necessary and consider using strontium in patients with combined osteoporosis and OA of the spine.

Vitamin D

Vitamin D has been used for many years for prevention of rickets and in the treatment of osteo-porosis. Recently, vitamin D has been recommended for cancer prevention and for reduction in all cause mortality.

The expression of vitamin D receptors is upregulated in human OA chondrocytes [83].

The Framingham study found a threefold increase in risk of OA progression for patients in the middle and lowest tertiles of serum levels of 25 OH vitamin D. Low serum levels of vitamin D also predicted osteophyte growth and loss of joint space [84]. Low vitamin D levels have been associated with an increased risk of falls in the elderly population [85]. Vitamin D receptors have been found in muscle. It is recommended that clinicians check serum 25 OH vitamin D levels in their patients with OA. It is recommended based on the physiology and clinical research that clinicians use supple-mental vitamin D3 to increase the serum level of vitamin D to well within the normal range (above 32 ng/ml). Preliminary results of a study that is ongoing at Tufts University on the relationship of vitamin D deficiency and symptoms of knee OA were presented in the Fall 2007 meeting of the American College of Rheumatology. Having a low vitamin D level was associated with more knee pain and greater functional limitations. This information is convincing enough to support serum testing and supplementation of vitamin D in patients with OA.

Selenium

Low selenium levels have been reported as a risk for osteoarthritis [86]. The primary organic forms of selenium are the amino acid–based selenocysteine and selenomethionine. Selenium is used in the body in a number of enzyme systems. Selenium can be obtained from dietary sources, although the soils are deficient in selenium in many countries; 100 mcg per day is usually recommended either in dietary or supplement sources.

Devils Claw

There have been a number of studies assessing the effectiveness of supplementing with devils claw (*Harpagophytum procumbens*) for low back pain or for OA. These studies have been reviewed recently [87]. Most of the studies are short term or lack controls. A recent study of patients with hip or knee OA using an aqueous extract of devils claw used 2400 mg of extract daily, corresponding to 50 mg of harpagoside, showed efficacy in pain reduction and improvement in function but was carried out for only 12 weeks [88]. The long-term safety of devils claw needs more investigation before it can be recommended for long-term use.

Taking devils claw orally alone or in conjunction with nonsteroidal anti-inflammatory drugs (NSAIDs) seems to help decrease osteoarthritis-related pain.

Green Tea Extracts

There is evidence to suggest that compounds found in green tea, including the polyphenol epigallocatechin gallate (EGCG), can interfere with the some of the inflammatory cytokines involved in the progression of osteoarthritis. During osteoarthritis, IL-1(b) causes an inflammatory response that enhances the expression and activity of matrix metalloproteinases, which are known to degrade cartilage. Studies are suggesting that EGCG can also inhibit the expression of IL-1(b) and matrix metalloproteinases [91]. In a study of osteoarthritis, researchers found that EGCG was a potent inhibitor of IL-1(b)–induced cartilage damage [92]. Additional studies have found that EGCG from green tea inhibits both IL-1(b) and the inflammatory cytokines COX-2 and inducible nitric oxide synthase, which are induced by IL-1(b) [93]. Overall, laboratory studies have found that EGCG was nontoxic and that green tea consumption may benefit patients who have osteoarthritis by reducing inflammation and slowing the breakdown of cartilage [94].

Hops Extracts

In an eight-week trial, the effectiveness of a combination of alpha acids from hops, rosemary extract, and oleanolic acid were tested in subjects with osteoarthritis. The results were that osteoarthritis subjects showed a 50% decrease in pain [95]. A different type of hops extract, tetrahydro-iso-alpha acids (THIAA), was used in research and showed inhibition of the MMP 13 enzyme. This appears to have potential in OA patients.

Hydration

It is important to recommend to patients that they remain well hydrated. There is evidence that chronic low-grade dehydration may contribute to OA of the knee and low back. The clinician can recommend a minimum intake of fluid with most of it in the form of filtered water. Water may also be obtained from juices low in sugar and in higher water content fruits and vegetables. Figure 36.1 demonstrates in visual form some of the effects of dehydration on the joint.

Duration of Joint Support Supplementation

The duration of supplementation depends on the pathology that the clinician is treating. If you are treating an acutely injured joint (knee, hip, or spinal joint) it is reasonable to start supplementation immediately upon diagnosis and continue treatment for approximately 12 weeks. It is also reasonable to consider an X-ray of the joint six months after the original injury to make sure that no significant OA changes have occurred. If OA has developed consider the guidelines that follow. If you

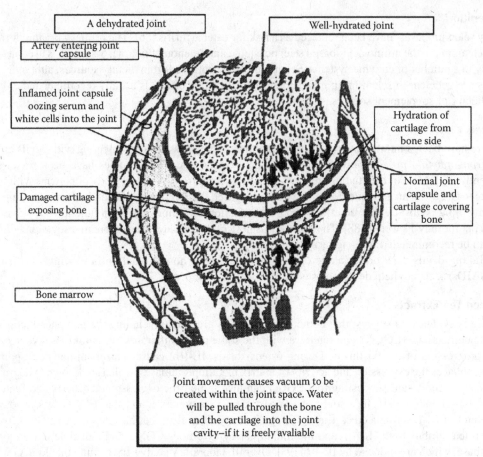

FIGURE 36.1   A well-hydrated joint is contrasted with a dehydrated joint. (Reprinted with permission from Taylor & Francis from *Scientific Basis for Musculoskeletal, Bariatric and Sports Nutrition*).

are treating a joint with osteoarthritis that has articular cartilage remaining you will need to make a long-term plan for nutritional joint support.

CHOICE AND TIMING OF NUTRITIONAL SUPPORT SUPPLEMENTS FOR OSTEOARTHRITIS

The choice of nutritional support for patients with osteoarthritis can be based on a number of factors including the monthly cost of an individual supplement, the efficacy of each nutritional intervention, current clinical studies, and side-effect profiles. It is also related to the pathology and clinical progression of OA in the joint or joints being treated. In general, patients with very severe OA are not likely to respond to glucosamine or chondroitin. The clinician should always make recommendations for exercise, posture, stable shoe wear, physical therapy, ligament laxity, and manipulative therapies when appropriate to normalize joint mechanics and forces. Although most of the research has been in regard to OA of the knee and hip one can use the following nutritional approach with OA of any joint including the spine.

In the patient with OA:

* Recommend that the patient drink two to three glasses of green tea per day or take a supplement with green tea extract.
* Recommend initiating a trial of a nightshade-free diet for about eight to 10 weeks to see if there is a reduction of pain or an improvement in function.

- A clinician should also run a food allergy panel on a patient with more diffuse OA to consider eliminating food allergens from the patient's diet.
- Initiate a balanced and well-formulated multivitamin mineral formula because of the information on selenium, vitamin D, and vitamin C. This formula should contain at least 100 ug of selenium, at least 200 mg of vitamin C, and at least 600–800 IU of vitamin D3. Vitamin D levels should be tested and patients should be supplemented appropriately to bring their level up to at least 32 ng/ml.

Supplement approaches can block proteases and inflammatory cytokines and also augment sulfur and chondrocyte nutrients and anabolic agents. When starting or adding any supplement for joint support it is important to inform the patient that they should monitor their pain level and functional abilities in a journal, wait at least eight to 10 weeks before starting any new supplement, and compare pain and function to just before they started the new product.

It is reasonable to start a patient on a supplement to reduce joint inflammation as a first-line agent. A combination of EPA/DHA of 3–4 grams per day with GLA 250–500 mg per day can be an appropriate starting dose in most patients. An EPA product formulated with the triglyceride form would be preferable. If there is evidence for a lot of inflammation such as joint swelling one can consider adding to this a combination of anti-inflammatories such as a readily absorbable formulation of curcumin, ginger, and boswellian. With NSAIDs and natural anti-inflammatories, one should monitor for symptoms of GI bleeding through CBC and kidney and liver function every three to four months. An alternative to the anti-inflammatories would be SAMe at doses of 600 to 800 mg per day in two divided doses. This would be preferable for a patient with depression but could be used in any patient with OA. Niacinamide would be a useful second-line agent in doses of 1500–4000 mg per day. Monitor liver enzymes intermittently if the patient stays on niacinamide.

For patients already using glucosmaine or chondroitin products with positive results, it is prudent to continue these products. For patients not already on these products that have OA one can consider a 10-week trial at the 1500 mg per day dose and continuing at a dose to be determined only if significant efficacy in pain reduction or improvement in function were observed. Glucosamine and chondroitin would be viewed as second- or third-line agents given the 2010 meta-analysis and the GALT study results. Glucosamine sulfate should be used instead of glucosamine hydrochloride. Vegan sources of glucosamine sulfate appear to have less lead contamination. However, vegan sources are usually derived from corn and thus a corn-sensitive patient should use the shell-based forms instead. At approximately 10 weeks, assess the patient's functional abilities and pain level. At this point, the clinician has a number of options on what to do. If there has been no decrease in pain or improvement in function, the clinician could stop the glucosamine sulfate. The clinician can consider adding chondroitin sulfate (unless the patient is a vegetarian) at the 1200 mg dose to see if there is an added benefit in symptoms and function after eight to 12 weeks. It would be reasonable to use the low molecular weight form for better absorption. If there is no significant additive effect after 10 weeks, it is not reasonable to continue chondroitin sulfate unless the patient is already on a CS product and feels it is working well for them.

Avocado/soybean unsaponifiable (ASU) residues would be a reasonable next agent because of research regarding ASU's utility in blocking cytokines as well as blocking metalloproteinases. One could use 300 mg of ASU per day.

Intraarticular hyaluronic acid should be considered for advanced knee and hip OA. This would be added to nutritional support; and, if it is efficacious can be repeated approximately every nine months. It is reasonable to consider it for moderate OA as well as chondromalacia patella. Long-term use of glucosamine, chondroitin, SAMe, and vitamin D appear safe, and patients can be maintained on any combination of these for long periods of time. ASU has not been used long-term, but it should be safe unless there is an allergy to soy.

Nutritional Support for Sprains and Osteoarthritis Prevention

There is a rationale for the use of joint support nutrients after traumatic injury that involves meniscus or articular cartilage including moderate to severe sprains or contusions to a joint. This would include motor vehicle injuries to the facets of the neck, thoracic and lumbar spine, and contusions to the patella, ankle, knee meniscus, and other extremity sprains. No long-term studies document the prevention of osteoarthritis with joint support nutrients after traumatic injury but the rationale of nutritionally supporting the healing and biochemical substrates of cartilage healing are very sound. EPA/DHA with glucosamine sulfate with or without chondroitin sulfate may be started at the time of the diagnosis and continued for a minimum of eight weeks and preferably for 12 weeks after the sprain. There is a definite preventative indication here with low chance of side effects. In addition to traumatic injuries, there appears to be good clinical response to the use of glucosamine sulfate in problems involving the articular cartilage of the patella in both patellofemoral tracking syndrome and chondromalacia. The clinician can recommend starting joint support nutrients six to eight weeks before high use of the knee in sports. If the problem and use of the knee are ongoing, then nutritional support should be continuous.

Limit higher-risk activities such as contact sports and sports with a high risk of falling. Limit running in patients with moderate OA of the knee or hip. Encourage cross training for exercise. Limit work- and household-related activities of squatting, kneeling, and excessive stair climbing.

SUMMARY

A nutritional approach to osteoarthritis is theoretically justified and has been overwhelmingly validated in laboratory and clinical trials. Whereas conventional therapeutics may offer the most effective short-term pain relief in OA, long-term pain relief, improvement in function, and regeneration of the joint is better accomplished with nutritional therapies with fewer side effects. Nutritional support when combined with assessment and optimization of biomechanics, strength, and balance can offer both immediate and long-term improvements in function and in pain relief of OA. It may also offer a slowing or stopping of joint surface loss.

REFERENCES

1. Lawrence, R. C., et al., National Arthritis Data Workgroup. *Estimates of the prevalence of arthritis and other rheumatic conditions in the United States. Part II.* Arthritis Rheum, 2008 Jan; 58(1): 26–35.
2. Felson, D.T. and D. J. Schurman, *Risk factors for osteoarthritis: Understanding joint vulnerability.* Clin Orthop, 2004. (427 Suppl): S16–21.
3. Brandt, K. D., Osteoarthritis, in *Harrison's Principles of Internal Medicine*, A.S. Fauci, et al., eds. New York: McGraw-Hill, 1935–41.
4. Hungin, A. P. and W. F. Kean, *Nonsteroidal anti-inflammatory drugs: Overused or underused in osteoarthritis?* Am J Med, 2001. 110(1A): 8S–11S.
5. Gartner, L. and J. Hiatt, Cartilage and Bone, in *Color Textbook of Histology*. Philadelphia: W.B. Saunders Company, 1997, 112.
6. Lorenzo, P., M. T. Bayliss, and D. Heinegard, *Altered patterns and synthesis of extracellular matrix macromolecules in early osteoarthritis.* Matrix Biol, 2004. 23(6): 381–91.
7. Schwartz, E. R. and L. Adamy, *Effect of ascorbic acid on arylsulfatase activities and sulfated proteoglycan metabolism in chondrocyte cultures.* J Clin Invest, 1977. 60(1): 96–106.
8. Goldring, S. R., M. B. Goldring, and J. Buckwalter, *The role of cytokines in cartilage matrix degeneration in osteoarthritis.* Clin Orthop, 2004. (427 Suppl): S27–36.
9. Dozin, B., et al., *Response of young, aged and osteoarthritic human articular chondrocytes to inflammatory cytokines: Molecular and cellular aspects.* Matrix Biol, 2002. 21(5): 449–59.
10. Henrotin, Y. E., et al., *Effects of three avocado/soybean unsaponifiable mixtures on metalloproteinases, cytokines and prostaglandin E2 production by human articular chondrocytes.* Clin Rheumatol, 1998. 17(1): 31–39.

11. Dean, D. D., J. Martel-Pelletier, J. P. Pelletier, D. S. Howell, J. F. Woessner, Jr. *Evidence for metallo-proteinase and metalloproteinase inhibitor imbalance in human osteoarthritic cartilage.* J Clin Invest, 1989. 84(2): 678–85.

12. Badley, E.M., *The effect of osteoarthritis on disability and health care use in Canada.* J Rheumatol Suppl, 1995. 43: 19–22.

13. Di Cesare, P. and S. Abramson, Pathogenesis of Osteoarthritis, in *Kelly's Textbook of Rheumatology,* E.J. Harris, et al., eds. Elsevier, 2005; 1493–1537.

14. Jadelis, K., et al., *Strength, balance, and the modifying effects of obesity and knee pain: Results from the Observational Arthritis Study in Seniors (oasis).* J Am Geriatr Soc, 2001. 49(7): 884–91.

15. Hart, D. J., and T. D. Spector. *The relationship of obesity, fat distribution and osteoarthritis in women in the general population: The Chingford study.* J Rheumatol, 1993. 20: 331.

16. Spector, T. D., D. J. Hart, and D. V. Doyle, *Incidence and progression of osteoarthritis in women with unilateral knee disease in the general population: The effect of obesity.* Ann Rheum Dis, 1994. 53: 565.

17. Bridges, A. J., E. Smith, and J. Reid, *Joint hypermobility in adults referred to rheumatology clinics.* J SOAnn Rheum Dis, 1992 Jun. 51(6): 793–96.

18. Bjordal, J. M., et al., *Non-steroidal anti-inflammatory drugs, including cyclo-oxygenase-2 inhibitors, in osteoarthritic knee pain: Meta-analysis of randomized placebo controlled trials.* BMJ, 2004. 329(7478): 1317.

19. Hungin, A. P. and W. F. Kean, *Nonsteroidal anti-inflammatory drugs: Overused or underused in osteoarthritis?* Am J Med, 2001. 110(1A): 8S–11S.

20. Brandt, K. D., *Effects of nonsteroidal anti-inflammatory drugs on chondrocyte metabolism in vitro and in vivo.* Am J Med, 1987. 83(5A): 29–34.

21. Brandt, K. D., *Nonsteroidal antiinflammatory drugs and articular cartilage.* J Rheumatol, 1987. 14 Spec No: 132–33.

22. Brandt, K. D. and S. Slowman-Kovacs, *Nonsteroidal antiinflammatory drugs in treatment of osteoarthritis.* Clin Orthop, 1986. (213): 84–91.

23. Rashad, S., et al., *Effect of non-steroidal anti-inflammatory drugs on the course of osteoarthritis.* Lancet, 1989. 2(8662): 519–22.

24. El Hajjaji, H., et al., *Celecoxib has a positive effect on the overall metabolism of hyaluronan and proteoglycans in human osteoarthritic cartilage.* J Rheumatol, 2003. 30(11): 2444–51.

25. Schnitzer, T. J., M. Posner, I. D. J. Lawrence, *High strength capsaicin cream for osteoarthritis pain: Rapid onset of action and improved efficacy with twice daily dosing.* Clin Rheumatol, 1995. 1(5): 268.

26. Soeken, K. L., et al., *Safety and efficacy of S-adenosylmethionine (SAMe) for osteoarthritis.* J Fam Pract, 2002. 51(5): 425–30.

27. Curtis, C. L., et al., *Pathologic indicators of degradation and inflammation in human osteoarthritic cartilage are abrogated by exposure to n-3 fatty acids.* Arthritis Rheum, 2002. 46(6): 1544–53.

28. Wandel, S., P. Jüni, B. Tendal, E. Nüesch, P. M. Villiger, N. J. Welton, S. Reichenbach, and S. Trelle, *Effects of glucosamine, chondroitin, or placebo in patients with osteoarthritis of hip or knee: Network meta-analysis.* BMJ, 2010. 341: c4675.

29. Sawitzke, A. D., et al., *Clinical efficacy and safety of glucosamine, chondroitin sulphate, their combination, celecoxib or placebo taken to treat osteoarthritis of the knee: 2-year results from GAIT.* Ann Rheum Dis, 2010 Aug. 69(8): 1459–64. Epub 2010 Jun 4.

30. Matheson, A. J. and C. M. Perry, *Glucosamine: A review of its use in the management of osteoarthritis.* Drugs Aging, 2003. 20(14): 1041–60.

31. Setnikar, I., et al., *Pharmacokinetics of glucosamine in man.* Arzneimittelforschung, 1993. 43(10): 1109–13.

32. Cohen, M., et al., *A randomized, double blind, placebo controlled trial of a topical cream containing glucosamine sulfate, chondroitin sulfate, and camphor for osteoarthritis of the knee.* J Rheumatol, 2003. 30(3): 523–28.

33. Pavelka, K., et al., *Glucosamine sulfate use and delay of progression of knee osteoarthritis: A 3-year, randomized, placebo-controlled, double-blind study.* Arch Intern Med, 2002. 162: 2113–23.

34. Reginster, J. Y., et al., *Long-term effects of glucosamine sulfate on osteoarthritis progression: A randomized, placebo-controlled trial.* Lancet, 2001. 357: 251–56.

35. Bruyere, O., et al., *Glucosamine sulfate reduces osteoarthritis progression in postmenopausal women with knee osteoarthritis: Evidence from two 3-year studies.* Menopause, 2004. 11(2): 138–43.

36. Christgau, S., et al., *Osteoarthritic patients with high cartilage turnover show increased responsiveness to the cartilage protecting effects of glucosamine sulphate.* Clin Exp Rheumatol, 2004. 22(1): 36–42.

37. Anderson, J. W., R. J. Nicolosi, and J. F. Borzelleca, *Glucosamine effects in humans: A review of effects on glucose metabolism, side effects, safety considerations and efficacy.* Food Chem Toxicol, 2005. 43(2): 187–201.

38. Scroggie, D. A., A. Albright, and M. D. Harris, *The effect of glucosamine-chondroitin supplementation on glycosylated hemoglobin levels in patients with type 2 diabetes mellitus: A placebo-controlled, double-blinded, randomized clinical trial.* Arch Intern Med, 2003. 163(13): 1587–90.

39. Tannis, A. J., J. Barban, and J. A. Conquer, *Effect of glucosamine supplementation on fasting and non-fasting plasma glucose and serum insulin concentrations in healthy individuals.* Osteoarthritis Cartilage, 2004. 12(6): 506–11.

40. Virkamaki, A., et al., *Activation of the hexosamine pathway by glucosamine in vivo induces insulin resistance in multiple insulin sensitive tissues.* Endocrinology, 1997. 138(6): 2501–07.

41. Gray, H. C., P. S. Hutcheson, and R. G. Slavin, *Is glucosamine safe in patients with seafood allergy?* J Allergy Clin Immunol, 2004. 114(2): 459–60.

42. Reichenbach, S., et al., *Meta-analysis: Chondroitin for osteoarthritis of the knee or hip.* Ann Intern Med, 2007. 146: 580–90.

43. Morreale, P., et al., *Comparison of the antiinflammatory efficacy of chondroitin sulfate and diclofenac sodium in patients with knee osteoarthritis.* J Rheumatol, 1996. 23(8): 1385–91.

44. Rovetta, G., et al., *Chondroitin sulfate in erosive osteoarthritis of the hands.* Int J Tissue React, 2002. 24(1): 29–32.

45. Reginster, J. Y., et al., *Naturocetic (glucosamine and chondroitin sulfate) compounds as structure-modifying drugs in the treatment of osteoarthritis.* Curr Opin Rheumatol, 2003. 15(5): 651–55.

46. Kahan A. *STOPP (STudy on Osteoarthritis Progression Prevention): A new two-year trial with chondroitin 4&6 sulfate (CS).* Available at: www.ibsa-ch.com/eular_2006_amsterdam_vignon-2.pdf.

47. Uebelhart, D., et al., *Effects of oral chondroitin sulfate on the progression of knee osteoarthritis: A pilot study.* Osteoarthritis Cartilage, 1998. 6: 39–46.

48. Uebelhart, D., et al., *Intermittent treatment of knee osteoarthritis with oral chondroitin sulfate: A one-year, randomized, double-blind, multicenter study versus placebo.* Osteoarthritis Cartilage, 2004. 12: 269–76.

49. Barthe, L., et al., *In vitro intestinal degradation and absorption of chondroitin sulfate, a glycosaminoglycan drug.* Arzneimittelforschung, 2004. 54(5): 286–92.

50. Conte, A., et al., *Biochemical and pharmacokinetic aspects of oral treatment with chondroitin sulfate.* Arzneimittelforschung, 1995. 45(8): 918–25.

51. Najm, W. I., et al., *S-adenosyl methionine (SAMe) versus celecoxib for the treatment of osteoarthritis symptoms: A double-blind cross-over trial. [ISRCTN36233495].* BMC Musculoskelet Disord, 2004. 5(1): 6.

52. Jacobsen, S., B. Danneskiold-Samsoe, and R. B. Andersen, *Oral S-adenosylmethionine in primary fibromyalgia. Double-blind clinical evaluation.* Scand J Rheumatol, 1991. 20: 294–302.

53. Usha, P. R., and M. U. R. Naidu, *Randomised, double-blind, parallel, placebo-controlled study of oral glucosamine, methylsulfonylmethane and their combinations.* Clin Drug Invest, 2004. 24: 353–63.

54. Kim, L. S., L. J. Axelrod, P. Howard, N. Buratovich, and R. F. Waters. *Efficacy of methylsulfonylmethane (MSM) in osteoarthritis pain of the knee: A pilot clinical trial.* Osteoarthritis Cartilage, 2006. 14: 286–29.4

55. Kelly, M. A., P. R. Kurzweil, and R. W. Moskowitz, *Intra-articular hyaluronans in knee osteoarthritis: Rationale and practical considerations.* Am J Orthop, 2004. 33(2 Suppl): 15–22.

56. Aggarwal, A. and I. P. Sempowski, *Hyaluronic acid injections for knee osteoarthritis. Systematic review of the literature.* Can Fam Physician, 2004. 50: 249–56.

57. Kelly, M. A., et al., *Osteoarthritis and beyond: A consensus on the past, present, and future of hyaluronans in orthopedics.* Orthopedics, 2003. 26(10): 1064–79; quiz 1080–81.

58. Hammesfahr, J. F., A. B. Knopf, and T. Stitik, *Safety of intra-articular hyaluronates for pain associated with osteoarthritis of the knee.* Am J Orthop, 2003. 32(6): 277–83.

59. Curtis, C. L., et al., *Pathologic indicators of degradation and inflammation in human osteoarthritic cartilage are abrogated by exposure to n-3 fatty acids.* Arthritis Rheum, 2002. 46(6): 1544–53.

60. Kremer, J. M., *Effects of modulation of inflammatory and immune parameters in patients with rheumatic and inflammatory disease receiving dietary supplementation of n-3 and n-6 fatty acids.* Lipids, 1996. 31 Suppl: S243–47.

61. Ariza-Ariza, R., M. Mestanza-Peralta, and M. H. Cardiel, *Omega-3 fatty acids in rheumatoid arthritis: An overview.* Semin Arthritis Rheum, 1998. 27(6): 366–70.

62. Cho, S. H., et al., *Clinical efficacy and safety of Lyprinol, a patented extract from New Zealand green-lipped mussel (Perna Canaliculus) in patients with osteoarthritis of the hip and knee: A multicenter 2-month clinical trial.* Allerg Immunol (Paris), 2003. 35(6): 212–16.
63. Hesslink, R. Jr., D. Armstrong, III, M. V. Nagendran, S. Sreevatsan, and R. Barathur. *Cetylated fatty acids improve knee function in patients with osteoarthritis,* JRheumatol, 2002 Aug. 29(8): 1708–12
64. Kraemer, W. J., et al., *Effect of a cetylated fatty acid topical cream on functional mobility and quality of life of patients with osteoarthritis.* J Rheumatol, 2004 Apr. 31(4): 767–74.
65. Kraemer, W. J., et al., *A cetylated fatty acid topical cream with menthol reduces pain and improves functional performance in individuals with arthritis.* J Strength Cond Res, 2005 May. 19(2): 475–80.
66. Peterkofsky, B., *Ascorbate requirement for hydroxylation and secretion of procollagen: Relationship to inhibition of collagen synthesis in scurvy.* Am J Clin Nutr, 1991. 54(6 Suppl): 1135S–40S.
67. Spanheimer, R. G., T. A. Bird, and B. Peterkofsky, *Regulation of collagen synthesis and mRNA levels in articular cartilage of scorbutic guinea pigs.* Arch Biochem Biophys, 1986. 246(1): 33–41.
68. McAlindon, T. E., et al., *Do antioxidant micronutrients protect against the development and progression of knee osteoarthritis?* Arthritis Rheum, 1996. 39(4): 648–56.
69. Hauselmann, H. J., *Nutripharmaceuticals for osteoarthritis.* Best Pract Res Clin Rheumatol, 2001. 15(4): 595–607.
70. Lequesne, M., et al., *Structural effect of avocado/soybean unsaponifiables on joint space loss in osteoarthritis of the hip.* Arthritis Rheum, 2002. 47(1): 50–58.
71. Boumediene, K., et al., *Avocado/soya unsaponifiables enhance the expression of transforming growth factor beta1 and beta2 in cultured articular chondrocytes.* Arthritis Rheum, 1999. 42(1): 148–56.
72. Ernst, E., *Avocado-soybean unsaponifiables (ASU) for osteoarthritis—a systematic review.* Clin Rheumatol, 2003. 22(4–5): 285–88.
73. Henrotin. Y. E., et al., *Avocado/soybean unsaponifiables increase aggrecan synthesis and reduce catabolic and proinflammatory mediator production by human osteoarthritic chondrocytes.* J Rheumatol, 2003. 30: 1825–34.
74. Kaufman, W., *The use of vitamin therapy to reverse certain concomitants of aging.* J Am Geriatr Soc, 1955. 3: 927.
75. Kaufman, W., *Niacinamide: A most neglected vitamin.* J Int Acad Prev Med, 1983. (Winter): 5–25.
76. Jonas, W. B., C. P. Rapoza, and W. F. Blair, *The effect of niacinamide on osteoarthritis: A pilot study.* Inflamm Res, 1996. 45(7): 330–34.
77. McCarty, M. F. and A. L. Russell, *Niacinamide therapy for osteoarthritis—does it inhibit nitric oxide synthase induction by interleukin 1 in chondrocytes?* Med Hypotheses, 1999. 53(4): 350–60.
78. Lampeter, E. F., A. Klinghammer, and W. A. Scherbaum, *The Deutsche Nicotinamide Intervention Study: An attempt to prevent type 1 diabetes.* Diabetes, 1998. 47: 980–84.
79. Knip, M., et al., *Safety of high-dose nicotinamide: A review.* Diabetologia, 2000. 43(11): 1337–45.
80. Henrotin, Y., et al., *Strontium ranelate increases cartilage matrix formation.* J Bone Miner Res, 2001. 16: 299–308.
81. Alexanderson, P., M. Karsdal, P. Qvist, J. Y. Reginster, and C. Christiansen, *Strontium ranelate reduces the urinary level of cartilage degradation biomarker CTX-II in postmenopausal women.* Bone, 2007. 40: 218–22.
82. Bruyere, O., et al., *Effects of strontium ranelate on spinal osteoarthritis progression.* Annals of the Rheumatic Diseases, 2008. 67: 335–39.
83. Tetlow, L. C., and D. E. Woolley. *Expression of vitamin D receptors and matrix metalloproteinases in osteoarthritic cartilage and human articular chondrocytes in vitro.* Osteoarthritis Cartilage, 2001. 9: 423–31.
84. McAlindon, T. E., D. T. Felson, Y. Zhang, M. T. Hannan, P. Aliabadi, B. Weissman, D. Rush, P. W. Wilson, and P. Jacques, *Relation of dietary intake and serum levels of vitamin D to progression of osteoarthritis of the knee among participants in the Framingham Study.* Ann Intern Med, 1996. 125: 353–59.
85. Flicker, L., et al., *Serum vitamin D and falls in older women in residential care in Australia.* J Am Geriatr Soc, 2003. 51: 1533–38.
86. Jordan, J. M., et al., *Low selenium levels are associated with increased risk for osteoarthritis of the knee.* American College of Rheumatology Annual Meeting. San Diego November 12–17, 2005. Abstract 1189.
87. Brien, S., G. T. Lewith, and G. McGregor. *Devil's claw (Harpagophytum procumbens) as a treatment for osteoarthritis: A review of efficacy and safety.* J Altern Complement Med, 2006 Dec. 12(10): 981–93.
88. Wegener, T., and N. P. Lüpke, *Treatment of patients with arthrosis of hip or knee with an aqueous extract of devil's claw.* Phytother Res, 2003 Dec. 17(10): 1165–72.
89. Ostojic, S. M., M. Arsic, S. Prodanovic, J. Vukovic, and M. Zlatanovic, *Glucosamine administration in athletes: Effects on recovery of acute knee injury.* Res Sports Med, 2007. 15(2): 113–24.

90. Herrero-Beaumont, G., et al., *Glucosamine sulfate in the treatment of knee osteoarthritis symptoms: A randomized, double-blind, placebo-controlled study using acetaminophen as a side comparator.* Arthritis Rheum, 2007. 56(2): 555–67.

91. Ahmed, S., et al., *Green tea polyphenol epigallocatechin-3-gallate (EGCG) differentially inhibits interleukin-1 beta-induced expression of matrix metalloproteinase-1 and -13 in human chondrocytes.* J Pharmacol Exp Ther, 2004 Feb. 308(2): 767–73.

92. Singh, R., et al., *Epigallocatechin-3-gallate selectively inhibits interleukin-1beta-induced activation of mitogen activated protein kinase subgroup c-Jun N-terminal kinase in human osteoarthritis chondrocytes.* J Orthop Res, 2003 Jan. 21(1): 102–9.

93. Ahmed, S., et al., *Green tea polyphenol epigallocatechin-3-gallate inhibits the IL-1 beta-induced activity and expression of cyclooxygenase-2 and nitric oxide synthase-2 in human chondrocytes.* Free Radic Biol Med, 2002 Oct. 15. 33(8): 1097–1105.

94. Adcocks, C., et al., *Catechins from green tea (Camellia sinensis) inhibit bovine and human cartilage proteoglycan and type II collagen degradation in vitro.* J Nutr, 2002 Mar. 132(3): 341–46.

95. Lukaczer, D. O., R. H. Lerman, G. K. Darland, D. J. Liska, B. C. Schiltz, M. L. Tripp, and J. S. Bland, *Benefits of a proprietary reduced iso-alpha acids (hops), rosemary extract, and oleanolic acid supplement on pain in subjects with osteoarthritis.* FASEB Journal, 2004. 18: 4–5.

Section VIII

Neoplasms

37 Cancer and Insulin

Targeting the Insulin-IGF System for Risk Reduction and Survival

D. Barry Boyd, M.D., M.S.

INTRODUCTION

For many years, researchers have sought to explain the rising incidence of malignancies in Western countries, including breast, colorectal, prostate, and other epithelial cancers. In a seminal article in 1981, Doll and Peto [1] evaluated the causes of cancer in the United States. The two leading causes were tobacco use and diet and lifestyle. They speculated that diet played a role in between one-third and two-thirds of all cancers. Early epidemiologic studies, based largely on international ecologic and case-control studies, suggested associations between cancer risk and per capita dietary fat, fiber, other dietary components, and micronutrients, as well as dietary fruit and vegetable intake [2–7]. Over the last decade, many of these factors have been shown to be only weakly associated with cancer risk based on longer term prospective cohort studies as well as randomized control trials [8–11].

There is a growing recognition that cancer, cardiovascular disease, and diabetes mellitus (DM) share overlapping metabolic features linked to the metabolic syndrome and insulin resistance. The importance of obesity, a feature of lifelong abnormal energy balance, as both a risk and prognostic factor for many cancers, is becoming more widely accepted [12].

There is increased awareness of the role of positive energy balance throughout the life course, from prenatal periods through adulthood, in both the origins as well as outcome of many cancers. The growing worldwide epidemic of obesity and diabetes has raised concerns about future cancer risks in these populations. The metabolic syndrome, characterized by dyslipidemia, hypertension, and insulin resistance associated with abdominal and visceral obesity, is reaching epidemic proportions at younger ages, in both western countries and the developing world [13]. There is growing recognition of the connection between the insulin resistant state associated with hyperglycemia and hyperinsulinemia as a risk factor for many cancers [14], as an important predictor of adverse prognosis in cancer [15], and, importantly, as a consequence of cancer treatment in the growing cancer survivor population [16]. A recent consensus statement of the American Diabetic Association and the American Cancer Society has called attention to this important association and raised important questions for future research [17].

This chapter presents the epidemiologic data and pathophysiologic mechanisms linking obesity and the insulin-insulin growth factor (IGF) system to cancer. Building on this scientific foundation, the chapter provides interventions to both reduce cancer risk and improve long-term outcomes in cancer survivors. Improving insulin sensitivity among cancer survivors is a major research focus that holds the potential for breakthrough therapies in the near future [18], including food and nutrient interventions.

EPIDEMIOLOGY

PRENATAL AND CHILDHOOD ORIGINS OF ADULT DISEASE AND CANCER RISK: THE ROLE OF ENERGY BALANCE IN EARLY LIFE

There is growing awareness that both the pre- and early postnatal environment influence risk of later adult disease [19]. A prominent feature of modern populations as well as developing populations in the nutrition transition is increasing per-capita height [20]. While overall population height is associated with increasing adult health and reduced overall and cardiovascular mortality, studies indicate an increase in risk as well as mortality for multiple cancers, including colon, breast, prostate, pancreas, liver, and lung. This relationship has been noted in Asian [21] as well as Caucasian populations [22]. Leg length, a marker of prepubertal growth, is the measure most highly correlated with adult cancer risk and is a marker of both prenatal and early childhood nutritional influences [23, 24]. The Boyd Orr Cohort Study [25,26], a survey of 1352 families from pre-WW II Britain followed into adulthood has documented the important role of early childhood growth and nutrition on adult health, confirming the relationship between early nutrition, childhood leg length, and adult cancer risk. The dietary component most closely linked to height is dairy—in particular dairy protein [27]. In addition, increased childhood energy intake has been associated with increased adult cancer risk [28]. These effects are felt to be partly mediated by nutritional influences on increasing levels of insulin-like growth factors, both prenatally and during early childhood [29, 30]. Recent research [31–33] has noted the association between higher cord blood IGF-1 levels and a higher number of circulating stem cells, suggesting that an important mediator of this early nutrition/ adult cancer relationship may be its effect on increasing tissue stem cell numbers. Increased adult height may simply be a surrogate for this effect and the heightened tissue vulnerability to the genotoxic, initiating events occurring later in life. In addition to height, increased birth weight is associated with adolescent and adult obesity as well as a higher risk of multiple adult cancers [34–35]. Birth weight has also been linked to higher risk of childhood cancers, including acute lymphocytic leukemia [36].

ADULT ENERGY BALANCE, INSULIN, AND CANCER RISK

Increasing body mass index (BMI), overweight, and obesity are increasingly linked to adult cancer risk. In an important review of multiple cohort studies, increasing adult BMI was linked to risk of colorectal, postmenopausal breast, kidney, pancreatic, liver, esophageal, gallbladder, endometrial, and ovarian cancer, multiple myeloma, non-Hodgkins lymphoma, and leukemia. In contrast, premenopausal breast cancer, prostate cancer, and several smoking-related cancers are inversely related to BMI [37]. Despite the inverse relationship with body weight, abdominal obesity is strongly associated with premenopausal breast cancer [38], aggressive prostate cancer [39], and non–small cell lung cancer in nonsmoking women [40,41].

The metabolic syndrome (MS), as well as individual components of the MS, including hypertriglyceridemia, low HDL cholesterol, and diastolic hypertension, has been associated with higher cancer risk. Hyperglycemia and hyperinsulinemia as well as c-peptide are associated with higher risk in multiple cancers, including breast, colon, prostate, liver, endometrial, and pancreas, independent of diabetes [42] and BMI [22,43,44]. Higher circulating IGF-1 levels have been linked with multiple adult cancers including breast, colorectal, prostate, and lung [45]. Increasing levels of physical activity [46], including both occupational and recreational forms of activity, have been associated with lower cancer risks, reinforcing the importance of activity in the energy balance equation.

Type 2 diabetes mellitus has been associated with an increased risk of numerous cancers, including colon, liver, pancreas, kidney, breast, and endometrium [47]. In a large cohort study from Korea, increasing glucose levels were associated with higher cancer risks at multiple sites, including pancreas, liver, colorectal, gall bladder, and esophagus. This relationship has been confirmed by additional large population studies [48,49]. In both the Korean [42] and the European Me-Can studies [50], there was a graded increase in risk with increasing fasting glucose levels above the normal range, independent of weight. There was a similar increase in mortality from cancer with increasing glucose levels.

The antidiabetic drug, metformin, a biguanide derived from the French lilac, limits hepatic gluconeogenesis and results in lower circulating insulin levels [51]. Multiple observation studies have documented a reduction in cancer risk in diabetics on metformin in contrast to those on sulfonylurea agents or insulin [52,53].

Adult Energy Balance and Outcomes in Cancer

Adult obesity, in the prospective ACS cohort study of over 900,000 adults (CPSI,II) was associated with increased mortality from a variety of cancers including breast, prostate, colorectal, kidney, pancreas, liver, esophageal, gallbladder, endometrial, cervical, ovarian, myeloma, NHL, and leukemia [54]. Despite lower risk for premenopausal breast and prostate cancer with increasing weight, mortality is increased with higher BMI for both pre- and postmenopausal breast cancer as well as prostate cancer [55,56]. There is evidence that abdominal obesity and concurrent insulin resistance is associated with more advanced-stages at diagnosis in both pre- and postmenopausal breast cancer and associated with advanced stage prostate cancer [57,58]. Weight gain, both preceding as well as subsequent to breast cancer diagnosis, is associated with adverse prognosis [59,60], while prediagnosis weight is associated with colorectal cancer mortality [61].

Type 2 DM appears to be associated with increased all-cause mortality in multiple cancers and cancer-specific mortality from some cancers. In a systematic review and meta-analysis, diabetes was associated with an increased mortality risk (HR = 1.41) compared to normoglycemic individuals for all cancer types [62]. In a review of the Swedish Cancer Registry [63], cancer-specific mortality was higher (HR = 1.38) in diabetic cancer patients compared to those without diabetes. In a companion study [64], Liu et al. noted that type 2 DM in cancer patients was associated with a higher risk of death from multiple causes, including myocardial infarction, hypertensive disease, bacterial infection, and urinary tract disorders.

Extensive research has documented multiple links between type 2 DM, hyperglycemia, hyperinsulinemia, and breast cancer. In the Women's Health, Eating and Living (HEAL) study [65] of early-stage breast cancer—those women with chronic hyperglycemia (HbA1C > 7.0%)—had a 2.4-fold increase in risk of all-cause mortality as well as a 26% increase in new breast cancer events. In a follow-up evaluation of the HEAL study, Irwin et al. [66] assessed the prognostic effect of measures of glucose intolerance and breast cancer mortality. In this population, a 1 ng/ml increase in serum c-peptide was associated with a 31% increase in overall mortality and a 35% increase in breast cancer mortality. This study reinforces the findings of Goodwin et al. [67] that serum insulin at diagnosis is a predictor of both breast cancer recurrence and mortality in early-stage breast cancer. In this pivotal study, those women in the upper quartile of insulin had more than twice the risk of distant recurrence (HR = 2.1) and three times the mortality (HR = 3.3) of women in the lowest quartile of insulin.

Multiple studies have documented the higher risk of recurrence with increasing weight after prostatectomy in prostate cancer [68]. Hyperinsulinemia has been associated with both more aggressive prostate cancers as well as adverse outcomes [69]. In contrast, diabetes is less consistently associated with adverse outcomes [70].

The critical role of obesity and insulin resistance in both the risk and survival from colorectal cancer is increasingly recognized [71]. Obesity and, in particular, abdominal obesity, including waist size and waist hip ratio are associated with higher colon cancer risk [72,73]. Both high c-peptide and hyperinsulinemia as well as diabetes mellitus have been closely associated with higher risk [74–77] as have various dietary features (low glycemic load, low-fat dairy and calcium, and high-dietary fiber and whole grains) commonly linked to increased insulin sensitivity and reduced risk of metabolic syndrome [78–81]. Similarly, studies indicate a higher risk of colon polyps in individuals with obesity and the metabolic syndrome [82,83]. Importantly, obesity, insulin resistance, and diabetes are associated with a higher colon cancer recurrence risk, cancer-specific, and overall mortality [84–86]. The prudent diet, characterized by limited red meat, high complex carbohydrate, and low concentrated carbohydrates and sweets, low-fat dairy, and high vegetable and fruits is associated, in contrast to the typical Western diet, with a lower all-cause and colorectal-specific mortality [87]. Interestingly, abdominal and visceral obesity is a marker of poor outcome in metastatic colorectal cancer patients on first-line treatment with both systemic chemotherapy [88] and the angiogenesis inhibitor, bevacizumab [89].

There is growing recognition of the role of increased physical activity with cancer prognosis. Early observational studies in the Nurses' Health Study [90] noted a reduction in breast cancer recurrence and mortality with increasing levels of activity, over 9 met/hrs weekly (the equivalent of three hours of vigorous walking). This association has been confirmed in multiple cohorts, and is associated with lower c-peptide and insulin levels, independent of body weight. Similar associations between physical activity and increased colorectal cancer survival have been noted in several cohorts, including an improved prognosis when assessing activity after diagnosis [91–93]. The level of activity linked to improved prognosis in colorectal cancer has been higher, at 18 met/hrs (the equivalent of six hours of vigorous walking per week). The risk of prostate cancer progression after diagnosis as well as overall and prostate cancer mortality may also be reduced with vigorous physical activity [94]. In the case of prostate cancer progression, the intensity rather than duration of activity appeared important. In a follow-up study of 1455 men with clinically localized prostate cancer, men who walked briskly for three or more hours per week had a 57% lower rate of progression than men who walked at an easy pace. This was independent of duration of walking alone.

There have been very few randomized control trials completed to date assessing the effect of targeting weight, metabolic syndrome, and cancer risk and outcome. Multiple nonrandomized cohorts have documented the significant reduction in long-term cancer risk as well as cardiovascular risk with bariatric surgery for morbid obesity [95,96]. This is associated with multiple metabolic changes but is consistently associated with a reversal of diabetes mellitus and hyperinsulinemia. A recent study [97] has noted a reduction in IGF-1 levels post–bariatric surgery.

The two large dietary adjuvant trials in early stage breast cancer, the WIN Study [98]—focusing on a reduction in total dietary fat, and the WHEL Study [99]—targeting an increase in dietary fruit and vegetable intake, led to apparent contradictory results. The WIN Study was associated, in the estrogen receptor (ER) negative subgroup, with a substantial reduction in breast cancer recurrence and mortality while the WHEL study noted no difference in the recurrence risk. A noteworthy difference between these two studies was a small though significant weight loss in the WIN cohort compared to a slight weight gain in the experimental arm of the WHEL study. The level of weight loss was equivalent to the reduction in weight seen in the Diabetes Prevention Program [100] associated with both lower diabetic risk and reduced insulin levels.

In addition to the observation that metformin is associated with a reduction in cancer risk in diabetic populations, there is evidence for lower cancer and overall mortality in diabetic patients on metformin [101]. In a cohort of patients with early-stage breast cancer on neoadjuvant chemotherapy from the MD Anderson Cancer Center, those women with diabetes who were on metformin had a significantly higher partial and complete response rate than diabetic women not on metformin, though not on overall survival [102]. Follow-up studies from the same group noted improved breast cancer specific survival in diabetic breast cancer patients with Her-2 positive disease on metformin or thiazolidinediones [103] compared to other diabetic medications and reduced distant recurrence in triple negative breast cancer [104]. Recent evidence suggests improved cancer specific survival in non–small cell lung cancer in diabetic patients on metformin [105].

There are more than 50 ongoing trials in progress or in planning targeting weight as well as metabolic mediators such as insulin and IGF through lifestyle, pharmacologic, and molecularly targeted interventions on cancer survival in multiple cancers. The Transdisciplinary Research on Energetic and Cancer (TREC) initiative, a multicenter collaboration established by the NCI in 2005 is tasked with fostering collaboration across multiple disciplines; it encompasses projects that cover the biology, genomics, and genetics of energy balance to behavioral, socio-cultural, and environmental influences upon nutrition, physical activity, weight, energetics, and cancer risk.

OBESITY, INSULIN RESISTANCE, AND THE METABOLIC SYNDROME IN CANCER SURVIVORS

While attention is increasingly focused on the role of obesity and insulin resistance on cancer prognosis, there has been growing awareness of the effects of cancer treatment on the risk of developing the metabolic syndrome and the long-term impact on cardiovascular as well as cancer-related morbidity and mortality in the cancer survivor population. The majority of early-stage breast, colon, and prostate cancer patients as well as more than 80% of childhood cancer patients will survive their disease without recurrence but may suffer from the consequences of their treatment.

Talvensaari et al. [106] have documented the increased incidence of the metabolic syndrome on adult survivors of childhood cancer, including hematologic cancers, central nervous system tumors, and testicular cancer. Breast cancer patients on systemic adjuvant chemotherapy as well as endocrine therapy have a higher incidence of weight gain [107] and higher recurrence risk and mortality [108]. Androgen deprivation therapy in advanced prostate cancer is associated with weight gain and a high risk of the metabolic syndrome and obesity, with a significantly higher risk of cardiovascular disease [109]. Concerns have also been raised about an adverse risk of resistant prostate cancer secondary to hyperinsulinemia that accompanies androgen deprivation therapy.

Systemic chemotherapy in early-stage disease may enhance the risk of both hyperglycemia and hyperinsulinemia, in part as a consequence of the frequent use of high-dose steroids, contributing to the long-term risk of the metabolic syndrome. In a study of early stage, nondiabetic breast cancer patients treated with adjuvant chemotherapy with FEC (fluorouracil, epirubicin, cyclophosphamide), followed by docetaxel accompanied by high-dose dexamethasone premedication reported by Hickish et al. [110], women developed increasing hyperglycemia consistent with insulin resistance as treatment cycles progressed. Similarly, in a study of 91 locally advanced head and neck cancer patients treated with combined modality therapy with radiation and concurrent fluorouracil and cisplatin chemotherapy, nondiabetic patients developed significant hyperglycemia with progressive treatment [111]. Recent studies [112] raise concern that this higher glucose may reduce the efficacy of chemotherapy either directly or indirectly through higher insulin/IGF-1 levels.

Even in the absence of increased body weight, many advanced cancer patients develop progressive sarcopenia (reduced lean body mass) coupled with higher abdominal and visceral obesity, so-called "metabolically obese, normal weight" [113]. This is a less commonly appreciated phenotype in adults with metabolic syndrome without cancer but appears more prevalent in the advanced cancer population as a consequence of therapy, alterations in diet and activity, as well as the advanced cancer itself. Despite an apparent normal or even low BMI, these patients possess many features of the metabolic syndrome with hyperinsulinemia and have higher morbidity and adverse outcomes [114,115]. Because they may not be overweight, this metabolic abnormality may not be recognized and their management differs from patients with weight-related metabolic syndrome.

PATHOPHYSIOLOGY

The mechanisms underlying the obesity-cancer relationship remain poorly understood. The growth and progression of tumors is highly dependent on the host microenvironment, balancing factors that inhibit cell proliferation and induce apoptosis with those that enhance cell growth, angiogenesis, and cancer cell survival. Tumors are influenced by local autocrine and paracrine factors but also respond to systemic factors, such as hormones, inflammatory cytokines, and growth factors. The last decade has seen a confluence of research from studies on obesity, caloric restriction, longevity, and cancer; the mechanisms of insulin-related growth signaling as well as the growing understanding of cancer cell energetics and metabolism, providing a more holistic understanding of the role of insulin and IGF in cancer development and progression [116]. The critical role of the metabolic syndrome, associated with dyslipidemia, hypertension, and impaired insulin tolerance with elevated glucose and insulin, is the central feature underlying many of these associations.

ADIPOSITY AND CANCER

The central feature of adult obesity is increasing adiposity, in particular, dysfunctional adipose (Figure 37.1), associated with both visceral and ectopic fat deposition [117]. Excess adipose tissue is associated with abnormalities in adipokine levels and activity, increased oxidative stress, and local and systemic inflammation. It is associated with increasing levels of insulin as well as estrogen and other hormones. Increased adipose stores are associated with an alteration in adipokine levels, including leptin, adiponectin, and resistin. Increasing adiposity is associated with high leptin levels and a state of relative leptin resistance. In contrast, adiponectin is inversely related to adiposity and insulin resistance [118]. Excess adipose tissue is also associated with inflammation, with increasing local and systemic inflammatory cytokines (such as IL-1, IL-6, and TNF-a), accompanying an increasing infiltration into adipose stores of proinflammatory M-1 macrophages [119]. This inflammatory state, coupled with high circulating levels of free fatty acids, increased oxidative stress, and lower adiponectin levels contributes to the insulin-resistant state characteristic of the metabolic syndrome. Adipose tissue shows a nearly linear relationship to circulating insulin levels and is the second leading source of IGF-1 after the liver. In addition, adipose-related aromatase (Figure 37.2) is a major source of estrogen in the postmenopausal setting. Increasing insulin levels will contribute to increasing estrogen through enhanced aromatase activity as well as a reduction in plasma levels of sex-hormone–binding globulin, leading to an increase in free sex-hormone levels [116].

The relative role of each of these factors in cancer remains uncertain. Animal models have helped to uncouple the separate effects of the adipose stores and the accompanying insulin resistant state. In the A-ZIP/F-1 mouse model [120], animals lack adipose tissue with negligible circulating adipokines but have both insulin resistance and an associated inflammatory state. In two

1. Proinflammatory state (Preadipocyte, macrophage)
   ↑TNF-α, ↑IL-6, ↑VEGF, ↑MCP-1

2. Abnormal adipokine expression
   ↑Leptin, ↓Adiponectin, ↑Resistin

3. Insulin resistance (↑FFA, ↓Adiponectin, ↑TNF-α)
   ↑Insulin, ↑Glucose

4. Oxidative stress (↑ROS, ↑HIF-1α)

(TNF-α = tumor necrosis factor-α; IL-6 = Interleukin-6; VEGF = vascular endothelial growth factor; MCP-1 = Monocyte attractant protein; FFA = free fatty acids; ROS = reactive oxygen species; HIF-1α = hypoxia inducible factor-1 α)

FIGURE 37.1 Dysfunctional adipose tissue.

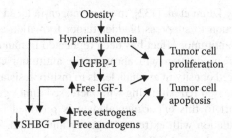

FIGURE 37.2 Insulin-endocrine interactions and cancer.

cancer models, a two-stage skin cancer carcinogenesis protocol and a transgenic mammary tumor model, the A-ZIP/F-1 mice demonstrated increased tumor incidence, greater tumor multiplicity, and shorter tumor latency than wild type mice, despite the absence of adipokines. Nonetheless, a direct effect of adipocytes has been suggested by other studies. In an acute lymphocytic leukemia murine model [121], diet-induced obesity was associated with a higher risk of leukemic progression. Direct in vitro coculture of adipocytes with leukemic cells resulted in impaired effectiveness of chemotherapy, independent of direct cell-cell contact, supporting an adipocyte paracrine factor in chemotherapy resistance.

CALORIC RESTRICTION, AGING, AND CANCER

Caloric restriction has long been recognized as a means of increasing lifespan across a spectrum of organisms, from yeast, nematodes, and drosophila to rodents and nonhuman primates [122,123]. A similar lifespan extension has been demonstrated by mutations affecting elements of the insulin/ IGF signaling cascade or its downstream regulators [124]. Caloric restriction leads to a reduction in insulin and IGF signaling, resulting in decreased PI3K/Akt activation [125]. Activation of PI3K through its second lipid messenger, phosphatidyl-inositol-3,4,5 triphosphate, recruits and anchors Akt to the cell membrane for further phosphorylation and activation. Akt, a cyclic AMP, cyclic GMP-dependent protein kinase C, when activated, stimulates cell-cycle progression, cell prolif- eration, and resistance to apoptosis through mTOR activation; mTOR is a highly conserved serine/ threonine protein kinase that, through phosphorylation of its downstream mediators, S6K, and eukaryotic translation initiation factor 4E-binding protein exerts translational control over new protein synthesis [126]. Inhibition of PI3k/Akt leads to suppression of mTOR, resulting in reduc- tion in cell growth, proliferation, and increased apoptosis. In addition, in the presence of reduced energy availability, with low glucose, decreased amino acids, and a high ADP:ATP ratio, the AMP- activated protein kinase (AMPK) pathway is activated, resulting in mTOR inhibition. AMP-kinase is an evolutionarily conserved energy-sensing enzyme activated in the presence of low cellular energy (high AMP-ADP/ATP ratio) that, when activated, stimulates fatty acid oxidation, increased insulin sensitivity, and reduced cell proliferation [127]. AMP-kinase has an important mediator of the effects of calorie restriction and is activated by the tumor suppressor gene, LKB1 [128]. These adaptations to caloric deprivation represent a highly conserved adaptive mechanism providing sur- vival benefit in the face of environmental stress and nutrient inadequacy [129].

The role of caloric balance and the importance of the insulin-IGF system in cancer is exemplified by the value of calorie restriction as an anticarcinogenesis strategy. Research, beginning in the early twentieth century with the work of Rous [130], followed by the seminal research of Tannenbaum [131], demonstrated the inhibitory effect of calorie restriction, without malnutrition and independent of macronutrient composition, on both spontaneous and induced epithelial cancers in animal mod- els. More recent research has confirmed the consistent effect of varying levels of calorie restriction in multiple animal models including mice, rats, as well as nonhuman primates, on lower cancer risk [124]. IGF-1 appears to mediate many of the effects of calorie restriction on cancer cell growth and proliferation. A study by Dunn et al. [132], in a carcinogen-induced tumor model, documented the ability of calorie restriction to suppress bladder tumor formation and the ability of IGF-1 to reverse this effect. The CR antitumor effect has been replicated in multiple animal models, where constitutively increased IGF production will abrogate the antitumor effect of calorie restriction [124]. Conversely, diet-induced obesity in animals leads to insulin resistance, increased insulin, and higher IGF-1 levels and increased IGF signaling with increased tumor growth [133,134].

A noteworthy counterpart to this experimental data is provided by the observations in the Centenarian Project, a population with extreme longevity and health. They are characterized by short stature, frequent longevity beyond 100 years, and a marked reduction in cancer incidence. One genetic characteristic of this population is a functionally significant mutation in the IGF-1 receptor and reduced IGF signaling, supporting the critical role of IGF signaling in cancer [135].

Mechanisms of Insulin/Insulin Growth Factor Signaling

The IGF system includes three ligands—IGF-1, IGF-2, and insulin—their surface receptors (IGF-1R, IGF-2R, the insulin receptor [IR], the hybrid IR/IGFR), six high-affinity binding proteins (IGFBP1-6), and their respective proteases (Figure 37.3). The insulin receptor (IR) and the IGF-1 receptor (IGF-1R) have both evolved from a common ancestral gene in invertebrates, combining both their metabolic and growth functions [124]. With vertebrate evolution, these functions diverged with the insulin receptor acquiring a largely metabolic function while IGF-1R signaling became the principal cell growth and proliferation effector pathway. It has long been recognized that insulin, acting primarily through activation of the insulin receptor (IR-B) in specific target tissues (liver, muscle, adipose), mediates its predominant metabolic effects, including maintaining glucose homeostasis, and lipid and protein synthesis. In contrast, IGF-1 is the most important paracrine and endocrine regulator of cell growth [136], with potent mitogenic effects in both normal and neoplastic cells. IGF-1 is synthesized predominantly in the liver, under the control of growth hormone, with a smaller contribution from adipose stores. There is emerging evidence that IGF-1 may also be synthesized locally in epithelial tissues in the stromal cell compartment [137]. The

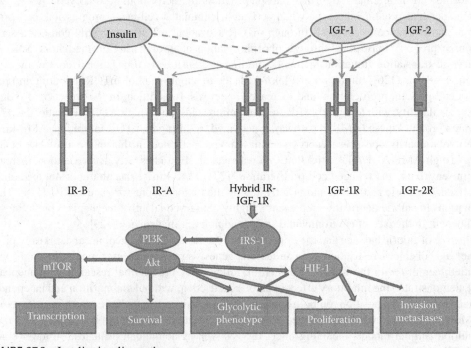

FIGURE 37.3   Insulin signaling pathways.

availability of IGF-1 for signaling is influenced by the level of its binding proteins with only free IGF-1 capable of binding and activating the IGF-1 receptor. Insulin may indirectly influence tumor cell proliferation through an insulin-mediated reduction in hepatic IGFBP-1, leading to higher free IGF levels [136].

Recent research [138] supports a more direct effect of insulin on cell proliferation in neoplastic cells. It has long been recognized that most tumor cell cultures require the addition of insulin to the medium, while many normal epithelial cells can survive, with adequate nutrients and other growth factors, in the absence of insulin. Withdrawal of insulin will result in loss of cell viability of these tumor cells. Alternative signaling receptors may mediate this mitogenic effect. In addition to the traditional IR-B receptor, insulin as well as IGF-1 can bind and activate hybrid receptors between IGF-1 and insulin receptor (IGF-1R/IR) [139]. Both obesity and diabetes are associated with an upregulation in the level of these hybrid receptors on muscle and adipocytes. They have also been identified on malignant cells [140]. In addition, the more recently described insulin receptor-A (IR-A), an alternate splice variant of the IR-B, is present in both embryonic cells [141] as well as in malignant cells and may play an important role in the mitogenic effect of IGF-2 and insulin in tumor progression. Thus, not only does increased exposure to higher levels of insulin and IGF influence cell growth and proliferation but the overexpression of these receptors may change target tissue responsiveness. The systemic effects of obesity and the insulin resistant state appear to influence both the levels of these growth factors and the receptor status of normal as well as neoplastic cells.

The downstream targets of IGF-1 and insulin signaling act predominantly through the induction of the PI3K/Akt pathway [136] with an increase in cell growth, proliferation, and decreased apoptosis.

Insulin, Insulin Growth Factor, and Tumor Cell Metabolism

For many years, the focus of cancer research has been on the effect of somatic mutations in oncogenes and tumor suppressor genes on cell growth and proliferation, diverting attention from the important role of cellular metabolism and cancer. Studies on oncogene activation through increased growth factor synthesis, increased expression of growth factor receptors, and constitutive activation of downstream signal transduction pathways and nuclear transcription regulators as well as loss of tumor suppressor gene function resulting in enhanced cell proliferation and reduced apoptosis has dominated the research in cancer cell biology. The last decade has seen a reawakening of interest in cancer cell metabolism and energetics and its regulation [142,143], with a renewed focus on the Warburg effect. There is growing evidence that growth factor activation of the PI3K/Akt pathway not only promotes cell growth and proliferation but coordinately upregulates the nutrient pathways associated with aerobic glycolysis, a central feature of the Warburg effect [144]. The critical role of insulin and IGF-1 signaling in this adaptive response is now emerging.

The original understanding of the Warburg effect, the shift to a more energy-inefficient aerobic glycolysis with increased lactate generation, from oxidative phosphorylation in normal, differentiated cells, was attributed by Warburg to a defect in mitochondrial function [144]. More recently [143], this has been recognized as an adaptive shift in proliferating cells, both normal and malignant, toward an anabolic state allowing for increased cellular biomass, with increased lipid, protein, and nucleotide biosynthesis. Activation of PI3K/Akt through growth factor pathways (insulin, IGF) leads to an upregulation in glucose transporters (GLUT-1) as well as increased hexokinase and phosphofructokinase, increasing glycolytic flux (Figure 37.4). Downstream activation of mTOR, by PI3K/Akt, increases amino acid transporters and activates protein synthesis. Tumor cells are unique in the high levels of lactate generated, resulting in increasing acidosis, even in the absence of low tumor oxygen levels [145]. This is accompanied by increased production of hypoxia inducible factors (HIF) [146] that reinforces the upregulation of the glycolytic pathway and contributes to tumor progression through increased cell proliferation, reduced apoptosis, increased invasiveness, and enhanced angiogenesis. The accompanying acidosis has been shown to directly enhance both

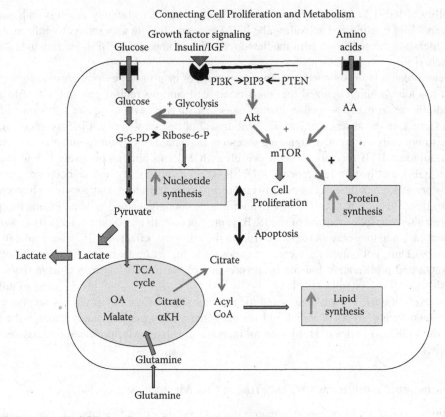

FIGURE 37.4   Insulin/IGF signaling and cancer cell metabolism.

tumor invasiveness and metastatic potential [147]. An additional adaptation to this metabolic shift is increased utilization of glutamine, accompanied by increased glutaminase expression, important in supporting glucose in the generation of NADPH and acetyl CoA for lipid as well as nucleotide synthesis [148].

Regulation of this metabolic adaptive response to the needs of a rapidly proliferating cell population is mediated through the PI3K/AKt downstream pathway, coordinating both cell proliferation and increased glucose metabolism [143]. The presence of high levels of IGF-R and IR signaling through the PI3K/AKt pathway may be critical in activating both this adaptive metabolic response as well as the stimulus to increased cell proliferation involved in tumor progression.

The critical role of the insulin/IGF–mediated activation of the PI3K/Akt pathway has been reinforced by the finding that one of the most commonly mutated genes in epithelial cancers involves the PIK3CA catalytic subunit of PI3k, in a variety of cancers, including colorectal, breast, lung, gastric, and glioblastoma, usually present in later in tumorigenesis [149]. This is an important effector in the activation pathway, as noted, for many TK receptors, including estrogen, ERBB2 (Her-2), in addition to insulin and IGF-1. Activating mutations of PI3k have been shown to be associated with resistance to endocrine therapy of breast cancer [150]. More recently, Kalaany and Sabatini [151] documented the central role of this pathway in mediating the effect of calorie restriction on suppression of tumor growth. In a tumor xenograft mouse model, dietary caloric restriction (DR) resulted in marked reduction in tumor growth, mediated by reduced IGF1 activation of the PI3k pathway in several tumor cell lines. In other cell lines, DR-mediated IGF1 suppression had no effect on tumor growth. The DR-resistant cell lines carried mutations associated with either constitutive activation of PI3K or loss of PTEN, a tumor suppressor gene that inhibits PI3K activation of Akt. In contrast to the DR-sensitive cells, the DR-resistant cells were able to proliferate in cell culture in the absence of either insulin or IGF. This provides a molecular model for the central role of insulin and IGF in the control of both cell proliferation and metabolism in many tumors, as well as an insight into an important mechanism of resistance of some cancers to dietary manipulation. Tumors with downstream activation of PI3K or inhibition of the PTEN tumor suppressor that inactivates this pathway may not have the same benefit in regard to lifestyle-mediated reduction in insulin and IGF.

METFORMIN: INSIGHTS INTO THE ROLE OF ENERGY BALANCE AND CANCER

Metformin has been in widespread use in the treatment of diabetes. In contrast to sulfonylurea medications, which enhance pancreatic insulin production, metformin improves insulin sensitivity, in part through reduction in hepatic gluconeogenesis, leading to lower insulin levels in patients [152]. In addition, it has been shown to reduce the development of diabetes in individuals at risk in several large trials [81] and is associated with lower all-cause and cardiovascular mortality compared to both sulfonylurea and insulin in diabetic populations [152].

Recent population-based studies have documented a significant reduction in both cancer risk as well as cancer mortality in diabetic populations on metformin, compared to alternate antidiabetic medication [82]. In a meta-analysis of 11 studies, Decensi et al. reported a 31% reduction in overall cancer risk in subjects on metformin, including a significant decrease in pancreatic, hepatocellular, as well as colon, breast, and prostate [153]. In a review of population-based mortality rates from Saskatchewan [154] of overall 12,272 newly diagnosed diabetics, cancer-related mortality was increased significantly in those using sulfonylureas or insulin, with an increasing mortality risk with increasing dose and duration of insulin use. While controversy continues to exist regarding the cancer risk and mortality with exogenous insulin use [155], the anticancer effect has been consistent in all studies. Of interest, this effect has also been observed in multiple cancers. In a Taiwan population-based study [156], 19,624 cases of newly diagnosed diabetics were identified. The use of metformin was associated with a decreased lung cancer risk of 39–45%. In newly diagnosed early stage breast cancer patients treated with neoadjuvant chemotherapy between 1990 and 2007 at MD Anderson Cancer Center, diabetic patients treated with metformin had a pathologic complete remission (pCR) rate of 24%, compared to an 8% pCR in diabetic patients not on metformin and a 16% pCR in nondiabetic individuals [102]. More recently, a review of 1983 patients with HER2+ breast cancer treated between 1998 and 2010 at MD Anderson [103], noted that breast cancer–specific mortality in diabetic patients was decreased with metformin (53%) as well as thiazolidinediones (58%) compared to nonusers.

Several mechanisms for this anticancer effect have been proposed. As noted, metformin, through reduction in insulin resistance, improves the hyperinsulinemic state, reducing insulin signaling. In addition, metformin activates the AMP-activated protein kinase (AMPK) pathway via the tumor suppressor LKB1, reducing downstream activation of mTOR, the effector of growth factor signaling [157]. In animal models, metformin has been shown to attenuate tumor growth induced by high-energy diet, associated with a reduction in insulin receptor activation as well as increased AMPK phosphorylation [157]. Metformin also interferes with cross talk between insulin/IGF receptor and G protein coupled receptor signaling, important in promotion of multiple tumor types [158]. In breast cancer, low-dose metformin has been shown, in combination with chemotherapy, to selectively target the chemotherapeutically resistant breast cancer stem cell population and prevent relapse in a mouse xenograft model [159]. The same group [160] has documented a synergy between metformin and multiple chemotherapeutic agents (doxorubicin, carboplatin, paclitaxel), with increased efficacy in combination compared to either agent alone and with enhanced effect at lower doses of chemotherapy and in multiple cancer subtypes (breast, prostate, and lung).

The potential importance of insulin signaling as well as targeting energy balance in cancers not traditionally associated with obesity is reflected in the observations on lung cancer. As noted earlier, in nonsmokers (compared to an inverse association in smokers), BMI may be associated with an increase in lung cancer risk [40]. A positive association with type 2 DM has been associated with both a higher risk and an adverse prognosis in lung cancer [156]. Lung cancer cells express increased receptors for both IFG-1 as well as insulin. A recent trial of inhaled insulin (exubera) was halted after a documented increase in lung cancer rates in the experimental arm compared to placebo. In a recent observational study [161] from five hospitals in China between 2004 and 2009, the influence of metformin on tumor response in diabetic lung cancer patients was assessed. Those patients on metformin had a significant improvement in both progression-free as well as overall survival compared to those patients on insulin or other diabetic medication. In an animal model of tobacco carcinogen–induced lung cancer with NNK, metformin reduced lung tumorigenesis [162]. The study noted that metformin reduced insulin/IGFR receptor phosphorylation with downstream decrease in mTOR but had did not activate AMPK in lung epithelial cells, suggesting an insulin-specific effect.

Multiple studies of metformin are now in progress including a large, multicenter trial of metformin in early stage breast cancer [163]. More importantly, the research on metformin highlights the critical role of energy balance and insulin-related signaling on cancer risk and survival in all cancer populations. It is important to note that the Diabetes Prevention Program randomized trial [100] demonstrated that the lifestyle intervention was more effective than metformin in preventing both type 2 diabetes and the development of the metabolic syndrome. This reinforces the critical importance that lifestyle change may have in cancer prevention and survival.

Stress, Obesity, and Cancer

The relationship between stress and cancer risk and survival continues to be controversial. One of the presumed mediators of this effect has been the impact of chronic stress on immunity as a result of altered hypothalamic-pituitary-adrenal function. A well-recognized effect of acute stress is impaired glycemic control in diabetic patients, resulting from increased glucocorticoid and cathecholamine production. Chronic hypercorticolism related to Cushing's Syndrome is associated with central obesity, insulin resistance, and diabetes. There is increasing evidence that long-term stress also induces hyperactivity within the hypothalamic-pituitary-adrenal axis, associated with abnormal cortisol secretory patterns, altered sex steroid and GH production, and visceral fat accumulation as well as central sympathetic system increases in blood pressure [164]. Chronic stress-related alterations in glucocorticoid production may contribute to altered appetite and increased food intake further promoting the risk [165]. Thus, stress may play an important, indirect role in cancer risk and survival, through a higher risk of the visceral obesity, insulin resistance, and the metabolic syndrome.

A common consequence of cancer-related stress is altered sleep and insomnia, affecting up to 60% of cancer patients. This is accompanied by fatigue, depression, and altered quality of life [166]. Sleep duration and quality have been associated with increased risk of a variety of cancers and precancerous lesions, including colorectal adenomas, colon cancer, and breast cancer. Shift work with nighttime light exposure is associated with altered circadian rhythm and diminished melatonin production. Several studies have documented an increase in risk of breast, colorectal, prostate, and endometrial cancer in night shift workers [167–170]. One important consequence of altered sleep is an increased risk of obesity [171]. Sleep deprivation increases plasma ghrelin and reduces leptin, resulting in increased hunger and appetite [172]. Long-term sleep deprivation increases BMI, insulin resistance, and measures of systemic inflammation, including higher C-RP and IL-6 levels [173]. The role of chronic sleep deprivation in increased risk of metabolic syndrome and diabetes is increasingly recognized. Its role as a mediator of stress-related cancer outcomes remains inadequately unexplored.

EVALUATION

The central role of the insulin/IGF system in both the origins and outcome of cancer, as well as the growing recognition that it has effects in many malignancies, supports the need to identify multiple populations likely to benefit from lifestyle interventions. While weight has been an important discriminator for population risk, it is important to recognize the role of metabolic status, independent of weight, as a determinant of risk, in part through abnormal body composition, with lower lean body mass and higher fat mass reflecting an adverse body phenotype, even in normal weight individuals. The target populations are broad as presented in Table 37.1.

PATIENT HISTORY

The initial evaluation should elicit a detailed history of both cancer and noncancer background, including onset and risk factors for cancer, prior and current treatments, as well as a detailed family history of malignancy, cardiovascular disease, and diabetes. In addition to the personal history of cancer, the noncancer history (hyperlipidemia, hypertension, DM, gestational DM, depression, psychiatric illness) is important for insights into risks of metabolic syndrome as well as competing noncancer morbidity risk critical in weighing lifestyle intervention benefits, including detailed medication history for drugs associated with weight gain, insulin resistance, and diabetes risk (antidepressant and antipsychotic medication, corticosteroids, thiazide diuretics, etc.). Patient perceptions, including their understanding and beliefs about the origins and risk factors for their illness, which may be inaccurate but drive their health behavior are critical for compliance with effective interventions. Assess the patient's weight history, including recent and long-term weight change, prior weight loss diets, as well as effectiveness. A detailed diet history, including food preferences,

---

TABLE 37.1
Target Populations for Weight Reduction

1. Children and Adolescents—at risk for obesity and the metabolic syndrome

    The rising epidemic of obesity, metabolic syndrome and early onset, type 2 diabetes mellitus are a critical population for long term risk reduction.

2. Overweight Adults (BMI 25–29) with evidence of the metabolic syndrome and insulin resistance

    Individuals with BMI 25 to 29, who are metabolically normal may have lower diabetes, cardiovascular, and cancer risk, compared to individuals who are metabolically obese with evidence for the metabolic syndrome. This is, in part reflected in the "obesity paradox"—the u-shaped curve for long-term survival with optimal survival between BMI 22 and 28.

    Individuals with BMI below 25, with evidence of the metabolic syndrome, have a significant CV risk and possibly higher cancer risk, despite lower weight.

3. Obese Adults (BMI ≥30)

    Obese individuals have a higher overall mortality and cancer risk.

    Individuals without evidence of the metabolic syndrome (metabolically normal, obese) may remain at increased risk due to increased sex hormone levels despite an absence of metabolic dysfunction.

    Obese individuals with the metabolic syndrome are at high risk for all-cause, cardiovascular, and cancer risk and mortality.

4. Early-Stage Cancer Patients, on curative therapy (adjuvant hormone, chemotherapy)

    Increased risk in overweight, obesity, insulin resistant, and diabetic individuals at diagnosis for recurrence, cancer, and noncancer mortality.

    Treatment-related weight gain and metabolic syndrome—adverse risk for cancer recurrence, second cancers, CV, and diabetes.

    Majority of research has focused on breast, colon, and prostate cancer. Effects may extend to multiple other cancers (lung, endometrial, kidney, liver, pancreas, gall bladder, myeloma, non-Hodgkins lymphoma, leukemia).

5. Cancer Survivors—post-treatment, without recurrence

    Long-term cancer survivors—post-treatment weight gain, obesity, and insulin resistance—increased risk second cancers, CV disease, and diabetes

6. Advanced-Cancer Patients

    High incidence of insulin resistance, sarcopenia, and adverse outcomes secondary to cancer cachexia, impaired nutrition and inactivity

    Reduces quality of life, increased overall mortality

intolerances, cravings, as well as eating behavior (home meals versus restaurant and fast food meals, ethnic food intake, etc.) and financial and geographic constraints on food choices are important for dietary counseling. A detailed sleep history (insomnia, daytime fatigue, drowsiness, sleep apnea) and prior sleep studies should be obtained. The patient should be asked about stressors, including personal, family, and work-related issues as well as perceptions about prognosis and coping issues (helpless, hopeless feelings) and the social support network available to the patient.

PHYSICAL EXAM

Initial weight and BMI should be calculated. In addition, waist circumference at the bending line, hip circumference at point of maximal girth, and waist-hip ratio, should be determined. These are more valid indicators of central obesity than BMI and they should be followed throughout a patient's course.

Body composition analysis should be obtained initially to assess baseline lean body mass and fat mass and should be monitored periodically. This may be accomplished by bioelectrical impedance analysis, which is affordable but somewhat inaccurate due to variations in technique. Anthropometric methods, including skin fold thickness or pinch test, measure subcutaneous fat at multiple locations with skin calipers but are limited by variations in body fat distribution and observer variation. The most accurate approach is the dual energy X-ray absorptiometry, or DXA scan. This provides measures of fat mass, lean mass, bone mineral content, percent fat and lean mass as well as regional fat distribution, important in distinguishing visceral related abdominal or android adiposity ("apple" shape) from gynoid ("pear" shape) adiposity at lower risk for insulin resistance.

LABORATORY ASSESSMENT

Assessment of metabolic status, including fasting glucose, HgbA1C, C-peptide, and fasting insulin, along with fasting lipid profile are important for evaluation of the metabolic syndrome (Table 37.2). A measure of insulin resistance, the homeostasis model assessment (HOMA), is a useful clinical tool, requiring only a single measure of fasting glucose and insulin. HOMA is calculated by the following formula: HOMA = [insulin (pg/ml) X glucose (mg/dl)]/405.

Measures of systemic inflammation, including C-reactive protein, thyroid function, and 25-OH vitamin D levels are additionally useful. Periodic measurements during and following completion of therapy are important in monitoring the development of insulin resistance, particularly in patients who develop post-treatment weight gain.

MANAGEMENT

The American Cancer Society has recently published their updated 2012 Nutrition and Physical Activity Guidelines [174] that serve as an important basis for management recommendations. They

---

TABLE 37.2
Metabolic Syndrome Criteria (NCEP ATP III)

	Females	Males
Waist Circumference	> 88 cm (35″)	> 102 cm (40″)
Hypertriglyceridemia	> 150 mg/dl	> 150 mg/dl
Low HDL-C	< 50 mg/dl	< 40 mg/dl
High Blood Pressure	> 130/85 mm/Hg (or treated HTN)	> 130/85 mm/Hg (or treated HTN)
High Fasting Glucose	> 110 mg/dl	

---

reflect the growing consensus of the cancer research community on the need to address abnormal energy balance, as manifest by obesity and the metabolic syndrome, as the central focus of public health efforts to reduce cancer risk, improve cancer survival, as well as improve cardiovascular and overall health. Several large cohort studies [175,176] confirm the benefit of following these lifestyle guidelines in lowering overall mortality, cardiovascular mortality, as well as cancer risk and mortality. While most research has focused on breast, colorectal, and prostate cancer, there is evidence that many other cancers are influenced by obesity, hyperinsulinemia, and the metabolic syndrome. These cancers include endometrial, liver and gall bladder, pancreas, ovarian, non–small cell lung cancer, as well as sarcoma and hematologic malignancies including non-Hodgkins lymphoma and chronic lymphocytic leukemia. The following suggestions should be considered for all cancer survivors and patients and are appropriate for overall health and possible risk reduction. The ACS guidelines are presented in Table 37.3. The following is a commentary on these guidelines, specific nutrients, and stress reduction.

WEIGHT CONTROL

- For individuals with increased BMI and features of the metabolic syndrome, a reduction of weight of 5–7% of baseline weight produces substantial improvement in metabolic parameters. Setting realistic goals enhances compliance with diet recommendations. Improving body composition (increased LBM, lower body fat) through concurrent exercise (both resistance and aerobic training) is critical.
- For overweight or obese individuals without evidence of hyperglycemia, hyperinsulinemia, or other features of the metabolic syndrome, similar weight reductions may still

---

TABLE 37.3

American Cancer Society Guidelines on Nutrition and Physical Activity for Cancer Prevention

Achieve and maintain a healthful weight throughout life.
- Be as lean as possible throughout life without being overweight.
- Avoid excess weight gain at all ages. For those who are currently overweight or obese, losing even a small amount of weight has health benefits and is a good place to start.
- Engage in regular physical activity and limit consumption of high-calorie foods and beverages as key strategies for maintaining a healthful weight.

Adapt a physically active lifestyle.
- Adults should engage in at least 150 minutes of moderate intensity or 75 minutes of vigorous intensity exercise each week, or an equivalent combination, preferably spread throughout the week.
- Children and adolescents should engage in a least one hour of moderate or vigorous activity each day, with vigorous activity occurring at least three days each week.
- Limit sedentary activity such as sitting, lying down, watching television, or other forms of screen-based activity.
- Doing some physical activity above usual activities, no matter what one's level of activity, can have many health benefits.

Consume a healthful diet, with an emphasis on plant foods.
- Choose foods and beverages in amounts that help achieve and maintain a healthful weight.
- Limit consumption of processed meat and red meat.
- Eat at least 2.5 servings of vegetables and fruits each day.
- Choose whole grains instead of refined grain products.

If you drink alcoholic beverages, limit consumption.
- Drink no more than one drink per day for women and two per day for men.

---

be beneficial in cancer and cardiovascular risk reduction as well as limiting the development of the metabolic syndrome.

- Patients who are metabolically obese but normal weight (increased WC, low LBM). should focus on improving body composition through resistance training to improve muscle mass as well as aerobic exercise, coupled with a diet focused on moderate to high protein, lower carbohydrate (low glycemic index, limited concentrated carbohydrate), but not calorie restricted. These individuals may benefit from pharmacologic interventions such as metformin or thiazolidenediones to manage their insulin-resistant state.

- Patients on active systemic therapy, particularly curative adjuvant chemotherapy for breast and colorectal cancer, and other malignancies should limit weight gain through careful diet and maintenance of physical activity, if possible. Attention to the potential risk of concurrent hyperglycemia should be noted, particularly in the setting of high-dose steroid premedication, now routine in chemotherapy regimens. Avoid high-dose steroids unless clearly indicated and for short periods, if feasible.

- An important principle derived from recent research and critical for practitioners and patients alike to understand is the recognition that *no single nutrient or food has been shown to change cancer survival in the absence of an influence on energy balance*, though weight management and exercise reflect a more holistic view of diet, lifestyle, and cancer.

DIET

The Prudent Diet—A Traditional Diet Approach

- The "prudent" diet pattern, contrasted with a "Western-style" diet, consistently has been associated with lower risk and improved survival from multiple cancers as well as cardiovascular risk (plant-based, low red and processed meat, limited refined grain, limited high-fat dairy, limited processed foods) and is associated with reduced risk of obesity and the metabolic syndrome. This pattern is common to many traditional diets (Mediterranean, Asian, etc.) that have been associated with low chronic disease risk.

- However, excess caloric intake, even of healthful foods, can lead to weight gain, and risk of adverse metabolic effects. Thus, a prudent diet pattern should be accompanied by adequate but not excess total calories.

Macronutrient Composition

- All calorie-restricted diets will lead to lower weight and improved metabolic status but low-carbohydrate, higher-protein diets are more effective in reducing adverse metabolic features, particularly in individuals with the metabolic syndrome and hyperinsulinemia.

- Concentrated carbohydrates, such as refined grains and sugars, should be limited. There is now evidence that lower overall carbohydrate intake itself, independent of calorie intake, may reduce tumor growth, through lower glucose and insulin levels [177]. This is preliminary but reinforces the common belief about the adverse effect of high-carbohydrate diets.

- Long-term population studies favor low carbohydrate, moderate fat and protein, higher in plant versus animal protein, with high legume, nut, whole grain, and modest poultry and fish intake.

Specific Foods

- Limit red and processed meat as well as high-fat dairy, whole milk, butter, and high saturated fat plant oils (palm, coconut oil). The high saturated fat of red meat and high-fat dairy increases risk of insulin resistance and the metabolic syndrome and is associated with higher risk of multiple cancers.

- Avoid trans fats, replace saturated and trans fat–containing foods with healthful oils rather than increased carbohydrate intake.
- Encourage moderate intake of monounsaturated fat (olive oil, canola, high oleic acid oils).
- Choose fat-rich cold-water fish (salmon, sardines, mackerel, rainbow trout) rich in long chain polyunsaturated fatty acids (omega-3 fatty acids). Limit farm-raised salmon intake. Chronic consumption with high PCB levels is associated with increased adiposity, insulin resistance and diabetic risk [178].
- Both flaxseed and walnuts are excellent plant sources of omega-3 fatty acids (alpha-linoleic acid).
- Low-fat dairy is not clearly linked to adverse cancer outcomes in adults. It is associated with lower weight gain and reduced insulin resistance. The association between dairy protein and cancer risk may reflect its association with early childhood growth in height rather than an effect of adult intake on risk.
- Low-fat dairy food intake has, in some studies, been associated with increased cancer survival. This may reflect the high quality protein or its micronutrient content (calcium, conjugated linoleic acid, etc.).
- Fermented dairy products, such as yogurt, may have benefits in part through a shift in the gut flora or microbiome.
- Increasing evidence supports the role of the gut bacterial composition in the risk of obesity and the metabolic syndrome. A high saturated fat diet coupled with an adverse gut floral composition (low *Bacteroidetes*, high *Firmicutes*, with low levels of *Bifidobacter* and *Lactobacillus sp.*) induces intestinal mucosal inflammation and systemic insulin resistance.
- A largely unexplored area is the potential adverse impact of systemic cancer treatments on the composition of the gut flora and whether it may mediate some of the adverse metabolic effects of chemotherapy.
- Patients should consume daily probiotic-containing food or supplement coupled with a fiber supplement (prebiotic) that supports healthy gut flora.
- Both green tea and coffee have been associated with lower diabetic risk. Each contains phytonutrients (EGCG, chlorogenic acid) associated with improved insulin resistance and, in observational studies, potential antitumor effects.
- Coffee has been consistently linked to lower risk of insulin resistance and diabetes, independent of caffeine.
- Coffee, particularly caffeinated, may acutely raise glucose levels in individuals with diabetes and insulin resistance.
- Coffee has been associated with a reduced risk of multiple cancers, including hepatocellular carcinoma, head and neck cancer, and colorectal cancer.
- Green tea, with a high content of polyphenol compounds, including epicathechin, epigallocatechin, and EGCG, has been associated with a reduction in adipogenesis and obesity, as well as improved insulin sensitivity and significantly lower risk of diabetes mellitus in observational studies.
- Green tea has potential activity as a chemopreventive agent for multiple cancers.

Choose Low Glycemic Index Foods

- Low glycemic index carbohydrate-containing foods (whole grains, legumes, whole vegetable, whole fruits) are beneficial and linked to lower risk of the metabolic syndrome, cardiovascular disease, and cancer. They are nutrient dense and, because they are often less calorie dense and tend to be high in bulk, they lead to feelings of fullness, reducing overall calorie intake.

- Avoid processed grains higher in both glycemic index and load (white breads, pasta, rice, etc.) and significantly lower in nutrient density (versus whole grains).

Limit Fructose, Fructose-Based Products, as Well as Sucrose

- In contrast to glucose, fructose does not stimulate insulin and, thus, has a low glycemic index. However, high intake of fructose will increase visceral obesity and the risk of metabolic syndrome. In addition, high fructose levels may activate tumor growth by increasing nucleotide synthesis for cell proliferation via increased transketolase activation [179].
- Despite the common perception, even natural, high-fructose foods (honey, agave, concentrated fruit juices) may have adverse metabolic effects and should be limited.
- There is no metabolic difference between table sugar and manufactured fructose-based corn syrup. Intake of both should be limited (sugar and high-fructose-sweetened beverages, etc.), particularly in individuals with evidence of insulin resistance and the metabolic syndrome.
- Very modest intakes of unrefined, natural sweeteners are probably safe as a sweetener in coffee or tea.
- Artificial sweeteners may increase caloric intake through increased preference for sweet foods and altered appetite drive and do not help to limit or reduce weight.

Limit Alcohol Consumption

- Alcohol is a both a cocarcinogen and tumor promoter for head and neck, esophageal, liver, colorectal, pancreas, and breast cancer when consumed on a regular basis in excess quantities, particularly coupled with a poor diet and tobacco use.
- Excess alcohol intake contributes to weight gain, obesity, and insulin resistance.
- Modest intake (two drinks/day for men, one drink/day for women) may be associated with cardiovascular benefit.

When Possible, Choose Organic Foods

- The relationship between persistent organic pollutants (POPs) and cancer risk remains speculative though early age of exposure (childhood, preadolescence) may play a role.
- Increasing evidence for the role of organochlorine pesticides and multiple health outcomes, including insulin resistance, diabetes, and hypertension is emerging [180].
- Early exposures to a variety of compounds (bisphenol A, phthalates, POPs, organotins) may act as developmental obesogens [181], increasing long-term risk of obesity through pre- and perinatal epigenetic programming effects on adipocytes as well as neural circuitry involved in appetite control.
- The most critical time to limit exposures to environmental toxins is during pregnancy and early childhood, through consumption of organic foods as well as care regarding other sources of exposure.
- The importance of a diverse, plant-based diet remains critical for both weight control and cancer prevention and, if organic food availability or cost is an issue, intake of conventional vegetables and fruit should not be limited.

Exercise

- Observational studies suggest increased levels of physical activity have been associated with reduced risk of many cancers as well as improvement in survival in breast, colorectal, and other cancers.
- Mixed exercise (aerobic endurance combined with progressive resistance training) improves insulin sensitivity, reduces circulating insulin and IGF-1, and increases SHBG, leading to lower free sex hormones, reduced measures of systemic inflammation (IL-6, C-RP),

as well as reduced fatigue, depression, and improved quality of life. In addition, increased cardiovascular fitness predicts improved overall survival, independent of weight.

- There may be a dose response by cancer site, with the recommended range of moderate activity weekly of at least 150 minutes of moderate activity (brisk walk) or 75 minutes of vigorous activity. Survival benefit has been observed for three or more hours of brisk walking in breast cancer and six or more hours in colorectal cancer.
- The optimal range for weight maintenance and increased risk reduction may be higher (300 minutes of moderate activity or 150 minutes of vigorous activity).
- Shorter bursts of activity (20–30 minutes) appear to be equivalent to fewer, longer sessions.
- Limit sedentary active. Individuals who intermittently exercise, then spend significant sedentary time (> 1–2 hr/day) remain at higher mortality risk. Limit television, computer, and video game time.
- Consider use of a pedometer: they are associated with increased levels of physical activity and weight control. Increase incremental steps by 2000 daily as tolerated. Pedometers provide useful feedback, improve motivation, and reduce sedentary lifestyle. Guidelines are shown in Table 37.4.

Micronutrients/Dietary Supplements

Adequate intake of dietary micronutrients has been associated with both reduced cancer risk and improved outcome as well as lower risk of insulin resistance and the metabolic syndrome. Individuals with higher intake through food sources or higher circulating levels of carotenoids, vitamin C, vitamin D, folate B-6, and other micronutrients have reduced cancer risk. Similarly, increased dietary antioxidants are strongly associated with lower risk of both insulin resistance and diabetes.

In contrast, multiple studies have failed to demonstrate benefit from supplementation with most micronutrients, particularly in well-nourished individuals. Increased folic acid as well as vitamin E (as alpha-tocopherol) may increase cancer risk in adults, at higher doses. This remains controversial.

The following nutrients may have benefits and should be considered:

- Vitamin D + Calcium—800–1000 IU vitamin D3 + 1200 mg calcium
  - Vitamin D deficiency is associated with glucose intolerance.
  - Calcium + D may assist in weight loss.
  - Vitamin D deficiency (<10 ng) is associated with adverse cancer, CV survival.
  - Recent cohort studies raise concern about cancer risk at levels > 50–60 ng/ml, particularly upper gastrointestinal and pancreatic cancer.
  - Higher doses of vitamin D to achieve adequacy (> 32 ng/ml) may be necessary.
  - The optimal range remains controversial (safe range 35–45 ng/ml).
  - Include outdoor activity with added supplemental vitamin D. There may be additional photoproducts linked to sun exposure beyond vitamin D, as yet unidentified. Long-term, adequate but not excessive sun exposure with high levels of outdoor activity is highly correlated with low cancer risk.

TABLE 37.4

Pedometer Guidelines

< 5000 steps	sedentary
5000–7499 steps	low active
7500–9999 steps	somewhat active
10,000–12,499 steps	active
> 12,500 steps	highly active

- Magnesium—250–500 mg/day (dietary sources—whole grains, nuts, legumes)
  - Deficiency is common, associated with increased insulin resistance, DM.
- Chromium—200 mcg/day (dietary—Brewer's yeast, barley flour)
  - Enhances insulin sensitivity, glucose control
- Vanadium—up to 50 mg/day (dietary sources—whole grains, spices [dill, parsley], fish, and shellfish
  - Supplementation remains controversial and is currently not recommended by ADA.
- Omega-3 fatty acid—2–3 grams/day (fish or krill oil)
  - Most studies support a reduction in risk of insulin resistance, an important anti-inflammatory effect and well-recognized cardiovascular benefits.
  - Emerging data on improved cancer outcomes in small trials suggests anticancer benefits.
  - Fish oil is largely free of organic contaminants.
  - Antioxidants—vitamin C, E—limit high-dose supplemental intake.
  - Recent research suggests suppression of ROS during exercise with supplemental vitamin C (1000 MG) and E (400 IU) impairs exercise-induced improvement in insulin sensitivity via decreased mitochondrial biogenesis[160].
- Multivitamin
  - In individuals with inadequate, limited diets, a single daily multivitamin may be useful in supplementing dietary inadequacy.
  - In well-nourished individuals with a very diverse, plant-based diet, a multivitamin may not be necessary.
- Amino acid supplementation (glycine, cysteine [as N-acetyl cysteine], glutamine, leucine) replete glutathione, suppress oxidative damage (f-isoprostane, lipid peroxide), and improve efficiency of muscle protein synthesis [161].
- Herbal and phytonutrients—cinnamon, curry, curcumin, berberine, resveratrol bitter melon, fenugreek, and gymnema (gurar) have been associated with improved glucose control as well as other possible benefits. Trials of several of these nutrients are in progress.

Stress Reduction

- Mind-body therapies—yoga, massage, acupuncture, and meditation (mindfulness-based meditation) are cost-effective management strategies and help reduce disease-related symptoms, treatment-related side effects, and may lower metabolic parameters associated with insulin resistance.
- Disordered sleep (insomnia, shortened sleep duration, and obstructive sleep apnea) is a significant stressor. It is a common component of the pain-fatigue-sleep disorder triad in cancer patients. It also plays a significant role in weight gain, obesity, and the metabolic syndrome.
- Initial approaches should include behavioral and stress reduction techniques including sleep hygiene, meditation, cognitive behavioral therapy, massage, etc.
- Evaluation and formal treatment for sleep apnea should be considered.
- Role of melatonin and melatoninergic compounds (ramelton, agomelatine) is being explored both for disrupted day-night cycling, jet lag, and shift work sleep disorder.
- Melatonin may play an important role in mediating the effect of sleep and reduced risk of insulin resistance and metabolic syndrome.
- Low doses of melatonin (2–5 mg) may improve insomnia and disrupted sleep.
- Weight reduction, in the setting of obesity, remains the best treatment for sleep apnea.

SUMMARY

The critical importance of obesity, the metabolic syndrome, and insulin resistance in both cancer risk and outcome is increasingly recognized. While the underlying mechanisms remain complex, the central role of insulin and the IGF system appears critical. One of the most important approaches to both reducing cancer risk and treating most cancers is to improve the insulin resistant state common in this population. Importantly, while obesity and increased BMI are risk factors for insulin resistance, many individuals—particularly cancer survivors and those with advanced disease—will have insulin resistance and features of the metabolic syndrome, despite a normal BMI. Thus, identifying and targeting the insulin resistant state with dietary and nutrition therapies is a necessary part of all cancer patients' treatment plans.

In addition to the interventions outlined here, many new avenues of research hold great promise for further advances in the future, including:

- Trials on weight control and exercise in cancer survival: multiple, ongoing national trials of weight control, diet, and exercise will further define long-term benefits, quantify risk reduction, and better define biomarkers of efficacy.
- Define role of diet, nutrition, and exercise interventions in less common cancers, where potential benefit might be expected based on associations with obesity, DM, physical activity, etc., and where few current studies are active (endometrial, ovarian, lung, pancreatic, renal, and liver cancer, hematologic cancers—myeloma, lymphoma, chronic lymphocytic leukemia, etc.).
- Defining role of macronutrient composition, efficacy of very low carbohydrate diets, in a trial setting on cancer outcomes and metabolic correlates.
- Molecular profiling of cancers to identify predictive markers (e.g., PI3K, Wnt, IGF-R, mTOR) of response to weight control, diet, and exercise intervention.
- Role of pharmacologic interventions, such as metformin, in improving tumor response and outcome and, potentially, the impact of combining diet, nutrition, and exercise interventions with metformin to improve response through targeting of the insulin/IGF pathway.
- Role of other caloromimetic agents (2-deoxyglucose, resveratrol) in cancer outcomes.
- Role of calorie restriction strategies targeting IGF/insulin in trial settings to limit chemotherapy toxicity and efficacy as well developing longer term strategies for cancer risk reduction (pretreatment fasting, intermittent or alternate day fasting, etc.).
- Define systemic cancer treatment-mediated effects on risk of insulin resistance:
  - Role of medications as mediators of risk (steroids, chemotherapy agents, etc.)
  - Impact of treatment on gut microbiome and the metabolic consequences
  - Effect of treatment-mediated disruption in circadian cycling, sleep, and potential role of melatonin and melatonergic agents in reducing the adverse metabolic effects.
- Role of early life interventions (pre- and postnatal) on limiting risks of long-term adverse metabolic outcome (obesity, metabolic syndrome, adult cancer risk) including impact of maternal diet, nutrient intake, and environmental exposures on epigenetic programming.

REFERENCES

1. Doll R, Peto R. The causes of cancer: Quantitative estimates of avoidable risks of cancer in the United States today. J Natl Cancer Inst. 1981;66:1191–98.
2. Hulka BS. Dietary fat and breast cancer: Case-control and cohort studies. Prev Med. 1989 Mar;18(2): 180–93.
3. Talbot JM. Role of dietary fiber in diverticular disease and colon cancer. Fed Proc.1981 Jul;40(9):2337–42.
4. Block G, Patterson B, Subar A. Fruit, vegetables, and cancer prevention: A review of the epidemiological evidence. Nutr Cancer. 1992;18(1):1–29.
5. Mayne ST, Janerich DT, Greenwald P, et al. Dietary beta carotene and lung cancer risk in U.S. nonsmokers. J Natl Cancer Inst. 1994;86:33–38.
6. Hartman TJ, Albanes D, Pietinen P, Hartman AM, Rautalahti M, Tangrea JA, Taylor PR. The association between baseline vitamin E, selenium, and prostate cancer in the alpha-tocopherol, beta-carotene cancer prevention study. Cancer Epidemiol Biomarkers Prev. 1998 Apr;7(4):335–40.

7. Prentice RL, Caan B, Chlebowski RT, et al. Low-fat dietary pattern and risk of invasive breast cancer: The Women's Health Initiative Randomized Controlled Dietary Modification Trial. JAMA. 2006 Feb 8;295(6):629–42.

8. Boffetta P, Couto E, Wichmann J, Ferrari P, Fruit and vegetable intake and overall cancer risk in the European Prospective Investigation into Cancer and Nutrition (EPIC). J Natl Cancer Inst. 2010 Apr 21;102 (8):529–37

9. Alberts DS, Martinez ME, Roe DJ, et al. Lack of effect of a high-fiber cereal supplement on the recurrence of colorectal adenomas. Phoenix Colon Cancer Prevention Physicians' Network. N Engl J Med. 2000;342:1156–62.

10. Albanes D, Heinonen OP, Huttunen JK, et al. Effects of alpha-tocopherol and beta-carotene supplements on cancer incidence in the Alpha-Tocopherol Beta-Carotene Cancer Prevention Study. Am J Clin Nutr. 1995 Dec;62(6 Suppl):1427S–30S.

11. Klein EA, Thompson IM, Jr, Tangen CM, et al. Vitamin E and the risk of prostate cancer: The Selenium and Vitamin E Cancer Prevention Trial (SELECT). JAMA. 2011 Oct 12;306(14):1549–56.

12. Basen-Engquist K, Chang M. Obesity and cancer risk: Recent review and evidence. Curr Oncol Rep. 2011 Feb;13(1):71–76.

13. Calle EE, Kaaks R. Overweight, obesity and cancer: Epidemiological evidence and proposed mechanisms. Nat Rev Cancer. 2004;4:579–91.

14. Pothiwala P, Jain SK, Yaturu S. Metabolic syndrome and cancer. Metab Syndr Relat Disord. 2009;7: 279–88.

15. Jaggers JR, Sui X, Hooker SP, LaMonte MJ, Matthews CE, Hand GA, Blair SN. Metabolic syndrome and risk of cancer mortality in men. Eur J Cancer. 2009;45:1831–38.

16. Jung HS, Myung SK, Kim BS, Seo HG. Metabolic syndrome in adult cancer survivors: A meta-analysis. Diabetes Res Clin Pract. 2012 Feb;95(2):275–82.

17. Giovannucci E, Harlan DM, Archer MC, Bergenstal RM, Gapstur SM, Habel LA, Pollak M, Regensteiner JG, Yee D. Diabetes and cancer: A consensus report. CA Cancer J Clin. 2010 Jul-Aug;60(4):207–21.

18. McCullough ML, Patel AV, Kushi LH, et al. Following cancer prevention guidelines reduces risk of cancer, cardiovascular disease, and all-cause mortality. Cancer Epidemiol Biomarkers Prev. 2011;20: 1089–97.

19. Barker DJ The origins of the developmental origins theory. J Intern Med. 2007 May;261(5):412–17.

20. Roche AF. Secular trends in human growth, maturation, and development. Monogr Soc Res Child Dev. 1979;44(3–4):1–120.

21. Song YM, Davey Smith GD, Sung J. Adult height and cause-specific mortality: A large prospective study of South Korean men. Am J Epidemiol. 2003;158:479–85.

22. Giovannucci E, Rimm EB, Liu Y, Willett WC. Height, predictors of C-peptide and cancer risk in men. Int J Epidemiol. 2004;33:217–25.

23. Gunnell D, Okasha M, Smith, GD, et al. Height, leg length, and cancer risk: A systematic review. Epidemiol Rev. 2001;23:313–42.

24. Gunnell DJ, Smith GD, Frankel SJ, Nanchahal K, Braddon FEM, Peters TJ. Childhood leg length and adult mortality—follow up of the Carnegie survey of diet and growth in prewar Britain. J Epidemiol Community Health. 1996;50:580–81.

25. Gunnell DJ, Davey Smith G, Holly JM, Frankel S. Leg length and risk of cancer in the Boyd Orr cohort. BMJ. 1998;317:1350–51.

26. Whitley E, Martin RM, Smith GD, Holly JM, Gunnell D. Childhood stature and adult cancer risk: The Boyd Orr cohort. Cancer Causes Control. 2009 Mar;20(2):243–51.

27. Berkey CS, Colditz GA, Rockett HR, Frazier AL, Willett WC. Dairy consumption and female height growth: Prospective cohort study. Cancer Epidemiol Biomarkers Prev. 2009;18:1881–87.

28. Frankel S, Gunnell DJ, Peters TJ, Maynard M, Davey Smith G. Childhood energy intake and adult mortality from cancer: The Boyd Orr Cohort Study. BMJ. 1998;316:499–504.

29. Baker J, Liu JP, Robertson EJ, Efstratiadis A. Role of insulin-like growth factors in embryonic and postnatal growth. Cell. 1993;75:73–82.

30. Liu JL, LeRoith D. Insulin-like growth factor I is essential for postnatal growth in response to growth hormone. Endocrinology. 1999;140:5178–84.

31. Savarese TM, Strohsnitter WC, Low HP, et al. Correlation of umbilical cord blood hormones and growth factors with stem cell potential: Implications for the prenatal origin of breast cancer hypothesis. Breast Cancer Res. 2007;9(3):R29.

32. Trichopoulos D, Lagiou P, Adami HO. Towards an integrated model for breast cancer etiology: The crucial role of the number of mammary tissue-specific stemcells. Breast Cancer Res. 2005;7(1):13–17.

33. MaBaik I, Devito WJ, Ballen K, et al. Association of fetal hormone levels with stem cell potential: Evidence for early life roots of human cancer. Cancer Res. 2005 Jan 1;65(1):358–63.

34. Jeffrey's M, Smith GD, Martin RM, Frankel S, Gunnell D. Childhood body mass index and later cancer risk: A 50-year follow-up of the Boyd Orr study. Int J Cancer. 2004 Nov 1;112(2):348–51.

35. Capittini C, Bergamaschi P, De Silvestri A, et al. Birth-weight as a risk factor for cancer in adulthood: The stem cell perspective. Maturitas. 2011;69(1):91–93.

36. Ross JA. Birthweight and childhood leukemia: Time to tackle bigger lessons. Pediatr Blood Cancer. 2012 Jan;58(1):1–2.

37. Renehan AG, Tyson M, Egger M, Heller RF, Zwahlen M. Body-mass index and incidence of cancer: A systematic review and meta-analysis of prospective observational studies. Lancet. 2008;371: 569–78.

38. Connolly BS, Barnett C, Vogt KN, Li T, Stone J, Boyd NF. A meta-analysis of published literature on waist-to-hip ratio and risk of breast cancer. Nutr Cancer. 2002;44(2):127–38.

39. Zilli T, Chagnon M, Van Nguyen T, Bahary JP, Guay JP, Dufresne A, Taussky D. Influence of abdominal adiposity, waist circumference, and body mass index on clinical and pathologic findings in patients treated with radio therapy for localized prostate cancer. Cancer. 2010 Dec 15;116(24):5650–58.

40. Kabat GC, Miller AB, Rohan TE. Body mass index and lung cancer risk in women. Epidemiology. 2007 Sep;18(5):607–12.

41. Kabat GC, Kim M, Hunt JR, Chlebowski RT, Rohan TE Body mass index and waist circumference in relation to lung cancer risk in the Women's Health Initiative. Am J Epidemiol. 2008 Jul 15;168(2):158–69.

42. Jee SH, Ohrr H, Sull JW, et al. Fasting serum glucose level and cancer risk in Korean men and women. JAMA 2005;293:194–202.

43. Rapp K, Schroeder J, Klenk J, et al. Fasting blood glucose and cancer risk in a cohort of more than 140000 adults in Austria. Diabetologia. 2006;49(5):945–52.

44. Pisani P. Hyper-insulin aecia and cancer, meta-analyses of epidemiological studies. Arch Physiol Biochem. 2008 Feb;114(1):63–70.

45. Renehan AG, Zwahlen M, Minder C, et al. Insulin-like growth factor (IGF)-I, IGF binding protein-3, and cancer risk: Systematic review and meta-regression analysis. Lancet. 2004;363:1346–53.

46. Na HK, Oliynyk S. Effects of physical activity on cancer prevention. Ann N Y Acad Sci. 2011 Jul;1229:176–83.

47. Gallagher EJ, Fierz Y, Ferguson RD, LeRoith D. The pathway from diabetes and obesity to cancer, on the route to targeted therapy. Endocr Pract. 2010 Sep-Oct 16(5):864–73.

48. Grote VA, Becker S, Kaaks R. Diabetes mellitus type 2—an independent risk factor for cancer? Exp Clin Endocrinol Diabetes. 2010;118:4–8.

49. Pandey A, Forte V, Abdallah M, Alickaj A, Mahmud S, Asad S, McFarlane SI. Diabetes mellitus and the risk of cancer. Minerva Endocrinol. 2011 Sep;36(3):187–209.

50. Stocks T, Rapp K, Bjørge T, et al. Blood glucose and risk of incident and fatal cancer in the metabolic syndrome and cancer project (Me-Can): Analysis of six prospective cohorts. PLoS Med. 2009 Dec; 6(12):e1000201.

51. Hundal RS, Krssak M, Dufour S, et al. Mechanism by which metformin reduces glucose production in type 2 diabetes. *Diabetes*. 2000;49:2063–69.

52. Evans JM, Donnelly LA, Emslie-Smith AM, Alessi DR, Morris AD. Metformin and reduced risk of cancer in diabetic patients. *BMJ*. 2005;330:1304–5.

53. Decensi A, Puntoni M, Goodwin P, Cazzaniga M, Gennari A, Bonanni B, Gandini S. Metformin and cancer risk in diabetic patients: A systematic review and meta-analysis. Cancer Prev Res (Phila). 2010 Nov;3(11):1451–61.

54. Calle EE, Rodriguez C, Walker-Thurmond K, Thun MJ. Overweight, obesity, and mortality from cancer in a prospectively studied cohort of U.S. adults. N Engl J Med. 2003;348:1625–38.

55. McTiernan A, Irwin M, Vongruenigen V. Weight, physical activity, diet, and prognosis in breast and gynecologic cancers. J Clin Oncol. 2010;28:4074–80.

56. Freedland SJ, Aronson WJ, Kane CJ, et al. Impact of obesity on biochemical control after radical prostatectomy for clinically localized prostate cancer: A report by the Shared Equal Access Regional Cancer Hospital database study group. J Clin Oncol. 2004;22:446–53.

57. Ewertz M, Jensen MB, Gunnarsdóttir KÁ, et al. Effect of obesity on prognosis after early-stage breast cancer. J Clin Oncol. 2001;29:25–31.

58. Discacciati A, Orsini N, Andersson SO, Andrén O, Johansson JE, Wolk A. Body mass index in early and middle-late adulthood and risk of localised, advanced and fatal prostate cancer: A population-based prospective study. Br J Cancer. 2011 Sep 27;105(7):1061–68.

59. Abrahamson PE, Gammon MD, Lund MJ, Flagg EW, Porter PL, Stevens J, Swanson CA, Brinton LA, Eley JW, Coates RJ. General and abdominal obesity and survival among young women with breast cancer. Cancer Epidemiol Biomarkers Prev. 2006 Oct;15(10):1871–77.

60. Bastarrachea J, Hortobagyi GN, Smith TL, et al. Obesity as an adverse prognostic factor for patients receiving adjuvant chemotherapy for breast cancer. Ann Intern Med. 1993;119:18–25.

61. Meyerhardt JA, Catalano PJ, Haller DG, Mayer RJ, Benson AB, III, Macdonald JS, Fuchs CS. Influence of body mass index on outcomes and treatment-related toxicity in patients with colon carcinoma. Cancer. 2003 Aug 1;98(3):484–95.

62. Coughlin SS, Calle EE, Teras LR, Petrelli J, Thun MJ. Diabetes mellitus as a predictor of cancer mortality in a large cohort of US adults. Am J Epidemiol. 2004;159:1160–67.

63. Liu X, Ji J, Sundquist K, Sundquist J, Hemminki K. The impact of type 2 diabetes mellitus on cancer-specific survival: A follow-up study in Sweden. Cancer. 2012 Mar 1;118(5):1353–61.

64. Liu X, Ji J, Sundquist K, Sundquist J, Hemminki K. Mortality causes in cancer patients with type 2 diabetes mellitus. Eur J Cancer Prev. 2012 May;21(3):300–6.

65. Duggan C, Irwin ML, Xiao L, Henderson KD, Smith AW, Baumgartner RN, Baumgartner KB, Bernstein L, Ballard-Barbash R, McTiernan A. Associations of insulin resistance and adiponectin with mortality in women with breast cancer. J Clin Oncol. 2011 Jan 1;29(1):32–39.

66. Irwin ML, Duggan C, Wang CY, et al. Fasting C-peptide levels and death resulting from all causes and breast cancer: The Health, Eating, Activity, and Lifestyle Study. J Clin Oncol. 2011;29:47–53.

67. Goodwin PJ, Ennis M, Pritchard KI, et al. Fasting insulin and outcome in early-stage breast cancer: Results of a prospective cohort study. J Clin Oncol. 2002;20:42–51.

68. Ma J, Li H, Giovannucci E, Mucci L, Qiu W, Nguyen PL, Gaziano JM, Pollak M, Stampfer MJ. Prediagnostic body-mass index, plasma C-peptide concentration, and prostate cancer—specific mortality in men with prostate cancer: A long-term survival analysis. Lancet Oncol. 2008 Nov;9(11):1039–47.

69. Prabhat P, Tewari R, Natu SM, Dalela D, Goel A, Tandon P, Goel MM, Singh K. Is central obesity, hyperinsulinemia and dyslipidemia associated with high-grade prostate cancer? A descriptive cross-sectional study. Indian J Urol. 2010 Oct;26(4):502–6.

70. Shetti MB, Merrick GS, Butler WM, Galbreath R, Torlone A, Lief JH, Adamovich E, Wallner KE. The impact of diabetes mellitus on survival in men with clinically localized prostate cancer treated with permanent interstitial brachytherapy. Am J Clin Oncol. 2011 Nov 29.

71. Giovannucci, E. Metabolic syndrome, hyperinsulinemia, and colon cancer; A review. Am J Clin Nutr. 2007 Sept;86(3):836s–42s.

72. Moore LL, Bradlee ML, Singer MR, Splansky GL, Proctor MH, Ellison RC, Kreger BE. BMI and waist circumference as predictors of lifetime colon cancer risk in Framingham Study adults. Int J Obes Relat Metab Disord. 2004 Apr;28(4):559–67.

73. Dai Z, Xu YC, Niu L. Obesity and colorectal cancer risk: A meta-analysis of cohort studies. World J Gastroenterol. 2007 Aug 21;13(31):4199–206.

74. Kaaks R, Toniolo P, Akhmedkhanov A, Lukanova A, Biessy C, Dechaud H, Rinaldi S, Zeleniuch-Jacquotte A, Shore RE, Riboli E. Serum C-peptide, insulin-like growth factor (IGF)-I, IGF-binding proteins, and colorectal cancer risk in women. J Natl Cancer Inst. 2000 Oct 4;92(19):1592–600.

75. Schoen RE, Tangen CM, Kuller LH, Burke GL, Cushman M, Tracy RP, Dobs A, Savage PJ. Increased blood glucose and insulin, body size, and incident colorectal cancer. J Natl Cancer Inst. 1999 Jul 7;91(13):1147–54.

76. Ahmed RL, Schmitz KH, Anderson KE, Rosamond WD, Folsom AR. The metabolic syndrome and risk of incident colorectal cancer. Cancer. 2006 Jul 1;107(1):28–36.

77. Larsson SC, Orsini N, Wolk A. Diabetes mellitus and risk of colorectal cancer: A meta-analysis. J Natl Cancer Inst. 2005 Nov 16;97(22):1679–87.

78. Larsson SC, Giovannucci E, Wolk A. Dietary carbohydrate, glycemic index, and glycemic load in relation to risk of colorectal cancer in women. Am J Epidemiol. 2007 Feb 1;165(3):256–61.

79. Larsson SC, Bergkvist L, Rutegård J, Giovannucci E, Wolk A. Calcium and dairy food intakes are inversely associated with colorectal cancer risk in the Cohort of Swedish Men. Am J Clin Nutr. 2006 Mar;83(3):667–73.

80. Cho E, Smith-Warner SA, Spiegelman D, et al. Dairy foods, calcium, and colorectal cancer: A pooled analysis of 10 cohort studies. JNatlCancerInst. 2004 Jul 7;96(13):1015–22.

81. Fung T, Hu FB, Fuchs C, Giovannucci E, Hunter DJ, Stampfer MJ, Colditz GA, Willett WC. Major dietary patterns and the risk of colorectal cancer in women. ArchInternMed. 2003 Feb 10;163(3): 309–14.

82. Kim BC, Shin A, Hong CW, et al. Association of colorectal adenoma with components of metabolic syndrome. Cancer Causes Control. 2012 Mar 27 [epub ahead of print].

83. Kim JH, Lim YJ, Kim YH, et al. Is metabolic syndrome a risk factor for colorectal adenoma? Cancer Epidemiol Biomarkers Prev. 2007 Aug;16(8):1543–46.

84. Sinicrope FA, Foster NR, Sargent DJ, O'Connell MJ, Rankin C. Obesity is an independent prognostic variable in colon cancer survivors. Clin Cancer Res. 2010 Mar 15;16(6):1884–93.

85. Haydon AM, Macinnis RJ, English DR, Giles GG. Effect of physical activity and body size on survival after diagnosis with colorectal cancer. Gut. 2006 Jan;55(1):62–67.

86. Dehal AN, Newton CC, Jacobs EJ, Patel AV, Gapstur SM, Campbell PT. Impact of diabetes mellitus and insulin use on survival after colorectal cancer diagnosis: The Cancer Prevention Study-II Nutrition Cohort. J Clin Oncol. 2012 Jan 1;30(1):53–59.

87. Meyerhardt JA, Niedzwiecki D, Hollis D, et al. Association of dietary patterns with cancer recurrence and survival in patients with stage III colon cancer. JAMA. 2007 Aug 15;298(7):754–64.

88. Dignam JJ, Polite BN, Yothers G, Raich P, Colangelo L, O'Connell MJ, Wolmark N. Body mass index and outcomes in patients who receive adjuvant chemotherapy for colon cancer. J Natl Cancer Inst. 2006 Nov 15;98(22):1647–54.

89. Guiu B, Petit JM, Bonnetain F, et al. Visceral fat area is an independent predictive biomarker of outcome after first-line bevacizumab-based treatment in metastatic colorectal cancer. Gut. 2010 Mar;59(3):341–47.

90. Holmes MD, Chen WY, Feskanich D, Kroenke CH, Colditz GA. Physical activity and survival after breast cancer diagnosis. JAMA. 2005 May 25;293(20):2479–88.

91. Jeon JY, Meyerhardt JA. Energy in and energy out: What matters for survivors of colorectal cancer? J Clin Oncol. 2012 Jan 1;30(1):7–10.

92. Meyerhardt JA, Giovannucci EL, Holmes MD, Chan AT, Chan JA, Colditz GA, Fuchs CS. Physical activity and survival after colorectal cancer diagnosis. J Clin Oncol. 2006 Aug 1;24(22):3527–34.

93. Meyerhardt JA, Heseltine D, Niedzwiecki D, et al. Impact of physical activity on cancer recurrence and survival in patients with stage III colon cancer: Findings from CALGB89803. J Clin Oncol. 2006 Aug 1; 24(22):3535–41.

94. Richman EL, Kenfield SA, Stampfer MJ, Paciorek A, Carroll PR, Chan JM. Physical activity after diagnosis and risk of prostate cancer progression: Data from the cancer of the prostate strategic urologic research endeavor. Cancer Res. 2011 Jun 1;71(11):3889–95.

95. Adams TD, Gress RE, Smith SC, Halverson RC, Simper SC, Rosamond WD, LaMonte MJ, Stroup AM, Hunt SC. Long-term mortality after gastric bypass surgery. N Engl J Med. 2007;357:753–61.

96. Sjöström L, Gummesson A, Sjöström CD, Narbro K,; Swedish Obese Subjects Study. Effects of bariatric surgery on cancer incidence in obese patients in Sweden (Swedish Obese Subjects Study): A prospective, controlled intervention trial. Lancet Oncol. 2009 Jul;10(7):653–62.

97. Mitterberger MC, Mattesich M, Klaver E, Piza-Katzer H, Zwerschke W. Reduced insulin-like growth factor-I serum levels in formerly obese women subjected to laparoscopic-adjustable gastric banding or diet-induced long-term caloric restriction. J Gerontol A Biol Sci Med Sci. 2011 Nov;66(11):1169–77.

98. Chlebowski RT, Blackburn GL, Thomson CA, et al. Dietary fat reduction and breast cancer outcome: Interim efficacy results from the Women's Intervention Nutrition Study. J Natl Cancer Inst. 2006; 98:1767–76.

99. Pierce JP, Natarajan L, Caan BJ, Parker BA, Influence of a diet very high in vegetables, fruit, and fiber and low in fat on prognosis following treatment for breast cancer: The Women's Healthy Eating and Living (WHEL) randomized trial. JAMA. 2007 Jul 18;298(3):289–98.

100. Knowler WC, Barrett-Connor E, Fowler SE, et al. Reduction in the incidence of type 2 diabetes with lifestyle intervention or metformin. N Engl J Med. 2002;346:393–403.

101. Landman GW, Kleefstra N, van Hateren KJ, Groenier KH, Gans RO, Bilo HJ. Metformin associated with lower cancer mortality in type 2 diabetes: ZODIAC-16. Diabetes Care. 2010;33:322–26.

102. Jiralerspong S, Palla SL, Giordano SH, Meric-Bernstam F, Liedtke C, Barnett CM, Hsu L, Hung MC, Hortobagyi GN, Gonzalez-Angulo AM. Metformin and pathologic complete responses to neoadjuvant chemotherapy in diabetic patients with breast cancer. J Clin Oncol. 2009;27:3297–302.

103. He X, Esteva FJ, Ensor J, Hortobagyi GN, Lee MH, Yeung SC. Metformin and thiazolidinediones are associated with improved breast cancer-specific survival of diabetic women with HER2 + breast cancer. Ann Oncol. 2011 Nov 22.

104. Soley Bayraktar, Leonel F. Hernadez-Aya, Xiudong Lei, et al. Effect of metformin on survival outcomes in diabetic patients with triple receptor-negative breast cancer. Cancer. 2012;118:1202–11.

105. Tan BX, Yao WX, Ge J, et al. Prognostic influence of metformin as first-line chemotherapy for advanced non small cell lung cancer in patients with type 2 diabetes. Cancer. 2011 Nov 15;117(22):5103–11.

106. Talvensaari KK, Lanning M, Tapanainen P, Knip M. Long-term survivors of childhood cancer have an increased risk of manifesting the metabolic syndrome. J Clin Endocrinol Metab. 1996 Aug;81(8):3051–55.

107. Thivat E, Thérondel S, Lapirot O, et al. Weight change during chemotherapy changes the prognosis in nonmetastatic breast cancer for the worse. BMC Cancer. 2010 Nov 25;10:648.

108. Protani M, Coory M, Martin JH, et al. Effect of obesity on survival of women with breast cancer: Systematic review and meta-analysis. Breast Cancer Res Treat. 2010;123:627–35.

109. Collier A, Ghosh S, McGlynn B, Hollins G. Prostate cancer, androgen deprivation therapy, obesity, the metabolic syndrome, type 2 diabetes, and cardiovascular disease: A review. Am J Clin Oncol. 2011 Feb 3.

110. Hickish T, Astra's G, Thomas P, Pinfold S, Purandare L, Hickish TF, Kerr D. Glucose intolerance during adjuvant chemotherapy for breast cancer. J Natl Cancer Inst. 2009 Apr 1;101(7):537.

111. Nguyen NP, Vos P, Vinh-Hung V, et al. Altered glucose metabolism during hemoradiation for head and neck cancer. Anticancer Res. 2009 Nov;29(11):4683–87.

112. Zeng L, Biernacka KM, Holly JM, Jarrett C, Morrison AA, Morgan A, Winters ZE, Foulstone EJ, Shield JP, Perks CM. Hyperglycaemia confers resistance to chemotherapy on breast cancer cells: The role of fatty acid synthase. Endocr Relat Cancer. 2010 May 18;17(2):539–51.

113. Kuk JL, Ardern CI. Are metabolically normal but obese individuals at lower risk for all-cause mortality? Diabetes Care. 2009;32(12):2297–99.

114. Parsons HA, Baracos VE, Dhillon N, Hong DS, Kurzrock R Body composition, symptoms, and survival in advanced cancer patients referred to a phase I service. PLoS One. 2012;7(1):e29330.

115. Dodesini AR, Benedini S, Terruzzi I, Sereni LP, Luzi L. A review of cancer cachexia and abnormal glucose metabolism in humans with cancer. J Am Coll Nutr. 1992 Aug;11(4):445–56.

116. Boyd D. Insulin and cancer. Integr Cancer Ther. 2003;2(4):315–29.

117. Rajala MW, et al. Minireview: The adipocyte–at the crossroads of energy homeostasis, inflammation, and atherosclerosis. Endocrinology. 2003;144:3765–73.

118. Kershaw EE, Flier JS. Adipose tissue as an endocrine organ. J Clin Endocrinol Metab. 2004;89:2548–56.

119. Lumeng CN, et al. Increased inflammatory properties of adipose tissue macrophages recruited during diet-induced obesity. Diabetes. 2007;56:16–23.

120. Hursting SD, Nunez NP, Varticovski L, Vinson C The obesity-cancer link: Lessons learned from a fatless mouse. Cancer Res. 2007 Mar 15;67(6):2391–93.

121. Behan JW, Yun JP, Proektor MP, et al. Adipocytes impair leukemia treatment in mice. Cancer Res. 2009 Oct 1;69(19):7867–74.

122. Hursting SD, Smith SM, Lashinger LM, Harvey AE, Perkins SN. Calories and carcinogenesis: Lessons learned from 30 years of calorie restriction research. Carcinogenesis. 2010;31:83–89.

123. Longo VD, Finch CE. Evolutionary medicine: From dwarf model systems to healthy centenarians? Science. 2003;299(5611):1342–46.

124. Colman RJ, Anderson RM, Johnson SC, et al. Caloric restriction delays disease onset and mortality in rhesus monkeys. Science. 2009;325(59): 212–30.

125. Hursting SD, Lavigne JA, Berrigan D, Perkins SN, Barrett JC. Calorie restriction, aging, and cancer prevention: Mechanisms of action and applicability to humans. Annu Rev Med. 2003;54:131–52.

126. Moore T, Beltran L, Carbajal S, Strom S, Traag J, Hursting SD, DiGiovanni J. Dietary energy balance modulates signaling through the Akt/mammalian target of rapamycin pathways in multiple epithelial tissues. Cancer Prev Res (Phila Pa). 2008;1(1):65–76.

127. Kahn BB, Alquier T, Carling D, Hardie DG. AMP-activated protein kinase: Ancient energy gauge provides clues to modern understanding of metabolism. Cell Metab. 2005;1:15–25.

128. Shaw RJ, et al. The tumor suppressor LKB1 kinase directly activates AMP-activated kinase and regulates apoptosis in response to energy stress. Proc Natl Acad Sci USA. 2004;101:3329–35.

129. Towler MC, Hardie DG. AMP-activated protein kinase in metabolic control and insulin signaling. Circ Res. 2007;100:328–41.

130. Rous P. The influence of diet on transplanted and spontaneous mouse tumors. J Exp Med. 1914;20:433–51.

131. Tannenbaum A, Silverstone H. The influence of the degree of caloric restriction on the formation of skin tumors and hepatomas in mice. Cancer Res. 1949;9(12):724–27.

132. Dunn SE, et al. Dietary restriction reduces insulin-like growth factor I levels, which modulates apoptosis, cell proliferation, and tumor progression in p53-deficient mice. Cancer Res. 1997;57: (4667–7237):201–4.

133. Venkateswaran V, Haddad AQ, Fleshner NE, et al. Association of diet-induced hyperinsulinemia with accelerated growth of prostate cancer (LNCaP) xenografts. J Natl Cancer Inst. 2007;99:1793–800.

134. Novosyadlyy R, Lann DE, Vijayakumar A, et al. Insulin-mediated acceleration of breast cancer development and progression in a nonobese model of type 2 diabetes. Cancer Res. 2010;70:741–51.

135. Suh Y, Atzmon G, Cho MO, et al. Functionally significant insulin-like growth factor I receptor mutations in centenarians. Proc Natl Acad Sci USA. 2008;105:3438–42.

136. Pollak M. Insulin and insulin-like growth factor signalling in neoplasia. Nat Rev Cancer. 2008;8:915–28.
137. Kawada M, Inoue H, Masuda T, Ikeda D. Insulin-like growth factor I secreted from prostate stromal cells mediates tumor-stromal cell interactions of prostate cancer. Cancer Res. 2006 Apr 15;66(8):4419–25.
138. Gallagher EJ, LeRoith D. The proliferating role of insulin and insulin-like growth factors in cancer. Trends Endocrinol Metab. 2010;21:610–18.
139. Belfiore A, Frasca F, Pandini G, Sciacca L, Vigneri R. Insulin receptor isoforms and insulin receptor/insulin-like growth factor receptor hybrids in physiology and disease. Endocr Rev. 2009;30:586–623.
140. Pandini G, Vigneri R, Costantino A, et al. Insulin and insulin-like growth factor-I (IGF-I) receptor overexpression in breast cancers leads to insulin/IGF-I hybrid receptor overexpression: Evidence for a second mechanism of IGF-I signaling. Clin Cancer Res. 1999;5:1935–44.
141. Frasca F, Pandini G, Scalia P, et al. Insulin receptor isoform A, a newly recognized high-affinity insulin-like growth factor II receptor in fetal and cancer cells. Mol Cell Biol. 1999;19:3278–88.
142. Kroemer G, Pouyssegur J. Tumor cell metabolism: Cancer's Achilles' heel. Cancer Cell. 2008;13:472–82.
143. Vander Heiden MG, Cantley LC, Thompson CB. Understanding the Warburg effect: The metabolic requirements of cellproliferation. Science. 2009 May 22;324(5930):1029–33.
144. Warburg O. On the origin of cancer cells. Science. 1956;123:309–14.
145. Hirschhaeuser F, Sattler UG, Mueller-Klieser W. Lactate: A metabolic key player in cancer. Cancer Res. 2011 Nov 15;71(22):6921–25.
146. Keith B, Johnson RS, Simon MC. HIF1α and HIF2α: Sibling rivalry in hypoxic tumour growth and progression. Nat Rev Cancer. 2011 Dec 15;12(1):9–22.
147. Gatenby RA, Gawlinski ET, Gmitro AF, Kaylor B, Gillies RJ. Acid-mediated tumor invasion: A multidisciplinary study. Cancer Res. 2006;66:5216–23.
148. Wise DR, Thompson CB. Glutamine addiction: A new therapeutic target in cancer. Trends Biochem Sci. 2010 Aug;35(8):427–33.
149. Samuels Y, et al. High frequency of mutations of the PIK3CA gene in human cancers. Science. 2004;304:554.
150. Lee JW, Soung YH, Kim SY, Lee HW, Park WS, Nam SW, Kim SH, Lee JY, Yoo NJ, Lee SH. PIK3CA gene is frequently mutated in breast carcinomas and hepatocellular carcinomas. Oncogene. 2005;24:1477–80.
151. Kalaany NY, et al. Tumours with PI3K activation are resistant to dietary restriction. Nature. 2009; 458:725–31.
152. Bailey CJ, Turner RC. Metformin. N Engl J Med. 1996;334:574–79.
153. Decensi A, Puntoni M, Goodwin P, et al. Metformin and cancer risk in diabetic patients: A systematic review and meta-analysis. Cancer Prev Res. 2010;3:1451–61.
154. Libby G, Donnelly LA, Donnan PT, Alessi DR, Morris AD, Evans JM. New users of metformin are at low risk of incident cancer: A cohort study among people with type 2 diabetes. Diabetes Care. 2009 Sep;32(9):1620–25.
155. Ish-Shalom D, Christoffersen CT, Vorwerk P, Sacerdoti-Sierra N, Shymko RM, Naor D, De Meyts P. Mitogenic properties of insulin and insulin analogues mediated by the insulin receptor. Diabetologia. 1997;40(Suppl 2):S25–31.
156. Lai SW, Liao KF, Chen PC, et al. Antidiabetes drugs correlate with decreased risk of lung cancer: A population-based observation in Taiwan. Clin Lung Cancer. 2012 Mar;13(2):143–48.
157. Ben Sahra I, Le Marchand-Brustel Y, Tanti JF, Bost F. Metformin in cancer therapy: A new perspective for an old antidiabetic drug? Mol Cancer Ther. 2010;9:1092–99.
158. Kisfalvi K, Eibl G, Sinnett-Smith J, Rozengurt E. Metformin disrupts crosstalk between G protein-coupled receptor and insulin receptor signaling systems and inhibits pancreatic cancer growth. CancerRes. 2009 Aug 15;69(16):6539–45.
159. Iliopoulos D, Hirsch HA, Struhl K. Metformin decreases the dose of chemotherapy for prolonging tumor remission in mouse xenografts involving multiple cancer cell types. Cancer Res. 2011 May 1;71(9):3196–201.
160. Hirsch HA, Iliopoulos D, Tsichlis PN, Struhl K. Metformin selectively targets cancer stem cells, and acts together with chemotherapy to block tumor growth and prolong remission. Cancer Res. 2009;69: 7507–11.
161. Tan BX, Yao WX, Ge J, et al. Prognostic influence of metformin as first-line chemotherapy for advanced nonsmall cell lung cancer in patients with type 2 diabetes. Cancer. 2011 Nov 15;117(22):5103–11.
162. Memmott RM, Mercado JR, Maier CR, Kawabata S, Fox SD, Dennis PA. Metformin prevents tobacco carcinogen— induced lung tumorigenesis. Cancer Prev Res (Phila). 2010;3:1066–76.
163. Goodwin PJ, Ligibel JA, Stambolic V. Metformin in breast cancer: Time for action. J Clin Oncol. 2009 Jul 10;27(20):3271–73.

164. Rosmond R, Dallman MF, Björntorp P. Stress-related cortisol secretion in men: Relationships with abdominal obesity and endocrine, metabolic and hemodynamic abnormalities. J Clin Endocrinol Metab. 1998 Jun;83(6):1853–59.

165. Diz-Chaves Y. Ghrelin, appetite regulation, and food reward: Interaction with chronic stress. Int J Pept. 2011;2011:898450.

166. Grutsch JF, Ferrans C, Wood PA, et al. The association of quality of life with potentially remediable disruptions of circadian sleep/activity rhythms in patients with advanced lung cancer. BMC Cancer. 2011 May 23;11:193.

167. Schernhammer ES, Kroenke CH, Laden F, Hankinson SE. Night work and risk of breast cancer. Epidemiology. 2006 Jan;17(1):108–11.

168. Viswanathan AN, Hankinson SE, Schernhammer ES Night shift work and the risk of endometrial cancer. Cancer Res. 2007 Nov 1;67(21):10618–22.

169. Schernhammer ES, Laden F, Speizer FE, Willett WC, Hunter DJ, Kawachi I, Fuchs CS, Colditz GA. Night-shift work and risk of colorectal cancer in the nurses' health study. J Natl Cancer Inst. 2003 Jun 4;95(11):825–28.

170. Kubo T, Ozasa K, Mikami K, et al. Prospective cohort study of the risk of prostate cancer among rotating-shift workers: Findings from the Japan collaborative cohort study. Am J Epidemiol. 2006 Sep 15;164(6):549–55.

171. Brown MA, Goodwin JL, Silva GE, Behari A, Newman AB, Punjabi NM, Resnick HE, Robbins JA, Quan SF The impact of sleep-disordered breathing on body mass index(BMI): The Sleep Heart Health Study(SHHS). Southwest J Pulm Crit Care. 2011 Dec 8;3:159–68.

172. Schmid SM, Hallschmid M, Jauch-Chara K, Born J, Schultes B. A single night of sleep deprivation increases ghrelin levels and feelings of hunger in normal-weight healthy men. J Sleep Res. 2008 Sep;17(3):331–34.

173. Balkau B, Vol S, Loko S, Andriamboavonjy T, Lantieri O, Gusto G, Meslier N, Racineux JL, Tichet J. Epidemiologic study on the Insulin Resistance Syndrome Study Group high baseline insulin levels associated with 6-year incident observed sleep apnea. Diabetes Care. 2010 May;33(5):1044–49.

174. Kushi LH, Doyle C, McCullough M, Rock CL, Demark-Wahnefried W, Bandera EV, Gapstur S, Patel AV, Andrews K, Gansler T; American Cancer Society 2010. Nutrition and Physical Activity Guidelines Advisory Committee. American Cancer Society Guidelines on nutrition and physical activity for cancer prevention: Reducing the risk of cancer with healthy food choices and physical activity. CA Cancer J Clin. 2012 Jan–Feb;62(1):30–67.

175. Cerhan JR, Potter JD, Gilmore JM, et al. Adherence to the AICR cancer prevention recommendations and subsequent morbidity and mortality in the Iowa Women's Health Study cohort. Cancer Epidemiol Biomarkers Prev. 2004;13:1114–20.

176. McCullough ML, Patel AV, Kushi LH, Patel R, Willett WC, Doyle C, Thun MJ, Gapstur SM. Following cancer prevention guidelines reduces risk of cancer, cardiovascular disease, and all-cause mortality. Cancer Epidemiol Biomarkers Prev. 2011 Jun;20(6):1089–97.

177. Masko EM, Thomas JA, Antonelli JA, et al. Low-carbohydrate diets and prostate cancer: How low is "low enough"? Cancer Prev Res (Phila). 2010;3:1124–31.

178. Ibrahim MM, Fjære E, Lock EJ, et al. Chronic consumption of farmed salmon containing persistent organic pollutants causes insulin resistance and obesity in mice. PLoS One. 2011;6(9):e25170. Epub 2011 Sep 23.

179. Liu H, Huang D, McArthur DL, Boros LG, Nissen N, Heaney AP. Fructose induces transketolase flux to promote pancreatic cancer growth. Cancer Res. 2010 Aug 1;70(15):6368–76.

180. Lee D, Steffes MW Sjödin A, Jones RS, Needham LL, Jacobs DR. Low dose of some persistent organic pollutants predicts type 2 diabetes: A nested case–control study. Environ Health Perspect. 2010;118:1235–42.

181. Holdcamp W. Obesogens: An environmental link to obesity. Environ Health Perspect.120(2):A63–A68.

38 Breast Cancer

Nutrition to Promote Recovery and Diminish Recurrence Risk

Keith I. Block, M.D., and Charlotte Gyllenhaal, Ph.D.

INTRODUCTION

There are currently more than 2.6 million breast cancer survivors in the United States [1]. During intensive surgery, radiation, and chemotherapy treatments, these patients are mainly under the care of specialists. After completing surgery, radiation, and adjuvant chemotherapy as needed, patients commonly undergo long-term endocrine treatment, during which time the primary care physician may see the patient more regularly. The use of aromatase inhibitors and other new therapies has increased survival times in breast cancer and is leading to a growing population focused on survivorship after primary treatment. For many postmenopausal early breast cancer patients, risk of cardiovascular disease is now equivalent to risk of breast cancer recurrence [2]. Long-term supervision of breast cancer patients must therefore manage both cancer and cardiovascular risk.

Primary care physicians who provide long-term care for breast cancer survivors are well placed to implement nutritional strategies. Recent research in nutrition is leading toward a consensus that management of weight and dietary patterns may contribute substantially to breast cancer survival, limit recurrence risks, reduce comorbidities, and improve well-being.

EPIDEMIOLOGY

Breast cancer is a family of diseases, each of which must be treated distinctively. For example, patients with early breast cancers that have estrogen receptors (ER positive) are treated with tamoxifen and aromatase inhibitors, while those that are ER negative receive chemotherapy. A further distinction is made with those with Her2/*neu* positive breast cancer, which is treated with Herceptin®. Treatment guidelines for breast cancer constitute a complex decision tree with very different treatment protocols for different situations. Conventional breast cancer treatment is thus becoming increasingly individualized. Genetic data analysis of breast cancers is also increasingly available. In the future, nutrition recommendations may be specific to breast cancer subtype and genetics, but while such advice is possible, supporting data are not yet available.

PATHOPHYSIOLOGY

While breast cancer treatment has been perceived for many years to be related to nutrition, the relationships have been controversial. Recent advances in research appear to be clarifying the situation.

Dietary patterns and caloric intake influence inflammation and insulin responsiveness to ultimately improve breast cancer survival. Fruits and vegetables are phytochemically rich foods and may influence outcomes. There is also a new awareness of alcohol consumption as a breast cancer risk factor.

DIETARY PATTERNS

The evidence for nutritional impacts on breast cancer is growing, although further research is needed before the efficacy of nutritional treatment is proven. Two large trials of diet and breast cancer have been conducted: the Women's Healthy Eating and Living (WHEL) randomized trial of a low-fat diet high in vegetables, fruit, and fiber [3,4], and the Women's Intervention Nutrition Study (WINS) trial of a low-fat diet [5]. More recently, a number of cohort studies of postdiagnosis diet in breast cancer have become available. The high-quality evidence provided by these studies has added to our knowledge of breast cancer and diet.

In the WINS study, the intervention group had a lower risk of recurrence, most significantly in ER negative patients. In the WHEL study, there was no difference in breast cancer events or in mortality between the two groups. However, different adherence to the recommended low-fat (20%) diets may explain these results. Notably, the low-fat group in the WINS study lost weight during the study, while the WHEL group did not. Among the WHEL patients, however, those who did not have hot flashes at baseline (i.e., those with higher estrogen levels) were found to have low rates of recurrence on the study diet [6], suggesting that the diet did improve the hormonal status of these women.

Smaller diet intervention studies [7,8] that counseled weight loss or lower caloric intake generally observed reduced mortality. Our study of a cohort of 90 metastatic breast cancer patients on a low-fat, mostly vegetarian diet along with exercise and other integrative interventions recorded an extended median survival time of 38 months, in comparison with survivals in the general range of 18–24 months in contemporaneous research trials and studies of community data [9].

Data on cohorts of postdiagnosis breast cancer patients point to obesity as one of the nutritional factors most important in breast cancer prognosis. Obesity, especially abdominal obesity, is associated with chronic inflammation and insulin resistance, both of which are characteristic of the metabolic syndrome [10], and known to increase cancer risks. Obesity increases the risk of metastasis and reduces survival in breast cancer, independently of other factors [11,12] and weight gain after diagnosis may be associated with recurrence or reduced survival [13]. Breast cancer patients placed on low-fat or low-carbohydrate diets were able to lose weight and improve insulin-related variables such as insulin resistance and hemoglobin A1c [14–16].

Experimental studies of diet in breast cancer suggest that controlling weight may improve breast cancer prognosis, though clinical trials are needed to confirm this. Patients who are overweight or obese should be encouraged to consult with a nutritionist for meal planning. They should receive regular follow-up to encourage healthy weight loss to a normal weight, to reduce risks associated with both breast cancer and cardiovascular diseases. Exercise is important in weight control and is associated with reduced mortality in breast cancer patients [17]. Because of its strong relationship to insulin resistance [18,19], exercise is discussed in Chapter 37.

Other cohort studies have examined different aspects of diet. These studies typically distinguish breast cancer–related mortality and all-cause or overall mortality, which includes mortality from comorbid conditions as well and highlights the survivorship concerns with this cancer. Patients who were on a "prudent" diet, for instance, were observed to have a decreased overall and non-breast cancer mortality [20]. Saturated and trans fat intake significantly predicted all-cause mortality, and nonsignificantly predicted breast cancer mortality [21]. Intake of vegetables reduced breast cancer recurrences in tamoxifen users [22], while high serum carotenoid levels were associated with improved breast cancer–free survival [23].

Postmenopausal patients who had high intakes of fiber and lignans (found in flax, sesame, cereal grains, soy, and cruciferous vegetables) had significantly reduced overall mortality [24]; a study of prediagnosis diet also found an inverse correlation of lignans and (nonsignificantly) dried beans with overall mortality [25]. Dietary fiber, although not carbohydrates or glycemic index, was inversely associated with total mortality, breast cancer mortality, and recurrence [26].

A report by the Institute of Medicine has focused on moderate alcohol intake as a breast cancer risk factor. Cohort studies of postdiagnosis alcohol intake suggest that moderate intake (three to six drinks per week) increases breast cancer recurrence, especially among overweight patients. However, moderate alcohol intake also reduces all-cause mortality in breast cancer patients [27,28]. The relationship of alcohol to breast cancer events and overall mortality emphasizes the complexity of managing overall health and survival in breast cancer survivors, and suggests that low alcohol intake may be more suitable than abstinence for early breast cancer patients who are already accustomed to alcohol intake.

Patients on low-fat or low-calorie diets may lose muscle mass (lean body mass) as well as fat, although resistance exercise (strength training) may help to maintain muscle mass [29]. Chemotherapy may also provoke loss of lean body mass and increase of fat mass. This change in body composition is undesirable since it impairs activities of daily living and reduces immune competence. [30,31]. It is also important to maintain adequate protein in the diet. In the context of a low-fat diet based largely on plant proteins, suitable protein sources include legumes and beans, egg whites, fish, and protein supplements including sources of amino acids or whey protein. Along with excluding red meat, refined grains, and sugar, and increasing fruit and vegetable intake, a whole-foods diet is also suitable for reducing risks of cardiovascular disease. Healthful fats and whole grains help reduce metabolic syndrome [14,15]. Fruits and vegetables are also low in calories, potentially assisting weight loss by reducing caloric density of the diet (Chapter 18, Obesity). In addition to phytochemical effects, diets high in fruits and vegetables contribute to a more alkaline internal pH, which may help reduce cancer risks [32].

A whole-foods Mediterranean diet may be suitable for patients with metabolic syndrome and also reduces cardiovascular risk [33], although its specific effect on breast cancer is not known.

HORMONES AND INFLAMMATION

Fats both modulate the hormonal milieu and contribute to the inflammatory potential of the diet. Modification of hormonal levels may require major modification of fat intake. It is primarily saturated fats that modulate the hormonal milieu. Low saturated-fat diets may suppress estrogenic stimulation of breast cancer growth, and some studies of low-fat or high-fiber diets have observed lowering of estradiol levels. Other studies in healthy women observed that low-fat, high-fiber diets lowered serum estrogen, although changes were not always significant and were not maintained after intervention periods were concluded [34]. Long-term commitment to dietary change may thus be required to alter estrogen levels. The role of environmental xenoestrogens in breast cancer prognosis is not clear; detoxification of these estrogens can be supported through a diet high in fiber and vegetables and low in animal foods, as well as exercise and choosing organic foods where possible (or maintaining awareness and avoidance of the foods highest in pesticide residues).

Obesity is associated with chronic low-level inflammation that contributes to cancer growth, and should be addressed with weight loss. But dietary factors also promote inflammation. Nutrition and supplements may modulate production of prostaglandin E2 [35], which promotes cell proliferation, inhibits apoptosis, and increases angiogenesis and invasiveness and may thus contribute to the progression of cancer. Patients with low levels of omega-3 fatty acids tend to have higher proinflammatory markers, indicated by tests such as C-reactive protein (CRP), and lower anti-inflammatory cytokines [36]. Breast cancer patients with higher intakes of the omega-3 fatty acids EPA and DHA from food had significantly reduced breast cancer recurrences and other events, as well as reduced all-cause mortality, suggesting the importance of moderating inflammation for this population [37].

The inflammatory state may affect quality of life as well as cancer progression. Both persistent fatigue in breast cancer survivors [38] and chemotherapy-related symptoms such as anorexia, cachexia, sleep disturbance, and depression [39] have been linked to elevated levels of inflammatory cytokines. However, major dietary changes may be needed to successfully modify levels of these markers [40]. Breast cancer patients who ate more whole grains, leafy green vegetables, tomatoes, and anti-inflammatory nutrients were less likely to be fatigued than other patients [41]. High intake of *trans* fatty acids was found to be strongly correlated with such inflammatory markers as plasma CRP, interleukin-6, soluble tumor necrosis factor receptors, E-selectin, and soluble cell adhesion molecules in healthy women [42]. Exercise training (stationary bike) has been reported to reduce CRP [43,44], perhaps due to weight loss, although one study found this effect disappeared when adjusted for increased fiber intake. Fiber intake over 15 g/day was associated with a lower probability of elevated CRP [45].

The pineal hormone melatonin, which has multiple anticancer activities, is of great interest in breast cancer. Night shift work, which disrupts circadian rhythm and reduces melatonin levels, is associated with elevated breast cancer risk. Suggestions for normalizing circadian function have been presented by Block et al. [46].

PHYTOCHEMICALS AND OTHER SUPPLEMENTS

Rock and Demark–Wahnefried found that that higher fruit and vegetable intakes are associated with better survival in breast cancer [47]. This suggests that the numerous phytochemicals in plants may improve breast cancer outcomes. Meta-analyses of trials on single antioxidants, however, show that single vitamins or phytochemicals do not improve cancer mortality or recurrence [48,49], although a cohort study of breast cancer patients found that patients using vitamins C and E had lower recurrence rates, while those using vitamin E had lower all-cause mortality; patients using combination carotenoids, however, had higher breast cancer mortality [50].

A more strategic approach to supplementation, which targets known metabolic disturbances with multiple, targeted supplements is more likely to succeed in improving outcomes. Testing of the internal biochemical milieu, which we term the "terrain," can be used to individualize supplementation based on standard laboratory assays [32] (see "Patient Evaluation" section in this chapter). Phytochemicals and supplements of special interest in breast cancer are briefly reviewed in this section.

Advancing understandings on the potential impact of soy on breast cancer prognosis were recently summarized by Messina et al. [51]. Soy isoflavones, such as genistein, have a molecular structure similar to estrogens and bind to estrogen receptors. They exert estrogen-like effects in some animal models; however, the digestion of soyfoods in these models has been shown to result in much higher levels of genistein than in humans. Further, cohort studies in breast cancer patients, three in China and two in the United States, indicate no stimulation of breast cancer and, in fact, have a trend to better outcomes in patients with high soy intake, including those with estrogen-sensitive tumors [51–53]. A randomized trial of two years of soy isoflavones in healthy menopausal women found no effects on lymphocytes, serum free thyroxine, endometrial thickness, or fibroid occurrence, and a lower-than-expected breast cancer incidence in both groups [54]. Messina et al. feel that moderate intake of soy foods as part of the diet is reasonable for breast cancer patients, although soy isoflavone supplements need further evaluation in high-risk women, and sufficient data do not exist to encourage these for postmenopausal ER positive breast cancer patients. Traditional forms of soy foods are recommended, rather than highly processed products. Soy has been observed to increase serum IGF-1, an effect that was reduced by seaweed supplements [55]. The IGF-1 effect suggests that soy intake should be moderate and balanced with other protein sources.

Several herbal medicines also have phytoestrogenic effects and should likely not be taken in large amounts by postmenopausal women with ER positive tumors, including licorice, red clover, fennel, fenugreek, hops, yucca, alfalfa, and wild carrot. Black cohosh, used for hot flashes (though not yet demonstrated to be effective), is likely not estrogenic, but occasional liver damage related to intake has been reported. While some animal studies raise concerns about cancer stimulation, a cohort study found that women using black cohosh had lower recurrence risks than nonusers [56–58].

Flax is high in lignans, which are phytoestrogenic, and is also a fiber source that has cancer-suppressive potential. Breast cancer patients who took flax-supplemented muffins before diagnostic surgery had high levels of apoptosis in cancer cells [45]. Flax may increase the ratio of 2-hydroxyestrone, a less cancer-stimulating estrogen metabolite, to 16-alpha hydroxyestrone which is more cancer-stimulating, although trials are conflicting [59–62]. Flax did not improve hot flashes in a Phase III trial [61]; an observational study, however, found that high dietary fiber was associated with reduced vasomotor symptoms [63].

Cruciferous vegetable phytonutrients include indole-3-carbinol (I3C), which increased 2-hydroxyestrone relative to 16-alpha-hydroxyestrone [64], as did cruciferous vegetable powder [65] in small trials. A review suggests, however, that this ratio may oversimplify the effects of different estrogen metabolites [66]. Diindolylmethane (DIM) may potentiate Taxotere® effects by inhibiting NF-kappaB [67]. Sulforaphane, which inhibits breast cancer stem cells in vitro, has been found in breast tissue after women ate broccoli sprouts, supporting the use of foods as sources of this nutrient [68,69].

Besides foods that are high in phytochemicals, such as soy and crucifers, a number of herbs, isolated phytochemicals, and related substances are available as dietary supplements. Research findings on these supplements are summarized in Table 38.1.

MINERALS AND VITAMINS

Iodine occurs in dietary seaweeds, which are consumed frequently in Asia where breast cancer rates are low, and is attracting attention for its anticarcinogenic effects. Breast cancer patients have been observed to have lower tissue iodine levels than normal controls [70]. Optimal thyroid function also requires iodine. Patients undertaking low-salt, low-fat vegetarian, or vegan diets, or increasing cruciferous vegetable intake may inadvertently reduce their iodine intake below the recommended daily allowance (RDA). Iodized salt, seaweed from clean waters, kelp tablets, or iodine-containing supplements can optimize iodine status.

Vitamin D is currently of interest in reducing cancer risk and improving prognosis for several cancers, including breast cancer. A meta-analysis of studies on vitamin D and calcium indicated that reduced risk of breast cancer was found among women with the highest levels of vitamin D and calcium [71]. Calcium and vitamin D are of particular importance for patients taking aromatase inhibitors (Arimidex®, Letrozole®, Femara®), which cause bone loss, osteoporosis, and fractures. It is important that patients on these medications take calcium (1500 mg/day) and vitamin D (1000 IU/day) [72]. Vitamin D may also help reduce joint pain typical of aromatase inhibitors. The use of an alkaline diet high in fruits and vegetables is relevant to controlling bone loss as well as risk of recurrence.

PHARMACOLOGY

Certain dietary supplements can be sources of potential drug interactions with cancer treatments. We will discuss these positive and negative interactions by the type of treatment involved. Additionally, chemotherapy agents deplete important vitamins or minerals in some cases; such depletion may be addressed through diet or supplementation.

Oncologists express concern about the use of dietary supplements concurrently with chemotherapy. Antioxidants may ameliorate chemotherapy side effects, but there is concern that they may counteract the therapeutic effects of some chemotherapy drugs as well as radiation therapy, which have free-radical-based mechanisms of action. A review of antioxidants given concurrently with such chemotherapy agents did not find evidence for diminished tumor response or an adverse impact on survival, although the trials involved were small and of lower quality. Antioxidants also appeared to diminish a variety of side effects, suggesting that evidence to date leans toward the use of antioxidants with chemotherapy [80]. A review of antioxidants and radiation therapy found several small

TABLE 38.1

Research Summary on Widely Used Breast Cancer Phytochemical and Related Supplements. Type of Human Study Is Indicated (Cohort, Case-control, Phase II, Meta-analysis)

Supplement [References]	Mechanism	In Vitro	Animal Studies	Human Studies	Comments
Curcumin [73,74]	Anti-inflammatory; inhibits NF-kappaB	Sensitized cells to Taxol™	Reduced ER+ mammary cancer		Bioavailability is a challenge; address with novel formulations
Fish oil [37,75,76]	Anti-inflammatory; inhibits NF-kappaB	Proapoptotic, antiangiogenic effects on breast cancer cell lines	Reduce bone metastases	Dietary omega-3 reduced recurrence (cohort); DHA potentiated anthracyclines (Phase II)	
Green tea [77]	Multi-targeted	Proapoptotic effects and inhibited metalloproteinase (angiogenesis) in breast cancer cell lines	Sensitized mouse tumors to Taxol™	Intake > 3 cups per day associated with reduced recurrence (meta-analysis of cohorts)	
Resveratrol [69]	Multi-targeted	Sensitized cells to cyclophosphamide, not Taxol™	Induced apoptosis and inhibited angiogenesis in implanted human tumors	Resveratrol from grapes reduced breast cancer risk (case-control)	Inhibits CYP enzymes
Vitamin E [50,78,79]	Antiproliferative, proapoptotic, antioxidant	Tocotrienols: antiangiogenic, antiprolfierative and proapoptotic effects on breast cancer cells	Gamma-tocopherol inhibited growth of implanted breast cancer cells	Antioxidant use, including vitamin E, reduced recurrence (cohort)	Alpha-tocopherol alone is questionable. Mixed tocopherols, with tocotrienols, or alpha-toco-pheryl succinate may be more effective.

trials that showed potential positive effects, although there are still concerns with protection of tumors [81]. Vitamin E along with Trental® reduced radiation-induced fibrosis in the shoulder.

A large trial of beta-carotene and vitamin E supplements during radiation therapy for head and neck cancer observed excess recurrence and mortality risks with supplements, but improved side effects. Later analysis, however, showed that excess risks of recurrence and mortality were all among those patients who smoked tobacco during supplementation [82]. Analysis of dietary intakes and plasma beta-carotene showed that patients who had higher dietary beta-carotene intake had lower incidence of adverse radiation effects, and those with higher plasma levels had lower rates of recurrence [83]. An additional complication in this study was that the vitamin E intake was in the form of alpha-tocopherol, which, as noted in Table 38.1, reduces effects of other forms of natural vitamin E (a mixture of 8 tocopherols and tocotrienols) [79].

Some chemotherapy agents used in breast cancer treatment deplete critical nutrient stores. Vitamin or mineral supplements may be useful in avoiding deficiencies, although specific evidence is not available in most cases. The most likely potential interactions are the following:

- **Adriamycin—riboflavin (vitamin B2) and iron:** foods high in riboflavin, such as dark green vegetables, squash, and almonds can be advised. The interaction with iron may worsen cardiac toxicity, so iron supplements should be avoided except in the case of deficiency.
- **5-fluorouracil—niacin and thiamin:** deficiencies can arise. In addition to supplements, niacin- and thiamin-rich foods can be recommended (salmon, tuna, fortified cereals/bread for niacin and tuna, asparagus, and dried beans for thiamin).
- **Cisplatin used in some protocols for relapsed metastatic disease—magnesium, potassium, zinc, l-carnitine:** intravenous magnesium supplementation is commonly used with cisplatin due to the severe deficiencies it causes. Potassium depletion can be addressed through remedying magnesium deficiency. Foods containing zinc include oysters, cashews, and baked beans. L-carnitine can be obtained in supplements.
- **Methotrexate—folate:** folate supplementation should be avoided during treatment unless prescribed by an oncologist, due to the potential to interfere with methotrexate's mechanism of action.

Extended periods of nausea, vomiting, and diarrhea during chemotherapy may cause multinutrient deficiencies. Supplementation or careful dietary adjustments may need to be undertaken during or after chemotherapy for patients who experience poor control of these side effects.

St. John's wort is well known for causing pharmacokinetic herb-drug interactions based on its induction of the cytochrome P450 isoenzyme 3A4, which can cause the many drugs metabolized by this enzyme to drop to subtherapeutic levels in the blood [83]. St. John's wort should be avoided during chemotherapy and related therapies. These protocols involve many drugs metabolized by different isoenzymes, raising the possibility that a patient will encounter an adverse interaction. Additional herb and food interactions with drugs are shown in Table 38.2 [85–89].

Anticoagulant herbs may affect both patients who have low platelet counts due to chemotherapy and those who are taking warfarin, given to cancer patients to prevent thrombosis. For patients taking warfarin, which has a narrow therapeutic index and is prone to drug interactions, the use of these anticoagulant herbs is problematic, as is the ingestion of foods that contain large amounts of vitamin K. This may become clinically relevant for cancer patients who frequently consume leafy green vegetables as part of a low-fat diet or drink beverages based on green vegetables, often called "green drinks." If patients take anticoagulant foods and supplements consistently, warfarin dose can be adjusted to account for dietary characteristics, since INR is monitored regularly.

Selected herbs and supplements have the potential to reduce chemotherapy and radiation therapy side effects, as shown in randomized and open-label trials (Table 38.3). The medication Gelclair® combines a licorice phytochemical with hyaluronic acid and a bioadherent gel to assist the two compounds in adhering to the gums as a strategy to decrease mucositis. Milk thistle may be considered as a hepatoprotector in patients with existing liver damage who undergo breast cancer chemotherapy or who experience marked abnormalities in liver function tests [90]. Taxanes, Adriamycin®, and the CMF (cyclophosphamide, methotrexate, and fluorouracil 5FU) chemotherapy regimen have some potential to cause hepatotoxicity [91]. High doses of melatonin (20 mg/day at bedtime) have been demonstrated for some chemotherapy protocols to improve survival and decrease chemotherapy side effects, but the protocols in which it is useful for breast cancer are as yet not well defined.

COMORBID CONDITIONS

Obesity, type 2 diabetes, and cardiovascular disease are all important comorbidities in breast cancer. See Chapters 18 and 19 and Section II of this book. Cardiovascular disease is especially relevant

---

TABLE 38.2

Supplements and Foods That Induce or Inhibit Cytochrome P450 Isoenzymes Relevant to Drugs Used in Breast Cancer Treatment

Pharmacokinetic Interactions

CYP450 isoenzyme induced or inhibited by foods or supplements	*Breast cancer medications metabolized by CYP450 isoenzyme*
CYP450 3A4	
Goldenseal	Emend®
Grapefruit	Decadron®
Star fruit	Taxol®
St. John's wort	Taxotere®
Resveratrol	
CYP450 1A2	
Cruciferous vegetables	Zofran®
Chargrilled meat	Warfarin
Echinacea	
Resveratrol	
CYP450 2D6	
Goldenseal	Zofran®
Resveratrol	Tamoxifen

Sources: [85,86,87,88,89,110].

Note: Not all potential interactions have been shown to be clinically relevant. Grapefruit interactions apply only to medications taken orally.

---

in postmenopausal patients with early stage breast cancer who have completed treatment and are in remission. Dietary patterns that may raise risks of breast cancer recurrence are the same ones that increase cardiovascular risks. Additionally, patients who incur cardiotoxicity from Adriamycin® or Herceptin® will need closer monitoring and perhaps medication.

PATIENT EVALUATION

As part of the physical examination at the primary care visit, weight should be monitored and body mass index (BMI) calculated. Since breast cancer risk and recurrence rates increase markedly at higher BMIs, and since weight gain during chemotherapy may worsen prognosis, control of weight is a primary area of prevention and intervention. Body composition analysis is particularly important for the patient who loses or gains weight during chemotherapy. Patients may be at risk for loss of muscle mass due to inactivity and loss of appetite from chemotherapy drugs. This can lead to losses of lean muscle and gains in fat mass, especially in patients who gain weight. Patients should engage in some type of strength exercise to avoid losing muscle mass; loss of fat mass, however, is entirely appropriate for the overweight patient. Advanced cancer patients are at higher risk of weight loss due to cachexia, an inflammatory condition that triggers a loss of muscle tissue. Although cachexia is less common in breast cancer than in gastrointestinal and lung cancers, it can occur in some patients. Such muscle wasting is also associated with a worsened prognosis.

Ongoing assessment of inflammation and glycemic variables is part of routine laboratory workups in integrative oncology clinics, and is recommended [32]; it will assist in managing cardiovascular disease risks as well as cancer. C-reactive protein (healthful levels < 1.0), erythrocyte sedimentation rate (healthful level 0 to 30 mm/hour), and fibrinogen (healthful level < 300 mg/dL)

TABLE 38.3

Foods and Nutrients With Potential to Relieve Chemotherapy and Radiation Side Effects

Condition	Herb or Nutrient	Contra-indications	Evidence	Dosage	Reference
Delayed nausea and vomiting	Ginger	Low platelet counts; warfarin	RCT	0.5–1.0 g dried powder every 4 hours	[92]
Fatigue	L-carnitine	None	Open-label trials + RCT	0.5–2.0 mg/day	[93,94]
Fatigue	Ginseng (Korean or American)	Estrogen-receptor positive tumors	Pilot RCT	1–2 g/day take in AM	[95,96]
Cardiotoxicity from Adriamycin®	Coenzyme Q10	None	Small trials	60–200 mg/day	[97]
Peripheral neuropathy	Glutamine	None	Review	0.5 g/kg/day	[98]
Mucositis/ stomatitis	Glutamine	None	RCTs	0.5 g/kg/day "Swish and swallow"	[99–101]
Mucositis/ stomatitis	Acetyl-l-carnitine	Epilepsy, bipolar disorder	RCTs	500 mg tid	[102]
Radiation skin reaction	Calendula	Allergy to plants in daisy family	RCT	Calendula ointment 1X apply topically after each radiation session	[103]

RCT = Randomized Controlled Trial

are basic inflammatory measurements. Abnormally high inflammation can be addressed pharmaceutically, or by optimizing the omega-6 to omega-3 ratio and avoiding *trans* fats, and with herbal supplements such as boswellia, curcumin, and bromelain. For discussion of insulin resistance and related conditions, see Chapter 37.

SPECIAL CONDITIONS

BONE METASTASES

Recommendations to use diet and exercise to achieve or maintain normal weight apply to patients with bone metastases as well as to other patients. However, referral to a physical therapist may be warranted to help the patient develop safe exercise routines. For instance, high-impact exercises should be avoided, and exercises such as some yoga positions that involve twisting the spine or placing excessive torque on extremities should not be attempted by patients with spinal or other metastases.

CARDIOMYOPATHY

Patients with cardiomyopathy from Adriamycin® or Herceptin® also need exercise, but should be advised that interval training, in which short periods of exercise alternate with rest, may prevent exhaustion or stress on the heart and are thus preferable to continuous aerobic training. Nutrients involved in ATP production, including ribose, coenzyme Q10, l-carnitine, and magnesium may augment pharmacologic management. The herb hawthorn may be useful for symptom management [104].

NEUROPATHY

Peripheral neuropathy is a dose-limiting toxicity of taxane treatment, which is commonly used in breast cancer. Up to 88% of Taxol patients may experience mild or moderate neuropathy. Alpha-lipoic acid, glutamine, vitamin E, and acetyl-l-carnitine have undergone preliminary testing for taxane neuropathy [105,106].

HOT FLASHES

Hot flashes and night sweats are common in breast cancer patients with oophorectomy- or chemotherapy-induced menopause and in those taking tamoxifen. Management of hot flashes in ER positive breast cancer can be perplexing because of the need to avoid hormone therapy. Supplemental doses of black cohosh have yielded mixed results on efficacy and safety [107]. Gold and colleagues analyzed diet composition and hot flashes in women in the WHEL study [63]. Higher severity of symptoms was associated with increased BMI and smoking, while lower severity was associated with high fiber intake. Weight loss may ameliorate hot flashes.

LYMPHEDEMA

Arm lymphedema following surgical removal of lymph nodes as part of diagnostic assessment is particularly problematic for obese patients. Recent small trials have indicated that weight loss is likely to help manage lymphedema [108,109].

SUMMARY

- Intensive chemotherapy treatment or long-term endocrine treatment of breast cancer is now individualized according to disease characteristics and stage.
- Women who adhered to a low-fat diet and mildly reduced caloric intake had a reduced risk of disease recurrence, especially among ER-negative patients in a large recent study (WINS).
- Exercise is safe for breast cancer patients and may be needed in addition to reduction of caloric intake in order to lose or maintain weight and preserve lean mass. Patients with bone metastases and those who have not previously been physically active should be referred to a physical therapist or other specialist in cancer-related fitness to develop appropriate exercise regimens.
- Combining diet and exercise to maintain normal weight, or to lose weight for patients who are obese or overweight, is likely to improve prognosis. Gaining weight, especially during chemotherapy treatment, worsens prognosis.
- Diets low in saturated, trans, and omega-6 fats and high in fiber such as that from whole grains are likely to reduce levels of estrogen and inflammation.
- Nutrient deficiency states of micronutrients should be evaluated and treated.
- St. John's wort and a few other herbal supplements and foods listed in Table 38.2 alter the pharmacokinetics of pharmacologic agents used for breast cancer treatment. Clinicians should be aware of potential herb- and food-drug interactions.
- Certain herbs and nutrients taken in supplemental doses may alleviate side effects of cancer treatment (Table 38.3). These include glutamine, calendula, l-carnitine, acetyl-l-carnitine, hawthorn, coenzyme Q10, and ginger.

- Obesity, cardiovascular disease, and diabetes are all common comorbid conditions with breast cancer and can be managed appropriately, at least in part, through nutrition and lifestyle interventions.
- Aromatase inhibitors and ovarian ablation (surgical or chemotherapy related) may cause osteoporosis, and patients should receive appropriate dietary counseling to maintain bone health. Calcium and vitamin D supplements are needed and appropriate with aromatase inhibitors.
- Patient evaluations should include weight, BMI, and referral to a dietitian and/or physical therapist for weight management if needed. C-reactive protein, erythrocyte sedimentation rate, and fibrinogen are appropriate measures for inflammation.
- A low-fat, plant-based diet can be recommended, emphasizing monounsaturated and omega-3 fats, fiber-rich whole grains, high vegetable and fruit consumption, and protein primarily from plant sources, fish, and egg whites. Fiber intake of approximately 30 g/day can be considered. Soy foods (not supplements) are safe for breast cancer and can be used two to three times per week. Patients should minimize or eliminate refined flours and sugars, low-fiber or high-fat prepared foods. Caloric intake should be commensurate with need to lose, gain, or maintain weight.

REFERENCES

1. American Cancer Society. 2011. Breast cancer facts & figures, 2011–2012. Atlanta: American Cancer Society.
2. Bardia A, Arieas ET, Zhang Z, et al. Comparison of breast cancer recurrence risk and cardiovascular disease incidence risk among postmenopausal women with breast cancer. Breast Cancer Res Treat 2011 Nov 1. [Epub ahead of print].
3. Pierce JP, Natarajan L, Caan BJ et al. Influence of a diet very high in vegetables, fruit, and fiber and low in fat on prognosis following treatment for breast cancer. JAMA 2007;298(3):289–298.
4. Pierce JP, Stefanick ML, Flatt SW et al. Greater survival after breast cancer in physically active women with high vegetable-fruit intake regardless of obesity. Journal of Clinical Oncology 2007b;28(17): 2345–2351.
5. Chlebowski RT, Blackburn GL, Thomson CA, et al. Dietary fat reduction and breast cancer outcome: Interim efficacy results from the Women's Intervention Nutrition Study. Journal of the National Cancer Institute 2006;98(24):1767–1776.
6. Pierce, JP. Diet and breast cancer prognosis: making sense of the Women's Healthy Eating and Living and Women's Intervention Nutrition Study trials. Curr Opin Obstet Gynecol 2009; 21(1):86–91.
7. de Waard F, Ramlau R, Mulders Y, de Vries T, van Waveren S. A feasibility study on weight reduction in obese postmenopausal breast cancer patients. European Journal of Cancer Prevention 1993;12(3):233–238.
8. Sopotsinskaia EB, Balitskii KP, Tarutinov VI, Zhukova VM, Semenchuk DD, Kozlovskaia SG, Grigorov IG. Experience with the use of a low-calorie diet in breast cancer patients to prevent metastasis. Voprosy Onkologii 1992;38(5):592–599.
9. Block KI, Gyllenhaal C, Tripathy D, Freels S, Mead MN, Block PB, Steinmann WC, Newman RA, Shoham J. Survival impact of integrative cancer in advanced metastatic breast cancer. Breast J 2009 Jul–Aug;15(4):357–366.
10. Doyle SL, Donohoe CL, Lysaght J, Reynolds JV. Visceral obesity, metabolic syndrome, insulin resistance and cancer. Proc Nutr Soc 2011 Nov 3:1–9. [Epub ahead of print].
11. Majed B, Moreau T, Senouci K, Salmon RJ, Fourquet A, Asselain B. Is obesity an independent prognosis factor in woman breast cancer? Breast Cancer Research and Treatment 2007 October 16. [Epub ahead of print].
12. Nichols HB, Trentham-Dietz A, Newcomb PA, Titus-Ernstoff L, Holick CN, Egan KM. Post-diagnosis weight change, body mass index, and breast cancer survival. Presented at 6th Annual Conference on Frontiers in Cancer Prevention Research, December 7, 2007. Abstract B95.
13. McTiernan A, Irwin M, Vongruenigen V. Weight, physical activity, diet, and prognosis in breast and gynecologic cancers. J Clin Oncol 2010 Sep 10;28(26):4074–4080.
14. Riccardi G, Giacco R, Rivellese AA. Dietary fat, insulin sensitivity and the metabolic syndrome. Clinical Nutrition 2004;22(4):447–456.

15. Sahyoun NR, Jacques PF, Zhang XL, Juan W, McKeown NM. Whole-grain intake is inversely associated with the metabolic syndrome and mortality in older adults. American Journal of Clinical Nutrition 2006;83(1):124–131.

16. Thomson CA, Stopeck AT, Bea JW, Cussler E, Nardi E, Frey G, Thompson PA. Changes in body weight and metabolic indexes in overweight breast cancer survivors enrolled in a randomized trial of low-fat vs. reduced carbohydrate diets. Nutr Cancer 2010;62(8):1142–1152.

17. Holmes MD, Chen WY, Feskanich D et al. Physical activity and survival after breast cancer diagnosis. JAMA 2005;293:2479–2486.

18. Ligibel JA, Campbell N, Partridge A, Chen WY, Salinardi T, Chen H, Adloff K, Keshaviah A, Winer EP. Impact of a mixed strength and endurance exercise intervention on insulin levels in breast cancer survivors. Journal of Clinical Oncology 2008;26(6):907–912.

19. McAuley K, Mann J. Thematic review series: Patient-oriented research. Nutritional determinants of insulin resistance. Journal of Lipid Research 2006;47(8):1668–1676.

20. Kwan ML, Weltzien E, Kushi LH, Castillo A, Slattery ML, Caan BJ. Dietary patterns and breast cancer recurrence and survival among women with early-stage breast cancer. J Clin Oncol 2009 Feb 20;27(6):919–926.

21. Beasley JM, Newcomb PA, Trentham-Dietz A, et al. Post-diagnosis dietary factors and survival after invasive breast cancer. Breast Cancer Res Treat 2011 Jul;128(1):229–236.

22. Thomson CA, Rock CL, Thompson PA, Caan BJ, Cussler E, Flatt SW, Pierce JP. Vegetable intake is associated with reduced breast cancer recurrence in tamoxifen users: A secondary analysis from the Women's Healthy Eating and Living Study. Breast Cancer Res Treat 2011 Jan;125(2):519–527.

23. Rock CL, Natarajan L, Pu M, et al. Women's Healthy Eating and Living Study Group. Longitudinal biological exposure to carotenoids is associated with breast cancer-free survival in the Women's Healthy Eating and Living Study. Cancer Epidemiol Biomarkers Prev 2009 Feb;18(2):486–494.

24. Buck K, Zaineddin AK, Vrieling A, Heinz J, Linseisen J, Flesch-Janys D, Chang-Claude J. Estimated enterolignans, lignan-rich foods, and fibre in relation to survival after postmenopausal breast cancer. Br J Cancer 2011 Oct 11;105(8):1151–1157.

25. McCann SE, Thompson LU, Nie J, et al. Dietary lignan intakes in relation to survival among women with breast cancer: the Western New York Exposures and Breast Cancer (WEB) Study. Breast Cancer Res Treat 2010 Jul;122(1):229–235.

26. Belle FN, Kampman E, McTiernan A, Bernstein L, Baumgartner K, Baumgartner R, Ambs A, Ballard-Barbash R, Neuhouser ML. Dietary fiber, carbohydrates, glycemic index, and glycemic load in relation to breast cancer prognosis in the HEAL cohort. Cancer Epidemiol Biomarkers Prev 2011 May;20(5):890–899.

27. Flatt SW, Thomson CA, Gold EB, Natarajan L, Rock CL, Al-Delaimy WK, Patterson RE, Saquib N, Caan BJ, Pierce JP. Low to moderate alcohol intake is not associated with increased mortality after breast cancer. Cancer Epidemiol Biomarkers Prev 2010 Mar;19(3):681–688.

28. Kwan ML, Kushi LH, Weltzien E, Tam EK, Castillo A, Sweeney C, Caan BJ. Alcohol consumption and breast cancer recurrence and survival among women with early-stage breast cancer: The life after cancer epidemiology study. J Clin Oncol 2010 Oct 10;28(29):4410–4416.

29. Visovsky C. Muscle strength, body composition, and physical activity in women receiving chemotherapy for breast cancer. Integrative Cancer Therapies 2006;5(3):183–191.

30. Battaglini C, Bottaro M, Dennehy C, Rae L, Shields E, Kirk D, Hackney A. The effect of an individualized exercise intervention on body composition in breast cancer patients undergoing treatment. Sao Paulo Medical Journal 2007;125(1):22–28.

31. Courneya KS, Segal RJ, Mackey JR, et al. Effects of aerobic and resistance exercise in breast cancer patients receiving adjuvant chemotherapy: A multicenter randomized controlled trial. *Journal of Clinical Oncology* 2007;25(28):4344–4345.

32. Block KI. *Life Over Cancer*. New York: Bantam Press, 2009.

33. Kastorini CM, Milionis HJ, Esposito K, Giugliano D, Goudevenos JA, Panagiotakos DB. The effect of Mediterranean diet on metabolic syndrome and its components: A meta-analysis of 50 studies and 534,906 individuals. J Am Coll Cardiol 2011 Mar 15;57(11):1299–1313.

34. Forman MR. Changes in dietary fat and fiber and serum hormone concentrations: nutritional strategies for breast cancer prevention over the life course. Journal of Nutrition 2007;137:170S–174S.

35. Wallace JM. Nutritional and botanical modulation of the inflammatory cascade—eicosanoids, cyclooxygenases, and lipoxygenases—as an adjunct in cancer therapy. Integrative Cancer Therapies 2002;1(1):7–37.

36. Ferrucci L, Cherubini A, Bandinelli S, Bartali B, Corsi A, Lauretani F, Martin A, Andres-Lacueva C, Senin U, Guralnik JM. Relationship of plasma polyunsaturated fatty acids to circulating inflammatory markers. Journal of Clinical Endocrinology and Metabolism 2006;91(2):439–446.
37. Patterson RE, Flatt SW, Newman VA, Natarajan L, Rock CL, Thomson CA, Caan BJ, Parker BA, Pierce JP. Marine fatty acid intake is associated with breast cancer prognosis. J Nutr 2011 Feb;141(2): 201–206.
38. Collado-Hidalgo A, Bower JE, Ganz PA, Cole SW, Irwin MR. Inflammatory biomarkers for persistent fatigue in breast cancer survivors. Clinical Cancer Research 2006;12(9):2759–2766.
39. Wood LJ, Nail LM, Gilster A, Winters KA, Elsea CR. Cancer chemotherapy-related symptoms: Evidence to suggest a role for proinflammatory cytokines. Oncology Nursing Forum 2006;33(3): 535–542.
40. Simopoulos AP. The importance of the ratio of omega-6/omega-3 essential fatty acids. Biomedicine and Pharmacotherapy 2002;56(8):365–379.
41. Zick S, Sen A, Han-Markey T, Harris R. Examination of the association of diet on persistent cancer related fatigue. Abstract 69. Presented at the 8th International Conference of the Society for Integrative Oncology, November 10–12, 2011, Cleveland, Ohio.
42. Lopez-Garcia E, Schulze MB, Meigs JB, Manson JE, Rifai N, Stampfer MJ, Willett WC, Hu FB. Consumption of *trans* fatty acids is related to plasma biomarkers of inflammation and endothelial dysfunction. Journal of Nutrition 2005;135(3):562–566.
43. Fairey AS, Courneya KS, Field CJ, Bell GJ, Jones LW, Martin BS, Mackey JR. Effect of exercise training on C-reactive protein in postmenopausal breast cancer patients: a randomized controlled trial. Brain Behavior and Immunity 2005;19(5):381–388.
44. Friedenreich C, Neilson HK, Woolcott CG, Wang Q, Stanczyk FZ, McTiernan A, Jones CA, Irwin ML, Yasui Y, Courneya KS. Alberta Physical Activity and Breast Cancer Prevention Trial: Inflammatory marker changes in a year-long exercise intervention among postmenopausal women. Cancer Prev Res (Phila) 2011 Oct 7. [Epub ahead of print].
45. Thompson LU, Chen JM, Strasser-Weippl K, Goss PE. Dietary flaxseed alters tumor biological markers in postmenopausal breast cancer. Clinical Cancer Research 2005;11(10):3828–3835.
46. Block KI, Block PB, Fox SR, Birris JS, Feng AY, de la Torre M, Nathan D, Tothy P, Maki AK, Gyllenhaal C. Making circadian cancer therapy practical. Integr Cancer Ther 2009 Dec;8(4):371–386.
47. Rock CL, Demark-Wahnefried W. Nutrition and survival after the diagnosis of breast cancer: a review of the evidence. Journal of Clinical Oncology 2002;20(15):3302–3316.
48. Coulter IA, Hardy ML, Morton SC, Hilton LG, Tu W, Valentine D, Shekelle PG. Antioxidants vitamin C and vitamin E for the prevention and treatment of cancer. Journal of General Internal Medicine 2006;21:735–744.
49. Davies AA, Smith GD, Harbord R, Bekkering GE, Stern JAC, Beynon R, Thomas S. Nutritional interventions and outcomes in patients with cancer or preinvasive lesions: Systematic review. Journal of the National Cancer Institute 2006;98:961–973.
50. Greenlee H, Kwan ML, Kushi LH, Song J, Castillo A, Weltzien E, Quesenberry CP Jr, Caan BJ. Antioxidant supplement use after breast cancer diagnosis and mortality in the Life After Cancer Epidemiology (LACE) cohort. Cancer 2011 Sep 27. doi: 10.1002/cncr.26526. [Epub ahead of print].
51. Messina M, Abrams DI, Hardy M. Can clinicians now assure their breast cancer patients that soyfoods are safe? Women's Health. 2010;6(3):335–338.
52. Caan BJ, Natarajan L, Parker B, Gold EB, Thomson C, Newman V, Rock CL, Pu M, Al-Delaimy W, Pierce JP. Soy food consumption and breast cancer prognosis. Cancer Epidemiol Biomarkers Prev 2011 May;20(5):854–858.
53. Kang X, Zhang Q, Wang S, Huang X, Jin S. Effect of soy isoflavones on breast cancer recurrence and death for patients receiving adjuvant endocrine therapy. CMAJ 2010 Nov 23;182(17):1857–1862.
54. Steinberg FM, Murray MJ, Lewis RD, et al. Clinical outcomes of a 2-y soy isoflavone supplementation in menopausal women. Am J Clin Nutr 2011 Feb;93(2):356–367.
55. Teas J, Irhimeh MR, Druker S, Hurley TG, Hébert JR, Savarese TM, Kurzer MS. Serum IGF-1 concentrations change with soy and seaweed supplements in healthy postmenopausal American women. Nutr Cancer 2011;63(5):743–748.
56. Einbond LS, Shimizu M, Nuntanakorn P, Seter C, Cheng R, Jiang B, Kronenberg F, Kennelly EJ, Weinstein IB. Actein and a fraction of black cohosh potentiate antiproliferative effects of chemotherapy agents on human breast cancer cells. Planta Medica 2006;72(13):1200–1206.
57. Einbond LS, Wen-Cai Y, He K, Wu HA, Cruz E, Roller M, Kronenberg F. Growth inhibitory activity of extracts and compounds from *Cimicifuga* species on human breast cancer cells. Phytomedicine 2008;15(6–7):504–511.

58. Henneicke-von Zepelin HH, Meden H, Kostev K, Schröder-Bernhardi D, Stammwitz U, Becher H. Isopropanolic black cohosh extract and recurrence-free survival after breast cancer. Int J Clin Pharmacol Ther 2007 Mar;45(3):143–154.

59. Brooks JD, Ward WE, Lewis JE, Hilditch J, Nickell L, Wong E, Thompson LU. Supplementation with flaxseed alters estrogen metabolism in postmenopausal women to a greater extent than does supplementation with an equal amount of soy. American Journal of Clinical Nutrition 2004;79(2):318–325.

60. Laidlaw M, Cockerline CA, Sepkovic DW. Effects of a breast-health herbal formula supplement on estrogen metabolism in pre- and post-menopausal women not taking hormonal contraceptives or supplements: A randomized controlled trial. Breast Cancer (Auckl) 2010 Dec 16;4:85–95.

61. Pruthi S, Qin R, Terstreip SA, et al. A phase III, randomized, placebo-controlled, double-blind trial of flaxseed for the treatment of hot flashes: North Central Cancer Treatment Group N08C7. Menopause 2011 Sep 1. [Epub ahead of print].

62. Sturgeon SR, Volpe SL, Puleo E, Bertone-Johnson ER, Heersink J, Sabelawski S, Wahala K, Bigelow C, Kurzer MS. Effect of flaxseed consumption on urinary levels of estrogen metabolites in postmenopausal women. Nutr Cancer 2010;62(2):175–180.

63. Gold EB, Flatt SW, Pierce JP, Bardwell WA, Hajek RA, Newman VA, Rock CL, Stefanick ML. Dietary factors and vasomotor symptoms in breast cancer survivors: the WHEL study. Menopause 2006;13(3):423–433.

64. Anonymous. Indole-3-carbinol. Alternative Medicine Reviews 2005;10(4):337–342.

65. Morrison J, Mutell D, Pollock TA, Redmond E, Bralley JA, Lord RS. Effects of dried cruciferous powder on raising 2/16 hydroxyestrogen ratios in premenopausal women. Altern Ther Health Med 2009 Mar–Apr;15(2):52–53.

66. Obi N, Vrieling A, Heinz J, Chang-Claude J. Estrogen metabolite ratio: Is the 2-hydroxyestrone to 16α-hydroxyestrone ratio predictive for breast cancer? Int J Womens Health. 2011 Feb 8;3:37–51.

67. Rahman KM, Ali S, Aboukameel A, Sarkar SH, Wang Z, Philip PA, Sakr WA, Raz A. Inactivation of NF-kappaB by 3,3′-diindolylmethane contributes to increased apoptosis induced by chemotherapeutic agent in breast cancer cells. Molecular Cancer Therapies 2007;6(10):2757–2765.

68. Cornblatt BS, Ye L, Dinkova-Kostova AT, et al. Preclinical and clinical evaluation of sulforaphane for chemoprevention in the breast. Carcinogenesis. 2007 Jul;28(7):1485–1490.

69. Li Y, Wicha MS, Schwartz SJ, Sun D. Implications of cancer stem cell theory for cancer chemoprevention by natural dietary compounds. J Nutr Biochem 2011 Sep;22(9):799–806.

70. Smyth PPA. The thyroid, iodine and breast cancer. Breast Cancer Research 2003;5:235–238.

71. Chen P, Hu P, Xie D, Qin Y, Wang F, Wang H. Meta-analysis of vitamin D, calcium and the prevention of breast cancer. Breast Cancer Res Treat 2010 Jun;121(2):469–477.

72. Files JA, Ko MG, Pruthi S. Managing aromatase inhibitors in breast cancer survivors: Not just for oncologists. Mayo Clin Proc 2010 Jun;85(6):560–566.

73. Kang HJ, Lee SH, Price JE, Kim LS. Curcumin suppresses the paclitaxel-induced nuclear factor-kappaB in breast cancer cells and potentiates the growth inhibitory effect of paclitaxel in a breast cancer nude mice model. Breast J 2009 May-Jun;15(3):223–229.

74. Lai HW, Chien SY, Kuo SJ, Tseng LM, Lin HY, Chi CW, Chen DR. The potential utility of curcumin in the treatment of HER-2-overexpressed breast cancer: An in vitro and in vivo comparison study with herceptin. Evid Based Complement Alternat Med 2012;2012:486568.

75. Bougnoux P, Hajjaji N, Ferrasson MN, Giraudeau B, Couet C, Le Floch O. Improving outcome of chemotherapy of metastatic breast cancer by docosahexaenoic acid: a phase II trial. Br J Cancer 2009 Dec 15;101(12):1978–1985.

76. Mandal CC, Ghosh-Choudhury T, Yoneda T, Choudhury GG, Ghosh-Choudhury N. Fish oil prevents breast cancer cell metastasis to bone. Biochem Biophys Res Commun 2010 Nov 26;402(4):602–607.

77. Ogunleye AA, Xue F, Michels KB. Green tea consumption and breast cancer risk or recurrence: A meta-analysis. Breast Cancer Res Treat. 2010 Jan;119(2):477–484.

78. Nesaretnam K, Meganathan P, Veerasenan SD, Selvaduray KR. Tocotrienols and breast cancer: The evidence to date. Genes Nutr 2011 Apr 24. [Epub ahead of print].

79. Wu JH, Ward NC, Indrawan AP, Almeida CA, Hodgson JM, Proudfoot JM, Puddey IB, Croft KD. 2007. Effects of alpha-tocopherol and mixed tocopherol supplementation on markers of oxidative stress and inflammation in type 2 diabetes. Clinical Chemistry 2006;53(3):511–519.

80. Block KI, Koch A, Mead MN, Tothy PK, Newman RA, Gyllenhaal C. Impact of antioxidant supplementation on chemotherapeutic efficacy: a systematic review of the evidence from randomized controlled trials. Cancer Treatment Reviews 2007;33(5):407–418.

81. Moss RW. Do antioxidants interfere with radiation therapy for cancer? Integrative Cancer Therapies 2007;6(3):281–292.

82. Meyer F, Bairati I, Fortin A, Gélinas M, Nabid A, Brochet F, Têtu B. Interaction between antioxidant vitamin supplementation and cigarette smoking during radiation therapy in relation to long-term effects on recurrence and mortality: a randomized trial among head and neck cancer patients. International Journal of Cancer 2007a;122(7):1679–1683.

83. Meyer F, Bairati I, Jobin E, Gélinas M, Fortin A, Nabid A, Têtu B. Acute adverse effects of radiation therapy and local recurrence in relation to dietary and plasma beta carotene and alpha tocopherol in head and neck cancer patients. Nutrition and Cancer 2007b;59(1):29–35.

84. Chavez ML, Jordan MA, Chavez PI. Evidence-based drug—herbal interactions. Life Sciences 2006;78(18):2146–2157.

85. Chow HH, Garland LL, Hsu CH, Vining DR, Chew WM, Miller JA, Perloff M, Crowell JA, Alberts DS. Resveratrol modulates drug- and carcinogen-metabolizing enzymes in a healthy volunteer study. Cancer Prev Res (Phila) 2010 Sep;3(9):1168–1175.

86. Flockhart D. Drug Interactions. Version 4, August 2007. Available at: http://medicine.iupui.edu/flockhart/.

87. Gorski JC, Huang SM, Pinto A, Hamman MA, Hilligoss JK, Zaheer NA, Desai M, Miller M, Hall SD. The effect of echinacea (*Echinacea purpurea* root) on cytochrome P450 activity in mice. Clinical Pharmacology and Therapeutics 2004;75(1):89–100.

88. Gurley BJ, Gardner SF, Hubbard MA, Williams DK, Gentry WB, Carrier J, Khan IA, Edwards DJ, Shah A. In vivo assessment of botanical supplementation on human cytochrome P450 phenotypes: *Citrus aurantium, Echinacea purpurea*, milk thistle, and saw palmetto. Clinical Pharmacology and Therapeutics 2004;76(5):428–440.

89. Gurley BJ, Gardner SF, Hubbard MA, Williams DK, Gentry WB, Khan IA, Shah A. In vivo effects of goldenseal, kava kava, black cohosh and valerian on human cytochrome P450 1A2, 2D6, 2E1 and 3A4/5 phenotypes. Clinical Pharmacology and Therapeutics 2005;77(5):415–426.

90. Post-White J, Ladas EJ, Kelly KM. Advances in the use of milk thistle. Integrative Cancer Therapies 2007;6(2):104–109.

91. King PD, Perry MC. Hepatotoxicity of chemotherapy. Oncologist 2001;6(2):162–176.

92. Ryan JL, Heckler CE, Roscoe JA, Dakhil SR, Kirshner J, Flynn PJ, Hickok JT, Morrow GR. Ginger (Zingiber officinale) reduces acute chemotherapy-induced nausea: a URCC CCOP study of 576 patients. Support Care Cancer 2011 Aug 5. [Epub ahead of print].

93. Carroll JK, Kohli S, Mustian KM, Roscoe JA, Morrow GR. Pharmacologic treatment of cancer-related fatigue. Oncologist 2007;12 Suppl 1:43–51.

94. Cruciani RA, Dvorkin E, Homel P, Culliney B, Malamud S, Lapin J, Portenoy RK, Esteban-Cruciani N. L-carnitine supplementation in patients with advanced cancer and carnitine deficiency: A double-blind, placebo-controlled study. J Pain Symptom Manage 2009 Apr;37(4):622–631.

95. Barton DL, Soori GS, Bauer BA, et al. Pilot study of Panax quinquefolius (American ginseng) to improve cancer-related fatigue: A randomized, double-blind, dose-finding evaluation: NCCTG trial N03CA. Support Care Cancer 2010 Feb;18(2):179–187.

96. King ML, Adler SR, Murphy LL. Extraction-dependent effects of American ginseng (*Panax quinquefolium*) on human breast cancer cell proliferation and estrogen receptor activation. Integrative Cancer Therapies 2006;5(3):236–264.

97. Conklin KA. Coenzyme Q10 for prevention of anthracycline-induced cardiotoxicity. Integrative Cancer Therapies 2005;4(2):110–130.

98. Amara S. Oral glutamine for the prevention of chemotherapy-induced peripheral neuropathy. Ann Pharmacother 2008 Oct;42(10):1481–1485.

99. Choi K, Lee SS, Oh SJ, Lim SY, Lim SY, Jeon WK, Oh TY, Kim JW. The effect of oral glutamine on 5-fluorouracil/leucovorin-induced mucositis/stomatitis assessed by intestinal permeability test. Clinical Nutrition 2007;26(1):57–62.

100. Peterson DE, Jones JB, Petit RG,II. Randomized, placebo-controlled trial of Saforis for prevention and treatment of oral mucositis in breast cancer patients receiving anthracycline-based chemotherapy. Cancer 2007 Jan 15;109(2):322–331.

101. Savarese DM, Savy G, Vahdat L, Wischmeyher PE, Corey B. Prevention of chemotherapy and radiation toxicity with glutamine. Cancer Treatment Reviews 2003;29(6):501–513.

102. de Grandis D. Acetyl-L-carnitine for the treatment of chemotherapy-induced peripheral neuropathy: A short review. CNS Drugs 2007;suppl 1:39–43.

103. Pommier P, Gomez F, Sunyach MP, D'Hombres A, Carrie C, Montbarbon X. Phase III randomized trial of *Calendula officinalis* compared with trolamine for the prevention of acute dermatitis during irradiation for breast cancer. Journal of Clinical Oncology 2004;22(8):1447–1453.

104. Holubarsch CJF, Colucci WS, Meinertz T, et al. Crataegus extract WS 1442 postpones cardiac death in patients with congestive heart failure class NYHA II-III: A randomized, placebo-controlled, double-blind trial in 2681 patients. American College of Cardiology 2007 Scientific Sessions March 27, 2007; New Orleans, LA. Late breaking clinical trials-3, Session 414–415.

105. Wischmeyer PE. Glutamine: Role in critical illness and ongoing clinical trials. Current Opinion in Gastroenterology 2008;24(2):190–197.

106. Wolf S, Barton D, Kottschade L, Grothey A, Loprinzi C. Chemotherapy-induced peripheral neuropathy: Prevention and treatment strategies. Eur J Cancer 2008 Jul;44(11):1507–1515.

107. Walji R, Boon H, Guns E, Oneschuck D, Younnus D. Black cohosh (*Cimicifuga racemosa* [L.] Nutt.): Safety and efficacy for cancer patients. Supportive Care in Cancer 2007;15(8):913–921.

108. Shaw C, Mortimer P, Judd PA. A randomized controlled trial of weight reduction as a treatment for breast cancer-related lymphedema. Cancer 2007a;110(8):1868–1874.

109. Shaw C, Mortimer P, Judd PA. Randomized controlled trial comparing a low-fat diet with a weightreduction diet in breast cancer-related lymphedema. Cancer 2007b;109(10):1949–1956.

110. Levi F, Pasche C, Lucchini F, Ghidoni R, Ferraroni M, La Vecchia C. Resveratrol and breast cancer risk. Eur J Cancer Prev. 2005 Apr;14(2):139–142.

39 Prostate Cancer

Food and Nutrients That May Slow Disease Progression

Geovanni Espinosa, N.D., Scott Quarrier,
M.P.H., and Aaron E. Katz, M.D.

INTRODUCTION

It is estimated that there will be more than 249,000 diagnoses of, and approximately 34,000 deaths from, prostate cancer (CaP) in 2012 [1]. Detection of this disease earlier, as a consequence of the introduction of the prostate specific antigen (PSA) blood test, has been recognized by the National Cancer Institute (NCI) as one factor contributing to lowering the CaP mortality rate in the past few years [2–5]. While PSA is routinely used for prostate cancer screening, concerns have emerged regarding the absence of evidence that screening itself directly decreases mortality. In 2011, the United States Preventive Services Task Force (USPSTF) recommended against screening for prostate cancer using PSA in healthy men. This USPSTF recommendation is based on studies concluding that PSA-based screening results in small or no reduction in CaP-specific mortality and is associated with harms related to subsequent evaluation and treatments [6]. However, the value of the PSA test may be increased by considering PSA velocity (PSAV) or a sustained rise in PSA rather than the absolute PSA value [7]. The prostate cancer gene 3 (PCA3) and the percentage free PSA (%fPSA) can also enhance the screening potential of CaP [8].

The PSA test has resulted in a dramatic increase in diagnosis of asymptomatic prostate cancer. Many of these patients have disease that is inherently different from the aggressive metastatic disease. These patients can be managed best by altering lifestyle, changing diet, and incorporating dietary supplements without radical surgical options. Patients with higher risk cancers can also benefit from augmenting standard therapies with nutrition.

Primary care physicians, treating both patients with prostate cancer and patients interested in reducing their risk of developing prostate cancer, are optimally situated to provide nutritional advice. There is increasing evidence that nutrition can slow the rate of CaP progression; conversely, poor nutrition may accelerate disease and reduce life and its quality dramatically. Weight management may also substantially reduce the risk of CaP and its recurrence. This chapter evaluates food, nutrients, and the role of dietary supplements in delaying CaP development and its progression.

EPIDEMIOLOGY

Although the rates of CaP vary widely between countries, it is least common in South and East Asia, more common in Europe, and most common in the United States [9]. In the United States, prostate cancer is least common among Asian American men and most common among black men, with figures for Caucasian men in-between [1,10]. However, these high rates may be affected by different rates of screening [11]. Ecologic studies have implicated a Western diet in CaP development. Asian immigrants who adopt a Western diet show an increased incidence of CaP thought to be related to environmental factors including variations in dietary pattern [12].

Two genes (BRCA1 and BRCA2) that are important risk factors for ovarian cancer and breast cancer in women have also been implicated in prostate cancer [13]. The possibility of specific nutrient-gene interactions merits further investigation. Meanwhile, men with these genes may wish to use food and nutrients as disease prophylaxis.

The role of nutrition and dietary supplements in CaP is of much interest. However several unresolved issues, which are discussed in this chapter, still linger:

- The expected time to achieve an effect is long, variable, and in need of further investigation. The impact of nutrition and dietary supplements on existing disease progression is difficult to research.
- Racial variation of risk of CaP and cross-cultural dietary variations may make it difficult to extend results across geographic and racial boundaries.
- The optimal dose and duration needed to test nutritional agents for cancer prevention are largely unidentified, making null findings hard to interpret.
- Baseline nutritional status can be critical [13]. For example, studies have shown that selenium supplements provided benefit for those individuals who had low levels of baseline plasma selenium, whereas subjects with normal or higher levels did not benefit and may have an increased risk for CaP [14].
- Particular nutrients may be effective only in subpopulations defined by genotypes or by nutritional status of another nutrient.

PATHOPHYSIOLOGY

Well-recognized precursor lesions in the peripheral zones of the prostate, including low-grade or high-grade prostatic intraepithelial neoplasia (PIN), are associated with the development of invasive cancer. Recently, proliferative inflammatory atrophy has been proposed as a precursor to PIN with merging of proliferative inflammatory atrophy and high-grade PIN seen in ~34% of proliferative inflammatory atrophy lesions [15]. Chronic inflammation may damage epithelial cells and result in proliferative lesions, likely precursors of PIN lesions and prostatic carcinomas; prostatitis has therefore been associated with a high risk of CaP [16]. The correlation between organ-specific inflammation and carcinoma is noteworthy. Reduction of inflammation is likely one route by which nutritional interventions influence disease.

FOODS IMPACT ON PROSTATE CANCER

MEAT

A recent prospective study of 1294 men with prostate cancer did not identify any association between increased meat consumption and prostate cancer recurrence or progression [17]. However, there is a correlation with consumption of meats cooked well done and the increase in CaP risk [18]. Charred meats and those cooked on an open flame contain heterocyclic amines (HCAs) and polycyclic aromatic hydrocarbons (PAH), carcinogenic chemicals formed from the cooking of muscle meats such as beef, pork, fowl, and fish. Researchers have identified 17 different HCAs resulting from the cooking of meats that may pose human cancer risk [18]. Cured and smoked meats should also be avoided because they contain nitrosamines. Lean meat from wild game or grass-fed animals is preferred, and eaten sparingly, cooked at low temperatures, and accompanied by fruits and vegetables. The meat of grass-fed animals contains high levels of carotenoid, vitamin E, glutathinone, conjugated linoleic acid (CLA), and low levels of saturated fat content relative to grain-fed livestock [19].

DIETARY FAT

The risk of prostate cancer correlates with dietary fat from country to country, a finding supported in some, [20,21] but not all [22], preliminary trials. In one study, prostate cancer patients consuming the most saturated fat (from meat and dairy), and followed for over five years, had over three times the risk of dying from prostate cancer compared with men consuming the least amount of saturated fat [23]. Men with higher serum levels of the short-chain omega-6 fatty acid linoleic acid have higher rates of prostate cancer and those with higher levels of the omega-3 fatty acids eicosapentaenoic acid (EPA) and docosahexaenoic acid (DHA) had lowered incidence. A long-term study reports that "blood levels of trans fatty acids, in particular trans fats resulting from the hydrogenation of vegetable oils, are associated with an increased prostate cancer risk" [24].

TABLE 39.1
Foods That May Be Beneficial in Prostate Cancer

Nutrient	Meat/Dairy Source	Vegetable/Fruit Source
Omega-3 fatty acids	Cold water fish (salmon, cod, herring, mackerel, anchovies, sardines), grass-fed beef, fish oils, eggs	Flax seeds (linseed), flax oil, krill oil, walnuts, canola, whole grains, legumes, green leafy vegetables, Acai palm fruit, kiwi fruit, black raspberries, wakame (sea vegetable)
Vitamin D	Cod liver oil, salmon, mackerel, sardines, liver, eggs	Green leafy vegetables, fortified cereals
Vitamin E	Sardines, Atlantic herring, blue crab	Almonds, sunflower seeds, safflower oil, hazelnuts, turnip greens, pine nuts, peanuts, peanut butter, tomato, wheat germ, avocado, carrot juice, olive oil, corn oil, peanut oil, spinach, dandelion greens, Brazil nuts
Zinc	Grass-fed beef, crabmeat, oysters, lamb, pork, turkey, salmon, chicken, clams, lobster	Brown rice, spinach, beans, rye bread, whole wheat bread, lentils, lima beans, oatmeal, peas, baked potato
Selenium	Dairy products, liver, cold water fish, shellfish	Asparagus, broccoli, garlic, onions, mushrooms, grains, sea vegetables
Indole-3-arbinol, 5 glucaric acid (calcium D-glucarate)	None	Arugula, broccoli, cauliflower, brussels sprouts, cabbage, watercress, bok choy, turnip greens, mustard greens, and collard greens, mizuna, tatsoi, rutabaga, napa or Chinese cabbage, daikon, horseradish, radishes, turnips, kohlrabi, and kale
Lycopene	None	Tomatoes, watermelon, pink grapefruit, pink guava, papaya, red bell pepper, and rosehip. Lycopene in tomato paste is four times more bioavailable than in fresh tomatoes
Genistein, daidzein	None	Soy products—especially fermented soy: miso, natto, sweet noodle sauce, tamari, tempeh, tofu (pickled), yellow soybean paste
Catechins	None	Camellia sinensis: including white tea, green tea, black tea, and oolong tea. Catechins are found in chocolate.

Alpha-linolenic acid (ALA) is the essential omega-3 fatty acid precursor of EPA and DHA, both known to have anti-inflammatory and possibly anticancer properties. Results indicate that people with measurably high ALA are at increased risk for prostate cancer. A significant portion of dietary alpha-linolenic acid often does come from meat. Therefore, in theory, alpha-linolenic acid may be a marker for meat consumption. When researchers have adjusted for the intake of meat or saturated fat, there remains a correlation between alpha-linolenic acid and prostate cancer risk [25,26]. Most [21,23], but not all [26] studies have found that high dietary or blood levels of alpha-linolenic acid correlate with an increased risk of prostate cancer. Another possible explanation is that the rate-limiting enzyme, which converts ALA to DHA and EPA, called delta-6-desaturase, is not functioning optimally. The ALA then accumulates and increased risk of prostate cancer is a result of inadequate enzyme activity. Elevated blood glucose, consumption of trans fats, and inadequate zinc impair delta-6-desaturase enzyme activity.

A high ratio of omega-6 to omega-3 fats increases inflammation. Eating meats and the ALA contained within can offset this balance. A study that investigated the balance between omega-6 and omega-3 fats investigated the supplementation of omega-3 fat and its impact on tumor growth. In a preliminary study of men with prostate cancer, supplementation with 30 grams per day for approximately one month of ground flaxseed, which is high in omega-3 fats, appeared to decrease the rate of tumor growth [27].

People that consume fish have been reported to have low risk for prostate cancer [28]. The omega-3 fatty acids EPA and DHA found in fish are thought by some researchers to be the components responsible for protection against cancer [29].

CRUCIFEROUS VEGETABLES

Cruciferous or brassica vegetables, such as broccoli, cauliflower, brussels sprouts, cabbage, bok choy, collard greens, and kale are rich in sulforaphane and indole-3 carbinol (I3C) [30]. These phytochemicals exhibit anticarcinogenic properties: induction of cell cycle arrest, inhibition of tumor invasion and angiogenesis, anti-inflammatory activity, inhibition of extracellular signal-regulated kinases, proteasome degradation, and alteration of phase I and phase II biotransformation enzyme expression [31,32]. Sulforaphane has also been shown to have proapoptotic properties in prostate cancer cells in vitro and in vivo [33] and I3C has antiproliferative and antimetastatic properties in animal models of CaP [34].

A preliminary study of men newly diagnosed with prostate cancer showed a 41% decreased risk of prostate cancer among men eating three or more servings of cruciferous vegetables per week, compared with those eating less than one serving per week [35]. Protective effects of cruciferous vegetables are thought to be due to their high concentration of the carotenoids, lutein, and zeaxanthin, as well as their stimulatory effects on the breakdown of environmental carcinogens associated with prostate cancer [35]. Cruciferous vegetables also contain phytoestrogens.

SOY

Phytoestrogens are fat-soluble nutrients found in a variety of foods, especially vegetables, which modulate the response of fat-soluble hormones especially estrogen. Phytoestrogens in food have been shown to be protective by helping the body metabolize estrogen-like toxins called xenoestrogens, which can be found in food, food packaging, water, and the environment at large.

Isoflavonoid phytoestrogens, such as genistein, daidzein, and glycitein, act as chemoprotectors by direct inhibition of DNA methyltransferase activity, reversal of DNA hypermethylation, and reactivation of methylation-silenced genes. Phytoestrogens are important regulators of proteins, such as 5α-reductase, tyrosine kinase, topoisomerase, and P450 aromatase, besides exerting an inhibitory effect on vitamin D metabolism in the prostate [36]. Isoflavonoid phytoestrogens, such as genistein, daidzein, and glycitein, show structural similarities with mammalian estrogens and are present in large amounts in soybean and soy products, such as miso and tofu. There is evidence that genistein, equol, and enterolactone inhibit the growth of LNCaP cells and reduce both intracellular and extracellular PSA concentrations. In addition, genistein is an effective inhibitor of angiogenesis and has been reported to decrease PSA levels and prevent metastatic disease in male rats [37]. Studies in animal models showed that rats fed on soy or rye bran exhibited a significant delay in the growth of implanted prostate tumors. Osteopontin, an extracellular matrix protein, may be involved in the transition from clinically insignificant tumors to metastatic CaP. A recent murine study using dietary genistein demonstrated improved survival, reduced expression of osteopontin, and inhibited progression to advanced CaP [38].

There is limited data on the effect of oral phytoestrogen supplements in prostate tissue itself. However, supplementation of oral phytoestrogen was able to increase plasma equol levels to detectable levels in 90% of patients after supplementation [39].

A 16-year-long prospective health study showed that men who consumed more than one glass of soy milk per day had a 70% lower risk of CaP [40]. More recently, two meta-analyses suggest that consumption of nonfermented soyfoods such as soy milk and tofu is associated with a 26% risk reduction of prostate cancer. An inverse trend between isoflavone intake and cancer risk has been observed [41], [42].

LYCOPENE

The primary dietary source of lycopene is tomatoes, though traces of lycopene can be found in watermelons, pink grapefruits, papaya, and guava. Cooked tomatoes and tomato sauce are actually better than raw tomatoes because cooking releases lycopene from storage sites enhancing absorption as does dietary fat. Lycopene has been reported to inhibit the proliferation of cancer cells and inflammatory markers in vivo [43].

In a preliminary human clinical trial, 26 men with prostate cancer were randomly assigned to receive lycopene (15 mg twice a day) or no lycopene for three weeks before undergoing prostate surgery. Prostate tissue was then obtained during surgery and examined. The men receiving supplemental lycopene were found to have significantly less aggressive growth of cancer cells [44].

In another trial, a three-week tomato intervention study in CaP patients demonstrated an increase in the apoptotic index of hyperplastic and neoplastic cells in the resected prostate tissue along with lower plasma levels of PSA [45]. Similar results were obtained when lycopene was given to patients undergoing orchidectomy with subsequent decrease in serum PSA level and reduction in the size of primary and secondary tumors [46]. In addition, a phase II study found that whole-tomato lycopene preventative supplementation reduced PSA significantly and maintained its effect on PSA over one year [47]. Similarly, there is some evidence to suggest that lycopene supplementation may also be of benefit in men with confirmed prostate cancer. A recent systematic review of eight interventional studies by Haseen et al. [48] has shown an inverse association between lycopene intake and serum PSA levels in six of the studies. However, more recently a small prospective open phase II study of daily lycopene supplementation (15 mg) in men with progressive advanced-stage prostate cancer did not result in any clinically significant benefit in this group of patients although 5 of 17 patients had a plateau-like stabilization in their PSA levels [49].

GREEN TEA

Evidence from a case-control study conducted in southeast China assessing 130 patients with histologically confirmed incidental prostate cancer and 274 patients without cancer matched by age, showed that the prostate cancer risk declined with increasing frequency, duration, and quantity of green tea consumed. The subjects in this trial drank three cups a day. This reduction was statistically significant, suggesting that green tea protects against prostate cancer [50].

In a double-blind trial, men with precancerous changes in the prostate received either a green tea extract providing 600 mg of catechins per day or a placebo for one year. After one year, prostate cancer had developed in 3.3% of the men receiving the green tea extract and in 30% of those given the placebo, a statistically significant difference. These results suggest that drinking green tea or taking green tea catechins may help prevent prostate cancer in men at high risk of developing the disease [51].

Similar results were seen in another clinical trial involving patients with hormone refractory CaP. Green tea extract capsules, prescribed at a dose level of 250 mg twice daily, showed minimal clinical activity against the disease [52]. Both these studies were conducted in end-stage disease, signifying that green tea may be more effective if used in the early stages of the disease or in patients at high risk.

In this context, Bettuzzi et al. have shown that after one year of oral administration of green tea catechins, only one man in a group of 32 with high-grade PIN developed CaP compared with nine of 30 in the control group; a rate of only 3% in men developing the disease versus the expected rate of 30% in men treated with placebo [51].

A large prospective cohort study of 49,920 men aged 40–69 years and their green tea consumption habits was conducted by the Japan Public Health Center between 1990 and 2004 [53]. During this time, there were 404 cases of newly diagnosed prostate cancer of which 114 cases were advanced, 271 were localized, and 19 were of an undetermined stage. The results indicate that there may be a dose-dependent decrease in the risk of advanced prostate cancer in men who consume more than five cups of green tea per day [53].

Based on all available evidence, green tea appears to markedly reduce the development of prostate cancer. The studies also demonstrate that this reduction may be attributed to several different pathways. Further study of green tea is needed including large-scale, prospective randomized trials. Nevertheless, based on existing research, clinicians should consider encouraging patients to change their hot beverage consumption to green tea [54]. There are several positive clinical studies of green tea's protective effects on the development of other types of cancer.

POMEGRANATE

Pomegranate is a rich source of polyphenolic compounds, including anthocyanins and hydrolyzable tannins, with a reportedly higher antioxidant activity than green tea and red wine. Studies show that anatomically discrete sections of the pomegranate fruit act synergistically to exert antiproliferative and antimetastatic effects against CaP cells.

Pomegranate fruit extract treatment of highly aggressive PC-3 cells resulted in a dose-dependent inhibition of cell growth/cell viability along with induction of apoptosis [55]. A two-year, single center study showed that pomegranate juice increased the mean PSA doubling time coupled with corresponding laboratory effects on CaP in vitro cell proliferation and apoptosis, as well as oxidative stress [56]. No serious adverse effects were reported, and the treatment was well tolerated. These results are being further tested in an ongoing randomized, double-blind, three-arm, placebo-controlled study [56].

SAW PALMETTO

Some in vivo studies have reported that saw palmetto may protect against prostate cancer [57,58]. Saw palmetto extract reduces the amount of dihydrotestosterone (DHT) (an active form of testosterone) binding in the part of the prostate surrounding the urethra. Test tube studies also suggest that saw palmetto weakly inhibits the action of 5-alpha-reductase, the enzyme responsible for converting testosterone to DHT [59].

There has, however, been no evidence in humans regarding the association with saw palmetto and prostate cancer in a clinical trial. In one prospective cohort study of 35,171 men aged 50–76 years, no association between commercial saw palmetto, which varied widely in dose and constituent ratios, and prostate cancer risk was found [60].

VITAMINS AND MINERALS IMPACT ON PROSTATE CANCER

VITAMIN D

Ecologic data that where sun exposure is low, prostate cancer rates increase [61] prompted a clinical study. Seven of 16 men who had prostate cancer that had spread to bone and who had been unresponsive to conventional treatment were found to have evidence of vitamin D deficiency [62]. All 16 were given 2000 IU of vitamin D per day for 12 weeks, and levels of pain were recorded for 14 of these men. Vitamin D supplementation led to reduced pain in four of the 14 men, and six showed evidence of increased strength. Those with vitamin D deficiency were more likely to respond, compared with those who were not deficient [62]. Osteomalacia may have been a previously overlooked component of the vitamin D deficient patients' pain.

In another preliminary study, men with prostate cancer that had relapsed after surgery or radiation therapy were treated with 2000 IU of vitamin D per day for nine months. In approximately half of the men, the prostate-specific antigen (PSA) level decreased, suggesting that the progression of the disease had been halted or reversed; this decrease was sustained for five to 17 months [63]. This study was performed in Toronto, Canada, where the amount of sunlight is limited and vitamin D status tends to be low. It is not known whether vitamin D supplementation would be as effective in geographical regions such as the southern United States, where the amount of sunlight is greater.

A normal vitamin D status may be an important precondition, via the local and autocrine synthesis of calcitriol (1,25[OH]2D) in the target tissues, for a lower risk of overall morality due to organ cancer [64]. A plethora of evidence that vitamin D and its synthetic analogues promote differentiation and inhibit the proliferation, invasiveness, and metastasis of human prostatic cancer cells both in in vitro and in vivo models exists [65]. In addition, data from various studies support the concept that adequate exposure to UV radiation results in reduced risk of various diseases, including cancer through a vitamin D–mediated mechanism. A recent analysis of mortality data over a 44-year period (1950–94) by Schwartz et al. confirmed their earlier findings that the geographic distribution of CaP mortality is the inverse of that of UV radiation [66].

In contrast, recent analysis of the available literature indicates a lack of evidence to support association between vitamin D receptor polymorphisms and risk of CaP [67]. Currently, more than 2000 vitamin D analogues have been evaluated, and several have entered phase I or phase II trials in patients with advanced cancer. A variety of drug administration schedules have been tried,

TABLE 39.2
Nutrients That May Be Beneficial in Prostate Cancer

Supplement	Dose	Regimen
Vitamin D (cholecalciferol)	2000 IU	Once to twice daily with food; monitor 25 hydroxy-vitamin D levels
Vitamin E (mixed tocopherols)	400 IU	Once a day with food
Selenium with mixed tocopherols	200 mcg	Once a day with food
Fish oil	1000 mg	Two times a day with food
Lycopene	15 mg	Two times a day with food
Green tea extract	250 mg	Two times a day with food
Curcumin	400 mg	Two to four times a day with food
Broccoli seed extract (sulforaphane glucosinolate)	500 mg	Two to four times a day with food

including daily or intermittent administration of oral calcitriol, subcutaneous. Injections, or combination with other chemotherapeutic agents [68], as the dose-limiting hypercalcemia associated with calcitriol has limited the use of natural vitamin D in cancer prevention. Clinical responses have been seen with the combination of high-dose calcitriol and dexamethasone, and in a large randomized trial in men with an androgen-independent CaP, calcitriol potentiated the antitumor effects of docetaxel and other antitumor chemotherapies [69]. Randomized phase III clinical trials are necessary to determine the optimal dose and preferred vitamin D analogue along with the route and schedule of administration.

It is appropriate to measure 25-hydroxyvitamin D (25[OH]D) in patients to ensure they are at an adequate level. Although normal ranges are 20–56 ng/ml, ideally vitamin D level should not fall below 32 ng/ml and any levels below 20 ng/ml are considered serious deficiency states [70].

Vitamin E

Among the tocopherols and tocotrienols included in the term vitamin E, α-tocopherol often exerts high antioxidant functions and is the predominant form of vitamin E found in plasma, whereas γ-tocopherol is the major form present in the diet. Besides its antioxidant function, vitamin E can regulate cell cycle through DNA synthesis arrest in LNCaP, PC-3, and DU-145 CaP cells [71]. Tocopherol metabolites have been reported to be as effective as their vitamin precursors in inhibiting PC-3 growth through down regulation of cyclin expression, with stronger inhibition seen with the γ forms [72].

Supplemental use of vitamin E has been associated with a reduced risk of prostate cancer in smokers. In a double-blind trial studying smokers, vitamin E supplementation (50 IU of α tocopherol per day for an average of six years) led to a 32% decrease in prostate cancer incidence and a 41% decrease in prostate cancer deaths [73].

A significant reduction in CaP was seen in men with normal PSA who received vitamin E supplements; however, in men with elevated PSA at baseline, the supplementation was associated with an increased incidence of CaP of borderline statistical significance [74]. Moreover, one serum-based study refuted any association between vitamin E levels and CaP risk [75]; six of seven prospective cohort studies based on questionnaire data failed to show a significant association suggestive of a nonsignificant protective trend among smokers. In addition, vitamin E (α-tocopherol) in doses > 400 IU/day has been associated with an increased mortality rate [76].

The SELECT trial (SELenium and vitamin E Cancer prevention Trial) focused on more than 35,000 subjects to see whether vitamin E and selenium might prevent prostate cancer. The participants were randomly assigned to receive one of four interventions between August 2001 and June 2004 for a planned minimum follow-up of seven years:

- L-selenomethionine (200 micrograms per day) and a vitamin E placebo
- α-tocopherol (400 IU/day) and a selenium placebo
- L-selenomethionine plus α-tocopherol, or
- Placebo

The results showed slightly more prostate cancers in men taking vitamin E alone, and slightly more diabetes in men taking only selenium. But neither finding was statistically significant, suggesting these findings were likely due to chance [77]. Recently, further review of the SELECT trial showed a 17% increase in prostate cancer among those taking vitamin E as α-tocopherol [78].

In contrast, in a case-control study of 10,456 men, higher blood levels of α-tocopherol and γ-tocopherol were each associated with a lower risk of developing prostate cancer, but the association with γ-tocopherol was stronger than that of α-tocopherol [79]. In addition to the finding that higher levels of γ-tocopherol significantly reduced prostate cancer risk, the study also showed that selenium and α-tocopherol also reduced prostate cancer incidence, but only when γ-tocopherol levels are high [79].

A surprising study found that men with the highest plasma γ-tocopherol concentrations had a highly significant fivefold lower risk of prostate cancer compared with men in the lowest quintile (lowest 20%). This effect was not significant for plasma α-tocopherol concentrations. Other researchers have also found that γ-tocopherol offers a protective effect against prostate cancer [80].

These observations raise the possibility that both α- and γ-tocopherol have protective effects against prostate cancer. However, when α-tocopherol is given by itself in large doses (such as ≥ 400 IU/d), depleting γ-tocopherol, the beneficial effect of α-tocopherol might be negated. Taking vitamin E as mixed tocopherols (containing all four forms of vitamin E) might not increase prostate cancer risk, and further research is needed to examine that possibility.

SELENIUM

Selenium is an essential micronutrient, and part of the body's antioxidant defense system. It has been shown to inhibit tumorigenesis in a variety of experimental models. Methylated selenium sensitizes CaP cells to apoptosis, effectively downregulating the expression of androgen receptor (AR) and PSA in the androgen-responsive LNCaP cells, and inhibiting the growth of LNCaP xenografts in nude mice [81,82].

The double-blind, randomized Nutritional Prevention of Cancer trial, designed to test whether selenium-fortified yeast could prevent the recurrence of nonmelanoma skin cancer in 1312 patients, showed a statistically significant increase in nonmelanoma skin cancer. A secondary end-point analysis revealed a striking reduction in CaP incidence in those with low-serum selenium levels. Furthermore, no evidence of selenium toxicity was seen at doses of 400 μg selenium daily in 424 people for 1220 person-years of observation [83].

Selenium may have a protective effect against mercury and other heavy metal toxicities [84,85]. Experimental findings have shown that selenium-deficient rodents are more susceptible to the prenatal toxicity of methyl mercury. In the neonate, significant alterations of the activities of selenoenzymes, such as glutathione peroxidase and iodothyronine deiodinases, were evident [86].

Selenium appears to antagonize cadmium, especially in acute exposures. In a mouse study, after acute cadmium exposure, a significant decrease in cadmium levels was observed in the kidneys and liver following an eight-week daily selenium supplementation [87].

Only one randomized controlled human trial has studied the effect of selenium on mortality of prostate cancer [77] compared with placebo group. The risk ratio for mortality of prostate cancer with selenium treatment was not changed. The reason for this null result may be caused by the lack of needed synergism between γ-tocopherol (not used in the SELECT Trial), α-tocopherol, and selenium [79].

ANTI-INFLAMMATORY CHEMOPREVENTION

Clinicians and researchers have long recognized that inflammatory processes play crucial roles in the development and progression of prostate cancer. COX-2 is overexpressed in many cancers, including prostate cancer, and is a well-established and significant target for efforts to forestall cancer growth. Benign prostate tissue in cancerous prostates has been found to have low COX-2, suggesting increased activity of the enzyme with disease progression. COX-2 overexpression is a predictor of worse prostate cancer outcome [88].

Other studies have suggested that angiogenesis is orchestrated in part by increased COX-2 activity and ensuing prostaglandin production. This hypothesis is supported by the effects of some COX-2 inhibitor drugs on the biochemical measures of apoptosis. COX-2 inhibitor drug celecoxib (Celebrex) has been found to be a promising chemotherapy. Inhibition of COX-2 in animals suppresses angiogenesis and prostate cancer growth and enhances sensitivity to radiation therapy.

Thus, the anti-inflammatory aspect of chemoprevention appears to be a pivotal one, particularly in cases of prostatic intraepithelial neoplasia (PIN). PIN, which can appear up to 10 years before diagnosable cancer, and which coexists with cancer in more than 85 percent of cases, offers investigators the opportunity to apply chemopreventive measures when dysplasia is present—the point at which prostate carcinogenesis may be at its earliest stages.

Proinflammatory eicosanoids can be reduced by balancing fatty acid intake, providing the body with increased substrate for the production of anti-inflammatory eicosanoids to competitively inhibit formation of proinflammatory eicosanoids. Manipulation of COX and LO enzyme isoforms can inhibit the inflammation found to encourage prostate carcinogenesis. To date, it appears that fatty acid intake is a safe and effective intervention in this regard. Manipulating COX and LO with pharmaceutical agents, however, has proven to be a less promising avenue for chemoprevention. Recent case-control studies have found significant risks with long-term COX-2 inhibitor therapy. Herbal anti-inflammatory agents have a broader, less-specific effect. As herbs are increasingly subjected to the rigors of modern studies, the research community is beginning to recognize their therapeutic value.

Many researchers have explored a variety of natural plant extracts and other natural products to elucidate their specific and nonspecific effects on COX and LO. Curcumin (turmeric), ginger, holy basil, resveratrol (concentrated in grape skins), and berberine (an alkaloid found in goldenseal, Oregon grape, barberry, and Chinese goldthread) are among the most promising candidates in the burgeoning field of herbal anti-inflammatories.

Zyflamend is a novel product comprised of several herbs in regulated concentrations. Components have anti-inflammatory, antioxidant, antiangiogenic, and/or antiproliferative effects. In 2005, Bemis et al. published the results of an analysis of Zyflamend's effects on LNCaP cells. The supplement brought about a dramatic drop in both COX-1 and COX-2 activity; increased p21 expression; attenuated cell growth; and induced apoptosis. Interestingly, the effect of the supplement on LNCaP cells appeared to be due to COX-independent mechanisms, including enhanced expression of p21 and reduced expression of AR, pStat3, and PKC alpha and beta [89].

A phase I clinical trial has been recently completed at Columbia in men with PIN to determine whether Zyflamend can influence the progression of biopsy-proven high-grade PIN to prostate cancer [90]. Of the 15 patients that finished the trial, 60% (8/15) had all benign tissue, 36% (5/15) had HGPIN in one core, and 14.3% (2/15) developed prostate cancer at the final 18-month biopsy. A statistically significant reduction in serum C-reactive protein (CRP) and reduction in nuclear factor kappa–B (NFkB) staining was also observed in the 18-month tissue samples [91].

Curcumin enhances radiation-induced clonogenic inhibition in tumor cells [92]. At Columbia, Dorai et al. found that curcumin modulates proteins that suppress apoptosis and interferes with growth factors that promote cancer progression [91].

Ginger root has been an herbal medicine since antiquity, used to treat nausea, motion sickness, upper respiratory infection, and intestinal parasites. Modern investigators have discovered in this rhizome more than 20 phytochemicals that inhibit COX-2 and 5-LO. Ginger constituents have potent antioxidant and anti-inflammatory activities; some, particularly shogaols and vallinoids [6]-gingerol and [6]-paradol, exhibit cancer preventive activity in experimental carcinogenesis [93].

NUTRIENT-DRUG INTERACTIONS

There are few studies observing the interactions between antioxidants and chemotherapy and/or radiation with prostate cancer patients. Simone et al. researched concomitant nutrient use with chemotherapy and/or radiation therapy (280 peer-reviewed articles including 62 in vitro and 218 in vivo) among different cancer patients from MEDLINE® and CANCERLIT® databases from 1965 to November 2003 [94]. These studies show that vitamin A, beta-carotene, and vitamin E do not interfere with and actually can enhance the activity of chemotherapeutic agents, decrease side effects, protect normal tissues, and, in some studies, prolong survival [94].

Five early studies showed that N-acetyl cysteine, an antioxidant, protects the heart from the cardiac toxicity of adriamycin without interfering with the tumor-killing capability of adriamycin [95]. Cellular, [96,97] animal studies, and human studies [98–101] have demonstrated that vitamins A, E, C, and K, as well as beta-carotene and selenium—as single agents or in combination—all protect against the toxicity of adriamycin and actually enhance its cancer-killing effects.

Cancer patients often suffer from caloric and nutritional malnutrition and have vitamin deficiencies, particularly of folic acid, vitamin C, and pyridoxine [102]. Chemotherapy and radiation therapy reduce serum levels of antioxidant vitamins and minerals due to lipid peroxidation and thus produce higher levels of oxidative stress. Iron may be the intermediate cause of this oxidative stress [103,104]. Therefore, supplemental iron should not be recommended to cancer patients who have anemia unless the anemia is caused by iron deficiency.

PATIENT EVALUATION

In primary care health maintenance exams in men over age 40, evaluation of the risk of CaP should include consideration of racial risk, genetic background, and in select patients, consideration of gene testing. Discussion of the benefits and disadvantages of PSA screening and the digital exam are also part of the standard of care. Review of urinary symptomatology in the context of BPH and prostate cancer is also important.

Men at risk for prostate cancer or who have prostate cancer should be weighed and body mass index (BMI) should be calculated since those with a high BMI are at risk of developing advanced prostate cancer and biochemical recurrence [105]. Tracking the patient's body composition is particularly important among patients with colon cancer given the added loss of muscle from androgen deprivation therapy.

A recommended complete biochemical workup includes CRP, fibrinogen, and erythrocyte sedimentation rate (ESR) to assess for inflammatory markers that may be associated with a higher risk of cancer progression; 25 hydroxy-vitamin D levels allow optimization of this nutrient associated with reduced risk of prostate cancer progression.

Although PSA screening has come under scrutiny, the PSA remains one of the premier tools to monitor progression of diagnosed prostate cancer. Patients attempting integrative approaches to control prostate cancer, including a nutritional regimen referred to in this chapter, should still be monitored for PSA increases suggestive of advancing disease.

SPECIAL CONDITION—HORMONE DEPRIVATION THERAPY

Hormone therapy for prostate cancer is also known as androgen deprivation therapy (ADT). Prostate cancer cannot grow or survive without androgens, which include testosterone and other male hormones. Hormone therapy decreases the amount of androgens in a man's body. Reducing androgens can slow the growth of the cancer and even shrink the tumor.

Men on ADT treatment generally require a total daily intake of 1200–1500 mg calcium with commensurate magnesium and 800–2000 IU vitamin D from food and supplements. This is crucial in men > 65 years of age and should be ensured even if the patient is on drug therapy for bone health. Some men need more calcium and vitamin D, and others need less, depending on the results of their bone density and laboratory tests. Ideally, keeping a weekly food/beverage intake diary can help determine how much calcium one is getting from his diet. Target serum level of 25-hydroxy vitamin D should be more than 35 ng/ml [106]. Calcium supplements should be taken in divided doses because the human body generally absorbs approximately 500 mg of elemental calcium at a time [107].

SUMMARY

Nutrient interventions can be synergistic with medical treatment of prostate cancer. Intensive dietary approaches should entail a plant-based diet that includes:

- Five servings of cruciferous vegetables
- Non-charred, low temperature cooked, lean meat from grass-fed or wild game (when possible), two servings a week
- Cold water fish
- Three to five cups of green tea a day
- Five servings of fermented and nonfermented organic soy a week
- Four ounces, two times a day, of diluted pomegranate juice
- Very low intake of simple carbohydrates
- Whole grains
- Multitude of multi-colored vegetables (in addition to crucifers)
- Multiple spices that include turmeric (contain curcumin), rosemary, garlic, and ginger

Food sources of nutrients are detailed in Table 39.1 and supplemental nutrients with dosing regiments can be found in Table 39.2.

Evaluation of vitamin D levels and supplementation with vitamin D is a general recommendation that is relevant for patients at risk for CaP, who have been diagnosed or treated for CaP, or who have metastatic disease. A complete work-up should include CRP and fibrinogen ESR to assess for inflammatory markers that seem to contribute to cancer progression.

REFERENCES

1. U.S. Cancer Statistics Working Group. United States Cancer Statistics: 1999–2008 Incidence and Mortality Web-based Report. Atlanta (GA): Department of Health and Human Services, Centers for Disease Control and Prevention, and National Cancer Institute; 2012. Available at: http://www.cdc.gov/uscs.
2. G. Bartsch, W. Horninger, H. Klocker, A. Reissigl, W. Oberaigner, D. Schönitzer, G. Severi, C. Robertson, and P. Boyle, "Prostate cancer mortality after introduction of prostate-specific antigen mass screening in the Federal State of Tyrol, Austria," *Urology*, vol. 58, no. 3, pp. 417–424, Sep. 2001.
3. R. Etzioni, J. M. Legler, E. J. Feuer, R. M. Merrill, K. A. Cronin, and B. F. Hankey, "Cancer surveillance series: Interpreting trends in prostate cancer—part III: Quantifying the link between population prostate-specific antigen testing and recent declines in prostate cancer mortality," *J. Natl. Cancer Inst.*, vol. 91, no. 12, pp. 1033–1039, Jun. 1999.
4. B. F. Hankey, E. J. Feuer, L. X. Clegg, R. B. Hayes, J. M. Legler, P. C. Prorok, L. A. Ries, R. M. Merrill, and R. S. Kaplan, "Cancer surveillance series: Interpreting trends in prostate cancer—part I: Evidence of the effects of screening in recent prostate cancer incidence, mortality, and survival rates," *J. Natl. Cancer Inst.*, vol. 91, no. 12, pp. 1017–1024, Jun. 1999.
5. F. H. Schröder and R. Kranse, "Verification bias and the prostate-specific antigen test—is there a case for a lower threshold for biopsy?," *N. Engl. J. Med.*, vol. 349, no. 4, pp. 393–395, Jul. 2003.
6. R. Chou, J. M. Croswell, T. Dana, C. Bougatsos, et al., "Screening for prostate cancer: A review of the evidence for the U.S. Preventive Services Task Force," *Ann. Intern. Med.*, vol. 155, no. 11, pp. 762–771, Dec. 2011.
7. S. Loeb, E. J. Metter, D. Kan, K. A. Roehl, and W. J. Catalona, "Prostate-specific antigen velocity (PSAV) risk count improves the specificity of screening for clinically significant prostate cancer," *BJU Int.*, vol. 109, no. 4, pp. 508–513; discussion 513–514, Feb. 2012.
8. M. Auprich, H. Augustin, L. Budäus, L. Kluth, S. Mannweiler, S. F. Shariat, M. Fisch, M. Graefen, K. Pummer, and F. K.-H. Chun, "A comparative performance analysis of total prostate-specific antigen, percentage free prostate-specific antigen, prostate-specific antigen velocity and urinary prostate cancer gene 3 in the first, second and third repeat prostate biopsy," *BJU Int.*, Sep. 2011.
9. IARC, "GLOBOCAN Cancer Fact Sheets: Prostate Cancer," 2008. [Online]. Available: http://globocan.iarc.fr/factsheets/cancers/prostate.asp. [Accessed: 18-Mar-2012.]
10. American Cancer Society, "What causes prostate cancer?" [Online]. Available: http://www.cancer.org/Cancer/ProstateCancer/OverviewGuide/prostate-cancer-overview-what-causes. [Accessed: 18-Mar-2012.]
11. A. L. Potosky, B. A. Miller, P. C. Albertsen, and B. S. Kramer, "The role of increasing detection in the rising incidence of prostate cancer," *JAMA*, vol. 273, no. 7, pp. 548–552, Feb. 1995.

12. M. A. Moyad and P. R. Carroll, "Lifestyle recommendations to prevent prostate cancer, part I: Time to redirect our attention?" *Urol. Clin. North Am.*, vol. 31, no. 2, pp. 289–300, May 2004.

13. J. Lorenzo Bermejo and K. Hemminki, "Risk of cancer at sites other than the breast in Swedish families eligible for BRCA1 or BRCA2 mutation testing," *Ann. Oncol.*, vol. 15, no. 12, pp. 1834–1841, Dec. 2004.

14. M. A. Moyad, "Selenium and vitamin E supplements for prostate cancer: Evidence or embellishment?" *Urology*, vol. 59, no. 4 Suppl 1, pp. 9–19, Apr. 2002.

15. W. G. Nelson, A. M. De Marzo, T. L. DeWeese, and W. B. Isaacs, "The role of inflammation in the pathogenesis of prostate cancer," *J. Urol.*, vol. 172, no. 5, Pt 2, pp. S6–11; discussion S11–12, Nov. 2004.

16. L. K. Dennis, C. F. Lynch, and J. C. Torner, "Epidemiologic association between prostatitis and prostate cancer," *Urology*, vol. 60, no. 1, pp. 78–83, Jul. 2002.

17. E. L. Richman, M. J. Stampfer, A. Paciorek, J. M. Broering, P. R. Carroll, and J. M. Chan, "Intakes of meat, fish, poultry, and eggs and risk of prostate cancer progression," *Am. J. Clin. Nutr.*, vol. 91, no. 3, pp. 712–721, Mar. 2010.

18. W. Zheng and S. A. Lee, "Well-done meat intake, heterocyclic amine exposure, and cancer risk," *Nutr. Cancer*, vol. 61, pp. 437–446, 2009.

19. C. A. Daley, A. Abbott, P. S. Doyle, G. A. Nader, and S. Larson, "A review of fatty acid profiles and antioxidant content in grass-fed and grain-fed beef," *Nutr. J.*, vol. 9, pp. 10–22, Mar. 2010.

20. K. J. Pienta and P. S. Esper, "Is dietary fat a risk factor for prostate cancer?" *J. Natl. Cancer Inst.*, vol. 85, no. 19, pp. 1538–1540, Oct. 1993.

21. E. Giovannucci, E. B. Rimm, G. A. Colditz, M. J. Stampfer, A. Ascherio, C. C. Chute, and W. C. Willett, "A prospective study of dietary fat and risk of prostate cancer," *J. Natl. Cancer Inst.*, vol. 85, no. 19, pp. 1571–1579, Oct. 1993.

22. L. Le Marchand, L. N. Kolonel, L. R. Wilkens, B. C. Myers, and T. Hirohata, "Animal fat consumption and prostate cancer: A prospective study in Hawaii," *Epidemiology*, vol. 5, no. 3, pp. 276–282, May 1994.

23. F. Meyer, I. Bairati, R. Shadmani, Y. Fradet, and L. Moore, "Dietary fat and prostate cancer survival," *Cancer Causes Control*, vol. 10, no. 4, pp. 245–251, Aug. 1999.

24. J. E. Chavarro, M. J. Stampfer, H. Campos, T. Kurth, W. C. Willett, and J. Ma, "A prospective study of trans-fatty acid levels in blood and risk of prostate cancer," *Cancer Epidemiol. Biomarkers Prev.*, vol. 17, no. 1, pp. 95–101, Jan. 2008.

25. A. G. Schuurman, P. A. van den Brandt, E. Dorant, and R. A. Goldbohm, "Animal products, calcium and protein and prostate cancer risk in The Netherlands Cohort Study," *Br. J. Cancer*, vol. 80, no. 7, pp. 1107–1113, Jun. 1999.

26. P. H. Gann, C. H. Hennekens, F. M. Sacks, F. Grodstein, E. L. Giovannucci, and M. J. Stampfer, "Prospective study of plasma fatty acids and risk of prostate cancer," *J. Natl. Cancer Inst.*, vol. 86, no. 4, pp. 281–286, Feb. 1994.

27. W. Demark-Wahnefried, T. J. Polascik, S. L. George, B. R. Switzer, et al., "Flaxseed supplementation (not dietary fat restriction) reduces prostate cancer proliferation rates in men presurgery," *Cancer Epidemiol. Biomarkers Prev.*, vol. 17, no. 12, pp. 3577–3587, Dec. 2008.

28. G. A. Kune, "Eating fish protects against some cancers: epidemiological and experimental evidence for a hypothesis," *Journal of Nutritional Medicine*, vol. 1, no. 2, pp. 139–144, 1990.

29. D. P. Rose and J. M. Connolly, "Omega-3 fatty acids as cancer chemopreventive agents," *Pharmacol. Ther.*, vol. 83, no. 3, pp. 217–244, Sep. 1999.

30. J. V. Higdon, B. Delage, D. E. Williams, and R. H. Dashwood, "Cruciferous vegetables and human cancer risk: Epidemiologic evidence and mechanistic basis," *Pharmacol. Res.*, vol. 55, no. 3, pp. 224–236, Mar. 2007.

31. A. R. Kristal and J. W. Lampe, "Brassica vegetables and prostate cancer risk: A review of the epidemiological evidence," *Nutr. Cancer*, vol. 42, no. 1, pp. 1–9, 2002.

32. S. V. Singh, S. K. Srivastava, S. Choi, K. L. Lew, et al., "Sulforaphane-induced cell death in human prostate cancer cells is initiated by reactive oxygen species," *J. Biol. Chem.*, vol. 280, no. 20, pp. 19911–19924, May 2005.

33. S. Choi, K. L. Lew, H. Xiao, A. Herman-Antosiewicz, D. Xiao, C. K. Brown, and S. V. Singh, "D,L-Sulforaphane-induced cell death in human prostate cancer cells is regulated by inhibitor of apoptosis family proteins and Apaf-1," *Carcinogenesis*, vol. 28, no. 1, pp. 151–162, Jan. 2007.

34. V. P. S. Garikapaty, B. T. Ashok, Y. G. Chen, A. Mittelman, M. Iatropoulos, and R. K. Tiwari, "Anti-carcinogenic and anti-metastatic properties of indole-3-carbinol in prostate cancer," *Oncol. Rep.*, vol. 13, no. 1, pp. 89–93, Jan. 2005.

35. J. H. Cohen, A. R. Kristal, and J. L. Stanford, "Fruit and vegetable intakes and prostate cancer risk," *J. Natl. Cancer Inst.*, vol. 92, no. 1, pp. 61–68, Jan. 2000.

36. M. Z. Fang, D. Chen, Y. Sun, Z. Jin, J. K. Christman, and C. S. Yang, "Reversal of hypermethylation and reactivation of p16INK4a, RARbeta, and MGMT genes by genistein and other isoflavones from soy," *Clin. Cancer Res.*, vol. 11, no. 19 Pt 1, pp. 7033–7041, Oct. 2005.

37. R. L. Schleicher, C. A. Lamartiniere, M. Zheng, and M. Zhang, "The inhibitory effect of genistein on the growth and metastasis of a transplantable rat accessory sex gland carcinoma," *Cancer Lett.*, vol. 136, no. 2, pp. 195–201, Mar. 1999.

38. R. Mentor-Marcel, C. A. Lamartiniere, I. A. Eltoum, N. M. Greenberg, and A. Elgavish, "Dietary genistein improves survival and reduces expression of osteopontin in the prostate of transgenic mice with prostatic adenocarcinoma (TRAMP)," *J. Nutr.*, vol. 135, no. 5, pp. 989–995, May 2005.

39. A. Rannikko, A. Petas, S. Rannikko, and H. Adlercreutz, "Plasma and prostate phytoestrogen concentrations in prostate cancer patients after oral phytoestogen supplementation," *Prostate*, vol. 66, no. 1, pp. 82–87, Jan. 2006.

40. B. K. Jacobsen, S. F. Knutsen, and G. E. Fraser, "Does high soy milk intake reduce prostate cancer incidence? The Adventist Health Study (United States)," *Cancer Causes Control*, vol. 9, no. 6, pp. 553–557, Dec. 1998.

41. Y. W. Hwang, S. Y. Kim, S. H. Jee, Y. N. Kim, and C. M. Nam, "Soy food consumption and risk of prostate cancer: A meta-analysis of observational studies," *Nutr. Cancer*, vol. 61, no. 5, pp. 598–606, 2009.

42. L. Yan and E. L. Spitznagel, "Soy consumption and prostate cancer risk in men: A revisit of a meta-analysis," *Am. J. Clin. Nutr.*, vol. 89, no. 4, pp. 1155–1163, Apr. 2009.

43. A. Herzog, U. Siler, V. Spitzer, N. Seifert, A. Denelavas, P. B. Hunziker, W. Hunziker, R. Goralczyk, and K. Wertz, "Lycopene reduced gene expression of steroid targets and inflammatory markers in normal rat prostate," *FASEB J.*, vol. 19, no. 2, pp. 272–274, Feb. 2005.

44. J. Levy, E. Bosin, B. Feldman, Y. Giat, A. Miinster, M. Danilenko, and Y. Sharoni, "Lycopene is a more potent inhibitor of human cancer cell proliferation than either alpha-carotene or beta-carotene," *Nutr. Cancer*, vol. 24, no. 3, pp. 257–266, 1995.

45. O. Kucuk, F. H. Sarkar, Z. Djuric, W. Sakr, M. N. Pollak, F. Khachik, M. Banerjee, J. S. Bertram, and D. P. Wood Jr., "Effects of lycopene supplementation in patients with localized prostate cancer," *Exp. Biol. Med. (Maywood)*, vol. 227, no. 10, pp. 881–885, Nov. 2002.

46. M. S. Ansari and N. P. Sgupta, "A comparison of lycopene and orchidectomy vs orchidectomy alone in the management of advanced prostate cancer," *BJU Int.*, vol. 95, no. 3, p. 453, Feb. 2005.

47. N. J. Barber, X. Zhang, G. Zhu, R. Pramanik, J. A. Barber, F. L. Martin, J. D. H. Morris, and G. H. Muir, "Lycopene inhibits DNA synthesis in primary prostate epithelial cells in vitro and its administration is associated with a reduced prostate-specific antigen velocity in a phase II clinical study," *Prostate Cancer Prostatic Dis.*, vol. 9, no. 4, pp. 407–413, 2006.

48. F. Haseen, M. M. Cantwell, J. M. O'Sullivan, and L. J. Murray, "Is there a benefit from lycopene supplementation in men with prostate cancer? A systematic review," *Prostate Cancer Prostatic Dis.*, vol. 12, no. 4, pp. 325–332, 2009.

49. C. Schwenke, B. Ubrig, P. Thürmann, C. Eggersmann, and S. Roth, "Lycopene for advanced hormone refractory prostate cancer: A prospective, open phase II pilot study," *J. Urol.*, vol. 181, no. 3, pp. 1098–1103, Mar. 2009.

50. L. Jian, L. P. Xie, A. H. Lee, and C. W. Binns, "Protective effect of green tea against prostate cancer: A case-control study in southeast China," *Int. J. Cancer*, vol. 108, no. 1, pp. 130–135, Jan. 2004.

51. S. Bettuzzi, M. Brausi, F. Rizzi, G. Castagnetti, G. Peracchia, and A. Corti, "Chemoprevention of human prostate cancer by oral administration of green tea catechins in volunteers with high-grade prostate intraepithelial neoplasia: a preliminary report from a one-year proof-of-principle study," *Cancer Res.*, vol. 66, no. 2, pp. 1234–1240, Jan. 2006.

52. E. Choan, R. Segal, D. Jonker, S. Malone, N. Reaume, L. Eapen, and V. Gallant, "A prospective clinical trial of green tea for hormone refractory prostate cancer: an evaluation of the complementary/alternative therapy approach," *Urol. Oncol.*, vol. 23, no. 2, pp. 108–113, Apr. 2005.

53. N. Kurahashi, S. Sasazuki, M. Iwasaki, M. Inoue, and S. Tsugane, "Green tea consumption and prostate cancer risk in Japanese men: A prospective study," *Am. J. Epidemiol.*, vol. 167, no. 1, pp. 71–77, Jan. 2008.

54. S. P. Patel, M. Hotston, S. Kommu, and R. A. Persad, "The protective effects of green tea in prostate cancer," *BJU Int.*, vol. 96, no. 9, pp. 1212–1214, Dec. 2005.

55. A. Malik, F. Afaq, S. Sarfaraz, V. M. Adhami, D. N. Syed, and H. Mukhtar, "Pomegranate fruit juice for chemoprevention and chemotherapy of prostate cancer," *Proc. Natl. Acad. Sci. U.S.A.*, vol. 102, no. 41, pp. 14813–14818, Oct. 2005.

56. A. J. Pantuck, J. T. Leppert, N. Zomorodian, W. Aronson, et al., "Phase II study of pomegranate juice for men with rising prostate-specific antigen following surgery or radiation for prostate cancer," *Clin. Cancer Res.*, vol. 12, no. 13, pp. 4018–4026, Jul. 2006.

57. Y. Yang, T. Ikezoe, Z. Zheng, H. Taguchi, H. P. Koeffler, and W.-G. Zhu, "Saw Palmetto induces growth arrest and apoptosis of androgen-dependent prostate cancer LNCaP cells via inactivation of STAT 3 and androgen receptor signaling," *Int. J. Oncol.*, vol. 31, no. 3, pp. 593–600, Sep. 2007.

58. F. Di Silverio, S. Monti, A. Sciarra, P. A. Varasano, C. Martini, S. Lanzara, G. D'Eramo, S. Di Nicola, and V. Toscano, "Effects of long-term treatment with Serenoa repens (Permixon) on the concentrations and regional distribution of androgens and epidermal growth factor in benign prostatic hyperplasia," *Prostate*, vol. 37, no. 2, pp. 77–83, Oct. 1998.

59. G. Strauch, P. Perles, G. Vergult, M. Gabriel, B. Gibelin, S. Cummings, W. Malbecq, and M. P. Malice, "Comparison of finasteride (Proscar) and Serenoa repens (Permixon) in the inhibition of 5-alpha reductase in healthy male volunteers," *Eur. Urol.*, vol. 26, no. 3, pp. 247–252, 1994.

60. R. M. Bonnar-Pizzorno, A. J. Littman, M. Kestin, and E. White, "Saw palmetto supplement use and prostate cancer risk," *Nutr. Cancer*, vol. 55, no. 1, pp. 21–27, 2006.

61. E. M. John, J. Koo, and G. G. Schwartz, "Sun exposure and prostate cancer risk: evidence for a protective effect of early-life exposure," *Cancer Epidemiol. Biomarkers Prev.*, vol. 16, no. 6, pp. 1283–1286, Jun. 2007.

62. P. J. Van Veldhuizen, S. A. Taylor, S. Williamson, and B. M. Drees, "Treatment of vitamin D deficiency in patients with metastatic prostate cancer may improve bone pain and muscle strength," *J. Urol.*, vol. 163, no. 1, pp. 187–190, Jan. 2000.

63. T. C. S. Woo, R. Choo, M. Jamieson, S. Chander, and R. Vieth, "Pilot study: potential role of vitamin D (Cholecalciferol) in patients with PSA relapse after definitive therapy," *Nutr. Cancer*, vol. 51, no. 1, pp. 32–36, 2005.

64. R. Krause, B. Matulla-Nolte, M. Essers, A. Brown, and W. Hopfenmüller, "UV radiation and cancer prevention: what is the evidence?" *Anticancer Res.*, vol. 26, no. 4A, pp. 2723–2727, Aug. 2006.

65. D. M. Peehl, A. V. Krishnan, and D. Feldman, "Pathways mediating the growth-inhibitory actions of vitamin D in prostate cancer," *J. Nutr.*, vol. 133, no. 7 Suppl, p. 2461S–2469S, Jul. 2003.

66. T. Kubota, K. Koshizuka, M. Koike, M. Uskokovic, I. Miyoshi, and H. P. Koeffler, "19-nor-26,27-bishomo-vitamin D3 analogs: A unique class of potent inhibitors of proliferation of prostate, breast, and hematopoietic cancer cells," *Cancer Res.*, vol. 58, no. 15, pp. 3370–3375, Aug. 1998.

67. G. G. Schwartz and C. L. Hanchette, "UV, latitude, and spatial trends in prostate cancer mortality: All sunlight is not the same (United States)," *Cancer Causes Control*, vol. 17, no. 8, pp. 1091–1101, Oct. 2006.

68. B. Mikhak, D. J. Hunter, D. Spiegelman, E. A. Platz, B. W. Hollis, and E. Giovannucci, "Vitamin D receptor (VDR) gene polymorphisms and haplotypes, interactions with plasma 25-hydroxyvitamin D and 1,25-dihydroxyvitamin D, and prostate cancer risk," *Prostate*, vol. 67, no. 9, pp. 911–923, Jun. 2007.

69. T. M. Beer and A. Myrthue, "Calcitriol in cancer treatment: from the lab to the clinic," *Mol. Cancer Ther.*, vol. 3, no. 3, pp. 373–381, Mar. 2004.

70. M. F. Holick, "Calcium and vitamin D. Diagnostics and therapeutics," *Clin. Lab. Med.*, vol. 20, no. 3, pp. 569–590, Sep. 2000.

71. A. Basu and V. Imrhan, "Vitamin E and prostate cancer: Is vitamin E succinate a superior chemopreventive agent?" *Nutr. Rev.*, vol. 63, no. 7, pp. 247–251, Jul. 2005.

72. T. J. Hartman, J. F. Dorgan, J. Virtamo, J. A. Tangrea, P. R. Taylor, and D. Albanes, "Association between serum alpha-tocopherol and serum androgens and estrogens in older men," *Nutr. Cancer*, vol. 35, no. 1, pp. 10–15, 1999.

73. M. Eichholzer, H. B. Stähelin, E. Lüdin, and F. Bernasconi, "Smoking, plasma vitamins C, E, retinol, and carotene, and fatal prostate cancer: Seventeen-year follow-up of the prospective basel study," *Prostate*, vol. 38, no. 3, pp. 189–198, Feb. 1999.

74. J. M. Chan, M. J. Stampfer, J. Ma, E. B. Rimm, W. C. Willett, and E. L. Giovannucci, "Supplemental vitamin E intake and prostate cancer risk in a large cohort of men in the United States," *Cancer Epidemiol. Biomarkers Prev.*, vol. 8, no. 10, pp. 893–899, Oct. 1999.

75. A. W. Hsing, G. W. Comstock, H. Abbey, and B. F. Polk, "Serologic precursors of cancer. Retinol, carotenoids, and tocopherol and risk of prostate cancer," *J. Natl. Cancer Inst.*, vol. 82, no. 11, pp. 941–946, Jun. 1990.

76. O. P. Heinonen, D. Albanes, J. Virtamo, P. R. Taylor, et al., "Prostate cancer and supplementation with alpha-tocopherol and beta-carotene: incidence and mortality in a controlled trial," *J. Natl. Cancer Inst.*, vol. 90, no. 6, pp. 440–446, Mar. 1998.

77. S. M. Lippman, E. A. Klein, P. J. Goodman, M. S. Lucia, et al., "Effect of selenium and vitamin E on risk of prostate cancer and other cancers: The Selenium and Vitamin E Cancer Prevention Trial (SELECT)," *JAMA*, vol. 301, no. 1, pp. 39–51, Jan. 2009.

78. E. A. Klein, I. M. Thompson Jr, C. M. Tangen, J. J. Crowley, et al., "Vitamin E and the risk of prostate cancer: The Selenium and Vitamin E Cancer Prevention Trial (SELECT)," *JAMA*, vol. 306, no. 14, pp. 1549–1556, Oct. 2011.

79. K. J. Helzlsouer, H. Y. Huang, A. J. Alberg, S. Hoffman, A. Burke, E. P. Norkus, J. S. Morris, and G. W. Comstock, "Association between alpha-tocopherol, gamma-tocopherol, selenium, and subsequent prostate cancer," *J. Natl. Cancer Inst.*, vol. 92, no. 24, pp. 2018–2023, Dec. 2000.

80. H.-Y. Huang, A. J. Alberg, E. P. Norkus, S. C. Hoffman, G. W. Comstock, and K. J. Helzlsouer, "Prospective study of antioxidant micronutrients in the blood and the risk of developing prostate cancer," *Am. J. Epidemiol.*, vol. 157, no. 4, pp. 335–344, Feb. 2003.

81. K. Yamaguchi, R. G. Uzzo, J. Pimkina, P. Makhov, K. Golovine, P. Crispen, and V. M. Kolenko, "Methylseleninic acid sensitizes prostate cancer cells to TRAIL-mediated apoptosis," *Oncogene*, vol. 24, no. 38, pp. 5868–5877, Sep. 2005.

82. S. O. Lee, J. Yeon Chun, N. Nadiminty, D. L. Trump, C. Ip, Y. Dong, and A. C. Gao, "Monomethylated selenium inhibits growth of LNCaP human prostate cancer xenograft accompanied by a decrease in the expression of androgen receptor and prostate-specific antigen (PSA)," *Prostate*, vol. 66, no. 10, pp. 1070–1075, Jul. 2006.

83. A. J. Duffield-Lillico, B. L. Dalkin, M. E. Reid, B. W. Turnbull, E. H. Slate, E. T. Jacobs, J. R. Marshall, and L. C. Clark, "Selenium supplementation, baseline plasma selenium status and incidence of prostate cancer: an analysis of the complete treatment period of the Nutritional Prevention of Cancer Trial," *BJU Int.*, vol. 91, no. 7, pp. 608–612, May 2003.

84. P. D. Whanger, 1981. Selenium and heavy metal toxicity. In: Spalhoz, J. E., Martin, J. L., Ganther, H. E. (Eds.), *Selenium in Biology and Medicine*. AVI: Westport, Conn, 230–255.

85. A. T. Diplock, W. J. Watkins, and M. Hewison, "Selenium and heavy metals," *Ann. Clin. Res.*, vol. 18, no. 1, pp. 55–60, 1986.

86. C. Watanabe, "Selenium deficiency and brain functions: the significance for methylmercury toxicity," *Nihon Eiseigaku Zasshi*, vol. 55, no. 4, pp. 581–589, Jan. 2001.

87. L. Jamba, B. Nehru, and M. P. Bansal, "Selenium supplementation during cadmium exposure: Changes in antioxidant enzymes and the ultrastructure of the kidney," *Journal of Trace Elements in Experimental Medicine*, vol. 10, no. 4, pp. 233–242, Jan. 1997.

88. No authors listed, "Study First: Over-expression of Cox-2 Can Predict Prostate Cancer Outcome," *Medical News Today*, 10-Nov-2006.

89. D. L. Bemis, J. L. Capodice, A. G. Anastasiadis, A. E. Katz, and R. Buttyan, "Zyflamend, a unique herbal preparation with nonselective COX inhibitory activity, induces apoptosis of prostate cancer cells that lack COX-2 expression," *Nutr. Cancer*, vol. 52, no. 2, pp. 202–212, 2005.

90. J. L. Capodice, P. Gorroochurn, A. S. Cammack, G. Eric, J. M. McKiernan, M. C. Benson, B. A. Stone, and A. E. Katz, "Zyflamend in men with high-grade prostatic intraepithelial neoplasia: Results of a phase I clinical trial," *J. Soc. Integr Oncol.*, vol. 7, no. 2, pp. 43–51, 2009.

91. T. Dorai, Y. C. Cao, B. Dorai, R. Buttyan, and A. E. Katz, "Therapeutic potential of curcumin in human prostate cancer. III. Curcumin inhibits proliferation, induces apoptosis, and inhibits angiogenesis of LNCaP prostate cancer cells in vivo," *Prostate*, vol. 47, no. 4, pp. 293–303, Jun. 2001.

92. D. Chendil, R. S. Ranga, D. Meigooni, S. Sathishkumar, and M. M. Ahmed, "Curcumin confers radio-sensitizing effect in prostate cancer cell line PC-3," *Oncogene*, vol. 23, no. 8, pp. 1599–1607, Feb. 2004.

93. Y. Shukla and M. Singh, "Cancer preventive properties of ginger: a brief review," *Food Chem. Toxicol.*, vol. 45, no. 5, pp. 683–690, May 2007.

94. M. Ciaccio, L. Tesoriere, A. M. Pintaudi, R. Re, S. Vallesi-Cardillo, A. Bongiorno, and M. A. Livrea, "Vitamin A preserves the cytotoxic activity of adriamycin while counteracting its peroxidative effects in human leukemic cells in vitro," *Biochem. Mol. Biol. Int.*, vol. 34, no. 2, pp. 329–335, Sep. 1994.

95. E. A. Ripoll, B. N. Rama, and M. M. Webber, "Vitamin E enhances the chemotherapeutic effects of adriamycin on human prostatic carcinoma cells in vitro," *J. Urol.*, vol. 136, no. 2, pp. 529–531, Aug. 1986.

96. K. Shimpo, T. Nagatsu, K. Yamada, T. Sato, H. Niimi, M. Shamoto, T. Takeuchi, H. Umezawa, and K. Fujita, "Ascorbic acid and adriamycin toxicity," *Am. J. Clin. Nutr.*, vol. 54, no. 6 Suppl, p. 1298S–1301S, Dec. 1991.

97. A. Geetha, R. Sankar, T. Marar, and C. S. Devi, "Alpha-tocopherol reduces doxorubicin-induced toxicity in rats— histological and biochemical evidences," *Indian J. Physiol. Pharmacol.*, vol. 34, no. 2, pp. 94–100, Apr. 1990.

98. A. Jotti, M. Maiorino, L. Paracchini, F. Piccinini, and F. Ursini, "Protective effect of dietary selenium supplementation on delayed cardiotoxicity of adriamycin in rat: Is PHGPX but not GPX involved?" *Free Radic. Biol. Med.*, vol. 16, no. 2, pp. 283–288, Feb. 1994.

99. C. E. Myers, W. McGuire, and R. Young, "Adriamycin: amelioration of toxicity by alpha-tocopherol," *Cancer Treat Rep*, vol. 60, no. 7, pp. 961–962, Jul. 1976.

100. P. K. Singal and J. G. Tong, "Vitamin E deficiency accentuates adriamycin-induced cardiomyopathy and cell surface changes," *Mol. Cell. Biochem.*, vol. 84, no. 2, pp. 163–171, Dec. 1988.

101. R. Lenzhofer, U. Ganzinger, H. Rameis, and K. Moser, "Acute cardiac toxicity in patients after doxorubicin treatment and the effect of combined tocopherol and nifedipine pretreatment," *J. Cancer Res. Clin. Oncol.*, vol. 106, no. 2, pp. 143–147, 1983.

102. T. H. Wasserman and D. M. Brizel, "The role of amifostine as a radioprotector," *Oncology (Williston Park, N.Y.)*, vol. 15, no. 10, pp. 1349–1354; discussion pp. 1357–1360, Oct. 2001.

103. K. Hellmann, "Anthracycline cardiotoxicity prevention by dexrazoxane: breakthrough of a barrier—sharpens antitumor profile and therapeutic index," *J. Clin. Oncol.*, vol. 14, no. 2, pp. 332–333, Feb. 1996.

104. P. Klein and F. M. Muggia, "Cytoprotection: Shelter from the storm," *Oncologist*, vol. 4, no. 2, pp. 112–121, 1999.

105. R. J. MacInnis and D. R. English, "Body size and composition and prostate cancer risk: Systematic review and meta-regression analysis," *Cancer Causes Control*, vol. 17, no. 8, pp. 989–1003, Oct. 2006.

106. M. A. Moyad, "Promoting general health during androgen deprivation therapy (ADT): A rapid 10-step review for your patients," *Urol. Oncol.*, vol. 23, no. 1, pp. 56–64, Feb. 2005.

107. P. R. Ebeling, "Clinical practice. Osteoporosis in men," *N. Engl. J. Med.*, vol. 358, no. 14, pp. 1474–1482, Apr. 2008.

Section IX

Reproductive Health and Toxicology

40 Male Infertility

Environmental and Nutritional Factors in Prevention and Treatment

*Leah Hechtman, M.Sci.Med (R.H.H.G.), BHSc
(Nat), N.D., and Roger Billica, M.D., FAAFP*

INTRODUCTION

Numerous epidemiological studies in recent decades have documented a decline in male fertility. Many of these studies propose a link between the deterioration in fertility with growing exposure to environmental toxins such as antiandrogenic pesticides and fungicides (e.g., DDT and vinclozolin), plasticizers (e.g., bisphenol-A and dibutyl phthalate), water disinfection by-products (e.g., dibromoacetic acid), heavy metals (e.g., lead, cadmium, and mercury), and common industrial contaminants in drinking water (e.g., benzene, phenol, and trichloroethylene). From a review of available literature, it is apparent that a variety of commonly used chemicals, now abundant in the environment, drinking water, and food chain, can have insidious and long-lasting effects on the male reproductive system.

The rising incidence of male infertility warrants a closer look at both preventable causes and potential solutions related to environmental and nutritional factors.

EPIDEMIOLOGY

Infertility is defined as an inability to conceive a child after 12 months of regular, unprotected intercourse (at least twice weekly) with the same female partner and in the absence of female causes. Male infertility is diagnosed from sperm abnormalities to either sperm count, morphology, motility, or other aspects confirmed by two properly performed semen analyses.

It affects approximately 7.3 million men and their partners in the United States, which equates to approximately 12% of the reproductive-age population [1]. One out of seven couples will experience difficulty conceiving. It affects men and women equally with approximately one-third of cases being responsible by male factors, one-third by female factors, and the remaining one-third by joint conception issues [2,3]. In the United States, it is estimated that as many as 18% of all couples have difficulty conceiving a child and current estimates suggest that about 6% of men between the ages of 15 and 50 years are infertile [4].

These infertility statistics have influenced the recent and dramatic decline in fertility rate that appears to be unrelated to the socioeconomic status of the country; however, deferred childbearing and improved contraceptive use are undoubtedly major factors. In the United States, some patients will require assisted reproductive technologies (ART) to enable them to conceive with statistics indicating that IVF and similar treatments account for less than 3% of infertility services and approximately 0.07% of US health care costs.

In 1992, Carlsen et al. reported a significant global decline in sperm density between 1938 and 1990 [5]. A few years later Swan et al. revisited the same issue with an analysis of 101 studies published between 1934–96 and concluded that there has been an overall decline in sperm density of approximately 1.5% per year in the United States and approximately 3% per year in Europe and Australia [6]. Their analysis controlled for variables such as abstinence time, age, percent of men with proven fertility, and specimen collection method. There was no decline trend in sperm density in non-Western countries, but the authors noted that data was very limited for these populations.

Skakkebaek et al. have found that at present, 30% of young Danish men seem to have sperm counts that are in the subnormal range according to World Health Organization guidelines and, in 10% of this population, the semen parameters are indicative of substantially reduced fertility prospects [7]. Furthermore, they have correlated that declining semen parameters correlate with increasing testicular cancer rates; leading researchers are suggesting that testicular dysgenesis syndrome (TDS) is environmentally triggered and warrants concern for population survival. The particularly low sperm counts recorded in Denmark are linked with other male reproductive pathologies, including one of the highest rates of testicular cancer in the world and an increasing occurrence of other male genital tract abnormalities such as cryptorchidism and hypospadias [8]. It has been proposed that environmental factors are involved in the etiology of TDS and that these factors have their effect during early fetal life, when the male genital tract is attempting to differentiate away from the default female condition [9]. Whether the outcome of TDS is impaired spermatogenesis or testicular cancer may depend on the timing and nature of the xenobiotic attack and the genetic background on which these factors are acting.

PATHOPHYSIOLOGY

Fertility is a reflection of one's general health and well-being and can also indicate latent or undiagnosed genetic abnormalities or other etiological considerations. There are many well-established known causes for male infertility [10,11], including:

- Primary hypogonadism (30–40%): androgen insensitivity, congenital or developmental testicular disorder (e.g., Klinefelter syndrome), cryptorchidism, medication (e.g., alkylating agents, antiandrogens, cimetidine [Tagamet], ketoconazole [Nizoral], spironolactone [Aldactone])
- Y chromosome defect: genetic defects, such as microdeletions on the long arm of the male determining Y chromosome and other yet to be discovered mutations, are responsible for some of the more severe defects of sperm production or function and these defects may be transmitted directly to sons or to future generations
- Altered sperm transport (10–20%): absent vas deferens or obstruction, prostate-related disorders or complications, postinfectious obstruction, epididymal absence or obstruction, erectile dysfunction and other coital disorders (defects in technique, premature withdrawal, infrequent intercourse, spinal cord injury), ejaculatory dysfunction (retrograde ejaculation, premature ejaculation), vasectomy or postvasectomy reversal
- Secondary hypogonadism (1–2%): androgen excess state (e.g., tumor, exogenous administration), congenital idiopathic hypogonadotropic hypogonadism, estrogen excess state (e.g., tumor), infiltrative disorder (e.g., sarcoidosis, tuberculosis), medication effect, multiorgan genetic disorder (e.g., Prader-Willi syndrome), pituitary adenoma, trauma
- Developmental or physiological: undescended testes, varicocele, torsion, testicular trauma, orchitis, including mumps orchitis
- Immunological: infection, inflammation, sperm antibodies, autoimmune diseases

- Unknown causes (40–50%): may be related to the following aspects—toxicity, oxidative damage to sperm, radiation exposure, excessive heat to testicles, poor nutritional status or nutritional deficiencies, heavy metal or environmental toxicity, systemic disorders, hormonal imbalances, xenobiotic exposure, hepatic cirrhosis, genito-urinary infections, cigarette smoking, recreational drug usage, age-related decline, obesity, others

The environmental impact cannot be underestimated. Industrial growth since the end of World War II has introduced many complex chemicals into the environment that are novel to biological detoxification systems. Some of these molecules are reproductive toxicants, capable of impairing fertility and inducing developmental abnormalities in the embryo, including errors in normal sexual differentiation.

Such compounds may exert their genetic or epigenetic effects on the germ line via several potential routes of exposure:

1. Women may be exposed to xenobiotics during pregnancy, thereby disrupting the normal differentiation of the germ line in the fetus.
2. Women exposed to toxicants may transmit xenobiotics to their offspring via breast milk.
3. Paternally mediated toxicity through effects on DNA integrity in the male germ line.

Toxicological studies in animal models reporting infertility, abortion, and birth defects as a result of male exposure to xenobiotics demonstrate that such associations are possible [12]. Epidemiological studies suggest that they are clinically significant [13,14].

As epidemiological studies have recognized the declining trend in male fertility, the discussion of etiology has included possible involvement of environmental factors. Since both men and women require a proper balance of estrogens in order to be successful reproductively, some of the more obvious considered causes have included exposures to estrogens [15] and xenoestrogens [16]. These estrogen mimics are known to be endocrine disrupters and are found in everyday personal care products and as the breakdown products from plastics used in items such as water jugs and baby bottles. The estrogen-mimic bisphenol-A (BPA) is used in the manufacture of polycarbonate plastics and epoxy resins from which food and beverage containers and dental materials are made. Perinatal exposure to environmentally relevant doses of BPA has been shown to cause morphological and functional changes of the male genital tract and reduced fertility [17]. Dibutyl phthalate is used widely in production as a plasticizer, in cosmetics such as nail polish, and as an additive to adhesives and print inks. Dibutyl phthalate is considered to be an endocrine disrupter and has been shown to impair spermatogenesis and induce lesions in the reproductive system in animal models [18,19].

Vinclozolin is a fungicide introduced in the 1970s that is used worldwide on fruits, vegetables, and vineyards, and thus is commonly ingested. Exposure to vinclozolin in rabbits during development stages induced presumably permanent changes in spermiogenesis and FSH secretion [20]; it disrupted the fertility in male rats [21]; and just one exposure of a pregnant female rat to this fungicide was found to disrupt spermatogenesis in more than 90% of the male offspring for at least four generations via an effect that was exclusively transmitted through the male germ line. Exposure to the fungicides tebuconazole and epoxiconazole were investigated for reproductive effects in rats and found disrupting effects to endocrine including disturbances of key enzymes involved with the synthesis of steroid hormones [22].

Reproductive disorders including sperm abnormalities, hypospadias, and decreased fertility have been linked to pesticide exposure [23–26]. In addition to the direct endocrine disrupting effects of the various pesticides, there is also evidence that long-term exposure to pesticides can cause changes in antioxidant enzymes with harmful consequences not only on the immune and nervous system but also with issues related to immunofertility [27,28].

Another environmental concern with infertility is the negative impact of heavy metals on sperm quality and production. Occupational exposure to lead, mercury, and cadmium has been shown to cause significant decrease in male fertility [29–33]. Of course, occupational contact with toxic metals is not the only risk of exposure due to the diffuse spread of these metals in the environment.

Other studies have examined the impact of the presence of heavy metals [34]. For example, the mechanism of lead toxicity on the testis involves several areas including spermatogenesis, steroidogenesis, and the reduction-oxidation system. Chronic lead exposure can induce decreased testosterone synthesis, decreased germ cell population, and peritubular fibrosis [35].

Male infertility issues have also been linked with a variety of common industrial and household chemicals [36–38]. These include:

- Dibromoacetic acid (a water disinfection by-product)
- Solvents (such as Trichlorethylene)
- Phenol
- Chloroform

In the presence of such widespread exposure to potentially harmful toxins, there is some question as to why the impacts on male fertility are not even more widespread than noted. A reasonable explanation could be related to the concept of biochemical individuality, wherein the level of function of the detoxification and elimination pathways necessary for neutralization and removal of these chemicals and heavy metals varies from person to person. One study showed that individuals with impaired methylation due to genetic polymorphisms have frequent alterations in fertility [39]. Other studies have found that disruption of glutathione S-transferases (enzymes that detoxify electrophillic compounds) interferes with fertilizing ability of spermatozoa [40]. So whether an individual has a genetic or acquired polymorphism, changes in cellular detoxification functions appear to be an additional risk factor for environmental impacts on male fertility.

Other important considerations include:

- Obesity: obese men are known to have lower sperm counts (up to 50%), reduced motility, reduced spermatogenesis, increased DNA fragmentation of sperm, and increased levels of erectile dysfunction. Additionally, extra abdominal weight can increase scrotal temperature [41].
- Increased scrotal temperature: the mean scrotal temperature of infertile men is significantly higher than that of fertile men and reduction of temperature can often resume fertility.
- Radiation: cell and cordless phones emit radiofrequency electromagnetic waves (EMW) and are implicated in DNA strand breaks [42]. Harmful EMW may interfere with normal spermatogenesis and result in a significant decrease in sperm quality, morphology and motility [43–45].
- Smoking: paternal cigarette smoking generates spermatozoa that suffer from high levels of DNA damage, largely as a result of oxidative stress. One of the consequences of this DNA damage is that the children of such men exhibit an increased incidence of childhood cancer [46]. Additionally, decreased sperm counts, decreased sperm motility, increased levels of abnormal sperm [47], increased miscarriage risk [48,49], and reduction in semen quality [50] are also noted.
- Marijuana: cannabinoids from marijuana have been found to inhibit mitochondrial respiration of human sperm [51], reduce testosterone production [52], decrease sperm motility, reduce sperm morphology, and decrease sperm function specifically capacitation and acrosome reactions [53].

PATIENT EVALUATION

When presented with a male patient expressing infertility, it is important to organize a general health screen and a specific fertility workup including a full hormone profile and semen analysis organized through a specialized andrology laboratory that reviews a standard semen analysis, testing for sperm antibodies (immunobead testing [IBT]), and DNA fragmentation. Scrotal ultrasonography and physical examination in instances of previous testicular trauma or a history of undescended testes and genetic screening (including karyotype) will be advisable in some cases.

Additionally, environmental assessments including those that assess PCBs, chlorinated pesticides, volatile solvents, phthalates, parabens, nutrient and toxic element screening (heavy metals), and other toxins should additionally be considered due to their deranging effects on reproductive function, endocrinology, gamete development, and thus embryological potential.

Since blood testing for levels of heavy metals is only accurate for fairly recent exposure, most evaluations for heavy metals should more appropriately focus on testing that indicates tissue impact of past or chronic exposures. These tests would include urinary porphyrins [54] and/or a urine provocative challenge test using clinical dosing of the appropriate chelating agent (such as EDTA or DMSA). A variety of laboratories perform these tests and can provide the clinician with detailed guides for test administration and assistance with interpretation of the results. Testing for organophosphate pesticide exposure within a few months of exposures can be accomplished with red blood cell cholinesterase determination [55].

As with most diagnostic endeavors, the clinician must take a careful history looking for potential exposures, family history of other potential manifestations of environmental toxicities (e.g., neurological and developmental disorders), and have a high index of suspicion. However, the chemicals and metals involved with increased risk of male infertility are so common and ubiquitous in today's world that it may not be necessary to find a specific or significant history of exposure. For example, one study demonstrated clinically significant human exposure to pesticides simply through the persistent presence of these chemicals on foods [56]. Another study demonstrated elevated pesticide urinary metabolites of children in farmworker households [57]. In many areas of the country, households receive routine treatments with pesticides, and a number of communities have reinstituted pesticide spraying due to the recent concerns with the West Nile virus.

TREATMENT

While the various treatment approaches for the more typical causes of male infertility are detailed elsewhere, the successful clinical intervention for environmental causes requires that the clinician be familiar with three areas of priority.

PREVENTION

Prevention basically consists of avoidance of exposure to the offending agents. This is not only important for men of reproductive age but also for women to prevent exposure to the fetus in utero and for children during growth and development. Due to the overwhelming presence of the identified chemicals and toxins in our environment, avoiding them may seem an impossible task. However there are feasible steps individuals can take to reduce their risk of exposure. For example:

- Knowing the source, quality, and content of household and workplace drinking water; and if necessary installing water filtration such as reverse osmosis sufficient to remove chemicals and heavy metals
- Reducing exposure to pesticides and fungicides on fruits and vegetables, either through purchase of trustworthy organic produce or use of vegetable wash soaps prior to consumption
- Being aware of and participating in efforts to reduce exposure to heavy metals that are still found in some vaccines, dental fillings, pharmacological agents, consumer products, certain fish and seafood, and other products
- Finding nontoxic alternatives for the use of household pesticides and cleaning agents
- Limiting exposure to plastics used in food preparation and storage. For example, use nonplastic containers and covers while heating food in microwave ovens. Discard scratched cookware with nonstick surfaces. Store food and beverages in glass instead of plastic containers

DETOXIFICATION

Detoxification of offending chemicals and heavy metals may involve a variety of therapies:

- The basic principles of clinical detoxification remain important when dealing with either heavy metals, pesticides, plastics, or other chemical toxins. Especially important are the maintenance of tissue hydration and avoidance of constipation. Correction of underlying metabolic and nutritional deficiencies such as impaired methylation and hypothyroidism should precede any focused detoxification protocols.
- Phospholipids and essential fatty acids: since the area of toxic impact often involves disruption of the cell membrane bi-lipid integrity, steps to restore the balance of essential fatty acids in the cell membranes are a foundation for recovery. The health of the cell membrane is a key determinant of the function of the tissue; therefore, detoxification requires that the membrane of the cell be supported with balanced essential fatty acids and supportive phospholipids. Phosphatidylcholine (PC) is the most abundant phospholipid of the cell membrane and plays a key role in detoxification. In addition to phosphatidylcholine, a ratio of balanced essential fatty acids (4:1 omega-6 to omega-3 oil) provides the cellular nourishment for healthy membrane function [58–60]. Typical adult dosing for phosphatidylcholine in support of cell membrane repair and detoxification is in the range of 1200 to 2500 mg daily in two divided doses. Essential fatty acids can be found in a balanced ratio of 4:1 omega-6 (such as sunflower or safflower oil) and omega-3 (flax oil) and are recommended in a therapeutic dose range of two to four tablespoons daily. It is very important that these oils be organic, cold pressed, and maintained in a refrigerated state to avoid rancidity.

Foods that are high in phosphatidylcholine are those that provide lecithin including eggs, soy, Brewer's yeast, grains, legumes, fish, and wheat germ. A word of caution is prudent concerning the inclusion of soy products with men being treated for infertility due to the possible estrogenic effects of soy proteins.

Glutathione (g-glutamylcysteinglycine [GSH]) performs a variety of vital physiological and metabolic functions within all cells affecting the preservation of tissue integrity. GSH plays a major role in detoxifying many reactive metabolites by either spontaneous conjugation or by a reaction catalyzed by the GSH S-transferases. As a result, its functions include a variety of areas such as:

- Maintenance olf protein structure and function by reducing disulfide linkages of proteins, including metallothioneins (involved with heavy metal detoxification)
- Stabilization of immune function
- Protection against oxidative damage
- Detoxification of reactive chemicals
- Formation of bile
- Leukotriene and prostaglandin metabolism
- Reduction of rebonucleotides to deoxyribonucleotides

The elevation of cellular levels of glutathione provides a key defense against toxic products of oxygen, particularly in the mitochondria [61], and serves to upregulate tissue detoxification [62]. Various strategies exist for repleting cellular glutathione:

- Glutathione given orally has been demonstrated in vivo to raise plasma levels [63]. Recently available formulations of acetyl-glutathione appear to have good absorption and bioavailability with recommended dosing of 100 mg once or twice daily.
- Intravenous glutathione (push) in doses ranging from 1500–2000 mg has been combined in series with IV phosphotidylcholine as a therapy for various neurodegenerative disorders [64].

- Glutathione precursors include N-acetyl-cysteine (NAC), L-methionine, L-glutamine, and L-taurine. Administration of precursors do not seem to raise glutathione levels it they are already in the normal range, but do appear to raise abnormally low GSH levels back to normal [65]. Following its intestinal absorption, NAC is converted to circulating cysteine and can effectively replenish GSH in depleted patients [66]. It is not recommended to use oral forms of plain L-cysteine because it is known to be highly unstable and potentially toxic. The activated counterpart of L-methionine, S-adenosylmethionine (SAMe), is well tolerated and has been shown to replenish erythrocyte GSH. Taurine is a sulfur amino acid that, given orally, can raise platelet GSH in healthy males [67].
- Alpha-lipoic acid (ALA) is a broad spectrum, fat- and water-phase antioxidant with potent electron-donating capacity and is another GSH repleter. Oral ALA raises GSH levels in HIV patients [68], and it has been demonstrated to improve biliary excretion of heavy metals as transported by reduced glutathione [69]. Typical therapeutic dosing is in the range of 100–300 mg twice a day.
- Far infrared sauna is a broad-spectrum detoxification modality that is available for home and clinical use. Far infrared wavelength is a section of the natural band of light that is not visible to the human eye but can be felt like heat. Rather than the traditional steam or dry saunas, far infrared saunas use that specific energy wavelength to penetrate the body tissues and stimulate cellular detoxification through the breakdown and release of fat-stored toxins and subsequent elimination through sweating. Although there are many claims regarding the ability of far infrared sauna to safely and effectively remove a variety of toxicants including heavy metals, there are few studies available to support these claims [70–72]. However, the data that is available suggests that this treatment warrants further attention and study given the scope of environmentally related illness.
- Detoxification of heavy metals is performed using chelation agents such as EDTA (IV and oral) and DMSA (oral) according to clinically established protocols.

NUTRITIONAL AND BIOCHEMICAL SUPPORT FOR MALE FERTILITY

Nutritional and biochemical support for a healthy male reproductive system is an important adjunctive strategy in any attempts to help a patient recover fertility. The following nutritional therapies have shown promise in this area:

- **L-Arginine:** the amino acid arginine is a precursor in the synthesis of putrescine, spermidine, and spermine, which are thought to be essential in sperm motility. Via its role as a precursor to nitric oxide synthesis, arginine is required for angiogenesis, spermatogenesis, and hormone secretion [73]. A number of studies have shown that arginine can improve sperm count and motility [74–77]. Researchers in Italy evaluated the efficacy of arginine in 40 infertile men. After six months of therapy, there was significantly improved sperm motility without any side effects [78].
- **L-Carnitine:** in the epididymis, carnitine serves as an energy substrate for spermatozoa, enhancing transport of fatty acids into the mitochondria. It is believed to have protective antioxidant effects and provides energy to the testicles and spermatozoa specifically [79]. In a study involving 124 infertile patients, a direct correlation between semen carnitine content and sperm motility was found [80]. Several studies comparing fertile men to infertile men found that fertile men had a statistically significant larger amount of carnitine in their seminal sample than the infertile men and that low levels of L-carnitine in the seminal plasma may be a potent marker for infertility [81–83]. Additionally, other studies have demonstrated improvements in sperm health parameters following administration of carnitine in the ranges of 3 to 4 grams per day [85–92].

- **Antioxidants:** key components of the sperm cell include polyunsaturated fatty acids and phospholipids, which are susceptible to oxidative damage. As with all cells, sperm metabolism results in production of reactive oxygen species, which can result in free radical–induced damage. A recent Cochrane review [93] assessed the impact of antioxidants and male subfertility by reviewing 34 trials and 2876 couples. Important findings included:
  - Antioxidant use was associated with a statistically significant increased pregnancy rate compared to control (pooled OR 4.18, 95% CI 2.65 to 6.59; $P < 0.00001$, I2 = 0%).
  - 1:20 males are affected by subfertility and 3–80% is believed to be due to oxidative stress [94].
  - Subfertile men are confirmed as having lower levels of antioxidants in their semen compared to fertile men [95].
  - ROS levels are significantly higher in infertile sperm samples when compared to healthy controls—high levels of free radicals are found in the semen of approximately 40% of infertile men [96–98]. Men exposed to higher levels of sources of free radicals are much more likely to have abnormal sperm and sperm counts [99–101].
- **Zinc:** zinc is found in high concentrations within the prostate, testes, and particularly high amounts are also found in the semen (approximately 2.5 mg of zinc is lost per ejaculate). It is involved in virtually every aspect of male reproduction, including hormone metabolism, spermatogenesis, and sperm motility [102]. Zinc deficiency is associated with decreased testosterone levels and sperm count. An adequate amount of zinc ensures proper sperm motility and production, while deficient levels are often found in infertile men with diminished sperm count [103–108].
- **Coenzyme Q10:** coQ_{10} found in the seminal fluid and the sperm [109] where it assists in optimal sperm motility [110,111]. Deceased levels have been found in the seminal plasma and spermatozoa of males with idiopathic and varicocele-associated asthenospermia [112].
- **Glutathione and Selenium:** in addition to its role in detoxification previously discussed, glutathione is vital to sperm antioxidant defenses and has demonstrated a positive effect on sperm motility [113]. Selenium and glutathione are essential to the formation of an enzyme present in spermatids that is necessary for spermatozoa maturation. Deficiencies in either substance can lead to defective sperm motility [114]. A variety of studies have shown improvement in male fertility parameters following administration of glutathione (600 mg daily IM) or selenium (200 mcg/day) [115,116].

  Selenium is involved in testosterone synthesis and sperm motility [117,118] and assists in the production of healthy spermatozoa [119]. Selenium is also required structurally as the sperm capsular selenoprotein involved in the stability and motility of the mature sperm and also forms part of the glutathione peroxidase antioxidant system that is paramount for spermatogenesis and protects the sperm against the effects of reactive oxygen species [120].
- **Vitamin C:** a marginal deficiency causes oxidative damage to sperm, resulting in reduced sperm motility and viability leading to infertility and increased damage to the sperm's genetic material [121]. Supplementation leads to improvement in both viability and motility, reduced numbers of abnormal sperm, and reduced sperm agglutination [122,123]. One study demonstrated significant improvements in sperm count in previously infertile but otherwise healthy men following administration of 1000 mg of vitamin C daily [124].
- **Vitamin A:** low concentrations of vitamin A are associated with abnormal semen parameters [125] and intake of beta-carotene is positively associated with a higher sperm concentration and improved sperm motility [126].
- **Vitamin E:** vitamin E has been shown to play an essential role in inhibiting free-radical damage to the unsaturated fatty acids of the sperm membrane [127] and to enhance the ability of sperm to fertilize an egg in an IVF setting. Additionally, it has been shown to protect DNA within the sperm from damage [128].

- **Alpha-Lipoic Acid (ALA):** in addition to its chelating functions, ALA is able to regenerate other antioxidants including vitamins C and E, coQ10, and glutathione [129]. It is a powerful antioxidant for sperm in animal studies [130–132] and protects the sperm against free-radical damage [132]. In animal studies, it has been shown to improve sperm motility and viability, minimize DNA damage [132], and assist with energy supply to the sperm [132],
- **Vitamin D3:** vitamin D3 has been found in the head and mid-piece (neck) of the sperm and is believed to be involved in protecting DNA with the head and assisting in movement of the sperm. Additionally, low serum levels are correlated with increased intracellular calcium concentration, reduced sperm motility, reduced acrosome reaction in mature spermatozoa, and reduced sperm function [133].
- **Vitamin B9 (Folate) and Vitamin B12:** the synthesis of RNA and DNA as part of cellular replication requires vitamin B9 and B12; deficiency states have been associated with decreased sperm count and motility. Both B9 and B12 facilitate spermatogenesis [134], which is reliant upon DNA synthesis [136] for germ cell growth and rapid division of cells. Multiple studies conclude similar findings that low levels of B9 in seminal plasma are associated with increased sperm DNA damage [135], while B12 deficiency is strongly associated with reduced sperm motility and count [137]. Studies have administered doses in the range of 1000 to 6000 mcg per day (the average dose being 1500 mcg daily) and have consistently shown improvements in sperm production [138,139].

SUMMARY

The decline in male fertility has been attributed in part to an increasing incidence of exposure to environmental factors such as pesticides and fungicides, heavy metals, plastics, and industrial and household chemicals. As part of a workup with patients who suffer from infertility, these environmental factors should be taken into consideration by the clinician. Testing for exposure could include:

- Urine panels for environmental pollutants and chemical exposures.
- Heavy metals testing using urine porphyrins and provocation with chelation agents.
- Red blood cell cholinesterase determination for pesticide exposure.

Treatment for these environmental factors in male infertility focuses first on prevention, with avoidance of exposures. Remediation of the toxicity can involve:

- Proper hydration and bowel elimination.
- Correction of underlying nutritional and metabolic deficiencies.
- Providing a therapeutic balance of phospholipids and essential fatty acids.
- Administration of glutathione and glutathione precursors.
- Removal of heavy metals via chelation.
- Encourage sweating through far infrared sauna, clay baths, exercise, and avoidance of aluminum containing deodorant.

Nutritional support for a healthy male reproductive system can be approached in various ways. Published research suggests benefit from food and supplement sourced nutrients: L-arginine, L-carnitine, antioxidants, zinc, coenzyme Q10, glutathione and selenium, vitamin C, vitamin A, vitamin E, alpha lipoic acid, vitamin D3, and vitamins B9 and B12.

REFERENCES

1. National Survey of Family Growth, CDC 2002.
2. MacLeod J. Human male infertility. *Obstet Gynecol Surv* 1979; 26:335.

3. Purvis K, Christiansen E. Male infertility: Current concepts. *Ann Med* 1992; 24:258–272.
4. Brugh VM,III, Lipshultz LI. Male factor infertility: Evaluation and management. *Med Clin North Am* 2004; 88:367–385.
5. Carlsen E, Giwercman A, Keiding N, Skakkebaek N. Evidence for decreasing quality of semen during past 50 years. *Br Med J* 1992; 305:609–613.
6. Swan S, Elkin E, Fenster L. The question of declining sperm density revisited: An analysis of 101 studies published 1934–1996. *Env Health Pers* 2000; 108:961–966.
7. Skakkebaek NE, Jorgensen N, Main NE, et al. Is human fecundity declining? *Int J Androl* 2006; 29 2–12.
8. Boisen K, Chellakooty M, Schmidt IM, et al. Hypospadias in a cohort of 1072 Danish newborn boys: Prevalence and relationship to placental weight, anthropometrical measurements at birth, and reproductive hormone levels at 3 months of age. *J Clin Endocrinol Metab* 2005; 90:4041–4046.
9. Skakkebaek NE, Jorgensen N, Main NE, et al. Is human fecundity declining? *Int J Androl* 2006; 29:2–12.
10. Matsumoto A. The Testis. In: Felig P and Frohman L, eds. *Endocrinology and Metabolism.* 4th ed. New York: McGraw Hill; 2001:635–705.
11. Jose-Miller, A., Boyden, JW, Frey, KA, Infertility, *Am Fam Physician* 2007; 75:849–856, 857–858.
12. Lewis SE, Aitken RJ. DNA damage to spermatozoa has impacts on fertilization and pregnancy. *Cell Tissue Res* 2005; 322:33–41.
13. Skakkebaek NE, Jorgensen N, Main NE, et al. Is human fecundity declining? *Int J Androl* 2006; 29:2–12.
14. Boisen K, Chellakooty M, Schmidt IM, et al. Hypospadias in a cohort of 1072 Danish newborn boys: Prevalence and relationship to placental weight, anthropometrical measurements at birth, and reproductive hormone levels at 3 months of age. *J Clin Endocrinol Metab* 2005; 90:4041–4046.
15. Sharpe R, Skakkebaek N. Are oestrogens involved in falling sperm counts and disorders of the male reproductive tract? *Lancet* 1993; 341:1392–1995.
16. Toppari J, et al. Male reproductive health and environmental xenoestrogens. *Environ Health Persp* 1996; 104:741–803.
17. Maffini M, Rubin B, Sonnenschein C, Soto A. Endocrine disruptors and reproductive health: The case of bisphenol-A. *Mol Cell Endocrinol* 2006; 25:254–255:179–186.
18. Higuchi T, Palmer J, Gray L, Veeramachaneni D. Effects of dibutyl phthalate in male rabbits following in utero, adolescent, or postpubertal exposure. *Toxicol Sci* 2003; 72:301–313.
19. Lee S, Veeramachaneni D. Subchronic exposure to low concentrations of Di-n-butyl phthalate disrupts spermatogenesis in Xenopus laevis frogs *Toxicol Sci* 2005; 84:394–407.
20. Veeramachaneni D, Palmer J, Amann R, Kane C, Higuchi T, Pau K. Disruption of sexual function, FSH secretion, and spermiogenesis in rabbits following development exposure to vinclozolin, a fungicide. Society for Reproduction and Fertility (paper) 2006.
21. Anway MD, Cupp AS, Uzumcu M, et al. Epigenetic transgenerational actions of endocrine disruptors and male fertility. *Science* 2005; 308:1466–1469.
22. Taxvig C, Hass U, Axelstad M, Dalgaarad M, Boberg J, Andeasen H, Vinggaard A. Endocrine-disrupting activities in vivo of the fungicides tebuconazole and epoxiconazole. *Toxicol Sci* 2007; 100(2):464–473.
23. Frazier L. Reproductive disorders associated with pesticide exposure. *J Agromedicine* 2007; 12(1): 227–237.
24. Peiris-John R, Wickremasinghe R. Impact of low-level exposure to organophosphates on human reproduction and survival. *Trans R Soc Trop Med Hyg* 2008; 102(3):239–245.
25. Fernandez M, Olmos B, Granada A, Lopez-Espinosa M, Molina-Molina J, Fernandez J, Cruz M, Olea-Serrano F, Olea N. Human exposure to endocrine-disrupting chemicals and prenatal risk factors for cryptorchodism and hypospadias: a nested case-control study. *Environ Health Perspect* 2007; 115:8–14.
26. Veeramachaneni D, Palmer J, Amann R, Pau K. Sequelae in male rabbits following developmental exposure to DDT or a mixture of DDT and vinclozolin : Cryptorchidism, germ cell atypia, and sexual dysfunction. *Reproductive Toxicology* 2007; 23:353–365.
27. Lopez O, Hernandez A, Rodrigo L, Gil F, Pena G, Serrano J, Parron T, Villanueva E, Pla A. Changes in antioxidant enzymes in humans with long-term exposure to pesticides. *Toxicol Lett* 2007; 171(3):146–153.
28. Palan P, Naz R. Changes in various antioxidant levels in human seminal plasma related to immunofertility. *Arch Androl* 1996; 36:139–143.
29. Shiau C, Wang J, Chen P. Decreased fecundity among male lead workers. *Occup Environ Med* 2004; 61(11):915–923.
30. Gennart J, Buchet J, Roels H, et al. Fertility of male workers exposed to cadmium, lead, or manganese. *Am J Epidemiol* 1992; 135:1208–1219.
31. Weber R, de Baat C. Male fertility: Possibly affected by occupational exposure to mercury *Ned Tijdschr Tandheelkd* 2000; 102(12):495–498.

32. Dickman M, Leung C, Leung M. Hong Kong male subfertility links to mercury in human hair and fish. *Sci Total Environ* 1998; 214:165–174.
33. Joffe M. Infertility and environmental pollutants. *Br Med Bull* 2003; 68:47–70.
34. Sinawat S. The environmental impact on male fertility. *J Med Assoc Thai* 2000; 83(8):880–885.
35. Martynowicz H, Andrzejak R, Medras M. The influence of lead on testis function. *Med Pr* 2005; 56(6): 495–500.
36. Veeramachaneni D, Palmer J, Amann R. Long-term effects on male reproduction of early exposure to common chemical contaminants in drinking water. *Hum Reprod* 2001; 16(5):979–987.
37. Feichtinger W. Environmental factors and fertility. *Hum Reprod* 1991; 6(8):1170–1175.
38. Veeramachaneni D. Impact of environmental pollutants on the male: Effects on germ cell differentiation. *Anim Reprod Sci* 2007, doi:10.1016/j.anireprosci.2007.11.020.
39. Dhillon V, Shahid M, Husain S. Associations of MTHFR DNMT3b 4977 bp deletion in mtDNA and GSTM1 deletion, aberrant CpG island hypermethylation of GSTM1 in non-obstructive infertility in Indian men. *Mol Hum Reprod* 2007; 13(4):213–222.
40. Hermachand T, Gopalakrishnan B, Slaunke D, Totey S, Shaha C. Sperm plasma-membrane-associated glutathione S-transferases as gamete recognition molecules. *J Cell Sci* 2002; 115:2053–2065.
41. Lighten A. A weighty issue: Managing reproductive problems in the obese, *Conceptions*, Sydney IVF, June 2009:9.
42. Lai H, Singh NP. Single- and double-strand DNA breaks in rat brain cells after acute exposure to radio-frequency electromagnetic radiation, *Int J Radiat Biol* 1996; 69:513–521.
43. Fejes I, Zavaczki Z, Szollosi J, et al. Is there a relationship between cell phone use and semen quality? *Arch Androl* 2005; 51:385–393.
44. Davoudi M, Brossner C, KuberW. The influence of electromagnetic waves on sperm motility, *Urol Urogynaecol* 2002; 19:18–22.
45. Agarwal A, Deepinder F, Sahrma RK, Ranga G, Li J. Effect of cell phone usage on semen analysis in men attending infertility clinic: An observational study, *Fert & Ster* 2008; 89(1), 124–128.
46. Ji BT, Shu XO, Linet MS, et al. Paternal cigarette smoking and the risk of childhood cancer among off-spring of nonsmoking mothers. *J Natl Cancer Inst* 1997; 89:238–244.
47. Saleh RA, Agarwal A, Sharma RK, et al. Effect of cigarette smoking on levels of seminal oxidative stress in infertile men: A prospective study. *Fertil Steril* 2002 Sep; 78:491–499.
48. Fuentes A, Munoz A, Barnhart K, Argüello B, Díaz M, Pommer R. Recent cigarette smoking and assisted reproductive technologies outcome. *Fertil Steril* 2010 Jan; 93(1):89–95. Epub 2008 Oct 29.
49. Aitken RJ, Skakkebaek NE, Roman SD. Male reproductive health and the environment. *Med J Aust* 2006; 185(8): 414–415.
50. Gaur DS, Talekar MS, Pathak VP. Alcohol intake and cigarette smoking:Iimpact of two major lifestyle factors on male fertility. *Indian J Pathol Microbiol* 2010 Jan-Mar; 53(1):35–40.
51. Badawy ZS, Chohan KR, Whyte DA, Penefsky HS, Brown OM, Souid AK. Cannabinoids inhibit the respiration of human sperm. *Fertil Steril* 2009 Jun; 91(6):2471–2476. Epub 2008 Jun 18.
52. Battista N, Pasquariello N, Di Tommaso M, Maccarrone M. Interplay between endocannabinoids, steroids and cytokines in the control of human reproduction *J Neuroendocrinol* 2008 May; 20 Suppl 1:82–89.
53. Rossato M. Endocannabinoids, sperm functions and energy metabolism *Mol Cell Endocrino*. 2008 Apr 16; 286(1–2 Suppl 1):S31–5. Epub 2008 Feb 29.
54. Geier D, Geier M. A prospective assessment of porphyrins in autistic disorders: A potential marker for heavy metal exposure. *Neurotox Res* 2006; 10(1):57–64.
55. Nigg H, Knaak J. Blood cholinesterases as human biomarkers of organophosphate pesticide exposure. *Rev Environ Contam Toxicol* 2000; 163:29–111.
56. Rivas A, Cerrillo I, Granada A, Mariscal-Arcas M, Olea-Serrano F. Pesticide exposure of two age groups of women and its relationship with their diet. *Sci Total Environ* 2007; 382(1):14–21.
57. Arcury T, Grzywacz J, Barr D, Tapia J, Chen H, Quandt S. Pesticide urinary metabolite levels of children in eastern North Carolina farmworker households. *Environ Health Perspect* 2007; 115(8):1254–1260.
58. Kalab M, Cervinka J. Essential Phospholipids in the treatment of cirrhosis of the liver. *Cas Lek Ces* 1983; 122:266–269.
59. Kuntz E. The "essential" phospholipids in hepatology—50 years of experimental and clinical experiences. *Gastroenterol* 1991; 29(2):7–19.
60. Rottini E, Brazzanella F. Marri D, et al. Therapy of different types of liver insufficiency using "essential" phospholipids. *Med Monatsschrift* 1963; 17:28–30.
61. Martensson J, Meister A. Mitochondrial damage in muscle occurs after marked depletion of glutathione and is prevented by giving glutathione monoester *Proc Natl Acad Sci USA* 1989; 86(2):471–475.

62. Ketterer B, Coles B, Meyer D. The role of glutathione in detoxification. *Environ Health Perspect* 1983; 49:59–60.

63. Lomaestro B, Malone M. Glutathione in health and disease: Pharmacotherapeutic issues. *Annals Pharmacother* 1976; 29:1263–1273(:

64. Kane PC, Foster JS, Speight N, Kane E. *The Detoxx Book: The PK Protocol for Chronic Neurotoxic Syndromes.*; Millville, NJ: BodyBio, 2009.

65. Tateishi N, Higashi T, Naruse A, et al. Relative contributions of sulfur atoms of dietary cysteine and methionine to rat liver glutathione and proteins. *J Biochem* 1981; 90:1603–1610.

66. Traber J, Suter M, Walter P, et al. In vivo modulation of total and mitochondrial glutathione in rat liver. *Biochem Pharmocol* 1992; 43:961–964.

67. Kidd P. Glutathione: systemic protectant against oxidative and free radical damage. *Altern Med Rev* 1997; 1:155–176.

68. Fuchs J, Schofer H, Milbradt R, et al. Studies on lipoate effects on blood redox state in human immuno-deficiency virus infected patients. *Arzneimittelforschung* 1993; 43:1359–1362.

69. Gregus Z, Stein A, Varga F, Klassen C. Effect of lipoic acid on bililary exretion of glutathione and metals. *Tox and Applied Pharmacol* 1992; 114:88–96 .

70. Cecchini M, Root D, Rachunow J, Gelb P. Use of the Hubbard sauna detoxification regimen to improve the health status of New York City rescue workers exposed to toxicants. *Townsend Ltr* 2006; 273:58–65.

71. Henderson G, Wilson B. Excretion of methadone and metabolites in human sweat. *Res Comm Chem Psthol Pharmacol* 1972; 5(1):1–8.

72. Masuda A, Munemoto T, Tei C. A new treatment: thermal therapy for chronic fatigue syndrome. *Nippon Rinsho* 2007; 65(6):1093–1098.

73. Wu G. Amino acids: Metabolism, functions, and nutrition *Amino Acids*. 2009 May; 37(1):1–17. Epub 2009 Mar 20.

74. Schachter A, Goldman J, Zukerman Z. Treatment of oligospermia with the amino acid arginine. *J Urol* 1973; 110:311–313.

75. Aydin, et al. The role of arginine, indomethacin and kallikrein in the treatment of oligoasthenospermia. *Int Urol Nephrol* 1995;27(2):199–202.

76. Fraga CG, et al. Ascorbic acid protects against endogenous oxidative DNA damage in human sperm. *Proc Natl Acad Sci* 1991; 88:11003–1106.

77. Sinclair S. *Altern Med Rev* 2000; 5(1):28–38.

78. Scibona M, Meschini P, Capparelli S, et al. L-arginine and male infertility. *Minerva Urol Nefrol* 1994; 46:251–253.

79. Kobayashi D, et al. Transport of carnitine and acetylcarnitine by carnitine/organic cation transporter (OCTN) 2 and OCTN3 into epididymal spermatozoa. *Reproduction* 2007; 134: 651–658.

80. Menchini-Fabris G, Canale D, Izzo P, et al. Free L-carnitine in human semen: its variability in different andrologic pathologies. *Fertil Steril* 1984; 42:263–267.

81. Gurbuz, et al. Relationship between semen quality and seminal plasma total carnitine in infertile men. *J Obstet Gynaecol* 2003;23: 653–56.

82. Dragomir D, et al. Distribution of steroidal saponins in Tribulus terrestris from different geographical regions. *Phytochemistry* 2008; 69(1): 1–288.

83. Khademi A et al. The effect of L-carnitine on sperm parameters in patients candidated for intracytoplasmic sperm injection. *Iranian Journal of Reproductive Medicine* 2004; 2(2):65–69.

84. Vitali G, Parente R, Melotti C. Carnitine supplementation in human idiopathic asthenospermia: clinical results. *Drugs Exp Clin Res* 1995; 21:157–159.

85. Costa M, Canale D, Filicori M, et al. L-carnitine in idiopathic astheno-zoospermia: a multi-center study. Italian Study Group on Carnitine and Male Infertility. *Andrologia* 1994; 26:155–159.

86. Vitali G, Parente R, Melotti C. Carnitine supplementation in human idiopathic asthenospermia. Clinical results. *Drugs Exp Clin Res* 1995; 21:157–159.

87. Vicari E, La Vignera S, Calogero AE. Antioxidant treatment with carnitines is effective in infertile patients with prostatovesiculoepididymitis and elevated seminal leukocyte concentrations after treatment with nonsteroidal anti-inflammatory compounds. *Fertil Steril* 2002; 78:1203–1208.

88. Lenzi A, Sgro P, Salacone P, et al. A placebo-controlled double-blind randomized trial of the use of combined-carnitine and -acetyl-carnitine treatment in men with asthenozoospermia. *Fertil Steril* 2004; 81:1578–1584.

89. Lenzi A, Lombardo F, Sgro P, et al. Use of carnitine therapy in selected cases of male factor infertility: A double-blind crossover trial. *Fertil Steril* 2003; 79:292–300.

90. Lenzi A, Sgro P, Salacone P, Paoli D, Gilio B, Lombardo F, Santulli M, Agarwal A, Gandini L: A placebo-controlled double-blind randomized trial of the use of combined L-carnitine and L-acetylcarnitine treatment in men with asthenozoospermia. *Fertil Steril* 2004; 81:1578–1584.

91. Balercia G, Regoli F, Armeni T, Koverech A, Mantero F, Boscaro M: Placebo-controlled, doubleblind, randomized trial on the use of L-carnitine, L-acetylcarnitine, or combined L-carnitine and L-acetylcarnitine in men with idiopathic astheno *Steril* 2005; 84:662–671.

92. Costa M, Canale D, Filicori M, et al. l-Carnitine in idiopathic asthenozoospermia: A multicenter study. Italian Study Group on Carnitine and Male Infertility. *Andrologia* 1994; 26:155–159.

93. Showell MG, Brown J, Tazdani A, Stankiewicz MT, Hart RJ. Antioxidants for male subfertility (Review). *The Cochrane Library*, 2011, Issue 2, Wiley Publishers.

94. Tremellen K, Miari G, Froilan D, Thompson J. A randomized control trial examining the effect of an antioxidant (Menevit) on pregnancy outcome during IVF-ICSI treatment. *Aust and New Zea J Ob & Gyn* 2007; 47:216–221.

95. Tremellen K, Miari G, Froilan D, Thompson J. A randomized control trial examining the effect of an antioxidant (Menevit) on pregnancy outcome during IVF-ICSI treatment. *Aust and New Zea J Ob & Gyn* 2007; 47:216-221.

96. Agarwal A, Nallella KP, Allamaneni SS, et al. Role of antioxidants in treatment of male infertility: An overview of the literature. *Reprod Biomed Online* 2004; 8:616–627.

97. Zini A, de Lamirande E, Gagnon C. Reactive oxygen species in semen of infertile patients: Levels of superoxide dismutase- and catalase-like activities in seminal plasma and spermatozoa. *Int J Androl* 1993; 16:183–188.

98. Pasqualotto FF, Sharma RK, Nelson DR, et al. Relationship between oxidative stress, semen characteristics, and clinical diagnosis in men undergoing infertility investigation. *Fertil Steril* 2000; 73:459–464.

99. Agarwal A, Nallella KP, Allamaneni SS, et al. Role of antioxidants in treatment of male infertility: an overview of the literature. *Reprod Biomed Online* 2004; 8:616–627.

100. Zini A, de Lamirande E, Gagnon C. Reactive oxygen species in semen of infertile patients: levels of superoxide dismutase- and catalase-like activities in seminal plasma and spermatozoa. *Int J Androl* 1993; 16:183–188.

101. Pasqualotto FF, Sharma RK, Nelson DR, et al. Relationship between oxidative stress, semen characteristics, and clinical diagnosis in men undergoing infertility investigation. *Fertil Steril* 2000; 73:459–464.

102. Wong WY, Thomas CM, Merkus JM, Zielhuis GA, Steegers-Theunissen RP. Male factor subfertility: Possible causes and the impact of nutritional factors. *Fertil Steril* 2000; 73:435–442

103. Madding C, Jacob M, Ramsay V, Sokol R. Serum and semen zinc levels in normozoospermic and oligospermic men. *Ann Nutr Metab* 1986; 30:213–218.

104. Tikkiwal M, Ajmera R, Mathur N. Effect of zinc administration on seminal zinc and fertility of oligospermic males. *Indian J Physiol Pharmacol* 1987; 31:30–34.

105. Takihara H, Cosentino MJ, Cockett AT. Zinc sulfate therapy for infertile males with or without varicocelectomy. *Urology* 1987; 29:638–641.

106. Netter A, Hartoma R, Nakoul K. Effect of zinc administration on plasma testosterone, dihydrotestosterone and sperm count. *Arch Androl* 1981; 7:69–73.

107. Wong WY, Merkus HM, Thomas CM, et al. Effects of folic acid and zinc sulfate on male factor subfertility: A double-blind, randomized, placebo-controlled trial. *Fertil Steril* 2002; 77:491–498.

108. Sandler B, Faragher B. Treatment of oligospermia with vitamin B12. *Infertility* 1984; 7:133–138.

109. Mancini A, De Marinis L, Oradei A, et al. Coenzyme Q10 concentration in normal and pathological human seminal fluid. *J Androl* 1994; 15: 591–559

110. Balercia G, Mosca F, Mantero F, et al. Coenzyme Q10 supplementation in infertile men with idiopathic asthenozoospermia: An open, uncontrolled pilot study. *Fertil Steril* 2004; 81:93–98

111. Balercia G, Buldreghini E, Vignini A, Tiano L, Paggi F, Amoroso S, Ricciardo-Lamonica G, Boscaro M, Lenzi A, Littarru G. Coenzyme Q10 treatment in infertile men with idiopathic asthenozoospermia: A placebo-controlled, double-blind randomized trial *Fertil Steril.* 2009 May; 91(5):1785–1792. Epub 2008 Apr 8.

112. Balercia G, Arnaldi G, Fazioli F, et al. Coenzyme Q10 levels in idiopathic and varicocele–associated asthenozoospermia. *Andrologia* 2002; 34:107–111.

113. Lenzi A, Lombardo F, Gandini L, et al. Glutathione therapy for male infertility. *Arch Androl* 1992; 29:65–68.

114. Hansen J, Deguchi Y. Selenium and fertility in animals and man—a review. *Acta Vet Scand* 1996; 37:19–30.

115. Lenzi A, Culasso f, Gandini L, et al. Placebo-controlled, double blind, cross-over trial of glutathione therapy in male infertility. *Hum Reprod* 1993; 8:1657–1662.

116. Scott R, MacPherson A, Yates R, et al. The effect of oral selenium supplementation on human sperm motility. *Br J Urol* 1998; 82:76–80.
117. Ursini F, Heim S, Kiess M, et al. Dual function of the selenoprotein PHGPx during sperm maturation. *Science* 1999; 285: 1393.
118. Hawkes, WC, Turek, PJ., Effects of dietary selenium on sperm motility in healthy men. *J Androl* 2001; Sep–Oct; 22(5): 764–72.
119. Vézina D, Mauffette F, Roberts KD, Bleau G. Selenium-vitamin E supplementation in infertile men. Effects on semen parameters and micronutrient levels and distribution *Biol Trace Elem Res* 1996 Summer; 53(1–3):65–83.
120. Rayman MP, Rayman MP. The argument for increasing selenium intake. *Proc Nutr Soc* 2002; 61:203–215.
121. Dabrowski K. Ciereszko A. Ascorbic acid protects against male infertility in teleost fish. *Experientia* 1996; 52:97–100.
122. Akmal M, Qadri JQ, Al-Waili NS, Thangal S, Haq A, Saloom KY. Improvement in human semen quality after oral supplementation of vitamin C. *J Med Food*. 2006 Fall; 9(3):440–442.
123. Colagar AH, Marzony ET. Ascorbic Acid in human seminal plasma: Determination and its relationship to sperm quality *J Clin Biochem Nutr* 2009 Sep; 45(2):144–149. Epub 2009 Aug 28.
124. Dawson E, Harris W, Rankin W, et al. Effect of ascorbic acid on male fertility. *Ann N Y Acad Sci* 1987; 498:312–323.
125. Al-Azemi MK, Omu AE, Fatinikun T, Mannazhath N, Abraham S. Factors contributing to gender differences in serum retinol and alpha-tocopherol in infertile couples. *Reprod Biomed Online* 2009 Oct; 19(4):583–590.
126. Eskenazi B, et al. Antioxidant intake is associated with semen quality in healthy men. *Human Reproduction* 2005; 20(4):1006–1012.
127. Aitken RJ, Clarkson JS, Hargreave TB, et al. Analysis of the relationship between defective sperm function and the generation of reactive oxygen species in cases of oligozoospermia. *J Androl* 1989; 10:214–220.
128. Greco E et al. Reduction of the incidence of sperm DNA fragmentation by oral antioxidant treatment. *J Andrology* 2005; 26(3):349–353.
129. Bilska A, Włodek L. Lipoic acid--the drug of the future? *Pharmacol Rep* 2005 Sep-Oct; 57(5):570–577.
130. Selvakumar E, Prahalathan C, Sudharsan PT, Varalakshmi P. Chemoprotective effect of lipoic acid against cyclophosphamide-induced changes in the rat sperm *Toxicology* 2006 Jan 5; 217(1):71–78. Epub 2005 Oct 3.
131. Prahalathan C, Selvakumar E, Varalakshmi P. Modulatory role of lipoic acid on adriamycin-induced testicular injury. *Chem Biol Interact* 2006 Mar 25; 160(2):108–114. Epub 2006 Jan 24.
132. Ibrahim SF, Osman K, Das S, Othman AM, Majid NA, Rahman MP. A study of the antioxidant effect of alpha lipoic acids on sperm quality.*Clinics* (Sao Paulo) 2008 Aug; 63(4):545–550.
133. Blomberg Jensen M, Bjerrum PJ, Jessen TE, Nielsen JE, Joensen UN, Olesen IA, Petersen JH, Juul A, Dissing S, Jorgensen N. Vitamin D is positively associated with sperm motility and increases intracellular calcium in human spermatozoa. *Human Reproduction* 2011, 26(6):1307–1317.
134. Boxmeer JC, Smit M, Weber RF, Lindemans J, Romijn JC, Eijkemans MJ, Macklon NS, Steegers-Theunissen RP. Seminal plasma cobalamin significantly correlates with sperm concentration in men undergoing IVF or ICSI procedures *J Androl* 2007 Jul-Aug; 28(4):521–527. Epub 2007 Feb 7.
135. Wong WY, Merkus HM, Thomas CM, Menkveld R, Zielhuis GA, Steegers-Theunissen RP. Effects of folic acid and zinc sulfate on male factor subfertility: A double-blind, randomized, placebo-controlled trial, *Fertil Steril* 2002; 77:491–498
136. Boxmeer JC, Smit M, Utomo E, Romijn JC, Eijkemans MJ, Lindemans J, Laven JS, Macklon NS, Steegers EA, Steegers-Theunissen RP. Low folate in seminal plasma is associated with increased sperm DNA damage. *Fertil Steril*. 2009 Aug; 92(2):548–556. Epub 2008 Aug 22.
137. Sinclair S. Male infertility: Nutritional and environmental considerations *Altern Med Rev* 2000 Feb; 5(1):28–38.
138. Kumamoto Y, Maruta H. Ishigami J, et al. Clinical efficacy of mecobalamin in the treatment of oligospermia–results of double-blind comparative clinical study. *Hinyokika Kiyo* 1988; 34:1109–1132.
139. Sandler B, Faragher B. Treatment of oligospermia with vitamin B-12. *Infertility* 1984; 7:133–138.

41 Asbestos

Profound Evidence for Disease Associations

Yoshiaki Omura, M.D., Sc.D., FACA, FICAE, FRSM

INTRODUCTION

"Asbestos" is derived from the Greek: α (a-: "not") + σ β ε σ τ ο ζ (–sbestos: "extinguishable") because flaming asbestos stone could not be doused with water. It is a naturally occurring fibrous silicate material often used in the past for its properties such as thermal insulation, chemical and thermal stability, fireproofing, part of cigarette or wine filters, and acoustic insulation [1]. Exposure to naturally occurring asbestos, food and water sources, and its lingering industrial uses result in asbestos deposition in humans, where the same physical properties of insulation implicate it in a broadening number of diseases. Until recently, clinical assessment of asbestosis has been difficult due to its nanoparticle size and inert chemical nature (not water soluble). In addition to avoiding any ongoing exposures such as those from food and water sources, methods involving nutritional strategies are presented in this chapter.

BACKGROUND

When we tried to find literature on the relationship between asbestos and various diseases, we found that very little work has been done in this field, with the exception of mesothelioma. We also found that very little is written about the kinds and amounts of asbestos involved in which of the three known pathological subtypes of malignant mesotheliomas (about 50–60% is epithelioid mesothelioma, about 10% is sarcomatoid mesothelioma, and about 30% is mixed/biphasic mesothelioma) [2,3]. The incidence of pleural mesothelioma in the lungs is 67–75%, and incidence of abdominal peritoneal mesothelioma is 25–33%, while less than 10% appears in the pericardium, brain, and other parts of the body. According to a study at Harvard University's Brigham Women's Hospital, the pathological diagnosis of one of the three specific subtypes of malignant mesothelioma made before biopsy had a relatively high percentage of errors [2].

No simple method of measuring asbestos is available for living systems, even in any major university hospitals or research institutes. The reason for this is that asbestos is not water soluble, and therefore, no simple, direct chemical method has been developed. Standard methods of detecting asbestos include either using high microscopic optical magnification or electron microscopy. Even simple detection of asbestos in drinking water requires a sample of at least 100 cc, and usually requires 1 liter of water. According to the Environmental Protection Agency's (EPA) requirement, when the length of asbestos crystal is over 10 microns, it needs to be reported. However, by the time asbestos in drinking water or bottled water is brought to a standard laboratory, most of the large crystals longer than 10 microns are usually already deposited on the bottom of the water bottle; and, if we can find them in the water, most of them are usually less than 2 microns. Particularly, most of them are less than 0.5 microns, which is generally considered to be grouped as dust. Therefore, if any water contains asbestos as small particles of less than 2 microns, particularly less than 0.5 microns, most of the water will erroneously be considered as nonasbestos containing water. Therefore, using Bi-Digital O-Ring Test (BDORT) electromagnetic field (EMF) resonance phenomenon between two identical molecules, we were able to measure any substances including asbestos even in small samples (less than 0.5 cc) noninvasively, as long as known different amounts of identical substances are available as reference control substances. For this method, a U.S. Patent was given in 1993 (U.S. Patent No. 5,188,107). We also semiquantitatively measured any asbestos inside of the body noninvasively from outside of the body [1,4]. In addition, we can measure the asbestos from X-ray film, MRI, CT-scan, and PET-scan photographs [1,4]. Using this method, we found asbestos plays a very important role not only in every type of cancer, but also in all types of malignancies as well as many intractable medical problems including Alzheimer's disease, autism, frequent intractable urination, amyotrophic lateral sclerosis, failing heart, varicose veins, and so on [1,4].

We describe potential sources of asbestos, the diseases associated with asbestos, and how to remove asbestos noninvasively and safely without surgical removal. As a practical solution to remove most of the asbestos accumulated in the body tissue noninvasively and safely, we have established two methods: 1) taking the herb cilantro, which increases the urinary excretion of asbestos; and 2) increasing normal cell telomere length from markedly reduced amounts as low as even 1 yg (= 10^{-24} g, which is practically 0) to 500–1300 ng BDORT units, which improves general circulation and increases urinary excretion of not only asbestos but also mercury (Hg), lead (Pb), aluminum (Al), and arsenic (As), in addition to enhanced excretion of pathogenic fungi, bacteria, and viruses.

In the 1980s, we developed a very quick, noninvasive method of detecting asbestos using electromagnetic field (EMF) resonance phenomenon between two identical molecules, and the fact that the EMF resonance is maximum when both molecules are identical and both molecules are present in the same amount. At least six types of asbestos are known as presented in Table 41.1 [5]. Most literature does not report which type of asbestos was identified. However, among those that do, the one most commonly found in human body pathological conditions is chrysotile asbestos, which is known as white asbestos. This is also the same asbestos commonly used in the past for ceilings and protection of heat transmission or even in the filter of cigarettes or wine and other alcoholic beverages. A rarer type of asbestos that can be more pathogenic is tremolite asbestos, sometimes contained in talcum powder. According to a cohort study, "vermiculite from a mine near Libby, Montana, was contaminated with tremolite asbestos and other amphibole fibers (winchite and richterite). Asbestos-contaminated Libby vermiculite was also used in loose-fill attic insulation that remains in millions of homes in the United States, Canada, and other countries. Libby workers

TABLE 41.1

Six Main Types of Asbestos and Their Chemical Formulas

Common Name	Additional Name	Chemical Formula
Chrysotile	White asbestos	$Mg_3(Si_2O_5)(OH)_4$
Amosite	Brown asbestos	$Fe_7Si_8O_{22}(OH)_2$
Crocidolite	Blue asbestos	$Na_2Fe^{2+}_3Fe^{3+}_2Si_8O_{22}(OH)_2$
Anthophyllite		$(Mg,Fe)_7Si_8O_{22}(OH)_2$
Tremolite		$Ca_2Mg_5Si_8O_{22}(OH)_2$
Actinolite		$Ca_2(Mg,Fe)_5Si_8O_{22}(OH)_2$

TABLE 41.2
Partial Listing of Potential Sources of Asbestos Exposure

1) Water coming through mechanically cracked asbestos surrounding cement water pipe used between cities' main water pipes and each building
2) Some bottled water
3) Ceiling or wall materials from room containing chrysotile asbestos
4) Living near old asbestos mine or asbestos-rich soil
5) Some ginger coming from parts of China or California/New Jersey/Montana (USA) where asbestos is found
6) Many almonds contain chrysotile asbestos, but also contain good nutritious components
7) Some egg yolk contains asbestos, but egg whites from the same egg do not contain asbestos
8) Dentures and other dental materials contaminated with asbestos (which often create headaches, astrocytoma response, or Alzheimer-like increases in β-Amyloid (1-42); can enhance cancer in the rest of the body and markedly reduce sirtuin 1 (the longevity gene)

frequently suffered or died from asbestosis, lung cancer, cancer of the pleura, and mesothelioma depending on the frequency of exposure to vermiculite" [6–8]. Sources of asbestos exposure are also often nonspecific, including food and water (Table 41.2).

EPIDEMIOLOGY

Through more than 10 years of our research on various cancers, we also found that the higher the amount of asbestos, the more malignant the cancer will be; for example, in brain tumors, when we compared the most benign astrocytoma with the more malignant anaplastic astrocytoma and the most malignant brain tumor, glioblastoma, the amount of chrysotile asbestos was highest in glioblastoma (0.135 mg BDORT units or higher); while in anaplastic astrocytoma it was 0.125–0.145 mg BDORT units, and in the benign astrocytoma it was 0.120–0.130 mg BDORT units. In mesothelioma, the amount of asbestos is often higher than 0.2–0.4 mg BDORT units, which is much higher than most other cancers; but integrin α5β1 or oncogene C-fos Ab2 usually do not exceed 50–60 ng BDORT units (which is the equivalent of the very early stage of any other malignancy). When the asbestos is successfully reduced, some of the malignant brain tumors can become less malignant when they are in the early stage and a relatively small size. In order to distinguish from standard magnification method, which is often not quantitative but descriptive (such as how big is the size, how many crystals are in the specific area of magnification), we use BDORT units for the estimated weight in mg, μg, or ng. Using EMF resonance phenomenon between two identical substances, we can not only measure noninvasively in humans or animals, but also more accurately, cost effectively, and quantitatively in in vivo and in vitro in the short time of less than 10 minutes. Using this method, we found involvement of asbestos in the diseases listed in Table 41.3 [4].

PATHOPHYSIOLOGY

What impairs nutrient delivery during common and serious diseases such as cancers? Anything that decreases normal cell telomere also reduces circulation throughout the body. Table 41.4 presents such substances and asbestos is one of them. While its presence in tumors has not been determined to be causal, a likely pathophysiologic role is to insulate the affected organ and region from circulation and nutrient delivery. Mesothelioma, a tumor with established asbestos exposure, is unlike other cancers in that it does not take up glucose. Mesotheliomas are associated with additional infections that the body is unable to clear largely due to the nutrient desert created by the asbestos deposition.

TABLE 41.3

Diseases and Organs Where Asbestos Is Markedly Increased

1) **Cancer**
   a) Mesothelioma and all four types of lung cancers, especially adenocarcinoma of the lung
   b) Brain tumors such as astrocytoma, anaplastic astrocytoma, and glioblastoma
   c) Malignant tumors including esophageal cancer, breast cancer, stomach cancer, pancreatic cancer, colon cancer, ovarian cancer, uterine cancer, prostate cancer, and kidney cancer

2) **Cardiovascular Diseases Including:**
   a) Left ventricle of failing heart
   b) Some myocardial infarcts
   c) Circulatory disturbance of brain
   d) Arteries supplying blood to malignant tumors
   e) Occluded part of inner lumen of arteries
   f) Varicose veins and spider veins

3) **Alzheimer's Disease**

4) **Autism**

5) **Infected Root Canal**
   This is usually combined with candida albicans, cytomegalovirus, and *Helicobacter pylori* (with or without mercury) and infections such as chlamydia trachomatis or borrelia burgdorferi, which usually require extraction of the infected tooth.

6) **Morgellons Disease (also known as Hair Disease or Fiber Disease)**
   First observed in 1544 as "the Hair Affection" (pilaris affection) of four infants with unusual hairs on their back who died in Languedoc (the old name of a province in southern France, whose capital city was Toulouse). This information was published in 1558 by a French doctor named Schenckius in the book *Halosis Febrium* as "a new affection of infants" [9]. The term "Morgellons" was first used in 1674 by Sir Thomas Browne, in reference to a mysterious disease of unknown cause [10]. During the seventeenth and eighteenth centuries, Morgellons disease was known under a variety of names including *Les Crinons* (meaning horse hair or coarse hair), masclous, and masquelons from which it is suggested the name Morgellons was derived [9]. Morgellons disease is not only found in infants and children, but also adults and, more frequently, in women. The hair-like substances can appear on any part of the body surface, but are more often prevalent on the legs of middle-aged women and are accompanied by severe itching, pain, and sleep interference. We found that thread-like excretions from the patient's skin often contain mixed fibers of different types of asbestos including chrysotile fibers. Some of the fibers were tangled with different colors of red, blue, black, and white [4, 9–15]. The condition can improve using our asbestos excretion enhancement methods.

7) **Some Cataracts**

8) **Intractable Pain**
   This includes fibromyalgia and intractable joint pain with mixed infections such as chlamydia trachomatis and borrelia burgdorferi.

9) **Electromagnetic Field Hypersensitivity**

10) **Some Postmenopausal Hot Flashes**

11) **Hair Loss from Regularly Showering with Hot Water Containing Asbestos**

12) **Intractable Skin Irritation**
    This includes atopic dermatitis and intractable itching where chlamydia trachomatis infection was accompanied by asbestos deposits.

13) **Some Dark Pigmentation Under the Eyes**

Source: [4].

Chromosome telomere length has been linked to longevity and health and a Nobel Prize was awarded for this work [16]. There is debate as to whether the blood tests and other DNA tests of telomere length can be used as an indicator of health or life expectancy. Our observations concur with the association with health and nutrient delivery, but that telomere length can be altered within a period too short to make laboratory testing of clinical relevance.

TABLE 41.4
Factors Reducing Normal Cell Telomeres and Increasing Cancer Cell Telomeres or Contributing to the Genesis of Cancer and Other Malignancies

1) Asbestos that entered human body via environmental air or was consumed as part of food or drinking water or part of some dentures containing asbestos
2) Electromagnetic fields from unprotected cellular phones, televisions, computers, keyboards, printers, and microwave ovens
3) BDORT negative underwear, accessories directly touching the skin, and contact lenses
4) Food and drinks containing the low-calorie artificial sweetener, aspartame, and other foods that test BDORT negative
5) Mixed infections such as candida albicans, cytomegalovirus, Simian vacuolating virus, and *Helicobacter pylori*, with or without chlamydia trachomatis or borrelia burgdorferi
6) Markedly reduced cesium levels of less than 1/5–1/100 of normal values (4–4.5 ng BDORT units) of normal and cancer tissue of the same cancer patient
7) Excessive deposits of mercury or arsenic; many BDORT negative cups or bowls with semitransparent decoration contain high amounts of mercury that can dissolve in water.
8) Frequently eating burned fish or meat with salty food.
9) Frequent snacking and excessive intake of vitamin D increased incidence of lung cancer.
10) Combination of above factors.

(BDORT = Bi-Digital O-Ring Test)

Not every person exposed to asbestos developed mesotheliomas; but in those who developed them, there was often viral infection of SV40. In fact, according to our previous study, in every cancer tissue, there is always some type of viral infection or multiple infections associated in addition to the abnormally increased amount of asbestos (usually chrysotile asbestos). Although the exact mechanisms are not known, mesothelioma-like changes were observed in research animals following intraperitoneal application of multi-walled carbon nanotubes [17,18]. Multi-walled nanotubes are used for many industrial purposes because of their light weight and stronger than steel properties; however, with unintended human exposure, they appear to act as an asbestos analog. Because of this, people working in this field are warned of potential toxicity similar to asbestos by a number of published articles [19–27].

Paraben (a para-hydroxybenzoate) is a preservative used in deodorants as well as foods, cosmetics, and drugs that has estrogen-like effects that may contribute to breast cancer [28–31]. It has, in fact, been found in most breast cancers. Similar to asbestos, there is an association combined with biologic plausibility, but causation cannot be established based on this.

PATIENT EVALUATION

Mesothelin as a Biomarker

For the standard laboratory tests using optical or electromicroscopic examination, it is practically useless for examining patients and identifying asbestos in any part of the body. Because there are no convenient noninvasive methods of quantitatively measuring asbestos currently available, some people use mesothelin by a blood test, which is considered to be a biomarker for mesothelioma, but its relationship with the amount of asbestos has not been studied [32–55]. It is also not specific for mesothelioma; it has been shown to increase in both ovarian and pancreatic cancer. Researchers have reported that in 71% of mesothelioma patients and 67% of ovarian cancer patients, mesothelin was increased [56]. Other researchers have also found an increase in pancreatic cancer patients.

Asbestos Can Be Detected by EMF Resonance Phenomenon between Asbestos in the Body and Projection of a Laser Beam Contains Molecular Information of Samples of Asbestos or Cancer-Related Substances to Eight Different Parts of the Body

Using the BDORT EMF resonance phenomenon, we can evaluate any abnormal deposits of asbestos in any part of the body noninvasively. Without knowing anything about the patient, as shown in Figure 41.1, we can screen by the use of indirect BDORT without directly touching the patient [57–90]. The third person holding a reference control substance of a known quantity of chrysotile asbestos holds a laser pointer with a red spectrum and, with the same hand, projects the red laser light beam directly onto the patient's body surface. The laser is projected onto each of eight different locations of the body surface as shown in Figure 41.1. During this time, the examiner performs BDORT with the other hand of the third person holding the laser and asbestos to determine EMF resonance phenomenon, which is characterized by an extreme reduction of muscle strength of not only the fingers, but also the entire body.

Use of Right and Left Mouthwriting, Handwriting, and Footwriting for Screening and Pathological Diagnosis (Specific Type of Malignancy Requires an Additional 10–20 Minutes for Each Type of Cancer)

In order to have a permanent record of these findings and evaluate any effects of the treatment including nutrition and specific drugs, we now use right and left mouthwriting, handwriting, and footwriting, as shown in Figure 41.2. In 15 years of research, mouthwriting, handwriting, and footwriting often have been found to provide more information than many of the standard laboratory tests long before imaging devices or a blood test for cancer markers can detect them. The entire procedure of mouthwriting, handwriting, and footwriting only usually takes about 10 minutes. Once this is completed, any malignancy in any part of the body can be screened for in less than five minutes. The degree and nature of the malignancy could be determined by the amount of integrin $\alpha_5\beta_1$ or oncogene C-fos Ab2, both of which increase more or less proportionally with the degree of

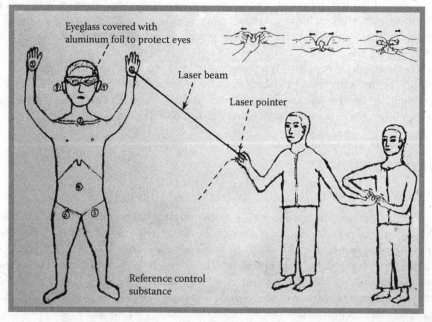

FIGURE 41.1 Noninvasive quick screening of cancer or asbestos: (1) right lobule, 2) left lobule, 3) suprasternal notch, 4) palm of the right hand, 5) palm of the left hand, 6) umbilicus, 7) right inguinal area, 8) left inguinal area.

Mouth, hand, and foot writing form
by Yoshiaki Omura, M.D., Sc.D., © 2010 and 2011

Name:_____ Age:_____ Sex:____ Weight :_____ Height:_____

Address:_____ Date:_____ Time completed:_____ am pm

_____ Profession _____ Questions? Call 212-781-6262

Phone #:_____ Cellular phone #:_____ Fax #:_____ E-mail:_____

Chief Complaint: _____

FAX TO DR. OMURA: 212-923-2279

BeforeTreatment: BP: /   Pulse: Resp. Rate: Body Temp:

Left Mouth write L-M	: Telomere : : Sirtuin 1, longevity gene : : Integrin $\alpha_5\beta_1$ (or Oncogene C-fos Ab2): : 8-OH-dG : : Pb; Al; Hg; Cs : : Chrysotile Asbestos; (Tremolite A.); Mesothelin : : Acetylcholine; Dopamine; Serotonin; GABA : : β-Amyloid (1-42); Tau Protein : : L- Homocysteine or CRP: : Chlamydia T.; Borrelia B. : : Mycobacterium TB; Helicobacter Pylori; C.A. : : Cytomegalovirus; Herpes Type : : Substance P : : DHEA :	Right Mouth write R-M
before treatment		before treatment
BDORT Grading:		BDORT Grading:
after treatment		after treatment
BDORT Grading:		BDORT Grading:
BDORT Grading:		BDORT Grading:

Left Hand write L-H	: Telomere : : Sirtuin 1, longevity gene : : Integrin $\alpha_5\beta_1$ (or Oncogene C-fos Ab2) : : 8-OH-dG : : CEA; CA-125; DUPAN-2: : Pb; Al; Hg; Cs : : Chrysotile Asbestos; (Tremolite A.); Mesothelin : : Acetylcholine : : Cardiac Troponin I; TXB_2; CRP : : Glucose : : Chlamydia T.; Borrelia B. : : Mycobacterium TB; Helicobacter Pylori; C.A. : : Cytomegalovirus; Herpes Type : : Substance P : : DHEA :	Right Hand write R-H
before treatment		before treatment
BDORT Grading:		BDORT Grading:
after treatment		after treatment
BDORT Grading:		BDORT Grading:

Left Foot write L-F	: Telomere : : Sirtuin 1, longevity gene : : Integrin $\alpha_5\beta_1$ (or Oncogene C-fos Ab2): : 8-OH-dG : : PSA;p CA-125; CEA : : Pb; Al; Hg; Cs : : Chrysotile Asbestos; (Tremolite A.); Mesothelin : : Acetylcholine : : Chlamydia T.; Borrelia B. : : Mycobacterium TB; Candida Albicans; H.P. : : Cytomegalovirus; Herpes Type : : Substance P : : DHEA :	Right Foot write R-F
before treatment		before treatment
BDORT Grading:		BDORT Grading:
after treatment		after treatment
BDORT Grading:		BDORT Grading:

After Treatment: BP:____/____,____/____Pulse:____,____Resp. Rate:____,____Body Temp:____,____

(All the measurement units used here are BDORT Units)

FIGURE 41.2 Mouth-, hand-, and footwriting form used for noninvasive, quick screening and diagnosis of malignancies and other intractable medical problems. It is extensively used to evaluate the effects of any treatment, including chemotherapy of cancers, by repeating before, and 30 minutes after, treatment to determine quantitatively if the given treatment is beneficial, has no effect, or is harmful. Reproduced with permission.

malignancy. However, in mesothelioma, these two factors increase moderately but not very significantly, unlike any other malignancies. From the mouthwriting, handwriting, and footwriting test, additional factors to evaluate the degree of malignancy include the amount of chrysotile asbestos and 8-OH-dG. If the malignant cell is active, 8-OH-dG is always increased. The normal value is less than 2 ng BDORT units; but if it is over 5 ng BDORT units, it indicates a presence of increased DNA mutation, and some may have a very early-stage malignancy. When it is over 10 ng BDORT units, the cancer is active. When it is over 15 ng BDORT units, the cancer is very active and can spread rapidly. In the presence of malignancy, sirtuin 1 and normal cell telomere are reduced significantly. If any treatment is effective, all of these values should improve.

A typical example of our chart used for "bilateral mouthwriting, handwriting, and footwriting" is shown in Figure 41.2. Using this recorded information, almost any type of malignancy in any part of the body can be screened in five minutes, but specific cell types of malignancy can be estimated by additional 10–20 minutes for each malignancy detected. If you have only one malignancy, it will take less than 10–20 minutes to identify which type of malignancy exists and at which part of the body. If there is a metastasis in a different part of the body, it will also be detected in early stage before any standard laboratory tests can detect it. Once the malignancy is screened and found to be positive and the pathological cell type of the malignancy is identified, the next step is to find what stage or what degree of malignancy exists with this newly discovered abnormal area.

The degree of abnormality can be estimated by the amount of the increase in integrin $\alpha_5\beta_1$ or oncogene C-fos Ab2 because these two substances are always less than 1 ng in normal tissue; but when there is a malignancy, the amount is increased. However, until the amount of integrin $\alpha_5\beta_1$ and oncogene C-fos Ab2 reach 100–150 ng BDORT units, standard laboratory tests often have difficulty in detection. Once these two parameters reach levels over 150 ng, standard laboratory tests including X-ray, CT scan, MRI, and PET scan can detect the tumor. Also, if the integrin $\alpha_5\beta_1$ is increased uniformly anywhere between 5–10 ng, and the value is always the same at any part of the body, this usually indicates the presence of leukemia or other bone-related malignancy. We can detect changes of almost any normal or abnormal substances, as long as we have a reference control substance with an exact known amount in addition to the list of the substances we often test as written in the chart.

PET Scan Findings with Appearance of Dark or Pitch-black Areas Due to Asbestos Deposits and Potential Risk of Misdiagnosis

In radiology, it is almost common sense that when there is a malignancy, uptake of radioactive glucose will increase significantly more than normal tissue depending on the degree and size of malignancies. However, our own research on the PET scan indicated that in the case of deposits of asbestos, unlike all other well-known cancers, glucose uptake reduces to one-thirtieth of normal tissue in the presence of asbestos (Figure 41.3). As a result, in a patient with excessive asbestos deposits as seen in epithelioid mesothelioma of the lung, instead of the PET scan becoming brighter with increased glucose uptake, it becomes dark or pitch-black if asbestos has a very high value of more than 0.2–0.3 mg BDORT units (higher asbestos than most cancers), and glucose uptake also often reduces to one-thirtieth of the normal part of tissue [91]. Before our work, no one has reported that in PET scan imaging the asbestos deposited area becomes darker instead of brighter because glucose uptake becomes markedly reduced in asbestos deposited areas. Since most radiologists were not taught this exceptionally unique finding, and despite these unusual abnormalities, radiologists often report this as within normal limits; as far as they are concerned, there is no malignancy since there is no significant uptake of radioactive glucose [92–94]. Therefore, the pitch-black area appearing in the PET scan is a very important diagnostic sign of mesothelioma and other asbestos-related diseases. By examining the black area appearing in PET scan imaging, using BDORT-EMF resonance phenomenon between two identical substances, we can confirm the very high asbestos and markedly reduced glucose within 30 minutes.

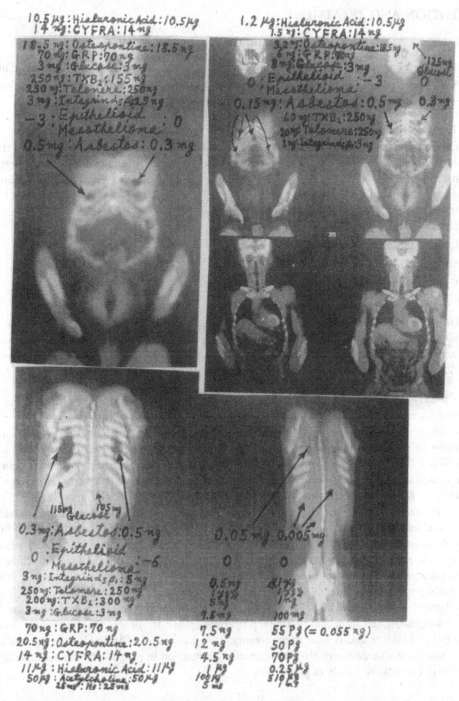

FIGURE 41.3 Omura's mesothelioma characteristic PET scan signs with the appearance of dark or pitch-black areas in chest or abdomen with decreased glucose uptake of less than one-thirtieth of normal tissue and excessive asbestos deposit at these dark areas. Analysis of epithelioid mesothelioma in FDG-PET scan images of a 65-year-old Japanese male dentist who would wake up due to chest tightness about four hours after he went to sleep almost every night in the past six months, without chest pain or coughing. Reproduced from: Omura, Y., Shimotsuura, Y., Duvvi, H., Ohata, N., and M. Ohki. "Reduced Glucose Uptake With Markedly Increased Gastrin Releasing Peptide, Osteopontine & Asbestos Found in Dark Black Areas of PET Scan of Chest Wall in Patient with Mesothelioma." *Acupuncture & Electro-Therapeutics Research, The International Journal.* Vol. 31, pp 247–257, 2006.

PREVENTION AND TREATMENT

STOP EXPOSURE TO ASBESTOS AND SYNERGISTIC CANCER RISK FACTORS

Anyone who has any cancer or other malignant tumor and wears dentures or any other dental material should be examined for asbestos to avoid ongoing exposure. Concurrent factors known to be associated with cancer should also be avoided. These include:

- Tobacco use.
- Eating burnt foods such as fish, meat, bread, and rice; heterocyclicamines and polycyclicaromatichydrocarbons are chemicals formed when muscle meat, including beef, pork, fish, and poultry, is cooked using high-temperature methods, such as pan frying or grilling directly over an open flame.
- Ingesting high salt-containing foods and drinks.
- Drinking liquor with high alcohol content.
- Ionizing radiation.
- Strong sunlight exposure.
- Viruses and bacteria.
- Chemical exposure.
- Hormones in certain forms.
- Combination of above factors; for example, in the past Japan had the highest incidence of stomach cancer due to a combination of eating burned surfaces of fish grilled on a direct flame and ingesting high salt-containing food and drinks or miso soup.

How food is sweetened may also require consideration. Since sugar and fructose promote insulin resistance, sugar substitutes are often chosen. Although a link between aspartame and cancer has been found in studies with rats and other animals, clinical studies have not confirmed a similar relationship in humans, although potential connections have been suspected [95,96]. According to Tollefson and Barnard, "There are many accounts of situations in which aspartame is believed to have caused negative effects on specific human functions. These include brain tumors, memory loss, seizures, headaches, confusion, personality disorders, visual difficulty and dizziness" [97]. Our most recent study [90] also indicates that aspartame reduces longevity gene sirtuin 1 as well as acetylcholine levels significantly with an increase in TXB2 due to a circulatory disturbance in the brain and can particularly be toxic to the hippocampus, which may interfere with memory and normal brain function. On the other hand, more people have started using Stevia, a sugar substitute that has zero calories and fewer recognized side effects. However, further studies regarding the effects on the brain are necessary. Stevioside, is extracted from the leaves of *Stevia rebaudiana Bertoni* [98]. Not only is it 300 times sweeter than sugar, it is also water soluble, resistant to high heat, can help with weight loss, has some antimicrobial properties against *Streptococcus mutans* (which often exist in the oral cavity), and is used in the treatment of gum disease. Stevia also has the tendency to lower blood pressure and may also cause an allergic reaction in people who are sensitive to the asteraceae or compositae family of plants [99].

CILANTRO FACILITES REMOVAL OF ASBESTOS AND HEAVY METALS

The therapeutic effect of excreting metals including Hg, Al, Pb, as well as asbestos was discovered while the author was trying to remove excessive deposits of mercury in the body. While going through a cardiac nuclear stress test at a safe limit of maximum heart rate, a radioactive substance (thallium) was injected intravenously. After radiation of the injected thallium disappeared, a large deposit of mercury was found in the endocrine organs as a byproduct. The author tried a variety of methods in order to remove the mercury from the body, however all of them failed. One day, he ate hot Vietnamese noodle soup with cilantro, and the next day, found that the amount of mercury was reduced significantly. The author then tried boiling cilantro leaves in water for about 10 minutes, and he found that by eating the leaves and drinking the water, mercury excretion in the urine was notably high. Eventually, the author found that lead, aluminum, and asbestos can be excreted in the urine efficiently and noninvasively. Cilantro is available as tablets and other extracts.

In order to find out the effectiveness of treatment for removing asbestos, we examined both the amount of asbestos in the body and in the urine. Usually, before treatment, excretion of asbestos in urine is practically zero, but within a half hour, after giving cilantro or increasing normal cell telomere to over 500 ng, we can detect very significant excretion of asbestos in urine and a gradual reduction of asbestos in the body, as long as the drug effect is maintained.

INCREASING NORMAL CELL TELOMERE LENGTH BY A SIGNIFICANT AMOUNT TO IMPROVE GENERAL CIRCULATION AND SIGNIFICANTLY INCREASE URINARY EXCRETION OF ASBESTOS AND HEAVY METALS

Through our research, the following different categories and methods or substances that significantly increase normal cell telomere levels were discovered. By increasing normal cell telomere levels very significantly, we can not only reduce or eliminate pain by reducing substance P, which is always increased in painful areas, and TXB_2 which is always increased in the presence of circulatory disturbances. When normal cell telomere increases significantly, excretion of asbestos, mercury, lead, arsenic, and aluminum can be significantly increased by markedly increased circulation all over the body. Therefore, we searched many substances that can potentially increase normal cell telomere levels. When we increased normal cell telomere to high levels of over 550 ng BDORT units, we also found that cancer cell telomere, which is always very high, practically becomes zero. As a result, cancer cells can no longer divide; thus, we discovered a safe method of inhibiting growth of cancer without side effects.

STIMULATION OF ACUPUNCTURE POINT TRUE ST 36 INDUCES TELOMERE LENGTHENING

The first method we discovered was mechanical or electrical stimulation of True ST 36 acupuncture point. After inserting a press-needle on True ST 36, simple mechanical stimulation of press and release procedure 250 times can always increase normal cell telomere from practically zero to over 500 ng. When normal cell telomere reaches over 500–550 ng BDORT units, cancer cell telomere (even if it was over a few hundred ng) becomes practically zero (1 yg = 10^{-24} g). In the case of advanced cancer patients, we usually recommend a minimum of 250–300 times for the press-release procedure on the press-needle inserted at True ST 36; repeat this at least four to five times a day.

The following is a case history that influenced the current research. About 10 years ago, we encountered a 28-year-old Chinese computer specialist who developed anaplastic astrocytoma of the brain, for which he had the surgical removal at one of the major teaching hospitals in Taipei, Taiwan. However, in spite of chemotherapy and radiation therapy, the tumor grew back, and his life was in danger. Since nothing was able to stop the recurrence of the tumor, he went to UCLA and underwent a second surgical removal of the tumor. But after this recurring anaplastic astrocytoma was removed, again both chemotherapy and radiation therapy failed to stop a recurrence of the tumor. When he was brought by a professor at NYU to our monthly seminar and workshop in New York City, he was having convulsions every day and could not walk or talk normally. When he came into the conference room, his parents were holding him to help him walk after he got out of his wheelchair. When doctors asked questions, he could not talk normally. We recommended the press-release procedure at True ST 36 for 200 times, four times a day. The next day when he came in, he was able to walk by himself and talk normally. By continuing ST 36 mechanical stimulation with supplement of optimal dose of EPA with DHA and cilantro tablets, he is alive and continues to work part-time 10 years later [87].

Since the 1980s, we found that by using BDORT resonance phenomenon between two identical substances, we were able to localize the exact location of the different meridians and acupuncture points on that meridian. Using a corresponding organ's microscopic slide, we can find the exact shape and diameter of the acupuncture point. When we examined the famous acupuncture point, traditional ST 36, using a slice of human fundus tissue in a microscope slide as a reference control substance, we found that in the location described in textbooks, there was no real acupuncture point. However, at a slightly different location, we found a new acupuncture point, which we called True ST 36; it is also known as Omura's ST 36. Using either simple mechanical stimulation of True ST 36 or electrical stimulation of 30 minutes with 1 pps (pulse per second), we were able to increase normal cell telomere to anywhere between 1000–1200 ng BDORT units. This not only improved the whole body's circulation, but it also reduced cancer cell telomere levels to practically zero, thus inhibiting the growth of the cancer. This also increased excretion of asbestos, mercury, lead, arsenic, and aluminum in the urine as long as high levels of normal cell telomere were maintained. Usually, the effects of each 30-minute session of transcutaneous electrical stimulation lasts at least one day. Since localizing the exact site of True ST 36 requires some anatomical knowledge and experience, we developed and taught a simple technique to replace press-needle stimulation or electrical stimulation so patients can do it by themselves [87,100].

DHEA PROMOTES TELOMERE LENGTHENING DEPENDING ON DOSE, ADMINISTRATION, AND COMPETING MEDICATIONS

Historically speaking, the second method we discovered was the use of optimal dose of DHEA. One dose of DHEA often lasted more than a few weeks as long as the patient did not drink orange juice or take high amounts of vitamin C, which cause food-drug-nutrient interactions. DHEA will improve circulation very significantly and also increase normal cell telomere levels to about 525 ng BDORT units or higher.

ASTROLAGUS AND BOSWELLIA SERRATA INCREASE CELL TELOMERE LENGTH

The third successful method is the use of Astragalus and *Boswellia serrata*. The optimal dose (which depends on the individual) of each increased normal cell telomere levels by 650 ng BDORT units. Both were very effective in inhibiting the activity of brain tumors and eventually reducing the size of benign astrocytoma (with headaches) as well as more malignant anaplastic astrocytoma (with headaches or nausea) and some of the early stages of glioblastoma, which is the most malignant brain tumor. Meanwhile, as a supplement, we also found that by eating bitter melon (average about 30–40 g) during each meal, normal cell telomere levels increased to about 500–550 ng BDORT units. We also found that ginger can increase normal cell telomere to 800 ng BDORT units, and an optimal dose of turmeric can increase telomere to over 850 ng BDORT units. In addition, maca supplement can increase cell telomere to 850 ng BDORT units (optimal dose for an average adult is between 350–400 mg). Eventually, we also found that using one optimal dose of haritaki (known as the "king of medicine" in Tibetan and Ayurvetic medicine) can increase normal cell telomere levels to 1350 ng BDORT units. However, it is only used in detoxification and rejuvenation and was supposedly contained in the pot Medicine Buddha is holding in his hand.

When one optimal dose induced an increase in telomere of 1300 ng in malignant brain tumors like anaplastic astrocytoma or glioblastoma with convulsions or headache, very high cancer cell telomere value of 500–1000 ng BDORT units in the tumor became less than 5 ng with a marked decrease of all the symptoms without chemotherapy or surgery. Haritaki, or acai, is highly beneficial in all types of cancers when the optimal dose is given, provided that no negative drug interaction from other drugs or cancelling effect due to drug and food or drink interactions exist.

In addition to this, we discovered a number of different methods of increasing normal cell telomere without taking any medicine. We also found electrical stimulation of ST 36 temporarily improved Alzheimer's disease by reducing abnormally increased β–Amyloid (1-42) and reduced asbestos and aluminum levels in the brain, and particularly in the hippocampus. Thirty-minute transcutaneous electrical stimulation (1 pulse/sec) of True ST 36 also improved cancer parameters and inhibited cancer activity of breast cancer because it often increases normal cell telomere levels to about 1200 ng BDORT units.

SELECT FOODS AND WATER INFLUENCE CELL TELEMERES

Certain fruits have been identified through our research to increase cell telemerase: bitter melon, mango, papaya, and pineapple. Certain fish may also increase cell telemeres: tuna, salmon, and eel.

Most notably, drinking water varies widely in its effects on cell telemeres. We evaluated famous water believed to be therapeutic such as Lourdes from France, Fatima from Portugal (increased telomere by 50 ng BDORT units per 100 cc of water), Salon-de-Provence in France (near the house where Nostradamus lived during his last years), which increased normal cell telomere by 75 ng BDORT units, and at an ancient palace of the Tan Dynasty at Xian, China, where the water increased normal cell telomere 35–50 ng BDORT units per 100 cc of water. Additionally, at the author's hometown, Asahi-machi, Toyama-ken, Japan, hot spring water of Ograwa Onsen Motoyu produced the highest telomere increase of 250–300 ng BDORT units per 100 cc of water; water at Mt. Tateyama at Toyama-ken also increased normal cell telomere to an average maximum of 150 ng per 100 cc. The author then found the number of centenarians who lived in the small town of Asahi-machi at the time (2009) was essentially the highest in Japan–even higher than Okinawa (where many centenarians used to live). However, the high rate of centenarians could be partly due to the fact that young people have a tendency to move out to larger cities. Among commercially available bottled water, Evian from France used to be very reliable with a BDORT strong positive response and cell telomere increased by about 25–35 ng BDORT units per 100 cc of water. Recently, we found many BDORT negative waters that can reduce normal cell telomere, but the most reliable and economical water where we consistently found BDORT positive response was bottled water by Crystal Geyser, for which normal cell telomere increases by about 25–35 ng BDORT units per 100 cc. Thus, it is very important to drink BDORT positive water with normal cell telomere increasing effects. Overall, we have examined the chemical components of many waters and eventually, we were able to reproduce high telomere increasing water.

USE SELECTIVE DRUG UPTAKE ENHANCEMENT METHOD TO SELECTIVELY DELIVER EFFECTIVE DRUGS AND NUTRIENTS TO THE PATHOLOGICAL AREAS MORE DIFFICULT TO REACH DUE TO ASBESTOS OR OTHER CAUSES

There has been much study of enhancing uptake of drugs, food, nutrients, water, and stem cell therapies. Asbestos, due to its inert state and failure to react in biochemical processes, impairs delivery of nutrients and medications to the areas where it is deposited. Asbestos in the brain is further challenged by transport of treatment across the blood brain barrier and using the body's innate strategies to remove asbestos.

By using the Selective Drug Uptake Enhancement Method (SDUEM), which was discovered by this author in the early 1990s, we can deliver the drug selectively to the inside of the brain by continuous stimulation (5–10 minutes) of organ representation areas corresponding to the area of the brain [67,70,72,75,76,81].

SDUEM can be confirmed using EMF resonance field phenomenon between two identical substances. For example, if the drug we want to deliver is amoxicillin and, by testing on the certain part of the head where the pathological condition exists and where we want to deliver the drug, there is no drug reaching there, the patient holds the same drug already taken in one hand and with the same hand's index finger touches the area where the drug should be delivered. If the drug is not reaching the area, when the same patient's other hand is examined with BDORT, the O-Ring will not open because there is no resonance between two identical substances—in this case amoxicillin in the brain and amoxicillin held in the hand. But during or after SDUEM, if the index finger of the hand holding the drug touches the part of the brain from outside the skull and the drug has reached the pathological

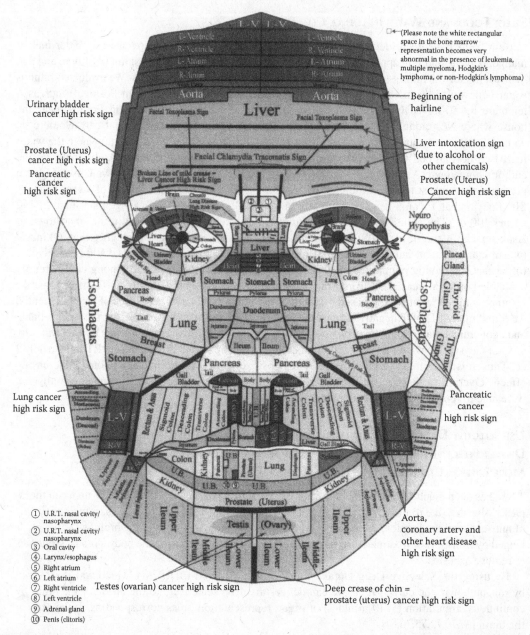

FIGURE 41.4 Accurate organ representation areas of the face localized by the use of the bi-digital O-ring test resonance phenomenon, used for both diagnosis and treatment with the selective drug uptake enhancement method. © Yoshiaki Omura, MD, ScD. This original diagram cannot be reproduced or copied without the written permission of Yoshiaki Omura, MD, SCD.

① Thymus gland
② Left lung
③ Right lung
④ Esophagus
⑤ S-A node
⑥ Right atrium
⑦ Right ventricle
⑧ Left atrium
⑨ Left ventricle

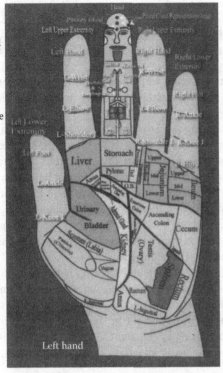
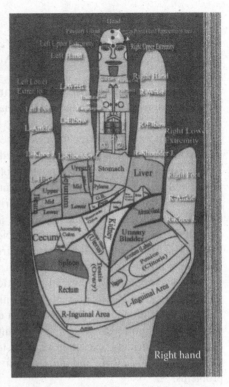

FIGURE 41.5 Accurate organ representation areas of the hands using the bi-digital O-ring test resonance phenomenon, where natural existing creases were often found to be the boundaries between various organ representation areas. © Yoshiaki Omura, MD, ScD. This original diagram cannot be reproduced or copied without the written permission of Yoshiaki Omura, MD, SCD.

area, there will be resonance between the identical molecules of the drug inside the brain and the same drug inside the hand of the individual. This EMF resonance phenomenon can be detected by BDORT. There will be a sudden marked decrease in the force of the fingers forming the O-ring and every ring can be opened. In order to enhance uptake to deliver a drug to a specific part of the organ, one can stimulate the accurate organ representation area corresponding to the pathological area.

Figure 41.4 shows the organ representation areas of the face used for both diagnosis and treatment with the selective drug uptake enhancement method. However, since stimulation of the face is more difficult without a mirror, we often use the more convenient organ representation areas of the hand (Figure 41.5), which do not require a mirror or any other device to identify the location of stimulation. For noninvasive and early diagnosis of the patient, abnormal signs appearing on the face as deep crease(s) corresponding to specific facial organ representation areas are shown. For diagnostic purposes, the facial chart is more convenient and powerful than the hand chart, without knowing anything about the patient's medical condition.

Figure 41.5 shows the accurate organ representation areas of the hands where natural existing creases were often found to be the boundaries between various organ representation areas. For example, most of the large intestines are represented between the two near-horizontal lines in the upper half of the palm (cecum, ascending colon, transverse colon, descending colon, to the anus). If an individual has diarrhea or a malignancy, when you touch the corresponding area, not only does the BDORT show a strong negative response by weakening and opening of the O-rings, but also, if you pinch the same area of the hand, one usually feels pain. If you want to deliver a drug to the abnormal area, you stimulate the area with tenderness (BDORT strong negative area) by pinching it for 5–10 minutes, and the drug will selectively be delivered to the pathological area. Furthermore, if you want a drug to reach the brain, stimulate the first segment of the middle finger, representing the head.

CLINICAL SUMMARY

Asbestos plays an important role in many chronic intractable medical problems including mesothelioma and other types of malignancies, Alzheimer's disease, autism, failing heart, varicose veins, and Morgellons disease.

The unique appearance of black areas in PET scans were found to be among the most important diagnostic signs of mesothelioma, which is characterized by markedly reduced glucose uptake and deposits of large amounts of asbestos.

Up until now, standard techniques of measuring asbestos have been very limited without taking a biopsy. We present a reproducible, patented method to assess asbestos. Potential sources of asbestos are several, and avoiding and removing potential ongoing asbestos exposure is important. Dentures and dental materials containing asbestos are an under-recognized source of human exposure.

Simple bilateral mouthwriting, handwriting, and footwriting, which takes less than 10 minutes, can often provide more clinically useful information than standard laboratory tests, which often miss the early stages of various malignancies and other serious medical problems. Using the form in Figure 41.2 before and after any medical treatment such as drugs, nutrition, or surgical procedures, the effects can be easily evaluated and permanently documented.

Asbestos' nonreactive physical properties make it difficult for the body to use its innate removal mechanisms. The author presents his clinical findings for increasing urine excretion of asbestos: Cilantro concentrated as tablets has been demonstrated effective. Raising normal cell telomere to significantly high levels results in a significant improvement in the entire body's circulation and enhances the urinary excretion of asbestos. Using organ representation areas, it is possible to selectively enhance drug and nutrient delivery to areas metabolically isolated by asbestos or other problems.

ACKNOWLEDGMENTS

The author wishes to acknowledge the help and advice received from the following individuals:

1. Ms. Kamila Paluch, MS, who studied biomedical engineering at Columbia University and is currently a part-time research assistant at the Heart Disease Research Foundation, for her devoted help in preparing and writing this manuscript.
2. Dr. Ingrid Kohlstadt, MD, MPH, who kindly invited this author to write about these new topics to be included in the field of nutrition and gave helpful suggestions.
3. Dr. Dominic P. Lu, DDS, FICAE, clinical professor of oral medicine, School of Dental Medicine, University of Pennsylvania; president, American Society for the Advancement of Anesthesia in Dentistry; visiting professor of holistic dentistry, International College of Acupuncture and Electro-Therapeutics, for his continued support and teaching of the Bi-Digital O-Ring Test in dentistry.
4. Dr. Marilyn Jones, MS, DDS, director, Holistic Dental Center of Houston; former assistant professor of chemistry, University of Houston, Texas; visiting associate professor of holistic dentistry, International College of Acupuncture and Electro-Therapeutics, for her continuous direct and indirect help for this research.
5. Dr. Andrew Pallos, DDS, director, Holistic Dental Clinic, Laguna Niguel, California; visiting associate professor, International College of Acupuncture and Electro-Therapeutics, for his continuous direct and indirect help for this research.
6. Dr. Giancarlo Ugazio, MD, professor emeritus of pathology, University of Turin, for his support of our asbestos research and translation of our original research articles in book form into Italian.

This research was supported by the Heart Disease Research Foundation.

REFERENCES

1. Omura, Y. "Asbestos as a possible major cause of not only malignant lung tumors (including small cell carcinoma, adenocarcinoma & mesothelioma), but also brain tumors (i.e. astrocytoma & glioblastoma multiforme), many other malignant tumors, some types of intractable pain including fibromyalgia, & some cardio-vascular pathology: Safe & effective methods of reducing asbestos from normal & pathological areas." *Acupuncture & Electro-Therapeutics Research, The International Journal*, Vol. 31, pp 61–125, 2006.

2. Bueno, R., et al. "Pleural biopsy: A reliable method for determining the diagnosis but not subtype in mesothelioma." *Annals of Thoracic Surgery*, Vol. 78, Nn. 5, pp. 1774–1776; 2004.

3. Johansson, L., and Lindén, C. "Aspects of histopathologic subtype as a prognostic factor in 85 pleural mesotheliomas." *Chest*, Vol. 109, no. 1, pp. 109–114, 1996.

4. Omura, Y. "Important role of asbestos in intractable medical problems including malignant tumors, cardiovascular diseases, alzheimer's disease, autism, cataracts, intractable painful substances, and morgellon's disease: how to remove asbestos and other harmful substances from the body safely and effectively by elevating normal cell telomere to more than 500 ng (BDORT Units) – updated in 2009. Program & Abstract of 19th Annual Symposium of Japan Bi-digital O-Ring Test Medical Society, Held at Tokyo University, during July 4th–5th, 2009, pp. 15–17.

5. Mesothelioma Research Foundation of America. "Types of asbestos," 2010. http://www.mesorfa.org/exposure/asbestos-types.php.

6. Sullivan, P.A. "Vermiculite, respiratory disease, and asbestos exposure in libby, montana: Update of a cohort mortality study." *Environmental Health Perspectives*, Vol. 115, no. 4, pp. 579–585, 2007.

7. Peipins, L.A. "Radiographic abnormalities and exposure to asbestos-contaminated vermiculite in the community of Libby, Montana, USA." *Environmental Health Perspectives*, Vol. 111, no., 14, pp. 1753–1759, 2003.

8. McDonald, J.C., Harris, J., and Armstrong, B.. "Mortality in a cohort of vermiculite miners exposed to fibrous amphibole in Libby, Montana." *Occupational and Environmental Medicine*, Vol. 61, pp. 363–366, 2004.

9. Kellett, C.E.. "Sir Thomas Browne and the disease called the Morgellons." *Annals of Medical History*, Vol. 7, pp. 467–479, 1935.

10. Koblenzer, C.S. "The challenge of Morgellons disease." *Journal of the American Academy of Dermatology*, Vol. 55, no. 5, pp. 920–922, 2006.

11. Savely, V.R., Leitao, M.M., Stricker, R.B. "The mystery of Morgellons Disease: Infection or delusion?" *American Journal of Clinical Dermatology*, Vol. 7, no. 1, pp. 1–5(5), 2006.

12. Greaves, M.W., Khalifa, N. "Itch: More than skin deep." *International Archives of Allergy and Immunology*, Vol. 135, pp. 166–172, 2004.

13. Morgellons Research Foundation Web site. Available at: http://www.morgellons.org/. Accessed January 10, 2012.

14. Savely, V.R., and Stricker, R.B. "Morgellons disease: Analysis of a population with clinically confirmed microscopic subcutaneous fibers of unknown etiology." *Clinical, Cosmetic and Investigational Dermatology*, Vol. 3, pp. 67–78, 2010.

15. Harvey, W.T., et al. "Morgellons disease, illuminating an undefined illness: A case series." *Journal of Medical Case Reports*, Vol. 3, no. 1, 8243, 2009.

16. Dreifus, C. "Finding clues to aging in the fraying tips of chromosomes." *New York Times*. July 3, 2007. http://www.nytimes.com/2007/07/03/science/03conv.html?pagewanted=all.

17. Takagi, A., et al. "Induction of mesothelioma in p53+/− mouse by intraperitoneal application of multiwall carbon nanotube." *Journal of Toxicological Sciences*, Vol. 33, no. 1, pp. 105–116, 2008.

18. Poland, C. A. et al. "Carbon nanotubes introduced into the abdominal cavity of mice show asbestos-like pathogenicity in a pilot study." *Nature Nanotechnology*, Vol. 3, pp. 423–428,(2008.

19. Chang, Kenneth. "In study, researchers find nanotubes may pose health risks similar to asbestos." *New York Times*. May 21, 2008.

20. Kane, A. B., and R. H. Hurt. "The asbestos analogy revisited." *Nature Nanotechnology*, Vol. 3, pp. 378–379, 2008.

21. Donaldson, K., and C. A. Poland. "New insights into nanotubes." *Nature Nanotechnology*, Vol. 4, pp. 708–710, 2009.

22. Service, R. F. "Nanotubes: The next asbestos?" *Science*, Vol. 281, pp. 941, 1998.

23. Poland, C. A., et al. "Carbon nanotubes introduced into the abdominal cavity of mice show asbestos-like pathogenicity in a pilot study." *Nature Nanotechnology*, Vol. 3, pp. 423–428, 2008.

24. Takagi, A., et al. "Induction of mesothelioma in p53+/– mouse by intraperitoneal application of multiwall carbon nanotube." *Journal of Toxicological Sciences,* Vol. 33, no. 1, pp. 105–116, 2008.

25. Fubini, B., and Otero-Areán, C. "Chemical aspects of the toxicity of inhaled mineral dusts." *Chemical Society Reviews,* Vol. 28, pp. 373–381, 1999.

26. IARC: Surgical Implants and Other Foreign Bodies. IARC Monographs on the Evaluation of Carcinogenic Risks to Humans. Vol. 74: pp. 313–322 (World Health Organization, Lyon, France, 1999).

27. Marsh, G.M., et al. "Cancer mortality among man-made vitreous fiber production workers." *Epidemiology,* Vol. 9, no. 2, pp. 218–220, 1998.

28. McGrath, K. "An earlier age of breast cancer diagnosis related to more frequent use of antiperspirants/ deodorants and underarm shaving." *European Journal of Cancer Prevention,* Vol. 12, no. 6, pp. 479–485, 2003.

29. Blue, L. "Do antiperspirants cause breast cancer?" TIME Healthland. http://healthland.time.com/2012/ 01/12/do-antiperspirants-cause-breast-cancer/ . January 12, 2012.

30. Doheny, K. "Does deodorant ingredient affect breast cancer risk?" HealthDay. http://consumer.health-day.com/Article.asp?AID=660647. January 12, 2012.

31. Mann, D. "Are fears that deodorant causes breast cancer unfounded?" WebMD Health News. http://www. webmd.com/breast-cancer/news/20120112/are-fears-that-deodorant-causes-breast-cancerunfounded. January 12, 2012.

32. Christensen, B.C. "Epigenetic profiles, asbestos burden, and survival in pleural mesothelioma." Dissertation/Thesis, Harvard University, 2008, 136 pages; AAT 3312317.

33. Roberts, H.C., et al. "Screening for malignant pleural mesothelioma and lung cancer in individuals with a history of asbestos exposure." *Journal of Thoracic Oncology,* Vol. 4; iss. 5, pp 620-628, May 2009.

34. Creaney, J., et al. "Serum mesothelin for early detection of asbestos-induced cancer malignant mesothelioma" *Cancer Epidemiology, Biomarkers & Prevention,* Vol. 19, no. 9, pp. 2238–2246, 2010.

35. Park, E., et al. "Soluble mesothelin-related protein in an asbestos-exposed population: The dust diseases board cohort study." *American Journal of Respiratory and Critical Care Medicine,* Vol. 178, no. 8, pp. 832–837, 2008.

36. Hollevoet, K. "Serial measurements of mesothelioma serum biomarkers in asbestos-exposed individuals: a prospective longitudinal cohort study." *Journal of Thoracic Oncology,* Vol. 6, no. 5, pp. 889–895, 2011.

37. Thurneysen, C., et al. "Functional inactivation of NF2/merlin in human mesothelioma." *Lung Cancer,* Vol. 64, pp. 140–147, 2009.

38. Eisenstadt, H.B. "Asbestos pleurisy." *Diseases of the Chest,* Vol 46, pp. 78–81, 1964.

39. Greillier, L. and P. Astoul. "Mesothelioma and asbestos-related pleural diseases." *Respiration,* Vol. 76, pp. 1–15, 2008.

40. Harber, P., Mohsenifar, Z., Oren, A., Lew, M. "Pleural plaques and asbestos-associated malignancy." *Journal of Occupational Medicine*, Vol. 29, pp. 641–644, 1987.

41. Weiss, W. "Asbestos-related pleural plaques and lung cancer." *Chest,* Vol. 103, pp. 1854–1859, 1993.

42. Solomon, A. "Radiological features of asbestos-related visceral pleural changes." *American Journal of Industrial Medicine,* Vol. 19, pp. 339–355, 1991.

43. Bianchi, C., Bianchi, T. "Malignant mesothelioma: Global incidence and relationship with asbestos." *Industrial Health,* Vol. 45, pp. 379–387, 2007.

44. Leigh, J., Davidson, P., Hendrie, L., Berry, D. "Malignant mesothelioma in Australia, 1945–2000." *American Journal of Industrial Medicine*, Vol. 41, pp. 188–201, 2002.

45. McElvenny, D.M., Darnton, A.J., Price, M.J., Hodgson, J.T. "Mesothelioma mortality in Great Britain from 1968 to 2001." *Occupational Medicine (London),* Vol. 55, pp. 79–87, 2005.

46. Benard, F., Sterman, D., Smith, R.J., Kaiser, L.R., Albelda, S.M., Alavi A. "Metabolic imaging of malignant pleural mesothelioma with fluorodeoxyglucose positron emission tomography." *Chest,* Vol. 114, pp. 713–722, 1998.

47. Flores, R.M., Akhurst, T., Gonen, M., Larson, S.M., Rusch, V.W. "Positron emission tomography defines metastatic disease but not locoregional disease in patients with malignant pleural mesothelioma." *Journal of Thoracic and Cardiovascular Surgery,* Vol. 126, pp. 11–16, 2003.

48. Flores, R.M., Akhurst, T., Gonen, M., Zakowski, M., Dycoco, J., Larson, S.M., Rusch, V.W. "Positron emission tomography predicts survival in malignant pleural mesothelioma." *Journal of Thoracic and Cardiovascular Surgery,* Vol. 132, pp. 763–768, 2006.

49. Ceresoli, G.L., Chiti, A., Zucali, P.A., Rodari, M., Lutman, R.F., Salamina, S., Incarbone, M., Alloisio, M., Santoro, A. "Early response evaluation in malignant pleural mesothelioma by positron emission tomography with [18f]fluorodeoxyglucose." *Journal of Clinical Oncology,* Vol. 24, pp. 4587–4593, 2006.

50. Bueno, R., Reblando, J., Glickman, J., Jaklitsch, M.T., Lukanich, J.M., Sugarbaker, D.J. "Pleural biopsy: a reliable method for determining the diagnosis but not subtype in mesothelioma." *Annals of Thoracic Surgery*, Vol. 78, pp. 1774–1776, 2004.

51. Alatas, F., Alatas, O., Metintas, M., Colak, O., Harmanci, E., Demir, S. "Diagnostic value of CEA, CA 15-3, CA 19-9, CYFRA 21-1, NSE and TSA assay in pleural effusions." *Lung Cancer*, Vol. 31, pp. 9–16, 2001.

52. van den Heuvel, M.M., Korse, C.M., Bonfrer, J.M., Baas, P. "Non-invasive diagnosis of pleural malignancies: The role of tumour markers. *Lung Cancer,* DOI: 10.1016/j.lungcan.2007.08.030.

53. Pass, H.I., Wali, A., Tang, N., Ivanova, A., Ivanov, S., Harbut, M., Carbone, M., Allard, J. "Soluble mesothelin-related peptide level elevation in mesothelioma serum and pleural effusions." *Annals of Thoracic Surgery,* Vol. 85, pp. 265–272, discussion 272, 2008.

54. Grigoriu, B.D., Scherpereel, A., Devos, P., Chahine, B., Letourneux, M., Lebailly, P., Gregoire, M., Porte, H., Copin, M.C., Lassalle, P. "Utility of osteopontin and serum mesothelin in malignant pleural mesothelioma diagnosis and prognosis assessment." *Clinical Cancer Research,* Vol. 13, pp. 2928–2935, 2007.

55. Herndon, J.E., Green, M.R., Chahinian, A.P., Corson, J.M., Suzuki, Y., Vogelzang, N.J. "Factors predictive of survival among 337 patients with mesothelioma treated between 1984 and 1994 by the Cancer and Leukemia Group B." *Chest,* Vol. 113, pp. 723–731, 1998.

56. Raffit, H., et al. "Detection and quantitation of serum mesothelin, a tumor marker for patients with mesothelioma and ovarian cancer." *Clinical Cancer Research,* Vol.12, pp. 447, 2006.

57. Omura, Y. "A new, simple, non-invasive imaging technique of internal organs and various cancer tissues using extended principles of the 'Bi-Digital O-Ring Test' without using expensive imaging instruments or exposing the patient to any undesirable radiation—Part 1." *Acupuncture & Electro-Therapeutics Research, The International Journal,* Vol. 10, pp. 255–277, 1985.

58. Omura, Y. "'Bi-Digital O-Ring Test Molecular Identification and Localization Method' and its application in imaging of internal organs and malignant tumors as well as identification and localization of neurotransmitters and micro-organisms—Part 1." *Acupuncture & Electro-Therapeutics Research, The International Journal,* Vol. 11, no. 2, pp. 65–100, 1986.

59. Omura, Y. "Re-evaluation of the classical acupuncture concept of meridians in oriental medicine by the new method of detecting meridian-like networks connected to internal organs using 'Bi-Digital O-Ring Test.'" *Acupuncture & Electro-Therapeutics Research, The International Journal,* Vol. 11, pp. 219–231, 1986.

60. Omura, Y. "Electro-magnetic resonance phenomenon as a possible mechanism related to the 'Bi-Digital O-Ring Test Molecular Identification and Localization Method.'" *Acupuncture & Electro-Therapeutics Research, The International Journal,* Vol. 11, no. 2, pp. 127–145, 1986.

61. Omura, Y. "Highlights of the forthcoming 1st International Symposium on Acupuncture & Electro-Therapeutics to celebrate the 10th anniversary of Acupuncture & Electro-Therapeutics Research, The International Journal., 1) Stress & Immunity and effects of stimulation of deep peroneal nerve at St.36 on ventricular arrhythmia, heart disease & sudden death. 2) New, simple, accurate and inexpensive imaging technique of internal organs and cancer tissue by a clinical application of "Bi-Digital O-Ring Test" and clinical significance of newly discovered networks of thymus glands in cancer treatment." *Acupuncture & Electro-Therapeutics Research, The International Journal,* Vol. 10, pp. 1–2, 1985.

62. Omura, Y. "Simple and quick non-invasive evaluation of circulatory condition of cerebral arteries by clinical application of the 'Bi-Digital O-Ring Test.'" *Acupuncture & Electro-Therapeutics Research, The International Journal,* Vol. 10, pp. 139–161, 1985.

63. Omura, Y. Editorial: "Effects of an electrical field and its polarity on an abnormal part of the body or organ representation point associated with a diseased internal organ, and its influence on the 'Bi-Digital O-Ring Test' (simple, non-invasive dysfunction localization method) & drug compatibility test—Part 1." *Acupuncture & Electro-Therapeutics Research, The International Journal,* Vol. 7, pp. 209–246, 1982.

64. Omura, Y., Nisteruk, C.J., Losco, Bro. M., Heller, S.I., Omura, A., Cook, A., Williams, G. "Noninvasive early diagnosis of cardiovascular diseases by the combined use of the 'Bi-Digital O-Ring Test Dysfunction Localization Method,' organ representation points & of wide frequency bandwidth ECG's & selective high frequency wide bandwidth ECG's." *Japanese Heart Journal,* Vol. 23, pp 564–566, supplement, 1982.

65. Omura, Y. "Application of the Bi-Digital O-Ring Test for diagnosis and effective treatment of intractable pain, infection, & cancer using selective drug-uptake enhancement methods, and the relationship between these intractable problems and harmful environmental electro-magnetic fields & localized deposits of heavy metal in the body." *6th Congress of the Japan Bi-Digital O-Ring Test Medical Society,* pp. 58–61, Tokyo University, Tokyo, Japan, 1996 Aug 8–10.

66. Shimotsura, Y., Omura, Y. "Standard laboratory test (x-ray with barium enema, colono-fiberscopic examination of the colon, and histopathological examination of pathological tissues) evaluation of 237 pathological areas of the colon where strong Bi-Digital O-Ring Test cancer positive response was found in 147 patients." *6th Congress of the Japan Bi-Digital O-Ring Test Medical Society*, p. 71, Tokyo University, Tokyo, Japan, 1996 Aug 8–10.

67. Omura, Y. "Early cancer screening and a new safe and effective cancer therapy using selective drug uptake enhancement methods, anti-viral agents, and the removal of mercury based on the Bi-Digital O-Ring Test evaluation." *3rd International Symposium on the Bi-Digital O-Ring Test*, pp. 127–128, Waseda University, Tokyo, Japan, 1997 Oct 3–5.

68. Omura, Y. "Long-term exposure to extremely high frequency electro-magnetic fields in the home or office environment, localized deposits of hg, and viral infection in individuals as major contributing factors to the genesis of cancer and cardiovascular disease." *3rd International Symposium on the Bi-Digital O-Ring Test*, pp. 129–130, Waseda University, Tokyo, Japan, 1997 Oct 3–5.

69. Omura, Y. "Major causes of intractable pain and their effective treatment using the Bi-Digital O-Ring Test." Combined use of effective anti-microbial agents, cilantro to remove heavy metals, and drug uptake enhancement method selectively deliver the drugs to the pathological areas." *3rd International Symposium on the Bi-Digital O-Ring Test*, pp. 147–148, Waseda University, Tokyo, Japan, 1997 Oct 3–5.

70. Omura, Y. "Early non-invasive cancer screening by detecting levels of integrin α5β1, oncogene C-fos Ab-2, Hg, acetylcholine, viral infection, NO, D-glucose, p53 (Ab-5) & Rb (Ab-8), and a new safe and effective cancer therapy using a mixture of EPA & DHA as an anti-viral agent, & cilantro to remove intracellular mercury and 'Selective Drug Uptake Enhancement Method' based on the Bi-Digital O-Ring Test evaluation." *8th Congress of the Japan Bi-Digital O-Ring Test Medical Society*, pp. 58–59, Showa University, Tokyo, Japan, 1998 Jul 19–20.

71. Omura, Y. "Electromagnetic field hypersensitivity, cancer, pre-cancer & abnormal pure (-) qi gong energy emission." *8th Congress of the Japan Bi-Digital O-Ring Test Medical Society*, pp. 60–61, Showa University, Tokyo, Japan, 1998 Jul 19–20.

72. Omura, Y. "Early non-invasive cancer screening by detecting levels of integrin α5β1, oncogene C-fos Ab-2, Hg, acetycholine, viral infection, NO, D-glucose, p53 (Ab-5) & Rb (Ab-8), and a new safe and effective cancer therapy using a mixture of EPA & DHA as an anti-viral agent, & cilantoro to remove intracellular mercury and 'Selective Drug Uptake Enhancement Method' based on the Bi-Digital O-Ring Test evaluation." Presented as a guest speaker at 8th Annual Congress of Japan Bi-Digital O-Ring Test Medical Society at Showa University, Tokyo, *Acupuncture & Electro-Therapeutics Research, The International Journal*, Vol. 23, nos. 3 and 4, pp. 229–230, 1998.

73. Omura, Y. "Accurate organ representation areas on the face, nose, lips, and tongue localized by Bi-Digital O-Ring Test and their clinical application for diagnosis and treatment." Presented as a guest speaker at 8th Annual Congress of Japan Bi-Digital O-Ring Test Medical Society at Showa University, Tokyo, *Acupuncture & Electro-Therapeutics Research, The International Journal*, Vol. 23, nos. 3 and 4, pg. 231, 1998.

74. Omura, Y., Shimotsuura, Y., Ooki, M., Noguchi, T. "Estimation of the amount of telomere molecules in different human age groups and the telomere increasing effect of acupuncture and Shiatsu on St.36, using synthesized basic units of the human telomere molecules as reference control substances for the Bi-Digital O-Ring Test resonance phenomenon." Presented as a guest speaker at 8th Annual Congress of Japan Bi-Digital O-Ring Test Medical Society at Showa University, Tokyo, *Acupuncture & Electro-Therapeutics Research, The International Journal*, Vol. 23, nos. 3 and 4, pp. 185–206, 1998.

75. Omura, Y. "Non-invasive diagnosis & effective treatment of chronic intractable lower back pain using the Bi-Digital O-Ring test resonance phenomenon & the Selective Drug Uptake Enhancement Method." Abstract published in Program and Abstract of the International Symposium: Satellite of the 9th Congress of the Pain Clinic, held in Tokyo, Japan, July 12–13, 2000, pg. 66; the paper was subsequently published in the hardcover book *Management of Pain: A World Perspective*, ed. H. Yanagida, K. Hanaoka, and O. Yuge, as part of the 9th International Symposium on Pain, organized by the International Association for the Study of Pain, by Monduzzi Editore, Bologna Italy, 2000, pp. 65–74.

76. Omura, Y. "Non-invasive and quick diagnostic method using the Bi-Digital O-Ring test resonance phenomenon between 2 identical substances for the early detection of cancer and effective treatment using the Selective Drug Uptake Enhancement Method." Presented at the 16th Annual Symposium on Acupuncture and Electro Therapeutics, October 19–22, 2000, at the School of International Affairs at Columbia University, abstract published in *Acupuncture & Electro-Therapeutics Research, The International Journal*, Vol. 25, nos. 3–4, pp. 211–213, 2000.

77. Duvvi, H., Omura, Y. "Evaluation of the Bi-Digital O-Ring Test for the detection of precancer from rat colon photographs." Presented at the 16th Annual Symposium on Acupuncture and Electro Therapeutics, October 19–22, 2000, at the School of International Affairs at Columbia University, abstract published in *Acupuncture & Electro-Therapeutics Research, The International Journal*, Vol. 25, nos. 3–4, pp. 249–250, 2000.

78. Omura, Y. "Transmission of molecular information on molecular structures and amounts of the molecules through the recorded traces of photons, sound waves, and electric currents coming through biological tissue and their clinical applications for new non-invasive diagnosis and treatment of intractable medical problems." Presented at the 4th Biennial International Symposium on the Bi-Digital O-Ring Test, July 21–23, 2001, at Waseda University, Tokyo, *Acupuncture & Electro-Therapeutics Research, The International Journal*, Vol. 26, nos. 1–2, pp. 77–79, 2001.

79. Omura, Y., Tobe, Y. "Marked beneficial effects obtained after acupuncture at True St. 36 compared with very little effects obtained from acupuncture on traditional St. 36—Localization of True St. 36 & traditional St. 36 and their acupuncture effects clarified using the Bi-Digital O-Ring Test." (In Japanese) Ido No Nippon, *The Japanese Journal of Acupuncture & Manual Therapies*, Serial No. 692, pp. 129–150, Oct. 2001.

80. Omura, Y., Shimotsuura, Y., Ohki, M. "2 minute non-invasive screening of heart disease and 2 minute non-invasive screening of cardio-vascular diseases, and their safe and effective treatment." Abstract of the 5th Biennial International Symposium on the Bi-Digital O-Ring Test, pp. 36–38, organized and published by Japan Bi-Digital O-Ring Test Medical Society, held at Ibuka International Auditorium, Waseda University, Tokyo, Japan, during July 19–21, 2002, reprinted in *Acupuncture & Electro-Therapeutics Research, The International Journal*, Vol. 27, nos. 3 and 4, pp. 219–221, 2002.

81. Omura, Y. "Non-invasive 6-minute screening of pre-alzheimer's disease by estimating amounts of Acetylcholine, b-Amyloid (1–42), Al, Hg & Pb of the brain, and the safe & effective treatment of pre-alzheimer's disease using the 'Selective Drug Uptake Enhancement Method.'" Abstract of 5th Biennial International Symposium on Bi-Digital O-Ring Test, pp. 75–76, organized and published by Japan Bi-Digital O-Ring Test Medical Society, held at Ibuka International Auditorium, Waseda University, Tokyo, Japan, during July 19–21, 2002, reprinted in *Acupuncture & Electro-Therapeutics Research, The International Journal*, Vol. 27, nos. 3 and 4, pp. 226–227, 2002.

82. Omura, Y., Tobe, Y. "Screening & effective treatment of alzheimer's disease & cancer, and correct location of acupuncture points St.36 (True St.36) and Li.4 (True Li.4) and their application for the treatment of intractable diseases by using Bi-Digital O-Ring Test." (In Japanese), Ido No Nippon. *The Japanese Journal of Acupuncture & Manual Therapies*, Vol 62, no. 10, pp. 81–92, Oct 2003.

83. Omura, Y. "Rapid screening & diagnosis of various cancers from human voice using Bi-Digital O-Ring Test resonance phenomenon between 2 identical substances i.e. between microscopic slide of specific cancer tissue & cancer information in the sound of human voice, and detection of myocardial damage & infection from human voice." *Acupuncture and Electro-Therapeutics Research, The International Journal*, Vol. 32, nos. 3/4, pp. 235–270, 2007.

84. Shimotsuura, Y., Omura, Y. "Case reports of clinical cancer found by standard laboratory tests several years after positive findings by Bi-Digital O-Ring Test." *Acupuncture and Electro-Therapeutics Research, The International Journal*, Vol. 33, nos. 1/2, pp. 54–55, 2008.

85. Omura, Y. "Organ representation areas of different internal organs localized on the eyebrows & eyelids by the Bi-Digital O-Ring Test electromagnetic resonance phenomenon between 2 identical molecules – part i: detection of increased markers for cancer & heart disease from white hairs on the eyebrows and marked decrease in the markers after taking one optimal dose of DHEA." *Acupuncture and Electro-Therapeutics Research, The International Journal*, Vol. 33, nos. 3/4, pp. 193–224, 2008.

86. Omura, Y. "Comparison of effects of press-needle acupuncture, moxibustion, (+) qigong energy stored paper or (+) solar energy stored paper on True ST-36 (Omura's ST-36) & traditional ST-36 on the amount of normal cell telomere & the anti-cancer, anti-aging & anti-alzheimer's effects of these treatments. To be presented in May 2011 at ICMART International congress on medical acupuncture in Holland (1-page abstract in press).

87. Omura, Y., Chen, Y., Lermand, O., Jones, M., Duvvi, H., Shimtosuura, Y. "Effects of transcutaneous electrical stimulation (1 pulse/sec) through custom-made disposable surface electrodes covering Omura's ST36 area of both legs on normal cell telomeres, oncogene C-fos Ab2, Integrin α5β1, chlamydia trachomatis, etc. in breast cancer & alzheimer patients." *Acupuncture & Electro-Therapeutics Research, The International Journal*, Vol. 35, nos. 3/4, pp. 147–186, 2010.

88. Omura, Y., O'Young, B., Jones, M., Pallos, A., Duvvi, H., Shimotsuura, Y. "Caprylic acid in the effective treatment of intractable medical problems of frequent urination, incontinence, chronic upper respiratory infection, root canalled tooth infection, ALS, etc., caused by asbestos & mixed infections of *Candida*

albicans, Helicobacter pylori, & *Cytomegalovirus* with or without other microorganisms & mercury." *Acupuncture & Electro-Therapeutics Research, The International Journal,* Vol. 36, nos. 1/2, pp. 19–64, 2011.

89. Omura, Y. "Beneficial effects of bitter melon (goya), which excretes toxic substances, including radioactive substances, and induces weight loss and anti-aging effect." *Soukai,* No. 8, pp. 148–149, 2011.

90. Omura, Y. Lu, DP., Jones, M., O'Young B., Duvvi, H., Paluch, K., Shimotsuura, Y., Ohki, M. "New clinical findings on the longevity gene in disease, health, & longevity: Sirtuin 1 often decreases with advanced age & serious diseases in most parts of the human body, while relatively high & constant sirtuin 1 regardless of age was first found in the hippocampus of supercentenarians." *Acupuncture & Electro-Therapeutics Research, The International Journal,* Vol. 36, nos. 3/4, 23 page article in press, 2011.

91. Omura, Y. "Reduced glucose uptake with markedly increased gastrin releasing peptide, osteopontine & asbestos found in dark black areas of PET scan of chest wall in patient with mesothelioma." *Acupuncture & Electro-Therapeutics Research, The International Journal,* Vol. 31, pp 247–257, 2006.

92. Francis, R.J., Byrne, M.J., van der Schaaf, A.A., Boucek, J.A., Nowak, A.K., Phillips, M., Price, R., Patrikeos, A.P., Musk, A.W., Millward, M.J. "Early prediction of response to chemotherapy and survival in malignant pleural mesothelioma using a novel semiautomated 3-dimensional volume-based analysis of serial 18F-FDG PET scans. *Journal of Nuclear Medicine,* Vol. 48, pp. 1449–1458, 2007.

93. Flores, R.M. "The role of PET in the surgical management of malignant pleural mesothelioma." *Lung Cancer,* Vol. 49, suppl 1, pp. S27–S32.

94. Steinert, H.C., Santos Dellea, M.M., Burger, C., Stahel, R. "Therapy response evaluation in malignant pleural mesothelioma with integrated PET-CT imaging." *Lung Cancer,* Vol. 49, suppl 1, pp. S33–S35, 2005.

95. Huff, J.; Ladou, J. "Aspartame bioassay findings portend human cancer hazards." *International Journal of Occupational and Environmental Health,* Vol 13: pp. 446–448; 2007.

96. Weihrauch, MR, Diehl, V. "Artificial sweeteners—do they bear a carcinogenic risk?" *Annals of Oncology,* Vol. 15, pp. 1460–1465, 2004.

97. Tollefson, L., Barnard, R.J. "An analysis of FDA passive surveillance reports of seizures associated with consumption of aspartame." *Journal of the American Dietetic Association,* Vol. 92, no. 5, pp. 598–601, 1992.

98. Kroyer, G. "Stevioside and Stevia-sweetener in food: application, stability and interaction with food ingredients." *Journal of Consumer Protection and Food Safety,* Vol. 5, no. 2: pp. 225–229, 2010.

99. "Stevia." WebMD. 2009. http://www.webmd.com/vitamins-supplements/ingredientmono-682-STEVIA. aspx?activeIngredientId = 682&activeIngredientName = STEVIA.

100. Omura, Y., Chen, Y., Duvvi, H. "Anatomical relationship between traditional acupuncture point ST 36 and Omura's ST 36(True ST 36) with their therapeutic effects: 1) inhibition of cancer cell division by markedly lowering cancer cell telomere while increasing normal telomere, 2) improving circulatory disturbances with reduction of abnormal increase in high triglyceride, L-Homocysstein, CRP, or Cardiac Troponin I & T in blood by the stimulation of Omura's ST 36—Part 1" *Acupuncture & Electro-Therapeutics Research, The International Journal,* Vol. 32, pp. 31–70, 2007.

42 Electromagnetic Hypersensitivity and Implications for Metabolism

John C. Cline, M.D., B.Sc., and
Beth Ellen DiLuglio, M.S., R.D., C.C.N.

INTRODUCTION

Over the past century, great discoveries in the biomolecular and biochemical nature and design of cells have led us to new understandings of how cells and systems of cells, such as the human being, work and exist [1]. Of equal importance, but less recognized, is that organisms are bioelectromagnetic beings. The human body can be visualized as an electromagnetic semiconductor matrix that allows for instantaneous communication among all cells within the system [2]. This living matrix is defined as "the continuous molecular fabric of the organism, consisting of fascia, the other connective tissues, extracellular matrices, integrins, cytoskeletons, nuclear matrices and DNA." Within the living matrix, extracellular, cellular, and nuclear biopolymers or ground substances constitute a body-wide reservoir of charge that can maintain electrical homeostasis and "inflammatory preparedness" throughout the organism [3]. Master control mechanisms such as the autonomic nervous system exist within the living matrix, with minute shifts in the established electrochemical gradients resulting in evoked changes within cells, tissues, and organs. Understanding that the body is bioelectromagnetic is important when considering the influence of external electromagnetic radiation (EMR), which has the potential to damage or threaten the health of the body as well as the potential to heal the body [2].

Electromagnetism and biochemistry are intertwined. Nutrition can reduce radiation exposure, block tissue uptake, provide antioxidant protection, and support repair, detoxification, and immune mechanisms. This chapter describes: the diverse types and sources of EMR, electromagnetic hypersensitivity (EHS) syndrome, implications for the impact on metabolic processes, and clinical approaches to mitigate and treat the effects of adverse EMR exposure.

BACKGROUND ON ELECTROMAGNETIC RADIATION AND IRRADIATED FOOD

Exposure to EMR comes in the form of high-frequency ionizing radiation and lower frequency non-ionizing radiation. The frequency of electromagnetic energy determines its properties and physiologic effects on the human body (Figure 42.1).

IONIZING RADIATION

Ionizing radiation (IR) is a known carcinogen, and its penetrative properties contribute to cell and organ damage (Figure 42.2). Sources of ionizing radiation include background radiation (solar,

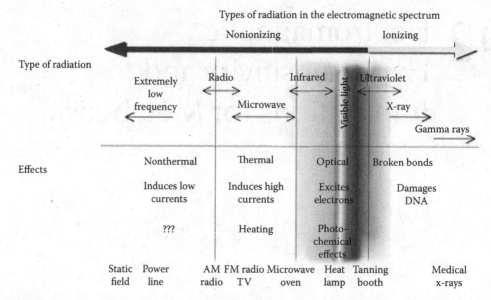

Types of radiation in the electromagnetic spectrum

FIGURE 42.1 Types of radiation in the electromagnetic spectrum and the physiologic effects they exert (Source: http://www.epa.gov/radiation/understand/index.html. Accessed November 25, 2011. Public domain.)

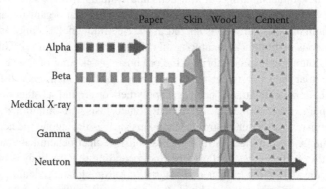

FIGURE 42.2 Penetrative properties of ionizing radiation (Source: http://www.nrc.gov/about-nrc/radiation/health-effects/radiation-basics.html. Accessed December 6, 2011. Public Domain.)

radon, uranium in soil); cosmic radiation (solar, air travel); medical radiation; and nuclear fission (nuclear weapons, nuclear power plants).

DIAGNOSTIC RADIATION

According to radiation expert John W. Gofman, MD, PhD, X-rays and CT scans are likely a principal cause of cancer mortality and ischemic heart disease [4,5]. Cumulative dose is seldom calculated for exposure from diagnostic X-rays, and iatrogenic complications may go unnoticed. Radiation from a single CT scan can be equal to that of several hundred chest X-rays [6] and can increase cancer risk, especially for children [7]. Excessive radiation exposure from mammograms has also created debate about the benefit-versus-risk ratio [8]. Cancer from unprotected exposure during X-ray administration was considered an "occupational disease" for dentists and physicians who performed their own X-rays. A safe X-ray radiation dose for one individual may increase relative risk of disease by up to 10 times in a susceptible individual [9]. The groundbreaking work of Alice Stewart, MD, shed light on the fact that an X-ray administered to a pregnant woman could subsequently cause cancer in the child [10–12].

MEDICAL RADIATION THERAPY

Radiation therapy (RT) is utilized in more than 50% of conventional treatment plans for cancer patients. External beam radiation and internal radioactive "seeds" affect nearby healthy cells as well as target cancer cells. Cardiac complications, including coronary artery and valvular disease, cardiomyopathy, and pericarditis, are known to occur following chest RT [13]. Additional complications of RT include thyroid cancer, renal dysfunction, GI dysfunction, hypertension, and severe anemia [14]. Unintentional RT overdose can occur due to human error, computer program flaws, and insufficient training and safety measures. A 43-year-old patient who received excessive doses of RT for three days suffered loss of hearing, vision, teeth, swallowing ability, and eventually death [15]. Experts predict that one in 20 patients will suffer injury from RT.

FOOD IRRADIATION

Food irradiation utilizes three types of ionizing radiation: gamma rays (from cobalt-60 and cesium-137), X-rays, and electron beam. Cobalt-60 and cesium-137 from military and commercial nuclear facilities are utilized as well as spent fuel rods, according to the Environmental Protection Agency (EPA). Food irradiation facilities also pose a danger to workers and surrounding communities due to spillage of radioactive waste water into municipal drains; hazardous transportation of radioactive material; creation of radioactive waste within the facility; and the potential for cobalt-60 pellets to be used in a "dirty bomb." Irradiation workers are at risk of exposure and the EPA concludes that "irradiation sources are very large and could prove lethal should a person accidentally be exposed to the beam" [16].

ENVIRONMENTAL SOURCES OF IONIZING RADIATION

Radioactive elements reach the body via air, food, and water. The EPA sets Maximum Contaminant Levels (MCLs) and Goals (MCLGs) for radionuclides in drinking water—including radioactive iodine, strontium, radium, and uranium—and violations are to be reported to customers "as soon as practical or within 30 days after a violation occurs." Radioactive isotopes (called radionuclides) are monitored in food and water following nuclear accidents and can persist in the environment due to variations in half-life from hours, to days, to millions of years. For example, with a half-life of 30 years, cesium-137 from Chernobyl continues to contaminate food and milk and is expected to do so for three more centuries [17]. Radioactive iodine-131 has an eight-day half-life but radioactive iodine-129 has a 15–17-million-year half-life and its potential for entering the food chain is frequently overlooked [18]. Traveling via atmospheric winds, radioactive iodine-131 was detected in Massachusetts rain water (a source of drinking water) within two weeks of the Fukushima Daiichi nuclear power plant melt-down [19]. Drinking water and food from provinces around the Fukushima plant were contaminated, and consumption was restricted [20].

Tracking radionuclides in the body is possible. Measurement of uranium in urine, hair, and nails can reflect ingestion of contaminated drinking water [21,22]. Measuring radioactive strontium-90 (Sr-90) in deciduous teeth has been utilized since the 1950s to assess exposure to nuclear fission by-products from weapons testing and nuclear power plants. The St. Louis Baby Teeth Survey demonstrated uptake of Sr-90 from nuclear bomb testing [23–25] while the more current Radiation and Public Health Project (RPHP) [26] demonstrated increased Sr-90 uptake in relation to nuclear power plant proximity [27,28]. RPHP was also able to analyze teeth from the 1950s study and found that Sr-90 levels were significantly higher (P < 0.04) in individuals diagnosed with cancer than for matched controls [29]. In 2011, the Nuclear Regulatory Commission (NRC) requested that the

National Academy of Sciences perform a comprehensive analysis in order to quantify cancer risk in relation to nuclear power plants.

Researcher Abram Petkau, PhD, discovered that chronic low-dose radiation was more damaging to cell membranes than high-dose, acute exposure (that the cell could quickly repair). The phenomenon became known as the "Petkau Effect" and appeared to be caused primarily by free radicals [30]. With regards to IR exposure, Dr. Gofman concludes "that there is no threshold dose (no risk-free dose). ...Therefore every exposure counts, and the consequences (including carcinogenic mutations) accumulate" [31]. The EPA concedes that it cannot set a "safe" level of IR exposure. The NRC limits the amount of IR a licensee can expose the public to, currently 0.1 rem (100 mrem) per year, excluding background radiation, medical radiation exposure, and "disposal of radioactive material into sanitary sewerage" [32].

Radiation is known to disrupt biological systems; severity of damage and symptoms tends to be dose and time related, particularly for IR. Listed as a "known human carcinogen" by the National Toxicology Program, IR can negatively affect humans throughout the lifespan, but critical periods of fetal development are particularly vulnerable. Exposure to radionuclides, particularly Sr-90, can lead to birth defects and prematurity, childhood cancer, and also learning disorders due to damage to the prefrontal cortex [33,34]. In adults, Sr-90 follows the path of calcium to bone where it irradiates bone marrow and can lead to cancer, immune disorders, and osteoporosis. Yttrium-90, the radioactive decay product of Sr-90, travels to soft tissues and hormone-producing glands, disrupting their function and integrity.

NONIONIZING RADIATION

Within the electromagnetic spectrum, nonionizing radiation (NR) produces enough energy to cause atoms to vibrate, but not enough to remove electrons from their orbits. Referring to Figure 42.3, low-frequency (LF) EMFs have very long wave lengths (one million meters or more) and frequencies of $1-3 \times 10^3$ Hz. Examples of LF EMF fields are electric power lines, medical devices such as ultrasound, electric motors (hair dryers, toothbrushes, power tools), fluorescent lights, home appliances, and electrical outlets. Radio frequencies (RF) have wave lengths between 1–100 meters and frequencies of $3 \times 10^2 - 3 \times 10^7$ Hz. Examples of RF include AM and FM radio, television, and medical magnetic resonance imaging. Microwaves have shorter wave lengths of about 1/100th of a meter with frequencies in the order of $3 \times 10^7 - 3 \times 10^{12}$ Hz. Examples of microwaves include cell phones and other wireless technologies (TV remotes, garage door openers, smart meters, two-way radios, baby monitors, etc.), cell phone and other telecommunications towers, microwave ovens, and so on [35]. Microwave ovens utilize molecular vibration to heat and cook food, and of course human tissue can be negatively affected by direct exposure. Of concern are the adverse effects from increased exposure from faulty microwave ovens. Exposure to microwaves is known to cause cytogenetic damage to human lymphocytes [36] and high-level exposure can induce cataracts, tissue burns, and sterility according to the FDA. Infrared fields have wavelengths in the 1 mm–750 nm range and a frequency range of 300–400 tHz (tera hertz). Examples of infrared fields include medical equipment such as thermography, saunas, infrared lamps, and spectroscopy (Figure 42.3).

The phenomenon "dirty electricity" occurs when a building is exposed to a compilation of the varous types of NR. Electrical wiring acts as an antenna and draws NR EMFs into a building from sources such as nearby buildings, cell phone and broadcast towers, as well as ground current produced by electric power substations. EMFs are also generated by items in buildings such as computers, plasma televisions, energy-efficient lighting (compact florescent lights), appliances, dimmer switches, cordless phones, and wireless routers (wi-fi and wi-max). The resulting high frequency voltage transients or electrical microsurges are known as dirty electricity. It has been postulated that the twentieth-century epidemic of the "diseases of civilization"—such as malignant neoplasms [37], leukemias [38], diabetes mellitus [39], coronary artery disease [40], and so on, are the result of the electrification of society [41].

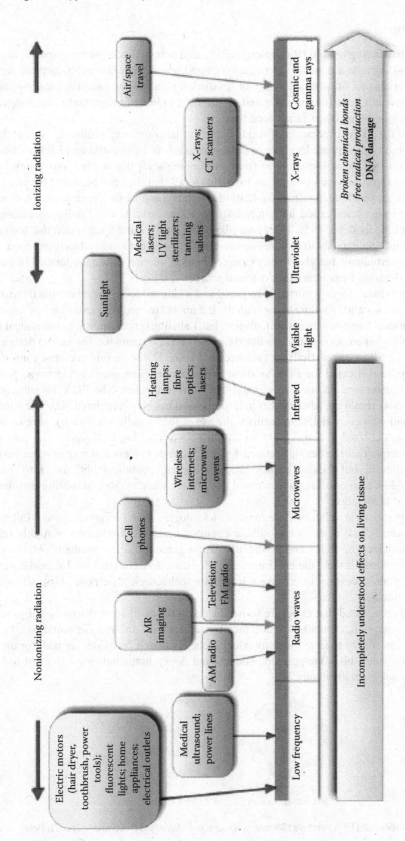

FIGURE 42.3 Electromagnetic spectrum exposures (Reprinted from: *Sci Total Environ*. 2012 Jan 1;414, Genuis SJ, Lipp CT, Electromagnetic hypersensitivity: Fact or fiction, pp.103–12. ©2012, with permission from Elsevier.)

IRRADIATED FOOD

The process of irradiating food to IR is described here as a potential occupational and environmental IR exposure. Concerns around food irradiation extend beyond the inherent hazards of handling radioactive materials and the primary safety of irradiation plant workers and the local community. Concerns that have not been fully investigated also pertain to loss of nutritional value and creation of harmful radiolytic by-products in the food itself.

According to the FDA, irradiation of foods (which utilizes ionizing radiation) is considered a safety measure used to eliminate food-borne pathogens (such as *Salmonella* and *Escherichia coli*); destroy organisms that can cause spoilage (hence extending shelf life of the food); control insect infestation; delay sprouting and ripening; and sterilize foods that then can be stored for years without refrigeration. As irradiation gained publicity through the Atoms for Peace program, Congress and administrative agencies called for safety testing, acknowledging that "radiation affected the characteristics of the food." In 1956, FDA commissioner George Lamck suggested that testing "be made clearly applicable not only to radioactive substances that might be introduced into food, either deliberately or unavoidably, but also to any changes in food, or new substance formed in food, by subjecting it to radiation from internal or external sources" [42].

Labeling of irradiated foods is currently required and irradiated foods must bear the international symbol for irradiation called a radura along with the statement "treated with radiation" or "treated by irradiation" in print at least the size of the ingredient list. Labeling is not required for individual ingredients in a multi-ingredient food or for irradiated food served in restaurants. The radura design bears resemblance to the EPA symbol. Both are presented in Figure 42.4 to prevent potential confusion.

In 2000, Congress directed the FDA to allow alternative labeling such as "electronic pasteurization" or "cold pasteurization" instead of using the word irradiation. The FDA has subsequently proposed completely removing labeling that indicates a food has been irradiated [43]. The American Medical Association's policy H-150.961 affirms the use of food irradiation with the stipulation that it be regulated and utilized in conjunction with proper food-handling techniques. The policy also affirms "the principle that the demonstration of safety requires evidence of a reasonable certainty that no harm will result but does not require proof beyond any possible doubt" (i.e., zero risk does not exist). The AMA also encourages continued use of the radura symbol indicating that the food has been exposed to radiation.

The current permissible radiation dose to meat (4.5 kilogray [kGy]—approximately 150 million times that of a chest X-ray) causes undesirable changes, including production of highly reactive free radicals, peroxides, benzene, and potentially carcinogenic radiolytic products [44,45]. Codex Alimentarius recommends that "the maximum absorbed dose delivered to a food should not exceed 10 kGy, except when necessary to achieve a legitimate technological purpose" [46], allowing for potentially unlimited exposure.

Early studies recognized that exposure to irradiated media resulted in disruption of growth as well as mitotic inhibition, chromosome aberrations, and forward and reverse mutations. In some cases, catalase was able to reverse the cytotoxic effects. Hydrogen peroxide, glyoxal, formic acid, hydroxyalkyl peroxides, histidine-peroxide adduct, and deoxycompounds were thought to be the cause of the physiological anomalies [47].

Irradiation Radura   EPA symbol

FIGURE 42.4   Radura and EPA symbols (Source: www.epa.gov. Accessed November 22, 2011. Public domain.)

By-products of food irradiation can now be traced as "radiation-induced detection markers," including radiolytic hydrocarbons and dimethyl disulfide [48]. Radiolytically produced hydrocarbons increased in concentration as radiation dose increased from 0–6 kGy [49], clearly below the threshold mentioned in Codex. Although concentration of radiolytic by-products increases with increasing radiation dose, higher doses are commonly used on herbs and spices as they are consumed in small quantities. Studies indicate that irradiation of herbs "produces formic acid, formaldehyde, and unique radiolytic byproducts with carcinogenic properties" [50].

Several radiolytic products were found to be mutagenic and carcinogenic with confirmed evidence of genotoxicity [51]. Unique radiolytic by-products called 2-alkylcyclobutanones (2-ACBs) (from the irradiation of dietary triglycerides) can be traced to adipose tissue in animals, reflecting their absorption and assimilation into the body [52]. After six months of exposure, experimental animals treated with 2-ACBs had three times the number of colon tumors than controls [53]. Human cell studies identified 2-dodecyclcyclobutanone (a radiolytic by-product of palmitic acid) as a potential promoter of colon carcinogenesis as it was "clearly genotoxic in healthy human colon epithelial cells and in cells representing preneoplastic colon adenoma" [54]; 2-tetradecyclobutanone from irradiation of stearic acid was associated with cytotoxicity when cells were incubated for greater than one to two days at concentrations greater than 50 mM [55].

The FDA has not required standard toxicological testing of irradiated food extracts, in spite of the recommendations of its own Irradiated Food Task Committee, and bases its safety claims on five studies that experts consider inherently flawed. Concerns also have been raised that irradiation will destroy odor-causing bacteria that otherwise would alert consumers that a food may be unfit for consumption. Although irradiation can destroy the pathogenic E. coli O157:H7, safer methods are available, such as grass feeding prior to slaughter.

Micronutrient losses (vitamins A, C, E, and B-complex) due to food irradiation are also of concern. Vitamin C content of green and red leaf lettuce was reduced by 24–53% following irradiation [56]. Irradiation damages plant cell membranes and increases permeability, causing electrolyte leakage that increases linearly with increasing radiation dose. All irradiated vegetables showed increased electrolyte leakage, while some were more sensitive (cilantro, celery, green onion, and carrot) than others (broccoli, endive, and red cabbage) [57].

PATHOGENESIS OF ELECTROMAGNETIC HYPERSENSITIVITY

There is a subset of the population who, if exposed to lower frequency electromagnetic radiation, develop various symptoms resulting in the syndrome known as electromagnetic hypersensitivity (EHS). The WHO working group has defined EHS as "… a phenomenon where individuals experience adverse health effects while using or being in the vicinity of devices emanating electric, magnetic, or electromagnetic fields (EMFs). …Whatever its cause, EHS is a real and sometimes a debilitating problem for the affected persons"[58]. The estimated number of people, who experience symptoms from NR EMFs, and go on to develop electromagnetic hypersensitivity, varies from 1.5% [59] to 8% [60] of the general population.

At this time, the exact pathogenesis of EHS is unknown but may be related to aberrant pathophysiological responses to the bioaccumulation of toxicants from various potential sources such as toxic chemicals/metals, surgical implants, infections, dental materials, and radioactive compounds—known as sensitivity-related illness (SRI)—as illustrated in Figure 42.4 [61].

The hyper-reactivity of the body toward EMFs may be triggered by seemingly unrelated toxicant exposure events leading to Toxicant Induced Loss of Tolerance (TILT) [62,63]. After surpassing a threshold of bioaccumulation, the body's immune system loses the normal adaptive responses (tolerance) and becomes sensitized to exposures from unrelated stimuli such as EMFs [64,65]. The nature of the body's reaction is individually unique based on the makeup of the bioaccumulated toxicant load and the distinctive genetic thumbprint of each person [61]. People who suffer with EHS often have defects in the genes affecting biotransformation/detoxification such as the phase

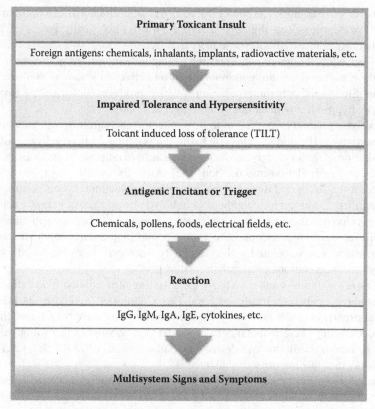

FIGURE 42.5 Pathogenic mechanism for development of sensitivity related illness (Reprinted from: *Sci Total Environ.* 2012 Jan 1;414, Genuis SJ, Lipp CT, Electromagnetic hypersensitivity: Fact or fiction, pp.103–12. ©2012, with permission from Elsevier.)

I cytochrome P450 enzymes and the phase II glutathione-S-transferases, superoxide dismutases, catalase, N-acetyl transferases, and so on [66]. Another pathophysiologic mechanism underlying EHS may be the impact of EMFs on catecholamine dysregulation. This has been demonstrated in those living in close proximity to cell phone base stations, manifesting as protracted alteration of norepinephrine, epinephrine, dopamine, and phenylethylamine biology [67]. These neurotransmitters are fundamental to a number of biological activities including autonomic nervous system regulation, neurotransmission and responses to stress, and so on. Other proposed pathophysiological mechanisms include heavy metal poisoning and the potential role that EMF exposure has on remobilization of the metals [68], alterations in heart rate and heart rate variability from exposure to microwave radiation from digital-enhanced cordless telecommunications (DECT) or "cordless" telephones [69], and finally, alterations in brain glucose metabolism with increased glucose uptake observed in regions of the brain closest to the radio frequencies produced by cell phones [70].

PATIENT EVALUATION

A patient history should include an environmental history. In order to prevent important items from being missed, a questionnaire can be used—as developed by the Agency for Toxic Substances & Disease Registry [71]. Patients can be equipped to measure EMR in the home and workplace by using tools such as a microsurge meter or a Gauss/RF/EMF meter. Resource materials are available [63]. Another option is to employ the services of a Bau biologist. Baubiologie or building biology is a recent discipline originating in Germany and defined as "the study of the holistic interrelationships between humans and their living environment" [72]. Bau biologists inspect buildings in regards to all aspects of electromagnetic radiation and environmental toxins such as heavy metals, chemicals, fungi, bacteria allergens, and so on [73].

Symptoms of EHS can vary and mimic those found in many other disease processes. Therefore, a high index of suspicion is required by the health practitioner when gathering historical information. Common signs and symptoms for EHS are listed as: general malaise, headache, thought-processing difficulties, memory impairment, heart palpitations, sleep disorder, immune dysfunction, inflammation, blurred vision, weakness, dizziness, chest discomfort, muscle pain, tinnitus, fatigue, nausea, night sweats, restless legs, and paresthesias [74–76]. Unfortunately, at the present time, there are no reliable biochemical markers to aid in the diagnosis of EHS and the diagnosis remains clinical [77].

The diagnosis of EHS is supported when symptoms improve with treatment. A clinical case (see text box) is presented to convey the clinical context of this emerging disease entity.

ELECTROMAGNETIC HYPERSENSITIVITY CASE HISTORY

The following case history is a compilation of two cases supervised by Dr. John Cline, MD, and utilizes the functional medicine approach to critical thinking looking at antecedent, triggering, and mediating factors [2]. This case also illustrates the Toxicant Induced Loss of Tolerance (TILT) model and approach to EHS [77]. A 58-year-old G2P1A1 married woman presented with fatigue, frequent respiratory infections, nightmares with sleep disturbance for many years, anxiety, sensitivities to fumes and fragrances, symptoms of allergic rhinitis, as well as paradoxical reactions to many medications. She had been a vegetarian for several decades. Taking an environmental history revealed that she had grown up in an old house that had lead-based paint and possibly lead water pipes. She had many mercury dental amalgams placed in her teeth as a child. Completing a degree in art/photography exposed her to many kinds of paints (containing organic chemicals and metals such as lead, cadmium, mercury, thallium, etc.). Working in the dark rooms for photographic development exposed her to various chemicals in an enclosed space. She and her husband had renovated several old houses, which would have exposed her to lead-based paint, solvents, glues, lacquers, and possibly asbestos. They built a new house seven years before our meeting. There were four cordless telephones as well as wireless internet in the house. She used a cell phone several times per day holding it to her head. She noticed that with prolonged cell phone conversations she would experience a burning sensation on the same side of her head. On examination, she appeared tired, nervous, and her skin was dry. BP 102/78 with pulse 72 BPM and regular. Nasal turbinates showed signs of chronic inflammation. Examination was otherwise unremarkable. Her lab work revealed normal CBC with suboptimal B12 = 328 pmol/l (N = 150 – 650 pmol/l), 25 (OH) Vitamin D suboptimal = 74 nmol/l (N = 75 – 150 nmol/l), low IgA = 0.6 g/l (N = 0.78 – 3.58 g/l), and normal tissue transglutaminase IgA antibody (TTG) = < 5 units (N = < 20 units). The normal appearing TTG could have been falsely low because of the low IgA. Skin testing for inhalant allergies revealed moderate reactions to house dust mite, dog and horse danders, and broom. She was advised to place dust mite covers on her pillows and mattress. She was placed on a therapeutic oral dose of pharmaceutical-grade fish oil, vitamin D3, sublingual methylcobalamin, and a B-complex.

Genomic analysis of her phase I and phase II biotransformation/detoxification pathways revealed single nucleotide polymorphisms (SNPs) present in phase I CYP1A1, CYP1B1, and CYP3A4 pathways. Analysis of the phase II pathways revealed SNPs present in two of the NAT2 (N-acetyl transferase) slow metabolizer pathways as well as the fast metabolizer pathway. Of great significance was the complete absence of GSTM1 (glutathione S-transferase), which is found in the liver and kidneys. This pathway is one of the major pathways for the biotransformation/detoxification of many environmental toxicants such as solvents, herbicides, fungicides, lipid peroxides, and heavy metals (mercury, cadmium lead, etc.). The patient was instructed to give a copy of the report to her pharmacist. Also, she was told to minimize exposure to the various chemicals/metals in her environment such as cigarette smoke, herbicides, fungicides, insecticides, industrial solvents, polycyclic aromatic hydrocarbons (cigarette smoke, vehicle exhaust, etc), polychlorinated biphenyls, and xenoestrogens such as organochlorines, and so on. Dietary advice was given in regards to the genetic SNPs that were discovered. This included eating a diet rich in antioxidants (colorful fruits and vegetables), emphasizing the cruciferous vegetables (broccoli, brussels sprouts, cauliflower, watercress, cabbage, and kale), garlic, onions, and berries. She was advised to avoid eating charbroiled food, fried foods, and red meat. She was advised to take nutritional supplements to redirect metabolism away from the 4-hydroxylation of estrogens with nutritional supplements such as diindoylmethane (DIM), indole 3-carbinol (I3C), fish oils, and rosemary. She was also encouraged to include glutathione precursors and cofactors such as methionine, N-acetylcysteine, L-glutamine, glycine, magnesium, and pyridoxal-5-phosphate as well as the use of alpha-lipoic acid, milk thistle, and taurine.

She was placed on a comprehensive elimination diet and discovered that she had significant reactions to gluten and dairy. Therefore, these were eliminated from her diet. She tested her home for dirty electricity using a Graham Stetzer microsurge meter and found fields in the order of 600–1000 dV/dt (N = <25 dV/dt) and placed a number of Graham Stetzer filters in the plug-ins throughout her home. She exchanged her cordless telephones for land-line telephones and obtained cable internet. She observed an immediate cessation of her chronic nightmares. She was advised to avoid placing cellular telephones and other like devices near her head. She went through a heavy metal detoxification program that involved dietary measures, nutritional supplements, dental work (replacing her mercury amalgams with BPA-free composites), and chelation therapy.

The treatment program resulted in renewed energy, cessation of nightmares with better quality sleep, no further anxiety, marked decrease in frequency of respiratory infections, improvement in allergic rhinitis symptoms and diminished reactions to fumes and fragrances.

TREATMENT

REDUCING EXPOSURE TO IONIZING RADIATION

Because EMR is not visible to the human eye, the extent and magnitude of exposure remains difficult to quantify. Recognizing all sources of EMR and assessing exposure is essential to a patient's care plan, because reducing exposure where possible is a central component to treatment.

Adequate nutrient intake and in some cases tissue saturation, is vital to reducing radionuclide uptake. "The principle of selective uptake is based on the demonstrable biological fact that when our cells are saturated with the nutrients they need, there is less chance for radioactive elements to move in" [78,79]. For example, iodine will block radioactive iodine-129 and -131, calcium will block strontium-90, potassium will block cesium-137, and iron will block plutonium-239. The NRC recommends that counties within a 10-mile radius around a nuclear power plant stock potassium iodide (KI) to block uptake of radioactive iodine in the event of a nuclear accident. Specific guidelines are set by the FDA for supplementation with potassium iodide and should be followed closely due to potential adverse reactions from higher doses. Some researchers suggest that KI be stocked within 200 miles of a potential nuclear meltdown [80]. Iodine deficiency appears to increase risk of thyroid cancer following exposure to radioactive iodine [81]. The RDA for nonpregnant, nonlactating adults is 150 mcg iodine per day. Good food sources include seaweed, cod fish, yogurt, milk, and iodized salt. One quarter teaspoon of iodized salt contains approximately 70 mcg iodine (and approximately 600 mg sodium).

Air, food, and water can be significant sources of IR exposure, particularly in the event of a nuclear accident or excessive routine releases. Radionuclides mimic their nutrient counterparts and are taken up and incorporated into biological tissue. For example, bone takes up Sr-90, plutonium, and phosphorus-32; kidney takes up cesium-137; liver takes up cesium-137, cobalt-60, and plutonium; muscle takes up cesium-137 and potassium-40; thyroid takes up iodine-129 and -131, and so on [78,79].

REDUCING EXPOSURE TO NONIONIZING RADIATION

In order to reduce the risk of developing EHS, the following principles are suggested by Genuis et al., 2011 (Table 42.1).

Minimizing radiation exposure is paramount to prevention. Reducing proximity to microwaves ovens, mobile devices, computer and television screens, wireless routers, and power lines, as well as curtailing excessive air travel, is recommended. The FDA notes that EMR from microwaves decreases as distance from the source increases; EMR at two inches is approximately 100 times greater than 20 inches away. Exposure to internal radiation can be minimized by consuming a diet rich in micronutrients, phytonutrients, and antioxidants, as well as utilizing targeted nutrition support to minimize

TABLE 42.1

Sources and Mitigation of Adverse EMR Exposure

Examples of Strategies to Reduce Electromagnetic Radiation

Sources of Adverse EMR	Considerations to Reduce EMR Exposure
Cell phones and cordless phones	• Minimize use of cell and cordless phones and use speaker phones when possible. • Leave cell or cordless phone away from the body rather than in pocket or attached at the hip.
Wireless internet	Use wired internet • Turn off the internet router when not in use (e.g., nighttime). • Use power line network kits to achieve internet access by using existing wiring and avoiding wireless emissions.
Computers releasing high EMR	• Limit the amount of time spent working on a computer. • Avoid setting a laptop computer on the lap. • Increase the distance from the transformer. • Stay a reasonable distance away from the computer.
Handheld electronics (electric toothbrush, hair dryer, smartphone, electronic tablets, etc.)	• Limit the use of electronics and/or revert to using power-free devices. • Turn devices off before going to sleep. • Minimize electronics in bedrooms.
Fluorescent lights	• Consider using alternate lighting such as incandescent. (Uncertainty exists about the safety of LED lights) • Rely on natural sunlight for reading.
Household power	• Measure levels of EMR and modify exposures as possible. • Avoid sleeping near sites of elevated EMR. • Filters can be used to mitigate dirty power.
High-voltage power lines and substations	• Consider relocating to an area not in close proximity to high-voltage power lines.
Transmission towers and emitters (cell phone tower, radar, etc.)	• Maintain considerable distance from emitters. • Consider forms of shielding (shielding paints; grounded metal sheets).
Utility neutral-to-ground bonded to water pipes	• Increase size of neutral-wire to substation and install dielectric coupling in water pipe.

Reprinted from: Genuis SJ, Lipp CT, Electromagnetic hypersensitivity: Fact or fiction. In *Sci Total Environ.* 2012 Jan 1;414; 103–112. ©2012, with permission from Elsevier.

radionuclide uptake. Consuming foods low on the food chain, especially plant-based foods, will decrease bioaccumulation and intake of toxicants and radionuclides. Purification of drinking water (specifically via reverse osmosis, ion exchange, or distillation) will diminish or remove radionuclides [82]. Applying the principle of selective uptake and consuming adequate amounts of blocking nutrients (especially iodine, calcium, potassium, magnesium, zinc, iron, sulfur, and cobalamin) and antioxidants is crucial. Government Dietary Guidelines provide a convenient listing of food sources of potassium, vitamin A, vitamin E, iron, magnesium, vitamin C, and fiber in Appendix B Food Sources of Selected Nutrients [83]. Supplementation following a thorough nutrition assessment may be warranted.

Reducing body burden of radiation is also possible to some extent. Dr. Hazel Parcells, ND, PhD, recommended "therapeutic baths" consisting of equal parts of Epsom salts and baking soda following radiation exposure. She also recommended sipping eight ounces of water mixed with one-quarter teaspoon each of sea salt, baking soda, and potassium hydrogen tartrate (cream of tartar) along with calcium lactate tablets [84]. Government guidance is available as well in the *2011 Complete Guide to Nuclear Power Plant Accidents, Meltdowns, and Radiation Emergencies: Practical, Authoritative Information on Health Effects and Treatment, Radioactive Decontamination.*

Consider Reducing Intake of Irradiated Foods

Avoiding irradiated foods completely may be difficult since labeling is not required for individual ingredients in a multi-ingredient food or for irradiated food served in restaurants. A closer look may be warranted at the several foods that have been approved for irradiation. These include: beef and pork; poultry; molluscan shellfish (oysters, clams, mussels, scallops); shell eggs; fresh fruit and vegetables; lettuce and spinach; spices and seasonings; and seeds for sprouting (e.g., alfalfa sprouts). Irradiation is prohibited for certified organic foods; small, local farms are unlikely to utilize it.

NUTRITION SUPPORT FOR DETOXIFICATION

As emphasized in the EHS case study, an individual's ability to detoxify plays an important role in overcoming the negative effects of EMR. Detoxification—the biotransformation of toxins into less harmful substances—is vital to the survival of an organism and plays a role in susceptibility to EMR. This complex process depends upon nutrient availability as well as genetic competence to carry out each step successfully. Research indicates that individuals deficient in the GSTM1 gene are unable to effectively carry out the phase II step of detoxifying heavy metal and chemical toxicants, contributing to the TILT phenomenon and EHS.

Nutrition therapy is fundamental to supporting metabolic detoxification and reversing EHS. Phase I detoxification (dependent upon cytochrome P450 enzymes) utilizes vitamins B2, B3, B6, B12, folic acid, glutathione, branched-chain amino acids, flavonoids, and phospholipids. Phase II conjugation pathways depend upon glycine, taurine, glutamine, N-acetylcysteine, cysteine, methionine, and methyl donors. Highly reactive intermediary metabolites, such as superoxide, are generated between the two phases and can cause free-radical damage if not countered by antioxidants. Nutrients specifically protective during the intermediary phase include carotenoids, vitamins C and E, selenium, copper, zinc, manganese, coenzyme Q10, thiols, bioflavonoids, silymarin, and pycnogenol [2]. Phase I P450 enzyme activity can be modified by dietary components, including macronutrients, micronutrients, phytonutrients, preservatives, alcohol, MSG, and aspartate [85]. If phase I is upregulated without adequate antioxidant protection or phase II completion, the resulting toxicants can be even more damaging.

Toxicant exposure and increased requirements for antioxidant protection and metabolic support amplify nutrient requirements. The Agency for Healthcare Research and Quality concludes that "multivitamin/mineral supplement use may prevent cancer in individuals with poor or suboptimal nutritional status" [86]. NASA is focusing current research on the role of antioxidants and phytonutrients in radiation protection, and administration of superoxide dismutase-plasmid/liposome (MnSOD-PL), antioxidants, and phytonutrients has yielded promising results [87,88].

Antioxidant protection is fundamental to mitigating the effects of radiation exposure. Though some level of free-radical activity plays a part in metabolism, excess free radicals must be countered by antioxidants to prevent damage to DNA and cellular integrity [89,90]. Viewed as "anti-carcinogens" and radioprotectants [91,92], antioxidants are produced endogenously (superoxide dismutase [SOD], catalase, alpha-lipoic acid, ubiquinol/CoQ10, glutathione, and glutathione peroxidase) and obtained exogenously (polyphenols, carotenoids, indoles, ascorbic acid [vitamin C], and tocopherols). Most mammals are able to synthesize ascorbic acid (e.g., 26–58 mg/kg/d in rat species) but humans lack one crucial enzyme [93]. For humans, 100–500 mg ascorbic acid per day is needed to saturate tissues and plasma [94], and Dr. Linus Pauling recommends 2300 mg/d per 2500 Kcals in divided doses to avoid osmotic diarrhea [93]. Radioprotective effects of ascorbic acid were observed in several studies and included decreased morbidity and mortality, improved wound healing, reduced GI damage, inhibition of lipid peroxidation, and enhanced recovery following stress [95–98].

Mounting evidence supports the use of antioxidant supplementation, demonstrating a statistically significant reduced risk of cancer mortality and all-cause mortality [99]. Radioprotective effects of an antioxidant cocktail consisting of l-selenomethionine, vitamin C, vitamin E succinate, alpha-lipoic acid, and N-acetylcysteine were observed in research. These effects included increased survival time, higher serum total white blood cell count and bone marrow cell count, and increased spleen mass [100]. Supplementing with antioxidants both before and after radiation exposure had protective effects through varying mechanisms [101]. Chemotherapy and RT cause mitochondrial oxidative stress that may lead to secondary malignancies in cancer patients. Researchers recommend that "medical oncologists should now re-consider the use of powerful anti-oxidants as a key component of patient therapy and cancer prevention" [102].

Antioxidant activity of foods can be measured via the oxygen radical absorbance capacity (ORAC) assay. High ORAC foods are listed in Table 42.2. Fruits, vegetables, herbs, and spices are excellent sources of antioxidants, particularly if grown using sustainable or organic methods [103–105]. Protection from radiation can be further enhanced with select nutrients, herbs, and supplements (Tables 42.3 and 42.4).

TABLE 42.2
USDA ORAC Top Antioxidant Foods

Top Antioxidant Foods
[Total ORAC* units per 100 grams**]

Fruits		Vegetables	
Raspberries, black, raw	19,220	Broccoli, boiled	2160
Blueberries, wild, raw	9621	Sweet potato, baked in skin	2115
Prunes, dried	8059	Beets, raw	1776
Plums, raw	6100	Asparagus, cooked	1644
Blackberries, raw	5905	Lettuce, green leaf, raw	1532
Strawberries, raw	4302	Onions, red, raw	1521
Cherries, sweet, raw	3747	Spinach, raw	1513
Raisins, seedless	3406	Alfalfa sprouts, raw	1510
Apples, Gala, raw with skin	2828	Mushrooms, portabella	968
Grapes, red, raw	1837	Peppers, sweet green, raw	935

* Total Oxygen Radical Absorbance Capacity, umol   **About 3.5 ounces
  TE/100 g. includes hydrophilic and lipophilic ORAC

Source: U.S. Department of Agriculture, A.R.S., Oxygen Radical Absorbance Capacity (ORAC) of Selected Foods, Release 2. May 2010. Public domain.

TABLE 42.3
Protective Foods in Radiation Exposure

	Well-nourished individuals are best equipped to block uptake of radioactive nutrients, excrete radionuclides, and repair DNA damage from EMR exposure. Nutrient deficiency can be detrimental while nutrient sufficiency and saturation have protective effects.
Alkalizing Diet	Goal: arterial blood pH 7.45, first morning urine pH 6.7–7.5; fruits and vegetables in general tend to be the most alkalizing foods, while sugar, meat, dairy, fried foods, and trans fats are most acid forming [106]. Mineral sufficiency is also crucial.
Antioxidants and Phytonutrients	**Antioxidants**: vitamins C and E, alpha-lipoic acid, ubiquinol, superoxide dismutases, glutathione **Phytonutrients from plant-based sources**: carotenoids, flavonoids, indoles and glucosinolates, phytic acid (inositol hexaphosphate—IP6) isoflavones, isothiocyanates, polyphenols, terpenes [107]
Detoxification Support	Phase I: B-complex, glutathione, branched-chain amino acids, flavonoids, phospholipids Phase II: glycine, taurine, glutamine, N-acetylcysteine, cysteine, methionine, methyl donors Intermediary: vitamins C and E, selenium, copper, zinc, manganese, CoQ10, thiols, bioflavonoids, silymarin, pycnogenol
Fiber	Insoluble (cellulose, lignin) and soluble (pectins, gums, gels) fiber plays an important role in radioprotection. Fiber adds bulk, speeds gastrointestinal transit time, absorbs toxicants, and promotes the growth of protective, probiotic bacteria.
Herbs and Spices	Herbs and spices are rich sources of antioxidants and phytonutrients that can inhibit carcinogen formation and activation, upregulate phase II detoxification enzymes, inhibit oxidation and inflammation, and demonstrate antitumor activity [108]. Herbs and spices studied for their protective antioxidant and anti-inflammatory effects include garlic, chives, onions, parsley, sage, rosemary, thyme, watercress, horseradish, dill, bay leaves, turmeric, and tea.
Legumes	Legumes (dried beans) contain minerals, chelating phytates, and radioprotective protease inhibitors [78,79].
Miso	Miso, a lactobacillus-fermented paste made from soybean and sea salt (aged ~18 months), has an alkalizing effect and is a source of calcium, iron, B vitamins, and zybicolin, which helps bind and eliminate radionuclides [78,79].
Nuts & Seeds	Nuts and seeds provide full spectrum vitamin E, B-complex, calcium, magnesium, potassium, iron, zinc, fiber, pectin, phytates, and omega-3 fatty acids. Sesamol from sesame seeds was also found to be radioprotective and exhibited a free-radical scavenging capacity 20 times that of melatonin [109].
Selective Uptake	Stable elements will block uptake of radionuclides: **Calcium** blocks Sr-90; **Cobalamin** blocks cobalt-60; **Iodine** blocks iodine-131; **Iron** blocks plutonium 238,239; **Potassium** blocks cesium-137; **Sulfur** blocks sulfur-35; **Zinc** blocks zinc-65.
Tempeh	Tempeh, a fermented soy product, contains beneficial bacteria, phytates, and analogues of B12 that can block cobalt-58,60.
Vegetables	Vegetables contain fiber, minerals, phytonutrients, and antioxidants. The *Brassicaceae* family (broccoli, cabbage, collard, kale, watercress, cauliflower, brussels sprouts, radish, etc.) contains sulfur compounds that protect cells from radiation.
Vegetables, Sea	Sea vegetables, (including agar, dulse, hijiki, irish moss, kelp, wakame, and nori from uncontaminated sources) are rich in minerals and found to reduce intestinal absorption of Sr-90.
Water Purification	Reverse osmosis, distillation, and ion exchange can remove radionuclides.
Whole Grains	Whole grains, as tolerated, provide vitamins, minerals, fiber, and phytates (which bind radionuclides but can also bind nutritive minerals).

Source: © 2012 Beth Ellen DiLuglio, MS, RD, CCN, Nutrition Is Your Best Health Insurance!® www.NutritionMission.org. Used with permission.

TABLE 42.4
Supplements Researched for Radiation Exposure

Adaptogens	Adaptogens (astragalus, ashwagandha, ginseng, eleutheroccus, schizandra, rhodiola, maitake and reishi mushrooms, holy basil, and boerhaavia diffusa) exert radioprotective effects and modulate neuroendocrine-immune communication.
AGE	AGE (aged garlic extract) protects against ionizing radiation, scavenges reactive oxygen species, enhances cellular antioxidant enzymes and cellular glutathione, protects DNA from free-radical damage, and inhibits multistep carcinogenesis [110].
Alpha-Lipoic Acid (ALA)	Alpha-lipoic acid, a potent antioxidant, regenerates vitamins C and E, increases intracellular glutathione, and protects the intracellular and extracellular environment [111]. "ALA may be beneficial to people exposed to high levels of radiation" [112]. The Linus Pauling Institute at OSU recommends 200–400 mg/d for healthy people.
Antioxidant Enzymes	Radiation depletes antioxidants and antioxidant enzymes such as glutathione peroxidase and glutathione reductase, superoxide dismutases (SODs), and catalase. SODs utilize the essential minerals copper, zinc, manganese, and iron. Manganese superoxide dismutase (MnSOD) and copper-zinc superoxide dismutase (CuZnSOD) are key intracellular antioxidants. Glutathione, a tri-peptide produced endogenously from glutamic acid, glycine, and cysteine, is also available in IV, topical, and oral form (as stable s-acetyl glutathione). Glutathione and MnSOD are particularly protective against ionizing radiation [113,114].
Ascorbic Acid	Ascorbic acid (vitamin C) is a primary antioxidant and regenerates other antioxidants. Radiation and heavy metal exposure, stress, infection, and temperature changes increase requirements. The Linus Pauling Institute at OSU recommends a base dose of 250 mg vitamin C BID. For optimal health, Dr. Pauling recommends 2.3 grams or more per 2500 Kcals [93].
Astaxanthin	Astaxanthin is a xanthophyll carotenoid primarily found in marine organisms such as microalgae (*Haematococcus pluvialis* and *Chlorella zofingiensis*) krill, trout, salmon, shrimp, crayfish, and crustaceans, as well as bee propolis [112]. Astaxanthin possesses radioprotective, antioxidant, and immune-stimulating effects [115].
Beta-glucans	Beta-glucans are plant and microbe-based polysaccharides found in barley, oats, baker's yeast, and mushrooms. Beta-glucans stimulate hematopoiesis following ionizing radiation [116], stimulate immune cells, and downregulate immunosuppressive cells [117]. Administration prior to, and within 24 hours of radiation exposure reduced signs of radiation sickness, enhanced immune cell response [118,119], and may be considered for use during nuclear emergencies and RT [120,121].
Chlorella	Chlorella species are a type of single-celled fresh water green algae known to bind and eliminate toxins and heavy metals [111]. Chlorella's radioprotective, bioprotective, and antioxidant effects have been documented in several studies [122–127]. Chlorella should be consumed in "broken cell wall" form to enhance its bioavailability. Dr. Joseph Mercola recommends at least 4 g daily (from uncontaminated sources) combined with fresh cilantro for a synergistic effect.
Fatty Acids	Conditionally essential omega-3 fatty acids EPA and DHA are considered anti-inflammatory and immune supportive with EPA specifically protective against UV radiation [128,129]. Cold water, oily fish such as mackerel, sardines, salmon, and purified fish oils are excellent source of EPA and DHA, while flaxseed, chia seeds, hemp seeds, and English walnuts are excellent sources of their precursor—alpha-linolenic acid. Flaxseeds were found to mitigate the negative effects of radiation, including inflammation, pulmonary fibrosis, and cytokine secretion [130]. USDA "adequate intake" of omega-3 fatty acids is 1.1–1.6 g/d for adults. Eating omega-3 rich seafood or consuming 2 g of high-quality fish oil is recommended several times per week by the Linus Pauling Institute at OSU.
Genistein	Genistein, a phytonutrient found in soybeans, exerts radioprotective, antioxidant, and antitumor effects [131]. Genistein applied following radiation was found to mitigate oxidative damage, lung fibrosis, and pneumonitis [132].
Melatonin	Melatonin, produced primarily in the pineal gland from serotonin, possesses radioprotective and antioxidant properties in addition to its role in circadian rhythm regulation [133,134]. Recommended doses range from 0.5–6 mg at bedtime [135].
Potassium Iodide	Potassium iodide protects the thyroid during acute exposure to radioactive iodine. FDA guidelines must be followed.

continued

TABLE 42.4 (*continued*)

Supplements Researched for Radiation Exposure

Seaweed, Sodium Alginate	Supplementing with sodium alginate from kelp and other sea vegetables was found to have a profound radioprotective effect as it blocks intestinal absorption and bone uptake of radioactive strontium and increases Sr-90 excretion without interfering with calcium metabolism [136,137].
Spirulina	*Spirulina plantensis*, a radioprotective, unicellular blue-green algae [138], was used extensively following the Chernobyl nuclear meltdown in workers and children with radiation sickness at a dose of 5 g per day for 45 consecutive days [50,139,140]. The phycocyanin content of Spirulina contributes to its radioprotective effects, complexing with heavy metals and radionuclides and facilitating their excretion. Spirulina inactivates superoxide and exerts dose-dependent anti-inflammatory effects [141]. Dr. Mercola recommends preventative doses of 3 g/d and increase to 10–20 g/d for therapeutic purposes [50].
Vitamin D (1,25-dihydroxy-vitamin D3)	Vitamin D, a hormone produced in the body from cholesterol in the presence of UV light, can be administered in supplement form to protect individuals from background radiation as well as nuclear accidents. Protective mechanisms include "cellular differentiation and communication. [In] Programmed Cell Death (PCD) (apoptosis and autophagy) and antiangiogenesis ... vitamin D... should be considered among the prime (if not the primary) nonpharmacological agents that offer protection against sublethal low radiation damage and, in particular, against radiation-induced cancer" [142]. Endogenous synthesis is inhibited by inadequate sunlight exposure, amount of body fat, skin pigmentation, amount of skin exposed, and use of sunblock. Deficiency occurs at a serum level less than 20 ng/mL and sufficiency occurs in the range of 33–80 ng/mL. "Studies indicate that intake of vitamin D in the range from 1,100 to 4,000 IU/d and a serum 25-hydroxyvitamin D concentration [25(OH)D] from 60–80 ng/mL may be needed to reduce cancer risk" [143], while a supplemental dose of 9600 IU/d was needed to achieve at least 40 ng/mL in 97.5% of a community-based cohort. Few foods contain vitamin D and supplementation may be indicated. The Linus Pauling Institute recommends that adults supplement with at least 2000 IU (50 mcg) daily and maintain a serum level of at least 80 nmol/L (32 ng/mL).
Zeolites	Zeolites, hydrated aluminum silicates with cation-exchange capacity, occur naturally but also can be synthesized and are frequently used as ion-exchange agents, filters, and water softeners. Both natural and synthetic zeolites have been utilized in the removal of radionuclides from biological tissues as well as from water supply systems [82,144].

Source: © 2012 Beth Ellen DiLuglio, MS, RD, CCN, Nutrition Is Your Best Health Insurance!® www.NutritionMission.org. Used with permission.

CLINICAL SUMMARY

The human being is bioelectromagnetic, responding to electromagnetic radiation (EMR) at the submolecular level. The electromagnetic spectrum consists of ionizing (IR) and nonionizing radiation (NR) and it has been known for many years that IR has enough energy to break chemical bonds and therefore disrupt molecular structures leading to various pathologies, especially neoplastic disease. There is emerging evidence that ongoing exposures to NR also results in a number of disease states including neoplastic disease.

Over the past half century, there has been an exponential rise in technologies exposing the general population to IR and NR. The risks of exposure to IR are well known and accepted, whereas the risks of exposure to NR are only now being elucidated. Electromagnetic hypersensitivity (EHS) is a syndrome that has recently been recognized as a distinct entity occurring in a subset of the population on a worldwide basis—wherever there has been a rise in the exposures to NR. The EHS diagnosis is strengthened by response to treatment.

The treatment of EHS used by the authors involves:

- Identifying and removing both ionizing and nonionizing radiation exposure where feasible;
- Optimizing the antioxidant potential of food;

- Avoiding irradiated food may be prudent given the limited safety data;
- Restoring the body's electrolytes and minerals;
- Employing detoxification strategies;
- Using supplemental foods and nutrients (see Tables 42.3 and 42.4).

REFERENCES

1. Alberts B, Johnson A, Lewis J, et al. 2008. *Molecular Biology of the Cell*. 5th ed. New York: Garland Science, Taylor & Francis Group.
2. Alexander BJ, Ames, BN, Baker SM, et al. 2010. *Textbook of Functional Medicine*, 153–156. Gig Harbor: The Institute for Functional Medicine.
3. Oschman JL. Charge transfer in the living matrix. *J Bodyw Mov Ther*. 2009 Jul;13(3):215–228. Review. PMID: 19524846.
4. Gofman, JW. 1981. *Radiation and Human Health*. www.archive.org/details/radiationhumanhe00gofm rich. Accessed November 25, 2011.
5. Gofman, JW. *Radiation from Medical Procedures in the Pathogenesis of Cancer and Ischemic Heart Disease: Dose-Response Studies with Physicians per 100,000 Population*. 1st Edition. San Francisco: C.N.R. Book Division Committee for Nuclear Responsibility, Inc.: 1999.
6. Redberg RF. Cancer risks and radiation exposure from computed tomographic scans: How can we be sure that the benefits outweigh the risks? *Arch Intern Med*. 2009 Dec 14;169(22):2049–2050. PMID: 20008685.
7. Brenner DJ, Hall EJ. Computed tomography—an increasing source of radiation exposure. *N Engl J Med*. 2007 Nov 29;357(22):2277–2284. Review. PMID: 18046031.
8. Brodersen J, Jørgensen KJ, Gøtzsche PC. The benefits and harms of screening for cancer with a focus on breast screening. *Pol Arch Med Wewn*. 2010 Mar;120(3):89–94. Review. PMID: 20332715.
9. Nguyen PK, Wu JC. Radiation exposure from imaging tests: Is there an increased cancer risk? *Expert Rev Cardiovasc Ther*. 2011 Feb;9(2):177–183. Review. PMID: 21453214.
10. Greene G. *The Woman Who Knew Too Much: Alice Stewart and the Secrets of Radiation*. Ann Arbor: University of Michigan Press, 2001.
11. Stewart A. Aetiology of childhood malignancies. *Br Med J*. 1961 Feb 18;1(5224):452–460. PMID: 20789069.
12. Stewart A, Kneale GW. Changes in the cancer risk associated with obstetric radiography. *Lancet*. 1968 Jan 20;1(7534):104–107. PMID: 4169702.
13. Adams MJ, Hardenbergh PH, Constine LS, Lipshultz SE. Radiation-associated cardiovascular disease. *Crit Rev Oncol Hematol*. 2003 Jan;45(1):55–75. Review. PMID: 12482572.
14. Cohen EP, Robbins ME. Radiation nephropathy. *Semin Nephrol*. 2003 Sep;23(5):486–499. PMID: 13680538.
15. Bogdanich W. Radiation offers new cures, and ways to do harm. January 23, 2010. *New York Times*. http://www.nytimes.com/2010/01/24/health/24radiation.html?pagewanted = all. Accessed November 9, 2011.
16. EPA. http://www.epa.gov/radiation/sources/facility_env.html. Accessed December 25, 2011.
17. Nesterenko AV, Nesterenko VB, Yablokov AV. Chernobyl's radioactive contamination of food and people. *Ann N Y Acad Sci*. 2009 Nov;1181:289–302. PMID: 20002056.
18. Magn, PJ, Reave TC, Apidianaki JC. Iodine-129 in the environment around a nuclear fuel reprocessing plant. Office of Radiation Programs, Washington, D.C. Report Number ORP/SDI-72-5. 1972. http://cfpub.epa.gov/ols/catalog/catalog_display.cfm?&FIELD1 = SUBJECT&INPUT1 = Nuclear%20 fuel%20reprocessing&TYPE1 = EXACT&item_count = 13. Accessed November 24, 2011.
19. Reuters 2011. http://www.reuters.com/article/2011/03/27/nuclear-japan-massachusetts-idUSN27137322 20110327. Accessed December 24, 2011.
20. Hamada N, Ogino H. Food safety regulations: what we learned from the Fukushima nuclear accident. *J Environ Radioact*. 2012 Sep;111:83–99. PMID: 21996550.
21. Karpas Z, Paz-Tal O, Lorber A, et al. Urine, hair, and nails as indicators for ingestion of uranium in drinking water. *Health Phys*. 2005 Mar;88(3):229–242. PMID: 15706143.
22. Li WB, Karpas Z, Salonen L, et al. A compartmental model of uranium in human hair for protracted ingestion of natural uranium in drinking water. *Health Phys*. 2009 Jun;96(6):636–645. PMID: 19430216.
23. Kalckar HM. An international milk teeth radiation census. *Nature*. 1958 Aug 2;182(4631):283–284. PMID: 13577816.

24. Rosenthal HL, Gilster JE, Bird JT. Strontium-90 content of deciduous human incisors. *Science*. 1963 Apr 12;140:176–177. PMID: 13974977.

25. Reiss LZ. Strontium-90 absorption by deciduous teeth. *Science*. 1961 Nov 24;134:1669–1673. PMID: 14491339.

26. RPHP. www.radiation.org. Accessed January 1, 2012.

27. Gould JM, Sternglass EJ, Sherman JD, Brown J, McDonnell W, Mangano JJ. Strontium-90 in deciduous teeth as a factor in early childhood cancer. *Int J Health Serv*. 2000;30(3):515–539. PMID: 11109179.

28. Mangano JJ, Sternglass EJ, Gould JM, Sherman JD, Brown J, McDonnell W. Strontium-90 in newborns and childhood disease. *Arch Environ Health*. 2000 Jul-Aug;55(4):240–244. PMID: 11005428.

29. Mangano JJ, Sherman JD. Elevated in vivo strontium-90 from nuclear weapons test fallout among cancer decedents: A case-control study of deciduous teeth. *Int J Health Serv*. 2011;41(1):137–158. PMID: 21319726.

30. Petkau A. Effect of 22 Na+ on a phospholipid membrane. *Health Phys*. 1972 Mar;22(3):239–244. PMID: 5015646.

31. Gofman, JW. 2001. http://ntp.niehs.nih.gov/ntp/roc/pbcarchive/11th/xradgammarad/gofman-09-11-01.pdf. Accessed September 18, 2011.

32. Nuclear Regulatory Commission. www.NRC.gov. Accessed December 26, 2011.

33. Sternglass EJ. Cancer: Relation of prenatal radiation to development of the disease in childhood. *Science*. 1963 Jun 7;140:1102–1104. PMID: 13983978.

34. Pauling L. Genetic and somatic effects of carbon-14. *Science*. 1958 Nov 14;128(3333):1183–1186. PMID: 13592303.

35. Goldman Lee, and Andrew I. Schafer. 2012. *Goldman's Cecil Medicine*, 24th ed. Philadelphia: Elsevier Saunders.

36. Zotti-Martelli L, Peccatori M, Scarpato R, Migliore L. Induction of micronuclei in human lymphocytes exposed in vitro to microwave radiation. *Mutat Res*. 2000 Dec 20;472(1–2):51–58. PMID: 11113697.

37. Carpenter DO. Electromagnetic fields and cancer: The cost of doing nothing. *Rev Environ Health*. 2010 Jan–Mar;25(1):75–80. Review. PMID: 20429163.

38. Maslanyj M, Lightfoot T, Schüz J, Sienkiewicz Z, McKinlay A. A precautionary public health protection strategy for the possible risk of childhood leukaemiafrom exposure to power frequency magnetic fields. *BMC Public Health*. 2010 Nov 5;10:673. PMID: 21054823.

39. Havas M. Dirty electricity elevates blood sugar among electrically sensitive diabetics and may explain brittle diabetes. *Electromagn Biol Med*. 2008;27(2):135–146. PMID: 18568931.

40. Goraca A, Ciejka E, Piechota A. Effects of extremely low frequency magnetic field on the parameters of oxidative stress in heart. *J Physiol Pharmacol*. 2010 Jun;61(3):333–338. PMID: 20610864.

41. Milham S. Historical evidence that electrification caused the 20th century epidemic of "diseases of civilization." *Med Hypotheses*. 2010 Feb;74(2):337–345. PMID: 19748187.

42. Pauli GH, Takeguchi CA. Irradiation of foods—FDA perspective. *Food Reviews International*. 1986;2(1). doi: 10.1080/87559128609540789.

43. Smith J L. Irradiation: It's what's for dinner and possibly even lunch. *Drake J Agric L*. 2008;Fall:561.

44. Schubert J. Mutagenicity and cytotoxicity of irradiated foods and food components. *Bull World Health Organ*. 1969;41(6):873–904. Review. PMID: 4908553.

45. Epstein SS, Hauter W. Preventing pathogenic food poisoning: Sanitation, not irradiation. *Int J Health Serv*. 2001;31(1):187–192. PMID: 11271643.

46. *Codex Alimentarius General Standard for Irradiated Foods*. STAN 106-1983, REV. 1-2003. www.codexalimentarius.net/download/standards/16/CXS_106e.pdf. Accessed January 5, 2012.

47. Kesavan PC, Swaminathan MS. Cytotoxic and mutagenic effects of irradiated substrates and food material. *Radiation Botany*. 1971;11(4):253–281.

48. Kwon JH, Akram K, Nam KC, Lee EJ, Ahn DU. Evaluation of radiation-induced compounds in irradiated raw or cooked chicken meat during storage. *Poult Sci*. 2011 Nov;90(11):2578–2583. PMID: 22010244.

49. Morehouse KM, Ku Y. Identification of irradiated foods by monitoring radiolytically produced hydrocarbons. *Radiation Physics and Chemistry*. 1993 July–Sept;42(1–3):359–362. doi:10.1016/0969-806X(93)90266-W.

50. Mercola. www.mercola.com. Accessed November 22, 2011.

51. Piccioni, R. Food irradiation: Contaminating our food. *Ecologist*. 1988;18(2):48–55.

52. Horvatovich P, Raul F, Miesch M, et al. Detection of 2-alkylcyclobutanones, markers for irradiated foods, in adipose tissues of animals fed with these substances. *J Food Prot*. 2002 Oct;65(10):1610–1613. PMID: 12380747.

53. Raul F, Gosse F, Delincee H, et al. Food-borne radiolytic compounds (2-alkylcyclobutanones) may promote experimental colon carcinogenesis. *Nutr Cancer*. 2002;44(2):189–191. PMID: 12734067.

54. Knoll N, Weise A, Claussen U, et al. 2-Dodecylcyclobutanone, a radiolytic product of palmitic acid, is genotoxic in primary human colon cells and in cells from preneoplastic lesions. *Mutat Res*. 2006 Feb 22;594(1–2):10–19. PMID: 16153665.

55. Delincee H, Soikaa C, Horvatovich P, et al. Genotoxicity of 2-alkylcyclobutanones, markers for an irradiation treatment in fat-containing food—Part I: Cyto- and genotoxic potential of 2-tetradecylcyclobutanone. *Radiation Physics and Chemistry*. 2002;63:431–435.

56. Fan X, Sokorai KJ. Retention of quality and nutritional value of 13 fresh-cut vegetables treated with low-dose radiation. *J Food Sci*. 2008 Sep;73(7):S367–372. PMID: 18803730.

57. Fan X, Sokorai KJB. Assessment of radiation sensitivity of fresh-cut vegetables using electrolyte leakage measurement. *Postharvest Biol Technol*. 2005 Dec;36:191–197.

58. Mild K, Repacholi M, van Deventer E. *Electromagnetic hypersensitivity*. Proceedings International Workshop on EMF Hypersensitivity Prague, Czech Republic, October 25–27, 2004; 196.

59. Hillert L, et al. Prevalence of self-reported hypersensitivity to electric or magnetic fields in a population-based questionnaire survey. *Scand J Work Environ Health*. 2002;28(1):33–41. PMID: 11871850.

60. Infas Institut für angewandte Sozialwissenschaft GmbH. In: Trahlenschutz Bf, editor. *Ermittlungen der Befürchtungen und Ängste der breiten Öffentlichkeit hinsichtlich möglicher Gefahren der hochfrequenten elektromagnetischen Felder des Mobilfunks—jährliche Umfragen*. Bonn: Institut für angewandte Sozialwissenschaft GmbH; 2003; 1–34.

61. Genuis SJ. Sensitivity-related illness: The escalating pandemic of allergy, food intolerance and chemical sensitivity. *Sci Total Environ*. 2010;408(24):6047–6061. PMID: 20920818.

62. Miller CS. Toxicant-induced loss of tolerance—an emerging theory of disease? *Environ Health Perspect*. 1997;105(Suppl 2):445–453. PMID: 9167978.

63. Cline J. *Detoxify for Life*. Stockton, CA: More Heart Than Talent Publishing, Inc., 2008; 18–19.

64. Hardell L, Carlberg M, Söderqvist F, et al. Increased concentrations of certain persistent organic pollutants in subjects with self-reported electromagnetic hypersensitivity—a pilot study. *Electromagn Biol Med*. 2008;27(2):197–203. PMID: 18568937.

65. Hardell L, Sage C. Biological effects from electromagnetic field exposure and public exposure standards. *Biomed Pharmacother*. 2008 Feb;62(2):104–109.PMID: 18242044.

66. Wormhoudt LW, Commandeur JN, Vermeulen NP. Genetic polymorphisms of human N-acetyltransferase, cytochrome P450, glutathione-S-transferase, and epoxide hydrolase enzymes: relevance to xenobiotic metabolism and toxicity. *Crit RevToxicol*. 1999;29(1):59–124. PMID: 10066160.

67. Buchner K, Eger H. Changes of clinically important neurotransmitters under the influence of modulated RF fields—a long-term study under real-life conditions. *Umwelt-Medizin-Gesellschaft*. 2011;24(1):44–57.

68. Costa A, Branca V, Minoia C, et al. Heavy metals exposure and electromagnetic hypersensitivity. *Sci Total Environ*. 2010; 408(20):4919–4920. Author reply 4921. PMID: 20643474.

69. Havas M, et al. Provocation study using heart rate variability shows microwave radiation from DECT phone affects atunomic nervous system. In: Giuliani L, Soffritti M, editors. Non-thermal effects and mechanisms of interaction between electromagnetic fields and living matter. *European J Oncology—Library*. National Institute for the Study and Control of Cancer and Environmental Disease. Bologna: Mattioli, 2010; 273–300.

70. Volkow ND, Tomasi D, Wang GJ, et al. Effects of cell phone radiofrequency signal exposure on brain glucose metabolism. *JAMA*. 2011;305(8):808–813. PMID: 21343580.

71. Agency for Toxic Substances and Disease Registry. www.atsdr.cdc.gov/csem. Accessed December 26, 2011.

72. Schneider A. Institute of Building Biology + Ecology Neubeuern IBN. www.baubiologie.de. Accessed January 25, 2012.

73. Bau biology. www.baubiologie.de. Accessed January 24, 2012.

74. Havas M. Electromagnetic hypersensitivity: Biological effects of dirty electricity with emphasis on diabetes and multiple sclerosis. *Electromagn Biol Med*. 2006;25(4):259–268. PMID: 17178585.

75. Johansson O. Electrohypersensitivity: State-of-the-art of a functional impairment. *Electromagn Biol Med*. 2006;25(4):245–258. PMID: 17178584.

76. Johansson O. Disturbance of the immune system by electromagnetic fields—A potentially underlying cause for cellular damage and tissue repair reduction which could lead to disease and impairment. *Pathophysiology*. 2009 Aug;16(2–3):157–177. PMID: 19398310.

77. Genuis SJ, Lipp CT. Electromagnetic hypersensitivity: Fact or fiction? *Sci Total Environ*. 2012 Jan 1;414:103–112. PMID: 22153604.

78. Shannon S. 1993. *Diet for the Atomic Age: How to Protect Yourself from Low-Level Radiation* (Revised Edition). New York: Instant Improvement, Inc.

79. Shannon S. 2012. *Radiation Protective Foods: A Menu For The Nuclear Age*. Bloomington: AuthorHouse.

80. Giovannelli G. Radioiodine and thyroid carcinoma: KI prophylaxis in children. *Acta Biomed.* 2004 Aug;75(2):I–XIII. PMID: 15481705.

81. Cardis E, Kesminiene A, Ivanov V, et al. Risk of thyroid cancer after exposure to 131I in childhood. *J Natl Cancer Inst.* 2005 May 18;97(10):724–732. PMID: 15900042.

82. Sato I, Kudo H, Tsuda S: Removal efficiency of water purifier and adsorbent for iodine, cesium, strontium, barium and zirconium in drinking water. *J Toxicol Sci.* 2011;36(6):829–834. PMID: 22129747.

83. Health.gov. http://www.health.gov/dietaryguidelines/dga2005/document/html/appendixb.htm. Accessed December 6, 2011.

84. Bodri B. 2004. *How to Help Support the Body's Healing after Intense Radioactive or Radiation Exposure.* Reno: Top Shape Publishing, LLC.

85. Guengerich FP. Influence of nutrients and other dietary materials on cytochrome P-450 enzymes. *Am J Clin Nutr.* 1995 Mar;61(3 Suppl):651S–658S. Review. PMID: 7879733.

86. AHRQ. Agency for Healthcare Research and Quality. http://www.ahrq.gov/clinic/tp/multivittp.htm. Accessed November 25, 2011.

87. Epperly MW, Wang H, Jones JA, et al. Antioxidant-chemoprevention diet ameliorates late effects of total-body irradiation and supplements radioprotection by MnSOD-plasmid liposome administration. *Radiat Res.* 2011 Jun;175(6):759–765. PMID: 21466381.

88. Rabin BM, Shukitt-Hale B, Joseph J, Todd P. Diet as a factor in behavioral radiation protection following exposure to heavy particles. *Gravit Space Biol Bull.* 2005 Jun;18(2):71–77. PMID: 16038094.

89. Halliwell B. Oxidants and antioxidants: Pathophysiologic determinants and therapeutic agents. Proceedings of a symposium. October 26-27, 1990, Marbella, Spain. *Am J Med.* 1991 Sep 30;91(3C):1S–145S. PMID: 1681730.

90. Bland, JS, Liska D, Lukaczer D, et al. 2004. *Clinical Nutrition: A Functional Approach.* 2nd edition. Gig Harbor: The Institute for Functional Medicine.

91. Ames BN. Dietary carcinogens and anticarcinogens. Oxygen radicals and degenerative diseases. *Science.* 1983 Sep 23;221(4617):1256–1264. Review. PMID: 6351251.

92. Ames BN. DNA damage from micronutrient deficiencies is likely to be a major cause of cancer. *Mutat Res.* 2001 Apr 18;475(1–2):7–20. Review. PMID: 11295149.

93. Pauling L. Evolution and the need for ascorbic acid. *Proc Natl Acad Sci* USA. 1970 Dec;67(4):1643–1648. PMID: 5275366.

94. Schlueter MS, Johnston CS. Vitamin C: Overview and update. *Journal of Evidence-Based Complementary & Alternative Medicine.* 2011;16(1):48–57.

95. Jagetia GC, Rajanikant GK, Baliga MS, Rao KV, Kumar P. Augmentation of wound healing by ascorbic acid treatment in mice exposed to gamma-radiation. *Int J Radiat Biol.* 2004 May;80(5):347–354. PMID: 15223767.

96. Kanter M, Akpolat M. Vitamin C protects against ionizing radiation damage to goblet cells of the ileum in rats. *Acta Histochem.* 2008;110(6):481–490. PMID: 19007656.

97. Chandra Jagetia G, Rajanikant GK, Rao SK, Shrinath Baliga M. Alteration in the glutathione, glutathione peroxidase, superoxide dismutase and lipid peroxidation by ascorbic acid in the skin of mice exposed to fractionated gamma radiation. *Clin Chim Acta.* 2003 Jun;332(1–2):111–121. PMID: 12763288.

98. Cai L, Koropatnick J, Cherian MG. Roles of vitamin C in radiation-induced DNA damage in presence and absence of copper. *Chem Biol Interact.* 2001 Jul 31;137(1):75–88. PMID: 11518565.

99. Li K, Kaaks R, Linseisen J, Rohrmann S. Vitamin/mineral supplementation and cancer, cardiovascular, and all-cause mortality in a German prospective cohort (EPIC-Heidelberg). *Eur J Nutr.* 2011 Jul 22. [Epub ahead of print] PMID: 21779961.

100. Wambi CO, Sanzari JK, Sayers CM, et al. Protective effects of dietary antioxidants on proton total-body irradiation-mediated hematopoietic cell and animal survival. *Radiat Res.* 2009 Aug;172(2):175–186. PMID: 19630522.

101. Alcaraz M, Acevedo C, Castillo J, et al. Liposoluble antioxidants provide an effective radioprotective barrier. *Br J Radiol.* 2009 Jul;82(979):605–609. PMID: 19188244.

102. Sotgia F, Martinez-Outschoorn UE, Lisanti MP. Mitochondrial oxidative stress drives tumor progression and metastasis: Should we use antioxidants as a key component of cancer treatment and prevention? *BMC Med.* 2011 May 23;9:62. PMID: 21605374.

103. Mitchell AE, Hong YJ, Koh E, et al. Ten-year comparison of the influence of organic and conventional crop management practices on the content of flavonoids in tomatoes. *J Agric Food Chem.* 2007 Jul 25;55(15):6154–6159. PMID: 17590007.

104. Asami DK, Hong YJ, Barrett DM, Mitchell AE. Comparison of the total phenolic and ascorbic acid content of freeze-dried and air-dried marionberry, strawberry, and corn grown using conventional, organic, and sustainable agricultural practices. *J Agric Food Chem.* 2003 Feb 26;51(5):1237–1241. PMID: 12590461.

105. Winters CK, Davis SF. Organic Foods. *J Food Sci*. Nov/Dec 2006;71(3):R117–R124. DOI: 10.1111/j.1750-3841.2006.00196.x.

106. Jaffe, RM. http://www.elisaact.com/pdfs/EAB_AlkalineWay.pdf. Accessed November 25, 2011.

107. American Institute for Cancer Research. www.aicr.org. Accessed November 13, 2011.

108. Craig WJ. Health-promoting properties of common herbs. *Am J Clin Nutr*. 1999 Sep;70(3 Suppl):491S–499S. Review. PMID: 10479221.

109. Mishra K, Srivastava PS, Chaudhury NK. Sesamol as a potential radioprotective agent: in vitro studies. *Radiat Res*. 2011 Nov;176(5):613–623. PMID: 21899433.

110. Borek C. Antioxidant health effects of aged garlic extract. *J Nutr*. 2001 Mar;131(3s):1010S–1015S. PMID: 11238807.

111. Packer L, Tritschler HJ, Wessel K. Neuroprotection by the metabolic antioxidant alpha-lipoic acid. *Free Radic Biol Med*. 1997;22(1–2):359–378. Review. PMID: 8958163.

112. Natural Standard Database. www.naturalstandard.com. Accessed November 6, 2011.

113. Morse ML, Dahl RH. Cellular glutathione is a key to the oxygen effect in radiation damage. *Nature*. 1978 Feb 16;271(5646):660–662. PMID: 342974.

114. Sun J, Chen Y, Li M, Ge Z. Role of antioxidant enzymes on ionizing radiation resistance. *Free Radic Biol Med*. 1998 Mar 1;24(4):586–593. PMID: 9559871.

115. Zhao W, Jing X, Chen C, Cui J, Yang M, Zhang Z. Protective effects of astaxanthin against oxidative damage induced by 60Co gamma-ray irradiation. *Wei Sheng Yan Jiu*. 2011 Sep;40(5):551–554. Chinese. PMID: 22043699.

116. Hofer M, Pospíšil M. Modulation of animal and human hematopoiesis by β-glucans: A review. *Molecules*. 2011 Sep 15;16(9):7969–7979. PMID: 21921869.

117. Qi C, Cai Y, Gunn L, et al. Differential pathways regulating innate and adaptive antitumor immune responses by particulate and soluble yeast-derived ß-glucans. *Blood*. 2011 Jun 23;117(25):6825–6836. PMID: 21531981.

118. Petruczenko A. Glucan effect on the survival of mice after radiation exposure. *Acta Physiol Pol*. 1984 May-Jun;35(3):231–236. PMID: 6537716.

119. Chertkov KS, Davydova SA, Nesterova TA, Zviagintseva TN, Eliakova LA. Efficiency of polysaccharide translam for early treatment of acute radiation illness. *Radiats Biol Radioecol*. 1999 Sep-Oct;39(5):572–577. Russian. PMID: 10576030.

120. Gu YH, Takagi Y, Nakamura T, et al. Enhancement of radioprotection and anti-tumor immunity by yeast-derived beta-glucan in mice. *J Med Food*. 2005 Summer;8(2):154–158. PMID: 16117606.

121. Rondanelli M, Opizzi A, Monteferrario F. The biological activity of beta-glucans. *Minerva Med*. 2009 Jun;100(3):237–245. Review. Italian. PMID: 19571787.

122. Mohd Azamai ES, Sulaiman S, Mohd Habib SH, et al. Chlorella vulgaris triggers apoptosis in hepatocarcinogenesis-induced rats. *J Zhejiang Univ Sci B*. 2009 Jan;10(1):14–21. PMID: 19198018.

123. Makpol S, Yaacob N, Zainuddin A, Yusof YA, Ngah WZ. Chlorella vulgaris modulates hydrogen peroxide-induced DNA damage and telomere shortening of human fibroblasts derived from different aged individuals. *Afr J Tradit Complement Altern Med*. 2009 Jul 3;6(4):560–572. PMID: 20606778.

124. Takekoshi H, Suzuki G, Chubachi H, Nakano M. Effect of chlorella pyrenoidosa on fecal excretion and liver accumulation of polychlorinated dibenzo-p-dioxin in mice. *Chemosphere*. 2005 Apr;59(2):297–304. PMID:15722102.

125. Li L, Li W, Kim YH, Lee YW. Chlorella vulgaris extract ameliorates carbon tetrachloride-induced acute hepatic injury in mice. *Exp Toxicol Pathol*. 2011 Jul 7. [Epub ahead of print] PMID: 21741806.

126. Shim JA, Son YA, Park JM, Kim MK. Effect of chlorella intake on cadmium metabolism in rats. *Nutr Res Pract*. 2009 Spring;3(1):15–22. PMID: 20016697.

127. Mercola J, Klinghardt D. Mercury toxicity and systemic elimination agents. *Journal of Nutritional & Environmental Medicine*. 2001; 11:53–62.

128. Moison RM, Beijersbergen Van Henegouwen GM. Dietary eicosapentaenoic acid prevents systemic immunosuppression in mice induced by UVB radiation. *Radiat Res*. 2001 Jul;156(1):36–44. PMID: 11418071.

129. Rhodes LE, Shahbakhti H, Azurdia RM, et al. Effect of eicosapentaenoic acid, an omega-3 polyunsaturated fatty acid, on UVR-related cancer risk in humans. An assessment of early genotoxic markers. *Carcinogenesis*. 2003 May;24(5):919–925. PMID: 12771037.

130. Christofidou-Solomidou M, Tyagi S, Tan KS, et al. Dietary flaxseed administered post thoracic radiation treatment improves survival and mitigates radiation-induced pneumonopathy in mice. *BMC Cancer*. 2011 Jun 24;11:269.PMID: 21702963.

131. Weiss JF, Landauer MR. Protection against ionizing radiation by antioxidant nutrients and phytochemicals. *Toxicology*. 2003 Jul 15;189(1–2):1–20. Review. PMID: 12821279.

132. Mahmood J, Jelveh S, Calveley V, Zaidi A, Doctrow SR, Hill RP. Mitigation of lung injury after accidental exposure to radiation. *Radiat Res*. 2011 Oct 20. PMID: 22013884.

133. El-Missiry MA, Fayed TA, El-Sawy MR, El-Sayed AA. Ameliorative effect of melatonin against gamma-irradiation-induced oxidative stress and tissue injury. *Ecotoxicol Environ Saf*. 2007 Feb;66(2):278–286. PMID:16793135.

134. Dreher F, Gabard B, Schwindt DA, Maibach HI. Topical melatonin in combination with vitamins E and C protects skin from ultraviolet-induced erythema: A human study in vivo. *Br J Dermatol*. 1998 Aug;139(2):332–339. PMID: 9767255.

135. Krinsky DL, LaValle JB, Hawkins EB, et al. 2003. *Natural Therapeutics Pocket Guide*. 2nd Edition. Hudson: Lexi-Comp, Inc.

136. Waldron-Edward D. Skoryna SC, Paul TM. Studies on the inhibition of intestinal absorption of radioactive strontium 3. The effect of administration of sodium alginate in food and in drinking water. *Can Med Assoc J*. 1964 Nov 7;91:1006–1010. PMID: 14222668.

137. Paul TM, Edward DW, Skoryna SC. Studies on inhibition of intestinal absorption of radioactive strontium II. Effects of administration of sodium alginate by orogastric intubation and feeding. *Can Med Assoc J*. 1964 Sep 5;91:553–557. PMID: 14176062.

138. Qishen P, Guo BJ, Kolman A. Radioprotective effect of extract from spirulina platensis in mouse bone marrow cells studied by using the micronucleus test. *Toxicol Lett*. 1989 Aug;48(2):165–169. PMID: 2505406.

139. Loseva, LP, Dardynskaya IV. 1993. Spirulina natural sorbent of radionucleides. Research Institute of Radiation Medicine, Minsk, Belarus. Paper presented at the 6th International Congress of Applied Algology, Czech Republic.

140. Loseva, LP. 1999. *Spirulina platensis* and specialties to support detoxifying pollutants and to strengthen the immune system. Paper presented at the 8th International Congress on Applied Algology, Italy.

141. Dartsch PC. Antioxidant potential of selected spirulina platensis preparations. *Phytother Res*. 2008 May;22(5):627–633. PMID: 18398928.

142. Hayes DP. The protection afforded by vitamin D against low radiation damage. *Int J Low Radiation*. 2008;5(4).

143. Garland CF, French CB, Baggerly LL, Heaney RP. Vitamin D supplement doses and serum 25-hydroxyvitamin D in the range associated with cancer prevention. *Anticancer Res*. 2011 Feb;31(2):607–611. PMID: 21378345.

144. Mizik P, Hrusovský J, Tokosová M. The effect of natural zeolite on the excretion and distribution of radiocesium in rats. *Vet Med* (Praha). 1989 Aug;34(8):467–474. Slovak. PMID: 2552638.

43 Mycotoxin-Related Illness

Diagnosis, Avoidance, and Nutritional Interventions

Neal Speight, M.D.

INTRODUCTION

Food contamination and water-damaged buildings represent two human exposures to mold bio-contaminants. Mycotoxins are associated with a variety of illness, including some cancers, rhinosinusitis, asthma, and inflammatory bowel disease. The primary challenge for clinicians is that while mycotoxins may influence the onset and progression of disease, the same diseases occur in the complete absence of mold. Except in the setting of massive food contamination (such as Balkan Endemic Nephropathy) or post-hurricane mold overgrowth (Hurricane Katrina in New Orleans, LA) the opportunity to treat patients' underlying mycotoxin-related illness is under-recognized. This chapter outlines the clinically relevant fungi and their mycotoxins, likely exposures, toxic effects, detection, and clinical management. Clinical approaches include detection, avoidance, toxin-binding therapy, and nutritional interventions, especially where underlying nutrient deficiencies increase vulnerability.

EPIDEMIOLOGY AND BACKGROUND

A mycotoxin is defined as a mold-produced secondary metabolite injurious to vertebrates upon ingestion, inhalation, or dermal contact [1]. The word mycotoxin is derived from Greek (mukos) and Latin (toxicum) roots. While by definition they are generally considered harmful to humans and animals, not all are classified as such. Penicillin is a notable example. In fact, the toxicity of these secondary metabolites varies greatly among the broad list of fungi. The term mycotoxin came into common use after the loss of more than 100,000 turkeys in the UK during the early 1960s; a series of subsequent experiments on poultry confirmed the relationship between moldy feed and necrotic changes leading to death in the birds [2,3]. Since then, more than 400 molecules have been classified, some of which exert adverse effects on human health [4].

CLINICAL MANIFESTATIONS

For classification purposes, mycotoxin-producing fungi are sometimes viewed by the diseases with which they are associated. Given the rapidly expanding clinical knowledge of mycotoxins and human disease this serves as but a classification framework (Table 43.1). Clinical manifestations are generalized here into three categories:

TABLE 43.1

Mycotoxins Produced by Toxic Molds.

Metabolite	Disease	Organisms	Health Concerns
Gliotoxin	Invasive aspergillosis	*Aspergillus fumigatus, terres, flavus, niger, Trichoderma virens, Penicillium spp, Candia albican*	Immune toxicity, immune suppression, neurotoxicity
Kojic acid; aspergillic acid; nitropropionic acid	Carcinogenesis	*Carcinogenesis*	Liver pathology and cancer; immune toxicity; neurotoxicity
Aflatoxins	Carcinogenesis Reye syndrome Kwashiorkor disease Hepatitis, Cirrhosis	*Aspergillus flavus Penicillium, Fusarium*	Liver pathology (including cirrhosis) and cancer, immune toxicity, neurotoxicity
Fumigaclavines; fumitoxins; fumitremorgens; verruculogen; gliotoxin	Aspergillosis	*Aspergillus fumigatus*	Lung disease; neurotoxicity; tremors; immune toxicity
Ochratoxin A (OTA)	BEN (implicated) Urinary tract tumors; Aspergillosis	*Aspergillus niger Penicillium verrucosum*	Immunosuppression lung disease
	Renal cell carcinoma (implicated)	*Aspergillus ochraceus*	Nephropathology including chronic kidney disease
Penicillic acid; xanthomegnin; viomellein; vioxanthin	Tumors	*Penicillium series Aspergillus*	Synergistic with OTA (penicillic acid) Nephropathology (penicillic acid)
Sterigmatocystin 5-methoxysterigmatocystin	Carcinogenesis	*Aspergillus versicolor*	Liver pathology and cancer
Chaetomiums; chaetoglobosum A and C	Unknown	*Chaetomium globosum*	Cytotoxicity Cell division
Griseofulvin; Dechlorogrseofulvins Trichodermin; Trichodermo	Unknown	*Memnoniella echinata*	Carcinogenesis, reproductive toxin, hypersensitivity, protein synthesis inhibition
Mycophenolic acid	Unknown	*Penicillium brevicompactum*	Cytotoxic; mutagen
Botryodiploidin	Unknown	*Penicillium expansum*	Immune toxicity; cytotoxic
Patulin (PAT); citrinin	Renal tumors (implicated)	*Penicillium expansum Penicillium griseofulvum Aspergillus*	Mitotoxicity Nephropathology (benign tumors- citrinin)
Chaetoglobosin Roquefortine C	Unknown	*Penicillium expansum*	Tremors
Verrucosidins	Unknown	*Penicillium planicium*	Tremors, cytotoxicity
Trichothecenes: Deoxynivalenol	Unknown IgA nephropathy	*Trichoderma species Fusarium, Penicillium*	Trichothecene toxicity Nausea, increased intestinal permeability
Trichodermol Trichodermin	Unknown		Immunotoxicity
Gliotoxin; viridin	Unknown		

TABLE 43.1 (*continued*)
Mycotoxins Produced by Toxic Molds.

Metabolite	Disease	Organisms	Health Concerns
Fumonisins	CNS birth defects	*Fusarium verticillioides (aka moniliforme)*	Neural tube defects in animals and humans, liver pathology, esophageal cancer
Spirocyclic drimanes roridin; satratoxins (F, G, H) hydroxyroridin E; verrucarin J Altrones B, C; stahybotrylactams	Pulmonary bleeding	*Stachybotrys chartarum*	Respiratory bleeding Protein synthesis inhibition Neurotoxicity, cytotoxicity, immune toxicity
Zearalenone	Implicated not proven in cryptorchidism, late term abortion, hypospadias	*Fusarium graminearum F. culmorum*	Hormone sensitive cancers, reproductive disruption

BEN: Balkan Endemic Nephropathy
Adapted from: Thrasher and Crawley; Gelderblom; Marasas; Williams; Pinton; Hocking.

- Infectious: mycoses are actively growing fungi on or within the tissues of the body (athlete's foot or invasive aspergillosis) and are typically either primary pathogens (*Coccidioides immitis, Histoplasma capsulatum, Histoplasma, Blastomyces,* and *Paracoccidioides*) or opportunists (*Aspergillus fumigatus, Candida albicans*) [4]. Mycoses are generally acquired by topical exposure or via inhalation of spores from an environmental reservoir or are secondary to overgrowth of commensal organisms in the setting of immunosuppression.
- Allergic: these include excessive pulmonary immune response secondary to fungal spore such as hypersensitivity pneumonitis, allergic rhinitis, and asthma [5], and bronchopulmonary aspergillosis [6,7].
- Toxic: mycotoxicoses are direct adverse effects due to fungal mycotoxin exposure via ingestion, topical exposure, or inhalation, and may cause insults to the human body [4]. Mycotoxicoses are generally thought to be secondary to the ingestion of contaminated foods but may occur with inhalation of mycotoxins. [4,8].

FUNGAL TAXONOMY

Classification of fungi is complex and based on a number of factors, including phylogeny, reproductive capabilities, cell structure, and morphology. Within the phyla *Ascomycota* and *Basidiomycota*, the genera relevant to this review include: *Aspergillus, Fusarium, Penicillium, Alternaria, Candida, Cryptococcus, Histoplasma, Penicillium, Stachybotrys, Cladosporium, Epicoccum, Geotrichum, Rhodotorula,* and *Chaetomium*. The first three genera (in bold) are the major mycotoxin-producing genera imposing significant concerns [9,10]. Multiple fungi produce the same or similar mycotoxins, thus one cannot necessarily infer the species of fungi based on identification of mycotoxin alone. The mycotoxins they produce depend on their nutrient base and will vary from building or agricultural source to that of the laboratory.

FOOD PRODUCTION

The Joint Expert Committee on Food Additives (JECFA), a scientific advisory body of the World Health Organization currently considers aflatoxins B1, B2, G1, and G2, aflatoxin M1; ochratoxin A; patulin; fumonisins B1, B2, and B3; zearalenone; T-2 and HT-2 toxins; and deoxynivalenol to be the mycotoxins of greatest concern based on their toxic effects (see Table 43.1) [11,12].

Molds and their metabolites are ubiquitous and thus not easily avoided. Twenty-five percent of the world's crops are estimated to be at risk of fungal infestation [13] with annual costs of crop loss in the United States alone between $0.5 million to $1.5 billion annually [14]. Some estimates place as many as 4.5 billion people at risk for chronic mycotoxin exposure and attribute as much as 40% of the disease in developing countries to food-borne exposure [15]. More than 100 countries currently regulate 40 or more mycotoxins in the food supply [16].

Despite the agricultural industry's efforts to control fungal contamination, toxic fungi are commonplace in the majority of the world's agricultural products. Low levels of mycotoxins are allowed to exist in marketable product as defined by nationally and internationally accepted levels of tolerability (see Table 43.2). The World Health Organization/Food and Agricultural Organization of the United Nations has listed tolerable daily intakes for a number of mycotoxins [12]. Others have summarized the association of specific mycotoxins with individual foods [17].

Genetic engineering and genotyping techniques allow growers to breed resistant strains of crops and improve surveillance for mycotoxins contamination of the food supply [18–20]. A representative sample of the world literature on mycotoxin assessment in the food supply is available [9]. An extensive review of food-based mycotoxin isolation and identification techniques is reviewed here [21].

INDOOR AIR

To the human body, innate mechanisms to manage toxins are similar whether the route of exposure is food or air, so both routes of exposure are presented here. Indoor mold growth occurs in 20–40% of northern European, 30% of Canadian, and as high as 50% of U.S. buildings. In Denmark, up to 50% of schools and daycare centers are contaminated with mold [22]. There is ongoing debate as to whether and to what extent indoor mold and microbial inhalation compromise health and contribute to human disease [6,23–25]. Representative molds in water-damaged buildings include *A. Versicolor, A. Sydowii, Trichoderma Viride, S. chartarum, Chaetomium globosum,* multiple species of *Penicillium, Acremonium, Cladosporium,* and *Aureobasidium* [26]. The indoor mycotoxins and metabolites include but are not limited to Gliotoxin, Aflatoxin B1, Ochratoxin A, Trichothecenes, Spirocyclic Drimanes, Saratoxins, and Stachybotrylactams. A more extensive list of these mycotoxins and the health concerns associated with them is located here (Figure 43.1) [27].

AIRBORNE FUNGAL CONTAMINANTS

HARMFUL ALGAE BLOOMS AND WATERBORNE ILLNESS

While dinoflagellates and fungi belong to different branches of the phylogenetic tree within the eukaryotic domain, the toxins of harmful algae blooms (HABs) deserve mention as they generate a number of neurologic manifestations, and in the case of *Pfiesteria piscicida* (Pp), may present with a chronic systemic inflammatory response syndrome (CIRS) similar to mold-induced illness. In 1992, Burkholder and others first identified *Pfiesteria* as the toxic dinoflagellate involved in fish kills with associated "punched out" lesions, in the estuaries of the Pamlico and Neuse on the Atlantic seaboard [28]. Gratton linked neuropsychological symptoms, such as increased forgetfulness, headache, and burning sensations of the skin with exposure to *Pfiesteria* toxins, and correlated degree of exposure with severity of symptoms [29].

Possible estuary-associated syndrome (PEAS) was defined by the Centers for Disease Control (CDC) in patients exposed to Pp if they met the following criteria: 1) developed symptoms within two weeks after exposure to coastal water, 2) reported certain cognitive or flu-like symptoms of a certain duration, and 3) the health-care provider cannot identify another cause for the symptoms.

In 2001, Shoemaker and Hudnell reported a case series of five people accidentally exposed to toxic pfiesteria complex (TPC) by direct immersion, exposure to spray, or inhalation of air at the water surface in areas of fish kills attributed to TPC. They delineated case symptoms, linked the

TABLE 43.2
Comparison of the Provisional Tolerable Daily Intake (PMTDI), Exposure Levels, and Doses of Particular Mycotoxins Required for Intestinal Effects.

Mycotoxin	PMTDI	Range of Exposure	Intestinal Effect/Species/Doses Required	Times PMTDI/Higher Dose
Aflatoxins	0.15 ng/kg	0.058 ng–2 µg/kg	Barrier defect/*human*/0.66 mg/kg[a]	$4.10^6/3.10^2$
			↑ Intestinal infection/*chicken*/750 µg/kg	$5.10^6/4.10^2$
DON	1 µg/kg	0.78–2.4 µg/kg	Microflora perturbation/*pig*/110–280 µg/kg	$1-10^2-3.10^2/5.10^1-1.10^2$
			↓ Mucus production/*pig*/1.48 µg/kg[b,d]	$1.10^0/6.10^{-1}$
			Barrier defect/*human*/10–90 µg/kg[a]	$1-10^1-1.10^2/4.10^0-4.10^1$
			↑ Bacterial translocation/*human*/48 µg/kg[a]	$5.10^1/2.10^1$
			↑ Intestinal infection/*mice*/10 mg/kg	$1.10^4/4.10^3$
			↑ IL-8 secretion/*human*/48 µg/kg[a]	$5.10^1/2.10^1$
			↓IL-8 secretion/*human*/480 µg/kg[a]	$5.10^2/2.10^2$
			Th2 > Th1 unbalance/*mice*/10 mg/kg	$1.10^4/4.10^3$
			Increased IgA secretion/*mice*/2.5 mg/kg	$3.10^3/1.10^3$
FB1	2 µg/kg	0.02–471 µg/kg	Barrier defect/*pig*/0.5 mg/kg[b]	$2.10^2/1.10^0$
			↑ Intestinal infection/*pig*/0.5 mg/kg	$2.10^2/1.10^0$
			↓ IL-8 secretion/*pig*/0.5 mg/kg[b]	$2.10^2/1.10^0$
			Th1 > Th2 unbalanced/*mice*/2.25 mg/kg	$1.10^3/5.10^0$
OTA	14 ng/kg	0.13–13 ng/kg	Barrier defect/*human*/30–170 µg/kg[a]	$2.10^3-12.10^3/2.10^3-12.10^3$
			↑ Bacterial translocation/*human*/5 µg/kg[a]	$4.10^2/4.10^2$
			↑ Intestinal infection/*chicken*/3 mg/kg	$2.10^5/2.10^5$
			↑ IL-8 secretion/*human*/5 µg/kg[a]	$4.10^2/4.10^2$
PAT	0.4 µg/kg	0.094–0.5 µg/kg	Barrier defect/*human*/20–90 µg/kg[a]	$5.10^1-2.10^2/4.10^1-2.10^2$
			↑ Bacterial translocation/*human*/2 µg/kg[a]	$5.10^0/4.10^0$
			↑ IL-8 secretion/*human*/20 µg/kg[a]	$5.10^1/4.10^1$
			↓ IL-8 secretion/*human*/210 µg/kg[a]	$5.10^2/4.10^2$
			TH2 > Th1 unbalance/*human* 3 µg/kg[c]	$7.10^0/6.10^0$
T-2 toxin	60 ng/kg	6–780 ng/kg	Microflora perturbation/*pig*/500 µg/kg	$8.10^3/6.10^2$
			↓ Mucus production/*pig*/0.59 µg/kg[b,d]	$1.10^1/7.10^{-1}$
			↑ intestinal infection/*mice*/1 mg/kg	$2.10^4/1.10^3$
ZEA	0.5 µg/kg	3–60 ng/kg	↓ Mucus production/*pig*/1.7 µg/kg[b,d]	$3.10^0/3.10^1$
			Barrier defect?/*human*/45 µg/kg	$9.10^1/7.10^2$

All doses are expressed in amount of mycotoxin per kg of human body weight per day.

[a] Doses used in vitro for enterocyte treatment (in µM) were converted assuming that the residual small intestine fluid content is 1 L for a human weighting 70 kg.

[b] Doses given to animals in mg/kg of food were converted accordingly to mycotoxin doses in food, amount of food ingested, and animal body weight.

[c] Doses used in vitro for PBMC treatment (µg/L) were converted assuming that the blood volume is 5 L for a human weighing 70 kg.

[d] Effect on mucus production in pigs was observed after exposure to mixture of DON, T-2 toxin, and ZEA at the indicated doses.

Source: Adapted from Murphy, 2006.

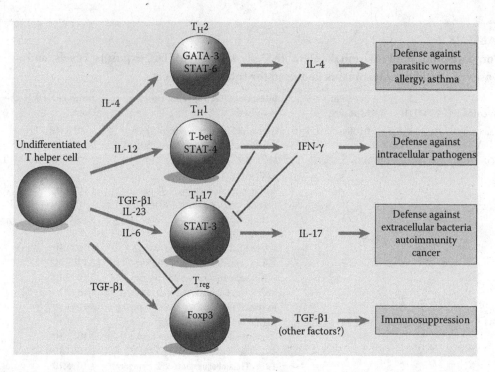

FIGURE 43.1 Th1, Th2, and Th17 response: various interleukins (IL) produced by dendritic cells and other sources induce undifferentiated T helper cells to develop into Th1 or Th2 lineages. In an inflammatory response, TGF-B1 and IL-6 induce the development of Th17 and its cytokine IL-17. Interferon gamma (IFN-gamma) and IL-5, products of Th1 and Th2 cells, inhibit Th17 differentiation. TGF-B1 increases expression of the IL-23 receptor and promotes expansion of Th17 cells by IL-23. However, TGF-B1 also promotes development of another line-regulatory T (Treg) cells by inducing the transcription factor Foxp3. This path is inhibited, however, by IL-6. Development of Th1 and Th2 cells depends on specific STAT proteins and other gene-transcription factors, such as T-bet and GATA-3. STAT-3 is likely involved in Th17 differentiation, but other Th17-lineage specific factors may well emerge. Adapted from Tato, 2006.

symptoms with abnormalities in visual contrast sensitivity and showed symptom resolution with CSM in a double-blinded, placebo-controlled, crossover trial [30]. Morris followed 107 cohort members over four seasons with regular occupational exposure to the Chesapeake Bay, collecting information on symptoms and data on the presence or absence of Pp based on PCR analysis of > 3500 water samples. No correlation was found between work areas where Pp was identified and specific symptomatology or changes in neuropsychological tests over four years of routine work exposure, though he acknowledged that PEAS could occur in heavily contaminated areas [31]. In 2007, Moeller characterized the metal-containing organic toxins produced by Pp corroborating data obtained from five different instrumental methods and confirmed that the high toxicity of its toxins was due to metal-mediated (Fe and primarily Cu species) free-radical production. These are highly labile toxins that may induce DNA damage, protein oxidation, and lipid peroxidation whose short-lived toxicity (two to five days) is dependent on pH variation and exposure to light [32,33]. HAB-induced illness is generated in many cases by a variety of dinoflagellates and responds to interventions recommended in the setting of mold induced CIRS. For representative neurologic symptoms see Table 43.3 [34].

WATER-DAMAGED BUILDINGS

WHO's 2009 report on Guidelines for Indoor Air Quality seemed to establish a stronger causal link to respiratory illness in water-damaged buildings than was previously acknowledged. "Although few

TABLE 43.3

Harmful Algal Bloom Illnesses Associated With Neuropsychological Symptoms

Disease	Amnesic Shellfish Poisoning (ASP)	Ciguatera Fish Poisoning (CPP)	Possible Estuarine-Associated Illness (PEAS)	Paralytic Shellfish Poisoning (PSP)	Neurotoxic Shellfish Poisoning (NSP)
Toxin	Domoic acid	Ciguatoxin maitotoxin	Unknown	Saxitoxin	Brevetoxin
Causative organism	Red tide diatom	Epibenthic dinoflagellate	Possibly pfiesteria piscicida	Red tide dinoflagellate	Red tide dinoflagellate
Route of exposure	Ingestion	Ingestion	Possibly dermal or respiratory	Ingestion	Ingestion
Major transvector	Shellfish	Fish, especially large reef fish	Possibly water or air	Shellfish	Shellfish
Molecular action	Glutamate receptor agonist	Na+, Ca2+ channel activator	Unknown	Na+ channel blocker	Na+ channel activator
Reported neuro-behavioral effects	Irreversible memory impairment	Memory impairment, hallucinations, paresthesias, hot/cold temperature reversal	Memory impairment	Numbness, incoordination, medullary disturbance, speech disturbance, paralysis, death (severe cases)	Vertigo, throat tightness, pupil dilation, ataxia, muscle twitching, paresthesias, hot/cold temperature reversal.

Adapted from Friedman and Levin, 2005.

interventions studies are available, their results show that remediation of dampness problems can reduce adverse health outcomes. There is clinical evidence that exposure to mold and other damp-ness-related microbial agents increases the risks of rare conditions, such as hypersensitivity pneumo-nitis, allergic alveolitis, chronic rhinosinusitis and allergic fungal sinusitis. Toxicological evidence obtained in vivo, and in vitro supports these findings, showing the occurrence of diverse inflamma-tory and toxic responses after exposure to microorganisms including their spores, metabolites, and components isolated from damp buildings" [35]. More recent evidence provides a stronger link [36].

Fatigue, rhinorrhea, dizziness, visual changes, wheezing, joint pain, and paresthesias are included in the more than 30 physical complaints related to water-damaged building exposure in some studies [37]. Occupants of water-damaged buildings are also exposed to toxic and immuno-genic byproducts of bacteria and molds [38] such as: 1) mycotoxins; 2) microbial and other volatile organic compounds (MVOC) and (VOC) produced during growth of bacteria and mold [22,27]; 3) 1–3 B-D-glucans that trigger inflammatory reactions similar to symptoms observed after exposure to endotoxins [8,22]; 4) extracellular polysaccharides (EPS) such as galactomannans [39]; 5) extra-cellular digestive enzymes (EDS) and hemolysins [40,41]; 6) bacterial endotoxin (LPS), which acts synergistically with fungal products; and 7) gram positive bacilli, actinomycetes, and others that produce exotoxins [27]. Repetitive damp-dry cycles in water-damaged buildings promote fungal growth and mycotoxin synthesis followed by dry periods that foster release of spores and hyphal fragments [22]. The impact of this large group of microbial products on immunity is well described [27,37].

These exposures may lead to one or more of the following illnesses or molecular injuries: 1) mycotic infections, 2) fungal rhino-sinusitis, 3) IgE mediated sensitivity and asthma, 4) non-IgE chronic rhinosinusitis (CRS), 5) hypersensitivity and related pulmonary inflammatory disease, 6) cytotoxicity, 7) immune suppression, 8) autoimmune disorders, 9) mitochondrial toxicity, 10) cancer, 11) renal toxicity, 12) neurotoxicity, and 13) formation of nuclear and mitochondrial DNA adducts [27,42,43].

In water-damaged buildings, inhalation represents the primary route of exposure for fungal spores, secondary metabolites such as mycotoxins and cell wall fragments. While most particles more than 8–10 um in size are stopped prior to reaching the lower respiratory tract, spores ranging from 3–7 um, hyphal fragments, and particulates as small as 0.05 um in size will likely reach the lower portions of the respiratory tree [5,37, 4]. Additionally, Gorny's work revealed that fungal fragments ≤ 0.03 um can be released from colonies in a 320-fold higher concentration compared to spore release [5]. Thus, relying on spore counts for total mold burden is less than ideal and does not necessarily give an accurate picture of the potential damage a mold-laden environment can inflict. Typical upper airway illness associated with molds and mycotoxins has included chronic rhinosinusitis, allergic rhinitis, and fungal sinusitis. However Islam and colleagues have demonstrated significant cytokine and neural aberrations, including olfactory sensory neuron apoptosis when mice are exposed to Saratoxin G, a macrocyclic trichothecene mycotoxin from *Stachybotrys chartarum* [45].

The criteria outlined in Table 43.4 were applied to WBS in 2006 [46]. Treatment with cholestyramine (CSM), a nonabsorbable anion-binding resin normally used in the treatment of hypercholesterolemia, which also binds many biologically produced toxins, led to resolution of symptoms [30,47]. The basis has been made for genetic vulnerability. HLA DR showed a strong relative risk (> 2.0) for illness for a selective genotypes considered to be specific, non-specific, or protective [48]. HLA susceptible patients were the quickest to succumb to symptoms on re-exposure. Other noted abnormalities were dysregulation of androgens, ADH:osmolality, and ACTH:cortisol ratios [49].

Laboratory markers of chronic systemic inflammatory response syndrome (CIRS) tend to be positive in patients and continue to be evaluated for clinical correlations. Among these are markers of autoimmunity (TGF-β1, antigliadin, and anticardiolipin antibodies), capillary hypoperfusion (C4a, TGF-β1 and VEGF), and deficiency of neuroregulatory peptides (MSH and VIP) now thought to be consistent with a chronic systemic inflammatory response syndrome (CIRS) [49]. In summary,

---

TABLE 43.4
Shoemaker's Criteria for Water-Damaged Building Syndrome.

1) Each of the following elements must be met:
   a) Potential for exposure to buildings with documented presence of toxigenic fungi, evident fungal growth, or a history of water intrusion with musty smells;
   b) Presence of multiple symptoms in at least four of eight system categories;
   c) Absence of confounders.
2) Three of the following six criteria must be met:
   a. Visual contrast sensitivity deficits;
   b. Melanocyte-stimulating hormone deficiency;
   c. Matrix metalloproteinase elevation;
   d. Human leukocyte antigen–associated genotype;
   e. Antidiuretic hormone/osmolality dysregulation, measured simultaneously;
   f. Adrenocorticotrophic/cortisol dysregulation, measured simultaneously.
3) Final criteria for case management include two of three of the following:
   a. Response to CSM, with abatement of symptoms and resolution of VCS deficit to control levels;
   b. Reduction of leptin if elevated, with treatment;
   c. Reduction in matrix metalloproteinase 9, if elevated, with treatment.
4) Clinical note to be made of
   a. Presence of Multiply Antibiotic Resistant Coagulase Negative Staph (MARCoNS) in deep nasal spaces;
   b. Elevated levels of myelin basic protein antibodies.

Source: Adapted from Shoemaker, Rash, and Simon.

the biocontaminants of indoor air that include mycotoxins appear to be contributing to chronic inflammation in a genetically susceptible group of patients.

PATHOPHYSIOLOGIC BASIS OF DISEASE

IMMUNE DYSFUNCTION ASSOCIATED WITH AIRBORNE EXPOSURE TO MYCOTOXINS

Exposure to WDBs has been associated with broad immune dysregulation and an associated inflammatory response. In Rand's work, rodent lungs exposed to proteases, isosatratoxin-F, and spores of *S. chartarum* resulted in the release of IL-1β, IL-6, IL-8, and TNF-α [50]. IL-6, in conjunction with TNF-α and γ-interferon, upregulate vascular cellular adhesion molecules (VCAMs), allowing T-helper cells to gain access to critical organs in autoimmune disease. VCAM-1 binds lymphocytes with alpha 4 integrin, which is a key tipping point in the genesis of several experimental autoimmune diseases, such as experimental autoimmune encephalomyelitis, type 1 diabetes mellitus, and collagen arthritis [51]. Spores from indoor *Aspergillus* and *Penicillium* have been associated with eosinophilia, neutrophilia, vascular permeability, raised IL-6, TNF-α, elevated LDH, and Th-2 inflammatory responses in a mouse model [27].

Until the last decade, the world of immunology neatly categorized the response of our immune system into one of two camps: Th1 or Th2. Th1 cells secrete cytokines such as IL-2 and IFN-γ, which help direct macrophage and natural killer cell activation. In contrast, Th2 CD4+ cells secrete cytokines (IL-4, IL-5, and IL-10) that inhibit the effects of Th1 and/or promote humoral immunity (i.e., synthesis of IgE). Autoimmune diseases do not fit into this simple picture. Other subsets of T helper cells such as Tregs and Th17 are clearly implicated. Treg cells act to keep immune hyperactivity in check, and Th17 cells (which secrete IL-17 and IL-21) in general promote an inflammatory response. TGF-β1 induces differentiation of Treg cells. However, in conjunction with IL-6, TGF-β1 appears to promote differentiation and propagation of Th17 cells, leading to an inflammatory response and inhibiting the expression of Foxp3, a gene-transcription factor essential for Treg differentiation (Figure 43.1) [52].

Additionally, IL-21 has been shown to promote the production of Th17, with or without the assistance of IL-6, though the response in murine models is not as strong without this cytokine [53]. In MS models, the blood-brain barrier endothelial cells (BBB-ECs) have receptors for IL-17 and IL-22. These cytokines have been shown now to disrupt BBB tight junctions in vitro and in vivo on binding to these receptors. Th-17 lymphocytes effectively transmigrate across the BBB-ECs, express granzyme B (a cytolytic enzyme), kill human neurons, and promote CNS inflammation as a result [54]. TGF-β1, IL-6, and Th17 now figure prominently in WDB-induced autoimmune illness. This research helps to validate the neurological deviations that many of those exposed to WDB air develop. Downregulating their influence appears to be one of the keys to restoring health in mold injured patients.

Allergic bronchopulmonary aspergillosis [55–57] is associated with types I and III immune responses and is most often caused by *A. fumigatus* (80% of clinical cases). It is associated with serum total IgE levels > 1000 IU/ml and immediate positive skin test to *A. fumigatus* > 3 mm, or positive specific IgE to the same. There is a higher incidence of chronic colonization in steroid-dependent asthma and cystic fibrosis patients where this fungus results in an augmented inflammatory Th17 response with increased production of Treg cells [58].

IMMUNE DYSFUNCTION—INFLAMMATORY BOWEL DISEASE AND INGESTED MYCOTOXINS

Mycotoxins may be responsible for inciting or exacerbating inflammatory bowel disease (IBD) in those who are genetically predisposed [59]. Normally, the mucosal immune system does not react to the intestinal content of microflora and food-based antigens. The development of oral tolerance includes induction of Treg cells expressing the Fox p3 transcription factor and the anti-inflammatory cytokines IL-10 and TGF-β1. In IBD, this pathway appears disrupted, leading to uncontrolled inflammation. In murine knockout models of IBD, removal of the genes responsible for the production of IL-2, IL-10, and TGF-β or their receptors is associated with spontaneous colitis or enteritis. The same is true when studies designed to interfere with, or to evaluate, compromised intestinal epithelial cell barrier function are performed. These include disruption of Toll receptors (TLRs) and organic cation transporters (OCTN1 and OCTN2). In most of these models, commensal microbes must be present to trigger inflammation. While it remains to be proven clinically, evidence points to a genetic predisposition associated with an inappropriate innate immune response to commensal bacteria in the setting of increased intestinal permeability (IP) and inadequate regulation of inflammatory cytokine pathways in the lamina propria [60]. This cytokine activity is responsible for the activation of macrophages and B cells, as well as the recruitment of other lymphocytes, leukocytes, and mononuclear cells to the gut via homing mechanisms involving leukocyte associated receptors, (Alpha4B7 integrin) and addressins on vascular endothelium (e.g., Mad CAM1).

Briefly the malfunctions of the immune system [61] with IBD include: compromised epithelial barrier leading to increased intestinal permeability, dysregulated toll-like receptors, disturbed antigen recognition and presentation by antigen-presenting calls (APC), atypical antigen-presenting cells become potent effector T-cell activators in the setting of elevated levels of INF-γ and TNF-α, overreactive or autoreactive T-cell populations leading to an overall immune "tone" of hypervigilance, and an imbalance of Treg versus T effector cells in IBD.

Macrophage release of TNF-α and IL-6 promotes: fibrinogenesis, activation of tissue MMPs, the coagulation cascade, and production of vWB factor. When these are not properly regulated, tissue damage ensues. As in WDB-induced disease, TGF-β is likely influential in determining the balance between a proinflammatory and anti-inflammatory response [62]. (See Figure 43.2.)

Microbial Imbalance

Studies have shown that the total number and composition of intestinal flora are altered in IBD, with an increase in aerobes and enterobacteria and a consequent decrease in anaerobic bacteria [63–66]. T-2 toxin and deoxynivalenol (DON), members of the trichothecene family, have been shown in porcine models to increase aerobic intestinal bacteria [67,68]. While the mechanism of microbial alteration is unclear, if the same process is at work in human subjects, variation in the microbial milieu may play a role in genetically susceptible patients. At present, DON and T-2 toxin are the only identified mycotoxins capable of altering the microbial balance of the intestine, but they are frequently present in our daily intake of grains.

Intestinal Permeability

Mycotoxins may predispose to IBD by compromising intestinal permeability (IP). Aflatoxin B1 (AFB1) has been shown to compromise intestinal permeability and induce DNA damage to caco-2 cells, a model of human enterocytes. Lactobacillus rhamnosus can reverse these effects. [69,70] Other contributors to increased intestinal permeability include DON, OTA, and PAT via altered expression or relocalization of tight junction proteins: claudins and occludins [71–74]. Fumonisin B1 (FB1) has been shown to increase permeability of porcine enterocytes [75]. This likely occurs via the inhibition of sphingolipid synthesis [76]. Because the mechanisms of cellular damage among mycotoxins often relate to DNA damage, inhibition of protein synthesis, and induction of cytotoxicity, it is likely that many mycotoxins increase intestinal permeability predisposing to immune dysregulation. However, there are other mechanisms at work that enable increased bacterial translocation, yet do not require an increase in intestinal permeability.

Bacterial Translocation without Permeability Changes

Historically, bacterial translocation (the movement of bacteria or its products across the intestinal membrane into the lymphatic or visceral circulation) has been assumed to be associated with increased intestinal permeability. Nazli and colleagues have demonstrated in vitro that under conditions of increased metabolic stress (via ox/phos uncoupling models), intestinal epithelia increase their rate of microtubule, microfilament-dependent internalization of nonpathogenic *E. coli* independent of a drop in transepithelial resistance (TER), a marker of paracellular permeability. Theoretically, this could lead to an inflammatory response by activation of resident immune cells [77]. Maresca has found that DON, OTA, and PAT at higher dosages can impact intestinal permeability and facilitate bacterial translocation. Surprisingly, however, even at doses that do not alter barrier function in terms of lower

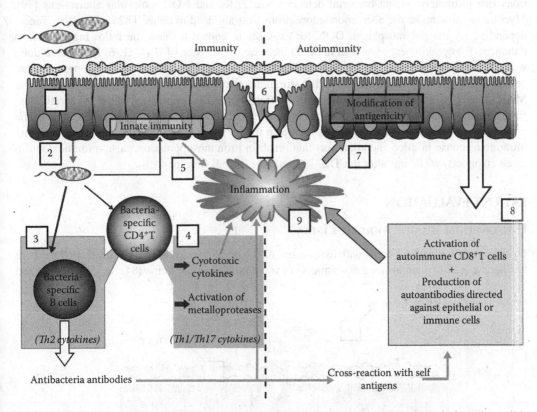

FIGURE 43.2 Inflammatory bowel disease, immunity, and autoimmunity: Crohn's and ulcerative colitis involve an immune response against bacteria, autoimmunity against self-antigens caused by cytokine dependent, and likely cytokine-independent reactions with predisposing factors. (1) Commensal bacteria gain access to the submucosa and its immune cells via damaged epithelium or through intact epithelium with the help of dendritic cells, M cells, and/or stressed enterocytes (IFN-gamma, metabolic stress, infection) with alteration of the tight junctions. (2) Once in the submucosa, bacteria stimulate innate immunity (linked to epithelial and immune cells) and CD4+ T-cells resulting in Th1/Th17 and Th2 immune responses. Importantly, gene mutations associated to IBD could modulate this critical step, resulting in loss of functions of TLRs and NODs proteins, leading to impaired innate immunity activation and stronger bacterial invasions; or gene mutations leading to gain of function of TLRs/NODs could induce inflammation independent of initial entry of gut bacteria. (3) The Th2 response aids specific B-cells in the production of antibodies directed against commensal bacteria, some of which present with cross-reactivity against self-antigens. (4) The Th1/Th17 response causes release of cytotoxic cytokines and metalloproteinase activation, both of which induce cell death and extracellular matrix destruction. (5) The combined action of innate immunity, cytotoxic cytokines, metalloproteinase, bacteria, and bacterial toxins such as LPS, antibodies, and autoantibodies, results in inflammation and tissue destruction. (6) Tissue destruction facilitates further bacterial entry via damaged epithelial cells. (7) Inflammation and tissue destruction associated with immunity toward bacteria lead to antigenic changes of epithelial and immune cells linking immunity and autoimmunity. (8) This results in production of autoantibodies and activation of autoimmune CD8 T+ cells directed against epithelial and/or immune cells antigens. (9) Autoimmunity leads to further inflammation, linking autoimmunity to immunity toward gut flora. (Adapted from Maresca 2010.)

TER, these three mycotoxins still induced a significant increase in bacterial translocation and a subsequent increase in inflammatory IL-8. At high doses of DON, IL-8 release was inhibited presumably due to a direct cytotoxic effect on the cell, a response not observed with OTA and PAT [78].

Intestinal Immunity

Both ulcerative colitis (UC) and Crohn's disease (CD) are associated with varying gene mutations that ultimately impact bacterial detection via TLRs and NOD molecular aberrations [79]. Mycotoxins may make the aberrations more prominent and lead to either Th2 or Th1 dominance, depending on the polymorphism. DON for example is known to have the following effects: 1) enhances T-2 cytokine expression in mice; 2) increases expression of IL-4, IL-6, IL-10, and along with T-2 toxins, suppresses TH1 immune and IFN-γ production in murine models; 3) potentiates the action of IL-1, TNF-alpha, and LPS; and 4) stimulates the production of IgA in Peyer's patches via MAP kinases, proinflammatory cytokine production, and COX-2 expression [59,78]. Altered intestinal immunity and infectious pathogens have long been theorized to play a role in IBD [80,81]. The probability of their pathogenic role is increased in the presence of mycotoxins. FB1 induces a Th1 immune response in mice and aflatoxins that result in immunosuppression, raise immunoglobulin levels in piglets, yet do not alter the Th1/Th2 balance [82,83] (Figure 43.3).

PATIENT EVALUATION

ENVIRONMENTAL RELATIVE MOLDINESS INDEX

Often patient evaluation begins with assessment of the home for exposures. However, to date there has been a lack of standardized assessments of mold burden in the home [84]. In 2002, Haugland

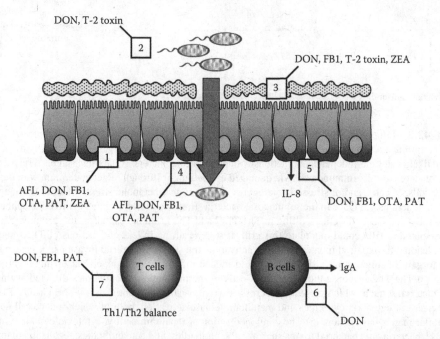

FIGURE 43.3 Proposed model of mycotoxin induced alterations: (1) mycotoxins induce mutations in enterocytes. (2) they may modify intestinal microflora, (3) alter composition of intestinal mucus and its production, (4) facilitate transepithelial passage of bacteria and luminal antigens secondary to increased transcellular passage of bacteria or increase in intestinal permeability linked to tight junction defect, (5) modulate secretion of proinflammatory cytokines such as IL-8 by IECs, (6) increase production of IgA against microflora and autoantigens, (7) disturb Th1/Th2 immune response balance. (Adapted from Maresca 2010.)

and the EPA were granted the patent describing the DNA sequences that make identification and quantification of various mold species possible [85]. The patent displays the DNA sequences used in distinguishing over 130 major indoor air fungi and has been licensed to firms in the United States, Germany, and the United Kingdom. The EPA and Department of Housing and Urban Development (HUD) researchers went on to develop the Environmental Relative Moldiness Index (ERMI) to objectively describe the mold burden inside water-damaged and persistently damp buildings. This technology utilizes mold specific quantitative polymerase chain reaction (MSQPCR) analysis of dust to measure indoor air mold burden. Samples are collected by vacuuming 2 m^2 living room and 2 m^2 bedroom spaces adjacent to the sofa and bed using a Mitest sampler-fitted vacuum [86]. Two groups composed of 36 species represent the molds analyzed in ERMI samples. Group 1 contains 26 species associated with water damaged homes, and Group 2 contains 10 species found in homes independent of water-damage. The ERMI value is calculated by subtracting the sum of the logs in Group 2 from the sum of the logs in Group 1. The scale ranges from -10 to 20 on average and is divided into quartiles. Homes in the lowest quartile have the lowest mold burden, with higher quartiles representing progressively higher mold burdens [86].

With the development of ERMI testing, home mold-burden estimates and correlations with disease will hopefully become more meaningful. This testing is recommended now for assessing suspicious homes and correlates well with moldy odors in homes. In one study, when ERMI was used in mold classification criterion, 26% of homes were rated in the high mold category as opposed to visible mold damage criterion (11%) or by moldy odor criterion (14%) [84]. While odor detection of mold isn't as high as ERMI, it does correlate with increased concentration of airborne *Aspergillus*, *Penicillium*, and *Cladosporium* [87]. Additionally it is associated with asthma, rhinitis, and eczema symptoms in children [88], and higher counts of total fungal DNA [89]. We should be listening when our patients complain of moldy odors in their home or workplace. For useful documents and websites with further information on ERMI-based mold assessment, mycotoxin factsheets, and fungal taxonomy please see this chapter's references [90–93].

PATIENT CLINICAL EVALUATION

Patient Medical History

The array of signs and symptoms in mycotoxin injured patients is quite extensive due to the molecular diversity of biotoxins. Aflatoxins induce hepatocellular disease with its associated symptoms; citrinin and ochratoxin A are nephrotoxic and implicated in renal cell carcinoma and chronic interstitial kidney disease with associated fatigue, weight loss, proteinuria, lumbar pain, renal colic, and rarely hematuria. IgA nephropathy is associated with DON. Pancytopenia, abdominal pain, nausea, vomiting, chills, and diarrhea occur in alimentary toxic aleukia induced by trichothecenes. Stachybotrys can be associated with leukopenia, irritation of the mouth, nose, and throat (in animals), tachycardia or bradycardia, and respiratory failure. Citreoviridin associated with stored yellow rice has induced paralysis and cardiac failure in animals. Chaetoglobosin is associated with tremors and, in the immunosuppressed, oral and intestinal candidiasis can be observed. Aspergillus can induce upper or lower respiratory symptoms as previously noted. WDB-SBS is associated with a constellation of symptoms increasingly associated with CIRS, but may be seen in other illnesses. Its manifestations include but are not limited to: dizziness, sinus congestion, fatigue, muscle aches, arthralgias, cough, shortness of breath, concentration difficulties, tingling, photophobia, night sweats, mood swings, and lancinating pain. As such, taking a thorough medical history means reviewing every organ system (particularly the gastrointestinal, renal, pulmonary, and neurologic systems) (Table 43.5). Assessing nutritional intake for proper amounts of antioxidants and foods rich in sulfhydryls found in cysteine and glutathione is important for poor nutritional status will increase susceptibility to mycotoxins (Table 43.6).

A good occupational, seasonal, and travel history should be elicited as mold-related risks are more likely in grain storage bins and damp: climates, seasons, buildings. Assessment of genetic

TABLE 43.5

Mycotoxin-Associated Symptoms

Organ or System	Symptom
General	Fatigue
	Weakness
Antidiuretic Hormone System	Excessive Thirst
	Frequent Urination
Central Nervous System	Decreased Assimilation of New Knowledge
	Decreased Focus or Concentration
	Decreased Word-Finding Ability
	Memory Deficits
	Vertigo
Eye	Blurred Vision
	Light Sensitivity
	Red Eye
	Tearing
Gastrointestinal	Abdominal Pain
	Diarrhea
Hypothalamic	Appetite Swings
	Mood Swings
	Nights Sweats
	Temperature Regulation
Musculoskeletal	Aches
	Ice-Pick Pain
	Joint Pain
	Lightning-Bolt Pain
	Morning Stiffness
Multifactorial	Headache
Pulmonary	Cough
	Shortness of Breath
Renal	Hematuria
	Proteinuria
Sinus	Sinus Congestion or Pressure
Skin	Photosensitivity

Source: Adapted from Shoemaker and House, 2006; Barceloux, 2008.

susceptibility is important. Methylene tetrahydrofolate reductase (MTHFR) polymorphisms may predispose to NTDs in pregnant women exposed to fumonisins. This polymorphism should be considered in anyone with a family history of neural tube defects, cardiovascular disease, and neurodegenerative diseases. Diarrhea is often associated with DON and this mycotoxin should be considered in the differential of anyone presenting with IBD or diarrhea of unexplained origin. Symptoms of chronic respiratory irritation (upper and lower) should be considered as well. As noted in Shoemaker's work, certain haplotypes appear predisposed to mold susceptibility, developing symptoms of chronic inflammatory response syndrome. Inquire if patients have already been screened or already have a history of autoimmune illness.

Visual Contrast Sensitivity

Visual contrast sensitivity (VCS) is an indicator of neurologic function of the visual system and is defined as a measure of the least amount of luminance contrast between darker and lighter areas of a defined pattern required for a viewer to distinguish the pattern from a homogeneous

TABLE 43.6
Antifungal Supportive Nutrients

Nutrient or Intervention	Proposed Role
Avoidance of gluten, corn, all grains	Grains contain a great deal of mold as they are stored in silos; corn, soft wheat, oat are soft and most prone to fungal growth.
Butyrate, Phenylbutyrate	Short chain anti-inflammatory fatty acid, hepatic detoxicant, stimulates the beta oxidation of very long chain fatty acids, peroxisomal function, formation of prostaglandin J2 and resolvins and is a PPAR agonist.
Cinnamon	Potent antimicrobial
Coenzyme Q10	Protects against cytotoxic effects of several mycotoxins
Essential Fatty Acids 4:1 omega 6 to omega 3 oil EPA, anchovies, evening primrose oil	Regulates the immune system, anti-inflammatory, precursors to resolvins and prostaglandins, antifungal
Folinic Acid, including Leucovorin, Isovorin, and Deplin (5-MTHF)	Fosters proper methylation, particularly in the setting of fumonisin exposure such as contaminated corn products
Glutathione, Branched Chain Amino Acids, N-Acetyl cysteine (NAC) and other therapeutic thiols	Lessen the risk for increased bacterial translocation (in the setting of patulin, gliotoxin and citrinin) and facilitate the production of glutathione-S-transferase in protection against aflatoxins
Low-carbohydrate, high-fat, high-protein diet	Controls Phospholipase A2 that stimulates the breakdown of membrane phospholipids, downregulates mycotoxin induced inflammation
Phosphatidylcholine (PC) (not choline, triple lecithin, or glycerophosphocholine)	Aids in downregulation of TNF-alpha mediated events, appears to clear mycotoxins from DNA adducts, stabilizes membrane architecture, key constituent in the production of surfactant; PC production is impaired by certain mold strains and their mycotoxins.
Saccharomyces Cerevisiae, Lactobaccillus Rhamnosus, Lb GG	Promotes mycotoxin binding and fosters production
Undecanoic acid, castor oil	Medium chain fatty acid with potent antifungal action
Vanillin	Potent antimicrobial
Vitamin D3	Anti-inflammatory, immunomodulator
Zinc	Potent antimicrobial, regulates immune function, necessary to prevent increased permeability of tight junctions

field [94]. The test measures contrast sensitivity for five special frequencies, as spatial vision is accomplished through neurons selectively tuned to different spatial frequencies. When it is abnormal, it is an indicator of neurologic dysfunction and has been correlated with the presence of: Lyme, Ciguatera, PEAS, and WDB SBS [46,94–96]. It can be used in part to determine if further laboratory evaluation of mold illness is warranted. It may also be used to help follow progress once treatment has been initiated as abnormalities in contrast detection should correct over time (Figure 43.4).

Toxicology Assays

A number of biomarkers and assays have been evaluated for efficacy in detecting mold and in vivo mycotoxins and mycotoxicosis (Table 43.7). For a review of the history of PCR-based diagnosis of mycotoxin producing fungi and their quantitative analysis see Niessen and Rahmani [21,97]. For a review of the benefits and limitations of fungal PCR assays, the reader is referred to Khot [98].

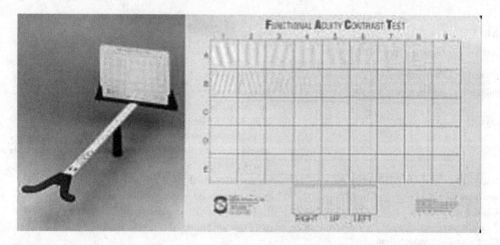

FIGURE 43.4 Visual contrast sensitivity (VCS) is an indicator of neurologic function of the visual system and is defined as a measure of the least amount of luminance contrast between darker and lighter areas of a defined pattern required for a viewer to distinguish the pattern from a homogeneous field. The test measures contrast sensitivity for five special frequencies, as spatial vision is accomplished via neurons selectively tuned to different spatial frequencies [42]. When abnormal, it is an indicator of neurologic dysfunction, but is not specific for a single neurologic insult, although it has been correlated with several, such as Lyme, Ciguatera, PEAS, and WDB-SBS. (Adapted from Hudnell 2005 and Shoemaker 2010.)

Laboratory Assessments

Tables 43.8 and 43.9 highlight laboratory tests utilized in the assessment of nutritional, endocrine, and immunologic status in patients suspected of mycotoxin-induced illness in our clinic [49,99,100]. The variety of symptomatology seen in mold illness may lead the physician to consider other conventional lab evaluations. While these are usually normal in mold illness, symptoms such as fatigue can be seen in illnesses such as iron deficiency, hypothyroidism, hepatitis, and so on. These illnesses and their lab evaluations should be considered in the process of evaluating patients suspected to have mold exposure. Additionally, these lab values can be used indirectly to help determine nutritional status (macrocytosis and folate deficiency for example). If VCS testing is positive or there is a history strongly suggestive of mold exposure then further evaluation for CIRS as denoted in Table 43.9 may be appropriate.

Imaging Studies

Functional Imaging of Mold-Injured Patients

Rea documented multiple immune abnormalities in 100 mold-exposed patients. Exposures to mold and mycotoxins were assessed by multiple methods: urine trichothecenes, serum antibodies, and intradermal skin testing. While obvious neurological symptoms were found in 70% of patients, autonomic nervous system abnormalities were seen in all 100 patients. A subgroup of 30 patients underwent triple-head single photon emission computed tomography (SPECT); 26 (86%) of these patients had abnormalities on SPECT scans consistent with a neurotoxicity pattern. In the glutathione-dependent areas of the cerebral hemispheres, the patterns were consistent with a decrease in flow and function and temporal lobe asymmetry. Neurological and psychological testing correlated well with triple SPECT scanning [101]. The severity of the neurological injury assessed clinically, however, did not correlate with severity of abnormalities on SPECT scan [102]. This study was limited in its application, but supports a more concerted effort to correlate SPECT imaging and brain injuries in mold-injured patients. Shoemaker has imaged mold-injured patients using MR spectroscopy, and compared to controls, findings suggest significant increases in lactate in the frontal lobes and hippocampus, thought to be secondary to capillary hypoperfusion and felt to correlate with reduced production of glutamate compared to glutamine in longstanding mold exposed patients [99].

TABLE 43.7

Mycotoxin Biomarkers and Assays

Mycotoxin or Mold	Assay and Marker	Tissue/Fluid	Comments	Ref
Aflatoxins	AFM1 AFB1-N7 guanine, AFB1-albumin.	Urine/Breast Milk :AFM1	9α-OH form of AFB1	Crews; Groopman
	ELISA DNA adducts: AFB1-N7-guanine	Urine	Indicator of acute exposure T1/2 9 hrs	Groopman
	AFB1-Albumin adducts	Serum	Indicator of exposure over 20 days	Crews
Aflatoxin B1,B2,G1,G2	Immunoaffinity and fluorometry	Urine	Moderate sensitivity (70.6%), specificity (100%)	Hooper
Blastomyces dermatitidis, Coccidioides immitis, Histoplasma capsulatum	Real Time Polymerase Chain Reaction Testing (PCR)	Serum or Body Fluids	Correlates well with conventional culture; more rapid diagnosis	Wengenack; Huang
Fumonisins	Sphinganine/ Sphingosine ratio	Urine and Blood	Elevation of Sphinganine; clear within three days of cessation of exposure: accurate in animals; efficacy questionable in humans; exposures do not correlate with levels, not recommended.	Sewram; Shephard
	HPLC coupled to electrospray ionization-mass spectrometry (HPLC-ESI-MS) for mycotoxins	Hair	Appears viable for Fumonisin B1, B2, and B3; limited clinical availability	Sewram
Ochratoxin A (OTA)	Reverse Phase Liquid Chromatography - OTA- Albumin	Serum/Urine	Serum levels two fold higher, but urine levels correlate better with actual exposure events	Huff; Russo; Scott
	Immunoaffinity and fluorometry	Urine	Poor sensitivity (17.5)	Hooper
Saratoxin G (SG)	Western Blot/Mass Spectrometry SG-Albumin adducts	Serum	Promising testing to date, but not clinically available	Yike
Trichothecenes	ELISA	Urine	Good sensitivity (94.5%) and specificity (100%)	Hooper

Source: Adapted from Huang et al., 2006; Sewram et al., 2003; Huff et al., 1979; Russo et al., 2005; Scott, 2005; Yike et al., 2006; Shephard et al., 2007; Crews et al., 2001; Groopman, 1994; Hooper, 2009; Wengenack and Binnicker, 2009.

TABLE 43.8

Laboratory Diagnostic Tests to Guide Nutritional Management during Mycotoxin-Related Illness

Screening Labs	Company	Notes	Rationale
Hormonal Assessment: DHEA, DHEA-S, Testosterone: Total and Free, Estradiol, Cortisol, Vitamin D, Pregnenolone, IGF-1	Lab Corp Quest Others	A screen for hormonal abnormalities often seen in patients: mycotoxins are disruptive to endocrine metabolism and have adverse influence on FSH, E2, cortisol receptors to name a few.	Mycotoxins may adversely influence hormonal function including FSH, estrogen, Vitamin D, IGF-1, pregnenolone and glucocorticoid activity. Basic assessment is considered prudent in adults. Proper management may result in relief of some symptoms.
Methylene Tetrahydrofolate (MTHFR) Gene Single Nucleotide Polymorphism	Lab Corp Quest Others	Genetic analysis of MTHFR polymorphisms known to influence activity of this	Methylation defects predispose to further membrane compromise in the presence of some mycotoxins, inducing further neurological damage, such as neural tube defects and susceptibility to toxic insult.
Nutritional Analysis	Lab Corp Quest Others	Functional nutritional analysis of standard chemistry analytes: CBC, lipid panel, CMP, SGGT, phosphorus, iron, etc.	Dysfunctional nutritional status plays a role in chronic inflammatory and neurodegenerative states, as is seen in mycotoxin-induced illness. Direct serum measurements of nutrients may be obtained as well if deemed necessary.
Red Cell Lipid Testing and Nutritional Analysis	Johns Hopkins Kennedy Krieger Institute with summary by BodyBio	Relative percentages of red blood cell (RBC) lipids; RBC lipid abnormalities and elevated levels of very long chain fats	An indirect representative measurement of cellular function via its delineation of the relative proportions of more than 40 fatty acids within cellular membranes: surface, mitochondrial, peroxisomal, etc. These lipids are crucial for signal transduction and proper organelle function. Once known, their relative percentages can be influenced with appropriate nutritional interventions. They may be altered in the setting of mycotoxin-induced illness.
Stool Analysis of Microbiome	Doctor's Data; Genova Diagnostics	Imbalanced flora leads to worsening of intestinal inflammatory states	Deficiencies in *Lactobacilli* predispose to compromised adsorption of some mycotoxins. Proper intestinal balance of the microbiome is important for modulating inflammatory cytokine production.

PROPOSED NUTRITIONAL INTERVENTIONS

GLUTATHIONE

Aflatoxins are common contaminants of nuts, corn, spices, copra (dried coconut), and figs. They are known to be human carcinogens, and AFB1 is metabolized through the liver via cytochrome P450 to AFB1-8,9 epoxide (AFBO) or to the less mutagenic forms AFM1, Q1, P1. The epoxy

TABLE 43.9

Laboratory Tests in Complications of Mycotoxin-Related Illness

Screening Labs	Laboratories	Notes	Rationale
Adrenocorticotrophic Hormone (ACTH)/ Cortisol	Lab Corp or Quest	ACTH–Lavender top cortisol–serum red-top or plasma lavender top	As MSH falls, elevated ACTH is associated with few symptoms. Marked increase in symptoms is seen when ACTH falls. Elevation of both ACTH and cortisol should correct with correction of dysregulated state; however, consider ACTH-secreting tumors.
Alpha Melanocyte Stimulating Hormone (α-MSH)	Lab Corp	Lavender-freeze with Trasylol preservative	Deficient in biotoxin illnesses and associated with impairment of cytokine and neurohormonal regulation; resulting symptoms: fatigue, unusual pain syndromes among others
Anticardiolipin Antibodies (ACLA) IgA, IgM, and IgG	Lab Corp or Quest	Citrated plasma (lt blue top); Alternate–serum	Seen in over 33% of children with biotoxin-associated illnesses; ACLAs are autoantibodies seen in collagen vascular diseases and predispose to coagulation abnormalities.
Antigliadin Antibodies (AGA) IgA and IgM	Lab Corp	Serum	While seen in patients with celiac disease, they are no longer felt to be specific for this illness. Ingestion of gliadin initiates a proinflammatory cytokine release and may cause cognitive symptoms shortly thereafter. They are seen in patients with low levels of MSH and in over 50% of Shoemaker's pediatric patients with biotoxin illness.
Antidiuretic Hormone (ADH)/osmolality	Lab Corp or Quest	ADH-Plasma in lavender-top; Osmolality-serum	Symptoms associated with dysregulation of ADH: dehydration, frequent urination, excessive thirst, and sensitivity to static electrical shocks.
Complement 3a (C3a) and Complement 4a (C4a) by RIA (not Futhan)	Quest or Lab Corp	Lavender-freeze	Elevations of C3a and C4a are seen in acute Lyme and, to a lesser degree, mold-induced illness; C4a elevations prominent in mold exposures. These are split products of complement activation. Sustained elevation in plasma levels seen within 12 hours of exposure. Results in increased vascular permeability, release of inflammatory components from leukocytes; induce vasospasm in capillaries
			Marker of capillary hypoperfusion from innate immune activation; consistent with ongoing activation of mannose binding lectin pathway of complement activation secondary to MASP2 enzyme (Wallis 2007)
Deep Aerobic Nasal Culture for multiply antibiotic resistant Coag Negative Staph (MARCoNS)	Lab Corp	Nasal swab	MARCoNS is seen in 80% of cases and none in controls. It is associated with elevations in cytokines that exacerbate neurologic function and must be addressed in the process of treatment to bring patients to recovery.

continued

TABLE 43.9 (*continued*)

Laboratory Tests in Complications of Mycotoxin-Related Illness

Screening Labs	Laboratories	Notes	Rationale
Human Leukocyte Antigen DR (HLA DR) by PCR	Lab Corp	Lavender–room temperature	The following haplotypes are found with much higher frequency in biotoxin-injured patients: DRB1-4, DQ3, DRB4-53, DRB1-11, DQ3-DRB3-52B.
Leptin	Lab Corp	Serum or plasma– refrigerate. stable for up to seven days	A adipocytokine produced by fat cells in the setting of elevated lipid levels; promotes storage of fat and influences hypothalamic function; elevated peripheral cytokines result in phosphorylation of the leptin receptor leading to leptin resistance and deficiency of MSH production.
Matrix Metalloproteinase 9 (MMP-9)	Lab Corp, Esoterix, or Quest	SST-freeze	Extracellular matrix zinc-dependent enzyme produced by neutrophils and macrophages involved in remodeling of the ECM; elevations associated with onset of COPD, atherosclerosis, demyelinating diseases, and others; stimulated by IL1, IL2, TNF, IL-1B, α and γ interferons; may be elevated
Vascular Endothelial Growth Factor (VEGF)	Quest	Plasma only; lavender–freeze	Low in mold illness and results in compromise of oxygen delivery secondary to degeneration of capillary growth and repair
Vasointestinal Peptide (VIP)	Lab Corp	Lav- freeze with Trasylol preservative	A neuroregulatory hormone which binds to receptors in the SCN of the hypothalamus; regulates peripheral cytokine responses, pulmonary artery pressure, and systemic inflammatory response; raises cAMP required for cell signaling; often deficient in mold exposed patients, which may be associated with dyspnea and depression
Transforming Growth Factor Beta 1 (TGF-β1)	Lab Corp or Quest	Lavender-freeze; use platelet poor plasma.	Plays a key role in directing immunity towards Th17 pathway. Elevated TGF-β1 and IL-6 are associated with manifestations of autoimmunity

Chronic Systemic Inflammatory Response Syndrome (CIRS) Labs as Delineated in Shoemaker's Hypothesis SCN: Suprachiasmatic Nucleus; IL: Interleukin; MASP2: Mannose-binding Protein Associated Serine Protease 2.

Source: Adapted from Shoemaker, 2007; Shoemaker and Maizel, 2009; Shoemaker, Rash, and Simon.

group readily binds to cellular macromolecules, including protein and DNA, to form adducts that may ultimately lead to cancer. AFB1-N7-guanine adduct is excreted in the urine of those affected. Animal models exposed to AFB1 stimulate the induction of glutathione S-transferase (GST), catalyzing the reaction that binds AFBO and renders it noncarcinogenic (Figure 43.5). Interestingly, mice are resistant to aflatoxin carcinogenesis and have GST activity three- to fivefold greater than rats, which are susceptible to carcinogenic aflatoxins. The activity of human GST is even lower than that of rats [9]. Johannessen's work shows that the depletion of intracellular glutathione, elevation of TGF-β1, IL-6, and IL-8 in a human alveolar model in the presence of citrinin and gliotoxin is consistent with a proinflammatory state. Fumonisin B1 exposed rats were found to have significantly increased number of placental GST + hepatocytes compared to nonexposed groups [103]. Intestinal epithelial cells exposed to patulin, a common fruit-based mycotoxin, rapidly lose

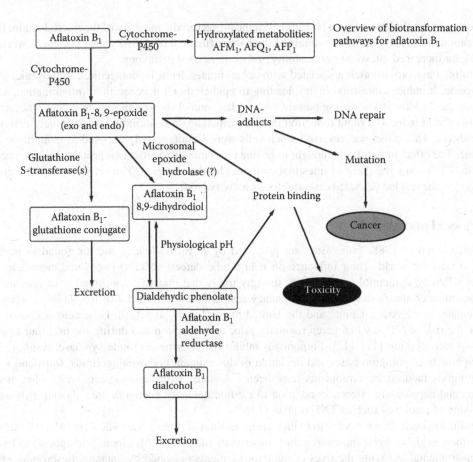

FIGURE 43.5 Aflatoxin B1 Metabolism. (Adapted from Murphy, 2006.)

organization of tight junctions, implying increased IP. Pre-exposure to cysteine and glutathione prevented intestinal epithelial cells (IECs) from patulin injury. Patulin toxicity was potentiated by the use of glutathione-depleting agents as well [104]. Finally, reduced glutathione administered to rats bearing aflatoxin B1-induced liver tumors saw regression of tumor growth and extension of survival times [105].

As noted earlier, the toxicity of Pp is copper dependent and involves lipid peroxidation. Glutathione-S-transferases are known to detoxify the endogenous products of lipid peroxidation [106]. In vitro studies have shown that glutathione binds copper, handing it off to metallothionein (MT) [107]. Additionally, depletion of cellular GSH results in a 50% reduction in incorporation of Cu into MT. Thus, elevating total body GSH may exert a protective mechanism in the setting of pfiesteria-induced illness.

Butenolide, a fusarium mycotoxin found in cereal grains, is known to deplete intracellular glutathione (GSH) and to induce cytotoxicity in human hepatic cells (HepG2). GSH depletion and ROS production were drastically reduced and cellular cytotoxicity was completely abated by GSH, N-acetylcysteine (NAC), and dithiothreitol (DTT) [109].

N-Acetyl Cysteine, Cysteine

Ochratoxin A (OTA) is a food-borne mycotoxin that significantly impairs the barrier function of the gut epithelia and appears to involve the loss of claudins 3 and 4 from the detergent-insoluble membrane microdomains of lipid rafts. These microdomains are responsible for tight junction integrity.

Incubation of the IEC model with N-acetyl cysteine preserved the integrity of the microdomain, the localization of the claudins and maintained the barrier function of caco-2 cells [73], thus lowering the risk for increased intestinal permeability and its associated pathology.

Patulin, a mycotoxin often associated with contaminated fruit, is mutagenic, carcinogenic, and teratogenic. It induces intestinal injury, leading to epithelial cell degeneration, inflammation, and hemorrhage. In vitro studies using patulin with an IEC model showed that micromolar concentrations of patulin induced a rapid reduction in TER, which again is an indirect reflection of cellular permeability. This effect was reversed when cells were simultaneously exposed to glutathione or cysteine. The effect of patulin is thought to be due to an inhibitory effect on protein tyrosine phosphatase (PTP) a key regulator of intestinal epithelial barrier function. The active site of PTP contains a cysteine residue (Cys215) essential for its activity [104].

FOLATE AND FUMONISINS

First discovered in 1988, fumonisins are produced by *F. Verticillioides* and are found in maize crops around the world. Their influence on neural tube defects (NTDs) is covered elsewhere in this text. Briefly, epidemiological studies strongly imply that maternal consumption of fumonisin B1-contaminated maize during early pregnancy results in an increased risk for NTDs in women (Guatemala, South Arica, China, and the United States/Texas) [108,110]. Folic acid is known to reduce the risk of NTDs when given regularly prior to conception and during the first four to six weeks postconception [111,112]. Fumonisins inhibit the enzyme ceramide synthase, resulting in elevation of free sphingoid bases and depletion of downstream glycosphingolipids. Imbalances in sphingolipids induced by fumonisins have been associated with carcinogenic, teratogenic, neurotoxic, and hepatotoxic effects, in addition to cardiopulmonary edema in animals and increased expression of cytokines such as TNF-α [108,113].

Patulin, has been shown in vitro to induce the generation of superoxide radicals [114]. DHLA, but not α-lipoic acid, has been shown to reduce superoxide radicals [116]. Lipoic acid appears to have been instrumental in saving the lives of numerous patients poisoned by amanita mushrooms who otherwise would have died [116]. Yet more recent evidence suggests that there may be great methylation demands placed on the body when α-lipoic acid or DHLA are utilized in an animal model. Evaluation of homocysteine and S-adenosylhomocysteine(SAH) levels may be warranted [117]. Chronic elevation of SAH is correlated with elevations of homocysteine and DNA hypomethylation in cellular studies [118]. Chronic nutritional deficiencies in folate, as is likely in fumonisin-induced illness, may predispose to elevations in SAH and homocysteine [119], suggesting that monitoring these levels is prudent during lipoic acid supplementation.

Folate plays an important role in DNA biosynthesis and amino acid metabolism. The primary receptors for cellular folate delivery are reduced folate carrier (RFC1) and receptor-mediated folate receptors (FR): α, β, δ, and γ. These receptors are characterized by the varying degrees of tissue expression and preferences for oxidized versus reduced folates [120]. Depletion of complex glycosphingolipids by fumonisins appears to disrupt GPI-anchored folate receptors and likely contributes to fumonisin-induced NTDs [120–122]. Martinez de Villarreal found that supplementation with 5 mg of folic acid once weekly cut the incidence of NTDs by 50% in two years along the Texas-Mexico border, where fumonisin contamination and corn intake were thought to contribute to NTDs, suggesting that folic acid may be capable of diminishing mycotoxin-induced neurologic defects [123].

VITAMIN B12

Anyanwu and Campbell report that the majority of patients presenting with chronic exposures to toxigenic molds were found to have persistent vitamin B12 deficiency in spite of adequate intake [124]. Unfortunately, data is not presented for this statement, nor is it referenced in Anyanwu's paper. However, Campbell published a review of *Mold and Mycotoxins* in the same year, referring to more than 200 patients who had symptoms including headache, fatigue, memory loss, and peripheral neuropathy with patterns suggestive of demyelination [37].These are all findings consistent with B12 deficiency, though certainly not exclusive of other etiologies. The case in support of mycotoxin-induced B12 deficiency is made biochemically at least in part by the number of one-carbon units in saccharomyces cerevisiae and the requirements of glycine, serine, and folate in maintaining the flow of these units [124] While B12 is certainly important in helping to resolve some cases of fatigue, memory loss, and peripheral neuropathy, additional research is required to establish the mechanism of B12 deficiency in mycotoxic patients. To the degree that B12 supports folate metabolism (which is more clearly associated with mycotoxin exposures), it is likely a beneficial nutrient in the mold toxic patient.

VITAMIN E

Citrinin, zearalenone, and T-2 toxin have been shown in vitro to induce Hsp 70, which exerts a protective effect regarding cytotoxicity. There was less expression of Hsp 70 when cells were pretreated with vitamin E (type unspecified), and likewise no relative loss of cell viability, implying a protective effect of vitamin E [125]. Zearalenone-treated mice develop DNA adducts in the kidney and liver. Pretreatment with alpha-tocopherol significantly reduces these DNA adducts [126].

ZINC

Ochratoxin A (OTA) is known to induce nephrotoxic, immunotoxic, and hepatotoxic effects. When intracellular zinc stores are depleted in cells exposed to OTA, tight junction permeability is increased, accompanied by an increase in apoptosis of intestinal epithelial cells. These effects are fully reversed with zinc supplementation. It is known that OTA upregulates zinc-dependent metallothionein gene activity and thus is postulated that perhaps this mycotoxin acts via generation of redox imbalance involving zinc [127].

BUTYRATE

Butyrate is a short-chain fatty acid produced by clostridia and a lactic acid bacterium. It has widening use in the treatment of cancer and neurodegenerative disorders. In vitro studies using sodium butyrate (SB) have shown strong inhibition of yeast in a concentration-dependent manner, resulting in a reduction of filamentation in *C. albicans* and melanization and capsule formation in *C. neoformans*. Additionally and most importantly, SB decreases yeast biofilm formation and enhances the activity of macrophages by increasing their production of reactive oxygen species. Both phagocytosis and antifungal activity of macrophages significantly increased in this study utilizing SB. While some strains of lactic acid bacteria are considered adsorbants for mycotoxins, an additional mechanism by which they discouraged mycotoxin production is downregulation of fungal overgrowth by the mechanisms noted here [128]. Other known roles of sodium butyrate include inhibition of tumorigenesis, promotion of healthy commensal bacteria, function as a key energy source for enterocytes, acceleration and proliferation of gastrointestinal epithelium, stimulation of digestive enzyme function, and suppression of IL-6, interferon gamma, and IL-1B. All of these qualities help improve gut integrity and reduce the degree of mycotoxin-induced risk.

UNDECANOIC ACID AND SYNTHETIC METABOLITES

Long-chain fatty acids have been long known to have antimycotic activity and have been in common use clinically for many years [129]. Undecanoic acid's properties are thought to be due to its ability to inhibit production of exocellular keratinase, lipase, and several phospholipids [130].

More recent synthetic derivatives of undecanoic acid have taken advantage of microbial dependence on iron for proper metabolism and have incorporated an iron-chelating hydroxamate to this 10-carbon-chain fat, resulting in more efficient growth-inhibition rates against *Aspergillus* and *Candida* species [129].

MYCOTOXIN BINDERS AND BIOTRANSFORMANTS

The literature is replete with studies reviewing mycotoxin adsorbents— hereafter known as mycotoxin binders (MB)— in animal feed and, to a lesser degree, the food supply [131–133]. They are summarized in Kolosova's paper. The bulk of these studies are performed using animals. With few exceptions, most agents have not been amply studied in humans. However, they are now being introduced to animal feed in Europe as adsorbents; thus they may be of clinical significance in coming years.

Key inorganic MBs include aluminosilicates, such as hydrated sodium calcium aluminosilicate (HSCAS), zeolites, bentonites, and activated carbons. HSCAS is a heat-processed, purified calcium montmorillonite clay known as NovaSil, and is the only MB in this group that has been tested in animals and humans for safety [135–137]. Kolosova reviews the aluminosilicates in detail. Calcium montmorillonite clay is highly effective at binding aflatoxins but appears limited in its ability to bind other mycotoxins. Activated charcoal may bind aflatoxin, zearalenone (ZER), and deoxynivalenol (DON). As of 2006, no adsorbent product was approved by the U.S. FDA for the prevention or treatment of mycotoxicosis, though several are recognized as safe feed additives (GRAS) [138]. Diatomaceous earth appears to bind aflatoxin, sterigmatocystin, T-2 toxin, zearalenone, and ochratoxin in vitro [139]. However, this does not necessarily translate to in vivo results.

Organic MBs include cholestyramine, divinylbenzene-styrene, and polyvinylpyrrolidone. As previously noted, CSM is an insoluble quaternary ammonium exchange resin that for many years has been in common use as a bile acid resin binder in the management of cholesterol. It is an effective binder in vitro for OTA, fumonisins, and ZEA [135], and has been used by Shoemaker and others with success, as noted elsewhere in this chapter.

Microorganism-derived MBs include *Saccharomyces cerevisiae* and lactic acid bacteria (LAB) [135]. These agents work on multiple levels and bind different mycotoxins to cell wall components. Various strains of lactobacillus produce antifungal metabolites that inhibit fungal growth in vitro. Their potential strength in animals and humans would be in their mycotoxin binding activity and, indeed, the cell walls of several strains have been reported to bind aflatoxin B1 in vitro and in vivo. Strains shown to be beneficial in vitro include the probiotics Lb. rhamnosus GG, and Lb. rhamnosus, with more than 80% of the toxin trapped in a 20 ug/ml solution [140].

CLINICAL SUMMARY

Mycotoxins are ubiquitous and are increasingly associated with the findings of chronic systemic inflammatory response syndrome and its related symptoms. While broad populations are affected subclinically, clinical manifestations occur in the genetically susceptible patient. While most certainly not the cause of all systemic inflammatory disease, they should be considered in patients presenting with signs and symptoms of unexplained fatigue, cognitive dysfunction, respiratory symptoms such as shortness of breath, gastrointestinal symptoms, muscle pain, headaches, and/or photophobia. It is very important to note that mycotoxins are only one of many contributors to mold illness seen in water-damaged buildings, but they very likely play a role in the genesis of WDB-SBS, and possibly inflammatory bowel disease. Clinical approaches are presented to assist in the recognition of common medical conditions exacerbated by food- and airborne mycotoxins. In addition to avoidance of further toxin exposure, nutritional support that may facilitate the body's innate mechanisms is presented (Table 43.6).

ACKNOWLEDGMENTS

The author wishes to thank Bill Cowhig, Tom Wnorowski, PhD, Reginald Scott, and Raymond Skinner for their assistance in the preparation of this manuscript.

REFERENCES

1. Robbins, C.A., et al., *Health effects of mycotoxins in indoor air: A critical review.* Applied Occupational and Environmental Hygiene, 2000. 15(10): p. 773–784.
2. Forgacs, J., et al., *Mycotoxicoses I. Relationship of toxic fungi to moldy-feed toxicosis in poultry.* Avian Diseases, 1962. 6(3): p. 363–380.
3. Blount, W., *Turkey "X" disease.* Turkeys, 1961. 9(2): p. 52.
4. Bennett, J. and M. Klich, *Mycotoxins, Clinical Microbiological Reviews 16.* Full text via CrossRefl View Record in Scopusl Cited By in Scopus (422), 2003: p. 497–516.
5. Górny, R.L., et al., *Fungal fragments as indoor air biocontaminants.* Applied and Environmental Microbiology, 2002. 68(7): p. 3522–3531.
6. Bush, R.K., et al., *The medical effects of mold exposure.* Journal of Allergy and Clinical Immunology, 2006. 117(2): p. 326–333.
7. Greenberger, P.A., *Allergic bronchopulmonary aspergillosis.* Journal of Allergy and Clinical Immunology, 2002. 110(5): p. 685–692.
8. Jarvis, B.B. and J.D. Miller, *Mycotoxins as harmful indoor air contaminants.* Applied Microbiology and Biotechnology, 2005. 66(4): p. 367–372.
9. Murphy, P.A., et al., *Food mycotoxins: An update.* Journal of Food Science, 2006. 71(5): p. R51–R65.
10. Bryden, W.L., *Mycotoxins in the food chain: Human health implications.* Asia Pac J Clin Nutr, 2007. 16(Suppl 1): p. 95–101.
11. van Egmond, H.P., R.C. Schothorst, and M.A. Jonker, *Regulations relating to mycotoxins in food.* Analytical and Bioanalytical Chemistry, 2007. 389(1): p. 147–157.
12. Joint, F., *WHO Expert Committee on Food Additives (JECFA)(2001) Evaluation of certain mycotoxins in food: 56th Report of the JECFA.* JECFA, Geneva (see http://www. who.int/gb/ebwha/pdf_files/EB110/eeb1106. pdf).
13. Mannon, J. and E. Johnson, *Fungi down on the farm.* New Scientist, 1985. 105: p. 12–16.
14. Robens, J. and K. Cardwell, *The costs of mycotoxin management to the USA: Management of aflatoxins in the United States.* Toxin Reviews, 2003. 22(2–3): p. 139–152.
15. Williams, J.H., et al., *Human aflatoxicosis in developing countries: A review of toxicology, exposure, potential health consequences, and interventions.* American Journal of Clinical Nutrition, 2004. 80(5): p. 1106.
16. Van Egmond, H. and M. Jonker, *Regulations and limits for mycotoxins in fruits and vegetables.* Mycotoxins in fruits and vegetables. Elsevier, Amsterdam, Netherlands, 2008: p. 45–74.
17. Weidenbörner, M., *Mycotoxins in Foodstuffs.* Springer Science + Business Media LLC, 2008.
18. Karlovsky, P., *Biological detoxification of fungal toxins and its use in plant breeding, feed and food production.* Natural Toxins, 1999. 7(1): p. 1–23.
19. Munkvold, G.P., *Cultural and genetic approaches to managing mycotoxins in maize.* Annual Review of Phytopathology, 2003. 41(1): p. 99–116.
20. Duvick, J., *Prospects for reducing fumonisin contamination of maize through genetic modification.* Environmental Health Perspectives, 2001. 109(Suppl 2): p. 337.
21. Rahmani, A., S. Jinap, and F. Soleimany, *Qualitative and quantitative analysis of mycotoxins.* Comprehensive Reviews in Food Science and Food Safety, 2009. 8(3): p. 202–251.
22. Fog Nielsen, K., *Mycotoxin production by indoor molds.* Fungal Genetics and Biology, 2003. 39(2): p. 103–117.
23. Shoemaker, R.C., L. Mark, and S. McMahon, *Research Committee Report on Diagnosis and Treatment of Chronic Inflammatory Response Syndrome Caused by Exposure to the Interior Environment of Water-Damaged Buildings.* 2010.
24. Strickland, M.H.V., *How solid is the Academy position paper on mold exposure?* Journal of Allergy and Clinical Immunology, 2006. 118(3): p. 763–764.
25. Lieberman, A., W. Rea, and L. Curtis, *Adverse health effects of indoor mold exposure.* Journal of Allergy and Clinical Immunology, 2006. 118(3): p. 763.
26. Vesper, S., et al., *Quantitative PCR analysis of molds in the dust from homes of asthmatic children in North Carolina.* J. Environ. Monit, 2007. 9(8): p. 826–830.

27. Thrasher, J.D. and S. Crawley, *The biocontaminants and complexity of damp indoor spaces: More than what meets the eyes.* Toxicology and Industrial Health, 2009. 25(9–10): p. 583–615.

28. Burkholder, J.M., et al., *New "phantom" dinoflagellate is the causative agent of major estuarine fish kills.* Nature, 1992. 358(6385):407–10.

29. Grattan, L.M., et al., *Learning and memory difficulties after environmental exposure to waterways containing toxin-producing Pfiesteria or Pfiesteria-like dinoflagellates.* Lancet, 1998. 352(9127): p. 532–539.

30. Shoemaker, R.C., *Residential and recreational acquisition of possible estuary-associated syndrome: A new approach to successful diagnosis and treatment.* Environmental Health Perspectives, 2001. 109(Suppl 5): p. 791.

31. Morris J.G. Jr., et al., *Occupational exposure to Pfiesteria species in estuarine waters is not a risk factor for illness.* Environmental Health Perspectives, 2006. 114(7): p. 1038.

32. Moeller, P.D.R., et al., *Metal complexes and free radical toxins produced by Pfiesteria piscicida.* Environmental Science & Technology, 2007. 41(4): p. 1166–1172.

33. Burkholder, J.A.M. and H.G. Marshall, *Toxigenic pfiesteria species—updates on biology, ecology, toxins, and impacts.* Harmful Algae, 2011.

34. Friedman, M.A. and B.E. Levin, *Neurobehavioral effects of harmful algal bloom (HAB) toxins: a critical review.* Journal of the International Neuropsychological Society, 2005. 11(03): p. 331–338.

35. World Health Organization, *WHO guidelines for indoor air quality: Dampness and mould.* 2009: World Health Organzation.

36. Park, J.H, and J.M. Cox–Ganser, *Mold exposure and respiratory health in damp indoor environments.* Frontiers in Bioscience (Elite edition), 2011. 3: p. 757.

37. Campbell, A.W., et al., *Mold and mycotoxins: effects on the neurological and immune systems in humans.* Advances in Applied Microbiology, 2004. 55: p. 375–406.

38. Johanning, E., et al., *Health and immunology study following exposure to toxigenic fungi (Stachybotrys chartarum) in a water-damaged office environment.* International Archives of Occupational and Environmental Health, 1996. 68(4): p. 207–218.

39. Douwes, J., et al., *Fungal extracellular polysaccharides in house dust as a marker for exposure to fungi: Relations with culturable fungi, reported home dampness, and respiratory symptoms.* Journal of Allergy and Clinical Immunology, 1999. 103(3): p. 494–500.

40. Monod, M., et al., *Secreted proteases from pathogenic fungi.* International Journal of Medical Microbiology: IJMM, 2002. 292(5–6): p. 405.

41. Birch, M., D.W. Denning, and G.D. Robson, *Comparison of extracellular phospholipase activities in clinical and environmental Aspergillus fumigatus isolates.* Medical Mycology, 2004. 42(1): p. 81–86.

42. Campbell, A., et al., *Neural autoantibodies and neurophysiologic abnormalities in patients exposed to molds in water-damaged buildings.* Archives of Environmental Health, 2003. 58(8): p. 464.

43. Thrasher, J.D., K. Kilburn, and N. Immers, *Indoor Environment Resulting From Water Intrusion, Part I.* 2006.

44. Górny, R.L., *Filamentous microorganisms and their fragments in indoor air–a review.* Ann Agric Environ Med, 2004. 11: p. 185–197.

45. Islam, Z., J.R. Harkema, and J.J. Pestka, *Satratoxin G from the black mold Stachybotrys chartarum evokes olfactory sensory neuron loss and inflammation in the murine nose and brain.* Environmental Health Perspectives, 2006. 114(7): p. 1099.

46. Shoemaker, R.C. and D.E. House, *Sick building syndrome (SBS) and exposure to water-damaged buildings: time series study, clinical trial and mechanisms.* Neurotoxicology and Teratology, 2006. 28(5): p. 573–588.

47. Shoemaker, R.C. and H.K. Hudnell, *Possible estuary-associated syndrome: Symptoms, vision, and treatment.* Environmental Health Perspectives, 2001. 109(5): p. 539.

48. Shoemaker, R.C., J.M. Rash, and E.W. Simon, *Sick building syndrome in water damaged buildings: Generalization of the chronic biotoxin-associated illness paradigm to indoor toxic fungi.* http://www.survivingmold.com/docs/Resources/Shoemaker%20Papers/Johanning_book_5_06.pdf.

49. Shoemaker, R. and M. Maizel, *Innate immunity, MR spectroscopy, HLA DR, TGF beta-1, VIP and capillary hypoperfusion define acute and chronic human illness acquired following exposure to water-damaged buildings.* http://www.survivingmold.com/products1/innate-immunity-mr-spectroscopy-hla-dr-tgf-beta-1-c4a-vip-and-capillary-hypoperfusion-define-acute-and-chronic-illness-acquired-after-exposure-to-wdb-product-details.

50. Rand, T., et al., *Microanatomical changes in alveolar type II cells in juvenile mice intratracheally exposed to Stachybotrys chartarum spores and toxin.* Toxicological Sciences, 2002. 65(2): p. 239–245.

51. Steinman, L., *A brief history of Th 17, the first major revision in the Th 1/Th 2 hypothesis of T cell–mediated tissue damage.* Nature Medicine, 2007. 13(2): p. 139.

52. Tato, C.M. and J.J. O'Shea, *Immunology: What does it mean to be just 17?* Nature, 2006. 441: p. 166–168.

53. Korn, T., et al., *IL-21 initiates an alternative pathway to induce proinflammatory TH17 cells.* Nature, 2007. 448(7152): p. 484–487.

54. Kebir, H., et al., *Human TH17 lymphocytes promote blood-brain barrier disruption and central nervous system inflammation.* Nature Medicine, 2007. 13(10): p. 1173–1175.

55. Lazarus, A.A., B. Thilagar, and S.A. McKay, *Allergic bronchopulmonary aspergillosis.* Disease A Month, 2008. 54(8): p. 547–564.

56. Nam, H.S., et al., *Clinical characteristics and treatment outcomes of chronic necrotizing pulmonary aspergillosis: A review of 43 cases.* International Journal of Infectious Diseases, 2010. 14(6): p. e479–e482.

57. Zmeili, O. and A. Soubani, *Pulmonary aspergillosis: A clinical update.* QJM, 2007. 100(6): p. 317.

58. Delhaes, L., E. Frealle, and C. Pinel, *Serum markers for allergic bronchopulmonary aspergillosis in cystic fibrosis: State of the art and further challenges.* Medical Mycology, 2010. 48(O1): p. 77–87.

59. Maresca, M. and Fantini, J, *Some food-associated mycotoxins as potential risk factors in humans predisposed to chronic intestinal inflammatory diseases.* Toxicon, 2010. 56: p. 282–294.

60. Friedman, S. and R. Blumberg, Chapter 295. *Inflammatory Bowel Disease.* Harrison's Principles of Internal Medicine, 18th Ed. McGraw Hill Medical, 2012.

61. Baumgart, D.C. and S.R. Carding, *Inflammatory bowel disease: Cause and immunobiology.* Lancet, 2007. 369(9573): p. 1627–1640.

62. Mangan, P.R., et al., *Transforming growth factor-β induces development of the TH17 lineage.* Nature, 2006. 441(7090): p. 231–234.

63. Bullock, N.R., J.C.L. Booth, and G.R. Gibson, *Comparative composition of bacteria in the human intestinal microflora during remission and active ulcerative colitis.* Current Issues in Intestinal Microbiology, 2004. 5(2): p. 59–64.

64. Fabia, R., et al., *Impairment of bacterial flora in human ulcerative colitis and experimental colitis in the rat.* Digestion, 1993. 54(4): p. 248–255.

65. Swidsinski, A., et al., *Mucosal flora in inflammatory bowel disease.* Gastroenterology, 2002. 122(1): p. 44–54.

66. Seksik, P., et al., *Alterations of the dominant faecal bacterial groups in patients with Crohn's disease of the colon.* Gut, 2003. 52(2): p. 237.

67. Tenk, I., E. Fodor, and C. Szathmary, *The effect of pure Fusarium toxins (T-2, F-2, DAS) on the microflora of the gut and on plasma glucocorticoid levels in rat and swine.* Zentralblatt für Bakteriologie, Mikrobiologie und Hygiene. 1. Abt. Originale A, Medizinische Mikrobiologie, Infektionskrankheiten und Parasitologie = *Medical microbiology, infectiousdiseases, parasitology.* International Journal of Microbiology and Hygiene, A, Medical microbiology, infectiousdiseases, parasitology, 1982. 252(3): p. 384.

68. Waché, Y.J., et al., *Impact of deoxynivalenol on the intestinal microflora of pigs.* International Journal of Molecular Sciences, 2009. 10(1): p. 1–17.

69. Gratz, S., et al., *Lactobacillus rhamnosus strain GG modulates intestinal absorption, fecal excretion, and toxicity of aflatoxin B1 in rats.* Applied and Environmental Microbiology, 2006. 72(11): p. 7398–7400.

70. Gratz, S., et al., *Lactobacillus rhamnosus strain GG reduces aflatoxin B1 transport, metabolism, and toxicity in Caco-2 Cells.* Applied and Environmental Microbiology, 2007. 73(12): p. 3958–3964.

71. Pinton, P., et al., *Deoxynivalenol impairs porcine intestinal barrier function and decreases the protein expression of claudin-4 through a mitogen-activated protein kinase-dependent mechanism.* Journal of Nutrition, 2010. 140(11): p. 1956.

72. Pinton, P., et al., *The food contaminant deoxynivalenol, decreases intestinal barrier permeability and reduces claudin expression.* Toxicology and Applied Pharmacology, 2009. 237(1): p. 41–48.

73. Lambert, D., et al., *Ochratoxin A displaces claudins from detergent resistant membrane microdomains.* Biochemical and Biophysical Research Communications, 2007. 358(2): p. 632–636.

74. McLaughlin, J., et al., *The mycotoxin patulin, modulates tight junctions in caco-2 cells.* Toxicology in Vitro, 2009. 23(1): p. 83–89.

75. Bouhet, S., et al., *The mycotoxin fumonisin B1 alters the proliferation and the barrier function of porcine intestinal epithelial cells.* Toxicological Sciences, 2004. 77(1): p. 165–171.

76. Loiseau, N., et al., *Fumonisin B1 exposure and its selective effect on porcine jejunal segment: Sphingolipids, glycolipids and trans-epithelial passage disturbance.* Biochemical Pharmacology, 2007. 74(1): p. 144–152.

77. Nazli, A., et al., *Enterocyte cytoskeleton changes are crucial for enhanced translocation of nonpathogenic Escherichia coli across metabolically stressed gut epithelia.* Infection and Immunity, 2006. 74(1): p. 192–201.

78. Maresca, M., et al., *Both direct and indirect effects account for the pro-inflammatory activity of entero-pathogenic mycotoxins on the human intestinal epithelium: Stimulation of interleukin-8 secretion, potentiation of interleukin-1β effect and increase in the transepithelial passage of commensal bacteria.* Toxicology and Applied Pharmacology, 2008. 228(1): p. 84–92.

79. Cario, E., *Bacterial interactions with cells of the intestinal mucosa: Toll-like receptors and NOD2.* Gut, 2005. 54(8): p. 1182.

80. Carroccio, A., et al., *Treatment of giardiasis reverses' active'coeliac disease to "latent"coeliac disease.* European Journal of Gastroenterology & Hepatology, 2001. 13(9): p. 1101.

81. De Hertogh, G., et al., *Evidence for the involvement of infectious agents in the pathogenesis of Crohn's disease.* World Journal of Gastroenterology: WJG, 2008. 14(6): p. 845.

82. Bhandari, N., C. Brown, and R. Sharma, *Fumonisin B1-induced localized activation of cytokine network in mouse liver.* Food and Chemical Toxicology, 2002. 40(10): p. 1483–1491.

83. Marin, D., et al., *Changes in performance, blood parameters, humoral and cellular immune responses in weanling piglets exposed to low doses of aflatoxin.* Journal of Animal Science, 2002. 80(5): p. 1250.

84. Reponen, T., et al., *Visually observed mold and moldy odor versus quantitatively measured microbial exposure in homes.* Science of the Total Environment, 2010. 408(22): p. 5565–5574.

85. Haugland, R. and S. Vesper, *Method of identifying and quantifying specific fungi and bacteria*, 2002, Google Patents.

86. Vesper, S., et al., *Development of an environmental relative moldiness index for US homes.* Journal of Occupational and Environmental Medicine, 2007. 49(8): p. 829.

87. Roussel, S., et al., *Characteristics of dwellings contaminated by moulds.* J Environ Monit, 2008. 10(6): p. 724–729.

88. Larsson, M., et al., *Can we trust cross-sectional studies when studying the risk of moisture-related problems indoor for asthma in children?* International Journal of Environmental Health Research, 2011. 21(4): p. 237–247.

89. Cai, G.H., et al., *Quantitative PCR analysis of fungal DNA in Swedish day care centers and comparison with building characteristics and allergen levels.* Indoor Air, 2009. 19(5): p. 392–400.

90. P&K, E.L., *Environmental Relative Moldiness Index (ERMI).* http://www.emlab.com.

91. *Classification of Fungi.* CABI databases 10th. [Available from: http://www.speciesfungorum.org/Names/fundic.asp.]

92. Lerda, D, *Mycotoxins Factsheet.* 4th ed. JRC Technical Notes, 2011. http://irmm.jrc.ec.europa.eu/EURLs/eurl_mycotoxins/Pages/index.aspx.

93. Database, C.-K.F. *CBS-KNAW Fungal Biodiversity Centre of the Netherlands.* Available from: www.cbs.knaw.nl/databases.

94. Hudnell, H.K., *Chronic biotoxin-associated illness: Multiple-system symptoms, a vision deficit, and effective treatment.* Neurotoxicology and Teratology, 2005. 27(5): p. 733–743.

95. Swinker, M. and W.A. Burke, *Visual contrast sensitivity as a diagnostic tool.* Environmental Health Perspectives, 2002. 110(3): p. A120.

96. Shoemaker, R.C., D. House, and J.C. Ryan, *Defining the neurotoxin derived illness chronic ciguatera using markers of chronic systemic inflammatory disturbances: A case/control study.* Neurotoxicology and Teratology, 2010. 32(6): p. 633–639.

97. Niessen, L., *PCR-based diagnosis and quantification of mycotoxin producing fungi.* International Journal of Food Microbiology, 2007. 119(1–2): p. 38–46.

98. Khot, P.D. and D.N. Fredricks, *PCR-based diagnosis of human fungal infections.* Expert Review of Anti-Infective Therapy, 2009. 7(10): p. 1201.

99. Shoemaker, R.C. and M.D.M.S. Maizel, *Exposure to interior environments of water-damaged buildings causes a CFS-like illness in pediatric patients: a case/control study.* Bulletin of the IACFS/ME, 2009. 17(2): p. 69–81.

100. Shoemaker, R., Letter to Barbara Shane PhD., Executive Secretary National Toxicology Program, NIEHS/NIH PO Box 12233-MD A3-01, 111 TW Alexander Dr., Research Triangle Park, NC 27709. 11/20/07.

101. Rea, W.J., et al., *Effects of toxic exposure to molds and mycotoxins in building-related illnesses.* Archives of Environmental Health, 2003. 58(7): p. 399–405.

102. Simon, T.R. and W.J. Rea, *Use of functional brain imaging in the evaluation of exposure to mycotoxins and toxins encountered in desert storm/desert shield.* Archives of Environmental Health, 2003. 58(7): p. 406–409.

103. Lebepe-Mazur, S., T. Wilson, and S. Hendrich, *Fusarium proliferatum-fermented corn stimulates development of placental glutathione S-transferase-positive altered hepatic foci in female rats.* Veterinary and Human Toxicology, 1995. 37(1): p. 55.

104. Mahfoud, R., et al., *The mycotoxin patulin alters the barrier function of the intestinal epithelium: Mechanism of action of the toxin and protective effects of glutathione.* Toxicology and Applied Pharmacology, 2002. 181(3): p. 209–218.

105. Novi, A.M., *Regression of aflatoxin B1-induced hepatocellular carcinomas by reduced glutathione.* Science, 1981. 212(4494): p. 541.

106. Eaton, D.L. and T.K. Bammler, *Concise review of the glutathione S-transferases and their significance to toxicology.* Toxicological Sciences: An Official Journal of the Society of Toxicology, 1999. 49(2): p. 156.

107. Freedman, J.H., M.R. Ciriolo, and J. Peisach, *The role of glutathione in copper metabolism and toxicity.* Journal of Biological Chemistry, 1989. 264(10): p. 5598.

108. Marasas, W.F.O., et al., *Fumonisins disrupt sphingolipid metabolism, folate transport, and neural tube development in embryo culture and in vivo: A potential risk factor for human neural tube defects among populations consuming fumonisin-contaminated maize.* Journal of Nutrition, 2004. 134(4): p. 711.

109. Wang, et al. *Depletion of intracellular glutathione mediates butenolide-induced cytoxicity in HepG2 cells.* Toxicology Letters, 2006. 164: p. 231–238.

110. Missmer, S.A., et al., *Exposure to fumonisins and the occurrence of neural tube defects along the Texas–Mexico border.* Environmental Health Perspectives, 2006. 114(2): p. 237.

111. Ray, J.G., et al., *Association of neural tube defects and folic acid food fortification in Canada.* Lancet, 2002. 360(9350): p. 2047–2048.

112. Berry, R.J., et al., *Prevention of neural-tube defects with folic acid in China.* New England Journal of Medicine, 1999. 341(20): p. 1485–1490.

113. Voss, K., G. Smith, and W. Haschek, *Fumonisins: Toxicokinetics, mechanism of action and toxicity.* Animal Feed Science and Technology, 2007. 137(3–4): p. 299–325.

114. Liu, B.H., et al., *Induction of oxidative stress response by the mycotoxin patulin in mammalian cells.* Toxicological Sciences, 2007. 95(2): p. 340.

115. Packer, L., E.H. Witt, and H.J. Tritschler, *Alpha-lipoic acid as a biological antioxidant.* Free Radical Biology and Medicine, 1995. 19(2): p. 227–250.

116. Becker, C.E., et al., *Diagnosis and treatment of Amanita phalloides-type mushroom poisoning: Use of thioctic acid.* Western Journal of Medicine, 1976. 125(2): p. 100.

117. Stabler, S.P., et al., *[alpha]-Lipoic acid induces elevated S-adenosylhomocysteine and depletes S-adenosylmethionine.* Free Radical Biology and Medicine, 2009. 47(8): p. 1147–1153.

118. Yi, P., et al., *Increase in plasma homocysteine associated with parallel increases in plasma S-adenosylhomocysteine and lymphocyte DNA hypomethylation.* Journal of Biological Chemistry, 2000. 275(38): p. 29318–29323.

119. James, S.J., et al., *Elevation in S-adenosylhomocysteine and DNA hypomethylation: Potential epigenetic mechanism for homocysteine-related pathology.* Journal of Nutrition, 2002. 132(8): p. 2361S.

120. Gelineau-van Waes, J., et al., *Maternal fumonisin exposure as a risk factor for neural tube defects.* Advances in Food and Nutrition Research, 2009. 56: p. 145–181.

121. Stevens, V.L. and J. Tang, *Fumonisin B1-induced sphingolipid depletion inhibits vitamin uptake via the glycosylphosphatidylinositol-anchored folate receptor.* Journal of Biological Chemistry, 1997. 272(29): p. 18020–18025.

122. Voss, K., J. Gelineau-van Waes, and R. Riley, *Fumonisins: Current research trends in developmental toxicology.* Mycotoxin Research, 2006. 22(1): p. 61–69.

123. Martínez de Villarreal, L., et al., *Decline of neural tube defects cases after a folic acid campaign in Nuevo Leon, Mexico.* Teratology, 2002. 66(5): p. 249–256.

124. Anyanwu, E.C., M. Morad, and A.W. Campbell, *Metabolism of Mycotoxins, Intracellular Functions of Vitamin B 12, and Neurological Manifestations in Patients with Chronic Toxigenic Mold Exposures. A Review.* ScientificWorld Journal, 2004. 4: p. 736–745.

125. El Golli, E., et al., *Induction of Hsp 70 in Vero cells in response to mycotoxins: Cytoprotection by sub-lethal heat shock and by Vitamin E.* Toxicology Letters, 2006. 166(2): p. 122–130.

126. Grosse, Y., et al., *Retinol, ascorbic acid and [alpha]-tocopherol prevent DNA adduct formation in mice treated with the mycotoxins ochratoxin A and zearalenone.* Cancer Letters, 1997. 114(1–2): p. 225–229.

127. Ranaldi, G., et al., *Intracellular zinc stores protect the intestinal epithelium from Ochratoxin A toxicity.* Toxicology in Vitro, 2009. 23(8): p. 1516–1521.

128. Nguyen, L.N., et al., *Sodium butyrate inhibits pathogenic yeast growth and enhances the functions of macrophages.* Journal of Antimicrobial Chemotherapy, 2011. 66(11): p. 2573–2580.

129. Ammendola, S., et al., *10-Undecanhydroxamic acid, a hydroxamate derivative of the undecanoic acid, has strong antimicrobial activity through a mechanism that limits iron availability.* FEMS Microbiology Letters, 2009. 294(1): p. 61–67.

130. Das, S. and A. Banerjee, *Effect of undecanoic acid on the production of exocellular lipolytic and keratinolytic enzymes by undecanoic acid-sensitive and-resistant strains of Trichophyton rubrum.* Medical Mycology, 1982. 20(3): p. 179–184.

131. Avantaggiato, G., R. Havenaar, and A. Visconti, *Evaluation of the intestinal absorption of deoxynivalenol and nivalenol by an* in vitro *gastrointestinal model, and the binding efficacy of activated carbon and other adsorbent materials.* Food and Chemical Toxicology, 2004. 42(5): p. 817–824.

132. Burel, S.D., et al., *Review of mycotoxin-detoxifying agents used as feed additives: Mode of action, efficacy and feed/food safety.* http://www.efsa.europa.eu/en/supporting/pub/22e.htm.

133. Diaz, D.E., *A review on the use of mycotoxin sequestering agents in agricultural livestock production.* Food Contaminants: Mycotoxins and Food Allergens, 2008. 1001: p. 125–150.

134. Jard, G., et al., *Review of mycotoxin reduction in food and feed: From prevention in the field to detoxification by adsorption or transformation.* Food Additives & Contaminants: Part A, 2011. Vol. 28: p. 1590–609.

135. Kolosova, A. and J. Stroka, *Substances for reduction of the contamination of feed by mycotoxins: A review.* World Mycotoxin Journal, 2011. 4(3): p. 225–256.

136. Afriyie-Gyawu, E., et al., *NovaSil clay intervention in Ghanaians at high risk for aflatoxicosis. I. Study design and clinical outcomes.* Food Additives and Contaminants, 2008. 25(1): p. 76–87.

137. Wang, J-S et al., *Short-term safety evaluation of processed calcium montmorillonite clay (NovaSil) in humans.* Food Additives and Contaminants, 2005. 22(3): p. 270–279.

138. Whitlow, L.W. *Evaluation of mycotoxin binders.* in *Proceedings of the 4th Mid-Atlantic Nutrition Conference.* Timonium, MD: Maryland Feed Industry Council University of Maryland, 2006.

139. Natour, R. and S. Yousef, *Adsorption efficiency of diatomaceous earth for mycotoxin.* Arab Gulf Journal of Scientific Research, 1998. 16(1): p. 113–127.

140. Dalié, D., A. Deschamps, and F. Richard-Forget, *Lactic acid bacteria-potential for control of mould growth and mycotoxins: A review.* Food Control, 2010. 21(4): p. 370–380.

141. Gelderblom, W., et al., *Fumonisins—novel mycotoxins with cancer-promoting activity produced by Fusarium moniliforme.* Applied and Environmental Microbiology, 1988. 54(7): p. 1806.

142. Hocking, A.D., *Advances in food mycology.* Vol. 571. 2006: Springer Science+Business Media, LLC.

143. Barceloux, D.G., *Medical Toxicology of Natural Substances: Foods, Fungi, Medicinal Herbs, Plants, and Venomous Animals.* Wiley and Sons: Hoboken, NJ, 2008.

144. Crews, H., et al., *A critical assessment of some biomarker approaches linked with dietary intake.* British Journal of Nutrition, 2001. 86(1): p. 5.

145. Groopman, J.D., *Molecular dosimetry methods for assessing human aflatoxin exposures.* The Toxicology of Aflatoxins: Human Health, Veterinary, and Agricultural Significance, 1994: p. 259–279.

146. Hooper, D.G., et al., *Mycotoxin detection in human samples from patients exposed to environmental molds.* International Journal of Molecular Sciences, 2009. 10(4): p. 1465–1475.

147. Wengenack, N.L. and M.J. Binnicker, *Fungal molecular diagnostics.* Clinics in Chest Medicine, 2009. 30(2): p. 391–408.

148. Huang, A., et al., *High-throughput identification of clinical pathogenic fungi by hybridization to an oligonucleotide microarray.* Journal of Clinical Microbiology, 2006. 44(9): p. 3299.

149. Sewram, V., et al., *Fumonisin mycotoxins in human hair.* Biomarkers, 2003. 8(2): p. 110–118.

150. Huff, W., et al., *Ochratoxin A-induced iron deficiency anemia.* Applied and Environmental Microbiology, 1979. 37(3): p. 601.

151. Russo, A., et al., *Ochratoxin A-induced DNA damage in human fibroblast: Protective effect of cyanidin 3-O-β-d-glucoside.* Journal of Nutritional Biochemistry, 2005. 16(1): p. 31–37.

152. Scott, P.M., *Biomarkers of human exposure to ochratoxin A.* Food Additives and Contaminants, 2005. 22(s1): p. 99–107.

153. Yike, I., et al., *Mycotoxin adducts on human serum albumin: Biomarkers of exposure to Stachybotrys chartarum.* Environmental Health Perspectives, 2006. 114(8): p. 1221.

154. Shephard, G., L. Van der Westhuizen, and V. Sewram, *Biomarkers of exposure to fumonisin mycotoxins: A review.* Food Additives and Contaminants, 2007. 24(10): p. 1196–1201.

44 Biotoxins

Supporting Removal via Intrinsic Pathways

Dietrich Klinghardt, M.D., Ph.D.

INTRODUCTION

The human body has evolved intrinsic mechanisms for the removal of toxicants from the body. Where medical advances have not provided effective therapies for biotoxin-related illness such as disease caused by typhoid toxins, mycotoxins, quinolinic acid from Lyme disease, and gangrene caused by three known staphylococcal toxins, pathophysiologic research and clinical experience suggest that patient improvement can occur when the body's intrinsic detoxification pathways are therapeutically activated. Nutrient depletion and epigenetic changes caused by exposures to toxins and trauma compromise one's ability to detoxify in general. This chapter premises how the body's natural detoxification mechanisms can be enhanced.

EPIDEMIOLOGY

What has changed at the population level regarding biotoxins that manifests what clinicians and their patients experience?

On one hand, advances in medicine, especially the use of some vaccines and antibiotics, have reduced morbidity. The fact that tetanus, typhoid, and streptococcal exposures are now rare represents a public health success.

On the other hand, some pathogens cause more disease on the population level. This can be from increased virulence factors adapted by the organism, spread to increasingly more populations, but can also be caused by increased population density and world travel or increased vulnerability on the part of the host. Possible causes include micronutrient depletion, synergistic effects of environmental pollutants accumulated in the body, and steadily increased exposure to electromagnetic radiation from cell phone broadcasting and other sources.

One organism increasingly attributed to disease in humans is *Borrelia burgdorferi*, the organism causing Lyme disease thought to have become a human pathogen more recently. However, in 2011, epidemiologic evidence emerged from an unlikely source, "Oetzi" the iceman. Spirochetes were identified in 5300-year-old cadaver whose body was preserved in the Alpine ice. The body was recently determined to be infected with *Borrelia* [1]. Oetzi was estimated to have been a healthy 20–45-year-old man at the time of his death (which has been attributed to trauma). *Borrelia* spirochetes have been around a long time and may have only recently developed their pathogenicity.

PATHOPHYSIOLOGY

The overarching principle relevant to this chapter and the treatments presented is that chronic illness is not caused by the presence of pathogens themselves but by their metabolic activity and the creation of potent biotoxins. The return to health is determined by appropriate immune reactions and the body's own ability to remove biotoxins, which can be enhanced in two key ways:

1. Using integrative nutritional and other approaches to restore the detoxification capacity or/ and upregulate the metabolic enzymes of the biotoxin pathway.
2. Reducing the easier-to-control harmful exposures that occupy the same detoxification pathways as those biotoxins that are less amenable to treatment and exposure reduction.

Genetic propensities play a major role in how well the toxin elimination pathways work to start with. This is demonstrated in the connection between apolipoprotein E (APO-E) subtypes and Alzheimer's disease [2]. The APO-E subtype 2 has two cysteine molecules that enable this compound to bind and eliminate sulfhydryl affinitive toxic metals from inside the cell. The subtype E-4 has no cysteine and is unable to participate in the constant clean up of the cell. The efficiency of the biotoxin pathway is also influenced by HLA system genotypes, which determine how the immune system responds to offending toxins and microbes. Several subtypes are significantly less able to eliminate toxins from the body, as illustrated in a case-control study of ciguatoxin fish poisoning [3].

Biotoxin exposures are diverse. They include tetanus toxin; botulinum toxin (botox); ascaridin from intestinal parasites; streptolysin toxins from *Streptococci*; toxins from *Staphylococci*, Lyme disease, chlamydia, *Babesia microti,* and tuberculosis; fungal toxins (also called mycotoxins); venom from brown recluse spiders; and toxins triggered by viral infections.

Biotoxins are minute molecules (200–1000 kilodaltons) containing nitrogen and sulfur. They belong to a group of chemical messengers that microorganisms use to control the host's immune system, host's behavior, and even the host's eating habits. Aggressive staphylococcus infections that cause tissue necrosis are caused by at least three potent biotoxins, not by the presence of the microbes themselves. The diversity of the biotoxins may be profound. For example *Candida albicans* produces 600 different known biotoxins.

Rationale for Reducing Neurotoxin Exposure in Patients with Chronic Lyme Disease

Biotoxins are neurotoxins as are heavy metals, xenobiotics (man-made environmental toxins such as dioxin, formaldehyde, insecticides, wood preservatives, polychlorinated biphenyls), and food additives. Neurotoxins are a subgroup of biotoxins attracted to the mammalian nervous system.

Neurotoxins act with synergy, making the fact that human pathophysiology surrounding Lyme disease and several other potentially chronic infections comes from nerve-damaging biotoxins clinically relevant. For example, in a rat toxicology study combining mercury and lead, each at doses lethal to 1 in 100 animals (LD1), all the rats died (LD100). The exponential effect of the combined neurotoxins can be expressed as: LD1 of Hg +LD1 lead = LD100. Similar applications have been made in marine ecosystems where combined toxicities are greater than individual ones [4].

The primary reason for the adverse effects being more than additive is that the human body experiences toxins every day and has common metabolic pathways to dispose of them. However, when several toxins are present at one time the pathways may become overwhelmed. Neurotoxins not promptly metabolized are absorbed by nerve endings and travel inside the neuron to the cell body. On their way, they disrupt vital functions of the nerve cell, such as axonal transport of nutrients, mitochondrial respiration, and proper DNA transcription.

The clinical corollary is that by reducing exposure to—and facilitating the elimination of—neurotoxins, the body can more effectively eliminate the biotoxins directly associated with medical illness.

RATIONALE FOR GASTROINTESTINAL SUPPORT

The body is constantly trying to eliminate neurotoxins via the available exit routes: the liver, kidney, skin, small intestine, and exhaled air. Detoxification mechanisms include acetylation, sulphation, glucoronidation, oxidation, and others. Figure 44.1 depicts how enzymes, cofactors, and toxicants interact in the metabolic pathways of detoxification. Detoxification occurs in three phases.

Phase 1 breaks the toxin into smaller particles, some of which may be more toxic than the original substance.

Phase 2 binds these toxic substances to the body's own molecules, which makes the toxin less toxic, soluble in bile as in the process of glucoronidation, or soluble in water so that it can be excreted by the kidney.

Phase 3 binds the substance to a transporter molecule shuttled out to kidney, skin, or liver.

Approximately 90% of the molecules are removed through the liver to the bile and then excreted in the stool. However, because of the lipophilic/neurotropic nature of the neurotoxins, most are reabsorbed by the abundant nerve endings of the enteric nervous system in the intestinal wall [5].

The exact mechanisms for the signaling from the gastrointestinal tract have not been determined, but the possible mechanisms are several since the reuptake of neurotoxins occurs in many pathways. Toxins undergoing neuronal uptake are transported via axons to the spinal cord (autonomic nervous system neurons) or brainstem (parasympathetics) and from there back to the brain. Venous uptake via the portal vein back to the liver occurs (enterohepatic circulation). Lymphatic uptake via the thoracic duct to the subclavian vein occurs. There is also uptake by bowel bacteria and tissues of the intestinal tract. The late Dr. Alfred Pischinger advanced the understanding of these mechanisms, which have been recently translated into English by those continuing his work [5].

In order to prevent the resorption of neurotoxins, we give binding agents such as chlorella species to act in the gut. That gives a feedback signal to the liver that more toxins can be eliminated. Binding toxins in the gut signal the liver and a successful phase 2 relays feedback to phase 1. To initiate a cascade of detoxification all the way from the interior of the cell to the inside of the bowel, it is most often not necessary to use intracellularly-acting, sophisticated toxin elimination agents. It is most often sufficient to use binding agents in the gastrointestinal tract.

FACILITATING PEROXISOMAL ACTIVITY

Detoxification occurs in every cell of the body, most prominently the liver followed by the kidney and skin. All are rich in these detoxification enzymes found in the peroxisomes. Peroxisomes are the "liver" of each cell and process neurotoxins. Therefore, detoxification can be facilitated when methods are used to increase peroxisomal function such as:

- Fever
- Hyperbaric oxygen
- Exercise
- Phosphatidyl choline
- Actos (acts as an agonist to the peroxisome proliferator activator receptor [PPAR]-gamma)
- Chlorophyll (PPAR-alpha and beta agonist)
- The omega-3 fatty acids eicosapentaenoic acid and docosahexaenoic acid activate PPAR

In contrast, excessive amounts of antioxidants, especially high doses of fat soluble vitamins, can inhibit the beta oxidation of fat that occurs within the peroxisomes.

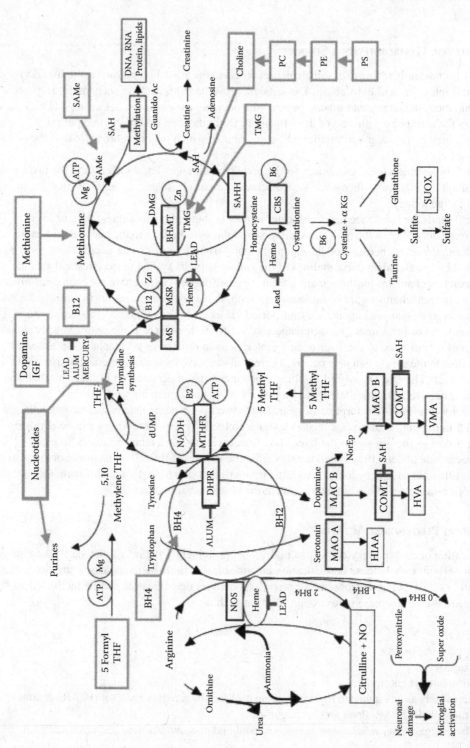

FIGURE 44.1 Metabolic pathways reflect the interference of neurotoxins in detoxification. Reproduced with permission from Amy Yasko, PhD.

RESTORING DETOXIFICATION NUTRIENTS WHEN THEY ARE DEPLETED THROUGH BACTERIAL AND FUNGAL VIRULENCE FACTORS

What are the mechanisms that the microbes are using to establish themselves in the human host? With a highly evolved human immune system, the mechanisms by which toxin-producing organisms evade the immune system are surprising in their complexity. One clinically significant, but less known, mechanism by which Lyme spirochetes evade host immune mechanisms is to deplete the host of nutrients integral to its defenses, by blocking one of the eight enzymes needed in the heme pathway, leading to the formation of hemopyrrollactams [6] and inefficient heme molecules. The heme molecule is part of the hemoglobin system and also used in the p450 liver detoxification system.

Hemopyrrollactamuria (HPU), formerly known as kryptopyrroluria, was identified in 1958 by Abrahm Hoffer, a psychiatrist researcher focusing his healing work on people with schizophrenia. He observed high concentrations of this substance in the urine of his patients and not in the general population. The HPU compound binds strongly to vitamin B6, zinc, and other micronutrients listed in Table 44.1 and illustrated in Figure 44.2. As the nutrients chaperone the hemopyrrollactams to be eliminated via the urine, the nutrients are also eliminated in excess of usual physiologic amounts, usually in direct proportion to the amount of hemopyrrollactams [7,8].

In HPU, nutrient deficiencies can arise from excess urine losses even when nutrient intake and absorption are adequate. The symptoms of this illness are related to the resulting depletion of the nutrients listed in Table 44.1. Treating with high doses of zinc and B6 reverses many of the symptoms.

HPU lowers serum levels of reduced glutathione. Glutathione levels and a variant of the glutathione peroxidase enzyme are correlated with longevity [9]. We therefore felt it clinically significant that our patients with Lyme consistently have presented with low glutathione levels. Once we began treating HPU we saw a steady increase in glutathione to levels of age-adjusted healthy patients, in keeping with earlier research findings [7,8].

Some patients with HPU experience reduction in their symptoms with antibiotics. Some Lyme patients convert from HPU positive to HPU negative as their condition improves with antimicrobial treatment [10]. It is not yet fully understood, but clinical observations suggest that HPU is reversible through different treatment mechanisms. Once HPU resolves, the nutrients losses abate, although without supplementation recovery of nutrient status is delayed.

PATIENT EVALUATION

Antibiotics successfully treat the acute infection with Lyme disease and a subset of patients with chronic Lyme disease. However, patients in integrative medical practices around the country

---

TABLE 44.1
Alphabetical Listing of Nutrients Known to Be Excreted in Patients with Hemopyrrollactamuria

Depleted Nutrient	Clinical and/or Metabolic Manifestations
Biotin	Cognitive processing difficulties such as short-term memory loss; skin aging; lowered immunity; impaired detoxification
Chromium	Glycemic instability; muscle loss
Glutathione	Antioxidant associated with longevity
Manganese	Needed for the antioxidant manganese superoxide dismutase, and when lacking it is associated with inflammation
Molybdenum	Difficulty processing sulfur
Vitamin B6	Difficulty with sleep; peripheral neuropathies
Zinc	Immune problems, impaired detoxification

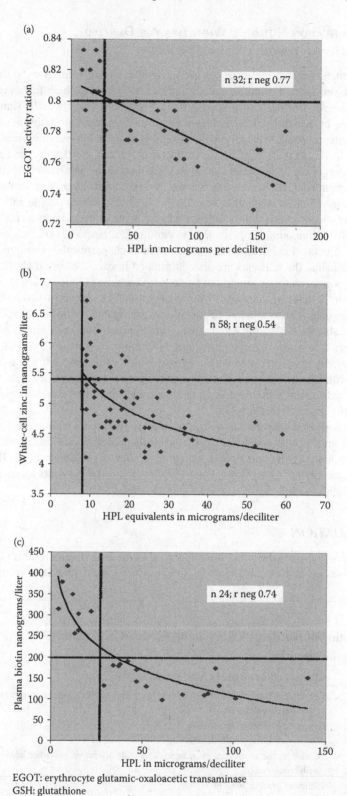

EGOT: erythrocyte glutamic-oxaloacetic transaminase
GSH: glutathione

FIGURE 44.2a–e   Correlation between hemopyrrollactams (HPL) in urine and nutrient status. Reproduced with permission from Dr. Tapan Audhya [7,8].

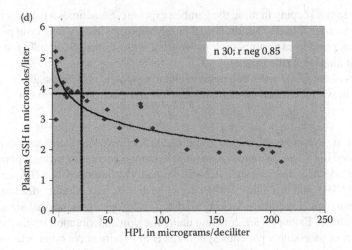

(d) n 30; r neg 0.85

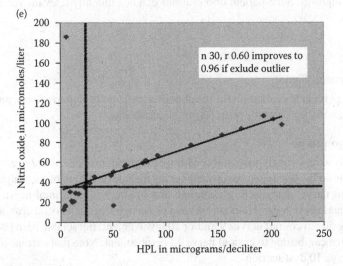

(e) n 30, r 0.60 improves to 0.96 if exlude outlier

FIGURE 44.2a–e (*continued*).

testing positive for Lyme disease tend to be the patients who did not sufficiently respond to antibiotic interventions. The fact that patients referred to my practice have not responded to prior conventional medical treatment greatly increases the probability of clinically significant neurotoxin exposure.

History

Exposure History

A patient history in my clinic emphasizes neurotoxin exposures. These include but are by no means limited to:

- Current or prior amalgam fillings, because of evaporation of metallic mercury, leaching of tin.
- Tick or other insect bites. Most so called "tick borne diseases" such as Lyme disease can also be carried by stinging flies, spiders, and insects other than ticks.
- Occupations such as working in machine shops with solvents; welding, which is associated with metal fume fever from aerosolized metal toxicants; veterinary clinic work; or working

in a beauty salon, keeping in mind the paraben exposure. Sometimes a parent's occupational exposures are transferred to children, so a family exposure history may be appropriate here.

- Hobbies can point to exposures such as working with stained glass, auto repair, or exposure to munitions at a rifle range.
- Long hours of computer work can point to electromagnetic radiation and also possible off-gassing of heavy metals and other toxicants from the electronic equipment.

Symptoms

Of particular note are symptoms of fatigue, insomnia, lack of zest, short-term memory loss, cognitive problems, and mood disorders. Symptoms can point to cranial nerve issues: facial paralysis (CN VII), facial pain (CN V), deteriorating eye sight (CNs II, IV, and VI), tinnitus (CN VIII), vertigo (CN VIII), hearing loss (CN VIII), and difficulty swallowing or gastroesophageal reflux disease (CN X). Some patients report neurological symptoms lacking a defined neurologic basis, but that are temporally associated with their illness. Examples are crawling under the skin and vibration inside the skull.

Another aspect of assessing a patient's symptoms is to inquire about what actions they took that improved their symptoms. Such patient observations can be clinically relevant and point to feasible treatment options.

Physical Exam

Upper Motor Neuron Signs

Neurologic findings include evaluation for the abnormal reflexes of hyperreflexia, ankle clonus, and the Babinski sign, which is common with *Bartonella henselae*.

Cranial Nerve Symptoms

Facial nerve paralysis is strongly associated with (pathognomonic) *Borrelia burgdorferi* infection. Other signs of neurotoxic damage to the cranial nerves include deviation of the tongue due to effects on the hypoglossus nerve; decreased or complete loss of smell from cranial nerve 1 involvement; lazy eye from cranial nerve 6 involvement; tinnitus or vertigo from effects on cranial nerve 8; difficulties swallowing due to cranial nerves 9 and/or 10 involvement; intractable pain in the lower neck/upper shoulders that can be due to cranial nerve 12 involvement. Note that cardiac arrhythmias can involve cranial nerve 10 dysfunction.

Skin Findings

Skin findings include pale translucent skin as commonly observed in HPU; cherry angiomata, which are associated with Babesia; striae in unusual areas in young nonpregnant clients—and furthermore these striae tend to be blue with Babesia and red with Bartonella; and skin tags associated with insulin resistance, which can be induced by Lyme and Bartonella in patients without other risk factors. Often the skin ages prematurely due to microbe-upregulated metallo-proteinases (MMP-9) from yet to be elucidated mechanisms.

Nail Findings

Nail findings include longitudinal ridges, which are a sign of a disturbed protein matrix of the nail often caused by underlying hypochlorhydria. Hypochlorhydria can be a sign of cranial nerve 10 dysfunction and is common in many chronic infections. Brittle nails and hair are often a sign of functional hypothyroidism, which may be more often associated with excessive exposure or sensitivity to electromagnetic radiation, rather than a direct effect of the microbial pathogens.

Autonomic Response Testing

Testing for autonomic response is a method to assess whether a food, medication, or biologic agent will be tolerated by the individual patient. When allergenic foods are placed on the patient's tongue or in proximity to the patient's skin the heart rate increases. The more rapid pulse indicates a withdrawal of parasympathetic activity and activation of the sympathetic nervous system. At the same time, the muscle tone of skeletal muscles changes throughout the body, which can be monitored by a trained practitioner [11]. Dr. Yoshiaki Omura, patented the Bi-Digital O-Ring Test from which autonomic response testing is built. Other related techniques are electrodermal screening and applied kinesiology.

Functional Acuity Contrast Test

In this test, also called visual contrast sensitivity, the ability of the client is tested to perceive different shades of contrast. Research has shown that the quality of contrast perception is directly related to intracranial arterial blood flow, sometimes diminished in chronic neurotoxicity from mold, Lyme, or exposure to tetrachloroethylene [12].

LABORATORY DIAGNOSTICS FOR HEAVY METALS

There is no direct way to assess the body burden of heavy metal neurotoxins. We start by establishing an experience-based general toxin metal elimination protocol. Six weeks into that we do a hair analysis of the proximal inch of hair that will reflect what was mobilized during those four to six weeks through the body's own activity. Over time, we use the urine porphyrin testing, red cell mineral tests, and urine and stool challenge tests.

Hair Analysis

The inch of hair proximal to the scalp reflects the last month of circulating metals in the blood. Metals get into the hair by circulating through the arterial supply of the hair root. Hair binds methyl mercury very well, but less so to metallic mercury or mercury salts. The major disadvantage is that toxic metals not only indicate high levels of toxins in the body. They also reflect the increased ability of the body to excrete metals. The hair test will not show what was not mobilized [13]. The same is true for hair mineral analysis. High levels of zinc, for example, in the hair analysis may reflect high plasma levels or high levels of loss. Patients with HPU may be severely depleted of zinc, yet in the early years may have very high levels of zinc in the hair analysis.

Porphyrin Testing for Hemopyrrollactamuria

Even though hemopyrrollactamuria (HPU) and porphyrin disorders are related, they are tested separately. The urine HPU test is available from a few diagnostic labs. It is a 24-hour urine collection with an approximately three-week turnaround time. One gram of ascorbate is added to the urine as a preservative. The urine collection container is wrapped with aluminum foil to avoid the chemical reaction of the HPU compound to light.

Urine porphyrin testing has been introduced by James Woods, PhD [14,15], and is also available via different labs in the United States and France. A few additional points: toxic metals and biotoxins damage metabolic enzymes, including those of the porphyrin synthesis. These enzymes are most sensitive to metal damage and respond with upregulation and increased urinary enzyme excretion. Since the porphyrin-related enzymes are intracellular, this test may reflect truly intracellular toxicity. However, since mercury, lead, and zinc are compartmentalized, that means they are present in some body compartments but not in others; it is never clear. If the test results reflect clearing or toxicity of one body compartment, while another is still extremely toxic, it may not be reflected by the test since porphyrins are not equally created in each cell of the body.

The Red Cell Toxic Metal Test

Erythrocytes actively absorb metals into their interior. The levels may reflect metal levels over the several month lifespan of the red blood cells. However, it is unclear, whether red cells were damaged by chronic illness or invaded by microbes because chronic infections can absorb levels of toxic metals equivalent to the average blood level.

Urine Challenge Test

A complexing or chelating agent is injected or ingested prior to urine collection, for the purpose of a urine heavy metal challenge test. A six- or 24-hour urine sample will accurately reflect what this particular agent mobilized via the kidneys, but not via the intestinal tract.

Detoxification agents that work via the intestinal tract are preferred for treatment apart from the challenge test. They avoid reabsorption by lining the gut with metal-binding agents. Agents that mobilize toxins only via the kidneys should be avoided. The kidney epithelium can be damaged by pushing too much of a concentration of toxic metals via the kidneys. The gut epithelium is less vulnerable to injury due to its large surface area and the high turnover rate of gastrointestinal epithelial cells.

Stool Analysis

This is the only test to reveal effectiveness of the hepatic and biliary pathway of excretion of metals. However, it is difficult to interpret, since different areas of stool may contain very different amounts of sequestered metal.

LABORATORY TESTING FOR BIOTOXIN-PRODUCING PATHOGENS AND METABOLIC SEQUELAE

Although there are few direct tests for pathogenic organisms and their associated biotoxins, many tests are available each with their respective shortcomings. Testing can include yeast and other fungal infections, stool analysis for ova and parasites, and bacterial infections including Lyme disease and mycoplasma.

Parasite tests are a deficient area in modern laboratory practice. Many species of worms autolyze and become undetectable 15–20 minutes after defecation. Typically the time from bowel movement to laboratory is several days. The PCR-based stool and saliva tests have a notoriously low detection rate. The most reliable test in our practice is the establishment of a reasonable diagnosis, including history (foreign travel, prior seeing of worms in stool, etc.), abdominal palpation, and indirect lab markers such as elevated eosinophils and macrophages. Improvement following a short medical trial with appropriate medication and dosages can also allow for a presumed diagnosis. The client is instructed to examine every bowel movement for signs of worms, larvae, or eggs. We had many patients send their delivered worms to our local laboratories, worms which were clearly still moving at the time of delivery, only to come back with the diagnosis taxonomy unavailable, or with the lab expressing doubts that the moving creature was really there.

Given the inadequate tools for detecting pathogenic organisms and metal toxins, metabolic tests are useful. There are several laboratory tests that are altered during neurotoxin exposures. Not only can they serve as a smoking guns for the presence of neurotoxins, they can also guide nutrient therapy and serve as biomarkers for patient recovery.

The inflammatory markers C4A, TGF beta 1, and matrix metalloproteinases (MMP9) are commonly upregulated in chronic illness. In that case, we use anti-inflammatory strategies such as the use of curcumin, ginger, and a variety of common medical drugs such as Actos, nonsteroidal anti-inflammatories, cholestyramine, and steroids.

The regulatory neuropeptides melanocyte stimulating hormone (MSH), oxytocin, antidiuretic hormone (ADH), and vasoactive intestinal polypeptide (VIP) can be evaluated and guide treatment. Diabetes insipidus from biotoxin-related reduction of antidiuretic hormone production in the pituitary gland may be underlying the electrolytes and minerals imbalances. The neuropeptide imbalances may also be the basis for the observation that hormonal deficiencies are common, especially progesterone in women and testosterone and growth hormone in men. When MSH is low, sinus and nasal treatments may be beneficial [16]. We also use water that has been imprinted with the physical structure of the neuropeptides in question [17]. This has been very effective and inexpensive to the patient.

The nagalase enzyme is upregulated by the intelligent activity of microbes in the client's system. Nagalase blocks the vitamin D receptors on the cell wall of macrophages, which effectively paralyzes the macrophages and therefore a significant portion of our immune system. An elevated (positive) nagalase enzyme test can be followed by the injection of Gc-MAF (vitamin D3-binding protein or Gc protein-derived macrophage activating factor) for several months. Initially the client often would observe a cytokine storm or other mild to severe immune reaction, which will be later followed by partial or complete recovery from their respective illness. Several sources of GcMAF are available [18].

IMAGING AND OTHER DIAGNOSTIC STUDIES

Cerebral magnetic resonance venography (MRV) can effectively evaluate for chronic cerebrospinal venous insufficiency. Single photon emission computed tomography (SPECT) and positron emission tomography (PET) imaging can be used to localize brain areas of increased or decreased metabolic activity. Results can inform decisions to either use drugs and nutrients that act, for example, on the monamine pathways, or to use mechanical means to open stenosed veins via a balloon catheter. For example, a child with autism and language delay with a SPECT that reveals that the frontal lobe has decreased uptake may benefit from low dose L-dopa. A patient with multiple sclerosis–like symptoms, cognitive deficits, and motor dysfunction may be treated with diagnosing and treating stenosed anterior neck veins referred to as chronic cerebrospinal venous insufficiency (CCSVI) [19].

ENVIRONMENT ASSESSMENT FOR ELECTROSMOG

Microwave radiation from cell phone broadcasting, wireless set-ups in homes, alarm systems, and the use of the cell phone itself have increasingly been shown to have adverse biological effects [20,21]. Microwave exposure can and should be measured in the home and workplace using a handheld device. Electrosensitivity is in part genetically determined, leaving some people more vulnerable than others. Astute practitioners have noticed significant illness causing effects in some of their chronically ill patients. Initial studies in this area drew heavily on comparative biology, such as sharks hunting with electromagnetic fields.

Electromagnetic radiation exposure has dramatically increased over the last few years. Electrosmog is likely to act directly on the host through a variety of mechanisms. It has been shown that microwave radiation from cell phones directly impairs intracellular signaling pathways. It is also likely to act indirectly by increasing biotoxin production. Fungi, when stressed by electrosmog, employ their own defense mechanisms to a greater extent. This has been demonstrated with fungal organisms that produce more potent mycotoxins when exposed to electrosmog [10].

TREATMENT

ALLOPATHIC AND BIOLOGICAL AGENTS

Opportunistic infections and infestations (i.e., roundworms, strongyloides, streptococcus, staphylococcus, clostridiae, etc.) are often best addressed in the early phase of treatment of the chronic illness with conventional medical drugs such as ivermectin, nitazoxanide, or Praziquantel, even though there are a variety of biological options. Parasites respond well to liposomal artemisinin—a wormwood extract—and bacterial infections to a plethora of plant substances such as allicin from garlic and curcumin from turmeric. In Lyme disease, coinfections can be acquired from the same insect bite as the primary *Borrelia* infection, most commonly *Babesia microti* and *Bartonella henselae*.

HPU may be managed with proprietary mineral and vitamins blends, containing high dosages of pyridoxal 5 phosphate (B6) and zinc. HPU treatment rearms the immune system, which then is more capable of dealing with the chronic infections such as Lyme.

Neurotransmitter imbalances are typically addressed with a cocktail of oral amino acids and diet changes (whey drink, chlorella, and nondairy, natural amino acid sources) but can also be treated conventionally with appropriate psychotropic medication.

Vitamin D deficiency disables many aspects of immunity and is addressed with medical doses of vitamin D (depending on 25-OH cholecalciferol blood levels), until the system has regained normal levels. The often-present circadian rhythm disturbance may have to be addressed with high doses of liposomal melatonin or psychotropic medication but may also respond to propolis tincture. Direct sunlight can raise both vitamin D and melatonin levels.

Heavy metal burden may be addressed initially with medical drugs such as sodium EDTA, DMSA, DMPS, and others but may also respond to biological agents such as curcumin, chlorella, cilantro, and garlic.

There are both biological detoxification protocols as well as pharmaceutical protocols. The most common medical agents used for intravenous therapy are as follows:

- A vitamin C drip mobilizes the heavy metals from the matrix and leads to excretion via the stool.
- DMPS (oral, i.v., i.m., s.c.) clears the vascular endothelium of the kidney. It often takes weeks before DMPS can "work" again after the initial dosing. It is used mostly for arsenic, lead, copper, and mercury.
- Desferal (s.c) is used for iron and aluminum excretion both via the stool and kidney.
- α-Lipoic acid (usually 600 mg/iv.) is a weak complexing agent for sulfhydryl affinitive metals such as mercury and lead.
- Glutahione (i.v., liposomal oral delivery) is a weak complexing agent. Together both α-Lipoic acid and glutathione given at the same time are an excellent tool to eliminate mycotoxins stored or trapped in the liver. The most natural sources of the precursor amino acids are goat and cow whey.
- Penicillamin (oral) might be the only effective medical detoxification agent working at the intracellular level.

Protein Intake

Proteins provide the important precursors to the endogenous metal detox and toxin-shuttle agents, such as coeruloplasmin, metallothionein, glutathione, and others. The branched-chain amino acids in cow and goat whey have valuable independent detoxification effects. The algae chlorella contains 50% amino acids and peptides, with a profile similar to human breast milk. Chlorella can be a significant dietary source of protein and a vegan source of vitamin B12 [22,23].

Adequate Minerals

Metals attach themselves in our tissues only in places that are programmed for attachment of metal ions. Mineral deficiency provides the opportunity for toxic metals to attach themselves to vacant binding sites. Repleted minerals including magnesium, selenium, zinc, manganese, germanium, and molybdenum are requisite for all metal detoxification attempts. Substituting minerals can detoxify the body by itself. We have observed that by giving supplemental zinc the body immediately starts pushing out lead from the storage sites in the bone marrow. Just as important are electrolytes, sodium, potassium, calcium, and magnesium, which regulate the physiological parameters of the body fluids and help to transport toxic waste across the extracellular space toward the lymphatic and venous vessels and across the filtrating membranes of the kidney.

IMPROVING LIPID INTAKE

Lipids made from fatty acids make up 60–80% of the central nervous system and need to be constantly replenished. Deficiency makes the nervous system vulnerable to the fat-soluble metals, such as metallic mercury constantly escaping as odorless and invisible vapor evaporating from amalgam fillings. Chlorella is 12% lipid. Its alpha- and gamma-linoleic acids help to balance the increased intake of fish oil during detoxification. Chlorella can normalize serum cholesterol and lipid composition and levels [24,25].

HYDRATION WITH ELECTROLYTE REPLETION

Without enough fluid intake, the kidneys may become contaminated with metals. The basal membranes swell up and the kidneys can no longer efficiently filter toxins [10]. Adding a balanced electrolyte solution in small amounts to water helps to restore intra- and extracellular fluid balance.

The autonomic nervous system in most toxic patients is dysfunctional. Electric messages in the organism are not received, are misunderstood, or are misinterpreted. Toxins cannot be shuttled through the extracellular space. Increased intake of natural ocean salt, such as Celtic sea salt, and avoidance of regular table salt has been found to be very effective in resolving some of these problems. Most common is the intravenous use of Ringer's Lactate. An oral solution pioneered by the American chemist Ketkovsky is effective in some clinical circumstances [26]. In patients who are sodium or chloride sensitive, caution must be taken to monitor the blood pressure, and dosing of the electrolyte solution may need to be adjusted downward; however, in these patients, the detoxification process takes longer and is more difficult.

Dosage: Use one to three tablespoons in a quart of water and titrate to slightly salty taste. During times of greater stress the dosage can be temporarily increased.

CILANTRO (CHINESE PARSLEY) IN SUPPLEMENTAL FORM

This kitchen herb is capable of mobilizing mercury, cadmium, lead, and aluminum in bones and the central nervous system [27]. It is probably the only effective biological agent in mobilizing mercury stored in the intracellular space that is attached to mitochondria, tubulin, and liposomes, and in the nucleus of the cell—where it can potentially reverse the DNA damage of mercury [28]. Because cilantro mobilizes more toxins than it can carry out of the body, it should be used with supplemental chlorella algae species that are effective binding agents.

Cilantro in an alcohol solution (elixir) can be initiated at an oral dose of five drops twice daily taken just before a meal. Gradually, the dose may be increased to 15 drops three times a day for full benefit. During the initial phase of the detoxification cilantro should be given one week on, followed by two to three weeks off.

Cilantro can be incorporated into the diet. The aforementioned cilantro solution can be consumed as a tea, by using 10 to 20 drops in a cup of hot water and sipped slowly. Another way of taking cilantro is to rub five drops twice a day into the ankles for mobilization of metals in all organs, joints, and structures below the diaphragm, and into the wrists for organs, joints, and structures above the diaphragm. The wrists have dense autonomic innervation that enables axonal uptake, and the wrists are crossed by the main lymphatic channels, allowing for lymphatic uptake.

CHLORELLA

The algae chlorella has a long history in the Chinese and Japanese medical literature for cleaning up the body after environmental disasters and offers a sustainable approach with well-studied safety data due to its extensive use. Chlorella is effective at biotoxin uptake, especially in the gastrointestinal tract.

Metal binding and elimination is facilitated by chlorella and parpachlorella species because the polysaccharide, sporopollenin, in the cell wall has unique toxic metal binding properties [22]. Many studies have identified specific metal binding: cadmium [29–31], uranium [32], lead [33], and mercury and methyl mercury [34,35].

- Chlorella species also facilitate the elimination of neuro- and immunotoxic chemicals [36–40]. Sporopollenin is as effective as cholestyramin in binding neurotoxins and more effective in binding toxic metals than any other natural substance found.
- Along similar lines, chlorella supplementation protects the fetus and newborn from maternal toxin transfer [41].
- There is support in the medical literature for an immune-system strengthening role [42–44]. Consistent with the immune-strengthening properties our personal observation is that chlorella supplementation increases reduced glutathione [10].
- Presumably mediated by the binding of neurotoxins, chlorella has been shown to delay cognitive decline [45].

Dosing is initiated with 1 gram (four tablets) three to four times a day. This is the standard maintenance dosage for adults for a six- to 24-month detoxification program. During the more active phase of the detoxification (one week every two to four weeks), whenever cilantro is given, the dose can be increased to 3 grams three to four times per day (one week on, two to four weeks back down to the maintenance dosage). Take 30 minutes before the main meals and at bedtime. The timing of 30 minutes before meals is to facilitate chlorella's presence in the small intestine when bile is released, since bile carries with it toxic metals and other toxic waste. These are bound by the chlorella cell wall and carried out via the digestive tract.

Some people have problems digesting the cell membrane of chlorella. The enzyme cellulase resolves this problem. Cellulase is available in many health food stores in digestive enzyme products. Taking chlorella together with food also helps in some cases, even though it is less effective that way. *C. pyreneidosa* has better absorption of toxins, but is harder to digest. *C. vulgaris* is easier to digest, but with less metal absorbing capability. Some manufacturers have created cell wall–free chlorella extracts that are more expensive, but more easily absorbed.

CHLORELLA GROWTH FACTOR

Chlorella growth factor (CGF) is a heat extract from chlorella that concentrates certain peptides, proteins, and other ingredients. CGF has been administered in various settings with salutary effects [46,47]. In our experience, CGF makes the detoxification process easier, shorter, and more effective. The recommended dosage is one capsule of CGF for each 10–20 tablets of chlorella.

GARLIC

Garlic (*Allium sativum*) has been shown to protect the white and red blood cells from the oxidative damage caused by metals in the bloodstream. It also has its own valid detoxification functions. Garlic contains sulphur components, including the most valuable sulfhydryl groups that oxidize mercury, cadmium, and lead and make these metals water soluble. This makes it easy for the organism to excrete these substances. Garlic also contains alliin, which is enzymatically transformed into allicin, a potent antimicrobial agent. Metal toxic patients almost always suffer from secondary infections, which are often responsible for part of the symptoms. Garlic also contains bioactive selenium that blocks mercury absorption and mercury's adverse neurologic effects. Industrial selenium products are often less absorbable than garlic and do not seem to reach those body compartments in need for it. Garlic is also protective against heart disease and cancer, as mentioned in the related chapters of this text. The half-life of allicin, after crushing garlic, is less than 14 days. Therefore, most commercial garlic products contain little allicin unless they have been freeze-dried.

The dosage is one to three capsules of freeze-dried garlic dissolved and stirred into water after each meal. Start with one capsule after the main meal per day, and slowly increase to the higher dosage. Initially, the patient may experience bloating or nausea as part of the pathogenic organism response.

PSYCHOLOGICAL APPROACHES

In the 1980s, amidst the genomics focus on medical research, Bruce Lipton instead focused his research on applying quantum physics to the inner workings of the cell. He theorized how cells, especially through their bilipid membranes, process and transmit information throughout the organism. In so doing, he laid the groundwork for several areas of research including the interface between the mind—thoughts, beliefs, memories—and the body's metabolic functioning.

Psychological resolution may favorably alter the epigenetic controls of the genome, deeply affecting metabolic enzymes (proteome) and their activity (metabolome), resulting in improved recovery and health. For example, chronically ill clients, who have not responded to reasonable prior therapies, may start responding to treatment only after significant progress has been made in the psychological area. A client who never produced significant amounts of toxic metals in the urine after a challenge test may start pouring out toxic metals in both stool and urine in large quantities after psychological treatment.

Healing occurs on many levels. Patients with chronic illness may feel they are at an impasse and want to have their treatment options presented to them in a way that allows them to prioritize and better understand their own approach. Figure 44.3 presents the model of healing we use to guide patients about underlying causes of illness and available treatment options. These options are detailed in Table 44.2. The model may help arrive at suggestions for appropriate referrals, prompt patients on paths of self-exploration, or broaden a practitioner's approach in a systematic way.

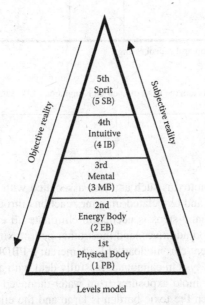

FIGURE 44.3 The five levels of healing: in this guide to diagnosis and treatment, the "emotional body" is a composite of levels 1 through 3 and the "soul" is a composite of levels 2 through 4. (Reproduced with permission from the work of Dietrich Klinghardt, MD, PhD.)

TABLE 44.2

The Five Levels of Healing as a Guide to Diagnosis and Treatment

Level Body/Sphere	Our experience at this level	Anatomical and conceptual designation	Related science	"Diagnostic" method	Related medical treatment and healing techniques
5th level spirit body	bliss, oneness with god, satori	spirit, higher consciousness	religion and spirituality	knowing and awareness	self-healing, prayer, true meditation, chanting
4th level intuitive body	intuition, symbols, trance, meditative states, dreams, magic, curses, spirit possession, out of body & near-death experiences, archetypes	collective unconscious, "no mind," the fourth level turiya	mathematics and quantum physics	Jungian approach, systemic family constellation, radiesthesia, dream analysis, psycho-kinesiology, sound and voice analysis, syntonic optometry, art therapy, shamanistic approaches	hypnotherapy, Jungian psychotherapy, music/singing, systemic family constellation, color and sound therapies, radionics, rituals, shamanism, induced drug states with psychotropics
3rd level mental body	toughts, beliefs, attitudes, long distance healing, healing effect from prayer, consensus reality language	mind and mental field [conscious and sub-conscious mind], morphic field, the will	psychology and homeopathy	conversation with client, observation, questionnaire-based interview–(MMP, etc.I), homeopathic repertorizing	most forms of psychotherapy, energy psychology: mental field technique, TFT, EMDR, PK, homeopathy
2nd level energy body	feelings [anger, excitement, etc.], chi [qigong energy], 6th sense and other "energetic perceptions"	nervous system, meridians, chakras, aura, bioelectric system	physiology and physics	thermogram, EEG, EKG, EMG, HRV, imaging studies: X-rays, MRI, CAT scan, ultrasound thermogram, kinesiology, Chinese pulses, Kirilian photography, autonomic response testing	ultrasound, heat/cold, radiation therapy, microcurrent therapies, acupuncture, laser therapy, photodynamic therapy, bodywork/touch, breath therapy, work with light, yoga, qigong, neural therapy
1st level physical body	sensations [touch, smell, etc.], action, movement	structure and biochemistry	mechanics and chemistry	physical exam, lab tests	diet, exercise, osteopathy and chiropractic, surgery, physical therapy, drugs and herbs, orthomolecular medicine, aromatherapy

EMDR: Eye movement desensitization and reprocessing
TFT: Thought field therapy
PK: Psychokinesis

Source: Reproduced with permission from the work of Dietrich Klinghardt, M.D., Ph.D.

CLINICAL SUMMARY

The human body eliminates biotoxins such as those associated with Lyme disease, streptococcal infections, food-borne illness, and associated immune reactions through a common detoxification pathway. This series of enzymatic steps is needed to eliminate all environmental toxins such as lead, benzene, mold toxins, food additives, and most other neurotoxins. When these pathways are already fully occupied by a silent chronic load of lead, mercury, PBDEs (polybrominated diphenyl ethers), and others, the client's system cannot successfully deal with a new biotoxin-producing illness, such as Lyme disease or mold exposures from water-damaged buildings. The system is on overload and shuts down. When the toxic burden is large and the elimination pathways are overloaded or constitutionally weak, healing will be impaired on all levels (see Figure 44.3). Optimizing epigenetic, metabolic, and nutritional support should be an essential part of a biotoxin-centered medical approach to chronic-illness.

ACKNOWLEDGMENTS

Many people worked together to develop this chapter. As the author, I wish to extend special thanks to: Ms. Deborah Floyd, director of the Klinghardt Academy, and Dr. Christine Schaffner, for sharing a vision for this contribution to practitioners of medicine globally; Drs. Tapan Audhya and Amy Yasko for sharing their work; Dr. Ingrid Kohlstadt for her editorial insights; and Dr. David Kennedy for his technical review of the manuscript.

REFERENCES

1. Hall, S.S. *Iceman Autopsy.* 2011 February 8, 2012.
2. Isoe, K., et al., *Apolipoprotein E in patients with dementia of the Alzheimer type and vascular dementia.* Acta Neurol Scand, 1996. 93(2-3): 133–7.
3. Shoemaker, R.C., D. House, and J.C. Ryan, *Defining the neurotoxin derived illness chronic ciguatera using markers of chronic systemic inflammatory disturbances: A case/control study.* Neurotoxicol Teratol, 2010. 32(6): 633–9.
4. Fernandez, N. and R. Beiras, *Combined toxicity of dissolved mercury with copper, lead and cadmium on embryogenesis and early larval growth of the Paracentrotus lividus sea-urchin.* Ecotoxicology, 2001. 10(5): 263–71.
5. Pischinger, A. and H. Heine, *The Extracellular Matrix and Ground Regulation: Basis for a Holistic Biological Medicine.* 2007, Berkeley, CA: North Atlantic Books. xix, 205 p.
6. Klinghardt, D., *Unpublished research: HPU positive in 8 out of 100 patients with a negative West Blot test, 74 out of 100 HPU pos in West Blot pos individuals,* 2009.
7. McGinnis, W.R., et al., *Discerning the mauve factor, part 2.* Altern Ther Health Med, 2008. 14(3): 56–62.
8. McGinnis, W.R., et al., *Discerning the mauve factor, part 1.* Altern Ther Health Med, 2008. 14(2): 40–50.
9. Soerensen, M., et al., *The Mn-superoxide dismutase single nucleotide polymorphism rs4880 and the glutathione peroxidase 1 single nucleotide polymorphism rs1050450 are associated with aging and longevity in the oldest old.* Mech Ageing Dev, 2009. 130(5): 308–14.
10. Klinghardt, D., *Clinical observation, unpublished data.* 2011.
11. Coca, A.F., *Familial nonreaginic food allergy (idioblapsis) practical management.* Int Arch Allergy Appl Immunol, 1950. 1(3): 173–89.
12. Storm, J.E., et al., *Visual contrast sensitivity in children exposed to tetrachloroethylene.* Arch Environ Occup Health, 2011. 66(3): 166–77.
13. Holmes, A.S., M.F. Blaxill, and B.E. Haley, *Reduced levels of mercury in first baby haircuts of autistic children.* Int J Toxicol, 2003. 22(4): 277–85.
14. Woods, J.S., et al., *Urinary porphyrin excretion in neurotypical and autistic children.* Environ Health Perspect, 2010. 118(10): 1450–7.
15. Woods, J.S., M.D. Martin, and B.G. Leroux, *Validity of spot urine samples as a surrogate measure of 24-hour porphyrin excretion rates. Evaluation of diurnal variations in porphyrin, mercury, and creatinine concentrations among subjects with very low occupational mercury exposure.* J Occup Environ Med, 1998. 40(12): 1090–101.
16. Shoemaker, R., *Personal communication.* 2009.
17. BioPure EU, LTD, www.biopure.eu.
18. www.gcmaf.eu.
19. Nicolaides, A.N., et al., *Screening for chronic cerebrospinal venous insufficiency (CCSVI) using ultrasound. Recommendations for a protocol.* Funct Neurol, 2011. 26(4): 229–48.
20. Fragopoulou, A.F., et al., *Brain proteome response following whole body exposure of mice to mobile phone or wireless DECT base radiation.* Electromagn Biol Med, Jan. 20 2012. Epub.
21. Hallberg, O. and LL Morgan, *The potential impact of mobile phone use on trends in brain and CNS tumors.* J Neurol Neurophysiol, 2011. S5.
22. Tamiya, N., et al. *Preliminary experiments in the use of chlorella as human food.* Food Technology, 1954. 8(4): 179–82.
23. Pratt, R., *Production of thiamine, riboflavin, folic acid and biotin by chlorella vulgaris und chlorella pyreneidosa* J of Pharmaceutical Sciences, 1965. 54(6).
24. Hidaka, S., Y. Okamoto, and M. Arita, *A hot water extract of chlorella pyrenoidosa reduces body weight and serum lipids in ovariectomized rats.* Phytother Res, 2004. 18(2): 164–8.

25. Wang, C.J., S.J. Shiow, and J.K. Lin, *Effects of chlorella on serum cholesterol levels in rats.* Taiwan Yi Xue Hui Za Zhi, 1981. 80(9): 929–33.

26. BioPure.com, Matrix electrolytes.

27. Omura, Y., *Preventative effects of Chinese parsley on aluminum deposits in ICR mice.* Acupuncture & Electro-Therapeutics Research, 2003. 28: 1–44.

28. D. Karunasagar, M.V. Balarama Krishna, S.V. Rao, and J. Arunachalam *Removal and preconcentration of inorganic and methyl mercury from aqueous media using a sorbent prepared from the plant Coriandrum sativum.* Journal of Hazardous Materials, 2005. B118: 133–9.

29. Hagino, N. and S. Ichimura, *Effect of chlorella on fecal and urinary cadmium excretion in "Itai-itai" disease.* Nihon Eiseigaku Zasshi, 1975. 30(1): 77.

30. Nagano, T., Y. Suketa, and S. Okada, *Absorption and excretion of chlorella ellipsoidea cadmium binding protein in rats.* Nihon Eiseigaku Zasshi, 1983. 38(4): 741–7.

31. Carr, H.P., et al., *Characterization of the cadmium-binding capacity of chlorella vulgaris.* Bull Environ Contam Toxicol, 1998. 60(3): 433–40.

32. Horikoshi, T., A. Nakajima, and T. Sakaguchi, *Uptake of uranium by various cell fractions of Chlorella regularis.* Radioisotopes, 1979. 28(8): 485–8.

33. Queiroz, M.L., et al., *Protective effects of chlorella vulgaris in lead-exposed mice infected with Listeria monocytogenes.* Int Immunopharmacol, 2003. 3(6): 889–900.

34. *Parachlorella beyerinckii CK-5 is found to accelerate excretion of methyl-mercury both into feces and urine.* Japan Society for Bioscience, Biotechnology and Agro-chemistry, (JSBBA: http://www.jsbba. or.jp) Meeting in Nagoya City, Japan, March 29~30, 2008.

35. Uchikawa, T., et al., *The influence of parachlorella beyerinckii CK-5 on the absorption and excretion of methylmercury (MeHg) in mice.* J Toxicol Sci, 2010. 35(1): 101–5.

36. Pore, R.S., *Detoxification of chlordecone poisoned rats with chlorella and chlorella derived sporopollenin.* Drug Chem Toxicol, 1984. 7(1): 57–71.

37. Urey, J.C., J.C. Kricher, and J.M. Boylan, *Bioconcentration of four pure PCB isomers by Chlorella pyrenoidosa.* Bull Environ Contam Toxicol, 1976. 16(1): 81–5.

38. Morita, K., et al., *Chlorella accelerates dioxin excretion in rats.* J Nutr, 1999. 129(9): 1731–6.

39. *Effect of chlorella pyreneidosa on fecal excretion and liver accumulastion of polychlorinated dibenzo-p-dioxin in mice.* Chemosphere, 2005. 59: 297–304.

40. Kunimasa M., M. Ogata, and T. Hasegawa, T, *Chlorophyll derived from chlorella inhibits dioxin absorption from the gastrointestinal tract and accelerates dioxin excretion in rats.* Environmental Health Perspectives, 2001. 109: 289.

41. Nakano, S., *Maternal-fetal distribution and transfer of dioxins in pregnant women in Japan, and attempts to reduce maternal transfer with chlorella (chlorella pyrenoidosa) supplements.* Chemosphere, April 2005.

42. Hasegawa, T., and K. Noda, *Chlorella vulgaris culture supernatant (CVE) reduces psychological stress-induced apoptosis in thymocytes in mice.* International Journal of Immunopharmacology, 2000. 22: 877–87.

43. Miyazawa, Y., et al., *Immunomodulation by a unicellular green algae (chlorella pyrenoidosa) in tumor-bearing mice.* J Ethnopharmacol, 1988. 24(2–3): 135–46.

44. Hasegawa, T., et al., *Augmentation of the resistance against listeria monocytogenes by oral administration of a hot water extract of chlorella vulgaris in mice.* Immunopharmacol Immunotoxicol, 1994. 16(2): 191–202.

45. Nakashima, Y., *Preventive effects of chlorella on cognitive decline in age-dependent dementia model of mice.* Neuroscience Letters, 2009. 464: 193–8.

46. Tokuyasu, M., *Examples of diets for infant's and children's nutritional guidance, and their effects of adding chlorella and C.G.F. to food schedule.* Totori City, Japan: Conference proceedings at the nutritional Illness Counseling Clinic, 1983, Jpn Nutr, 1983. 41(5): 275–83, (1980 u.) 1983.

47. Konishi, F.T., et al., *Anti-tumour effect induced by a hot water extract of chlorella vulgaris: Resistance to meth-A tumour growth mediated by CE-induced polymorphonuclear leucocytes.* Cancer Immunology and Immunotheraphy, 1985. 19: 73–8.

Index